The Renal Drug Handbook

The ultimate prescribing guide for renal practitioners

FOURTH EDITION

Edited by

Caroline Ashley and Aileen Dunleavy

UK Renal Pharmacy Group

Foreword by

Professor David C Wheeler

Professor of Kidney Medicine
University College London
President, Renal Association

Radcliffe Publishing
London • New York

Radcliffe Publishing Ltd
St Mark's House
Shepherdess Walk
London N1 7BQ
United Kingdom

www.radcliffehealth.com

British Library Cataloguing in Publication Data

A catalogue record for this book is available from the British Library.

ISBN-13: 978 190936 894 1

The paper used for the text pages of this book is FSC® certified. FSC (The Forest Stewardship Council®) is an international network to promote responsible management of the world's forests.

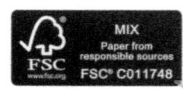

Typeset by Darkriver Design, Auckland, New Zealand
Manufacturing managed by 21six

Contents

x CONTENTS

Foreword to the fourth edition

I was delighted to learn that *The Renal Drug Handbook* was being updated and expanded. The book provides essential information on drug dosing in patients with different levels of kidney function. As in previous editions, the logical format makes it easy to use and simple to follow. Included in this update are 130 new drugs and a new section on drug metabolism and excretion in each drug monograph. As well as the familiar book, I was excited to find that this edition is also going to be available online, where it will be updated regularly.

Previous editions have always been readily available on our wards and 'Caroline's book' is frequently requested on our ward rounds. A copy of the Third Edition was at one time padlocked to the drugs trolley. Wide dissemination of this new Fourth Edition will help healthcare professionals who prescribe and, more importantly, protect their patients from avoidable harm. Well done to Caroline and Aileen for maintaining this amazing resource.

David C Wheeler
Professor of Kidney Medicine, University College London
President, Renal Association
April 2014

Preface to the fourth edition

Welcome to the fourth edition of *The Renal Drug Handbook*. The information contained in this book has been compiled from a wide range of sources and from the clinical experience of the editorial board of the UK Renal Pharmacy Group, all of whom are involved in the pharmaceutical care of renally impaired patients. As such, some of the information contained in the monographs may not be in accordance with the licensed indications or use of the drug.

The Handbook aims to:

- provide healthcare professionals with a single reference of easily retrievable, practical information relating to drug use, sourced from the practical experience of renal units throughout the UK. By referring to the monographs, the user is guided in how to prescribe, prepare and administer the drug with due regard to potentially serious drug interactions and to any renal replacement therapy the patient may be undergoing
- provide a practice-based review of drug utilisation in renal units across the UK, indicating, where appropriate, any local methods of use, licensed or otherwise.

In recent years, the classification for chronic kidney disease (CKD) has changed, now being described as CKD stages 1–5. Each stage is defined by the patient's eGFR (or estimated GFR), which is calculated using the MDRD (modification of diet in renal disease) equation. One point to note is that the eGFR is normalised to a standard body surface area of 1.73 m^2. There is relatively good correlation between the two equations for calculating renal function in patients of average weight, and either could be used for the majority of drugs. However, eGFR should not be used for calculating drug doses in patients at extremes of body weight nor for drugs with a narrow therapeutic window unless it is first corrected to the actual GFR for that patient. Actual GFR can be calculated from the following equation:

$$\text{Actual GFR} = (\text{eGFR} \times \text{BSA}/1.73)$$

At extremes of body weight neither the MDRD nor the Cockcroft-Gault equation is particularly accurate. If an accurate GFR is required, e.g. for chemotherapy, then an isotope GFR determination should be performed.

The information on dosage adjustments in renal impairment given in this book is based on Cockcroft-Gault creatinine clearance and not eGFR, since the majority of published information available is based on creatinine clearance.

The Handbook is not intended to offer definitive advice or guidance on how drugs should be used in patients with renal impairment, nor is it a comprehensive and complete list of all drugs licensed in the UK.

The range of drugs covered will continue to grow with subsequent editions. The

Handbook is not a guide to diagnosis nor to a drug's side-effect profile, except where adverse drug events are more pronounced in the presence of renal impairment. For more in-depth information, users are advised to refer to the Summary of Product Characteristics, the *British National Formulary*, package inserts or other product data.

The use of drugs in patients with impaired renal function can give rise to problems for several reasons:

- Altered pharmacokinetics of some drugs, i.e. changes in absorption, tissue distribution, extent of plasma protein binding, metabolism and excretion. In renal impairment these parameters are often variable and interrelated in a complex manner. This may be further complicated if the patient is undergoing renal replacement therapy.
- For many drugs, some or even all of the altered pharmacokinetic parameters and modified interrelationships are unknown. In such circumstances, the informed professional judgement of clinicians and pharmacists must be used to predict drug disposition. This must be based on knowledge of the drug, its class, chemistry and pharmacokinetics in patients with normal renal function.
- Sensitivity to some drugs is increased, even if elimination is unimpaired.
- Many side-effects are particularly poorly tolerated by renally impaired patients.
- Some drugs are ineffective when renal function is reduced.
- Renal function generally declines with age, and many elderly patients have a GFR less than 50 mL/min which, because of reduced muscle mass, may not be reflected by an elevated creatinine. Consequently, one can justifiably assume mild renal impairment when prescribing for the elderly.

Many of these problems can be avoided by careful choice and use of drugs. This Handbook seeks to assist healthcare professionals in this process.

Using the monographs

- **Drug name**: The approved (generic) name is usually stated.
- **Clinical use**: A brief account of the more common indications in renally impaired patients is given. Where an indication or route is unlicensed, this is usually stated.
- **Dose in normal renal function**: The doses quoted for patients with normal renal function are generally the licensed dosage recommendations stated in the Summary of Product Characteristics for each drug. Where a product is not licensed in the UK, dosage guidelines are provided by the relevant drug company.
- **Pharmacokinetics**: Basic pharmacokinetic data such as molecular weight, half-life, percentage protein-binding, volume of distribution and percentage excreted unchanged in the urine are quoted, to assist in predicting drug handling in both renal impairment and renal replacement therapy.
- **Metabolism**: Very few drugs are 100% excreted via either the liver or the kidneys. Many are metabolised by the liver to either active or inactive metabolites, and some of these may be excreted via the kidneys. Pharmacologically active metabolites that undergo renal excretion must be taken into account when prescribing the parent drug in patients with renal impairment.
- **Dose in renal impairment**: The level of renal function below which the dose of a drug must be reduced depends largely on the extent of renal metabolism and elimination, and on the drug's toxicity. Most drugs are relatively well tolerated, have a broad therapeutic index or are metabolised and excreted hepatically, so precise

dose modification is unnecessary. In such cases, the user is instructed to 'dose as in normal renal function'.

For renally excreted drugs with a narrow therapeutic index, the total daily maintenance dose may be reduced either by decreasing the dose or by increasing the dosing interval, or sometimes by a combination of both. Dosing guidelines for varying degrees of renal impairment are stated accordingly.

- **Dose in renal replacement therapy**: Details are given for dosing in continuous ambulatory peritoneal dialysis (CAPD), intermittent haemodialysis (HD), intermittent haemodiafiltration (HDF), continuous venovenous haemodialysis/haemodiafiltration (CVV HD/HDF), and continuous arteriovenous haemodialysis/haemodiafiltration (CAV HD/HDF), where known. Drugs are categorised into dialysable/not dialysable/dialysability unknown, to aid the practitioner in making an informed decision for dosing within a particular form of renal replacement therapy. Only a few specific guidelines are given for dosing in continuous arteriovenous/venovenous haemofiltration (CAV/VVH). In general, dosing schedules are the same as those quoted for CAV/VVHD, although it should be borne in mind that CAV/VVH may have a lower drug clearance capacity. Thus the clinician or pharmacist should use informed professional judgement, based on knowledge of the drug and its pharmacokinetics, when deciding whether to further modify dosing regimens.

It should be noted that HDF removes drugs more efficiently than HD, although there is limited information in this area.

The Intensive Care Group based at St Thomas' Hospital, London, has an extensive database on drug removal by haemofiltration and haemodiafiltration, so any extra information can be obtained from them (Tel. 020 7188 7188, pager 1863 or 1830).

- **Important drug interactions**: The interactions listed are those identified by a black spot in Appendix 1 of the *British National Formulary*. They are defined as those interactions which are potentially serious, and where combined administration of the drugs involved should be avoided, or only undertaken with caution and appropriate monitoring. Users of the monographs are referred to Appendix 1 of the *British National Formulary* for a more comprehensive list of interactions deemed to be not so clinically significant.
- **Administration**: Information is given on reconstitution, route and rate of administration, and other relevant factors. Much of the information relates to local practice, including information on the minimum volume that drugs can be added to. Only the most commonly used and compatible reconstitution and dilution solutions are stated. The product literature should always be consulted for the most up to date information.
- **Other information**: Details given here are only relevant to the use of that particular drug in patients with impaired renal function or on renal replacement therapy. For more general information, please refer to the Summary of Product Characteristics for that drug.

Your contribution to future editions is vital. Any ideas, comments, corrections, requests, additions, local practices, etc. on the drugs in the Handbook should be put in writing to the Editors-in-Chief: Caroline Ashley, Pharmacy Department, Royal Free Hospital, Hampstead, London NW3 2QG *or* Aileen Dunleavy, Pharmacy Department, Crosshouse Hospital, Kilmarnock KA2 0BE.

Caroline Ashley
Aileen Dunleavy
April 2014

The following texts have been used as reference sources for the compilation of the monographs in this book:

Electronic Medicines Compendium.
British National Formulary No. 66. London: BMJ Publishing Group/RPS Publishing; 2013.
Sweetman SC. *Martindale: The Complete Drug Reference.* 36th ed. Pharmaceutical Press; 2009. Accessed via www.knowledge.scot.nhs.uk
Bennett WM, *et al. Drug Prescribing in Renal Failure: dosing guidelines for adults.* 5th ed. American College of Physicians; 2007.
Drug Information Handbook. 22nd ed. Lexicomp; 2013. American Pharmacists Association.
Knoben JE, Anderson PO. *Clinical Drug Handbook.* 7th ed. Drug Intelligence Publications Inc.; 1993.
Schrier RW, Gambertoglio JG. *Handbook of Drug Therapy in Liver and Kidney Disease.* Little, Brown and Co.; 1991.
Dollery C. *Therapeutic Drugs.* 2nd ed. Churchill Livingstone; 1999.
Seyffart G. *Drug Dosage in Renal Insufficiency.* Kluwer Academic Publishers; 1991.
Cyclosporin Interaction File (Novartis Pharmaceuticals UK).
Drugdex Database. Micromedex 2.0 Inc., USA.
Drug company information.
www.rxlist.com
medsafe.govt.nz
www.medicinescomplete.com
www.drugbank.ca/drugs

About the editors

Caroline Ashley is the Lead Specialist Pharmacist for Renal Services at the University College London Centre for Nephrology and Transplantation, Royal Free Hospital. She has nearly 25 years' renal experience, and her major areas of interest are transplantation and auto-immune renal disease. Caroline was involved in the development of the Renal National Service Framework, and the NICE guidelines on Immunosuppression in Renal Transplantation, Renal Anaemia, and Acute Kidney Injury. She is the co-editor of both *The Renal Drug Handbook* and the *Introduction to Renal Therapeutics*, and sits on the editorial board of the *British Journal of Renal Medicine*. She has been the Chair of the UK Renal Pharmacy Group since 1996, and was made Associate Professor of Pharmacy Practice, UCL School of Pharmacy in 2011.

Aileen Dunleavy is the Senior Specialist Pharmacist for Renal Services at the University Hospital Crosshouse, NHS Ayrshire and Arran, with 20 years' renal experience. Her major areas of interest are dialysis, anaemia and CKD. She became an independent prescriber in 2008. She is the co-editor of *The Renal Drug Handbook* and has contributed to the *Introduction to Renal Therapeutics, Drugs in Use* and *Adverse Drug Reactions*. She has been a committee member of the UK Renal Pharmacy Group for more than 15 years.

List of abbreviations

ABC	advanced breast cancer	CRF	chronic renal failure
ACE	angiotensin-converting enzyme	CRIP	constant-rate infusion pump
ADH	antidiuretic hormone	CSF	cerebrospinal fluid
AIDS	acquired immunodeficiency syndrome	CSM	Committee on Safety of Medicines
AKI	acute kidney injury	CVVH	continuous venovenous haemofiltration
ALG	antilymphocyte immunoglobulin		
ALT	alanine transaminase	CVVHD	continuous venovenous haemodialysis
APTT	activated partial thromboplastin time		
		CyA	ciclosporin
ARF	acute renal failure	CYP	cytochrome pigment
5-ASA	5-aminosalicylic acid	DIC	disseminated intravascular coagulation
AST	aspartate transaminase		
ATG	antithymocyte immunoglobulin	DVT	deep-vein thrombosis
AT-II	angiotensin-II	E/C	enteric coated
ATN	acute tubular necrosis	ECG	electrocardiogram
AUC	area under the curve	ECT	electroconvulsive therapy
AV	atrioventricular	ED	erectile dysfunction
BD	twice daily	EDTA	edetic acid
BP	blood pressure British Pharmacopoeia	eGFR	estimated glomerular filtration rate
BSA	body surface area	ERF	established renal failure
BUN	blood urea nitrogen	ESA	erythropoiesis stimulating agents
BWt	body-weight	ESRD	end-stage renal disease
CAPD	continuous ambulatory peritoneal dialysis	ESRF	end-stage renal failure
		G-6-PD	glucose-6-phosphate dehydrogenase
CAVH	continuous arteriovenous haemofiltration		
		GFR	glomerular filtration rate
CAVHD	continuous arteriovenous haemodialysis	GI	gastrointestinal
		GTN	glyceryl trinitrate
CVVHDF	continuous venovenous haemodiafiltration	HCL	hairy-cell leukaemia
		HD	intermittent haemodialysis
CIVAS	centralised intravenous additive service	HDF	intermittent haemodiafiltration
		HIT	heparin-induced thrombocytopenia
CKD	chronic kidney disease	HMG CoA	3-hydroxy-3-methyl-glutaryl coenzyme A
CLL	chronic lymphocytic leukaemia		
CMV	cytomegalovirus	HUS	haemolytic uraemic syndrome
CNS	central nervous system	ICU	intensive care unit
COX-2	cyclo-oxygenase-2	IM	intramuscular
CRCL	creatinine clearance	INR	international normalised ratio

IP	intraperitoneal	PR	rectally
IV	intravenous	PRCA	pure red cell aplasia
LFT	liver function test	prn	when required
LHRH	luteinising hormone-releasing hormone	PTH	parathyroid hormone
LMWH	low molecular weight heparin	PTLD	post transplant lymphoproliferative disorder
LVF	left ventricular failure	PVC	polyvinyl chloride
MAO	monoamine oxidase	RA	rheumatoid arthritis
MAOI	monoamine oxidase inhibitor	RBC	red blood cells
MI	myocardial infarction	RhG-CSF	recombinant human granulocyte colony-stimulating factor
MMF	mycophenolate mofetil		
MPA	mycophenolic acid	RHuEPO	recombinant human erythropoietin
M/R	modified release	SBECD	sulphobutylether beta cyclodextrin sodium
mw	molecular weight		
NNRTI	non-nucleoside reverse transcriptase inhibitor	SC	subcutaneous
		SLE	systemic lupus erythematosus
NSAID	non-steroidal anti-inflammatory drug	SPC	Summary of Product Characteristics
NSLC	non-small-cell lung cancer	SR	sustained release
NYHA	New York Heart Association	SSRI	selective serotonin reuptake inhibitor
OA	osteoarthritis		
OC	ovarian carcinoma	SVT	symptomatic non-sustained ventricular tachy-arrhythmias
OD	daily		
PAH	primary arterial pulmonary hypertension	$T_{1/2}$	elimination half-life
		T_3	tri-iodothyronine (liothyronine)
PCA	patient-controlled analgesia	T_4	thyroxine (levothyroxine)
PCP	*Pneumocystis jiroveci* pneumonia	TDM	therapeutic-drug monitoring
PCR	polymerase chain reaction	TPN	total parenteral nutrition
PD	peritoneal dialysis Parkinson's disease	UTI	urinary tract infection
		VAP	ventilator associated pneumonia
PE	pulmonary embolism phenytoin equivalent	WM	Waldenström's macroglobulinaemia
PO	orally		

Abacavir

CLINICAL USE

Nucleoside reverse transcriptase inhibitor:
- Used for HIV infection in combination with other antiretroviral drugs

DOSE IN NORMAL RENAL FUNCTION

600 mg daily in 1 or 2 divided doses

PHARMACOKINETICS

Molecular weight (daltons)	286.3 (670.7 as sulphate)
% Protein binding	49
% Excreted unchanged in urine	2
Volume of distribution (L/kg)	0.8
Half-life – normal/ESRF (hrs)	1.5/Unchanged

METABOLISM

Abacavir is primarily metabolised by the liver with approximately 2% of the administered dose being renally excreted, as unchanged compound. The primary pathways of metabolism in man are by alcohol dehydrogenase and by glucuronidation to produce the 5'-carboxylic acid and 5'-glucuronide which account for about 66% of the administered dose. The metabolites are excreted in the urine.

DOSE IN RENAL IMPAIRMENT GFR (mL/MIN)

20–50	Dose as in normal renal function.
10–20	Dose as in normal renal function.
<10	Dose as in normal renal function.

DOSE IN PATIENTS UNDERGOING RENAL REPLACEMENT THERAPIES

CAPD	Unknown dialysability. Dose as in normal renal function.
HD	Unlikely to be dialysed. Dose as in normal renal function.
HDF/High flux	Not dialysed. Dose as in normal renal function.
CAV/VVHD	Unknown dialysability. Dose as in normal renal function.

IMPORTANT DRUG INTERACTIONS

Potentially hazardous interactions with other drugs
- Antivirals: possibly reduces effects of ribavirin; concentration reduced by tipranavir.

ADMINISTRATION

RECONSTITUTION

–

ROUTE
- Oral

RATE OF ADMINISTRATION

–

COMMENTS

–

Abatacept

CLINICAL USE

Treatment of moderate to severe rheumatoid arthritis in people who have not responded adequately to other treatment

DOSE IN NORMAL RENAL FUNCTION

Loading doses: <60 kg: 500 mg, 60–100 kg: 750 mg, >100 kg: 1000 mg Then 125 mg weekly

PHARMACOKINETICS

Molecular weight (daltons)	92 000
% Protein binding	No data
% Excreted unchanged in urine	No data
Volume of distribution (L/kg)	0.07
Half-life – normal/ ESRF (hrs)	13.1 days/–

METABOLISM

Abatacept is cleared via Fc-mediated phagocytosis.

DOSE IN RENAL IMPAIRMENT GFR (mL/MIN)

20–50	Dose as in normal renal function.
10–20	Dose as in normal renal function. Use with caution.
<10	Dose as in normal renal function. Use with caution.

DOSE IN PATIENTS UNDERGOING RENAL REPLACEMENT THERAPIES

CAPD	Unlikely to be dialysed. Dose as in GFR<10 mL/min.
HD	Unlikely to be dialysed. Dose as in GFR<10 mL/min.
HDF/High flux	Unlikely to be dialysed. Dose as in GFR<10 mL/min.
CAV/ VVHD	Unlikely to be dialysed. Dose as in GFR=10–20 mL/min.

IMPORTANT DRUG INTERACTIONS

Potentially hazardous interactions with other drugs
- Vaccines: avoid concomitant use with live vaccines.
- Avoid with certolizumab, etanercept, golimumab and infliximab.

ADMINISTRATION

RECONSTITUTION
- With 10 mL of water for injection per vial
ROUTE
- IV infusion
RATE OF ADMINISTRATION
- Over 30 minutes.
COMMENTS
- DO NOT SHAKE when reconstituting. Add dose to 100 mL of sodium chloride 0.9%.

OTHER INFORMATION

- Stable for 24 hours at 2–8°C if made under aseptic conditions.
- Administer with an infusion set with a low protein binding filter (pore size 0.2–1.2 μm).
- Manufacturer does not have any information on its use in renal impairment. Main side effects are infections and malignancies, to which renal patients may be at increased risk, therefore use with caution.

Abciximab

CLINICAL USE

Antiplatelet agent:
- Prevention of ischaemic cardiac complications in patients undergoing percutaneous coronary intervention
- Short-term prevention of myocardial infarction in patients with unstable angina not responding to treatment or awaiting percutaneous coronary intervention.

DOSE IN NORMAL RENAL FUNCTION

IV bolus: 250 mcg/kg then by infusion at 0.125 mcg/kg/minute for 12 hours after intervention (maximum 10 mcg/minute).

PHARMACOKINETICS

Molecular weight (daltons)	47 455.4
% Protein binding	Binds to platelets.
% Excreted unchanged in urine	Minimal (catabolised like other proteins)
Volume of distribution (L/kg)	0.118[1]
Half-life – normal/ ESRF (hrs)	<10 minutes/ Unchanged

METABOLISM

Following IV administration, abciximab rapidly binds to the platelet GPIIb/IIIa receptors, and remains in the circulation for 15 days or more in a platelet-bound state. Metabolism is via proteolytic cleavage.

DOSE IN RENAL IMPAIRMENT GFR (mL/MIN)

20–50	Dose as in normal renal function.
10–20	Dose as in normal renal function.
<10	Dose as in normal renal function. Use with caution. See 'Other information'.

DOSE IN PATIENTS UNDERGOING RENAL REPLACEMENT THERAPIES

CAPD	Unlikely to be dialysed. Dose as in GFR<10 mL/min.
HD	Unlikely to be dialysed. Dose as in GFR<10 mL/min.
HDF/High flux	Unlikely to be dialysed. Dose as in GFR<10 mL/min.
CAV/ VVHD	Unlikely to be dialysed. Dose as in normal renal function.

IMPORTANT DRUG INTERACTIONS

Potentially hazardous interactions with other drugs
- Heparin, anticoagulants, antiplatelets and thrombolytics: increased risk of bleeding.

ADMINISTRATION

RECONSTITUTION
–
ROUTE
- IV bolus, IV infusion
RATE OF ADMINISTRATION
- Bolus: 1 minute; infusion: 0.125 mcg/kg/minute (maximum 10 mcg/minute)
COMMENTS
- Dilute in sodium chloride 0.9% or glucose 5%. Give via a non-pyrogenic low-protein-binding 0.2, 0.22 or 5 micron filter.

OTHER INFORMATION

- Increased risk of bleeding in CKD 5, benefits of abciximab treatment may be reduced.
- In the UK the licence says use with caution in severe renal disease due to increased risk of bleeding and benefits may be reduced. It also advises to avoid in haemodialysis patients due to increased risk of bleeding (as on heparin for dialysis) but it is used in normal doses in the USA.
- Antibodies to abciximab develop 2–4 weeks post dose in 5.8% of patients so monitor for hypersensitivity reactions if re-administered.
- Abciximab remains in the body for at least 15 days, bound to platelets.
- Once infusion is stopped, the concentration of abciximab falls rapidly for 6 hours then decreases at a slower rate.

Reference:
1. Mager DE, Mascelli MA, Kleiman NS, et al. Simultaneous modelling of abciximab plasma concentrations and ex vivo pharmacodynamics in patients undergoing coronary angioplasty. *J. Pharmacol Exp Thera.* 2003; **307**(3): 969–76.

Abiraterone acetate

CLINICAL USE

Hormone antagonist:
- Treatment of metastatic prostate cancer

DOSE IN NORMAL RENAL FUNCTION

1000 mg daily

PHARMACOKINETICS

Molecular weight (daltons)	391.6
% Protein binding	99.8
% Excreted unchanged in urine	5
Volume of distribution (L/kg)	5630 litres
Half-life – normal/ ESRF (hrs)	15/Unchanged

METABOLISM

Abiraterone acetate is hydrolysed to abiraterone, which then undergoes metabolism including sulphation, hydroxylation and oxidation mainly in the liver to form inactive metabolites. About 88% of a dose is excreted in the faeces, of which about 55% is unchanged abiraterone acetate and about 22% is abiraterone; about 5% of a dose is excreted in the urine.

DOSE IN RENAL IMPAIRMENT GFR (mL/MIN)

20–50	Dose as in normal renal function.
10–20	Dose as in normal renal function.
<10	Dose as in normal renal function.

DOSE IN PATIENTS UNDERGOING RENAL REPLACEMENT THERAPIES

CAPD	Unlikely to be dialysed. Dose as in normal renal function.
HD	Not dialysed. Dose as in normal renal function.
HDF/High flux	Not dialysed. Dose as in normal renal function.
CAV/ VVHD	Unlikely to be dialysed. Dose as in normal renal function.

IMPORTANT DRUG INTERACTIONS

Potentially hazardous interactions with other drugs
- None known

ADMINISTRATION

RECONSTITUTION
–

ROUTE
- Oral

RATE OF ADMINISTRATION
–

COMMENTS
- Should be taken on an empty stomach

OTHER INFORMATION

- The manufacturer suggests using normal doses in renal patients although no formal studies have been done so use with caution.

Acamprosate calcium

CLINICAL USE

Maintenance of abstinence in alcohol
dependence

DOSE IN NORMAL RENAL FUNCTION

>60 kg: 666 mg 3 times a day; <60 kg: 666 mg
at breakfast, 333 mg at midday and 333 mg
at night

PHARMACOKINETICS

Molecular weight (daltons)	400.5
% Protein binding	0
% Excreted unchanged in urine	Majority
Volume of distribution (L/kg)	Approximately 1
Half-life – normal/ ESRF (hrs)	33/85.8

METABOLISM

Acamprosate is excreted in the urine and is
not metabolised significantly.

DOSE IN RENAL IMPAIRMENT GFR (mL/MIN)

30–50	333 mg 3 times daily.
10–30	333 mg, twice daily. See 'Other information'.
<10	333 mg once daily. See 'Other information'.

DOSE IN PATIENTS UNDERGOING RENAL REPLACEMENT THERAPIES

CAPD	Dialysed. Dose as in GFR<10 mL/min.
HD	Dialysed. Dose as in GFR<10 mL/min.
HDF/High flux	Dialysed. Dose as in GFR<10 mL/min.
CAV/ VVHD	Dialysed. Dose as in GFR=10–30 mL/min.

IMPORTANT DRUG INTERACTIONS

Potentially hazardous interactions with other
drugs
● None known

ADMINISTRATION

RECONSTITUTION
–
ROUTE
● Oral
RATE OF ADMINISTRATION
–
COMMENTS
–

OTHER INFORMATION

● Recommended treatment period is a year.
● In USA manufacturer advises to
  avoid if GFR<30 mL/min, in the UK
  it is contraindicated if creatinine
  >120 micromol/L.
● Doses estimated from evaluation of
  pharmacokinetic data, use with caution in
  moderate to severe renal impairment.
● After a single dose of 666 mg in patients
  with severe renal impairment, the average
  maximum concentration was 4 times that
  in healthy individuals.
● Bioavailability is reduced if administered
  with food.

Acarbose

CLINICAL USE

Antidiabetic agent

DOSE IN NORMAL RENAL FUNCTION

50–200 mg 3 times a day

PHARMACOKINETICS

Molecular weight (daltons)	645.6
% Protein binding	15
% Excreted unchanged in urine	1.7 (35% including inactive metabolites)
Volume of distribution (L/kg)	0.32
Half-life – normal/ ESRF (hrs)	3–9/Increased

METABOLISM

Oral bioavailability is 1–2%. After oral administration of the ^{14}C-labelled substance, on average, 35% of the total radioactivity was excreted by the kidneys within 96 hours. The proportion of drug excreted in the urine was 1.7% of the administered dose. 50% of the activity was eliminated within 96 hours in the faeces.

DOSE IN RENAL IMPAIRMENT GFR (mL/MIN)

25–50	Dose as in normal renal function.
10–25	Avoid
<10	Avoid

DOSE IN PATIENTS UNDERGOING RENAL REPLACEMENT THERAPIES

CAPD	Unknown dialysability. Avoid.
HD	Unknown dialysability. Avoid. See 'Other information'.
HDF/High flux	Unknown dialysability. Avoid. See 'Other information'.
CAV/ VVHD	Unknown dialysability. Avoid.

IMPORTANT DRUG INTERACTIONS

Potentially hazardous interactions with other drugs

- Antibacterials: hypoglycaemic effect possibly enhanced and increased gastrointestinal side effects with neomycin.
- Lipid lowering agents: hypoglycaemic effect possibly enhanced by cholestyramine.

ADMINISTRATION

RECONSTITUTION

–

ROUTE

- Oral

RATE OF ADMINISTRATION

–

OTHER INFORMATION

- Only 1–2% of active drug is absorbed.
- In renal impairment, peak concentrations are 5 times higher than in the general population and the AUC is 6 times higher.
- Manufacturer advises to avoid if GFR<25 mL/min due to lack of studies.
- One paper records the use of acarbose in a haemodialysis patient who had undergone a total gastrectomy to treat oxyhyperglycaemia: using a dose of 100 mg before meals. (Teno S, Nakajima-Uto Y, Nagai K, *et al*. Treatment with α-glucosidase inhibitor for severe reactive hypoglycemia. A case report. *Endocr J*. 2000; Aug; **47**(4): 437–42.)

Acebutolol

CLINICAL USE

Beta-adrenoceptor blocker:
- Hypertension
- Angina
- Arrhythmias

DOSE IN NORMAL RENAL FUNCTION

- Hypertension: 400 mg once a day or 200 mg twice a day, increased after 2 weeks to 400 mg twice daily if necessary
- Angina: 400 mg once a day, or 200 mg twice daily initially. Increase up to 300 mg 3 times daily; maximum 1200 mg.
- Arrhythmias: 400–1200 mg/day (in 2–3 divided doses)

PHARMACOKINETICS

Molecular weight (daltons)	336.4 (372.9 as hydrochloride)
% Protein binding	26
% Excreted unchanged in urine	55
Volume of distribution (L/kg)	1.2
Half-life – normal/ ESRF (hrs)	3–4 (8–13 for active metabolite)/Increased (32 for active metabolite)

METABOLISM

After oral administration, there is rapid formation of a major equiactive metabolite, diacetolol, which possesses a similar pharmacological profile to acebutolol. Peak plasma concentrations of active material (i.e. acebutolol plus diacetolol) are achieved within 2–4 hours and the terminal plasma elimination half-life is around 8–10 hours. Because of biliary excretion and direct transfer across the gut wall from the systemic circulation to the gut lumen, more than 50% of an oral dose of acebutolol is recovered in the faeces with acebutolol and diacetolol in equal proportions; the rest of the dose is recovered in the urine, mainly as diacetolol.

DOSE IN RENAL IMPAIRMENT GFR (mL/MIN)

25–50	50% of normal dose, but frequency should not exceed once daily.
10–25	50% of normal dose, but frequency should not exceed once daily.
<10	25–50% of normal dose, but frequency should not exceed once daily.

DOSE IN PATIENTS UNDERGOING RENAL REPLACEMENT THERAPIES

CAPD	Unknown dialysability. Dose as in GFR<10 mL/min.
HD	Dialysed. Dose as in GFR<10 mL/min.
HDF/High flux	Dialysed. Dose as in GFR<10 mL/min.
CAV/VVHD	Dialysed. Dose as in GFR=10–25 mL/min.

IMPORTANT DRUG INTERACTIONS

Potentially hazardous interactions with other drugs
- Anaesthetics: enhanced hypotensive effect.
- Analgesics: NSAIDs antagonise hypotensive effect.
- Anti-arrhythmics: increased risk of myocardial depression and bradycardia; increased risk of bradycardia, myocardial depression and AV block with amiodarone; increased risk of myocardial depression and bradycardia with flecainide.
- Antidepressants: enhanced hypotensive effect with MAOIs.
- Antihypertensives: enhanced hypotensive effect; increased risk of withdrawal hypertension with clonidine; increased risk of first dose hypotensive effect with post-synaptic alpha-blockers such as prazosin.
- Antimalarials: increased risk of bradycardia with mefloquine.
- Antipsychotics enhanced hypotensive effect with phenothiazines.
- Calcium-channel blockers: increased risk of bradycardia and AV block with diltiazem; hypotension and heart failure possible with nifedipine and nisoldipine; asystole, severe hypotension and heart failure with verapamil.
- Cytotoxics: possible increased risk of bradycardia with crizotinib.
- Diuretics: enhanced hypotensive effect.

- Fingolimod: possibly increased risk of bradycardia
- Moxisylyte: possible severe postural hypotension.
- Sympathomimetics: severe hypertension with adrenaline and noradrenaline and possibly with dobutamine.

ADMINISTRATION

RECONSTITUTION

–

ROUTE

- Oral

RATE OF ADMINISTRATION

–

COMMENTS

–

OTHER INFORMATION

- Administration of high doses in severe renal failure cautioned due to accumulation.
- Doses from Sani M. Clinical pharmacology in the ICU. 1994. Section 1: p. 64 and *Drug Prescribing in Renal Failure*, 5th edition, by Aronoff *et al.*
- Dose frequency should not exceed once daily in renal impairment.
- Has an active metabolite – diacetolol.

Aceclofenac

CLINICAL USE

NSAID and analgesic

DOSE IN NORMAL RENAL FUNCTION

100 mg twice daily

PHARMACOKINETICS

Molecular weight (daltons)	354.2
% Protein binding	>99
% Excreted unchanged in urine	66 (mainly as metabolites)
Volume of distribution (L/kg)	25 litres
Half-life – normal/ESRF (hrs)	4/Unchanged

METABOLISM

About two-thirds of a dose is excreted in the urine, mainly as hydroxymetabolites, the principal one being 4-hydroxyaceclofenac. A small amount is converted to diclofenac.

DOSE IN RENAL IMPAIRMENT GFR (mL/MIN)

20–50	Dose as in normal renal function but use with caution.
10–20	Dose as in normal renal function but avoid if possible.
<10	Dose as in normal renal function but only if on dialysis.

DOSE IN PATIENTS UNDERGOING RENAL REPLACEMENT THERAPIES

CAPD	Not dialysed. Dose as in normal renal function. See 'Other information'.
HD	Not dialysed. Dose as in normal renal function. See 'Other information'.
HDF/High flux	Unknown dialysability. Dose as in normal renal function. See 'Other information'.
CAV/VVHD	Not dialysed. Dose as in normal renal function.

IMPORTANT DRUG INTERACTIONS

Potentially hazardous interactions with other drugs

- ACE inhibitors and angiotensin-II antagonists: antagonism of hypotensive effect; increased risk of nephrotoxicity and hyperkalaemia.
- Analgesics: avoid concomitant use of 2 or more NSAIDs, including aspirin (increased side effects); avoid with ketorolac (increased risk of side effects and haemorrhage).
- Antibacterials: possible increased risk of convulsions with quinolones.
- Anticoagulants: effects of coumarins and phenindione enhanced; possibly increased risk of bleeding with heparins and dabigatran.
- Antidepressants: increased risk of bleeding with SSRIs and venlafaxine.
- Antidiabetic agents: effects of sulphonylureas enhanced.
- Anti-epileptics: possibly increased phenytoin concentration.
- Antivirals: increased risk of haematological toxicity with zidovudine; concentration possibly increased by ritonavir.
- Ciclosporin: may potentiate nephrotoxicity.
- Cytotoxic agents: reduced excretion of methotrexate; increased risk of bleeding with erlotinib.
- Diuretics: increased risk of nephrotoxicity; antagonism of diuretic effect, hyperkalaemia with potassium-sparing diuretics.
- Lithium: excretion decreased.
- Pentoxifylline: increased risk of bleeding.
- Tacrolimus: increased risk of nephrotoxicity.

ADMINISTRATION

RECONSTITUTION

–

ROUTE
- Oral

RATE OF ADMINISTRATION

–

OTHER INFORMATION

- Use with caution in uraemic patients predisposed to gastrointestinal bleeding or uraemic coagulopathies.
- Inhibition of renal prostaglandin synthesis by NSAIDs may interfere with renal function, especially in the presence of existing renal disease – avoid if possible; if not, check serum creatinine 48–72 hours after starting NSAID therapy – if raised, discontinue NSAID therapy.
- Use normal doses in patients with ESRD on dialysis if they do not pass any urine.
- Use with great caution in renal transplant recipients; it can reduce intrarenal autocoid synthesis.

Acenocoumarol (nicoumalone)

CLINICAL USE

Anticoagulant

DOSE IN NORMAL RENAL FUNCTION

4 mg on 1st day; 4–8 mg on 2nd day
Maintenance dose usually 1–8 mg daily
according to INR

PHARMACOKINETICS

Molecular weight (daltons)	353.3
% Protein binding	>98
% Excreted unchanged in urine	<0.2
Volume of distribution (L/kg)	0.16–0.18 R(+) enantiomer; 0.22–0.34 S(−) enantiomer
Half-life – normal/ ESRF (hrs)	8–11/Probably unchanged

METABOLISM

Acenocoumarol is extensively metabolised,
although the metabolites appear to be
pharmacologically inactive in man. Twenty-
nine per cent is excreted in the faeces and
60% in the urine, with less than 0.2% of the
dose renally excreted being unchanged.

DOSE IN RENAL IMPAIRMENT GFR (mL/MIN)

20–50	Dose as in normal renal function.
10–20	Dose as in normal renal function.
<10	Dose as in normal renal function.

DOSE IN PATIENTS UNDERGOING RENAL REPLACEMENT THERAPIES

CAPD	Unknown dialysability. Dose as in normal renal function.
HD	Unknown dialysability. Dose as in normal renal function.
HDF/High flux	Unknown dialysability. Dose as in normal renal function.
CAV/ VVHD	Unknown dialysability. Dose as in normal renal function.

IMPORTANT DRUG INTERACTIONS

Potentially hazardous interactions with other
drugs
- There Are Many Significant Interactions
  With Coumarins. Prescribe With Care
  With Regard To The Following:

- Anticoagulant effect enhanced by:
  alcohol, amiodarone, anabolic steroids,
  aspirin, aztreonam, bicalutamide,
  cephalosporins, chloramphenicol,
  cimetidine, ciprofloxacin, fibrates,
  clopidogrel, cranberry juice, danazol,
  dipyridamole, disulfiram, dronedarone,
  esomeprazole, ezetimibe, fluconazole,
  flutamide, fluvastatin, grapefruit juice,
  itraconazole, ketoconazole, levamisole,
  levofloxacin, macrolides, methylphenidate,
  metronidazole, miconazole, nalidixic
  acid, neomycin, norfloxacin, NSAIDs,
  ofloxacin, omeprazole, pantoprazole,
  paracetamol, penicillins, propafenone,
  ritonavir, rosuvastatin, SSRIs, simvastatin,
  sulfinpyrazone, sulphonamides, tamoxifen,
  testosterone, tetracyclines, levothyroxine,
  tigecycline, toremifene, tramadol,
  trimethoprim, valproate, vitamin E,
  voriconazole.
- Anticoagulant effect decreased by:
  acitretin, azathioprine, carbamazepine,
  griseofulvin, oral contraceptives,
  phenobarbital, phenytoin, rifamycins,
  St John's wort (avoid concomitant use),
  sucralfate, vitamin K.
- Anticoagulant effects enhanced/reduced
  by: anion exchange resins, corticosteroids,
  dietary changes, efavirenz, fosamprenavir,
  tricyclics.
- Analgesics: increased risk of bleeding
  with IV diclofenac and ketorolac – avoid
  concomitant use.
- Anticoagulants: increased risk of
  haemorrhage with apixaban, dabigatran
  and rivaroxaban – avoid concomitant use.
- Antidiabetic agents: enhanced
  hypoglycaemic effect with sulphonylureas
  also possible changes to anticoagulant
  effect.
- Ciclosporin: there have been a few reports
  of altered anticoagulant effect; decreased
  ciclosporin levels have been seen rarely.
- Cytotoxics: increased risk of bleeding with
  erlotinib; enhanced effect with etoposide,
  fluorouracil, ifosfamide and sorafenib;
  reduced effect with mercaptopurine and
  mitotane.

ADMINISTRATION

RECONSTITUTION

–

ROUTE
- Oral

RATE OF ADMINISTRATION
–

COMMENTS
–

OTHER INFORMATION

- Acenocoumarol prolongs the thromboplastin time within approximately 36–72 hours.
- Decreased protein binding in uraemia.
- Titrate dose to INR.
- Company advises to avoid in severe renal disease due to increased risk of haemorrhage if risk is greater than benefit.

Acetazolamide

CLINICAL USE

Carbonic anhydrase inhibitor:
- Glaucoma
- Diuretic
- Epilepsy

DOSE IN NORMAL RENAL FUNCTION

- Glaucoma/Epilepsy: 0.25–1 g daily in divided doses
- Diuretic: 250–375 mg daily

PHARMACOKINETICS

Molecular weight (daltons)	222.2
% Protein binding	70–90
% Excreted unchanged in urine	100
Volume of distribution (L/kg)	0.2
Half-life – normal/ESRF (hrs)	3–6/26

METABOLISM

Acetazolamide is tightly bound to carbonic anhydrase and accumulates in tissues containing this enzyme, particularly red blood cells and the renal cortex. It is also bound to plasma proteins. It is excreted unchanged in the urine, renal clearance being enhanced in alkaline urine.

DOSE IN RENAL IMPAIRMENT GFR (mL/MIN)

20–50	250 mg up to twice a day.
10–20	250 mg up to twice a day.
<10	Avoid. See 'Other information'.

DOSE IN PATIENTS UNDERGOING RENAL REPLACEMENT THERAPIES

CAPD	Not dialysed. Dose as in GFR<10 mL/min.
HD	Unlikely dialysability. Dose as in GFR<10 mL/min.
HDF/High flux	Unknown dialysability. Dose as in GFR<10 mL/min.
CAV/ VVHD	Unknown dialysability. Dose as in GFR=10–20 mL/min.

IMPORTANT DRUG INTERACTIONS

Potentially hazardous interactions with other drugs
- Analgesics: high dose aspirin reduces excretion (risk of toxicity).
- Anti-arrhythmics: increased toxicity if hypokalaemia occurs.
- Antibacterials: effects of methenamine antagonised.
- Anti-epileptics: increased risk of osteomalacia with phenytoin and phenobarbital; concentration of carbamazepine and possibly phenytoin increased.
- Antihypertensives: enhanced hypotensive effect.
- Antipsychotics: increased risk of ventricular arrhythmias due to hypokalaemia.
- Atomoxetine: increased risk of ventricular arrhythmias due to hypokalaemia.
- Beta-blockers: increased risk of ventricular arrhythmias due to hypokalaemia with sotalol.
- Cardiac glycosides: increased toxicity if hypokalaemia occurs.
- Ciclosporin: possibly increases ciclosporin concentration.
- Cytotoxics: alkaline urine increases methotrexate excretion; increased risk of ventricular arrhythmias due to hypokalaemia with arsenic trioxide; increased risk of nephrotoxicity and ototoxicity with platinum compounds.
- Lithium: lithium excretion increased.

ADMINISTRATION

RECONSTITUTION
- Add at least 5 mL of water for injection

ROUTE
- Oral, IM, IV

RATE OF ADMINISTRATION
- Give slow IV

COMMENTS
- Avoid IM due to alkaline pH.
- Monitor for signs of extravasation and skin necrosis during administration.

OTHER INFORMATION

- Manufacturer advises to avoid in severe renal failure.
- Doses in renal impairment from *Drug Prescribing in Renal Failure*, 5th edition, by Aronoff *et al*.
- Acetazolamide sodium (Diamox) parenteral contains 2.36 millimoles of sodium per vial.
- Severe metabolic acidosis may occur in the elderly and in patients with reduced renal function.
- May cause neurological side effects in dialysis patients.

Acetylcysteine

- Treatment of paracetamol overdose
- Renal protection during radiological scans involving contrast media (unlicensed)

DOSE IN NORMAL RENAL FUNCTION

- IV infusion: Dose varies according to patient's weight. See manufacturer's information.
- Renal protection – see 'Other information'.

PHARMACOKINETICS

Molecular weight (daltons)	163.2
% Protein binding	50
% Excreted unchanged in urine	20–30
Volume of distribution (L/kg)	0.33–0.47
Half-life – normal/ESRF (hrs)	2–6/–

METABOLISM

Acetylcysteine undergoes transformation in the liver, and may be present in plasma as the parent compound or as various oxidised metabolites such as N-acetylcystine, N, N-diacetylcystine, and cysteine either free or bound to plasma proteins Oral bioavailability is low (4–10%). It has been suggested that acetylcysteine's low oral bioavailability may be due to metabolism in the gut wall and first-pass metabolism in the liver.

DOSE IN RENAL IMPAIRMENT
GFR (mL/MIN)

20–50	Dose as in normal renal function.
10–20	Dose as in normal renal function.
<10	Dose as in normal renal function. See 'Other information'.

DOSE IN PATIENTS UNDERGOING
RENAL REPLACEMENT THERAPIES

CAPD	Likely to be dialysed. Dose as in normal renal function.
HD	Dialysed. Dose as in normal renal function.
HDF/High flux	Dialysed. Dose as in normal renal function.
CAV/ VVHD	Likely to be dialysed. Dose as in normal renal function.

IMPORTANT DRUG INTERACTIONS

Potentially hazardous interactions with other drugs
- None known.

ADMINISTRATION

RECONSTITUTION
- Glucose 5%

ROUTE
- IV, PO (PO route unlicensed in the UK)

RATE OF ADMINISTRATION
- See under Dose

COMMENTS
- Acetylcysteine has been administered neat or in a 1 to 1 dilution using an infusion pump. These are unlicensed methods of administration.
- Minimum dilutions can range from 100 to 250 mL. It is advised to give strong solutions centrally. (UK Critical Care Group, *Minimum Infusion Volumes for Fluid Restricted Critically Ill Patients*, 3rd edition, 2006).

OTHER INFORMATION

- Bennett recommends administering 75% of dose for patients with severe renal impairment; however, the manufacturer does not recommend a dose reduction for paracetamol poisoning and, from its records, neither does the National Poisons Centre.
- There is some evidence that acetylcysteine may have a renoprotective effect during scans involving the use of contrast media, in patients with already impaired renal function.
- Dose = 600 mg PO BD the day before the scan, repeated the day of the scan, together with IV or PO fluids. Injection may be taken orally, or tablets are available from IDIS.
- Alternatively, give 1 g acetylcysteine IV in 500 mL sodium chloride 0.9% or dextrose 5%, the day before the scan, repeated the day of the scan.

Aciclovir IV

CLINICAL USE

Antiviral agent:
- Herpes simplex and Herpes zoster infection

DOSE IN NORMAL RENAL FUNCTION

- Herpes simplex treatment: normal or immunocompromised 5 mg/kg every 8 hours
- Recurrent varicella zoster infection: normal immune status 5 mg/kg every 8 hours
- Primary and recurrent varicella zoster infection: immunocompromised 10 mg/kg every 8 hours
- Herpes simplex encephalitis: normal or immunocompromised 10 mg/kg every 8 hours

PHARMACOKINETICS

Molecular weight (daltons)	225.2
% Protein binding	9–33
% Excreted unchanged in urine	40–70
Volume of distribution (L/kg)	0.7
Half-life – normal/ ESRF (hrs)	2.9/19.5 (dialysis: 5.7)

METABOLISM

Most of the drug is excreted unchanged by the kidney. Renal clearance of aciclovir is substantially greater than creatinine clearance, indicating that tubular secretion, in addition to glomerular filtration, contributes to the renal elimination of the drug. 9-carboxymethoxy-methylguanine is the only significant metabolite of aciclovir and accounts for 10–15% of the dose excreted in the urine.

DOSE IN RENAL IMPAIRMENT GFR (mL/MIN)

25–50	5–10 mg/kg every 12 hours.
10–25	5–10 mg/kg every 24 hours (some units use 3.5–7 mg/kg every 24 hours)
<10	2.5–5 mg/kg every 24 hours.

DOSE IN PATIENTS UNDERGOING RENAL REPLACEMENT THERAPIES

CAPD	Not dialysed. Dose as in GFR<10 mL/min.
HD	Dialysed. Dose as in GFR<10 mL/min.
HDF/High flux	Dialysed. Dose as in GFR<10 mL/min.
CAV/ VVHD	Dialysed. Dose as in GFR = 10–25 mL/min.

IMPORTANT DRUG INTERACTIONS

Potentially hazardous interactions with other drugs
- Ciclosporin: reports of increased and decreased ciclosporin levels. Some editors report no experience of interaction locally; possibly increased risk of nephrotoxicity.
- Higher plasma levels of aciclovir and mycophenolate mofetil with concomitant administration.
- Tacrolimus: possibly increased risk of nephrotoxicity.

ADMINISTRATION

RECONSTITUTION
- Sodium chloride 0.9% or water for injection; 10 mL to each 250 mg vial; 20 mL to 500 mg vial. (Resulting solution contains 25 mg/mL.)

ROUTE
- IV

RATE OF ADMINISTRATION
- 1 hour; can worsen renal impairment if injected too rapidly!

COMMENTS
- Reconstituted solution may be further diluted to concentrations not greater than 5 mg/mL.
- Use 100 mL infusion bags for doses of 250–500 mg; use 2 × 100 mL bags for 500–1000 mg.
- Compatible with sodium chloride 0.9% and glucose 5%.
- DO NOT REFRIGERATE.
- Do not use turbid or crystal-containing solutions.
- Reconstituted solution very alkaline (pH 11).

OTHER INFORMATION

- Aciclovir clearance in CAVHD is approximately equivalent to urea clearance, i.e. lower clearance than in intermittent haemodialysis.
- Monitor aciclovir levels in critically ill patients. Reports of neurological toxicity at maximum recommended doses.
- Renal impairment developing during treatment with aciclovir usually responds rapidly to rehydration of the patient, and/ or dosage reduction or withdrawal of the drug. Adequate hydration of the patient should be maintained.
- Plasma aciclovir concentration is reduced by 60% during haemodialysis.

References:
1. Dose from CVVH Initial Drug Dosing Guidelines on www.thedrugmonitor.com.
2. Trotman RL, Williamson JC, Shoemaker DM, *et al*. Antibiotic dosing in critically ill adult patients receiving continuous renal replacement therapy. *Clin Infect Dis.* 2005 15 October; **41**: 1159–66.

Aciclovir oral

CLINICAL USE

Antiviral agent:
- Herpes simplex and Herpes zoster infection

DOSE IN NORMAL RENAL FUNCTION

- Simplex treatment: 200–400 mg 5 times daily
- Prophylaxis (immunocompromised): 200–400 mg every 6 hours
- Suppression: 200 mg every 6 hours, or 400 mg every 12 hours
- Zoster: 800 mg 5 times a day for 7 days

PHARMACOKINETICS

Molecular weight (daltons)	225.2
% Protein binding	9–33
% Excreted unchanged in urine	40–70
Volume of distribution (L/kg)	0.7
Half-life – normal/ ESRF (hrs)	2.9/19.5 (dialysis: 5.7)

METABOLISM

Most of the drug is excreted unchanged by the kidney. Renal clearance of aciclovir is substantially greater than creatinine clearance, indicating that tubular secretion, in addition to glomerular filtration, contributes to the renal elimination of the drug. 9-carboxymethoxy-methylguanine is the only significant metabolite of aciclovir and accounts for 10–15% of the dose excreted in the urine.

DOSE IN RENAL IMPAIRMENT GFR (mL/MIN)

25–50	Dose as in normal renal function.
10–25	Simplex: 200 mg 3–4 times daily Zoster: 800 mg every 8–12 hours
<10	Simplex: 200 mg every 12 hours Zoster: 400–800 mg every 12 hours

DOSE IN PATIENTS UNDERGOING RENAL REPLACEMENT THERAPIES

CAPD	Not dialysed. Dose as in GFR<10 mL/min.
HD	Dialysed. Dose as in GFR<10 mL/min. Give dose after dialysis.
HDF/High flux	Dialysed. Dose as in GFR<10 mL/min. Give dose after dialysis.
CAV/VVHD	Dialysed. Dose as in GFR=10–25 mL/min.

IMPORTANT DRUG INTERACTIONS

Potentially hazardous interactions with other drugs
- Ciclosporin: reports of increase and decrease in ciclosporin levels; some editors report no experience of interaction locally; possibly increased risk of nephrotoxicity.
- Higher plasma levels of aciclovir and mycophenolate mofetil with concomitant administration.
- Tacrolimus: possibly increased risk of nephrotoxicity.

ADMINISTRATION

RECONSTITUTION
–
ROUTE
- Oral
RATE OF ADMINISTRATION
–
COMMENTS
- Dispersible tablets may be dispersed in a minimum of 50 mL of water or swallowed whole with a little water.

OTHER INFORMATION

- Consider IV therapy for Zoster infection if patient severely immunocompromised.
- Plasma aciclovir concentration is reduced by 60% during haemodialysis.

Acipimox

CLINICAL USE

Hyperlipidaemia

DOSE IN NORMAL RENAL FUNCTION

250 mg 2 or 3 times daily

PHARMACOKINETICS

Molecular weight (daltons)	154.1
% Protein binding	0
% Excreted unchanged in urine	86–90
Volume of distribution (L/kg)	0.3–0.4
Half-life – normal/ ESRF (hrs)	2/Increased

METABOLISM

Acipimox is not significantly metabolised and is eliminated almost completely intact by the urinary route.

DOSE IN RENAL IMPAIRMENT GFR (mL/MIN)

40–80	250 mg daily.
20–40	250 mg alternate days. See 'Other information'.
<20	See 'Other information'.

DOSE IN PATIENTS UNDERGOING RENAL REPLACEMENT THERAPIES

CAPD	Likely dialysability. Dose as in GFR<20 mL/min.
HD	Dialysed. Dose as in GFR<20 mL/min.
HDF/High flux	Dialysed. Dose as in GFR<20 mL/min.
CAV/ VVHD	Dialysed. Dose as in GFR=20–40 mL/min.

IMPORTANT DRUG INTERACTIONS

Potentially hazardous interactions with other drugs
- None known

ADMINISTRATION

RECONSTITUTION
–
ROUTE
- Oral
RATE OF ADMINISTRATION
–
COMMENTS
- Take with or after meals.

OTHER INFORMATION

- Females are twice as likely as males to suffer from side effects, e.g. flushing, pruritis and skin rashes.
- Manufacturer advises to avoid if GFR <30 mL/min.
- Doses up to 1200 mg have been given safely for long periods.
- After a 5 hour dialysis 70% of the drug had been removed.
- Dollery advises the doses given in the table, down to 20 mL/minute, but nothing after that.
- Micromedex gives the following recommendations:
GFR: 30–60 mL/min 150 mg twice daily
GFR: 10–30 mL/min 150 mg once daily
GFR: <10 mL/min 150 mg alternate days

Acitretin

CLINICAL USE

- Severe extensive psoriasis, palmoplantar pustular psoriasis
- Severe congenital ichthyosis
- Severe Darier's disease

DOSE IN NORMAL RENAL FUNCTION

- Initially: 25–30 mg daily (Darier's disease 10 mg daily) for 2–4 weeks, adjusted according to response.
- Ongoing: usually 25–50 mg/day (maximum 75 mg) for further 6–8 weeks. (In Darier's disease and ichthyosis not more than 50 mg daily for up to 6 months.)

PHARMACOKINETICS

Molecular weight (daltons)	326.4
% Protein binding	>99 (<0.1% present as unbound drug in pooled human plasma)
% Excreted unchanged in urine	Excreted as metabolites.
Volume of distribution (L/kg)	9
Half-life – normal/ ESRF (hrs)	50/–

METABOLISM

Acitretin is metabolised by isomerisation into its 13-cis isomer (*cis* acitretin), which is also a teratogen, by glucuronidation and cleavage of the side chain. Acitretin is excreted entirely in the form of its metabolites, in approximately equal parts via the kidneys and the bile.

DOSE IN RENAL IMPAIRMENT GFR (mL/MIN)

20–50	No data available. Assume dose as in normal renal function. See 'Other information'.
10–20	No data available. Assume dose as in normal renal function. See 'Other information'.
<10	No data available. Assume dose as in normal renal function. See 'Other information'.

DOSE IN PATIENTS UNDERGOING RENAL REPLACEMENT THERAPIES

CAPD	Unlikely to be dialysed. Dose as in GFR<10 mL/min.
HD	Not dialysed. Dose as in GFR<10 mL/min.
HDF/High flux	Unlikely to be dialysed. Dose as in GFR<10 mL/min.
CAV/ VVHD	Unknown dialysability. Dose as in GFR=10–20 mL/min.

IMPORTANT DRUG INTERACTIONS

Potentially hazardous interactions with other drugs
- Alcohol: increased risk of teratogenicity in women.
- Antibacterials: possibly increased risk of benign intracranial hypertension with tetracyclines – avoid concomitant use.
- Anticoagulants: possible antagonism of the anticoagulant effect of coumarins.
- Cytotoxics: increased concentration of methotrexate (also increased risk of hepatotoxicity) – avoid concomitant use.
- Vitamin A: risk of hypervitaminosis – avoid concomitant use.

ADMINISTRATION

RECONSTITUTION
–
ROUTE
- Oral
RATE OF ADMINISTRATION
–
COMMENTS
- Take once daily with meals or with milk.

OTHER INFORMATION

- Manufacturer's literature contraindicates the use of acitretin in severe renal failure.
- Patients with renal impairment are at risk of hypervitaminosis. Monitor liver function closely.
- Start with the lowest dose possible and increase cautiously.

Acrivastine

CLINICAL USE

Antihistamine:
- Symptomatic relief of allergy such as hay fever, urticaria

DOSE IN NORMAL RENAL FUNCTION

8 mg 3 times a day

PHARMACOKINETICS

Molecular weight (daltons)	348.4
% Protein binding	50
% Excreted unchanged in urine	60
Volume of distribution (L/kg)	0.6–0.7
Half-life – normal/ ESRF (hrs)	1.5/–

METABOLISM

Acrivastine undergoes metabolism in the liver, and along with an active metabolite, is excreted principally in the urine.

DOSE IN RENAL IMPAIRMENT GFR (mL/MIN)

20–50	8 mg twice a day
10–20	8 mg 1–2 times a day
<10	8 mg 1–2 times a day

DOSE IN PATIENTS UNDERGOING RENAL REPLACEMENT THERAPIES

CAPD	Unknown dialysability. Dose as in GFR<10 mL/min.
HD	Unknown dialysability. Dose as in GFR<10 mL/min.
HDF/High flux	Unknown dialysability. Dose as in GFR<10 mL/min.
CAV/ VVHD	Unknown dialysability. Dose as in GFR=10–20 mL/min.

IMPORTANT DRUG INTERACTIONS

Potentially hazardous interactions with other drugs
- Antivirals: concentration possibly increased by ritonavir.

ADMINISTRATION

RECONSTITUTION

–

ROUTE
- Oral

RATE OF ADMINISTRATION

–

COMMENTS

–

OTHER INFORMATION

- Manufacturers do not recommend use in patients with significant renal impairment due to lack of data.
- Dose in severe renal impairment is from *Drug Prescribing in Renal Failure*, 5th edition, by Aronoff *et al.*

Adalimumab

CLINICAL USE

Tumour necrosis factor alpha inhibitor:
- Treatment of moderate to severe rheumatoid arthritis with or without methotrexate
- Psoriatic arthritis
- Ankylosing spondylitis
- Crohn's disease and ulcerative colitis
- Psoriasis

DOSE IN NORMAL RENAL FUNCTION

- 40 mg on alternate weeks increased to weekly if monotherapy for rheumatoid arthritis
- Crohn's disease and ulcerative colitis: see product literature
- Psoriasis: 80 mg initially then 40 mg on alternate weeks
- Other conditions: 40 mg on alternate weeks

PHARMACOKINETICS

Molecular weight (daltons)	148 000
% Protein binding	No data
% Excreted unchanged in urine	No data
Volume of distribution (L/kg)	5–6 litres
Half-life – normal/ESRF (hrs)	14 days/–

METABOLISM

Most likely removed by opsonisation via the reticuloendothelial system.

DOSE IN RENAL IMPAIRMENT GFR (mL/MIN)

20–50	Use with caution. See 'Other information'.
10–20	Use with caution. See 'Other information'.
<10	Use with caution. See 'Other information'.

DOSE IN PATIENTS UNDERGOING RENAL REPLACEMENT THERAPIES

CAPD	Unlikely to be dialysed. Dose as in GFR<10 mL/min.
HD	Unlikely to be dialysed. Dose as in GFR<10 mL/min.
HDF/High flux	Unlikely to be dialysed. Dose as in GFR<10 mL/min.
CAV/VVHD	Unlikely to be dialysed. Dose as in GFR=10–20 mL/min.

IMPORTANT DRUG INTERACTIONS

Potentially hazardous interactions with other drugs
- Anakinra: avoid concomitant use.
- Live vaccines: avoid concomitant use.

ADMINISTRATION

RECONSTITUTION
- SC

ROUTE
–

RATE OF ADMINISTRATION
–

COMMENTS
- Suitable injection sites are the thigh and abdomen

OTHER INFORMATION

- Contraindicated in patients with severe infections and moderate to severe heart failure.
- Bioavailability is 64%.
- After subcutaneous injection peak concentrations are reached in about 3 to 8 days.
- Manufacturer is unable to provide a dose in renal impairment due to lack of studies.
- A case study has been reported where a haemodialysis patient was successfully treated with adalimumab for psoriatic arthritis – initially at a dose of 80 mg followed by 40 mg on alternate weeks.[1]
- Case reports of glomerulonephritis have been reported with adalimumab.[2]

References:
1. Adalimumab monotherapy in a patient with psoriatic arthritis associated with chronic renal failure on hemodialysis: a case report and literature review. Shimojima Y, Matsuda M, Ishii W, Ikeda S. *Clin Med Insights Case Rep.* 2012; **5**: 13–17.
2. Development of glomerulonephritis during anti-TNF-α therapy for rheumatoid arthritis. Stokes MB, Foster K, Markowitz GS, Ebrahimi F, Hines W, KaufmanD, *et al. Nephrol Dial Transplant.* 2005; **20**(7): 1400–6.

Adefovir dipivoxil

CLINICAL USE

Treatment of chronic hepatitis B infection

DOSE IN NORMAL RENAL FUNCTION

10 mg once daily

PHARMACOKINETICS

Molecular weight (daltons)	501.5
% Protein binding	<4
% Excreted unchanged in urine	45
Volume of distribution (L/kg)	0.4
Half-life – normal/ ESRF (hrs)	7/15

METABOLISM

Following oral administration, the prodrug adefovir dipivoxil is rapidly converted to adefovir, which in turn is excreted renally by a combination of glomerular filtration and active tubular secretion.

DOSE IN RENAL IMPAIRMENT GFR (mL/MIN)

30–50	10 mg every 48 hours
10–30	10 mg every 72 hours
<10	10 mg every 72 hours. See 'Other information'.

DOSE IN PATIENTS UNDERGOING RENAL REPLACEMENT THERAPIES

CAPD	Unknown dialysability. Dose as in GFR<10 mL/min.
HD	Dialysed. 10 mg weekly or after a cumulative total of 12 hours dialysis. See 'Other information'.
HDF/High flux	Dialysed. Dose as in GFR<10 mL/min.
CAV/ VVHD	Unknown dialysability. Dose as in GFR=10–30 mL/min.

IMPORTANT DRUG INTERACTIONS

Potentially hazardous interactions with other drugs

- Use with caution in combination with other nephrotoxins.
- Antivirals: avoid concomitant administration with tenofovir.
- Interferons: use with caution with peginterferon alfa.

ADMINISTRATION

RECONSTITUTION

–

ROUTE

- Oral

RATE OF ADMINISTRATION

–

COMMENTS

–

OTHER INFORMATION

- Nephrotoxic in higher IV doses, but risk is lower with oral doses; although cases of raised creatinine and AKI have been reported.
- Manufacturer has no data for GFR<10 mL/min and other forms of dialysis apart from haemodialysis therefore has no information on dosing.
- Dose in severe renal impairment is from *Drug Prescribing in Renal Failure*, 5th edition, by Aronoff *et al.*
- Discontinue treatment if any of the following occur: lactic acidosis, rapid increase in aminotransferase, progressive hepatomegaly or steatosis.
- 35% of dose is removed with a 4 hour dialysis session.
- There is a case report of it being used at a dose of 10 mg 3 times a week post dialysis. (Tillmann HL, Bock CT, Bleck JS, *et al.* Successful treatment of fibrosing cholestatic hepatitis using adefovir dipivoxil in a patient with cirrhosis and renal insufficiency. *Liver Transpl.* 2003 Feb; **9**(2): 191–6.)

Adenosine

CLINICAL USE

- Rapid reversion to sinus rhythm of paroxysmal supraventricular tachycardias
- Diagnosis of broad or narrow complex supraventricular tachycardias

DOSE IN NORMAL RENAL FUNCTION

Initially: 6 mg over 2 seconds with cardiac monitoring followed, if necessary, by 12 mg after 1–2 minutes and then by 12 mg after a further 1–2 minutes.

PHARMACOKINETICS

Molecular weight (daltons)	267.2
% Protein binding	0
% Excreted unchanged in urine	<5
Volume of distribution (L/kg)	No data
Half-life – normal/ ESRF (hrs)	<10 seconds/ Unchanged

METABOLISM

It is impossible to study adenosine in classical pharmacokinetic studies, since it is present in various forms in all the cells of the body. An efficient salvage and recycling system exists in the body, primarily in erythrocytes and blood vessel endothelial cells. The half-life *in vitro* is estimated to be less than 10 seconds, and may be even shorter *in vivo*.

DOSE IN RENAL IMPAIRMENT GFR (mL/MIN)

20–50	Dose as in normal renal function.
10–20	Dose as in normal renal function.
<10	Dose as in normal renal function.

DOSE IN PATIENTS UNDERGOING RENAL REPLACEMENT THERAPIES

CAPD	Not dialysed. Dose as in normal renal function.
HD	Not dialysed. Dose as in normal renal function.
HDF/High flux	Unknown dialysability. Dose as in normal renal function.
CAV/ VVHD	Not dialysed. Dose as in normal renal function.

IMPORTANT DRUG INTERACTIONS

Potentially hazardous interactions with other drugs

- Anti-arrhythmics: increased risk of myocardial depression.
- Antipsychotics: increased risk of ventricular arrhythmias with antipsychotics that prolong the QT interval.
- Beta-blockers: increased risk of myocardial depression.
- Effect is enhanced and extended by dipyridamole; therefore if use of adenosine is essential, dosage should be reduced by a factor of 4 (i.e. initial dosage of 0.5–1 mg).
- Theophylline and other xanthines are potent inhibitors of adenosine.

ADMINISTRATION

RECONSTITUTION

–

ROUTE

- IV

RATE OF ADMINISTRATION

- Rapid IV bolus (see dose)

COMMENTS

- Do not refrigerate.
- Administer into central vein, large peripheral vein, or into an IV line. If IV line used, follow dose by rapid sodium chloride 0.9% flush.

OTHER INFORMATION

- Neither the kidney nor the liver are involved in the degradation of exogenous adenosine, so dose adjustments are not required in hepatic or renal insufficiency.
- Unlike verapamil, adenosine may be used in conjunction with a beta-blocker.
- Common side effects: facial flushing, chest pain, dyspnoea, bronchospasm, nausea and lightheadedness; the side effects are short-lived.

Adrenaline (epinephrine)

CLINICAL USE

Sympathomimetic and inotropic agent

DOSE IN NORMAL RENAL FUNCTION

0.01–1 mcg/kg/minute

PHARMACOKINETICS

Molecular weight (daltons)	183.2
% Protein binding	50
% Excreted unchanged in urine	1
Volume of distribution (L/kg)	No data
Half-life – normal/ ESRF (hrs)	Phase 1: 3 minutes; Phase 2: 10 minutes

METABOLISM

Most adrenaline that is either injected into the body or released into the circulation from the adrenal medulla is very rapidly inactivated by processes that include uptake into adrenergic neurones, diffusion, and enzymatic degradation in the liver and body tissues by catechol-O-methyltransferase (COMT) and monoamine oxidase (MAO). In general, adrenaline is methylated to metanephrine by COMT followed by oxidative deamination by MAO and eventual conversion to 4-hydroxy-3-methoxymandelic acid (formerly termed vanillylmandelic acid; VMA), or oxidatively deaminated by MAO and converted to 3,4-dihydroxymandelic acid which, in turn, is methylated by COMT, once again to 4-hydroxy-3-methoxymandelic acid; the metabolites are excreted in the urine mainly as their glucuronide and ethereal sulfate conjugates. Up to 90% of an IV dose is excreted in the urine as metabolites.

DOSE IN RENAL IMPAIRMENT GFR (mL/MIN)

20–50	Dose as in normal renal function.
10–20	Dose as in normal renal function.
<10	Dose as in normal renal function.

DOSE IN PATIENTS UNDERGOING RENAL REPLACEMENT THERAPIES

CAPD	Not dialysed. Dose as in normal renal function.
HD	Not dialysed. Dose as in normal renal function.
HDF/High flux	Unknown dialysability. Dose as in normal renal function.
CAV/ VVHD	Not dialysed. Dose as in normal renal function.

IMPORTANT DRUG INTERACTIONS

Potentially hazardous interactions with other drugs

- Alpha-blockers: avoid with tolazoline.
- Anaesthetics: increased risk of arrhythmias if given with volatile anaesthetics.
- Antidepressants: increased risk of arrhythmias and hypertension if given with tricyclics; MAOIs and moclobemide may cause hypertensive crisis.
- Beta-blockers: increased risk of severe hypertension.
- Clonidine: possible increased risk of hypertension.
- Dopaminergics: effects possibly increased by entacapone; avoid concomitant use with rasagiline.
- Sympathomimetics: effects possibly enhanced by dopexamine.

ADMINISTRATION

RECONSTITUTION
- 1 mg in 100 mL glucose 5%
- 6 mL/hour = 1 microgram/minute – according to local protocol

ROUTE
- IV, IM, SC

RATE OF ADMINISTRATION
- Monitor blood pressure and adjust dose according to response.

COMMENTS
–

OTHER INFORMATION

- Catecholamines have a high non-renal systemic clearance; therefore the effect of any renal replacement therapy is unlikely to be relevant.

Albendazole (unlicensed product)

CLINICAL USE

- Treatment of *Echinococcus granulosus* (hydatid disease), in combination with surgery
- Treatment of nematode infections

DOSE IN NORMAL RENAL FUNCTION

Echinococcus granulosus:
- >60 kg: 400 mg twice daily for 28 days
- <60 kg: 15 mg/kg in 2 divided doses to a maximum of 800 mg daily

Treatment of nematode infections: 400 mg as a single dose

PHARMACOKINETICS

Molecular weight (daltons)	265.3
% Protein binding	70
% Excreted unchanged in urine	<1
Volume of distribution (L/kg)	No data
Half-life – normal/ ESRF (hrs)	8–12 (metabolite)/ Probably unchanged

METABOLISM

Albendazole rapidly undergoes extensive first-pass metabolism. Its principal metabolite albendazole sulfoxide has anthelmintic activity and a plasma half-life of about 8.5 hours. Albendazole sulfoxide is widely distributed throughout the body including into the bile and the CSF. It is about 70% bound to plasma protein. Albendazole sulfoxide is eliminated in the bile; only a small amount appears to be excreted in the urine.

DOSE IN RENAL IMPAIRMENT GFR (mL/MIN)

20–50	Dose as in normal renal function.
10–20	Dose as in normal renal function.
<10	Dose as in normal renal function.

DOSE IN PATIENTS UNDERGOING RENAL REPLACEMENT THERAPIES

CAPD	Unlikely dialysability. Dose as in normal renal function.
HD	Not dialysed. Dose as in normal renal function.
HDF/High flux	Unknown dialysability. Dose as in normal renal function.
CAV/ VVHD	Unlikely dialysability. Dose as in normal renal function.

IMPORTANT DRUG INTERACTIONS

Potentially hazardous interactions with other drugs
- Anti-epileptics: metabolism increased by carbamazepine, phenobarbital and phenytoin.
- Dexamethasone: increased concentrations of metabolite of albendazole.

ADMINISTRATION

RECONSTITUTION
–
ROUTE
- Oral

RATE OF ADMINISTRATION
–
COMMENTS
–

OTHER INFORMATION

- Available on a named patient basis from IDIS (Zentel®).

Aldesleukin

CLINICAL USE

Recombinant Interleukin-2:
- Treatment of metastatic renal cell carcinoma

DOSE IN NORMAL RENAL FUNCTION

IV: 18×10^6 IU/m^2 for 5 days, followed by 2–6 days without treatment, then an additional 5 days with treatment and then 3 weeks without.
SC: 18×10^6 IU every day for 5 days, followed by 2 days without treatment. For the following 3 weeks, 18×10^6 IU is administered on days 1 and 2 of each week followed by 9×10^6 IU on days 3–5. On days 6 and 7 no treatment is administered. After 1 week of treatment this 4-week cycle should be repeated.
Or as per local policy.

PHARMACOKINETICS

Molecular weight (daltons)	15315
% Protein binding	No data
% Excreted unchanged in urine	0 (mainly as amino acids)
Volume of distribution (L/kg)	0.18
Half-life – normal/ ESRF (hrs)	IV: 85 minutes; SC: 3–5

METABOLISM

Greater than 80% of aldesleukin distributed to plasma, cleared from the circulation and presented to the kidney is metabolised to amino acids in the cells lining the proximal convoluted tubules. A secondary elimination pathway is IL-2 receptor-mediated uptake.

DOSE IN RENAL IMPAIRMENT GFR (mL/MIN)

20–50	Use with caution.
10–20	Use with caution.
<10	Use with caution.

DOSE IN PATIENTS UNDERGOING RENAL REPLACEMENT THERAPIES

CAPD	Not dialysed. Dose as in GFR<10 mL/min.
HD	Not dialysed. Dose as in GFR<10 mL/min.
HDF/High flux	Not dialysed. Dose as in GFR<10 mL/min.
CAV/ VVHD	Not dialysed. Dose as in GFR=10–20 mL/min.

IMPORTANT DRUG INTERACTIONS

Potentially hazardous interactions with other drugs
- Corticosteroids: avoid concomitant use.
- Cytotoxics: avoid concomitant use with cisplatin, dacarbazine and vinblastine.

ADMINISTRATION

RECONSTITUTION
- 1.2 mL water for injection per 22 million IU vial
ROUTE
- IV, SC
RATE OF ADMINISTRATION
- 24 hours
COMMENTS
- Dilute in up to 500 mL with glucose 5% containing 1 mg/mL (0.1%) human albumin.

OTHER INFORMATION

- No dosage from manufacturer due to lack of studies.
- Risk of toxicity may be greater in patients with renal impairment.
- Bioavailability is 31–47%.
- Can cause an increase in urea and creatinine.
- Clearance is preserved in patients with rising serum creatinine concentration.

Alemtuzumab (MabCampath) (unlicensed)

CLINICAL USE

- Treatment of chronic lymphocytic leukaemia not totally responsive to other treatment
- Induction therapy in renal transplantation

DOSE IN NORMAL RENAL FUNCTION

3 mg increasing to 30 mg
Maximum dose: 30 mg 3 times a week

PHARMACOKINETICS

Molecular weight (daltons)	150 000
% Protein binding	No data
% Excreted unchanged in urine	No data
Volume of distribution (L/kg)	0.15
Half-life – normal/ ESRF (hrs)	2–32 hours (single dose) 1–14 days (repeated dosing)

METABOLISM

The metabolic pathway of alemtuzumab has not been elucidated. Clearance decreases with repeated administration due to decreased receptor mediated clearance (loss of CD52 receptors in the periphery).

DOSE IN RENAL IMPAIRMENT GFR (mL/MIN)

20–50	Use with extreme caution. See 'Other information'.
10–20	Use with extreme caution. See 'Other information'.
<10	Use with extreme caution. See 'Other information'.

DOSE IN PATIENTS UNDERGOING RENAL REPLACEMENT THERAPIES

CAPD	Unlikely to be dialysed. Dose as in GFR<10 mL/min.
HD	Unlikely to be dialysed. Dose as in GFR<10 mL/min.
HDF/High flux	Unlikely to be dialysed. Dose as in GFR<10 mL/min.
CAV/ VVHD	Unlikely to be dialysed. Dose as in GFR=10–20 mL/min.

IMPORTANT DRUG INTERACTIONS

Potentially hazardous interactions with other drugs
- Other chemotherapy: do not give within 3 weeks of each other.
- Live vaccines: avoid for at least 12 months after treatment.

ADMINISTRATION

RECONSTITUTION
–
ROUTE
- IV infusion
RATE OF ADMINISTRATION
- 2 hours
COMMENTS
- Add to 100 mL sodium chloride 0.9% or glucose 5%.
- Once diluted protect from light and use within 8 hours.
- Add dose through a low protein binding 5 micron filter.

OTHER INFORMATION

- Patients should have a premedication of an antihistamine and paracetamol 30 minutes before treatment.
- Patients should also receive anti-herpes and anti-infective prophylaxis against PCP during, and up to 2 months after stopping, treatment.
- More than 80% of patients will experience side effects, usually during the first week of therapy.
- There have been no studies using alemtuzumab for CLL in patients with renal failure and there is no information on excretion, therefore if it must be used it should be with great care at the consultant's discretion.
- Doses of 20–30 mg given on the day of transplantation (and on day 1 according to local protocol) have been used for induction therapy in renal and combined kidney/pancreas transplantation.

Alendronic acid

CLINICAL USE

Bisphosphonate:
- Treatment and prophylaxis of osteoporosis

DOSE IN NORMAL RENAL FUNCTION

10 mg daily or 70 mg once weekly

PHARMACOKINETICS

Molecular weight (daltons)	249.1 (325.1 as sodium salt)
% Protein binding	78
% Excreted unchanged in urine	Approx 50
Volume of distribution (L/kg)	28 litres
Half-life – normal/ ESRF (hrs)	>10 years/Increased

METABOLISM

Alendronate transiently distributes to soft tissues but is then rapidly redistributed to bone or excreted in the urine. There is no evidence that alendronate is metabolised in animals or humans. Following a single intravenous dose of [^{14}C] alendronate, approximately 50% of the radioactivity was excreted in the urine within 72 hours and little or no radioactivity was recovered in the faeces.

DOSE IN RENAL IMPAIRMENT GFR (mL/MIN)

35–50	Dose as in normal renal function.
<35	Avoid. See 'Other information'.

DOSE IN PATIENTS UNDERGOING RENAL REPLACEMENT THERAPIES

CAPD	Unlikely to be dialysed. Dose as in GFR<35 mL/min.
HD	Not dialysed. Dose as in GFR<35 mL/min.
HDF/High flux	Unknown dialysability. Dose as in GFR<35 mL/min.
CAV/ VVHD	Unlikely to be dialysed. Dose as in GFR<35 mL/min.

IMPORTANT DRUG INTERACTIONS

Potentially hazardous interactions with other drugs
- Calcium salts: reduced absorption of alendronate.

ADMINISTRATION

RECONSTITUTION

–

ROUTE
- Oral

RATE OF ADMINISTRATION

–

COMMENTS

–

OTHER INFORMATION

- Swallow whole with a glass of water on an empty stomach, at least 30 minutes before breakfast and any other oral medication.
- Patient should stand or sit upright for at least 30 minutes after taking tablets.
- Combination therapy with alendronate and intravenous calcitriol, for the treatment of secondary hyperparathyroidism in haemodialysis patients, has been used at a dose of 10 mg alendronate plus IV calcitriol 2 mcg post dialysis to reduce PTH levels. (McCarthy JT, Kao PC, Demick DS, et al. Combination therapy with alendronate and intravenous calcitriol for the treatment of secondary hyperparathyroidism in hemodialysis patients. J Am Soc Nephrol. 1999; 10 Program, 81A–82A).
- Manufacturers do not recommend use of alendronate in severe renal impairment due to lack of data.
- One paper reviewed all the information available and concluded that 50% of the recommended dose may be possible in ESRD, but more trials are required and osteomalacia and adynamic bone disease must first be excluded. (Miller PD. Treatment of osteoporosis in chronic kidney disease and end-stage renal disease. Curr Osteoporos Rep. 2005; 3: 5–12.)
- Anecdotally, several renal units use either 70 mg weekly or standard doses of all preparations in patients with CKD 3, 4 and 5 to good effect.
- If used in patients with ESRD ensure the patient has an adequate PTH, e.g. at least 3 times the upper limit of normal.

Alfacalcidol

CLINICAL USE

Vitamin D analogue:
- Increase serum calcium levels
- Suppression of PTH production

DOSE IN NORMAL RENAL FUNCTION

0.25–1 micrograms daily according to response. Alternatively, up to 4 micrograms 3 times a week.

PHARMACOKINETICS

Molecular weight (daltons)	400.6
% Protein binding	Extensive plasma protein binding
% Excreted unchanged in urine	13
Volume of distribution (L/kg)	No data
Half-life – normal/ ESRF (hrs)	<3/–

METABOLISM

Alfacalcidol is hydroxylated in the liver by the enzyme vitamin D 25-hydroxylase to form the active 1.25-dihydroxycolecalciferol (calcitriol). Calcitriol is inactivated in both the kidney and the intestine, through the formation of a number of intermediates including the formation of the 1,24,25-trihydroxy derivatives. Vitamin D compounds and their metabolites are excreted mainly in the bile and faeces with only small amounts appearing in urine; there is some enterohepatic recycling but it is considered to have a negligible contribution to vitamin D status.

DOSE IN RENAL IMPAIRMENT GFR (mL/MIN)

20–50	Dose as in normal renal function.
10–20	Dose as in normal renal function.
<10	Dose as in normal renal function.

DOSE IN PATIENTS UNDERGOING RENAL REPLACEMENT THERAPIES

CAPD	Not dialysed. Dose as in normal renal function.
HD	Not dialysed. Dose as in normal renal function.
HDF/High flux	Not dialysed. Dose as in normal renal function.
CAV/ VVHD	Not dialysed. Dose as in normal renal function.

IMPORTANT DRUG INTERACTIONS

Potentially hazardous interactions with other drugs
- Carbamazepine, phenytoin, phenobarbital and primidone may increase metabolism of alfacalcidol, necessitating larger doses than normal to produce the desired effect.

ADMINISTRATION

RECONSTITUTION
–
ROUTE
- Oral, IV
RATE OF ADMINISTRATION
- Over 30 seconds
COMMENTS
–

OTHER INFORMATION

- Adjust dose according to response. Serum calcium ref range 2.1–2.6 mmol/L (total).
- An IV preparation (2 micrograms/mL) and an oral solution (2 micrograms/mL) are also available.
- Doses of 1 microgram daily for 5 days may need to be given prior to parathyroidectomy. Alternatively, give 5 micrograms immediately prior to parathyroidectomy.
- Capsules of One-Alfa (Leo) contain sesame oil.

Alfentanil

CLINICAL USE

Opioid analgesic:
- Short surgical procedures
- Intensive care sedation

DOSE IN NORMAL RENAL FUNCTION

- IV injection:
  — Spontaneous respiration: up to
    500 micrograms over 30 seconds;
    supplemental dose: 250 micrograms
  — Assisted ventilation:
    30–50 micrograms/kg; supplemental
    dose: 15 micrograms/kg
- By IV infusion with assisted ventilation:
  loading dose 50–100 micrograms/kg as
  bolus or fast infusion over 10 minutes,
  followed by 0.5–1 micrograms/kg/minute.
  Discontinue infusion 30 minutes before
  anticipated end of surgery.
- For analgesia and suppression of
  respiratory activity during intensive care
  with assisted ventilation: by IV infusion
  2 mg/hour, adjusted according to response
  (usual range 0.5–10 mg/hour).
- For more rapid initial control give 5 mg
  IV in divided portions over 10 minutes
  (slower if hypotension or bradycardia
  develops); additional doses of 0.5–1 mg
  may be given by IV injection during short
  painful procedures.

PHARMACOKINETICS

Molecular weight (daltons)	453 (as hydrochloride)
% Protein binding	92
% Excreted unchanged in urine	0.4
Volume of distribution (L/kg)	0.4–1
Half-life – normal/ ESRF (hrs)	1–2 (average 90 minutes)/Unchanged

METABOLISM

Alfentanil is metabolised in the liver;
oxidative N- and O-dealkylation by the
cytochrome P450 isoenzyme CYP3A4 leads
to inactive metabolites, which are excreted in
the urine.

DOSE IN RENAL IMPAIRMENT GFR (mL/MIN)

20–50	Dose as in normal renal function.
10–20	Dose as in normal renal function.
<10	Dose as in normal renal function.

DOSE IN PATIENTS UNDERGOING RENAL REPLACEMENT THERAPIES

CAPD	Not dialysed. Dose as in normal renal function.
HD	Not dialysed. Dose as in normal renal function.
HDF/High flux	Unknown dialysability. Dose as in normal renal function.
CAV/ VVHD	Not dialysed. Dose as in normal renal function.

IMPORTANT DRUG INTERACTIONS

Potentially hazardous interactions with other
drugs
- Antibacterials: concentration increased by
  erythromycin; metabolism accelerated by
  rifampicin.
- Antidepressants: possible CNS excitation
  or depression (hypertension or
  hypotension) in patients also receiving
  MAOIs (including moclobemide) – avoid
  concomitant use; possibly increased
  sedative effects with tricyclics.
- Antifungals: metabolism inhibited by
  fluconazole and ketoconazole (risk
  of prolonged or delayed respiratory
  depression); metabolism possibly inhibited
  by itraconazole; concentration increased
  by voriconazole, consider reducing
  alfentanil dose.
- Antihistamines: increased sedative effects
  with sedating antihistamines.
- Antipsychotics: enhanced hypotensive and
  sedative effects.
- Antivirals: concentration possibly
  increased by ritonavir; increased risk of
  ventricular arrhythmias with saquinavir
  – avoid.
- Cytotoxics: use crizotinib with caution.
- Dopaminergics: avoid with selegiline.
- Sodium oxybate: enhanced effect of
  sodium oxybate – avoid concomitant use.

ADMINISTRATION

RECONSTITUTION
–
ROUTE
- IV bolus, IV infusion

RATE OF ADMINISTRATION
- See dose

COMMENTS
- Alfentanil can be mixed with sodium chloride 0.9%, glucose 5%, or compound sodium lactate injection (Hartmann's solution) at a concentration of 0.5 mg/ mL, but can be used at 2 mg/mL or even undiluted at 5 mg/mL. (UK Critical Care Group, *Minimum Infusion Volumes for Fluid Restricted Critically Ill Patients*, 3rd edition, 2006).

OTHER INFORMATION

- Free fraction of drug is increased in renal failure, hence dose requirements may be reduced.
- IV administration: 500 micrograms alfentanil has peak effect in 90 seconds, and provides analgesia for 5–10 minutes (in unpremedicated adults).
- Transient fall in BP and bradycardia may occur on administration.
- Analgesic potency = 1/4 that of fentanyl
- Duration of action = 1/3 that of an equi-analgesic dose of fentanyl.
- Onset of action = 4 times more rapid than an equi-analgesic dose of fentanyl.

Alfuzosin hydrochloride

CLINICAL USE

Alpha Blocker:
- Treatment of benign prostatic hyperplasia
- Treatment of acute urinary retention

DOSE IN NORMAL RENAL FUNCTION

2.5 mg 2–3 times daily, maximum 10 mg daily
XL: 10 mg once daily

PHARMACOKINETICS

Molecular weight (daltons)	425.9
% Protein binding	90
% Excreted unchanged in urine	11
Volume of distribution (L/kg)	3.2
Half-life – normal/ ESRF (hrs)	3–5; XL:8–9.1/ Unchanged

METABOLISM

Extensively metabolised in the liver, mainly by the cytochrome P450 isoenzyme CYP3A4, to inactive metabolites that are mainly excreted in faeces via the bile.

DOSE IN RENAL IMPAIRMENT GFR (mL/MIN)

30–50	Dose as in normal renal function.
10–30	Initially 2.5 mg twice daily. See 'Other information'.
<10	Initially 2.5 mg twice daily. See 'Other information'.

DOSE IN PATIENTS UNDERGOING RENAL REPLACEMENT THERAPIES

CAPD	Not dialysed. Dose as in GFR<10 mL/min.
HD	Not dialysed. Dose as in GFR<10 mL/min.
HDF/High flux	Unlikely to be dialysed. Dose as in GFR<10 mL/min.
CAV/ VVHD	Not dialysed. Dose as in GFR=10–30 mL/min.

IMPORTANT DRUG INTERACTIONS

Potentially hazardous interactions with other drugs
- Anaesthetics: enhanced hypotensive effect.
- Antidepressants: enhanced hypotensive effect with MAOIs.
- Antivirals: concentration possibly increased by ritonavir – avoid; avoid with telaprevir.
- Beta-blockers: enhanced hypotensive effect; increased risk of first dose hypotensive effect.
- Calcium-channel blockers: enhanced hypotensive effect; increased risk of first dose hypotensive effect.
- Diuretics: enhanced hypotensive effect; increased risk of first dose hypotensive effect.
- Moxisylyte: possibly severe postural hypotension.
- Vardenafil, sildenafil and tadalafil: enhanced hypotensive effect, separate administration by 4–6 hours.

ADMINISTRATION

RECONSTITUTION
–

ROUTE
- Oral

RATE OF ADMINISTRATION
–

COMMENTS
–

OTHER INFORMATION

- Bioavailability is 64%.
- Bioavailability and C_{max} are increased by approximately 50% in moderate to severe renal impairment.
- Manufacturer advises to avoid XL in severe renal impairment due to lack of studies but a study by Marbury has found it to be safe (Marbury TC, Blum RA, Rauch C, Pinquier JL. Pharmacokinetics and safety of a single oral dose of once-daily alfuzosin, 10 mg, in male subjects with mild to severe renal impairment. *J Clin Pharmacol* 2002; **42**: 1311–17).

Alimemazine tartrate (trimeprazine)

CLINICAL USE

- Urticaria and pruritus
- Pre-med in children

DOSE IN NORMAL RENAL FUNCTION

10 mg every 8–12 hours, maximum 100 mg/day
Elderly: 10 mg once or twice daily

PHARMACOKINETICS

Molecular weight (daltons)	747
% Protein binding	>90
% Excreted unchanged in urine	>70
Volume of distribution (L/kg)	Large
Half-life – normal/ESRF (hrs)	4.8/–

METABOLISM

Undergoes biotransformation in the liver to hydroxy, N-dealkyl, S-oxide, and sulfone derivatives. The hydroxy compounds, which are the main metabolites (greater than 50%), are partly conjugated. Five to 10 per cent of metabolites are sulfones. Some of the metabolites were detected in the faeces, too. The relationship of the excretion products in urine and faeces is 75:25%.

DOSE IN RENAL IMPAIRMENT GFR (mL/MIN)

20–50	Dose as in normal renal function.
10–20	Reduce frequency to every 12–24 hours.
<10	Reduce frequency to every 12–24 hours.

DOSE IN PATIENTS UNDERGOING RENAL REPLACEMENT THERAPIES

CAPD	Unlikely to be dialysed. Dose as in GFR<10 mL/min.
HD	Unlikely to be dialysed. Dose as in GFR<10 mL/min.
HDF/High flux	Unlikely to be dialysed. Dose as in GFR<10 mL/min.
CAV/VVHD	Unlikely to be dialysed. Dose as in GFR=10–20 mL/min.

IMPORTANT DRUG INTERACTIONS

Potentially hazardous interactions with other drugs

- Analgesics: sedative effects possibly increased with opioid analgesics.

ADMINISTRATION

RECONSTITUTION
–
ROUTE
- Oral
RATE OF ADMINISTRATION
–
COMMENTS
–

OTHER INFORMATION

- Significant amounts of alimemazine are excreted in urine. It is therefore contraindicated by the manufacturer in renal failure; reduced clearance and elevated serum levels will occur in patients with impaired renal function.
- However, it can be used at a dose of 10 mg at night to treat uraemic pruritis.

Aliskiren fumarate

CLINICAL USE

Renin inhibitor:
- Hypertension

DOSE IN NORMAL RENAL FUNCTION

150–300 mg once daily

PHARMACOKINETICS

Molecular weight (daltons)	1219.6
% Protein binding	47–51
% Excreted unchanged in urine	0.6
Volume of distribution (L/kg)	135 litres
Half-life – normal/ ESRF (hrs)	34–41/Unchanged

METABOLISM

Aliskiren is mainly eliminated as unchanged compound in the faeces (78%). Approximately 1.4% of the total oral dose is metabolised by CYP3A4. Approximately 0.6% of the dose is recovered in urine following oral administration.

DOSE IN RENAL IMPAIRMENT GFR (mL/MIN)

20–50	Dose as in normal renal function.
10–20	Dose as in normal renal function.
<10	Dose as in normal renal function.

DOSE IN PATIENTS UNDERGOING RENAL REPLACEMENT THERAPIES

CAPD	Unlikely to be dialysed. Dose as in normal renal function.
HD	Unlikely to be dialysed. Dose as in normal renal function.
HDF/High flux	Unlikely to be dialysed. Dose as in normal renal function.
CAV/ VVHD	Unlikely to be dialysed. Dose as in normal renal function.

IMPORTANT DRUG INTERACTIONS

Potentially hazardous interactions with other drugs
- Other antihypertensive agents: enhanced antihypertensive effect; concentration possibly reduced by irbesartan.
- Antifungals: concentration of aliskiren increased by ketoconazole; concentration increased by itraconazole – avoid.
- Ciclosporin: concentration of aliskiren increased – avoid concomitant use.
- Diuretics: may reduce concentration of furosemide; hyperkalaemia with potassium-sparing diuretics.
- Grapefruit juice: concentration of aliskiren reduced – avoid concomitant administration.
- Heparins: increased risk of hyperkalaemia.
- Potassium salts: increased risk of hyperkalaemia.

ADMINISTRATION

RECONSTITUTION
–
ROUTE
- Oral
RATE OF ADMINISTRATION
–
COMMENTS
–

OTHER INFORMATION

- Potassium should be monitored in patients with renal impairment, diabetes or heart failure.
- Manufacturer advises to avoid if GFR<30 mL/min and should not be used in combination with ACE-I or ARBs if GFR<60 mL/min due to risk of hyperkalaemia.
- Oral bioavailability is only 2–3%.

Allopurinol

CLINICAL USE

- Gout prophylaxis
- Hyperuricaemia

DOSE IN NORMAL RENAL FUNCTION

100–900 mg/day (usually 300 mg/day)
Doses above 300 mg should be given in
divided doses.

PHARMACOKINETICS

Molecular weight (daltons)	136.1
% Protein binding	<5
% Excreted unchanged in urine	<10
Volume of distribution (L/kg)	1.6
Half-life – normal/ESRF (hrs)	1–2/Increased

METABOLISM

Approximately 20% of ingested allopurinol
is excreted in the faeces. Elimination of
allopurinol is mainly by metabolic conversion
to oxipurinol by xanthine oxidase and
aldehyde oxidase, with less than 10% of the
unchanged drug excreted in the urine.

Oxipurinol is a less potent inhibitor
of xanthine oxidase than allopurinol, but
the plasma half-life of oxipurinol is far
more prolonged. Estimates range from 13
to 30 hours in man. Therefore effective
inhibition of xanthine oxidase is maintained
over a 24 hour period with a single daily
dose.

Oxipurinol is eliminated unchanged in
the urine but has a long elimination half-life
because it undergoes tubular reabsorption.

DOSE IN RENAL IMPAIRMENT GFR (mL/MIN)

20–50	200–300 mg daily
10–20	100–200 mg daily
<10	100 mg daily or 100 mg on alternate days

DOSE IN PATIENTS UNDERGOING RENAL REPLACEMENT THERAPIES

CAPD	Dialysed. Dose as in GFR<10 mL/min.
HD	Dialysed. Dose as in GFR<10 mL/min or 300–400 mg post dialysis on dialysis days only.
HDF/High flux	Dialysed. Dose as in GFR<10 mL/min.
CAV/VVHD	Dialysed. Dose as in GFR=10–20 mL/min.

IMPORTANT DRUG INTERACTIONS

Potentially hazardous interactions with other
drugs

- ACE inhibitors: increased risk of toxicity with captopril.
- Antivirals: concentration of didanosine increased – avoid.
- Ciclosporin: isolated reports of raised ciclosporin levels (risk of nephrotoxicity).
- Cytotoxics: effects of azathioprine and mercaptopurine enhanced with increased toxicity; avoid concomitant use with capecitabine and ideally azathioprine.

ADMINISTRATION

RECONSTITUTION

–

ROUTE

- Oral

RATE OF ADMINISTRATION

–

COMMENTS

- In all grades of renal impairment commence with 100 mg/day and increase if serum and/or urinary urate response is unsatisfactory. Doses less than 100 mg/day may be required in some patients.
- Take as a single daily dose, preferably after food.

OTHER INFORMATION

- A parenteral preparation is available from Glaxo Wellcome on a named patient basis.
- HD patients may be given 300 mg post dialysis, i.e. on alternate days.
- Increased incidence of skin rash in patients with renal impairment.
- Efficient dialysis usually controls serum uric acid levels.
- If a patient is prescribed azathioprine or 6-mercaptopurine concomitantly, reduce azathioprine or 6-mercaptopurine dose by 66–75%. Preferably avoid concomitant use.
- Main active metabolite: oxipurinol – renally excreted; plasma protein binding 17%; half-life: Normal/ESRF = 13–30/>125 hours – 1 week.

Almotriptan

CLINICAL USE

$5HT_1$ receptor agonist:
- Acute relief of migraine

DOSE IN NORMAL RENAL FUNCTION

12.5 mg repeated after 2 hours if migraine recurs (do not take 2nd dose for the same attack)
Maximum 25 mg in 24 hours

PHARMACOKINETICS

Molecular weight (daltons)	469.6 (as malate)
% Protein binding	35
% Excreted unchanged in urine	40–50
Volume of distribution (L/kg)	195 litres
Half-life – normal/ ESRF (hrs)	3.5/7

METABOLISM

More than 75% of a dose is eliminated in urine, and the remainder in faeces. Approximately, 50% of the urinary and faecal excretion is unchanged almotriptan. The major biotransformation route is via monoamine oxidase (MAO-A) mediated oxidative deamination to the indole acetic metabolite. Cytochrome P450 (3A4 and 2D6 isozymes) and flavin mono-oxygenase are other enzymes involved in the metabolism of almotriptan. None of the metabolites are significantly active pharmacologically.

DOSE IN RENAL IMPAIRMENT GFR (mL/MIN)

30–50	Dose as in normal renal function.
10–30	6.25 mg; maximum daily dose 12.5 mg. Use with caution.
<10	6.25 mg; maximum daily dose 12.5 mg. Use with caution.

DOSE IN PATIENTS UNDERGOING RENAL REPLACEMENT THERAPIES

CAPD	Unknown dialysability. Dose as in GFR<10 mL/min.
HD	Likely dialysability. Dose as in GFR<10 mL/min.
HDF/High flux	Likely dialysability. Dose as in GFR<10 mL/min.
CAV/ VVHD	Unknown dialysability. Dose as in GFR=10–30 mL/min.

IMPORTANT DRUG INTERACTIONS

Potentially hazardous interactions with other drugs
- Antidepressants: increased risk of CNS toxicity with citalopram – avoid; possibly increased serotonergic effects with duloxetine or venlafaxine; increased serotonergic effects with St John's wort – avoid concomitant use.
- Antifungals: concentration increased by ketoconazole (increased risk of toxicity).
- Ergot alkaloids: increased risk of vasospasm – avoid.

ADMINISTRATION

RECONSTITUTION
–
ROUTE
- Oral
RATE OF ADMINISTRATION
–
COMMENTS
–

Alteplase (rt-PA) (recombinant human tissue-type plasminogen activator)

CLINICAL USE

Fibrinolytic drug:
- Acute myocardial infarction
- Pulmonary embolism
- Acute ischaemic stroke
- To unblock dialysis lines (unlicensed indication)

DOSE IN NORMAL RENAL FUNCTION

- Myocardial infarction: accelerated regimen (initiated within 6 hours) 15 mg IV bolus, 50 mg over 30 minutes, then 35 mg over 1 hour (total dose 100 mg); or (if initiated within 6–12 hours) 10 mg over 1–2 minutes followed by IV infusion of 50 mg over 1 hour, then 4 infusions each of 10 mg over 30 minutes (total dose – 100 mg over 3 hours).
- Reduce dose if patient <65 kg
- Pulmonary embolism: 10 mg by IV injection over 1–2 minutes, followed by an infusion of 90 mg over 2 hours. Total dose should not exceed 1.5 mg/kg in patients who weigh <65 kg.
- Acute ischaemic stroke: 0.9 mg/kg over 60 minutes, 10% of dose as initial bolus; maximum 90 mg. Must start within 4.5 hours of symptoms.

PHARMACOKINETICS

Molecular weight (daltons)	65 000 (non-glycosylated protein)
% Protein binding	No data
% Excreted unchanged in urine	Minimal
Volume of distribution (L/kg)	0.1
Half-life – normal/ ESRF (hrs)	α: 4–5 minutes; β: 40 minutes

METABOLISM

Alteplase appears to be cleared principally by the liver, which subsequently releases degradation products into the blood. The excretion characteristics of alteplase and its degradation products have not been fully elucidated. There is limited evidence from healthy adults receiving radiolabelled human melanoma cell t-PA that exogenously administered t-PA is excreted mainly in urine, with about 80% of total radioactivity being excreted within 18 hours.

DOSE IN RENAL IMPAIRMENT GFR (mL/MIN)

20–50	Dose as in normal renal function.
10–20	Dose as in normal renal function.
<10	Dose as in normal renal function.

DOSE IN PATIENTS UNDERGOING RENAL REPLACEMENT THERAPIES

CAPD	Not dialysed. Dose as in normal renal function.
HD	Not dialysed. Dose as in normal renal function.
HDF/High flux	Unknown dialysability. Dose as in normal renal function.
CAV/ VVHD	Not dialysed. Dose as in normal renal function.

IMPORTANT DRUG INTERACTIONS

Potentially hazardous interactions with other drugs
- Risk of haemorrhage can be increased by the use of coumarin derivatives, platelet aggregation inhibitors, heparin, and other agents influencing coagulation.

ADMINISTRATION

RECONSTITUTION
- 50 mg vial: dissolve in 50 mL water for injection.
- 20 mg vial: dissolve in 20 mL water for injection.
- The reconstituted solutions can be further diluted (minimum concentration 0.2 mg/mL) with sterile sodium chloride 0.9%.

ROUTE
- IV

RATE OF ADMINISTRATION
- See under dose.

COMMENTS
- Water or glucose solution must NOT be used for dilution.
- 50 mg vial = 29 mega units/vial
- 20 mg vial = 11.6 mega units/vial

OTHER INFORMATION

- Patients weighing less than 65 kg should receive a total dose of 1.5 mg/kg according to dose schedule.
- Allergic reactions are less likely with alteplase than streptokinase and repeated administration is possible.
- 1.7 g arginine in the 50 mg vial, 0.7 g arginine in 20 mg vial – may lead to hyperkalaemia in renal failure.
- Pay attention to potential bleeding sites during treatment.
- To unblock dialysis lines, use 2 mg in 2 mL down each lumen and leave in situ for at least 60 minutes or until the next dialysis session.
- Alternative regimens for unblocking dialysis lines: an infusion of 20 mg over 20 hours, or 50 mg over 12 hours, or 8 mg over 4 hours down each lumen.

Aluminium hydroxide

CLINICAL USE

- Phosphate binding agent
- Antacid

DOSE IN NORMAL RENAL FUNCTION

- Phosphate binder: 4–20 capsules daily in divided doses
- Antacid: 1 capsule 4 times daily and at bedtime

PHARMACOKINETICS

Molecular weight (daltons)	78
% Protein binding	70–90
% Excreted unchanged in urine	No data
Volume of distribution (L/kg)	No data
Half-life – normal/ ESRF (hrs)	No data

METABOLISM

Aluminium hydroxide or oxide is slowly solubilised in the stomach and reacts with hydrochloric acid to form aluminium chloride and water. In addition to forming aluminium chloride, dihydroxyaluminium sodium carbonate and aluminium carbonate form carbon dioxide, and aluminium phosphate forms phosphoric acid. About 17–30% of the aluminium chloride formed is absorbed and is rapidly excreted by the kidneys in patients with normal renal function.

Aluminium-containing antacids also combine with dietary phosphate in the intestine forming insoluble, nonabsorbable aluminium phosphate which is excreted in the faeces.

DOSE IN RENAL IMPAIRMENT GFR (mL/MIN)

20–50	Dose as in normal renal function.
10–20	Dose as in normal renal function.
<10	Dose as in normal renal function.

DOSE IN PATIENTS UNDERGOING RENAL REPLACEMENT THERAPIES

CAPD	Unknown dialysability. Dose as in normal renal function.
HD	Unknown dialysability. Dose as in normal renal function.
HDF/High flux	Unknown dialysability. Dose as in normal renal function.
CAV/ VVHD	Unknown dialysability. Dose as in normal renal function.

IMPORTANT DRUG INTERACTIONS

Potentially hazardous interactions with other drugs

- Cytotoxics: concentration of erlotinib possibly reduced – give at least 4 hours before or 2 hours after erlotinib.

ADMINISTRATION

RECONSTITUTION

–

ROUTE

- Oral

RATE OF ADMINISTRATION

–

COMMENTS

- Take/administer with or immediately before meals.

OTHER INFORMATION

- K/DOQI guidelines caution that CKD 5 patients on chronic therapy may develop aluminium toxicity; therefore best avoided in all but short term therapy (calcium carbonate, calcium acetate, lanthanum or sevelamer are used in chronic therapy).
- In patients undergoing chronic therapy with aluminium hydroxide, serum aluminium levels should be monitored using the Desferrioxamine Test (5 mg/kg); see local protocol.

Amantadine hydrochloride

CLINICAL USE

- Parkinson's disease (but not drug-induced extrapyramidal symptoms)
- Post-herpetic neuralgia
- Prophylaxis and treatment of influenza A

DOSE IN NORMAL RENAL FUNCTION

- Parkinson's disease: 100 mg once a day, increased after one week to 100–200 mg twice a day.
- Post-herpetic neuralgia: 100 mg twice a day for 14 days.
- Influenza A: treatment – 100 mg once a day for 4–5 days; prophylaxis – 100 mg once a day.

PHARMACOKINETICS

Molecular weight (daltons)	187.7
% Protein binding	67
% Excreted unchanged in urine	90
Volume of distribution (L/kg)	5–10
Half-life – normal/ ESRF (hrs)	15/500

METABOLISM

Amantadine is metabolised in the liver to a minor extent, principally by N-acetylation. The renal amantadine clearance is much higher than the creatinine clearance, suggesting renal tubular secretion in addition to glomerular filtration. After 4 to 5 days, 90% of the dose appears unchanged in urine. The rate is considerably influenced by urinary pH: a rise in pH brings about a fall in excretion.

Haemodialysis does not remove significant amounts of amantadine, possibly due to extensive tissue binding.

DOSE IN RENAL IMPAIRMENT GFR (mL/MIN)

35–50	100 mg every 24 hours
15–35	100 mg every 48–72 hours
<15	100 mg every 7 days. See 'Other information'.

DOSE IN PATIENTS UNDERGOING RENAL REPLACEMENT THERAPIES

CAPD	Not dialysed. Dose as in GFR<15 mL/min.
HD	Not dialysed. Dose as in GFR<15 mL/min.
HDF/High flux	Unknown dialysability. Dose as in GFR<15 mL/min.
CAV/ VVHD	Unknown dialysability. Dose as in GFR=15–35 mL/min.

IMPORTANT DRUG INTERACTIONS

Potentially hazardous interactions with other drugs

- Memantine: increased risk of CNS toxicity – avoid concomitant use; effects of amantadine possibly enhanced.

ADMINISTRATION

RECONSTITUTION

–

ROUTE

- Oral

RATE OF ADMINISTRATION

–

COMMENTS

–

OTHER INFORMATION

- Manufacturer in the UK advises to avoid if GFR<15 mL/min but in the USA a dose of 200 mg every 7 days is given for treatment of Parkinson's disease.
- Peripheral oedema may occur in some patients; should be considered when the drug is prescribed for those with congestive heart failure.
- Side effects are often mild and transient; usually appear within 2–4 days of treatment and disappear 24–48 hours after discontinuation of the drug.
- Due to extensive tissue binding, <5% of a dose is removed by a 4 hour haemodialysis session.
- A reduction in creatinine clearance to 40 mL/min may result in a 5-fold increase in elimination half-life.

Ambrisentan

CLINICAL USE

Endothelin A (ETA) receptor antagonist
● Treatment of pulmonary arterial
  hypertension

DOSE IN NORMAL RENAL FUNCTION

5–10 mg once daily

PHARMACOKINETICS

Molecular weight (daltons)	378.4
% Protein binding	98.8
% Excreted unchanged in urine	3.3
Volume of distribution (L/kg)	Low to moderate[1]
Half-life – normal/ ESRF (hrs)	13.6–16.5

METABOLISM

Ambrisentan is glucuronidated via several
UGT isoenzymes (UGT1A9S, UGT2B7S
and UGT1A3S) to form ambrisentan
glucuronide (13%). Ambrisentan also
undergoes oxidative metabolism mainly by
CYP3A4 and to a lesser extent by CYP3A5
and CYP2C19 to form 4-hydroxymethyl
ambrisentan (which has little activity) which
is further glucuronidated to 4-hydroxymethyl
ambrisentan glucuronide.
    Ambrisentan is excreted mainly by
the liver, although the contribution of
hepatic metabolism and biliary excretion is
unknown.

DOSE IN RENAL IMPAIRMENT GFR (mL/MIN)

30–50	Dose as in normal renal function.
10–30	Dose as in normal renal function. Use with care.
<10	Dose as in normal renal function. Use with care.

DOSE IN PATIENTS UNDERGOING RENAL REPLACEMENT THERAPIES

CAPD	Unlikely to be dialysed. Dose as in GFR<10 mL/min.
HD	Unlikely to be dialysed. Dose as in GFR<10 mL/min.
HDF/High flux	Unlikely to be dialysed. Dose as in GFR<10 mL/min.
CAV/ VVHD	Unlikely to be dialysed. Dose as in GFR=10–30 mL/min.

IMPORTANT DRUG INTERACTIONS

Potentially hazardous interactions with other
drugs
● Ciclosporin: concentration of ambrisentan
  doubled with an increased risk of side
  effects; maximum dose 5 mg daily.

ADMINISTRATION

RECONSTITUTION
–
ROUTE
● Oral
RATE OF ADMINISTRATION
–

OTHER INFORMATION

● Renal clearance is reduced by 20–40% in
  moderate renal impairment.
● Manufacturer advises to use with care in
  severe renal impairment and to increase
  up to 10 mg cautiously due to lack of
  studies.

Reference:
1. www.ema.europa.eu/docs/en_GB/
document_library/EPAR_-_Public_
assessment_report/human/000839/
WC500053063.pdf

Amifostine

Aminothiol compound
- Cytoprotective agent

DOSE IN NORMAL RENAL FUNCTION

- 30 minutes before chemotherapy: $910 \, mg/m^2$
- Subsequent doses should be reduced to $740 \, mg/m^2$ in patients unable to tolerate the full dose
- Reduction of cisplatin toxicity if doses of cisplatin of less than $100 \, mg/m^2$ are used: $740 \, mg/m^2$
- Prevention of xerostomia during radiotherapy for head and neck cancer: $200 \, mg/m^2$ daily as a 3-minute intravenous infusion starting 15 to 30 minutes before radiotherapy.

PHARMACOKINETICS

Molecular weight (daltons)	214.2
% Protein binding	4
% Excreted unchanged in urine	0.69
Volume of distribution (L/kg)	3.5 litres[1]
Half-life – normal/ ESRF (hrs)	8 minutes

METABOLISM

Amifostine is rapidly cleared from the plasma after intravenous doses and is dephosphorylated by alkaline phosphatase to the active metabolite WR-1065, a free thiol compound. This is further metabolised to a less active disulfide metabolite (WR-33278).

Renal excretion of amifostine and its metabolites is minimal.

DOSE IN RENAL IMPAIRMENT GFR (mL/MIN)

20–50	Dose as in normal renal function.
10–20	Dose as in normal renal function.
<10	Dose as in normal renal function.

DOSE IN PATIENTS UNDERGOING RENAL REPLACEMENT THERAPIES

CAPD	Dialysed. Dose as in normal renal function.
HD	Dialysed. Dose as in normal renal function.
HDF/High flux	Dialysed. Dose as in normal renal function.
CAV/ VVHD	Dialysed. Dose as in normal renal function.

IMPORTANT DRUG INTERACTIONS

Potentially hazardous interactions with other drugs
- None known

ADMINISTRATION

RECONSTITUTION
- 9.7 mL of sodium chloride 0.9%

ROUTE
- IV

RATE OF ADMINISTRATION
- 3 or 15 minutes (depending on indication)

OTHER INFORMATION

- Manufacture advises to avoid due to lack of studies.

Reference:
1. rxindex.ru/generic/gen-a/30554-amifostine.html

Amikacin

CLINICAL USE

Antibacterial agent

DOSE IN NORMAL RENAL FUNCTION

15 mg/kg/day in 2 divided doses (maximum dose: 1.5 g/day; maximum cumulative dose: 15 g)

PHARMACOKINETICS

Molecular weight (daltons)	585.6
% Protein binding	<20
% Excreted unchanged in urine	94–98
Volume of distribution (L/kg)	0.22–0.29
Half-life – normal/ ESRF (hrs)	2–3/17–150

METABOLISM

Amikacin diffuses readily through extracellular fluids and has been found in cerebrospinal fluid, pleural fluid, amniotic fluid and in the peritoneal cavity following parenteral administration. It is excreted in the urine unchanged, primarily by glomerular filtration.

DOSE IN RENAL IMPAIRMENT GFR (mL/MIN)

20–50	5–6 mg/kg every 12 hours or as per local protocol.
10–20	3–4 mg/kg every 24 hours or as per local protocol.
<10	2 mg/kg every 24–48 hours or as per local protocol.

DOSE IN PATIENTS UNDERGOING RENAL REPLACEMENT THERAPIES

CAPD	Dialysed. Dose as in GFR<10 mL/min.
HD	Dialysed. Give 5 mg/kg after dialysis.
HDF/High flux	Dialysed. Give 5 mg/kg after dialysis.
CAV/ VVHD	Dialysed. 7.5 mg/kg every 24 hours and monitor levels.[1]

IMPORTANT DRUG INTERACTIONS

Potentially hazardous interactions with other drugs

- Antibacterials: increased risk of nephrotoxicity with colistimethate or polymyxins and possibly cephalosporins; increased risk of ototoxicity and nephrotoxicity with capreomycin or vancomycin.
- Ciclosporin: increased risk of nephrotoxicity.
- Cytotoxics: increased risk with platinum compounds of nephrotoxicity and possibly of ototoxicity.
- Diuretics: increased risk of ototoxicity with loop diuretics.
- Muscle relaxants: enhanced effects of non-depolarising muscle relaxants and suxamethonium.
- Parasympathomimetics: antagonism of effect of neostigmine and pyridostigmine.
- Tacrolimus: increased risk of nephrotoxicity.

ADMINISTRATION

RECONSTITUTION
–
ROUTE
- IM/IV
RATE OF ADMINISTRATION
- IV bolus – over 2–3 minutes
- Infusion – at concentration 2.5 mg/mL over 30 minutes
- (Diluents: sodium chloride 0.9%, glucose 5% and others)
COMMENTS
- May be used intraperitoneally.
- Can be given in 50 mL. (UK Critical Care Group, Minimum Infusion Volumes for Fluid Restricted Critically Ill Patients, 3rd edition, 2006).
- Do not mix physically with any other antibacterial agents.

OTHER INFORMATION

- Nephrotoxic and ototoxic; toxicity no worse when hyperbilirubinaemic.
- Serum levels must be measured for efficacy and toxicity.
- Peritoneal absorption increases in the presence of inflammation.
- Volume of distribution increases with oedema, obesity and ascites.
- Peak serum concentration should not exceed 30 mg/L.
- Trough serum concentration should be less than 5 mg/L.
- Amikacin affects auditory function to a greater extent than gentamicin.

- Doses in renal impairment from *Drug Dosing in Renal Insufficiency* by Seyffart G.

Reference:
1. CVVH Initial Drug Dosing Guidelines on www.thedrugmonitor.com

Amiloride hydrochloride

CLINICAL USE

- Oedema
- Potassium conservation with thiazide and loop diuretics

DOSE IN NORMAL RENAL FUNCTION

5–10 mg daily; maximum 20 mg daily

PHARMACOKINETICS

Molecular weight (daltons)	302.1
% Protein binding	30–40
% Excreted unchanged in urine	50
Volume of distribution (L/kg)	5
Half-life – normal/ESRF (hrs)	6–20/100

METABOLISM

Amiloride is excreted unchanged in the urine. In two studies in which single doses of ^{14}C-amiloride were used, approximately 50% was recovered in urine and 40% in the faeces within 72 hours.

DOSE IN RENAL IMPAIRMENT GFR (mL/MIN)

20–50	Use 50% of dose.
10–20	Use 50% of dose.
<10	Avoid.

DOSE IN PATIENTS UNDERGOING RENAL REPLACEMENT THERAPIES

CAPD	Not applicable. Avoid
HD	Not applicable. Avoid
HDF/High flux	Not applicable. Avoid
CAV/ VVHD	Unknown dialysability. Dose as in GFR=10–20 mL/min.

IMPORTANT DRUG INTERACTIONS

Potentially hazardous interactions with other drugs

- ACE inhibitor and angiotensin-II antagonists: increased risk of hyperkalaemia and hypotension.
- Antibacterials: avoid concomitant use with lymecycline.
- Antidepressants: increased risk of postural hypotension with tricyclics; enhanced hypotensive effect with MAOIs.
- Antihypertensives: enhanced hypotensive effect.
- Ciclosporin: increased risk of hyperkalaemia and nephrotoxicity.
- Cytotoxics: increased risk of nephrotoxicity and ototoxicity with platinum compounds.
- Lithium excretion reduced.
- NSAIDs: increased risk of hyperkalaemia; increased risk of nephrotoxicity; antagonism of diuretic effect.
- Potassium salts: increased risk of hyperkalaemia.
- Tacrolimus: increased risk of hyperkalaemia.

ADMINISTRATION

RECONSTITUTION
–
ROUTE
- Oral
RATE OF ADMINISTRATION
–
COMMENTS
–

OTHER INFORMATION

- Monitor for hyperkalaemia.
- Greatly increased risk of hyperkalaemia in patients with a GFR<30 mL/min, especially in diabetics.
- Increased risk of hyperchloraemic metabolic acidosis in patients with reduced GFR.
- Bioavailability is 50% and can be reduced by administering with food.
- Reduced natriuretic effect once the GFR<50 mL/min.
- Diuretic effect starts 2 hours after administration, peaks after 6–10 hours and can last up to 24 hours.

Aminophylline

CLINICAL USE

- Reversible airways obstruction
- Acute severe asthma

DOSE IN NORMAL RENAL FUNCTION

- Modified release: 225–450 mg twice daily
- IV loading dose: 5 mg/kg (250–500 mg)
- Maintenance dose: 0.5–0.7 mg/kg/hour adjusted according to levels

PHARMACOKINETICS

Molecular weight (daltons)	420.4
% Protein binding	40–60 (theophylline)
% Excreted unchanged in urine	<10
Volume of distribution (L/kg)	0.4–0.7 (theophylline)
Half-life – normal/ ESRF (hrs)	4–12/Unchanged (theophylline)

METABOLISM

Aminophylline is metabolised to theophylline *in vivo*.

Theophylline is excreted in the urine as metabolites, mainly 1,3-dimethyluric acid and 3-methylxanthine, and about 10% is excreted unchanged.

DOSE IN RENAL IMPAIRMENT GFR (mL/MIN)

20–50	Oral: Dose as in normal renal function and adjust in accordance with blood levels. IV: Dose as in normal renal function and adjust in accordance with blood levels.
10–20	Oral: Dose as in normal renal function and adjust in accordance with blood levels. IV: Dose as in normal renal function and adjust in accordance with blood levels.
<10	Oral: Dose as in normal renal function and adjust in accordance with blood levels. IV: Dose as in normal renal function and adjust in accordance with blood levels.

DOSE IN PATIENTS UNDERGOING RENAL REPLACEMENT THERAPIES

CAPD	Not dialysed. Dose as in GFR<10 mL/min. Monitor blood levels. See 'Other information'.
HD	Not dialysed. Dose as in GFR<10 mL/min. Monitor blood levels. See 'Other information'.
HDF/High flux	Not dialysed. Dose as in GFR<10 mL/min. Monitor blood levels. See 'Other information'.
CAV/ VVHD	Not dialysed. Dose as in GFR=10–20 mL/min. Monitor blood levels. See 'Other information'.

IMPORTANT DRUG INTERACTIONS

Potentially hazardous interactions with other drugs

- Antibacterials: increased concentration with azithromycin, clarithromycin, erythromycin, ciprofloxacin, norfloxacin and isoniazid; decreased erythromycin levels if erythromycin is given orally; increased risk of convulsions if given with quinolones; rifampicin accelerates metabolism of theophylline.
- Antidepressants: concentration increased by fluvoxamine – avoid concomitant use or halve theophylline dose and monitor levels; concentration reduced by St John's wort – avoid concomitant use.
- Anti-epileptics: metabolism increased by carbamazepine and phenobarbital; concentration of both drugs increased with phenytoin.
- Antifungals: concentration increased by fluconazole and ketoconazole.
- Antivirals: metabolism of theophylline increased by ritonavir; concentration possibly increased by aciclovir.
- Calcium-channel blockers: concentration increased by diltiazem and verapamil and possibly other calcium-channel blockers.
- Deferasirox: concentration of theophylline increased.
- Febuxostat: use with caution.
- Interferons: reduced metabolism of theophylline.
- Tacrolimus: may increase tacrolimus levels.
- Ulcer-healing drugs: metabolism inhibited by cimetidine; absorption possibly reduced by sucralfate.

ADMINISTRATION

RECONSTITUTION

–

ROUTE

- IV, Oral

RATE OF ADMINISTRATION

- Loading dose over 20 minutes by slow IV injection.

COMMENTS

- Can be added to glucose 5%, sodium chloride 0.9% and compound sodium lactate.
- Minimum volumes range from 2–25 mg/mL, give concentrated solution via central line. (UK Critical Care Group, *Minimum Infusion Volumes for Fluid Restricted Critically Ill Patients*, 3rd edition, 2006).

OTHER INFORMATION

- Aminophylline: 80% theophylline + 20% ethylenediamine.
- In bodily fluids, aminophylline rapidly dissociates from ethylenediamine and releases free theophylline in the body. It is therefore not present in the body long enough to be dialysed, whereas theophylline is dialysed, see theophylline monograph.
- Optimum response obtained at plasma theophylline levels of 10–20 mg/L (55–110 micromol/L).
- Increased incidence of GI and neurological side effects in renal impairment at plasma levels above optimum range.

Amiodarone hydrochloride

CLINICAL USE

Cardiac arrhythmias

DOSE IN NORMAL RENAL FUNCTION

- Oral: 200 mg 3 times a day for 1 week, then twice a day for 1 week, then 200 mg daily maintenance dose or minimum required to control arrhythmia
- IV: via central catheter – 5 mg/kg (maximum 1.2 g in 24 hours)
- Ventricular arrhythmias or pulseless ventricular tachycardias: 300 mg over at least 3 minutes

PHARMACOKINETICS

Molecular weight (daltons)	681.8
% Protein binding	96
% Excreted unchanged in urine	<5
Volume of distribution (L/kg)	70–140
Half-life – normal/ ESRF (hrs)	20–100 days/ Unchanged

METABOLISM

Amiodarone is metabolised in the liver; the major metabolite, desethylamiodarone, also has antiarrhythmic properties. There is very little urinary excretion of amiodarone or its metabolites, the major route of excretion being in faeces via the bile; some enterohepatic recycling may occur.

DOSE IN RENAL IMPAIRMENT GFR (mL/MIN)

20–50	Dose as in normal renal function.
10–20	Dose as in normal renal function.
<10	Dose as in normal renal function.

DOSE IN PATIENTS UNDERGOING RENAL REPLACEMENT THERAPIES

CAPD	Not dialysed. Dose as in normal renal function.
HD	Not dialysed. Dose as in normal renal function.
HDF/High flux	Unknown dialysability. Dose as in normal renal function.
CAV/ VVHD	Not dialysed. Dose as in normal renal function.

IMPORTANT DRUG INTERACTIONS

Potentially hazardous interactions with other drugs

- Anti-arrhythmics: additive effect and increased risk of myocardial depression; increased risk of ventricular arrhythmias with disopyramide or dronedarone – avoid; increased flecainide concentration – halve flecainide dose; increased procainamide concentration – avoid.
- Antibacterials: increased risk of ventricular arrhythmias with parenteral erythromycin, co-trimoxazole levofloxacin and moxifloxacin – avoid concomitant use; possibly increased risk of ventricular arrhythmias with telithromycin.
- Anticoagulants: metabolism inhibited (increased anticoagulant effect); increased dabigatran concentration (reduce dabigatran dose).
- Antidepressants: increased risk of ventricular arrhythmias with tricyclic antidepressants – avoid concomitant use.
- Anti-epileptics: phenytoin metabolism inhibited (increased concentration).
- Antihistamines: increased risk of ventricular arrhythmias with mizolastine – avoid.
- Antimalarials: increased risk of ventricular arrhythmias with chloroquine, hydroxychloroquine, mefloquine and quinine and possibly with piperaquine with artenimol – avoid concomitant use; avoid concomitant use with artemether/ lumefantrine.
- Antimuscarinics: increased risk of ventricular arrhythmias with tolterodine.
- Antipsychotics: increased risk of ventricular arrhythmias with antipsychotics that prolong the QT interval; increased risk of ventricular arrhythmias with amisulpride, benperidol, droperidol, haloperidol, phenothiazines, pimozide or zuclopenthixol – avoid; increased risk of ventricular arrhythmias with sulpiride.
- Antivirals: increased risk of ventricular arrhythmias with fosamprenavir ritonavir, saquinavir and telaprevir – avoid concomitant use; concentration possibly increased by atazanavir; avoid with indinavir.

- Atomoxetine: increased risk of ventricular arrhythmias.
- Beta-blockers, diltiazem, verapamil: Increased risk of bradycardia, AV block and myocardial depression; increased risk of ventricular arrhythmias with sotalol – avoid.
- Ciclosporin: increased levels of ciclosporin possible.
- Colchicine: possibly increased colchicine toxicity.
- Cytotoxics: possibly increased risk of ventricular arrhythmias with vandetanib – avoid; increased risk of ventricular arrhythmias with arsenic trioxide.
- Digoxin: increased concentration (halve digoxin maintenance dose).
- Fingolimod: possible increased risk of bradycardia.
- Ivabradine: increased risk of ventricular arrhythmias – avoid concomitant use.
- Lipid-lowering drugs: increased risk of myopathy with simvastatin – do not exceed 20 mg of simvastatin.[1]
- Lithium: increased risk of ventricular arrhythmias – avoid concomitant use.
- Pentamidine: increased risk of ventricular arrhythmias – avoid concomitant use.
- Grapefruit juice: may increase concentration of amiodarone – avoid concomitant use.

ADMINISTRATION

RECONSTITUTION
–
ROUTE
- Oral, IV via central catheter or peripherally in veins with good blood flow.

RATE OF ADMINISTRATION
- 20–120 minutes (max 1.2 g in up to 500 mL glucose 5% in 24 hours).

COMMENTS
- Add dose to 250 mL glucose 5%.
- Solutions containing less than 300 mg in 500 mL glucose 5% should not be used, as unstable.
- Minimum volumes for central use only are up to 900 mg in 48–50 mL. (UK Critical Care Group, *Minimum Infusion Volumes for Fluid Restricted Critically Ill Patients*, 3rd edition, 2006).
- Volumetric pump should be used as amiodarone can reduce drop size.

OTHER INFORMATION

- Amiodarone and desethylamiodarone levels can be monitored to assess compliance.
- In extreme clinical emergency, may be given by slow IV bolus using 150–300 mg in 10–20 mL glucose 5% over a minimum of 3 minutes with close monitoring. This should not be repeated for at least 15 minutes.
- Incompatible with sodium chloride 0.9%.
- Rapid IV administration has been associated with anaphylactic shock, hot flushes, sweating, and nausea.

Reference:
1. MHRA. *Drug Safety Update*. 2012 August; 1(6).

Amisulpride

CLINICAL USE

Treatment of acute and chronic
schizophrenia

DOSE IN NORMAL RENAL FUNCTION

50–1200 mg daily (in divided doses if
>300 mg); varies according to indication

PHARMACOKINETICS

Molecular weight (daltons)	369.5
% Protein binding	16
% Excreted unchanged in urine	50
Volume of distribution (L/kg)	5.8
Half-life – normal/ ESRF (hrs)	12/Unchanged

METABOLISM

Amisulpride is weakly metabolised: two
inactive metabolites, accounting for
approximately 4% of the dose, have been
identified. Amisulpride is eliminated
unchanged in the urine. Fifty per cent of an
intravenous dose is excreted via the urine, of
which 90% is eliminated in the first 24 hours.
  The AUC of amisulpride in people with
a GFR 30–60 mL/min is increased 2-fold,
and almost 10-fold in people with a GFR
10–30 mL/min.

DOSE IN RENAL IMPAIRMENT GFR (mL/MIN)

30–60	Reduce dose by 50%.
10–30	Use a third of the dose. See 'Other information'.
<10	Use with caution. Start with minimum dose and increase according to patient's response.

DOSE IN PATIENTS UNDERGOING RENAL REPLACEMENT THERAPIES

CAPD	Not dialysed. Dose as in GFR<10 mL/min.
HD	Poorly dialysed. Dose as in GFR<10 mL/min.
HDF/High flux	Unknown dialysability. Dose as in GFR<10 mL/min.
CAV/ VVHD	Poorly dialysed. Dose as in GFR=10–30 mL/min.

IMPORTANT DRUG INTERACTIONS

Potentially hazardous interactions with other
drugs
- Alcohol: may enhance CNS effects of
  alcohol.
- Anaesthetics: enhanced hypotensive effect.
- Analgesics: increased risk of convulsions
  with tramadol; enhanced hypotensive and
  sedative effects with opioids; increased
  risk of ventricular arrhythmias with
  methadone – avoid.
- Anti-arrhythmics: increased risk of
  ventricular arrhythmias with anti-
  arrhythmics that prolong the QT interval;
  avoid concomitant use with amiodarone,
  disopyramide and procainamide (risk of
  ventricular arrhythmias).
- Antibacterials: avoid concomitant use with
  erythromycin (increased risk of ventricular
  arrhythmias).
- Antidepressants: increased level of tricyclics.
- Anti-epileptics: antagonises anticonvulsant
  effect.
- Antihypertensives: increased risk of
  hypotension.
- Antimalarials: avoid concomitant use with
  artemether/lumefantrine.
- Antipsychotics: increased risk of
  ventricular arrhythmias with droperidol,
  sertindole – avoid concomitant use.
- Antivirals: concentration possibly
  increased by ritonavir.
- Anxiolytics & hypnotics: increased
  sedative effects.
- Atomoxetine: increased risk of ventricular
  arrhythmias.
- Beta-blockers: increased risk of ventricular
  arrhythmias with sotalol.
- Cytotoxics: increased risk of ventricular
  arrhythmias with vandetanib – avoid;
  increased risk of ventricular arrhythmias
  with arsenic trioxide.
- Diuretics: increased risk of ventricular
  arrhythmias due to hypokalaemia.
- Pentamidine: increased risk of ventricular
  arrhythmias – avoid.

ADMINISTRATION

RECONSTITUTION
–
ROUTE
- Oral
RATE OF ADMINISTRATION
–
COMMENTS
–

OTHER INFORMATION

- Elimination half-life is unchanged in patients with renal insufficiency, while systemic clearance is reduced by a factor of 2.5–3. The area under the curve of amisulpride in mild renal failure is increased 2-fold, and almost 10-fold in moderate renal failure. Experience is limited and there is no data with doses >50 mg.
- Manufacturer advises to avoid if GFR<10 mL/min due to lack of data.

Amitriptyline hydrochloride

CLINICAL USE

Tricyclic antidepressant:
- Depression, used especially where sedation is required
- Neuropathic pain

DOSE IN NORMAL RENAL FUNCTION

10–200 mg daily depending on indication

PHARMACOKINETICS

Molecular weight (daltons)	313.9
% Protein binding	96
% Excreted unchanged in urine	<2
Volume of distribution (L/kg)	6–36
Half-life – normal/ ESRF (hrs)	9–25/Unchanged

METABOLISM

Amitriptyline undergoes extensive first-pass metabolism and is demethylated in the liver by the cytochrome P450 isoenzymes CYP3A4, CYP2C9, and CYP2D6 to its primary active metabolite, nortriptyline. Other paths of metabolism of amitriptyline include hydroxylation (possibly to active metabolites) by CYP2D6 and N-oxidation; nortriptyline follows similar paths. Amitriptyline is excreted in the urine, mainly in the form of its metabolites, either free or in conjugated form.

DOSE IN RENAL IMPAIRMENT GFR (mL/MIN)

20–50	Dose as in normal renal function.
10–20	Dose as in normal renal function.
<10	Dose as in normal renal function.

DOSE IN PATIENTS UNDERGOING RENAL REPLACEMENT THERAPIES

CAPD	Not dialysed. Dose as in normal renal function.
HD	Not dialysed. Dose as in normal renal function.
HDF/High flux	Unknown dialysability. Dose as in normal renal function.
CAV/ VVHD	Not dialysed. Dose as in normal renal function.

IMPORTANT DRUG INTERACTIONS

Potentially hazardous interactions with other drugs
- Alcohol: increased sedative effect.
- Analgesics: increased risk of CNS toxicity with tramadol; possibly increased risk of side effects with nefopam; possibly increased sedative effects with opioids.
- Anti-arrhythmics: increased risk of ventricular arrhythmias with amiodarone – avoid concomitant use; increased risk of ventricular arrhythmias with disopyramide, flecainide or propafenone; avoid with dronedarone.
- Antibacterials: increased risk of ventricular arrhythmias with moxifloxacin and possibly telithromycin – avoid concomitant use with moxifloxacin.
- Anticoagulants: may alter anticoagulant effect of coumarins.
- Antidepressants: possibly increased serotonergic effects with duloxetine; enhanced CNS excitation and hypertension with MAOIs and moclobemide; concentration possibly increased with SSRIs; concentration reduced by St John's wort.
- Anti-epileptics: convulsive threshold lowered; concentration reduced by carbamazepine, phenobarbital and possibly phenytoin.
- Antimalarials: avoid concomitant use with artemether/lumefantrine and piperaquine with artenimol.
- Antipsychotics: increased risk of ventricular arrhythmias especially with droperidol and pimozide – avoid; increased antimuscarinic effects with clozapine and phenothiazines; concentration increased by antipsychotics.
- Antivirals: increased risk of ventricular arrhythmias with saquinavir – avoid; concentration possibly increased with ritonavir.
- Atomoxetine: increased risk of ventricular arrhythmias and possibly convulsions.
- Beta-blockers: increased risk of ventricular arrhythmias with sotalol.
- Clonidine: tricyclics antagonise hypotensive effect; increased risk of hypertension on clonidine withdrawal.
- Cytotoxics: increased risk of ventricular arrhythmias with arsenic trioxide.

- Dopaminergics: avoid use with entacapone; CNS toxicity reported with selegiline and rasagiline.
- Pentamidine: increased risk of ventricular arrhythmias.
- Sympathomimetics: increased risk of hypertension and arrhythmias with adrenaline and noradrenaline; metabolism possibly inhibited by methylphenidate.

ADMINISTRATION

RECONSTITUTION

–

ROUTE

- Oral

RATE OF ADMINISTRATION

–

COMMENTS

–

OTHER INFORMATION

- Introduce treatment gradually in renal impairment due to dizziness and postural hypotension.
- Withdraw treatment gradually.
- Anticholinergic side effects: causes urinary retention, drowsiness, dry mouth, blurred vision and constipation.

Amlodipine

CLINICAL USE

Calcium-channel blocker:
- Hypertension
- Angina prophylaxis

DOSE IN NORMAL RENAL FUNCTION

5–10 mg daily

PHARMACOKINETICS

Molecular weight (daltons)	567.1 (as besilate)
% Protein binding	>95
% Excreted unchanged in urine	<10
Volume of distribution (L/kg)	20
Half-life – normal/ ESRF (hrs)	35–50/50

METABOLISM

Amlodipine is extensively metabolised by the liver to inactive metabolites with 10% of the parent compound and 60% of metabolites excreted in the urine.

DOSE IN RENAL IMPAIRMENT GFR (mL/MIN)

20–50	Dose as in normal renal function.
10–20	Dose as in normal renal function.
<10	Dose as in normal renal function.

DOSE IN PATIENTS UNDERGOING RENAL REPLACEMENT THERAPIES

CAPD	Not dialysed. Dose as in normal renal function.
HD	Not dialysed. Dose as in normal renal function.
HDF/High flux	Unlikely to be dialysed. Dose as in normal renal function.
CAV/ VVHD	Not dialysed. Dose as in normal renal function.

IMPORTANT DRUG INTERACTIONS

Potentially hazardous interactions with other drugs
- Anaesthetics: enhanced hypotensive effect.
- Antibacterials: metabolism possibly inhibited by clarithromycin, erythromycin & telithromycin.
- Antidepressants: enhanced hypotensive effect with MAOIs, concentration possibly reduced by St John's wort.
- Antifungals: negative inotropic effect possibly increased with itraconazole.
- Antihypertensives: enhanced hypotensive effect; increased risk of first dose hypotensive effect of post-synaptic alpha-blockers.
- Antivirals: concentration increased by telaprevir and possibly by ritonavir.
- Lipid lowering agents: possibly increased risk of myopathy – do not exceed 20 mg of simvastatin.[1]
- Theophylline: possibly increased theophylline concentration.

ADMINISTRATION

RECONSTITUTION
–
ROUTE
- Oral
RATE OF ADMINISTRATION
–
COMMENTS
–

OTHER INFORMATION

Reference:
1. MHRA. *Drug Safety Update*. 2012 August; **1**(6).

Amoxicillin

CLINICAL USE

Antibacterial agent

DOSE IN NORMAL RENAL FUNCTION

250 mg – 1 g every 8 hours (maximum 6 g per day, up to 12 g in endocarditis)

PHARMACOKINETICS

Molecular weight (daltons)	365.4
% Protein binding	20
% Excreted unchanged in urine	60
Volume of distribution (L/kg)	0.3
Half-life – normal/ ESRF (hrs)	1–1.5/7–20

METABOLISM

Amoxicillin is metabolised to a limited extent to penicilloic acid which is excreted in the urine. About 60% of an oral dose of amoxicillin is excreted unchanged in the urine by glomerular filtration and tubular secretion. Probenecid reduces renal excretion. High concentrations have been reported in bile; some may be excreted in the faeces.

DOSE IN RENAL IMPAIRMENT GFR (mL/MIN)

20–50	Dose as in normal renal function.
10–20	Dose as in normal renal function.
<10	250 mg – 1 g every 8 hours (Maximum 6 g per day in endocarditis.)

DOSE IN PATIENTS UNDERGOING RENAL REPLACEMENT THERAPIES

CAPD	Not dialysed. Dose as in GFR<10 mL/min.
HD	Dialysed. Dose as in GFR<10 mL/min.
HDF/High flux	Dialysed. Dose as in GFR<10 mL/min.
CAV/ VVHD	Dialysed. Dose as in normal renal function.

IMPORTANT DRUG INTERACTIONS

Potentially hazardous interactions with other drugs
- Amoxicillin can reduce the excretion of methotrexate (increased risk of toxicity).

ADMINISTRATION

RECONSTITUTION
- IV: Dissolve each 250 mg in 5 mL water for injection
- IM: Dissolve 250 mg in 1.5 mL water for injection; 500 mg in 2.5 mL water for injection; 1 g in 2.5 mL water for injection or 1% sterile lidocaine hydrochloride

ROUTE
- Oral, IV, IM

RATE OF ADMINISTRATION
- Slow bolus IV over 3–4 minutes
- Infusion over 30–60 minutes

COMMENTS
- IV Infusion: Dilute in 100 mL glucose 5% or sodium chloride 0.9%
- Stability in infusion depends upon diluent

OTHER INFORMATION

- Sodium – 3.3 mmol/g vial of Amoxil.
- Do not mix with aminoglycosides.

Amphotericin IV – Abelcet (lipid complex)

CLINICAL USE

Antifungal agent:
- Systemic fungal infections (yeasts and yeast-like fungi including *Candida albicans*)

DOSE IN NORMAL RENAL FUNCTION

5 mg/kg/day for at least 14 days (see individual product data sheet)

PHARMACOKINETICS

Molecular weight (daltons)	924.1
% Protein binding	90
% Excreted unchanged in urine	<1
Volume of distribution (L/kg)	2286
Half-life – normal/ ESRF (hrs)	173.4/Unchanged

METABOLISM

The metabolic fate of amphotericin B in humans has not been fully elucidated. Conventional amphotericin B is eliminated very slowly (over weeks to months) by the kidneys; slow release of the drug from the peripheral compartment may account for the long elimination half-life. Over a 7-day period, the cumulative urinary excretion of a single dose of conventional amphotericin B is about 40% of the administered drug. It has been estimated that only about 2–5% of a total dose of amphotericin B is excreted in urine unchanged. When conventional IV amphotericin B therapy is discontinued, the drug can be detected in blood for up to 4 weeks and in urine for up to 4–8 weeks.

Abelcet is Amphotericin B complexed to phospholipids; the pharmacokinetic properties of Abelcet and conventional amphotericin B are different. Pharmacokinetic studies showed that, after administration of Abelcet, amphotericin B levels were highest in the liver, spleen and lung.

DOSE IN RENAL IMPAIRMENT GFR (mL/MIN)

20–50	Dose as in normal renal function.
10–20	Dose as in normal renal function.
<10	Dose as in normal renal function.

DOSE IN PATIENTS UNDERGOING RENAL REPLACEMENT THERAPIES

CAPD	Not dialysed. Dose as in normal renal function.
HD	Not dialysed. Dose as in normal renal function.
HDF/High flux	Unknown dialysability. Dose as in normal renal function.
CAV/ VVHD	Not dialysed. Dose as in normal renal function.

IMPORTANT DRUG INTERACTIONS

Potentially hazardous interactions with other drugs
- Ciclosporin: increased nephrotoxicity.
- Tacrolimus: increased nephrotoxicity.
- Increased risk of nephrotoxicity with aminoglycosides and other nephrotoxic agents and cytotoxics.
- Cardiac glycosides: increased toxicity if hypokalaemia occurs.
- Corticosteroids: increased risk of hypokalaemia (avoid concomitant use unless corticosteroids are required to control reactions).
- Cytotoxics: increased risk of ventricular arrhythmias with arsenic trioxide.
- Flucytosine: enhanced toxicity in combination with amphotericin.

ADMINISTRATION

RECONSTITUTION
- See individual data sheet. Prepare intermittent infusion in glucose 5% (incompatible with sodium chloride 0.9%, electrolytes or other drugs).
- Dilute to a concentration of 1–2 mg/mL.

ROUTE
- IV infusion

RATE OF ADMINISTRATION
- 2.5 mg/kg/hour

COMMENTS

- Paracetamol and parenteral pethidine may alleviate rigors associated with amphotericin administration. Can also use antihistamines to control reactions.
- Flush existing IV line with glucose 5% before and after infusion administration.
- For patients on CAV/VVHD, amphotericin should be given into the venous return of the dialysis circuit.
- Should be given post dialysis.

OTHER INFORMATION

*** AMPHOTERICIN IS HIGHLY NEPHROTOXIC ***

- Can cause distal tubular acidosis.
- May cause polyuria, hypovolaemia, hypokalaemia and acidosis.
- Amphotericin and flucytosine act synergistically when co-administered enabling lower doses to be used effectively.
- A test dose of amphotericin is recommended at the beginning of a new course (1 mg over 15 minutes).
- Monitor renal function, full blood count, potassium, magnesium and calcium levels.
- Liposomal amphotericin is considerably less nephrotoxic compared with conventional amphotericin B, but is considerably more expensive.

Amphotericin IV – AmBisome (liposomal)

CLINICAL USE

Antifungal agent:
- Systemic fungal infections (yeasts and yeast-like fungi including *Candida albicans*)
- Treatment of visceral leishmaniasis

DOSE IN NORMAL RENAL FUNCTION

- 1–3 mg/kg/day, maximum 5 mg/kg (unlicensed dose)
- Visceral leishmaniasis: total dose of 21–30 mg/kg given over 10–21 days

PHARMACOKINETICS

Molecular weight (daltons)	924.1
% Protein binding	90
% Excreted unchanged in urine	2–5
Volume of distribution (L/kg)	0.1–0.44
Half-life – normal/ESRF (hrs)	6.3–10.7/ Unchanged

METABOLISM

The metabolic fate of amphotericin B in humans has not been fully elucidated. Conventional amphotericin B is eliminated very slowly (over weeks to months) by the kidneys; slow release of the drug from the peripheral compartment may account for the long elimination half-life. Over a 7-day period, the cumulative urinary excretion of a single dose of conventional amphotericin B is about 40% of the administered drug. It has been estimated that only about 2–5% of a total dose of amphotericin B is excreted in urine unchanged. When conventional IV amphotericin B therapy is discontinued, the drug can be detected in blood for up to 4 weeks and in urine for up to 4–8 weeks.

AmBisome has a significantly different pharmacokinetic profile from that reported in the literature for conventional presentations of amphotericin B, with higher amphotericin B plasma concentrations (C_{max}) and increased exposure (AUC_{0-24}). Due to the size of the liposomes, there is no glomerular filtration and renal elimination of AmBisome, thus avoiding interaction of amphotericin B with the cells of the distal tubuli and reducing the potential for nephrotoxicity seen with conventional amphotericin B presentations.

DOSE IN RENAL IMPAIRMENT GFR (mL/MIN)

20–50	Dose as in normal renal function.
10–20	Dose as in normal renal function.
<10	Dose as in normal renal function.

DOSE IN PATIENTS UNDERGOING RENAL REPLACEMENT THERAPIES

CAPD	Not dialysed. Dose as in normal renal function.
HD	Not dialysed. Dose as in normal renal function.
HDF/High flux	Unknown dialysability. Dose as in normal renal function.
CAV/ VVHD	Not dialysed. Dose as in normal renal function.

IMPORTANT DRUG INTERACTIONS

Potentially hazardous interactions with other drugs
- Ciclosporin: increased nephrotoxicity.
- Tacrolimus: increased nephrotoxicity.
- Increased risk of nephrotoxicity with aminoglycosides and other nephrotoxic agents and cytotoxics.
- Cardiac glycosides: increased toxicity if hypokalaemia occurs.
- Corticosteroids: increased risk of hypokalaemia (avoid concomitant use unless corticosteroids are required to control reactions).
- Cytotoxics: increased risk of ventricular arrhythmias with arsenic trioxide.
- Flucytosine: enhanced toxicity in combination with amphotericin.

ADMINISTRATION

RECONSTITUTION
- See SPC. Prepare intermittent infusion in glucose 5% (incompatible with sodium chloride 0.9%, electrolytes or other drugs). Reconstitute vial contents with water for injection.
- Dilute to a concentration of 0.2–2 mg/mL.

ROUTE
- IV infusion

RATE OF ADMINISTRATION
- 30–60 minutes (doses >5 mg/kg over 2 hours)

COMMENTS
- Paracetamol and parenteral pethidine may alleviate rigors associated with amphotericin administration. Antihistamines can also be administered to control reactions.
- Flush existing IV line with glucose 5% before and after infusion administration.
- For patients on CAV/VVHD, amphotericin should be given into the venous return of the dialysis circuit.
- Should be given post dialysis.

OTHER INFORMATION

*** AMPHOTERICIN IS HIGHLY NEPHROTOXIC ***
- Can cause distal tubular acidosis.
- May cause polyuria, hypovolaemia, hypokalaemia and acidosis.
- Amphotericin and flucytosine act synergistically when co-administered enabling lower doses to be used effectively.
- A test dose of amphotericin is recommended at the beginning of a new course (1 mg over 10 minutes then stop and observe for next 30 minutes).
- Monitor renal function, full blood count, potassium, magnesium and calcium levels.
- Liposomal amphotericin is considerably less nephrotoxic compared with amphotericin, but is considerably more expensive.

Amphotericin IV – Fungizone

CLINICAL USE

Antifungal agent:
- Systemic fungal infections (yeasts and yeast-like fungi including *Candida albicans*)

DOSE IN NORMAL RENAL FUNCTION

250 micrograms – 1.5 mg/kg/day
Can be given on alternate days if using a higher dose.

PHARMACOKINETICS

Molecular weight (daltons)	924.1
% Protein binding	>90
% Excreted unchanged in urine	2–5
Volume of distribution (L/kg)	4
Half-life – normal/ESRF (hrs)	24–48 (up to 15 days with long term use)/Unchanged

METABOLISM

The metabolic fate of amphotericin B in humans has not been fully elucidated. Conventional amphotericin B is eliminated very slowly (over weeks to months) by the kidneys; slow release of the drug from the peripheral compartment may account for the long elimination half-life. Over a 7-day period, the cumulative urinary excretion of a single dose of conventional amphotericin B is about 40% of the administered drug. It has been estimated that only about 2–5% of a total dose of amphotericin B is excreted in urine unchanged. When conventional IV amphotericin B therapy is discontinued, the drug can be detected in blood for up to 4 weeks and in urine for up to 4–8 weeks.

DOSE IN RENAL IMPAIRMENT GFR (mL/MIN)

20–50	Dose as in normal renal function.
10–20	Dose as in normal renal function.
<10	Dose as in normal renal function.

DOSE IN PATIENTS UNDERGOING RENAL REPLACEMENT THERAPIES

CAPD	Not dialysed. Dose as in GFR<10 mL/min.
HD	Not dialysed. Dose as in GFR<10 mL/min.
HDF/High flux	Not dialysed. Dose as in GFR<10 mL/min.
CAV/VVHD	Not dialysed. Dose as in GFR=10–20 mL/min.

IMPORTANT DRUG INTERACTIONS

Potentially hazardous interactions with other drugs
- Ciclosporin: increased nephrotoxicity.
- Tacrolimus: increased nephrotoxicity.
- Increased risk of nephrotoxicity with aminoglycosides and other nephrotoxic agents and cytotoxics.
- Cardiac glycosides: increased toxicity if hypokalaemia occurs.
- Corticosteroids: increased risk of hypokalaemia – avoid concomitant use unless corticosteroids are required to control reactions.
- Cytotoxics: increased risk of ventricular arrhythmias with arsenic trioxide.
- Flucytosine: enhanced toxicity in combination with amphotericin.

ADMINISTRATION

RECONSTITUTION
- See SPC. Prepare intermittent infusion in glucose 5% (incompatible with sodium chloride 0.9%, electrolytes or other drugs). Reconstitute vial contents with water for injection. pH should be adjusted to >4.2.
- Dilute to a concentration of 10 mg in 100 mL.

ROUTE
- IV infusion

RATE OF ADMINISTRATION
- 2–6 hours
- If given over 12–24 hours there is a reduced incidence of side effects.

COMMENTS
- Minimum volume peripherally 0.2 mg/mL, centrally 0.5 mg/mL. (UK Critical Care Group, *Minimum Infusion Volumes for Fluid Restricted Critically Ill Patients*, 3rd edition, 2006).
- Higher rates of infusion are associated with greater risk of adverse reactions. Administration over less than 1 hour, particularly in renal failure, has been

- associated with hyperkalaemia and arrhythmias.
- Paracetamol and parenteral pethidine may alleviate rigors associated with amphotericin administration. Can also give antihistamines and corticosteroids to control reactions.
- Flush existing IV line with glucose 5% before and after infusion administration.
- For patients on CAV/VVHD, amphotericin should be given into the venous return of the dialysis circuit.

OTHER INFORMATION

*** AMPHOTERICIN IS HIGHLY NEPHROTOXIC ***

- Permanent renal impairment may occur, particularly in patients receiving conventional amphotericin B at doses >1 mg/kg/day, or with pre-existing renal impairment, prolonged therapy, sodium depletion or concurrent nephrotoxic drugs.
- Nephrotoxicity may be reduced by giving an IV infusion of sodium chloride 0.9% 250–500 mL over 30–45 minutes immediately before administering amphotericin B.
- Can cause distal tubular acidosis.
- May cause polyuria, hypovolaemia, hypokalaemia and acidosis.
- Amphotericin and flucytosine act synergistically when co-administered enabling lower doses to be used effectively.
- A test dose of amphotericin is recommended at the beginning of a new course (1 mg over 20–30 minutes then stop and observe for 30 minutes).
- Monitor renal function, full blood count, potassium, magnesium and calcium levels.
- Liposomal amphotericin is considerably less nephrotoxic compared with conventional amphotericin B, but is considerably more expensive.
- There are reports of the use of amphotericin in 20% lipid solution being as well tolerated as liposomal amphotericin.

Ampicillin

CLINICAL USE

Antibacterial agent

DOSE IN NORMAL RENAL FUNCTION

- Oral: 250 mg – 1 g every 6 hours
- IM/IV: 500 mg – 2 g every 4–6 hours

PHARMACOKINETICS

Molecular weight (daltons)	349.4
% Protein binding	20
% Excreted unchanged in urine	Oral: 20–60; Parenteral: 60–80
Volume of distribution (L/kg)	0.17–0.31
Half-life – normal/ ESRF (hrs)	1–1.5/7–20

METABOLISM

Ampicillin is metabolised to some extent to penicilloic acid which is excreted in the urine.

Renal clearance of ampicillin occurs partly by glomerular filtration and partly by tubular secretion; it is reduced by probenecid. About 20–40% of an oral dose and 60–80% of an IV dose may be excreted unchanged in the urine in 6 hours. High concentrations are reached in bile; it undergoes enterohepatic recycling and some is excreted in the faeces.

DOSE IN RENAL IMPAIRMENT GFR (mL/MIN)

20–50	Dose as in normal renal function.
10–20	250 mg – 2 g every 6 hours
<10	250 mg – 1 g every 6 hours

DOSE IN PATIENTS UNDERGOING RENAL REPLACEMENT THERAPIES

CAPD	Not dialysed. Dose as in GFR<10 mL/min.
HD	Dialysed. Dose as in GFR<10 mL/min.
HDF/High flux	Dialysed. Dose as in GFR<10 mL/min.
CAV/ VVHD	Dialysed. Dose as in GFR=10–20 mL/min.

IMPORTANT DRUG INTERACTIONS

Potentially hazardous interactions with other drugs

- Ciclosporin: may increase ciclosporin levels.
- Reduces excretion of methotrexate (increased risk of toxicity).

ADMINISTRATION

RECONSTITUTION
- Use water for injection: 5 mL for each 250 mg (1.5 mL for 250 mg or 500 mg for IM administration).

ROUTE
- Oral, IV, IM

RATE OF ADMINISTRATION
- Slow IV bolus over 3–4 minutes. Doses greater than 500 mg should be given by infusion
- Infusion: 30–60 minutes

COMMENTS
- Can be diluted in 100 mL glucose 5% or sodium chloride 0.9%.

OTHER INFORMATION

- Rashes more common in patients with renal impairment.
- Can cause nephrotoxicity if dose not reduced in renal impairment.
- Sodium content of injection 1.47 mmol/500 mg vial.
- Ampicillin may be used in peritoneal dialysis fluids for treatment of peritonitis.
- Do not mix with aminoglycosides.
- Doses in renal impairment estimated from evaluation of pharmacokinetics.

Amsacrine

CLINICAL USE

Antineoplastic agent:
● Acute leukaemias

DOSE IN NORMAL RENAL FUNCTION

● Induction of remission: 90–120 mg/m^2 daily for 5–8 days, repeated at 2–4 week intervals according to response
● Maintenance: 150 mg/m^2 as a single dose or divided over 3 consecutive days every 3–4 weeks
● Or according to local policy

PHARMACOKINETICS

Molecular weight (daltons)	393.5
% Protein binding	96–98
% Excreted unchanged in urine	2–10
Volume of distribution (L/kg)	1.67
Half-life – normal/ ESRF (hrs)	5–8/Unchanged

METABOLISM

Amsacrine is extensively metabolised in the liver. The principal metabolites, produced via microsomal oxidation, are much more cytotoxic than the parent drug. Excretion is via the bile; >50% excreted in faeces within 2 hours; 35% in urine.

DOSE IN RENAL IMPAIRMENT GFR (mL/MIN)

20–50	60–75 mg/m^2 daily
10–20	60–75 mg/m^2 daily.
<10	60–75 mg/m^2 daily.

DOSE IN PATIENTS UNDERGOING RENAL REPLACEMENT THERAPIES

CAPD	Unlikely to be dialysed. Dose as in GFR<10 mL/min.
HD	Unlikely to be dialysed. Dose as in GFR<10 mL/min.
HDF/High flux	Unlikely to be dialysed. Dose as in GFR<10 mL/min.
CAV/ VVHD	Unknown dialysability. Dose as in GFR=10–20 mL/min.

IMPORTANT DRUG INTERACTIONS

Potentially hazardous interactions with other drugs
● None known

ADMINISTRATION

RECONSTITUTION
–
ROUTE
● IV
RATE OF ADMINISTRATION
● 60–90 minutes
COMMENTS
● Dilute in 500 mL of glucose 5%.
● Use glass syringes.
● Incompatible with sodium chloride.

OTHER INFORMATION

● Increased risk of side effects in renal impairment.

Anagrelide

CLINICAL USE

Platelet-reducing agent

DOSE IN NORMAL RENAL FUNCTION

1–10 mg daily in divided doses; maximum single dose 2.5 mg; normal range 1–3 mg daily

PHARMACOKINETICS

Molecular weight (daltons)	292.5 (as hydrochloride)
% Protein binding	No data
% Excreted unchanged in urine	<1
Volume of distribution (L/kg)	12
Half-life – normal/ ESRF (hrs)	1.3 days/–

METABOLISM

Anagrelide is primarily metabolised by CYP1A2; less than 1% is recovered in the urine as anagrelide. Two major urinary metabolites, 2-amino-5, 6-dichloro-3, 4-dihydroquinazoline and 3-hydroxy anagrelide (pharmacologically active) have been identified. The mean recovery of 2-amino-5, 6-dichloro-3, 4-dihydroquinazoline in urine is approximately 18–35% of the administered dose.

DOSE IN RENAL IMPAIRMENT GFR (mL/MIN)

30–50	Dose as in normal renal function.
10–30	Dose as in normal renal function, but use with caution and keep to lowest dose possible.
<10	Dose as in normal renal function, but use with caution and keep to lowest dose possible.

DOSE IN PATIENTS UNDERGOING RENAL REPLACEMENT THERAPIES

CAPD	Unknown dialysability. Dose as in GFR<10 mL/min.
HD	Unknown dialysability. Dose as in GFR<10 mL/min.
HDF/High flux	Unknown dialysability. Dose as in GFR<10 mL/min.
CAV/ VVHD	Unknown dialysability. Dose as in GFR=10–30 mL/min.

IMPORTANT DRUG INTERACTIONS

Potentially hazardous interactions with other drugs
- Cilostazol: avoid concomitant use.
- Phosphodiesterase inhibitors: avoid concomitant use with milrinone and enoximone.
- Aspirin: potential risks and benefits must first be assessed, additive antiplatelet effect.
- Grapefruit juice: may reduce clearance of anagrelide.

ADMINISTRATION

RECONSTITUTION
–
ROUTE
- Oral
RATE OF ADMINISTRATION
–
COMMENTS
–

OTHER INFORMATION

- Manufacturer has no data in renal impairment so use with caution.
- May cause fluid retention, tachycardia and various cardiac complications.
- Rarely can increase creatinine levels.
- High doses can cause a drop in blood pressure.

Anakinra

CLINICAL USE

Interleukin-1 inhibitor
- Treatment of rheumatoid arthritis with methotrexate

DOSE IN NORMAL RENAL FUNCTION

100 mg once daily

PHARMACOKINETICS

Molecular weight (daltons)	17 300
% Protein binding	No data
% Excreted unchanged in urine	Majority
Volume of distribution (L/kg)	No data
Half-life – normal/ ESRF (hrs)	4–6/9.7[1]

METABOLISM

Renally metabolised and excreted.

DOSE IN RENAL IMPAIRMENT GFR (mL/MIN)

30–50	Dose as in normal renal function.
<30	100 mg on alternate days.

DOSE IN PATIENTS UNDERGOING RENAL REPLACEMENT THERAPIES

CAPD	Not dialysed. Dose as in GFR<30 mL/min.
HD	Unlikely to be dialysed. Dose as in GFR<30 mL/min.
HDF/High flux	Unlikely to be dialysed. Dose as in GFR<30 mL/min.
CAV/ VVHD	Unlikely to be dialysed. Dose as in GFR<30 mL/min.

IMPORTANT DRUG INTERACTIONS

Potentially hazardous interactions with other drugs
- Live vaccines: avoid concomitant use.
- Adalimumab, certolizumab, etanercept, golimumab & infliximab: avoid concomitant use.

ADMINISTRATION

RECONSTITUTION
–
ROUTE
- SC
RATE OF ADMINISTRATION
–

OTHER INFORMATION

- Bioavailability is 95%.
- UK data sheet advises to avoid in severe renal impairment (GFR<30 mL/min) but American data sheet advises to administer on alternate days.
- In severe renal insufficiency and end stage renal disease (creatinine clearance <30 mL/min), mean plasma clearance declined by 70% and 75%, respectively.
- Less than 2.5% of the administered dose was removed by haemodialysis or continuous ambulatory peritoneal dialysis.

Reference:
1. *Drug Information Handbook*. 22nd ed. American Pharmacists Association. Lexicomp.

Anastrozole

Treatment of breast cancer in post menopausal women

DOSE IN NORMAL RENAL FUNCTION

1 mg daily

PHARMACOKINETICS

Molecular weight (daltons)	293.4
% Protein binding	40
% Excreted unchanged in urine	<10
Volume of distribution (L/kg)	No data
Half-life – normal/ ESRF (hrs)	40–50/Probably unchanged

METABOLISM

Anastrozole is extensively metabolised by postmenopausal women with less than 10% of the dose excreted in the urine unchanged within 72 hours of dosing. Metabolism of anastrozole occurs by N-dealkylation, hydroxylation and glucuronidation via CYP 3A4 & 3A5, and UGT1A4. The metabolites are excreted primarily via the urine. Triazole, the major metabolite in plasma, does not inhibit aromatase.

DOSE IN RENAL IMPAIRMENT GFR (mL/MIN)

20–50	Dose as in normal renal function.
10–20	Dose as in normal renal function.
<10	Dose as in normal renal function.

DOSE IN PATIENTS UNDERGOING RENAL REPLACEMENT THERAPIES

CAPD	Dialysed. Dose as in normal renal function.
HD	Dialysed. Dose as in normal renal function.
HDF/High flux	Dialysed. Dose as in normal renal function.
CAV/ VVHD	Dialysed. Dose as in normal renal function.

IMPORTANT DRUG INTERACTIONS

Potentially hazardous interactions with other drugs

- Oestrogen-containing therapies: avoid concomitant administration as would negate pharmacological action.
- Tamoxifen: avoid concomitant administration

ADMINISTRATION

RECONSTITUTION

–

ROUTE

- Oral

RATE OF ADMINISTRATION

–

COMMENTS

–

OTHER INFORMATION

- Although renal clearance of anastrozole decreases proportionally with creatinine clearance, the reduction in renal clearance does not affect total body clearance of anastrozole.
- According to the American SPC a dose reduction is not required in renal impairment.
- In the UK, the SPC recommends avoiding the use of anastrozole in patients with GFR<20 mL/min.

Anidulafungin

CLINICAL USE

Antifungal agent:
- Invasive candidiasis

DOSE IN NORMAL RENAL FUNCTION

200 mg loading dose then 100 mg daily

PHARMACOKINETICS

Molecular weight (daltons)	1140.2
% Protein binding	>99
% Excreted unchanged in urine	<1
Volume of distribution (L/kg)	30–50 litres
Half-life – normal/ ESRF (hrs)	40–50/Unchanged

METABOLISM

Hepatic metabolism of anidulafungin has not been observed. Anidulafungin is not a clinically relevant substrate, inducer, or inhibitor of cytochrome P450 isoenzymes.

Anidulafungin undergoes slow chemical degradation at physiologic temperature and pH to a ring-opened peptide that lacks antifungal activity. The ring-opened product is subsequently converted to peptidic degradants and eliminated mainly through biliary excretion.

In a single-dose clinical study, radiolabelled (^{14}C) anidulafungin (~88 mg) was administered to healthy subjects. Approximately 30% of the administered radioactive dose was eliminated in the faeces over 9 days, of which less than 10% was intact drug. Less than 1% of the administered radioactive dose was excreted in the urine, indicating negligible renal clearance.

DOSE IN RENAL IMPAIRMENT GFR (mL/MIN)

20–50	Dose as in normal renal function.
10–20	Dose as in normal renal function.
<10	Dose as in normal renal function.

DOSE IN PATIENTS UNDERGOING RENAL REPLACEMENT THERAPIES

CAPD	Not dialysed. Dose as in normal renal function.
HD	Not dialysed. Dose as in normal renal function.
HDF/High flux	Unlikely to be dialysed. Dose as in normal renal function.
CAV/ VVHD	Unlikely to be dialysed. Dose as in normal renal function.

IMPORTANT DRUG INTERACTIONS

Potentially hazardous interactions with other drugs
- None known

ADMINISTRATION

RECONSTITUTION
- With diluent provided

ROUTE
- IV infusion

RATE OF ADMINISTRATION
- 1.1 mg/minute (3 mL/minute)

COMMENTS
- Can be further diluted in sodium chloride 0.9% or glucose 5%.
- Add 100 mg to 250 mL or 200 mg to 500 mL of fluid.

Apixaban

CLINICAL USE

Factor Xa inhibitor:
- Prevention of venous thromboembolism in adult patients undergoing elective hip or knee replacement surgery
- Prophylaxis of stroke and systemic embolism in AF

DOSE IN NORMAL RENAL FUNCTION

- Surgery: 2.5 mg twice daily
- AF: 2.5–5 mg twice daily (depending on weight and age)

PHARMACOKINETICS

Molecular weight (daltons)	459.5
% Protein binding	87
% Excreted unchanged in urine	27
Volume of distribution (L/kg)	21 litres
Half-life – normal/ESRF (hrs)	12/–

METABOLISM

Apixaban is metabolised in the liver mainly via the P450 cytochromes CYP3A4 and CYP3A5.

Apixaban has multiple routes of elimination. Of the administered apixaban dose in humans, approximately 25% was recovered as metabolites, with the majority recovered in faeces. Renal excretion of apixaban accounts for approximately 27% of total clearance. There are also additional contributions from biliary and direct intestinal excretion.

DOSE IN RENAL IMPAIRMENT GFR (mL/MIN)

20–50	Dose as in normal renal function. Use with caution.
15–20	Dose as in normal renal function. Use with caution.
<15	Use with caution.

DOSE IN PATIENTS UNDERGOING RENAL REPLACEMENT THERAPIES

CAPD	Unlikely to be dialysed. Dose as in GFR<15 mL/min.
HD	Not Dialysed. Dose as in GFR<15 mL/min.
HDF/High flux	Unknown dialysability. Dose as in GFR<15 mL/min.
CAV/ VVHD	Unknown dialysability. Dose as in GFR =15–20 mL/min.

IMPORTANT DRUG INTERACTIONS

Potentially hazardous interactions with other drugs
- Analgesics: increased risk of haemorrhage with IV diclofenac and ketorolac – avoid concomitant use.
- Anticoagulants: increased risk haemorrhage with other anticoagulants – avoid.
- Antifungals: concentration increased by ketoconazole – avoid concomitant use; avoid concomitant use with itraconazole, posaconazole and voriconazole.
- Antivirals: avoid concomitant use with atazanavir, boceprevir, darunavir, fosamprenavir, indinavir, lopinavir, ritonavir, saquinavir, telaprevir and tipranavir.

ADMINISTRATION

RECONSTITUTION
–
ROUTE
- Oral
RATE OF ADMINISTRATION
–

OTHER INFORMATION

- Oral bioavailability is 50%.
- Manufacturer doesn't recommend use in severe renal impairment due to lack of data and the potential of an increased risk of bleeding.
- The American Heart Association/ American Stroke Association do not recommend its use in severe renal impairment for stroke/embolism prevention.
- There was no impact of impaired renal function on peak concentration of apixaban. There was an increase in apixaban exposure correlated to a decrease in renal function, as assessed via measured CRCL. In individuals with mild (CRCL=51–80 mL/min), moderate (CRCL=30–50 mL/min) and severe (CRCL=15–29 mL/min) renal impairment, apixaban plasma concentrations (AUC) were increased by 16%, 29%, and 44% respectively, compared to individuals with normal creatinine clearance. Renal impairment had no evident effect on the relationship between apixaban plasma concentration and anti-Xa activity.

Apomorphine hydrochloride

CLINICAL USE

Treatment of refractory motor fluctuations in Parkinson's disease

DOSE IN NORMAL RENAL FUNCTION

3–30 mg daily in divided doses (maximum single dose 10 mg); infusion: 1–4 mg/hour during waking hours
Maximum dose 100 mg daily

PHARMACOKINETICS

Molecular weight (daltons)	312.8
% Protein binding	90
% Excreted unchanged in urine	<2
Volume of distribution (L/kg)	2–19
Half-life – normal/ ESRF (hrs)	29.1–36.9 minutes

METABOLISM

After subcutaneous injection its fate can be described by a two-compartment model, with a distribution half-life of 5 (±1.1) minutes and an elimination half-life of 33 (±3.9) minutes. Clinical response correlates well with levels of apomorphine in the cerebrospinal fluid.

Apomorphine is extensively metabolised in the liver, mainly by conjugation with glucuronic acid or sulfate; the major metabolite is apomorphine sulfate. It is also demethylated to produce norapomorphine. Most of a dose is excreted in urine, mainly as metabolites.

DOSE IN RENAL IMPAIRMENT GFR (mL/MIN)

20–50	Dose as in normal renal function. Start with 1 mg.
10–20	Dose as in normal renal function. Start with 1 mg.
<10	Dose as in normal renal function. Start with 1 mg.

DOSE IN PATIENTS UNDERGOING RENAL REPLACEMENT THERAPIES

CAPD	Unlikely to be dialysed. Dose as in GFR<10 mL/min.
HD	Unlikely to be dialysed. Dose as in GFR<10 mL/min.
HDF/High flux	Unlikely to be dialysed. Dose as in GFR<10 mL/min.
CAV/ VVHD	Unlikely to be dialysed. Dose as in GFR=10–20 mL/min.

IMPORTANT DRUG INTERACTIONS

Potentially hazardous interactions with other drugs
- Nitrates: enhanced hypotensive effect
- Antihypertensives: enhanced hypotensive effect
- $5HT_3$-receptor antagonists: possibly increased hypotensive effects with ondansetron.

ADMINISTRATION

RECONSTITUTION
–
ROUTE
- SC
RATE OF ADMINISTRATION
- 1–4 mg/hour
COMMENTS
- Change site every 4 hours for SC administration

OTHER INFORMATION

- Pre-treatment with domperidone is required for at least 2 days before and at least 3 days after treatment.
- Bioavailability by subcutaneous administration is 17–18%.

Aprepitant

CLINICAL USE

Prevention of acute and delayed nausea and vomiting associated with moderate and highly emetogenic cancer chemotherapy

DOSE IN NORMAL RENAL FUNCTION

125 mg once daily on day 1 followed by 80 mg once daily on days 2 and 3

PHARMACOKINETICS

Molecular weight (daltons)	534.4
% Protein binding	>95
% Excreted unchanged in urine	0
Volume of distribution (L/kg)	66 litres
Half-life – normal/ ESRF (hrs)	9–13/Unchanged

METABOLISM

Aprepitant undergoes extensive metabolism. Following a single IV 100 mg dose of [^{14}C]-fosaprepitant, a prodrug for aprepitant, aprepitant accounts for approximately 19% of the radioactivity in plasma over 72 hours. 12 metabolites of aprepitant have been identified in human plasma. The metabolism of aprepitant, primarily by CYP3A4 and potentially with minor contribution by CYP1A2 and CYP2C19, occurs largely via oxidation at the morpholine ring and its side chains and the resultant metabolites were only weakly active. Aprepitant is not excreted unchanged in urine. Metabolites are excreted in urine (57%) and via biliary excretion in faeces (45%).

DOSE IN RENAL IMPAIRMENT GFR (mL/MIN)

20–50	Dose as in normal renal function.
10–20	Dose as in normal renal function.
<10	Dose as in normal renal function.

DOSE IN PATIENTS UNDERGOING RENAL REPLACEMENT THERAPIES

CAPD	Not dialysed. Dose as in normal renal function.
HD	Not dialysed. Dose as in normal renal function.
HDF/High flux	Unlikely to be dialysed. Dose as in normal renal function.
CAV/ VVHD	Not dialysed. Dose as in normal renal function.

IMPORTANT DRUG INTERACTIONS

Potentially hazardous interactions with other drugs
- Avoid concurrent administration with pimozide or St John's wort.
- Oestrogens and progestogens: may cause contraceptive failure.

ADMINISTRATION

RECONSTITUTION
–
ROUTE
- Oral
RATE OF ADMINISTRATION
–
COMMENTS
–

OTHER INFORMATION

- Less than 0.2% of a dose is recovered in dialysate after haemodialysis.

Argatroban

CLINICAL USE

Anticoagulant:
- Prophylaxis or treatment of thrombosis in patients with heparin-induced thrombocytopenia (HIT)
- Adjunct in patients at risk of HIT undergoing percutaneous coronary intervention

DOSE IN NORMAL RENAL FUNCTION

- Anticoagulant for prophylaxis or treatment of thrombosis: Infusion of 2 mcg/kg/min; adjust according to response (APTT); maximum 10 mcg/kg/min.
- Anticoagulant for patients undergoing percutaneous coronary intervention: Initially a bolus of 350 mcg/kg administered via a large bore IV line over 3–5 minutes, followed by an infusion of 25 mcg/kg/min. Additional IV bolus doses of 150 mcg/kg may be given if required and the infusion rate changed to 15–40 mcg/kg/min.

PHARMACOKINETICS

Molecular weight (daltons)	508.6
% Protein binding	54
% Excreted unchanged in urine	16
Volume of distribution (L/kg)	0.17
Half-life – normal/ESRF (hrs)	39–51 minutes/ Unchanged

METABOLISM

The metabolism of argatroban has not yet been fully characterised. The metabolites identified (M-1, M-2, and M-3) are formed by hydroxylation and aromatisation of the 3-methyltetrahydroquinoline ring in the liver. The primary metabolite (M1) exerts 40-fold weaker antithrombin effect than argatroban. Metabolites M-1, M-2 and M-3 were detected in the urine, and M-1 was detected in plasma and faeces.

Argatroban is excreted mainly in the faeces, presumably through biliary secretion. Following intravenous infusion of ^{14}C-radiolabelled argatroban 21.8±5.8% of the dose was excreted in urine and 65.4±7.1% in the faeces.

DOSE IN RENAL IMPAIRMENT GFR (mL/MIN)

20–50	Dose as in normal renal function.
10–20	Dose as in normal renal function.
<10	Dose as in normal renal function.

DOSE IN PATIENTS UNDERGOING RENAL REPLACEMENT THERAPIES

CAPD	Unlikely to be dialysed. Dose as in normal renal function.
HD	Not dialysed. Dose as in normal renal function.
HDF/High flux	Not dialysed. Dose as in normal renal function.
CAV/ VVHD	Not dialysed. Dose as in normal renal function.

IMPORTANT DRUG INTERACTIONS

Potentially hazardous interactions with other drugs
- Heparin: avoid concomitant administration.
- Urokinase: may increase the risk of bleeding.
- Thrombolytics: may increase risk of bleeding complications; enhance effect of argatroban.
- Antiplatelets and anticoagulants: increased risk of bleeding complications.

ADMINISTRATION

RECONSTITUTION
–

ROUTE
- IV

RATE OF ADMINISTRATION
- Bolus: over 3–5 minutes
- Infusion: 2–25 mcg/kg/min

COMMENTS
- Physically and chemically stable for up to 96 hours if refrigerated or at controlled room temperature and protected from light.
- Dilute to 1 mg/mL with sodium chloride 0.9%, glucose 5% or Lactated Ringer's solution, i.e. 250 mg (2.5 mL) into 250 mL of diluent. The solution must be mixed by inversion for 1 minute.

OTHER INFORMATION

- Can also be used for haemodialysis anticoagulation: 0.1 mg/kg bolus, followed by a continuous infusion of 0.1–0.2 mg/kg/hour, dosing being adjusted to maintain an APTT 1.5–3 times normal.

- For CVVHD a dose of 0.5–1 mcg/kg/min was suggested, dosing being adjusted to maintain an APTT 1.5–2 times normal. (O Shea SI, Ortel TL, Kovalik EC. Alternative methods of anticoagulation for dialysis-dependent patients with heparin-induced thrombocytopenia. *Seminars in Dialysis*. 2003. **16**(1): 61–7.)
- 20% of argatroban is removed during a 4 hour dialysis session.
- There is no specific antidote.
- Contraindicated in patients with overt major bleeding.

Aripiprazole

CLINICAL USE

Atypical antipsychotic:
- Treatment of schizophrenia
- Depression in bipolar disorder

DOSE IN NORMAL RENAL FUNCTION

- Oral: 10–30 mg daily
- IM: 5.25–15 mg followed by 5.25–15 mg after 2 hours, max 3 injections daily
- Combined route daily dose: 30 mg

PHARMACOKINETICS

Molecular weight (daltons)	448.4
% Protein binding	>99
% Excreted unchanged in urine	<1
Volume of distribution (L/kg)	4.9
Half-life – normal/ ESRF (hrs)	75 (146 in poor metabolisers)/ Unchanged

METABOLISM

Aripiprazole is extensively metabolised by the liver primarily by three biotransformation pathways: dehydrogenation, hydroxylation, and N-dealkylation. Based on *in vitro* studies, CYP3A4 and CYP2D6 enzymes are responsible for dehydrogenation and hydroxylation of aripiprazole, and N-dealkylation is catalysed by CYP3A4. Aripiprazole is the predominant medicinal product moiety in systemic circulation. At steady state, dehydro-aripiprazole, the active metabolite, represents about 40% of aripiprazole AUC in plasma.

Following a single oral dose of [^{14}C]-labelled aripiprazole, approximately 27% of the administered radioactivity was recovered in the urine and approximately 60% in the faeces. Less than 1% of unchanged aripiprazole was excreted in the urine and approximately 18% was recovered unchanged in the faeces.

DOSE IN RENAL IMPAIRMENT GFR (mL/MIN)

20–50	Dose as in normal renal function.
10–20	Dose as in normal renal function.
<10	Dose as in normal renal function.

DOSE IN PATIENTS UNDERGOING RENAL REPLACEMENT THERAPIES

CAPD	Not dialysed. Dose as in normal renal function.
HD	Not dialysed. Dose as in normal renal function.
HDF/High flux	Unlikely to be dialysed. Dose as in normal renal function.
CAV/ VVHD	Not dialysed. Dose as in normal renal function.

IMPORTANT DRUG INTERACTIONS

Potentially hazardous interactions with other drugs
- Anaesthetics: enhanced hypotensive effect.
- Analgesics: increased risk of convulsions with tramadol; enhanced hypotensive and sedative effects with opioids.
- Antihypertensives: may enhance antihypertensive effect.
- Alcohol and other CNS drugs: increased sedation and other related side effects.
- Anti-arrhythmics: increased risk of ventricular arrhythmias with anti-arrhythmics that prolong the QT interval.
- Antibacterials: concentration possibly reduced by rifabutin and rifampicin – increase dose of aripiprazole.
- Antidepressants: fluoxetine and paroxetine possibly inhibit metabolism – reduce dose of aripiprazole; concentration possibly reduced by St John's wort – increase aripiprazole dose; increased concentration of tricyclics.
- Anti-epileptics: antagonises anticonvulsant effect; concentration reduced by carbamazepine and possibly reduced by phenytoin and phenobarbital – increase dose of aripiprazole.
- Antifungals: metabolism inhibited by ketoconazole and possibly by itraconazole – reduce dose of aripiprazole.
- Antimalarials: avoid concomitant use with artemether/lumefantrine.
- Antivirals: metabolism possibly inhibited by atazanavir, fosamprenavir, indinavir, lopinavir, ritonavir and saquinavir – reduce dose of aripiprazole; concentration possibly reduced by efavirenz and nevirapine – increase dose of aripiprazole.
- Anxiolytics and hypnotics: increased sedative effects.

ADMINISTRATION

RECONSTITUTION

–

ROUTE

- Oral, IM

RATE OF ADMINISTRATION

–

COMMENTS

–

OTHER INFORMATION

- Can cause QT prolongation.

Arsenic trioxide

CLINICAL USE

Antineoplastic agent:
- Acute promyelocytic leukaemia (APL)

DOSE IN NORMAL RENAL FUNCTION

150 mcg/kg daily until remission occurs
Consolidation: 150 mcg/kg daily for 5 days
per week for 25 doses spread over up to
5 weeks (to start 3–4 weeks after completion
of induction).

PHARMACOKINETICS

Molecular weight (daltons)	197.8
% Protein binding	96% bound to haemoglobin
% Excreted unchanged in urine	1–8
Volume of distribution (L/kg)	4 litres
Half-life – normal/ESRF (hrs)	92/Increased

METABOLISM

When placed into solution, arsenic
trioxide immediately forms the hydrolysis
product arsenious acid (As^{III}), which is the
pharmacologically active species of arsenic
trioxide.

The metabolism of arsenic trioxide
involves oxidation of arsenious acid (As^{III}),
the active species of arsenic trioxide, to
arsenic acid (As^V), as well as oxidative
methylation to monomethylarsonic acid
(MMA^V) and dimethylarsinic acid (DMA^V)
by methyltransferases, primarily in the liver.
Approximately 15% of the administered
arsenic trioxide dose is excreted in the
urine as unchanged As^{III}. The methylated
metabolites of As^{III} (MMA^V, DMA^V) are
primarily excreted in the urine.

Plasma clearance of As^{III} was not altered
in patients with mild renal impairment
(CRCL=50–80 mL/min) or moderate renal
impairment (CRCL=30–49 mL/min). The
plasma clearance of As^{III} in patients with
severe renal impairment (CRCL <30 mL/
min) was 40% lower when compared with
patients with normal renal function. Systemic
exposure to MMA^V and DMA^V tended to be
larger in patients with renal impairment; the
clinical consequence of this is unknown but
no increased toxicity was noted.

DOSE IN RENAL IMPAIRMENT GFR (mL/MIN)

20–50	Reduce dose, use with caution.
10–20	Reduce dose, use with caution.
<10	Reduce dose, use with caution.

DOSE IN PATIENTS UNDERGOING RENAL REPLACEMENT THERAPIES

CAPD	Unknown dialysability. Dose as in GFR<10 mL/min.
HD	Dialysed. Dose as in GFR<10 mL/min.
HDF/High flux	Dialysed. Dose as in GFR<10 mL/min.
CAV/ VVHD	Unknown dialysability. Dose as in GFR=10–20 mL/min.

IMPORTANT DRUG INTERACTIONS

Potentially hazardous interactions with other
drugs
- Use with care in combination with
  other drugs known to cause QT interval
  prolongation.
- Anti-arrhythmics: increased risk of
  ventricular arrhythmias with amiodarone
  and disopyramide.
- Antibacterials: increased risk of ventricular
  arrhythmias with erythromycin,
  levofloxacin and moxifloxacin.
- Antidepressants: increased risk of
  ventricular arrhythmias with amitriptyline
  or clomipramine.
- Antifungals: increased risk of ventricular
  arrhythmias with amphotericin.
- Antimalarials: increased risk of ventricular
  arrhythmias with piperaquine with
  artenimol – avoid.
- Antipsychotics: increased risk
  of ventricular arrhythmias with
  antipsychotics that prolong the
  QT interval and haloperidol; avoid
  with clozapine, increased risk of
  agranulocytosis.
- Beta-blockers: increased risk of ventricular
  arrhythmias with sotalol.
- Cytotoxics: increased risk of ventricular
  arrhythmias with vandetanib – avoid.
- Diuretics: increased risk of ventricular
  arrhythmias if hypokalaemia occurs due to
  acetazolamide, loop diuretics or thiazide
  diuretics.
- Lithium: increased risk of ventricular
  arrhythmias.

ADMINISTRATION

RECONSTITUTION

–

ROUTE

- IV

RATE OF ADMINISTRATION

- Over 1–4 hours

COMMENTS

- Dilute with 100–250 mL glucose 5% or sodium chloride 0.9%.

OTHER INFORMATION

- Manufacturer advises to use with caution in renal impairment due to lack of data.
- Renal excretion is the main route of elimination; can accumulate in renal impairment.
- Can cause QT interval prolongation and hypokalaemia.
- Arsenic trioxide is under investigation for other conditions, e.g. multiple myeloma, acute myeloid leukaemias and myelodysplastic syndromes.
- Intensive monitoring is required.
- Arsenic is stored mainly in liver, kidney, heart, lung, hair and nails. Trivalent forms of arsenic are methylated in humans and mostly excreted in urine. In APL patients, daily administration of 0.15 mg/kg/day of arsenic trioxide resulted in an approximate 4-fold increase in the urinary excretion of arsenic after 2 to 4 weeks of continuous dosing, when compared to baseline values.

Artemether with lumefantrine

CLINICAL USE

Treatment of malaria

DOSE IN NORMAL RENAL FUNCTION

>35 kg: 6 doses of 4 tablets, i.e. 24 tablets
given over 60 hours.
Give 4 tablets at 0, 8, 24, 36, 48 and 60 hours.

PHARMACOKINETICS

Molecular weight (daltons)	Artemether: 298.4; Lumefantrine: 528.9
% Protein binding	Artemether: 95.4; Lumefantrine: 99.9
% Excreted unchanged in urine	No data
Volume of distribution (L/kg)	Artemether: 5.4–8.6; Lumefantrine: 3.8
Half-life – normal/ ESRF (hrs)	Artemether 0.8–7; Lumefantrine: 48–72 (4–6 days in people with falciparum malaria)

METABOLISM

Human liver microsomes metabolise
artemether to the biologically active
main metabolite dihydroartemisinin
(demethylation), predominantly through the
isoenzyme CYP3A4/5. Dihydroartemisinin is
further converted to inactive metabolites.

Lumefantrine is N-debutylated, mainly by
CYP3A4, in human liver microsomes, and is
excreted in the faeces.

DOSE IN RENAL IMPAIRMENT GFR (mL/MIN)

20–50	Dose as in normal renal function.
10–20	Dose as in normal renal function.
<10	Dose as in normal renal function. Use with caution

DOSE IN PATIENTS UNDERGOING RENAL REPLACEMENT THERAPIES

CAPD	Unknown dialysability. Dose as in GFR<10 mL/min.
HD	Unknown dialysability. Dose as in GFR<10 mL/min.
HDF/High flux	Unknown dialysability. Dose as in GFR<10 mL/min.
CAV/ VVHD	Unknown dialysability. Dose as in normal renal function.

IMPORTANT DRUG INTERACTIONS

Potentially hazardous interactions with other
drugs
- Anti-arrhythmics: avoid concomitant use with amiodarone, disopyramide, flecainide and procainamide – risk of ventricular arrhythmias.
- Antibacterials: avoid concomitant use with macrolides and quinolones.
- Antidepressants: avoid concomitant use.
- Antifungals: avoid concomitant use with imidazoles and triazoles.
- Antimalarials: avoid with antimalarials; increased risk of ventricular arrhythmias with quinine – avoid concomitant use.
- Antipsychotics: avoid concomitant use.
- Antivirals: use atazanavir, fosamprenavir, indinavir, lopinavir, ritonavir, saquinavir and tipranavir with caution; avoid with boceprevir; concentration of lumefantrine increased by darunavir.
- Beta-blockers: avoid concomitant use with metoprolol and sotalol.
- Cytotoxics: possible increased risk of ventricular arrhythmias with vandetanib – avoid.
- Grapefruit juice: may increase bioavailability and inhibit metabolism – avoid concomitant use.
- Ulcer-healing drugs: avoid concomitant use with cimetidine.

ADMINISTRATION

RECONSTITUTION
–
ROUTE
- Oral
RATE OF ADMINISTRATION
–
COMMENTS
- Take with food to increase absorption.
- If patient vomits within 1 hour of taking the tablet the dose should be repeated.

OTHER INFORMATION

- In renal impairment monitor ECG and potassium levels.
- Manufacturer advises to use with caution in severe renal impairment due to lack of studies.

Ascorbic acid

CLINICAL USE

- Acidification of urine
- Vitamin C deficiency

DOSE IN NORMAL RENAL FUNCTION

- Up to 4 g daily in divided doses
- Prophylaxis: 25–75 mg daily
- Therapeutic: 250 mg daily in divided doses
- IV: 0.5–1 g daily
- Preventative therapy: 200–500 mg daily

PHARMACOKINETICS

Molecular weight (daltons)	176.1
% Protein binding	25
% Excreted unchanged in urine	Minimal[1]
Volume of distribution (L/kg)	No data
Half-life – normal/ ESRF (hrs)	3–4/Unchanged

METABOLISM

Ascorbic acid is reversibly oxidised to dehydroascorbic acid; some is metabolised to ascorbate-2-sulfate, which is inactive, and oxalic acid which are excreted in the urine. Ascorbic acid in excess of the body's needs is also rapidly eliminated unchanged in the urine; this generally occurs with intakes exceeding 100 mg daily.

DOSE IN RENAL IMPAIRMENT GFR (mL/MIN)

20–50	Dose as in normal renal function.
10–20	Dose as in normal renal function.
<10	Dose as in normal renal function.

DOSE IN PATIENTS UNDERGOING RENAL REPLACEMENT THERAPIES

CAPD	Dialysed. Dose as in normal renal function.
HD	Dialysed. Dose as in normal renal function.
HDF/High flux	Dialysed. Dose as in normal renal function.
CAV/ VVHD	Dialysed. Dose as in normal renal function.

IMPORTANT DRUG INTERACTIONS

Potentially hazardous interactions with other drugs
- None known

ADMINISTRATION

RECONSTITUTION

–

ROUTE
- Oral, IV

RATE OF ADMINISTRATION

–

COMMENTS

–

OTHER INFORMATION

- No scientific evidence from clinical trial of efficacy in reducing UTI via acidification of urine.
- In CKD 5 on dialysis, requirements are usually about 75–90 mg per day. (Kalanter-Zadeh K, Kopple JD. Trace elements and vitamins in maintenance dialysis patients. *Adv Ren Replace Ther.* 2003; **10**(3): 170–82.)
- Try to use lower doses in CKD 5 patients due to risk of oxalate formation.

Reference:
1. Ching-San CL, Marbury TC. Drug therapy in patients undergoing haemodialysis: clinical pharmacokinetic considerations. *Clin Pharmacokinet.* 1984; **9**: 42–66.

Asenapine

CLINICAL USE

Atypical antipsychotic:
- Treatment of schizophrenia & bipolar disorder

DOSE IN NORMAL RENAL FUNCTION

5–10 mg twice daily

PHARMACOKINETICS

Molecular weight (daltons)	401.8 (as maleate)
% Protein binding	95
% Excreted unchanged in urine	50 (small amount unchanged)
Volume of distribution (L/kg)	20–25
Half-life – normal/ ESRF (hrs)	24/–

METABOLISM

Metabolism is by direct glucuronidation by UGT1A4 and oxidative metabolism by cytochrome P450 isoenzymes (predominantly CYP1A2) are the primary metabolic pathways for asenapine.

Excretion is 50% renal and 50% via the faeces.

DOSE IN RENAL IMPAIRMENT GFR (mL/MIN)

20–50	Dose as in normal renal function.
15–20	Dose as in normal renal function.
<15	Dose as in normal renal function. Use with caution.

DOSE IN PATIENTS UNDERGOING RENAL REPLACEMENT THERAPIES

CAPD	Unlikely to be dialysed. Dose as in GFR<15 mL/min.
HD	Unlikely to be dialysed. Dose as in GFR<15 mL/min.
HDF/High flux	Unlikely to be dialysed. Dose as in GFR<15 mL/min.
CAV/ VVHD	Unlikely to be dialysed. Dose as in normal renal function.

IMPORTANT DRUG INTERACTIONS

Potentially hazardous interactions with other drugs
- Anaesthetics: enhanced hypotensive effect.
- Analgesics: increased risk of convulsions with tramadol; enhanced hypotensive and sedative effects with opioids.
- Anti-arrhythmics: increased risk of ventricular arrhythmias with anti-arrhythmics that prolong the QT interval; avoid concomitant use with amiodarone, disopyramide and procainamide (risk of ventricular arrhythmias).
- Antidepressants: concentration possibly increased by fluvoxamine; possibly increased paroxetine concentration; concentration of tricyclics possibly increased.
- Anti-epileptics: antagonises anticonvulsant effect.
- Antimalarials: avoid concomitant use with artemether/lumefantrine.
- Antivirals: concentration possibly increased by ritonavir.
- Anxiolytics & hypnotics: increased sedative effects.

ADMINISTRATION

RECONSTITUTION
–
ROUTE
- Sublingual
RATE OF ADMINISTRATION
–
COMMENTS
- Avoid eating and drinking for 10 minutes after taking tablet as affects bioavailability.

OTHER INFORMATION

- Manufacturer has no information in GFR<15 mL/min but does not advise a dose reduction.

Aspirin

CLINICAL USE

NSAID:
- Analgesic and antipyretic
- Prophylaxis of cerebrovascular disease or myocardial infarction

DOSE IN NORMAL RENAL FUNCTION

- Analgesia: Oral: 300–900 mg every 4 hours. Maximum 8 g daily in acute conditions
- PR: 450–900 mg every 4 hours
- Prophylaxis of cerebrovascular disease or myocardial infarction: 75–300 mg daily

PHARMACOKINETICS

Molecular weight (daltons)	180.2
% Protein binding	80–90
% Excreted unchanged in urine	2 (acidic urine); 30 (alkaline urine)
Volume of distribution (L/kg)	0.1–0.2
Half-life – normal/ ESRF (hrs)	2–3/Unchanged

METABOLISM

After oral doses, absorption of non-ionised aspirin occurs in the stomach and intestine. Some aspirin is hydrolysed to salicylate in the gut wall. Once absorbed, aspirin is rapidly converted to salicylate, but during the first 20 minutes after an oral dose aspirin is the main form of the drug in the plasma. Both aspirin and salicylate have pharmacological activity although only aspirin has an anti-platelet effect. Salicylate is extensively bound to plasma proteins and is rapidly distributed to all body parts.

Salicylate is mainly eliminated by hepatic metabolism; the metabolites include salicyluric acid, salicyl phenolic glucuronide, salicylic acyl glucuronide, gentisic acid, and gentisuric acid. The formation of the major metabolites, salicyluric acid and salicyl phenolic glucuronide, is easily saturated and follows Michaelis–Menten kinetics. As a result, steady-state plasma-salicylate concentrations increase disproportionately with dose. Salicylate is also excreted unchanged in the urine; the amount excreted by this route increases with increasing dose and also depends on urinary pH, about

30% of a dose being excreted in alkaline urine compared with 2% of a dose in acidic urine. Renal excretion involves glomerular filtration, active renal tubular secretion, and passive tubular reabsorption.

DOSE IN RENAL IMPAIRMENT GFR (mL/MIN)

20–50	Dose as in normal renal function. See 'Other information'.
10–20	Dose as in normal renal function. See 'Other information'.
<10	Dose as in normal renal function. See 'Other information'.

DOSE IN PATIENTS UNDERGOING RENAL REPLACEMENT THERAPIES

CAPD	Dialysed. Dose as in normal renal function.
HD	Dialysed. Dose as in normal renal function.
HDF/High flux	Dialysed. Dose as in normal renal function.
CAV/ VVHD	Dialysed. Dose as in normal renal function.

IMPORTANT DRUG INTERACTIONS

Potentially hazardous interactions with other drugs
- ACE inhibitors and angiotensin-II antagonists: antagonism of hypotensive effect, increased risk of nephrotoxicity and hyperkalaemia.
- Analgesics: avoid concomitant use of 2 or more NSAIDs, including aspirin – increased side effects; avoid with ketorolac – increased risk of side effects and haemorrhage.
- Antibacterials: possibly increased risk of convulsions with quinolones.
- Anticoagulants: effects of coumarins enhanced; possibly increased risk of bleeding with heparins and coumarins.
- Antidepressants: increased risk of bleeding with SSRIs and venlafaxine.
- Antidiabetic agents: effects of sulphonylureas enhanced.
- Anti-epileptics: possibly increased phenytoin concentration.
- Antivirals: increased risk of haematological toxicity with zidovudine; concentration possibly increased by ritonavir.
- Ciclosporin: may potentiate nephrotoxicity.

- Cytotoxic agents: reduced excretion of methotrexate; increased risk of bleeding with erlotinib.
- Diuretics: increased risk of nephrotoxicity; antagonism of diuretic effect, hyperkalaemia with potassium-sparing diuretics.
- Lithium: excretion decreased.
- Pentoxifylline: increased risk of bleeding.
- Tacrolimus: increased risk of nephrotoxicity.

ADMINISTRATION

RECONSTITUTION

–

ROUTE

- Oral

RATE OF ADMINISTRATION

–

COMMENTS

–

OTHER INFORMATION

- Aspirin at analgesic/antipyretic dose is best avoided in patients with renal impairment, especially if severe.
- Antiplatelet effect may add to uraemic gastrointestinal and haematological symptoms.
- Degree of protein binding reduced in ESRD.

Atazanavir

CLINICAL USE

Protease inhibitor:
- HIV infection, in combination with other antiretroviral drugs

DOSE IN NORMAL RENAL FUNCTION

300 mg once daily with ritonavir 100 mg once daily

PHARMACOKINETICS

Molecular weight (daltons)	802.9 (as sulphate)
% Protein binding	86
% Excreted unchanged in urine	7
Volume of distribution (L/kg)	No data
Half-life – normal/ESRF (hrs)	7/No data

METABOLISM

Atazanavir is principally metabolised by CYP3A4 isozyme to oxygenated metabolites. Metabolites are then excreted in the bile as either free or glucuronidated metabolites. Additional minor metabolic pathways consist of N-dealkylation and hydrolysis. Two minor metabolites of atazanavir in plasma have been characterised. Neither metabolite demonstrated *in vitro* antiviral activity. Following a single 400 mg dose of ^{14}C-atazanavir, 79% and 13% of the total radioactivity was recovered in the faeces and urine, respectively. Unchanged drug accounted for approximately 20% and 7% of the administered dose in the faeces and urine, respectively.

DOSE IN RENAL IMPAIRMENT GFR (mL/MIN)

20–50	Dose as in normal renal function.
10–20	Dose as in normal renal function.
<10	Dose as in normal renal function.

DOSE IN PATIENTS UNDERGOING RENAL REPLACEMENT THERAPIES

CAPD	Unlikely to be dialysed. Dose as in normal renal function.
HD	Unlikely to be dialysed. Dose as in normal renal function.
HDF/High flux	Unlikely to be dialysed. Dose as in normal renal function.
CAV/VVHD	Unknown dialysability. Dose as in normal renal function.

IMPORTANT DRUG INTERACTIONS

Potentially hazardous interactions with other drugs
- Anti-arrhythmics: possibly increased levels of amiodarone and lidocaine.
- Antibacterials: concentration of both drugs increased when given with clarithromycin; rifabutin concentration increased – reduce dose of rifabutin; rifampicin reduces atazanavir concentration – avoid concomitant use; avoid concomitant use with telithromycin in severe renal and hepatic impairment.
- Antidepressants: concentration reduced by St John's wort – avoid concomitant use.
- Antifungals: concentration increased by posaconazole.
- Antimalarials: avoid concomitant administration with artemether/lumefantrine; may increase quinine concentration.
- Antipsychotics: possibly inhibits metabolism of aripiprazole – reduce dose of aripiprazole; possibly increased concentration of pimozide and quetiapine – avoid concomitant use.
- Antivirals: concentration reduced by boceprevir; concentration reduced by efavirenz – avoid; concentration possibly reduced by nevirapine – avoid concomitant use; increased risk of ventricular arrhythmias with saquinavir – avoid; concentration reduced by tenofovir and tenofovir concentration possibly increased; avoid concomitant use with indinavir; concentration of maraviroc increased, consider reducing dose of maraviroc; possibly reduces telaprevir concentration, also concentration of atazanavir increased; concentration of tipranavir increased, also concentration of atazanavir reduced.
- Anxiolytics and hypnotics: possibly increases concentration of midazolam – avoid with oral midazolam.
- Calcium-channel blockers: concentration of diltiazem increased – reduce dose of diltiazem; possibly increased verapamil concentration.

- Ciclosporin: possibly increased concentration of ciclosporin.
- Colchicine: possibly increases risk of colchicine toxicity, avoid in hepatic or renal impairment.
- Cytotoxics: possibly increases concentration of axitinib, reduce dose of axitinib; possibly increases concentration of crizotinib and everolimus – avoid; avoid with cabazitaxel and pazopanib; possibly inhibits metabolism of irinotecan – increased risk of toxicity.
- Ergot alkaloids: possibly increased concentration of ergot alkaloids – avoid concomitant use.
- Ranolazine: possibly increases ranolazine concentration – avoid.
- Sildenafil: possibly increased side effects of sildenafil.
- Sirolimus: possibly increased concentration of sirolimus.
- Statins: avoid concomitant use with simvastatin – increased risk of myopathy; possibly increased risk of myopathy with atorvastatin, pravastatin and rosuvastatin – avoid with rosuvastatin.
- Tacrolimus: possibly increased concentration of tacrolimus.
- Ticagrelor: possibly increases concentration of ticagrelor – avoid.
- Ulcer-healing drugs: concentration significantly reduced by omeprazole and esomeprazole and possibly other proton pump inhibitors – avoid concomitant use; concentration possibly reduced by histamine H_2 antagonists.

ADMINISTRATION

RECONSTITUTION

–

ROUTE

- Oral

RATE OF ADMINISTRATION

- Take with food.

COMMENTS

- Take didanosine 2 hours after atazanavir if used in combination.

Atenolol

CLINICAL USE

Beta-adrenoceptor blocker:
- Hypertension
- Angina
- Arrhythmias

DOSE IN NORMAL RENAL FUNCTION

Oral:
- Hypertension: 25–50 mg daily
- Angina: 100 mg daily in 1 or 2 divided doses
- Arrhythmias: 50–100 mg daily
- Migraine prophylaxis (unlicensed): 50–200 mg daily in divided doses.

IV:
- Arrhythmias: 2.5 mg at a rate of 1 mg/min repeated at 5 minute intervals to a maximum of 10 mg.

Infusion:
- 150 mcg/kg, repeated every 12 hours if required.

PHARMACOKINETICS

Molecular weight (daltons)	266.3
% Protein binding	3
% Excreted unchanged in urine	>90
Volume of distribution (L/kg)	1.1
Half-life – normal/ESRF (hrs)	6–7/15–35

METABOLISM

Atenolol has low lipid solubility. It crosses the placenta and is distributed into breast milk where concentrations higher than those in maternal plasma have been achieved. Only small amounts are reported to cross the blood-brain barrier. Atenolol undergoes little or no hepatic metabolism and more than 90% of that absorbed reaches the systemic circulation unaltered; it is excreted mainly in the urine.

DOSE IN RENAL IMPAIRMENT GFR (mL/MIN)

20–50	Dose as in normal renal function.
10–20	Dose as in normal renal function.
<10	Dose as in normal renal function.

DOSE IN PATIENTS UNDERGOING RENAL REPLACEMENT THERAPIES

CAPD	Not dialysed. Dose as in normal renal function.
HD	Dialysed. Dose as in normal renal function.
HDF/High flux	Dialysed. Dose as in normal renal function.
CAV/VVHD	Dialysed. Dose as in normal renal function.

IMPORTANT DRUG INTERACTIONS

Potentially hazardous interactions with other drugs
- Anaesthetics: enhanced hypotensive effect.
- Analgesics: NSAIDs antagonise hypotensive effect.
- Anti-arrhythmics: increased risk of myocardial depression and bradycardia; increased risk of bradycardia, myocardial depression and AV block with amiodarone; increased risk of myocardial depression and bradycardia with flecainide.
- Antidepressants: enhanced hypotensive effect with MAOIs.
- Antihypertensives: enhanced hypotensive effect; increased risk of withdrawal hypertension with clonidine; increased risk of first dose hypotensive effect with post-synaptic alpha-blockers such as prazosin.
- Antimalarials: increased risk of bradycardia with mefloquine.
- Antipsychotics: enhanced hypotensive effect with phenothiazines.
- Calcium-channel blockers: increased risk of bradycardia and AV block with diltiazem; hypotension and heart failure possible with nifedipine and nisoldipine; asystole, severe hypotension and heart failure with verapamil.
- Cytotoxics: possible increased risk of bradycardia with crizotinib.
- Diuretics: enhanced hypotensive effect.
- Fingolimod: possibly increased risk of bradycardia.
- Moxisylyte: possible severe postural hypotension.
- Sympathomimetics: severe hypertension with adrenaline and noradrenaline and possibly with dobutamine.

ADMINISTRATION

RECONSTITUTION

–

ROUTE

- Oral, IV

RATE OF ADMINISTRATION

- Infusion: 20 minutes
- IV Injection: 1 mg/minute

COMMENTS

- Dilute with glucose 5% or sodium chloride 0.9%

OTHER INFORMATION

- CSM advise that beta-blockers are contraindicated in patients with asthma or history of obstructive airway disease.

ATG (Rabbit) (Thymoglobuline)

CLINICAL USE
Prophylaxis and treatment of acute or steroid resistant transplant rejection

DOSE IN NORMAL RENAL FUNCTION
Prophylaxis:
- Kidney 1–1.5 mg/kg/day for 3–9 days
- Heart 1–2.5 mg/kg/day for 3–5 days

Treatment: 1.5 mg/kg/day for 7–14 days
NB: In obese patients use ideal body-weight to avoid overdosage.

PHARMACOKINETICS

Molecular weight (daltons)	No data
% Protein binding	No data
% Excreted unchanged in urine	No data
Volume of distribution (L/kg)	0.12
Half-life – normal/ ESRF (hrs)	48–72/–

METABOLISM
Total rabbit IgG remains detectable in 81% of patients at 2 months. Active ATG (that is IgG which is available to bind to human lymphocytes and which causes the desired immunological effects) disappears from the circulation faster, with only 12% of patients having detectable active ATG levels at day 90.

Significant immunisation against rabbit IgG is observed in about 40% of patients. In most cases, immunisation develops within the first 15 days of treatment initiation. Patients presenting with immunisation show a faster decline in total but not active rabbit IgG levels.

DOSE IN RENAL IMPAIRMENT GFR (mL/MIN)
20–50	Dose as in normal renal function.
10–20	Dose as in normal renal function.
<10	Dose as in normal renal function.

DOSE IN PATIENTS UNDERGOING RENAL REPLACEMENT THERAPIES
CAPD	Not dialysed. Dose as in normal renal function.
HD	Not dialysed. Dose as in normal renal function.
HDF/High flux	Unknown dialysability. Dose as in normal renal function.
CAV/ VVHD	Not dialysed. Dose as in normal renal function.

IMPORTANT DRUG INTERACTIONS
Potentially hazardous interactions with other drugs
- Risk of over-immunosuppression with concomitant prescribing of standard maintenance immunosuppressive regimens.
- Safety of immunisation with attenuated live vaccines following Thymoglobuline therapy has not been studied; therefore, immunisation with attenuated live vaccines is not recommended for patients who have recently received ATG.

ADMINISTRATION
RECONSTITUTION
–
ROUTE
- IV via central line or via peripheral vein with good blood flow rates.

RATE OF ADMINISTRATION
- 4–16 hours

COMMENTS
- Dilute dose in 250 mL sodium chloride 0.9%, maximum concentration 5 mg/mL for peripheral administration.
- To minimise risk of adverse effects, chlorphenamine (10 mg IV) and hydrocortisone (100 mg IV) may be given 15–60 minutes before administration of full dose ATG.
- Chlorphenamine, hydrocortisone and adrenaline should be immediately available in case of severe anaphylaxis.

OTHER INFORMATION
- Aim to keep total lymphocyte count below 3% of total white cell count or 50 cells/μL. Alternatively, keep absolute T cell count below 50 cells/μL, and only dose when above this.
- The manufacturers advise that overdosage of Thymoglobuline may result in leucopenia (including lymphopenia and neutropenia) and/or thrombocytopenia.
- The dose of ATG should be reduced by one-half if the WBC count is between 2000

and 3000 cells/mm^3 or if the platelet count is between 50000 and 75000 cells/mm^3.

- Stopping ATG treatment should be considered if the WBC count falls below 2000 cells/mm^3 or platelets below 50000 cells/mm^3.
- Avoid simultaneous transfusions of blood or blood derivatives and infusions of other solutions, particularly lipids.
- The recommended route of administration for ATG is IV infusion using a high-flow vein; however, it may be administered through a peripheral vein. In this instance, concomitant use of heparin and hydrocortisone in an infusion solution of 0.9% sodium chloride may minimise the potential for superficial thrombophlebitis and deep vein thrombosis.
- The combination of ATG, heparin and hydrocortisone in a dextrose infusion solution has been noted to precipitate and is not recommended.
- ATG should not be administered in presence of: fluid overload, allergy to rabbit protein, pregnancy or acute viral illness.

Atorvastatin

CLINICAL USE

Hyperlipidaemia and hypercholesterolaemia

DOSE IN NORMAL RENAL FUNCTION

10–80 mg daily

PHARMACOKINETICS

Molecular weight (daltons)	558.6 (1209.4 as calcium salt)
% Protein binding	>98
% Excreted unchanged in urine	Negligible
Volume of distribution (L/kg)	381 litres
Half-life – normal/ ESRF (hrs)	14 (active metabolite 20–30)/Unchanged

METABOLISM

Atorvastatin undergoes extensive presystemic clearance in gastrointestinal mucosa and/or hepatic first-pass metabolism. Atorvastatin is metabolised by cytochrome P450 3A4 to ortho- and parahydroxylated derivatives and various beta-oxidation products. These products are further metabolised via glucuronidation. Approximately 70% of circulating inhibitory activity for HMG-CoA reductase is attributed to active metabolites.

Atorvastatin is eliminated primarily in bile as active metabolites following hepatic and/or extrahepatic metabolism, but does not appear to undergo significant enterohepatic recirculation.

DOSE IN RENAL IMPAIRMENT GFR (mL/MIN)

20–50	Dose as in normal renal function.
10–20	Dose as in normal renal function.
<10	Dose as in normal renal function.

DOSE IN PATIENTS UNDERGOING RENAL REPLACEMENT THERAPIES

CAPD	Not dialysed. Dose as in normal renal function.
HD	Not dialysed. Dose as in normal renal function.
HDF/High flux	Unknown dialysability. Dose as in normal renal function.
CAV/ VVHD	Not dialysed. Dose as in normal renal function.

IMPORTANT DRUG INTERACTIONS

Potentially hazardous interactions with other drugs

- Anti-arrhythmics: concentration possibly increased by dronedarone.
- Antibacterials: erythromycin, clarithromycin or fusidic acid possibly increased risk of myopathy; concentration increased by clarithromycin – do not exceed 20 mg of atorvastatin[1]; avoid concomitant use with telithromycin; increased risk of myopathy with daptomycin; concentration possibly reduced by rifampicin.
- Anticoagulants: may transiently reduce anticoagulant effect of warfarin.
- Antifungals: increased risk of myopathy with itraconazole – do not exceed 40 mg of atorvastatin,[1] posaconazole and possibly other imidazoles and triazoles – avoid concomitant use.
- Antivirals: increased risk of myopathy with atazanavir, boceprevir (reduce atorvastatin dose), darunavir, fosamprenavir, indinavir, lopinavir, ritonavir, saquinavir or tipranavir (max dose of atorvastatin 10 mg); concentration reduced by efavirenz and possibly etravirine; avoid with telaprevir.
- Calcium-channel blockers: concentration increased by diltiazem – increased risk of myopathy.
- Ciclosporin: increased risk of myopathy – do not exceed 10 mg of atorvastatin.[1]
- Colchicine: possible increased risk of myopathy.
- Grapefruit juice: concentration possibly increased.
- Lipid lowering agents: increased risk of myopathy with fibrates, gemfibrozil (avoid) and nicotinic acid.

ADMINISTRATION

RECONSTITUTION

–

ROUTE

- Oral

RATE OF ADMINISTRATION

–

COMMENTS

–

OTHER INFORMATION

- Rhabdomyolysis with renal dysfunction secondary to myoglobinaemia has been reported with other statins.

Reference:
1. MHRA. *Drug Safety Update.* Statins: interactions and updated advice. August 2012; **6**(1): 2–4.

Atovaquone

CLINICAL USE

Treatment of PCP if intolerant to co-trimoxazole

DOSE IN NORMAL RENAL FUNCTION

750 mg twice daily for 21 days

PHARMACOKINETICS

Molecular weight (daltons)	366.8
% Protein binding	99.9
% Excreted unchanged in urine	<1
Volume of distribution (L/kg)	0.62±0.19
Half-life – normal/ ESRF (hrs)	2–3 days/No data

METABOLISM

There is indirect evidence that atovaquone may undergo limited metabolism, although no specific metabolites have been identified. It has a long plasma half-life, thought to be due to enterohepatic recycling. It is excreted almost exclusively in faeces as unchanged drug.

DOSE IN RENAL IMPAIRMENT GFR (mL/MIN)

20–50	Dose as in normal renal function.
10–20	Dose as in normal renal function.
<10	Dose as in normal renal function. Use with caution.

DOSE IN PATIENTS UNDERGOING RENAL REPLACEMENT THERAPIES

CAPD	Not dialysed. Dose as in normal renal function.
HD	Not dialysed. Dose as in normal renal function.
HDF/High flux	Unknown dialysability. Dose as in normal renal function.
CAV/ VVHD	Unlikely to be dialysed. Dose as in normal renal function.

IMPORTANT DRUG INTERACTIONS

Potentially hazardous interactions with other drugs

- Antibacterials: avoid with rifabutin, concentration of both drugs reduced; avoid with rifampicin, concentration reduced and rifampicin concentration increased; concentration reduced by tetracycline.
- Antivirals: concentration reduced by efavirenz – avoid; concentration of indinavir possibly reduced; concentration of zidovudine increased.
- Metoclopramide: significant reduction in plasma atovaquone levels.

ADMINISTRATION

RECONSTITUTION

–

ROUTE

- Oral

RATE OF ADMINISTRATION

–

COMMENTS

–

OTHER INFORMATION

- Manufacturer advises to use with caution due to lack of data.
- Administer with food. The presence of food, particularly high fat food, increases bioavailability 2 or 3-fold.
- The most commonly reported abnormalities in laboratory parameters are increased liver function tests and amylase levels, and hyponatraemia.

Atracurium besilate

CLINICAL USE

Non-depolarising muscle relaxant of short to medium duration

DOSE IN NORMAL RENAL FUNCTION

- Initially: 300–600 mcg/kg, depending on duration of full block required.
- Maintenance: 100–200 mcg/kg as required or IV infusion: 300–600 mcg/kg/hour
- Intensive care: Initially, 300–600 mcg/kg then by infusion: 270–1770 mcg/kg/hour (usual dose: 650–780 mcg/kg/hour).

PHARMACOKINETICS

Molecular weight (daltons)	1243.5
% Protein binding	82
% Excreted unchanged in urine	0
Volume of distribution (L/kg)	0.16
Half-life – normal/ ESRF (hrs)	Approx 20 minutes/ Unchanged

METABOLISM

Atracurium besilate undergoes spontaneous degradation via Hofmann elimination (a non-enzymatic breakdown process occurring at physiological pH and temperature) to produce laudanosine and other metabolites. There is also ester hydrolysis by non-specific plasma esterases. The metabolites have no neuromuscular blocking activity. Excretion of atracurium is in urine and bile, mostly as metabolites.

DOSE IN RENAL IMPAIRMENT GFR (mL/MIN)

20–50	Dose as in normal renal function.
10–20	Dose as in normal renal function.
<10	Dose as in normal renal function.

DOSE IN PATIENTS UNDERGOING RENAL REPLACEMENT THERAPIES

CAPD	Unlikely to be dialysed. Dose as in normal renal function.
HD	Unlikely to be dialysed. Dose as in normal renal function.
HDF/High flux	Unknown dialysability. Dose as in normal renal function.
CAV/ VVHD	Unlikely to be dialysed. Dose as in normal renal function.

IMPORTANT DRUG INTERACTIONS

Potentially hazardous interactions with other drugs
- Anaesthetics: effects enhanced by ketamine; enhanced effect with volatile liquid general anaesthetics.
- Anti-arrhythmics: procainamide enhances muscle relaxant effect.
- Antibacterials: aminoglycosides, clindamycin, polymyxin, piperacillin enhance effect of atracurium.
- Anti-epileptics: muscle relaxant effects antagonised by carbamazepine; effects reduced by long-term use of phenytoin but might be increased by acute use.
- Atracurium enhances the neuromuscular block produced by botulinum toxin (risk of toxicity).

ADMINISTRATION

RECONSTITUTION
–
ROUTE
- IV bolus, IV infusion
RATE OF ADMINISTRATION
- IV infusion: Initial bolus dose of 0.3–0.6 mg/kg over 60 seconds, then administer as a continuous infusion at rates of 0.3–0.6 mg/kg/hour.
COMMENTS
- Stable in sodium chloride 0.9% for 24 hours, and glucose 5% for 8 hours when diluted to concentrations of 0.5 mg/mL or above.

Axitinib

CLINICAL USE

Tyrosine kinase inhibitor:
- Treatment of advanced renal cell carcinoma

DOSE IN NORMAL RENAL FUNCTION

2–10 mg twice daily

PHARMACOKINETICS

Molecular weight (daltons)	368.5
% Protein binding	>99
% Excreted unchanged in urine	23 (as metabolites)
Volume of distribution (L/kg)	160 litres
Half-life – normal/ ESRF (hrs)	2.5–6.1/Unchanged

METABOLISM

Axitinib is metabolised primarily in the liver by CYP3A4/5 and to a lesser extent by CYP1A2, CYP2C19, and UGT1A1.

Most of the drug is excreted via the faeces and urine as metabolites.

DOSE IN RENAL IMPAIRMENT GFR (mL/MIN)

20–50	Dose as in normal renal function.
15–20	Dose as in normal renal function.
<15	Dose as in normal renal function. Use with caution.

DOSE IN PATIENTS UNDERGOING RENAL REPLACEMENT THERAPIES

CAPD	Unlikely dialysability. Dose as in GFR<15 mL/min.
HD	Unlikely dialysability. Dose as in GFR<15 mL/min.
HDF/High flux	Unlikely dialysability. Dose as in GFR<15 mL/min.
CAV/ VVHD	Unlikely dialysability Dose as in normal renal function.

IMPORTANT DRUG INTERACTIONS

Potentially hazardous interactions with other drugs
- Antipsychotics: avoid concomitant use with clozapine (increased risk of agranulocytosis); avoid concomitant use with pimozide.

ADMINISTRATION

RECONSTITUTION

–

ROUTE
- Oral

RATE OF ADMINISTRATION

–

COMMENTS

–

OTHER INFORMATION

- No experience in GFR<15 mL/min hence use with caution.
- Bioavailability of 58%.

Azacitidine

CLINICAL USE

Antineoplastic agent:
- Treatment of people not eligible for stem cell transplants with myelodysplastic syndromes, chronic myelomonocytic leukaemia or acute myeloid leukaemia.

DOSE IN NORMAL RENAL FUNCTION

$75\,mg/m^2$ daily for 7 days followed by a rest period of 21 days.
Following doses may be altered depending on bone marrow toxicity.

PHARMACOKINETICS

Molecular weight (daltons)	244.2
% Protein binding	No data
% Excreted unchanged in urine	50–85
Volume of distribution (L/kg)	50–102
Half-life – normal/ ESRF (hrs)	33–49 minutes/No data

METABOLISM

Azacitidine undergoes spontaneous hydrolysis and deamination mediated by cytidine deaminase.

Following IV administration of radioactive azacitidine to 5 cancer patients, the cumulative urinary excretion was 85% of the radioactive dose. Faecal excretion accounted for <1% of administered radioactivity over three days. Mean excretion of radioactivity in urine following SC administration of ^{14}C-azacitidine was 50%.

DOSE IN RENAL IMPAIRMENT GFR (mL/MIN)

20–50	Dose as in normal renal function. See 'Other information'.
10–20	Dose as in normal renal function. See 'Other information'.
<10	Dose as in normal renal function. See 'Other information'.

DOSE IN PATIENTS UNDERGOING RENAL REPLACEMENT THERAPIES

CAPD	Unknown dialysability. Dose as in GFR<10 mL/min.
HD	Unknown dialysability. Dose as in GFR<10 mL/min.
HDF/High flux	Unknown dialysability. Dose as in GFR<10 mL/min.
CAV/ VVHD	Unknown dialysability. Dose as in GFR=10–20 mL/min.

IMPORTANT DRUG INTERACTIONS

Potentially hazardous interactions with other drugs
- None known

ADMINISTRATION

RECONSTITUTION
- 4 mL water for injection

ROUTE
- SC

RATE OF ADMINISTRATION
–

COMMENTS
- The reconstituted suspension must be administered within 45 minutes. If made up in advance it can be in a refrigerator (2°C to 8°C) immediately after reconstitution, and kept for a maximum of 8 hours. The syringe with reconstituted suspension should be allowed up to 30 minutes prior to administration to reach a temperature of approximately 20°C–25°C.

OTHER INFORMATION

- Clearance was 147±47 l/h.
- If unexplained reductions in serum bicarbonate levels <20 mmol/L occur, the dose should be reduced by 50% on the next cycle. If unexplained elevations in serum creatinine or BUN to ≥2-fold above baseline values occur, the next cycle should be delayed until values return to normal or baseline and the dose should be reduced by 50% on the next treatment cycle.
- Patients with renal impairment should be closely monitored for toxicity since azacitidine and/or its metabolites are primarily excreted by the kidney.

Azathioprine

CLINICAL USE

Immunosuppressive:
- Prophylaxis of transplant rejection
- Treatment of various autoimmune conditions

DOSE IN NORMAL RENAL FUNCTION

1–5 mg/kg/day

PHARMACOKINETICS

Molecular weight (daltons)	277.3
% Protein binding	<30
% Excreted unchanged in urine	<2
Volume of distribution (L/kg)	0.55–0.8
Half-life – normal/ESRF (hrs)	3–5/Increased

METABOLISM

Azathioprine is extensively metabolised to its active moiety mercaptopurine, which in turn is activated intracellularly by conversion to nucleotide derivatives. Mercaptopurine is rapidly and extensively metabolised in the liver, by methylation, oxidation and by the formation of inorganic sulfates. Thiol methylation is catalysed by the enzyme thiopurine methyltransferase (TPMT). TPMT activity is highly variable in patients because of a genetic polymorphism in the TPMT gene. About 10% of a dose of azathioprine is reported to be split between the sulfur and the purine ring to give 1-methyl-4-nitro-5-thioimidazole. The proportion of different metabolites is reported to vary between patients. Metabolites and small amounts of unchanged azathioprine and mercaptopurine are eliminated in the urine.

DOSE IN RENAL IMPAIRMENT GFR (mL/MIN)

20–50	Dose as in normal renal function.
10–20	75–100%
<10	50–100%

DOSE IN PATIENTS UNDERGOING RENAL REPLACEMENT THERAPIES

CAPD	Dialysed. Dose as in normal renal function.
HD	Dialysed. Dose as in normal renal function.
HDF/High flux	Dialysed. Dose as in normal renal function.
CAV/VVHD	Dialysed. Dose as in normal renal function.

IMPORTANT DRUG INTERACTIONS

Potentially hazardous interactions with other drugs
- Allopurinol: enhances effect with increased toxicity. Reduce azathioprine dose by 50–75% if administered concomitantly – ideally avoid.
- Antibacterials: increased risk of haematological toxicity with co-trimoxazole.
- Anticoagulants: possibly reduced anticoagulant effect of coumarins.
- Antipsychotics: avoid concomitant use with clozapine.
- Antivirals: myelosuppressive effects enhanced by ribavirin.
- Ciclosporin: decreased ciclosporin absorption and bioavailability.
- Cytotoxic agents may be additive or synergistic in producing toxicity, particularly on the bone marrow.
- Febuxostat: avoid concomitant use.

ADMINISTRATION

RECONSTITUTION
- Add 5 mL water for injection to each vial (50 mg).

ROUTE
- Oral, IV

RATE OF ADMINISTRATION
- Over not less than 1 minute.

COMMENTS
- Some units dilute to 100 mL sodium chloride or glucose 5% and infuse over 1 hour. (UK Critical Care Group, *Minimum Infusion Volumes for Fluid Restricted Critically Ill Patients*, 3rd edition, 2006).
- IV bolus peripherally, preferably in the side arm of a fast-running infusion.
- Very irritant to veins. Flush with 50 mL sodium chloride 0.9% after administration.
- Take tablets with or after food.

OTHER INFORMATION

- 1 mg by IV injection is equivalent to 1 mg by oral route.
- 6-mercaptopurine levels can be monitored in patients with low urate clearance.
- Monitor white cell and platelet counts.
- Cytotoxic Drug – Do Not Handle.
- Can be given as an intermittent infusion (up to 250 mg in 100 mL).
- About 40–60% is removed by haemodialysis.

Azilsartan medoxomil

CLINICAL USE

Angiotensin-II antagonist:
- Hypertension

DOSE IN NORMAL RENAL FUNCTION

20–80 mg once daily

PHARMACOKINETICS

Molecular weight (daltons)	568.5
% Protein binding	>99
% Excreted unchanged in urine	15
Volume of distribution (L/kg)	16 litres
Half-life – normal/ ESRF (hrs)	11/–

METABOLISM

Azilsartan is metabolised in the liver by CYP2C9 to two inactive metabolites. The major metabolite is formed by O-dealkylation (M-II), and the minor metabolite is formed by decarboxylation (M-I).

Approximately 55% of radioactivity was recovered in faeces and approximately 42% in urine, with 15% of the dose excreted in urine as azilsartan.

DOSE IN RENAL IMPAIRMENT GFR (mL/MIN)

20–50	Dose as in normal renal function.
10–20	Initial dose 20 mg and increase according to response.
<10	Initial dose 20 mg and increase according to response.

DOSE IN PATIENTS UNDERGOING RENAL REPLACEMENT THERAPIES

CAPD	Not dialysed. Dose as in GFR<10 mL/min.
HD	Not dialysed. Dose as in GFR<10 mL/min.
HDF/High flux	Not dialysed. Dose as in GFR<10 mL/min.
CAV/ VVHD	Unlikely to be dialysed. Dose as in GFR=10–20 mL/min.

IMPORTANT DRUG INTERACTIONS

Potentially hazardous interactions with other drugs
- Anaesthetics: enhanced hypotensive effect.
- Analgesics: antagonism of hypotensive effect and increased risk of renal impairment with NSAIDs; hyperkalaemia with ketorolac and other NSAIDs.
- Ciclosporin: increased risk of hyperkalaemia and nephrotoxicity.
- Diuretics: enhanced hypotensive effect; hyperkalaemia with potassium-sparing diuretics.
- ESAs: increased risk of hyperkalaemia; antagonism of hypotensive effect.
- Lithium: reduced excretion, possibility of enhanced lithium toxicity.
- Potassium salts: increased risk of hyperkalaemia.
- Tacrolimus: increased risk of hyperkalaemia and nephrotoxicity.

ADMINISTRATION

RECONSTITUTION
–
ROUTE
- Oral
RATE OF ADMINISTRATION
–
COMMENTS
–

OTHER INFORMATION

- Oral bioavailability is 60%.
- In patients with mild, moderate, and severe renal impairment azilsartan total exposure (AUC) was +30%, +25% and +95% increased.
- Adverse reactions, especially hyperkalaemia, are more common in patients with renal impairment.
- Renal failure has been reported in association with angiotensin-II antagonists in patients with renal artery stenosis, post renal transplant, and in those with congestive heart failure.
- Close monitoring of renal function during therapy is necessary in those with renal insufficiency.

Azithromycin

CLINICAL USE

Antibacterial agent

DOSE IN NORMAL RENAL FUNCTION

- Genital chlamydia/uncomplicated gonorrhoea infections: 1 g as single dose
- All other indications: 500 mg daily for 3 days or 500 mg on day 1 followed by 250 mg daily for 4 days
- Typhoid (unlicensed)/Lyme disease: 500 mg daily for 7–10 days (7 days for typhoid)

PHARMACOKINETICS

Molecular weight (daltons)	785
% Protein binding	12–52
% Excreted unchanged in urine	6–12
Volume of distribution (L/kg)	31.1
Half-life – normal/ESRF (hrs)	48–96/–

METABOLISM

In pharmacokinetic studies it has been demonstrated that the concentrations of azithromycin measured in tissues are noticeably higher (as much as 50 times) than those measured in plasma, which indicates that the agent strongly binds to tissues. Azithromycin is excreted in bile mainly as unchanged drug. Ten metabolites have also been detected in bile, which are formed through N- and O-demethylation in the liver, hydroxylation of desosamine – and aglycone rings and cleavage of cladinose conjugate. The metabolites of azithromycin are not microbiologically active.

DOSE IN RENAL IMPAIRMENT GFR (mL/MIN)

20–50	Dose as in normal renal function.
10–20	Dose as in normal renal function.
<10	Dose as in normal renal function. See 'Other information'.

DOSE IN PATIENTS UNDERGOING RENAL REPLACEMENT THERAPIES

CAPD	Not dialysed. Dose as in GFR<10 mL/min.
HD	Unknown dialysability. Dose as in GFR<10 mL/min.
HDF/High flux	Unknown dialysability. Dose as in GFR<10 mL/min.
CAV/VVHD	Unknown dialysability. Dose as in normal renal function.

IMPORTANT DRUG INTERACTIONS

Potentially hazardous interactions with other drugs

- Anti-arrhythmics: increased toxicity with disopyramide; increased risk of ventricular arrhythmias with dronedarone – avoid
- Antibacterials: possibly increased rifabutin concentration (increased risk of uveitis & neutropenia) – reduce dose of rifabutin.
- Anticoagulants: effect of coumarins may be enhanced.
- Antidepressants: the manufacturer of reboxetine advises to avoid concomitant use.
- Antihistamines: may inhibit the metabolism of mizolastine (risk of hazardous arrhythmias) – avoid concomitant use.
- Antimalarials: avoid concomitant administration with artemether/lumefantrine; increased risk of ventricular arrhythmias with piperaquine with artenimol – avoid.
- Antipsychotics: increased risk of ventricular arrhythmias with droperidol – avoid concomitant use.
- Antivirals: concentration possibly increased by ritonavir.
- Ciclosporin: may inhibit the metabolism of ciclosporin (increased ciclosporin levels).
- Colchicine: treatment with both agents has been shown in a study to increase the risk of fatal colchicine toxicity, especially in patients with renal impairment – avoid.
- Ergot alkaloids: increased risk of ergotism – avoid concomitant use.

ADMINISTRATION

RECONSTITUTION
- Powder for oral suspension to be reconstituted with water (200 mg/5 mL strength)

ROUTE
- Oral

RATE OF ADMINISTRATION
–

COMMENTS
- Administer as a once daily dose 1 hour before food or 2 hours after food.

OTHER INFORMATION

- In patients with a GFR<10 mL/min a 33% increase in systemic exposure to azithromycin was seen therefore the manufacturer advises to use with caution.
- Dose in severe renal impairment is from *Drug Prescribing in Renal Failure*, 5th edition, by Aronoff *et al.*
- May be used safely in patients on tacrolimus who require treatment with a macrolide.

Aztreonam

CLINICAL USE

Antibacterial agent

DOSE IN NORMAL RENAL FUNCTION

- 1 g every 8 hours or 2 g every 12 hours
- Severe infections: 2 g every 6–8 hours
- UTI: 0.5–1 g every 8–12 hours
- Nebulised: 75 mg three times per day for 28 days

PHARMACOKINETICS

Molecular weight (daltons)	435.4
% Protein binding	60
% Excreted unchanged in urine	60–70
Volume of distribution (L/kg)	0.5–1
Half-life – normal/ESRF (hrs)	1.7/6–8

METABOLISM

Aztreonam is not extensively metabolised. The principal metabolite, SQ-26992, is inactive and is formed by opening of the beta-lactam ring; it has a much longer half-life than the parent compound. Aztreonam is excreted as unchanged drug with only small quantities of metabolites, mainly in the urine, by renal tubular secretion and glomerular filtration. Only small amounts of unchanged drug and metabolites are excreted in the faeces.

DOSE IN RENAL IMPAIRMENT GFR (mL/MIN)

30–50	Dose as in normal renal function.
10–30	IV: 1–2 g loading dose, then maintenance of 50% of appropriate normal dose; Nebulised: Dose as in normal renal function.
<10	1–2 g loading dose, then maintenance of 25% of appropriate normal dose; Nebulised: Dose as in normal renal function.

DOSE IN PATIENTS UNDERGOING RENAL REPLACEMENT THERAPIES

CAPD	Not dialysed. Dose as in GFR<10 mL/min.
HD	Dialysed. Dose as in GFR<10 mL/min.
HDF/High flux	Dialysed. Dose as in GFR<10 mL/min.
CAV/VVHD	Dialysed. Loading dose of 2 g then 1–2 g every 12 hours.[1,2]
CVVHD/HDF	Dialysed. 2 g every 12 hours.[2]

IMPORTANT DRUG INTERACTIONS

Potentially hazardous interactions with other drugs
- Possibly enhanced anticoagulant effect of coumarins.

ADMINISTRATION

RECONSTITUTION
- 3 mL of water for injection per 1 g vial
ROUTE
- IM, IV bolus, IV infusion, Nebulised
RATE OF ADMINISTRATION
- IM injection: Give by deep injection into a large muscle mass.
- IV: Slowly inject directly into the vein over a period of 3–5 minutes.
- IV infusion: Give over 20–60 minutes.
COMMENTS
- Suitable infusion solutions: glucose 5%, sodium chloride 0.9%, compound sodium lactate.
- Dilute to a concentration of not less than 20 mg/mL.
- Once reconstituted aztreonam can be stored in a refrigerator for 24 hours.
- IV route recommended for single doses >1 g.

OTHER INFORMATION

- Manufacturers recommend that patients with renal impairment be given the usual initial dose followed by a maintenance dose adjusted according to creatinine clearance. The normal dose interval should not be altered.

References:
1. CVVH Initial Drug Dosing Guidelines on www.thedrugmonitor.com
2. Trotman RL, Williamson JC, Shoemaker DM, et al. Antibiotic dosing in critically ill adult patients receiving continuous renal replacement therapy. Clin Infect Dis. 2005 Oct 15; 41: 1159–66.

Baclofen

CLINICAL USE

Chronic severe spasticity of voluntary muscles

DOSE IN NORMAL RENAL FUNCTION

Oral: 5 mg, 3 times a day; increase dose gradually up to 100 mg/day

PHARMACOKINETICS

Molecular weight (daltons)	213.7
% Protein binding	30
% Excreted unchanged in urine	70
Volume of distribution (L/kg)	0.7
Half-life – normal/ ESRF (hrs)	3–4/–

METABOLISM

After oral doses some baclofen crosses the blood-brain barrier, with concentrations in CSF about 12% of those in the plasma. Baclofen is metabolised to only a minor extent. Deamination yields the main metabolite, β-(p-chlorophenyl)-4-hydroxybutyric acid, which is pharmacologically inactive. Approximately 70–80% of a dose is excreted in the urine mainly as unchanged drug; about 15% is metabolised in the liver.

DOSE IN RENAL IMPAIRMENT GFR (mL/MIN)

20–50	5 mg, 3 times a day and titrate according to response.
10–20	5 mg, twice a day and titrate according to response.
<10	5 mg, once a day and titrate according to response.

DOSE IN PATIENTS UNDERGOING RENAL REPLACEMENT THERAPIES

CAPD	Unknown dialysability. Dose as in GFR<10 mL/min.
HD	Dialysed. Dose as in GFR<10 mL/min.
HDF/High flux	Dialysed. Dose as in GFR<10 mL/min.
CAV/ VVHD	Unknown dialysability. Dose as in GFR=10–20 mL/min.

IMPORTANT DRUG INTERACTIONS

Potentially hazardous interactions with other drugs
- Anti-arrhythmics: enhanced muscle relaxant effect with procainamide.
- Antidepressants: enhanced muscle relaxant effect with tricyclics.
- Antihypertensives: enhanced hypotensive effect.
- Lithium: use with caution.

ADMINISTRATION

RECONSTITUTION

–

ROUTE
- Oral, intrathecal injection

RATE OF ADMINISTRATION

–

COMMENTS
- Take with or after food.
- Baclofen can be given intrathecally (at doses greatly reduced compared with oral dose), by bolus injection, or continuous infusion. Individual titration of dosage is essential due to variability in response. Test doses must be given. Maintenance dose: 300–800 micrograms/day but doses up to 2000 mcg have been used but experience is limited in doses >1000 mcg.

OTHER INFORMATION

- Withdraw treatment gradually over 1–2 weeks to avoid anxiety and confusional state, etc.
- Drowsiness and nausea frequent at the start of therapy.
- Signs of overdose have been seen in renal patients given doses >5 mg.
- Use with caution as a case report of encephalopathy has been reported in a haemodialysis patient. (Wu VC, Lin SM, Fang CC. Treatment of baclofen overdose by haemodialysis: a pharmacokinetic study. *Nephrol Dial Transplant*. 2005 Feb; **20**(2): 441–3.)
- Another report has seen reduced conscious levels in a haemodialysis patient who was receiving baclofen 5 mg three times a day, within 12 hours she became disorientated and by 36 hours had a GCS of 8. (Su W, Yegappan C, Carlisle EJ, Clase CM. Reduced level of consciousness from baclofen in people with low kidney function. *BMJ*. 2009 Dec 31; **339**: 4559.)

Balsalazide sodium

CLINICAL USE

Treatment and maintenance of remission, in mild to moderate ulcerative colitis.

DOSE IN NORMAL RENAL FUNCTION

- Acute treatment: 2.25 g, 3 times a day
- Maintenance: 1.5 g twice daily, maximum 6 g/day

PHARMACOKINETICS

Molecular weight (daltons)	437.3
% Protein binding	40 (similar to mesalazine), (NASA – 80%)
% Excreted unchanged in urine	25 (as metabolites)
Volume of distribution (L/kg)	No data
Half-life – normal/ ESRF (hrs)	No data ($T_{1/2}$ NASA = 6–9)

METABOLISM

Very little of an oral dose of balsalazide is absorbed via the upper gastrointestinal tract, and almost the entire dose reaches its site of action in the colon intact. It is broken down by the colonic bacterial flora into 5-aminosalicylic acid (mesalazine), which is active, and 4-aminobenzoylalanine, which is considered to be an inert carrier. Most of a dose is eliminated via the faeces, but about 25% of the released mesalazine is absorbed and acetylated. A small proportion of 4-aminobenzoylalanine is absorbed and acetylated by first-pass metabolism through the liver. The acetylated metabolites are excreted in the urine.

DOSE IN RENAL IMPAIRMENT GFR (mL/MIN)

20–50	Dose as in normal renal function.
10–20	Use with caution and only if necessary.
<10	Start with low doses and monitor closely.

DOSE IN PATIENTS UNDERGOING RENAL REPLACEMENT THERAPIES

CAPD	Unlikely to be dialysed. Dose as in GFR<10 mL/min.
HD	Unlikely to be dialysed. Dose as in GFR<10 mL/min.
HDF/High flux	Unlikely to be dialysed. Dose as in GFR<10 mL/min.
CAV/ VVHD	Unknown dialysability. Dose as in GFR=10–20 mL/min.

IMPORTANT DRUG INTERACTIONS

Potentially hazardous interactions with other drugs
- None known

ADMINISTRATION

RECONSTITUTION
–

ROUTE
- Oral

RATE OF ADMINISTRATION
–

COMMENTS
–

OTHER INFORMATION

- Balsalazide is a prodrug of mesalazine (5-amino-salicylic acid).
- Manufacturer advises to avoid in moderate to severe renal impairment.
- Mesalazine is best avoided in patients with established renal impairment, but if necessary should be used with caution and the patient carefully monitored.
- Serious blood dyscrasias have been reported with mesalazine – monitor full blood count closely.

Basiliximab

CLINICAL USE

Chimeric murine/human monoclonal anti CD25 antibody:
- Prophylaxis of acute allograft rejection in combination with maintenance immunosuppression

DOSE IN NORMAL RENAL FUNCTION

20 mg 2 hours before transplant and 20 mg 4 days after transplant.

PHARMACOKINETICS

Molecular weight (daltons)	Approx 144 000
% Protein binding	See 'Other information'.
% Excreted unchanged in urine	No data
Volume of distribution (L/kg)	4.5–12.7 litres
Half-life – normal/ ESRF (hrs)	4–10.4 days/ Unchanged

METABOLISM

In vitro studies using human tissues indicate that basiliximab binds only to activated lymphocytes and macrophages/monocytes. It is most likely removed by opsonisation via the reticuloendothelial system when bound to lymphocytes, or by human antimurine antibody production.

DOSE IN RENAL IMPAIRMENT GFR (mL/MIN)

20–50	Dose as in normal renal function.
10–20	Dose as in normal renal function.
<10	Dose as in normal renal function.

DOSE IN PATIENTS UNDERGOING RENAL REPLACEMENT THERAPIES

CAPD	Not dialysed. Dose as in normal renal function.
HD	Not dialysed. Dose as in normal renal function.
HDF/High flux	Unknown dialysability. Dose as in normal renal function.
CAV/ VVHD	Not dialysed. Dose as in normal renal function.

IMPORTANT DRUG INTERACTIONS

Potentially hazardous interactions with other drugs
- Ciclosporin: may alter ciclosporin requirements.
- Tacrolimus: may alter tacrolimus requirements.

ADMINISTRATION

RECONSTITUTION
- Reconstitute each vial with 5 mL water for injection then dilute to 50 mL or greater with sodium chloride 0.9% or glucose 5%.

ROUTE
- IV infusion

RATE OF ADMINISTRATION
- 20–30 minutes

COMMENTS
–

OTHER INFORMATION

- Basiliximab is detectable in serum for up to 3 months after 15–25 mg doses.
- Use with caution in patients who have previously had basiliximab due to increased risk of developing hypersensitivity reactions.

Belatacept

CLINICAL USE

Prevents T-cell activation
- Prophylaxis of renal transplant rejection

DOSE IN NORMAL RENAL FUNCTION

10 mg/kg
Reduces to 5 mg/kg once in maintenance phase

PHARMACOKINETICS

Molecular weight (daltons)	90 000
% Protein binding	No data
% Excreted unchanged in urine	No data
Volume of distribution (L/kg)	0.11–0.12
Half-life – normal/ ESRF (hrs)	8.2–9.8 days (depends on dose)/–

METABOLISM

Because the drug is a protein, belatacept is degraded into smaller peptides and amino acids by proteolytic enzymes.

DOSE IN RENAL IMPAIRMENT GFR (mL/MIN)

20–50	Dose as in normal renal function.
10–20	Dose as in normal renal function.
<10	Dose as in normal renal function.

DOSE IN PATIENTS UNDERGOING RENAL REPLACEMENT THERAPIES

CAPD	Not dialysed. Dose as in normal renal function.
HD	Not dialysed. Dose as in normal renal function.
HDF/High flux	Not dialysed. Dose as in normal renal function.
CAV/ VVHD	Not dialysed. Dose as in normal renal function.

IMPORTANT DRUG INTERACTIONS

Potentially hazardous interactions with other drugs
- Vaccines: avoid concomitant use with live vaccines.

ADMINISTRATION

RECONSTITUTION
- 10.5 mL of sodium chloride 0.9%, glucose 5% or water for injection

ROUTE
- IV infusion

RATE OF ADMINISTRATION
- 30 minutes
- Use an infusion set and a sterile, non-pyrogenic, low protein binding filter (pore size of 0.2 μm to 1.2 μm)

COMMENTS
- Make up to 100 mL with sodium chloride 0.9% or glucose 5% (volumes may vary between 50 mL and 250 mL depending on dose).
- Use the silicone free syringes supplied and do not shake to minimise foaming.

OTHER INFORMATION

- MPA exposure is approximately 40% higher with belatacept co-administration than with ciclosporin co-administration.
- There was a trend toward higher clearance of belatacept with increasing body weight.

Belimumab

CLINICAL USE

Anti-lymphocyte monoclonal antibody:
- Treatment of systemic lupus erythematosus

DOSE IN NORMAL RENAL FUNCTION

10 mg/kg repeated 2 & 4 weeks after initial infusion then every 4 weeks

PHARMACOKINETICS

Molecular weight (daltons)	147 000
% Protein binding	No data
% Excreted unchanged in urine	Negligible
Volume of distribution (L/kg)	5.29 litres
Half-life – normal/ ESRF (hrs)	19.4 days/Slightly increased

METABOLISM

Belimumab is a protein for which the expected metabolic pathway is degradation to small peptides and individual amino acids by widely distributed proteolytic enzymes. Classical biotransformation studies have not been conducted.

DOSE IN RENAL IMPAIRMENT GFR (mL/MIN)

30–50	Dose as in normal renal impairment.
10–30	Dose as in normal renal impairment. Use with caution.
<10	Dose as in normal renal impairment. Use with caution.

DOSE IN PATIENTS UNDERGOING RENAL REPLACEMENT THERAPIES

CAPD	Unlikely to be dialysed. Dose as in GFR<10 mL/min.
HD	Unlikely to be dialysed. Dose as in GFR<10 mL/min.
HDF/High flux	Unlikely to be dialysed. Dose as in GFR<10 mL/min.
CAV/ VVHD	Unlikely to be dialysed. Dose as in GFR=10–30 mL/min.

IMPORTANT DRUG INTERACTIONS

Potentially hazardous interactions with other drugs
- Live vaccines: avoid concomitant use.

ADMINISTRATION

RECONSTITUTION
- 120 mg vial with 1.5 mL water for injection; 400 mg vial with 4.8 mL water for injection. To provide 80 mg/mL dilution

ROUTE
- IV infusion

RATE OF ADMINISTRATION
- Over 1 hour

COMMENTS
- Further dilute to 250 mL with sodium chloride 0.9%.

OTHER INFORMATION

- Use with caution in severe renal impairment due to lack of studies.
- During clinical development belimumab was studied in patients with SLE and renal impairment (261 subjects with moderate renal impairment, creatinine clearance ≥30 and <60 mL/min; 14 subjects with severe renal impairment, creatinine clearance ≥15 and <30 mL/min). The reduction in systemic clearances were 1.4% for mild (75 mL/min), 11.7% for moderate (45 mL/min) and 24% for severe (22.5 mL/min) renal impairment. Although proteinuria (≥ 2 g/day) increased belimumab clearance and decreases in creatinine clearance decreased belimumab clearance, these effects were within the expected range of variability. Therefore, no dose adjustment is recommended for patients with renal impairment.

Bendamustine hydrochloride

CLINICAL USE

Alkylating agent:
- CLL, NHL & multiple myeloma

DOSE IN NORMAL RENAL FUNCTION

- CLL: 100 mg/m^2 on days 1 & 2 every 4 weeks
- NHL: 120 mg/m^2 on days 1 & 2 every 3 weeks
- Multiple myeloma: 120–150 mg/m^2 on days 1 & 2 every 4 weeks
- Or according to local protocol

PHARMACOKINETICS

Molecular weight (daltons)	394.7
% Protein binding	>95
% Excreted unchanged in urine	3 (20% as unchanged drug & metabolites)
Volume of distribution (L/kg)	15.8–20.5 litres
Half-life – normal/ ESRF (hrs)	28.2 minutes/–

METABOLISM

A major route of clearance of bendamustine is the hydrolysis to monohydroxy- and dihydroxy-bendamustine. Formation of N-desmethyl-bendamustine and gamma-hydroxy-bendamustine by hepatic metabolism involves cytochrome P450 (CYP) 1A2 isoenzyme. Another major route of bendamustine metabolism involves conjugation with glutathione.

Excreted in the urine and faeces as unchanged drug and metabolites.

DOSE IN RENAL IMPAIRMENT GFR (mL/MIN)

20–50	Dose as in normal renal function.
10–20	Dose as in normal renal function.
<10	Dose as in normal renal function. Use with caution.

DOSE IN PATIENTS UNDERGOING RENAL REPLACEMENT THERAPIES

CAPD	Unlikely to be dialysed. Dose as in GFR<10 mL/min.
HD	Unlikely to be dialysed. Dose as in GFR<10 mL/min.
HDF/High flux	Unlikely to be dialysed. Dose as in GFR<10 mL/min.
CAV/ VVHD	Unlikely to be dialysed. Dose as in normal renal function.

IMPORTANT DRUG INTERACTIONS

Potentially hazardous interactions with other drugs
- Antipsychotics: avoid concomitant use with clozapine (increased risk of agranulocytosis).

ADMINISTRATION

RECONSTITUTION
- 10 mL water for injection per 25 mg
- 40 mL water for injection per 100 mg
ROUTE
- IV infusion
RATE OF ADMINISTRATION
- 30–60 minutes
COMMENTS
- Add to 500 mL sodium chloride 0.9%

OTHER INFORMATION

- Manufacturer advises to use with caution in severe renal impairment due to lack of studies although there is little renal clearance.

Bendroflumethiazide

CLINICAL USE

Thiazide diuretic:
- Hypertension
- Oedema

DOSE IN NORMAL RENAL FUNCTION

- Oedema: 5–10 mg in the morning or alternate days
- Maintenance: 5–10 mg, 1–3 times weekly
- Hypertension: 2.5 mg daily

PHARMACOKINETICS

Molecular weight (daltons)	421.4
% Protein binding	94
% Excreted unchanged in urine	30
Volume of distribution (L/kg)	1.2–1.5
Half-life – normal/ESRF (hrs)	3–9/–

METABOLISM

There are indications that bendroflumethiazide is fairly extensively metabolised. About 30% is excreted unchanged in the urine with the remainder excreted as uncharacterised metabolites.

DOSE IN RENAL IMPAIRMENT GFR (mL/MIN)

30–50	Dose as in normal renal function.
10–30	Dose as in normal renal function.
<10	Unlikely to work.

DOSE IN PATIENTS UNDERGOING RENAL REPLACEMENT THERAPIES

CAPD	Unlikely to be dialysed. Unlikely to work.
HD	Not dialysed. Unlikely to work.
HDF/High flux	Unknown dialysability. Unlikely to work.
CAV/VVHD	Probably not dialysed. Unlikely to work.

IMPORTANT DRUG INTERACTIONS

Potentially hazardous interactions with other drugs
- Analgesics: increased risk of nephrotoxicity with NSAIDs; antagonism of diuretic effect.
- Anti-arrhythmics: hypokalaemia leads to increased cardiac toxicity; effects of lidocaine and mexiletine antagonised.
- Antibacterials: avoid administration with lymecycline.
- Antidepressants: increased risk of hypokalaemia with reboxetine; enhanced hypotensive effect with MAOIs; increased risk of postural hypotension with tricyclics.
- Anti-epileptics: increased risk of hyponatraemia with carbamazepine.
- Antifungals: increased risk of hypokalaemia with amphotericin.
- Antihypertensives: enhanced hypotensive effect; increased risk of first dose hypotension with post-synaptic alpha-blockers like prazosin; hypokalaemia increases risk of ventricular arrhythmias with sotalol.
- Antipsychotics: hypokalaemia increases risk of ventricular arrhythmias with amisulpride; enhanced hypotensive effect with phenothiazines; hypokalaemia increases risk of ventricular arrhythmias with pimozide – avoid concomitant use.
- Atomoxetine: hypokalaemia increases risk of ventricular arrhythmias.
- Cardiac glycosides: increased toxicity if hypokalaemia occurs.
- Ciclosporin: increased risk of nephrotoxicity and hypomagnesaemia.
- Cytotoxics: increased risk of ventricular arrhythmias due to hypokalaemia with arsenic trioxide; increased risk of nephrotoxicity and ototoxicity with platinum compounds.
- Lithium excretion reduced, increased toxicity.

ADMINISTRATION

RECONSTITUTION
–
ROUTE
- Oral
RATE OF ADMINISTRATION
–
COMMENTS
–

OTHER INFORMATION

- Monitor for hypokalaemia.
- Manufacturer advises to avoid in severe renal impairment.
- Thiazide diuretics are unlikely to be of use once GFR<30 mL/min.

- There are anecdotal reports of bendroflumethiazide being used in combination with loop diuretics for a synergistic effect in resistant oedema.

Benzbromarone (unlicensed product)

CLINICAL USE

Treatment of hyperuricaemia, chronic gout and tophaceous gout.

DOSE IN NORMAL RENAL FUNCTION

50–200 mg daily
(Usual dose 50–100 mg daily)

PHARMACOKINETICS

Molecular weight (daltons)	424.1
% Protein binding	>99
% Excreted unchanged in urine	6–18 (as metabolites)
Volume of distribution (L/kg)	19 litres
Half-life – normal/ ESRF (hrs)	2–4/–

METABOLISM

Benzbromarone is metabolised to 1'-hydroxy BBR and 6-hydroxy BBR in the liver. 6-hydroxy BBR is further metabolised to 5,6-dihydroxy BBR. Benzbromarone and its metabolites are excreted mainly in the faeces; a small amount appears in the urine.

DOSE IN RENAL IMPAIRMENT GFR (mL/MIN)

40–60	50–200 mg daily[1]
20–40	50–100 mg daily[1]
<20	Avoid. Ineffective

DOSE IN PATIENTS UNDERGOING RENAL REPLACEMENT THERAPIES

CAPD	Avoid. Ineffective.
HD	Avoid. Ineffective.
HDF/High flux	Avoid. Ineffective.
CAV/ VVHD	Use with caution. Dose as in GFR=20–40 mL/min.

IMPORTANT DRUG INTERACTIONS

Potentially hazardous interactions with other drugs
- Aspirin and salicylates: antagonise uricosuric effects of benzbromarone.
- Anticoagulants: may enhance effect of warfarin.
- Pyrazinamide, sulfinpyrazone and thiazide diuretics: antagonise uricosuric effects of benzbromarone.
- Hepatotoxic agents: enhanced hepatotoxicity.

ADMINISTRATION

RECONSTITUTION
–
ROUTE
- Oral
RATE OF ADMINISTRATION
–
COMMENTS
–

OTHER INFORMATION

- Monitor LFTs while on benzbromarone as can cause fulminant liver failure.
- Benzbromarone has been withdrawn in a number of countries due to hepatoxicity.
- As with other uricosurics, treatment with benzbromarone should not be started during an acute attack of gout.
- Maintain an adequate fluid intake to reduce the risk of uric acid renal calculi.
- Biological effect of 100 mg benzbromarone is equivalent to 1.5 g probenecid or greater than 300 mg of allopurinol. (Masbernard A. Ten years' experience with benzbromarone in the management of gout and hyperuricaemia. *SAMJ.* 1981 May 9; 701–6.)
- Benzbromarone is considered unsafe in patients with acute porphyria.

Reference:
1. Perez-Ruiz F. Treatment of chronic gout in patients with renal function impairment. *J Clin Rheumatol.* 1999; **5**: 49–55.

Benzylpenicillin

CLINICAL USE

Antibacterial agent

DOSE IN NORMAL RENAL FUNCTION

2.4–14.4 g daily in 4–6 divided doses

PHARMACOKINETICS

Molecular weight (daltons)	334.4
% Protein binding	60
% Excreted unchanged in urine	60–90
Volume of distribution (L/kg)	0.3–0.42
Half-life – normal/ESRF (hrs)	0.5/10

METABOLISM

Benzylpenicillin is metabolised to a limited extent and the penicilloic acid derivative has been recovered in the urine.

Benzylpenicillin is rapidly excreted in the urine; about 20% of an oral dose appears unchanged in the urine; about 60–90% of an IM dose of benzylpenicillin undergoes renal elimination, 10% by glomerular filtration and 90% by tubular secretion, mainly within the first hour.

Significant concentrations occur in bile, but in patients with normal renal function only small amounts are excreted via the bile.

Renal tubular secretion is inhibited by probenecid, which can be given to increase plasma-penicillin concentrations and prolong half-life.

DOSE IN RENAL IMPAIRMENT GFR (mL/MIN)

20–50	Dose as in normal renal function.
10–20	600 mg – 2.4 g every 6 hours depending on severity of infection.[1]
<10	600 mg – 1.2 g every 6 hours depending on severity of infection.[1]

DOSE IN PATIENTS UNDERGOING RENAL REPLACEMENT THERAPIES

CAPD	Dialysed. Dose as in GFR<10 mL/min.
HD	Dialysed. Dose as in GFR<10 mL/min.
HDF/High flux	Dialysed. Dose as in GFR<10 mL/min.
CAV/VVHD	Dialysed. Dose as in GFR=10–20 mL/min.

IMPORTANT DRUG INTERACTIONS

Potentially hazardous interactions with other drugs
- Reduced excretion of methotrexate

ADMINISTRATION

RECONSTITUTION
- IV Bolus: 600 mg in 5 mL water for injection
- IV Infusion: 600 mg in at least 10 mL sodium chloride 0.9%
- IM: 600 mg in 1.6 mL water for injection
- 600 mg displaces 0.4 mL

ROUTE
- IV Bolus, IV Infusion, IM

RATE OF ADMINISTRATION
- IV bolus: over 3–4 minutes
- IV infusion: over 30–60 minutes

COMMENTS
- IV doses in excess of 1.2 g must be given slowly at minimum rate of 300 mg/minute.

OTHER INFORMATION

- Dose in normal renal function: meningitis up to 14.4 g daily; bacterial endocarditis 4.8 g daily.
- Maximum dose in severe renal impairment: 4.8 g per day.
- 600 mg of benzylpenicillin sodium (1 mega unit) contains 1.68 mmol of sodium.
- 600 mg of benzylpenicillin potassium contains 1.7 mmol potassium.
- Increased incidence of neurotoxicity in renal impairment (seizures).
- False positive urinary protein reactions may be caused by benzylpenicillin therapy.

Reference:
1. Foster P, Gordon F, Holloway S. Drug dosage adjustment during continuous renal replacement therapy. *Br J Int Care.* April 1996; 120–4.

Betahistine dihydrochloride

CLINICAL USE

Treatment of vertigo, tinnitus and hearing loss associated with Ménière's syndrome

DOSE IN NORMAL RENAL FUNCTION

8–16 mg, 3 times a day

PHARMACOKINETICS

Molecular weight (daltons)	209.1
% Protein binding	0–5
% Excreted unchanged in urine	85–90
Volume of distribution (L/kg)	No data
Half-life – normal/ ESRF (hrs)	3.4/–

METABOLISM

Betahistine is excreted almost exclusively in the urine as 2-pyridylacetic acid within 24 hours of administration. No unchanged betahistine has been detected.

DOSE IN RENAL IMPAIRMENT GFR (mL/MIN)

20–50	Dose as in normal renal function.
10–20	Dose as in normal renal function.
<10	8–16 mg, 2–3 times a day.

DOSE IN PATIENTS UNDERGOING RENAL REPLACEMENT THERAPIES

CAPD	Likely dialysability. Dose as in GFR<10 mL/min.
HD	Likely dialysability. Dose as in GFR<10 mL/min.
HDF/High flux	Likely dialysability. Dose as in GFR<10 mL/min.
CAV/ VVHD	Likely dialysability. Dose as in normal renal function.

IMPORTANT DRUG INTERACTIONS

Potentially hazardous interactions with other drugs
• None known

ADMINISTRATION

RECONSTITUTION
–
ROUTE
• Oral
RATE OF ADMINISTRATION
–
COMMENTS
–

OTHER INFORMATION

• Betahistine is rapidly and completely absorbed after oral administration.
• Manufacturer has no data in renal impairment.

Betamethasone

CLINICAL USE

Corticosteroid:
- Suppression of inflammatory and allergic disorders
- Congenital adrenal hyperplasia

DOSE IN NORMAL RENAL FUNCTION

- Oral: 0.5–5 mg daily
- Injection: 4–20 mg repeated up to 4 times in 24 hours

PHARMACOKINETICS

Molecular weight (daltons)	392.5
% Protein binding	65
% Excreted unchanged in urine	5
Volume of distribution (L/kg)	1.4
Half-life – normal/ ESRF (hrs)	5.5/–

METABOLISM

Corticosteroids are metabolised mainly in the liver but also in other tissues, and are excreted in the urine. The slower metabolism of the synthetic corticosteroids with their lower protein-binding affinity may account for their increased potency compared with the natural corticosteroids.

DOSE IN RENAL IMPAIRMENT GFR (mL/MIN)

20–50	Dose as in normal renal function.
10–20	Dose as in normal renal function.
<10	Dose as in normal renal function.

DOSE IN PATIENTS UNDERGOING RENAL REPLACEMENT THERAPIES

CAPD	Unknown dialysability. Dose as in normal renal function.
HD	Unknown dialysability. Dose as in normal renal function.
HDF/High flux	Unknown dialysability. Dose as in normal renal function.
CAV/ VVHD	Unknown dialysability. Dose as in normal renal function.

IMPORTANT DRUG INTERACTIONS

Potentially hazardous interactions with other drugs
- Aldesleukin: avoid concomitant use.
- Antibacterials: metabolism accelerated by rifampicin; metabolism possibly inhibited by erythromycin; concentration of isoniazid possibly reduced.
- Anticoagulants: efficacy of coumarins and phenindione may be altered.
- Anti-epileptics: metabolism accelerated by carbamazepine, phenobarbital and phenytoin.
- Antifungals: increased risk of hypokalaemia with amphotericin – avoid concomitant use; metabolism possibly inhibited by itraconazole and ketoconazole.
- Antivirals: concentration possibly increased by ritonavir.
- Ciclosporin: rare reports of convulsions in patients on ciclosporin and high-dose corticosteroids.
- Diuretics: enhanced hypokalaemic effects of acetazolamide, loop diuretics and thiazide diuretics.
- Vaccines: high dose corticosteroids can impair immune response to vaccines; avoid concomitant use with live vaccines.

ADMINISTRATION

RECONSTITUTION
–
ROUTE
- Oral, IV, IM, topical
RATE OF ADMINISTRATION
- IV bolus: over half to one minute.
COMMENTS
- Can be added to glucose 5% or sodium chloride 0.9%.

OTHER INFORMATION

- 750 micrograms betamethasone ≡ 5 mg prednisolone.
- Even when applied topically, sufficient corticosteroid may be absorbed to give a systemic effect.
- Effects of betamethasone on sodium and water retention are less than those of prednisolone and approximately equal to those of dexamethasone.

Betaxolol hydrochloride

CLINICAL USE

Beta-adrenoceptor blocker:
● Topical use in glaucoma

DOSE IN NORMAL RENAL FUNCTION

Apply twice daily

PHARMACOKINETICS

Molecular weight (daltons)	343.9
% Protein binding	50
% Excreted unchanged in urine	15
Volume of distribution (L/kg)	5–10
Half-life – normal/ESRF (hrs)	16–22/30–35

METABOLISM

Betaxolol is highly lipophilic which results in good permeation of the cornea, allowing high intraocular levels of the drug. The elimination of betaxolol is primarily by the renal rather than faecal route. The major metabolic pathways yield two carboxylic acid forms plus unchanged betaxolol in the urine (approximately 16% of the administered dose).

DOSE IN RENAL IMPAIRMENT GFR (mL/MIN)

20–50	Dose as in normal renal function.
10–20	Dose as in normal renal function.
<10	Dose as in normal renal function.

DOSE IN PATIENTS UNDERGOING RENAL REPLACEMENT THERAPIES

CAPD	Not dialysed. Dose as in normal renal function.
HD	Not dialysed. Dose as in normal renal function.
HDF/High flux	Unknown dialysability. Dose as in normal renal function.
CAV/VVHD	Unknown dialysability. Dose as in normal renal function.

IMPORTANT DRUG INTERACTIONS

Potentially hazardous interactions with other drugs
● Anaesthetics: enhanced hypotensive effect.
● Analgesics: NSAIDs antagonise hypotensive effect.
● Anti-arrhythmics: increased risk of myocardial depression and bradycardia; increased risk of bradycardia, myocardial depression and AV block with amiodarone.
● Antidepressants: enhanced hypotensive effect with MAOIs.
● Antihypertensives: enhanced hypotensive effect; increased risk of withdrawal hypertension with clonidine; increased risk of first dose hypotensive effect with post-synaptic alpha-blockers such as prazosin.
● Antimalarials: increased risk of bradycardia with mefloquine.
● Antipsychotics: enhanced hypotensive effect with phenothiazines.
● Calcium-channel blockers: increased risk of bradycardia and AV block with diltiazem; hypotension and heart failure possible with nifedipine and nisoldipine; asystole, severe hypotension and heart failure with verapamil.
● Cytotoxics: possible increased risk of bradycardia with crizotinib.
● Diuretics: enhanced hypotensive effect.
● Fingolimod: possibly increased risk of bradycardia.
● Moxisylyte: possible severe postural hypotension.
● Sympathomimetics: severe hypertension with adrenaline and noradrenaline, and possibly with dobutamine.

ADMINISTRATION

RECONSTITUTION
–
ROUTE
● Topical
RATE OF ADMINISTRATION
–
COMMENTS
–

OTHER INFORMATION

● Use with caution in patients with asthma, or a history of obstructive airways disease or diabetes.
● Systemic absorption may follow topical administration to the eye.

Bevacizumab

CLINICAL USE

Monoclonal antibody:
- Treatment of colorectal cancer
- Treatment of breast cancer
- Treatment of renal cell carcinoma
- Treatment of lung cancer
- Treatment of ovarian, fallopian tube or peritoneal cancer

DOSE IN NORMAL RENAL FUNCTION

5–10 mg/kg every 14 days
Or 7.5–15 mg/kg every 3 weeks
Dose varies according to indication
Consult local protocol

PHARMACOKINETICS

Molecular weight (daltons)	149 000
% Protein binding	No data
% Excreted unchanged in urine	No data
Volume of distribution (L/kg)	0.046
Half-life – normal/ ESRF (hrs)	11–50 days (average 20 days)/–

METABOLISM

Assessment of bevacizumab metabolism in rabbits following a single IV dose of ^{125}I-bevacizumab indicated that its metabolic profile was similar to that expected for a native IgG molecule which does not bind VEGF. The metabolism and elimination of bevacizumab is similar to endogenous IgG, i.e. primarily via proteolytic catabolism throughout the body, including endothelial cells, and does not rely primarily on elimination through the kidneys and liver. Binding of the IgG to the FcRn receptor results in protection from cellular metabolism and the long terminal half-life.

DOSE IN RENAL IMPAIRMENT GFR (mL/MIN)

20–50	Use with caution. See 'Other information'.
10–20	Use with caution. See 'Other information'.
<10	Use with caution. See 'Other information'.

DOSE IN PATIENTS UNDERGOING RENAL REPLACEMENT THERAPIES

CAPD	Not dialysed. Use with caution. See 'Other information'.
HD	Not dialysed. Use with caution. See 'Other information'.
HDF/High flux	Not dialysed. Use with caution. See 'Other information'.
CAV/ VVHD	Not dialysed. Use with caution. See 'Other information'.

IMPORTANT DRUG INTERACTIONS

Potentially hazardous interactions with other drugs
- Bisphosphonates: increased risk of osteonecrosis of the jaw.

ADMINISTRATION

RECONSTITUTION
–
ROUTE
- IV infusion
RATE OF ADMINISTRATION
- 30–90 minutes depending on how the patient tolerates it
COMMENTS
- Dilute in 100 mL of sodium chloride 0.9%.
- DO NOT mix with glucose solutions.

OTHER INFORMATION

- Increased incidence of hypertension has been seen with treatment.
- Manufacturer advises to use with caution due to lack of data.
- MHRA/CHM advice: may increase risk of developing osteonecrosis of the jaw.
- Necrotising fasciitis has also been reported, discontinue if suspected.
- People with a history of hypertension may be at an increased risk of proteinuria. Discontinue therapy in patients with Grade 4 proteinuria (nephrotic syndrome).
- Can delay wound healing.
- Bevacizumab has been used in a haemodialysis patient at a dose of 5 mg/ kg every 14 days. (Garnier-Viogeat N, Rixe O, Paintaud G, et al. Pharmacokinetics of bevacizumab in haemodialysis. *Nephrol Dial Transplant.* 2007; **22**: 975.)

Bexarotene

CLINICAL USE

Antineoplastic agent:
* Treatment of skin manifestations of cutaneous T-cell lymphoma

DOSE IN NORMAL RENAL FUNCTION

$300\,mg/m^2$ daily as a single dose

PHARMACOKINETICS

Molecular weight (daltons)	348.5
% Protein binding	>99
% Excreted unchanged in urine	<1
Volume of distribution (L/kg)	1^1
Half-life – normal/ ESRF (hrs)	1–3/Unchanged

METABOLISM

Hepatic metabolism. Studies suggest glucuronidation as a metabolic pathway, and that cytochrome P450 3A4 is the major cytochrome P450 isozyme responsible for formation of the oxidative metabolites. Bexarotene metabolites have little pharmacological activity.

No studies have been done in renal failure although the pharmacokinetic data indicates that renal elimination is a minor excretory pathway.

DOSE IN RENAL IMPAIRMENT GFR (mL/MIN)

20–50	Dose as in normal renal function.
10–20	Dose as in normal renal function.
<10	Dose as in normal renal function. See 'Other information'.

DOSE IN PATIENTS UNDERGOING RENAL REPLACEMENT THERAPIES

CAPD	Not dialysed. Dose as in GFR<10 mL/min.
HD	Not dialysed. Dose as in GFR<10 mL/min.
HDF/High flux	Not dialysed. Dose as in GFR<10 mL/min.
CAV/ VVHD	Not dialysed. Dose as in normal renal function.

IMPORTANT DRUG INTERACTIONS

Potentially hazardous interactions with other drugs
* Antipsychotics: avoid concomitant use with clozapine (increased risk of agranulocytosis)
* Lipid-regulating drugs: concentration increased by gemfibrozil – avoid concomitant use.

ADMINISTRATION

RECONSTITUTION
–
ROUTE
* Oral
RATE OF ADMINISTRATION
–

OTHER INFORMATION

Reference:
1. www.ema.europa.eu/docs/en_GB/document_library/EPAR_-_Scientific_Discussion/human/000326/WC500034204.pdf

Bezafibrate

CLINICAL USE

Hyperlipidaemia

DOSE IN NORMAL RENAL FUNCTION

200 mg, 3 times a day
Modified release: 400 mg daily

PHARMACOKINETICS

Molecular weight (daltons)	361.8
% Protein binding	95
% Excreted unchanged in urine	50
Volume of distribution (L/kg)	0.24–0.35
Half-life – normal/ ESRF (hrs)	1–2 (MR: 3.4)/7.8–20

METABOLISM

Fifty per cent of the administered bezafibrate dose is recovered in the urine as unchanged drug and 20% in the form of glucuronides.

Elimination is rapid, with excretion almost exclusively renal. Ninety-five per cent of the activity of the ^{14}C-labelled drug is recovered in the urine and 3% in the faeces within 48 hours.

DOSE IN RENAL IMPAIRMENT GFR (mL/MIN)

40–60	400 mg daily
15–40	200 mg every 24–48 hours
<15	Avoid

DOSE IN PATIENTS UNDERGOING RENAL REPLACEMENT THERAPIES

CAPD	Not dialysed. 200 mg every 72 hours.
HD	Not dialysed. 200 mg every 72 hours.
HDF/High flux	Unknown dialysability. 200 mg every 72 hours.
CAV/ VVHD	Unknown dialysability. Dose as in GFR=15–40 mL/min.

IMPORTANT DRUG INTERACTIONS

Potentially hazardous interactions with other drugs
- Antibacterials: increased risk of myopathy with daptomycin – try to avoid concomitant use.
- Anticoagulants: enhances effect of coumarins and phenindione; dose of anticoagulant should be reduced by up to 50% and adjusted by monitoring INR.
- Antidiabetics: may improve glucose tolerance and have an additive effect with insulin or sulphonylureas.
- Ciclosporin: may increase nephrotoxicity and reduce ciclosporin levels.
- Colchicine: possible increased risk of myopathy.
- Lipid-regulating drugs: increased risk of myopathy in combination with statins and ezetimibe – avoid with ezetimibe; do not exceed 10 mg of simvastatin and 20 mg of rosuvastatin.[1]

ADMINISTRATION

RECONSTITUTION
–

ROUTE
- Oral

RATE OF ADMINISTRATION
–

COMMENTS
–

OTHER INFORMATION

- Take dose with or after food.
- Contraindicated in nephrotic syndrome.
- There should be an interval of 2 hours between intake of ion exchange resin and bezafibrate.
- Modified-release preparation is not appropriate in renal impairment.

Reference:
1. MHRA. *Drug Safety Update*. 2012 August; **1**(6).

Bicalutamide

CLINICAL USE

Treatment of prostate cancer

DOSE IN NORMAL RENAL FUNCTION

50–150 mg daily
(with orchidectomy or gonadorelin therapy)

PHARMACOKINETICS

Molecular weight (daltons)	430.4
% Protein binding	96
% Excreted unchanged in urine	approx 50
Volume of distribution (L/kg)	No data
Half-life – normal/ ESRF (hrs)	6–7 days/Unchanged

METABOLISM

The (S)-enantiomer is rapidly cleared relative to (R)-enantiomer, the latter having a plasma elimination half-life of about 1 week.

On daily administration of Casodex 150 mg, the (R)-enantiomer accumulates about 10-fold in plasma as a consequence of its long half-life.

At steady state, the predominantly active (R)-enantiomer accounts for 99% of the total circulating enantiomers.

Bicalutamide is highly protein bound (racemate 96%, (R)-enantiomer >99%) and extensively metabolised (oxidation and glucuronidation); its metabolites are eliminated via the kidneys and bile in approximately equal proportions.

DOSE IN RENAL IMPAIRMENT GFR (mL/MIN)

20–50	Dose as in normal renal function.
10–20	Dose as in normal renal function.
<10	Dose as in normal renal function.

DOSE IN PATIENTS UNDERGOING RENAL REPLACEMENT THERAPIES

CAPD	Unlikely to be dialysed. Dose as in normal renal function.
HD	Unlikely to be dialysed. Dose as in normal renal function.
HDF/High flux	Unknown dialysability. Dose as in normal renal function.
CAV/ VVHD	Unlikely to be dialysed. Dose as in normal renal function.

IMPORTANT DRUG INTERACTIONS

Potentially hazardous interactions with other drugs
- Anticoagulants: possibly enhances anticoagulant effect of coumarins.
- See 'Other information'.

ADMINISTRATION

RECONSTITUTION
–
ROUTE
- Oral
RATE OF ADMINISTRATION
–
COMMENTS
–

OTHER INFORMATION

- *In vitro* studies have shown that bicalutamide is an inhibitor of CYP450 3A4. For drugs eliminated by this route, e.g. ciclosporin, tacrolimus, sirolimus, it is recommended that plasma concentrations and clinical condition be monitored following initiation or cessation of bicalutamide therapy.

Bilastine

CLINICAL USE

Non-sedating antihistamine:
● Symptomatic relief of allergy such as hay fever, urticaria

DOSE IN NORMAL RENAL FUNCTION

20 mg once daily

PHARMACOKINETICS

Molecular weight (daltons)	463.6
% Protein binding	84–90
% Excreted unchanged in urine	28.3
Volume of distribution (L/kg)	1.29
Half-life – normal/ ESRF (hrs)	14.5/–

METABOLISM

Not significantly metabolised.
   Almost 95% of the administered dose was recovered in urine (28.3%) and faeces (66.5%) as unchanged bilastine.

DOSE IN RENAL IMPAIRMENT GFR (mL/MIN)

20–50	Dose as in normal renal function.
10–20	Dose as in normal renal function.
<10	Dose as in normal renal function.

DOSE IN PATIENTS UNDERGOING RENAL REPLACEMENT THERAPIES

CAPD	Unlikely to be dialysed. Dose as in normal renal function.
HD	Unlikely to be dialysed. Dose as in normal renal function.
HDF/High flux	Unlikely to be dialysed. Dose as in normal renal function.
CAV/ VVHD	Unlikely to be dialysed. Dose as in normal renal function.

IMPORTANT DRUG INTERACTIONS

Potentially hazardous interactions with other drugs
● Antivirals: concentration possibly increased by ritonavir.
● Grapefruit juice: concentration of bilastine reduced.

ADMINISTRATION

RECONSTITUTION
–
ROUTE
● Oral
RATE OF ADMINISTRATION
–

OTHER INFORMATION

● Oral bioavailability is 61%.

Bisacodyl

CLINICAL USE

Laxative

DOSE IN NORMAL RENAL FUNCTION

- Oral: 5–10 mg at night
- Rectal: 10 mg in the morning
- Bowel evacuation: 10 mg orally in the morning and 10 mg at night the day before the procedure followed by 10 mg as suppositories the next morning

PHARMACOKINETICS

Molecular weight (daltons)	361.4
% Protein binding	Negligible
% Excreted unchanged in urine	30
Volume of distribution (L/kg)	See 'Other information'.
Half-life – normal/ ESRF (hrs)	See 'Other information'.

METABOLISM

Bisacodyl is rapidly hydrolysed to the active principle bis-(p-hydroxyphenyl)-pyridyl-2-methane (BHPM), mainly by esterases of the enteric mucosa. After oral and rectal administration, only small amounts of the drug are absorbed and are almost completely conjugated in the intestinal wall and the liver to form the inactive BHPM glucuronide. Following the administration of bisacodyl coated tablets, an average of 51.8% of the dose was recovered in the faeces as free BHPM and an average of 10.5% of the dose was recovered in the urine as BHPM glucuronide. Following the administration as a suppository, an average of 3.1% of the dose was recovered as BHPM glucuronide in the urine. Stool contained large amounts of BHPM (90% of the total excretion) in addition to small amounts of unchanged bisacodyl.

DOSE IN RENAL IMPAIRMENT GFR (mL/MIN)

20–50	Dose as in normal renal function.
10–20	Dose as in normal renal function.
<10	Dose as in normal renal function.

DOSE IN PATIENTS UNDERGOING RENAL REPLACEMENT THERAPIES

CAPD	Unknown dialysability. Dose as in normal renal function.
HD	Unknown dialysability. Dose as in normal renal function.
HDF/High flux	Unknown dialysability. Dose as in normal renal function.
CAV/ VVHD	Unknown dialysability. Dose as in normal renal function.

IMPORTANT DRUG INTERACTIONS

Potentially hazardous interactions with other drugs
- None known

ADMINISTRATION

RECONSTITUTION
–
ROUTE
- Oral, rectal
RATE OF ADMINISTRATION
–
COMMENTS
–

OTHER INFORMATION

- Absorption is <5% orally or rectally.

Bisoprolol fumarate

CLINICAL USE

Beta-1 adrenoceptor blocker:
- Hypertension
- Angina
- Adjunctive treatment for heart failure

DOSE IN NORMAL RENAL FUNCTION

5–20 mg daily
Heart failure: 1.25 mg daily increasing to
10 mg daily

PHARMACOKINETICS

Molecular weight (daltons)	767
% Protein binding	30
% Excreted unchanged in urine	50
Volume of distribution (L/kg)	3.5
Half-life – normal/ESRF (hrs)	9–12/18–24

METABOLISM

Bisoprolol is excreted from the body by two
routes. Fifty per cent is metabolised by the
liver to inactive metabolites which are then
excreted by the kidneys. The remaining
50% is excreted by the kidneys in an
unmetabolised form.

DOSE IN RENAL IMPAIRMENT GFR (mL/MIN)

20–50	Dose as in normal renal function.
10–20	Dose as in normal renal function.
<10	Dose as in normal renal function.

DOSE IN PATIENTS UNDERGOING RENAL REPLACEMENT THERAPIES

CAPD	Not dialysed. Dose as in normal renal function.
HD	Not dialysed. Dose as in normal renal function.
HDF/High flux	Unknown dialysability. Dose as in normal renal function.
CAV/ VVHD	Unknown dialysability. Dose as in normal renal function.

IMPORTANT DRUG INTERACTIONS

Potentially hazardous interactions with other
drugs
- Anaesthetics: enhanced hypotensive effect.
- Analgesics: NSAIDs antagonise hypotensive effect.
- Anti-arrhythmics: increased risk of myocardial depression and bradycardia; increased risk of bradycardia, myocardial depression and AV block with amiodarone; increased risk of myocardial depression and bradycardia with flecainide.
- Antibacterials: concentration reduced by rifampicin.
- Antidepressants: enhanced hypotensive effect with MAOIs.
- Antihypertensives; enhanced hypotensive effect; increased risk of withdrawal hypertension with clonidine; increased risk of first dose hypotensive effect with post-synaptic alpha-blockers such as prazosin.
- Antimalarials: increased risk of bradycardia with mefloquine.
- Antipsychotics enhanced hypotensive effect with phenothiazines.
- Calcium-channel blockers: increased risk of bradycardia and AV block with diltiazem; hypotension and heart failure possible with nifedipine and nisoldipine; asystole, severe hypotension and heart failure with verapamil.
- Cytotoxics: possible increased risk of bradycardia with crizotinib.
- Diuretics: enhanced hypotensive effect.
- Fingolimod: possibly increased risk of bradycardia.
- Moxisylyte: possible severe postural hypotension.
- Sympathomimetics: severe hypertension with adrenaline and noradrenaline, and possibly with dobutamine.

ADMINISTRATION

RECONSTITUTION
–

ROUTE
- Oral

RATE OF ADMINISTRATION
–

COMMENTS
–

OTHER INFORMATION

- Use with caution in patients with chronic obstructive airways disease, asthma or diabetes.

Bivalirudin

CLINICAL USE

Anticoagulant:
- Percutaneous coronary intervention (PCI)
- Unstable angina or non-ST elevation MI

DOSE IN NORMAL RENAL FUNCTION

- PCI: Initially bolus of 750 mcg/kg then an infusion of 1.75 mg/kg/hour
- Unstable angina or non-ST elevation MI: 100 mcg/kg bolus then 250 mcg/kg/hour – see product literature

PHARMACOKINETICS

Molecular weight (daltons)	2180.3
% Protein binding	0
% Excreted unchanged in urine	20
Volume of distribution (L/kg)	0.1
Half-life – normal/ ESRF (hrs)	13–37 minutes/ 57 minutes (310 minutes in dialysis patients on non-HD days)

METABOLISM

As a peptide, bivalirudin is expected to undergo catabolism to its constituent amino acids, with subsequent recycling of the amino acid in the body pool. Bivalirudin is metabolised by proteases, including thrombin. The primary metabolite resulting from the cleavage of Arg_3-Pro_4 bond of the N-terminal sequence by thrombin is not active because of the loss of affinity to the catalytic active site of thrombin.

DOSE IN RENAL IMPAIRMENT GFR (mL/MIN)

30–50	Dose as in normal renal function.
10–29	Normal bolus dose. Reduce infusion dose by 20% (1.4 mg/kg/hour). See 'Other information'.
<10	Normal bolus dose. Reduce infusion dose by 80% and monitor ACT. See 'Other information'.

DOSE IN PATIENTS UNDERGOING RENAL REPLACEMENT THERAPIES

CAPD	Unknown dialysability. Dose as in GFR<10 mL/min.
HD	Dialysed. Dose as in GFR<10 mL/min.
HDF/High flux	Dialysed. Dose as in GFR<10 mL/min.
CAV/ VVHD	Unknown dialysability. Dose as in GFR=10–29 mL/min.

IMPORTANT DRUG INTERACTIONS

Potentially hazardous interactions with other drugs
- Antiplatelets and anticoagulants: increased risk of bleeding.
- Thrombolytics: may increase risk of bleeding complications; enhance effect of bivalirudin.

ADMINISTRATION

RECONSTITUTION
- Reconstitute each 250 mg vial with 5 mL water for injection

ROUTE
- IV

RATE OF ADMINISTRATION
- 1.75 mg/kg/hour

COMMENTS
- Further dilute with 50 mL sodium chloride 0.9% or glucose 5% if for infusion.
- Stable for 24 hours at room temperature.

OTHER INFORMATION

- Monitor ACT in renal impairment.
- Can start bivalirudin 30 minutes after stopping unfractionated heparin and 8 hours after stopping LMWH.
- No known antidote.
- Dose recommendations vary from country to country; doses above are from New Zealand.
- UK doses:
  — GFR=30–59 mL/min: Normal bolus dose then reduce infusion to 1.4 mg/ kg/hour
  — GFR<30 mL/min: contraindicated.
- USA doses:
  — Normal dose: 0.75 mg/kg bolus then 1.75 mg/kg/hr infusion
  — GFR=30–59 mL/min: Normal bolus dose then reduce infusion to 1.75 mg/ kg/hr
  — GFR<30 mL/min: Normal bolus dose then reduce infusion to 1 mg/kg/hr
  — Dialysis dependent: Normal bolus dose then reduce infusion to 0.25 mg/kg/hr
- Lobo BL. Use of newer anticoagulants in patients with chronic kidney disease. *Am J Health-Syst Pharm.* 2007 Oct 1; **64**: 2017–26:
  — GFR=30–50 mL/min: 1.75 mg/kg/hour
  — GFR<30 mL/min: 1 mg/kg/hour
  — On haemodialysis: 0.25 mg/kg/hour

Bleomycin

CLINICAL USE

Antineoplastic agent

DOSE IN NORMAL RENAL FUNCTION

Squamous cell carcinoma and testicular teratoma:
- range 45–60 × 10³ IU per week IM/IV (total cumulative dose up to 500 × 10³ IU)
- OR, continuous IV infusion 15 × 10³ IU/24 hours for up to 10 days
- OR, 30 × 10³ IU/24 hours for up to 5 days

Malignant lymphomas:
- 15–30 × 10³ IU/week IM to total dose of 225 × 10³ IU
- Lower doses required in combination chemotherapy.

Malignant effusions:
- 60 × 10³ IU in 100 mL sodium chloride 0.9% intrapleurally (total cumulative dose of 500 × 10³ IU).

PHARMACOKINETICS

Molecular weight (daltons)	Approximately 1500
% Protein binding	<1
% Excreted unchanged in urine	60–70
Volume of distribution (L/kg)	0.3
Half-life – normal/ ESRF (hrs)	4 (bolus), 9 (continuous infusion)/20

METABOLISM

The mechanism for biotransformation is not yet fully known. Inactivation takes place during enzymatic breakdown by bleomycin hydrolase, primarily in plasma, liver and other organs and, to a much lesser degree, in skin and lungs.

About 60–70% of the administered drug is excreted unchanged in the urine, probably by glomerular filtration. Approximately 50% is recovered in the urine in the 24 hours following an IV or IM injection. The rate of excretion, therefore, is highly influenced by renal function; concentrations in plasma are greatly elevated if usual doses are given to patients with renal impairment with only up to 20% excreted in 24 hours.

DOSE IN RENAL IMPAIRMENT GFR (mL/MIN)

30–50	Dose as in normal renal function.
10–30	75% of normal dose (100% for malignant effusions).
<10	50% of normal dose (100% for malignant effusions).

DOSE IN PATIENTS UNDERGOING RENAL REPLACEMENT THERAPIES

CAPD	Not dialysed. Dose as in GFR<10 mL/min.
HD	Not dialysed. Dose as in GFR<10 mL/min.
HDF/High flux	Unknown dialysability. Dose as in GFR<10 mL/min.
CAV/ VVHD	Unknown dialysability. Dose as in GFR=10–30 mL/min.

IMPORTANT DRUG INTERACTIONS

Potentially hazardous interactions with other drugs
- Antipsychotics: avoid concomitant use with clozapine, increased risk of agranulocytosis.
- Cytotoxics: increased pulmonary toxicity with cisplatin and brentuximab, avoid with brentuximab; in combination with vinca alkaloids can lead to Raynaud's syndrome and peripheral ischaemia.

ADMINISTRATION

RECONSTITUTION
- IM: dissolve required dose in up to 5 mL sodium chloride 0.9% (or 1% solution of lidocaine if pain on injection).
- IV: dissolve dose in 5–200 mL sodium chloride 0.9%.
- Intracavitary: 60 × 10³ IU in 100 mL sodium chloride 0.9%.
- Locally: dissolve in sodium chloride 0.9% to make a 1–3 ×10³ IU/mL solution.

ROUTE
- IM, IV, also intra-arterially, intrapleurally, intraperitoneally, locally into tumour.

RATE OF ADMINISTRATION
- Give by slow IV injection, or add to reservoir of a running IV infusion.

COMMENTS
- Avoid direct contact with the skin.

OTHER INFORMATION

- Lesions of skin and oral mucosa common after full course of bleomycin.
- Pulmonary toxicity: interstitial pneumonia and fibrosis – most serious delayed effect.
- Dose in severe renal impairment is from *Drug Prescribing in Renal Failure*, 5th edition, by Aronoff *et al.*
- Rapid distribution to body tissues (highest concentration is in skin, lungs, peritoneum and lymph).

Boceprevir

CLINICAL USE

HCV-protease inhibitor:
- Treatment of chronic hepatitis C (HCV) genotype 1 infection, in combination with peginterferon alfa and ribavirin

DOSE IN NORMAL RENAL FUNCTION

800 mg three times a day with food

PHARMACOKINETICS

Molecular weight (daltons)	519.7
% Protein binding	75
% Excreted unchanged in urine	9
Volume of distribution (L/kg)	772 litres
Half-life – normal/ ESRF (hrs)	3.4/Unchanged

METABOLISM

Boceprevir mainly undergoes metabolism through the aldo-ketoreductase mediated pathway to ketone-reduced metabolites that are inactive against HCV. After a single 800 mg oral dose of ^{14}C-boceprevir, the most abundant circulating metabolites were a diasteriomeric mixture of ketone-reduced metabolites with a mean exposure approximately 4-fold greater than that of boceprevir. Boceprevir also undergoes, to a lesser extent, oxidative metabolism mediated by CYP3A4/5.

Mainly excreted by the liver – approximately 79% and 9% of the dose was excreted in faeces and urine, respectively, with approximately 8% and 3% eliminated as boceprevir in faeces and urine.

DOSE IN RENAL IMPAIRMENT GFR (mL/MIN)

20–50	Dose as in normal renal function.
10–20	Dose as in normal renal function.
<10	Dose as in normal renal function.

DOSE IN PATIENTS UNDERGOING RENAL REPLACEMENT THERAPIES

CAPD	Not dialysed. Dose as in normal renal function.
HD	Not dialysed. Dose as in normal renal function.
HDF/High flux	Not dialysed. Dose as in normal renal function.
CAV/ VVHD	Not dialysed. Dose as in normal renal function.

IMPORTANT DRUG INTERACTIONS

Potentially hazardous interactions with other drugs
- Antibacterials: concentration possibly reduced by rifampicin – avoid concomitant use.
- Antiepileptics: concentration possibly reduced by carbamazepine, phenobarbital & phenytoin avoid.
- Antifungals: concentration increased by ketoconazole.
- Antimalarials: avoid concomitant use with artemether & lumefantrine.
- Antipsychotics: avoid concomitant use with pimozide; possibly increases quetiapine concentration avoid.
- Antivirals: reduces concentration of atazanavir; avoid with darunavir, fosamprenavir and lopinavir; concentration of both drugs reduced with ritonavir.
- Anxiolytics & hypnotics: increased oral midazolam concentration – avoid concomitant use.
- Ciclosporin: concentration of ciclosporin increased.
- Cytotoxics: avoid concomitant use with dasatinib, erlotinib, gefitinib, imatinib, lapatinib, nilotinib, pazopanib, sorafenib & sunitinib; reduce dose of ruxolitinib.
- Ergot alkaloids: avoid concomitant use.
- Lipid-regulating drugs: enhances effects and toxicity of atorvastatin, reduce atorvastatin dose; increases pravastatin concentration; avoid with simvastatin.
- Oestrogens: possibly causes contraception failure.
- Sirolimus: possibly increases sirolimus concentration.
- Tacrolimus: concentration of tacrolimus increased, reduce tacrolimus dose.

ADMINISTRATION

RECONSTITUTION
–
ROUTE
- Oral
RATE OF ADMINISTRATION
–

OTHER INFORMATION

- Absorption is increased by 60% when given with food.
- Boceprevir is administered as an approximately equal mixture of two diastereomers which rapidly interconvert in plasma. At steady-state, the exposure ratio for the two diastereomers is approximately 2:1, with the predominant diastereomer being pharmacologically active.

Bortezomib

CLINICAL USE

Proteasome inhibitor:
- Treatment of multiple myeloma for people who have already tried at least 2 prior therapies and have disease progression

DOSE IN NORMAL RENAL FUNCTION

$1.3 \, mg/m^2$ twice weekly for 2 weeks (days 1, 4, 8 and 11) followed by a 10 day rest period

PHARMACOKINETICS

Molecular weight (daltons)	384.2
% Protein binding	82.9
% Excreted unchanged in urine	Small amount
Volume of distribution (L/kg)	>500 litres
Half-life – normal/ ESRF (hrs)	5–15/Unknown

METABOLISM

In vitro studies with human liver microsomes and human cDNA-expressed cytochrome P450 isozymes indicate that bortezomib is primarily oxidatively metabolised via cytochrome P450 enzymes, 3A4, 2C19, and 1A2. The major metabolic pathway is deboronation to form two deboronated metabolites that subsequently undergo hydroxylation to several metabolites. Deboronated-bortezomib metabolites are inactive as 26S proteasome inhibitors.

DOSE IN RENAL IMPAIRMENT GFR (mL/MIN)

20–50	Dose as in normal renal function.
10–20	Dose as in normal renal function. Monitor carefully. See 'Other information'.
<10	A reduced dose may be required. Monitor carefully.

DOSE IN PATIENTS UNDERGOING RENAL REPLACEMENT THERAPIES

CAPD	Unlikely to be dialysed. Dose as in GFR<10 mL/min.
HD	Unlikely to be dialysed. Dose as in GFR<10 mL/min.
HDF/High flux	Unknown dialysability. Dose as in GFR<10 mL/min.
CAV/ VVHD	Unlikely to be dialysed. Dose as in GFR=10–20 mL/min.

IMPORTANT DRUG INTERACTIONS

Potentially hazardous interactions with other drugs
- Antipsychotics: avoid with clozapine, increased risk of agranulocytosis.

ADMINISTRATION

RECONSTITUTION
- 3.5 mL sodium chloride 0.9%

ROUTE
- SC, IV bolus

RATE OF ADMINISTRATION
- 3 to 5 seconds

COMMENTS
- Administer within 8 hours of reconstitution

OTHER INFORMATION

- Consecutive doses should be at least 72 hours apart.
- Normal doses have been used in patients with a GFR of 10–30 mL/min but there is an increased risk of adverse effects. (Jagannath S, Barlogie B, Berenson JR, *et al.* Bortezomib in recurrent and/or refractory multiple myeloma. *Cancer.* 2005; **103**(6): 1195–1200.)
- Some trials have used doses of $1 \, mg/m^2$ in patients with a GFR of 10–30 mL/min, with similar efficacy and incidence of side effects.
- Both hypokalaemia and hyperkalaemia have been reported with bortezomib as has hypophosphataemia and hypomagnesaemia.
- There have been incidences of renal impairment, renal colic, proteinuria, dysuria, urinary frequency, urinary hesitation and haematuria.
- Anecdotally, has been used at normal doses in a few haemodialysis patients; in some of the patients platelet infusions have been required.
- In patients with peripheral neuropathy then bortezomib has a high probability of exacerbating it.

Bosentan

CLINICAL USE

Treatment of primary arterial pulmonary hypertension (PAH), and PAH secondary to scleroderma without significant interstitial pulmonary disease.
Treatment of systemic sclerosis with ongoing digital ulcer disease.

DOSE IN NORMAL RENAL FUNCTION

- PAH: 62.5–250 mg twice daily
- Systemic sclerosis: 62.5–125 mg twice daily

PHARMACOKINETICS

Molecular weight (daltons)	551.6
% Protein binding	>98
% Excreted unchanged in urine	<3
Volume of distribution (L/kg)	18 litres
Half-life – normal/ ESRF (hrs)	5–8/Unchanged

METABOLISM

Upon multiple dosing, plasma concentrations of bosentan decrease gradually to 50–65% of those seen after single dose administration. This decrease is probably due to auto-induction of metabolising liver enzymes. Steady-state conditions are reached within 3–5 days.

Bosentan is eliminated by biliary excretion following metabolism in the liver by the cytochrome P450 isoenzymes, CYP2C9 and CYP3A4. Less than 3% of an administered oral dose is recovered in urine.

Bosentan forms three metabolites and only one of these is pharmacologically active. This metabolite is mainly excreted unchanged via the bile. In adult patients, the exposure to the active metabolite is greater than in healthy subjects. In patients with evidence of the presence of cholestasis, the exposure to the active metabolite may be increased.

In patients with severe renal impairment (creatinine clearance 15–30 mL/min), plasma concentrations of bosentan decreased by approximately 10%. Plasma concentrations of bosentan metabolites increased about 2-fold in these patients as compared to subjects with normal renal function.

DOSE IN RENAL IMPAIRMENT GFR (mL/MIN)

20–50	Dose as in normal renal function.
10–20	Dose as in normal renal function.
<10	Dose as in normal renal function.

DOSE IN PATIENTS UNDERGOING RENAL REPLACEMENT THERAPIES

CAPD	Not dialysed. Dose as in normal renal function.
HD	Not dialysed. Dose as in normal renal function.
HDF/High flux	Not dialysed. Dose as in normal renal function.
CAV/ VVHD	Not dialysed. Dose as in normal renal function.

IMPORTANT DRUG INTERACTIONS

Potentially hazardous interactions with other drugs
- Antibacterials: concentration reduced by rifampicin – avoid concomitant use.
- Antidiabetics: increased risk of hepatoxicity with glibenclamide – avoid concomitant use.
- Antifungals: fluconazole, ketoconazole and itraconazole cause large increases in concentration of bosentan – avoid concomitant use.
- Antivirals: ritonavir causes greatly increased bosentan levels – avoid concomitant use; telaprevir concentration reduced and bosentan concentration possibly increased; avoid concomitant use with tipranavir.
- Ciclosporin: co-administration of ciclosporin and bosentan is contraindicated. When ciclosporin and bosentan are co-administered, initial trough concentrations of bosentan are 30 times higher than normal. At steady state, trough levels are 3–4 times higher than normal. Blood concentrations of ciclosporin decreased by 50%.
- Lipid lowering agents: concentration of simvastatin reduced by 45% – monitor cholesterol levels and adjust dose of statin.
- Oestrogens and progestogens: may be failure of contraception – use alternative method.

ADMINISTRATION

RECONSTITUTION

–

ROUTE

● Oral

RATE OF ADMINISTRATION

−

COMMENTS

−

OTHER INFORMATION

● Bosentan should only be used if the systemic systolic blood pressure is >85 mm/Hg.
● Treatment with bosentan is associated with a dose-related, modest decrease in haemoglobin concentration.
● Bosentan is an inducer of CYP 3A4 and CYP 2C9.
● Bosentan has been associated with dose-related elevations in liver aminotransferases.
● Side effects include leg oedema and hypotension.

Brentuximab vedotin

CLINICAL USE

Monoclonal antibody:
- Hodgkin's lymphoma
- Systemic anaplastic large cell lymphoma

DOSE IN NORMAL RENAL FUNCTION

1.8 mg/kg every 3 weeks
Maximum weight calculation 100 kg

PHARMACOKINETICS

Molecular weight (daltons)	153 000
% Protein binding	68–82 (MMAE)
% Excreted unchanged in urine	24 (MMAE) – in urine & faeces
Volume of distribution (L/kg)	6–10 litres
Half-life – normal/ ESRF (hrs)	4–6 days/Increased

METABOLISM

Brentuximab vedotin consists of a monoclonal antibody conjugated with monomethyl auristatin E (MMAE). Only a small fraction of MMAE released from brentuximab vedotin is metabolised; this metabolism is mainly via oxidation by cytochrome P450 isoenzyme CYP3A4/5.
   MMAE is eliminated in the faeces (72% unchanged) and urine.

DOSE IN RENAL IMPAIRMENT GFR (mL/MIN)

20–50	Use with caution.
10–20	Use with caution.
<10	Use with caution.

DOSE IN PATIENTS UNDERGOING RENAL REPLACEMENT THERAPIES

CAPD	Unlikely to be dialysed. Dose as in GFR<10 mL/min.
HD	Not dialysed. Dose as in GFR<10 mL/min.
HDF/High flux	Unlikely to be dialysed. Dose as in GFR<10 mL/min.
CAV/ VVHD	Unknown dialysability. Dose as in GFR=10–20 mL/min.

IMPORTANT DRUG INTERACTIONS

Potentially hazardous interactions with other drugs
- Antifungals: possible increased risk of neutropenia with ketoconazole.
- Antipsychotics: avoid with clozapine, increased risk of agranulocytosis.
- Cytotoxics: increased risk of pulmonary toxicity with bleomycin – avoid.

ADMINISTRATION

RECONSTITUTION
- 10.5 mL water for injection
ROUTE
- IV infusion
RATE OF ADMINISTRATION
- Over 30 minutes
COMMENTS
- Add to 150 mL sodium chloride 0.9%, glucose 5% or Lactated Ringer's solution to achieve a concentration of 0.4–1.2 mg/mL.

OTHER INFORMATION

- Manufacturer has no data in renal impairment therefore advises to monitor carefully.
- Population analysis indicated that MMAE clearance might be affected by moderate and severe renal impairment. MMAE clearance was reduced about 2-fold in patients with severe renal impairment (creatinine clearance <30 mL/min).
- A premedication of paracetamol and an antihistamine before infusion may be required.

Bromocriptine

CLINICAL USE

- Parkinsonism (but not drug-induced extrapyramidal symptoms)
- Endocrine disorders

DOSE IN NORMAL RENAL FUNCTION

- Parkinson's disease:
  — Week 1: 1–1.25 mg at night
  — Week 2: 2–2.5 mg at night
  — Week 3: 2.5 mg twice daily
  — Week 4: 2.5 mg, 3 times daily
  — then increasing by 2.5 mg every 3–14 days according to response – usual range 10–30 mg daily
- Hypogonadism/galactorrhoea, infertility: 1–1.25 mg at night, increased gradually; usual dose 7.5 mg daily in divided doses (maximum 30 mg daily); infertility without hyperprolactinaemia: 2.5 mg twice daily
- Cyclical benign breast disease and cyclical menstrual disorders: 1–1.25 mg at night increased gradually; usual dose 2.5 mg twice daily
- Acromegaly: 1–1.25 mg at night increased gradually to 5 mg every 6 hours
- Prolactinoma: 1–1.25 mg at night increased gradually to 5 mg every 6 hours (maximum 30 mg daily)

PHARMACOKINETICS

Molecular weight (daltons)	750.7 (as mesilate)
% Protein binding	90–96
% Excreted unchanged in urine	2.5–5.5
Volume of distribution (L/kg)	1–3
Half-life – normal/ ESRF (hrs)	8–20/–

METABOLISM

Bromocriptine is extensively metabolised. It undergoes extensive first-pass biotransformation in the liver, reflected by complex metabolite profiles and by almost complete absence of parent drug in urine and faeces. In plasma the elimination half life is 3–4 hours for the parent drug and 50 hours for the inactive metabolites. The parent drug and its metabolites are also completely excreted via the liver with only 6% being eliminated via the kidney.

DOSE IN RENAL IMPAIRMENT GFR (mL/MIN)

20–50	Dose as in normal renal function.
10–20	Dose as in normal renal function.
<10	Dose as in normal renal function.

DOSE IN PATIENTS UNDERGOING RENAL REPLACEMENT THERAPIES

CAPD	Not dialysed. Dose as in normal renal function.
HD	Not dialysed. Dose as in normal renal function.
HDF/High flux	Unknown dialysability. Dose as in normal renal function.
CAV/ VVHD	Not dialysed. Dose as in normal renal function.

IMPORTANT DRUG INTERACTIONS

Potentially hazardous interactions with other drugs
- Increased risk of toxicity with bromocriptine and isometheptene.

ADMINISTRATION

RECONSTITUTION
–
ROUTE
- Oral
RATE OF ADMINISTRATION
–
COMMENTS
- Take with food

OTHER INFORMATION

- Hypotensive reactions may occur during the first few days of treatment. Tolerance may be reduced by alcohol.
- Digital vasospasm can occur.
- Concomitant administration of macrolide antibiotics may elevate bromocriptine levels.

Budesonide

CLINICAL USE

- Asthma
- Allergic and vasomotor rhinitis
- Inflammatory skin disorders

DOSE IN NORMAL RENAL FUNCTION

- Inhaler/Turbohaler: 200–1600 micrograms daily in divided doses
- Respules: 1–2 mg twice daily; half doses for maintenance
- Nasal spray: depends on preparation.
- Topical preparations: apply 1–2 times daily
- Capsules: 3 mg, 3 times a day, CR: 9 mg once daily
- Enema: 2 mg/100 mL at bedtime

PHARMACOKINETICS

Molecular weight (daltons)	430.5
% Protein binding	85–90
% Excreted unchanged in urine	0
Volume of distribution (L/kg)	3
Half-life – normal/ ESRF (hrs)	1.8–2.2 (inhaled), 3–4 (oral)/–

METABOLISM

Budesonide is rapidly and almost completely absorbed after oral administration, but has poor systemic availability (about 10%) due to extensive first-pass metabolism in the liver, mainly by the cytochrome P450 isoenzyme CYP3A4. The major metabolites, 6-β-hydroxybudesonide and 16-α-hydroxyprednisolone have less than 1% of the glucocorticoid activity of unchanged budesonide.

DOSE IN RENAL IMPAIRMENT GFR (mL/MIN)

20–50	Dose as in normal renal function.
10–20	Dose as in normal renal function.
<10	Dose as in normal renal function.

DOSE IN PATIENTS UNDERGOING RENAL REPLACEMENT THERAPIES

CAPD	Unlikely to be dialysed. Dose as in normal renal function.
HD	Unlikely to be dialysed. Dose as in normal renal function.
HDF/High flux	Unlikely to be dialysed. Dose as in normal renal function.
CAV/ VVHD	Unlikely to be dialysed. Dose as in normal renal function.

IMPORTANT DRUG INTERACTIONS

Potentially hazardous interactions with other drugs
- Antifungals: concentration of inhaled budesonide increased by itraconazole and ketoconazole.
- Antivirals: concentration of inhaled and intranasal budesonide increased by ritonavir.

ADMINISTRATION

RECONSTITUTION
- Respules: may be diluted up to 50% with sterile sodium chloride 0.9%
ROUTE
- Inhalation, topical, oral
RATE OF ADMINISTRATION
–
COMMENTS
–

OTHER INFORMATION

- Special care is needed in patients with quiescent lung tuberculosis, fungal and viral infections in the airways.

Bumetanide

CLINICAL USE

Loop diuretic

DOSE IN NORMAL RENAL FUNCTION

- Oral: 1–10 mg daily, may be given in 2 divided doses.
- Injection: IV 1–2 mg repeated after 20 minutes; IM if necessary, 1 mg then adjust according to response.
- IV infusion: 2–5 mg over 30–60 minutes

PHARMACOKINETICS

Molecular weight (daltons)	364.4
% Protein binding	95
% Excreted unchanged in urine	50
Volume of distribution (L/kg)	0.2–0.5
Half-life – normal/ ESRF (hrs)	0.75–2.6/1.5

METABOLISM

About 80% of a dose of bumetanide is excreted in the urine, about 50% as unchanged drug, and 10–20% in the faeces. No active metabolites are known. In patients with chronic renal failure the liver takes more importance as an excretory pathway although the duration of action is not markedly prolonged.

DOSE IN RENAL IMPAIRMENT GFR (mL/MIN)

20–50	Dose as in normal renal function.
10–20	Dose as in normal renal function.
<10	Dose as in normal renal function.

DOSE IN PATIENTS UNDERGOING RENAL REPLACEMENT THERAPIES

CAPD	Not dialysed. Dose as in normal renal function.
HD	Not dialysed. Dose as in normal renal function.
HDF/High flux	Unknown dialysability. Dose as in normal renal function.
CAV/ VVHD	Not dialysed. Dose as in normal renal function.

IMPORTANT DRUG INTERACTIONS

Potentially hazardous interactions with other drugs

- Analgesics: increased risk of nephrotoxicity with NSAIDs; antagonism of diuretic effect with NSAIDs.
- Anti-arrhythmics: risk of cardiac toxicity with anti-arrhythmics if hypokalaemia occurs; effects of lidocaine and mexiletine antagonised.
- Antibacterials: increased risk of ototoxicity with aminoglycosides, polymyxins and vancomycin; avoid concomitant use with lymecycline.
- Antidepressants: increased risk of hypokalaemia with reboxetine; enhanced hypotensive effect with MAOIs; increased risk of postural hypotension with tricyclics.
- Anti-epileptics: increased risk of hyponatraemia with carbamazepine.
- Antifungals: increased risk of hypokalaemia with amphotericin.
- Antihypertensives: enhanced hypotensive effect; increased risk of first dose hypotensive effect with alpha-blockers; increased risk of ventricular arrhythmias with sotalol if hypokalaemia occurs.
- Antipsychotics: increased risk of ventricular arrhythmias with amisulpride or pimozide if hypokalaemia occurs – avoid with pimozide; enhanced hypotensive effect with phenothiazines.
- Atomoxetine: increased risk of ventricular arrhythmias if hypokalaemia occurs.
- Cardiac glycosides: increased toxicity if hypokalaemia occurs.
- Cytotoxics: increased risk of ventricular arrhythmias due to hypokalaemia with arsenic trioxide; increased risk of nephrotoxicity and ototoxicity with platinum compounds.
- Lithium: risk of toxicity.

ADMINISTRATION

RECONSTITUTION

–

ROUTE

- Oral, IV, IM

RATE OF ADMINISTRATION

- IV infusion: 2–5 mg in 500 mL of infusion fluid over 30–60 minutes
- IV bolus: 1–2 mg over 3–4 minutes

COMMENTS

- Compatible with glucose 5% or sodium chloride 0.9%

OTHER INFORMATION

- 1 mg bumetanide ≡ 40 mg furosemide at low doses, but avoid direct substitution at high doses.
- In patients with severe chronic renal failure given high doses of bumetanide there are reports of musculoskeletal pain and muscle spasm.
- Orally: diuresis begins within 30 minutes, peaks after 1–2 hours, lasts 3 hours.
- IV: diuresis begins within few minutes and ceases in about 2 hours.
- Use with caution in patients receiving nephrotoxic or ototoxic drugs.
- Smaller doses may be sufficient in the elderly and cirrhotics (500 micrograms).
- Use twice daily for higher doses.

Buprenorphine

CLINICAL USE

Opioid analgesic

DOSE IN NORMAL RENAL FUNCTION

Sublingual: 200–400 mcg every 6–8 hours
IM, Slow IV: 300–600 mcg every 6–8 hours
Transdermal:
- Transtec: 35–140 mcg/hour every 96 hours
- Butrans: 5–40 mcg/hour, change patch every 7 days

PHARMACOKINETICS

Molecular weight (daltons)	467.6
% Protein binding	96
% Excreted unchanged in urine	Minimal
Volume of distribution (L/kg)	2.5
Half-life – normal/ ESRF (hrs)	20–25 (Transdermal 30 hours)/Unchanged

METABOLISM

Elimination of buprenorphine is bi- or triphasic; metabolism takes place in the liver by oxidation via the cytochrome P450 isoenzyme CYP3A4 to the pharmacologically active metabolite N-dealkylbuprenorphine (norbuprenorphine), and by conjugation to glucuronide metabolites. Buprenorphine is subject to considerable first-pass metabolism after oral doses. However, when given by the usual routes buprenorphine is excreted mainly unchanged in the faeces; there is some evidence for enterohepatic recirculation. Metabolites are excreted in the urine, but very little unchanged drug is excreted in this way.

DOSE IN RENAL IMPAIRMENT GFR (mL/MIN)

20–50	Dose as in normal renal function.
10–20	Dose as in normal renal function, but avoid very large doses.
<10	Reduce dose by 25–50% initially and increase as tolerated; avoid very large single doses. Transdermal: dose as in normal renal function.

DOSE IN PATIENTS UNDERGOING RENAL REPLACEMENT THERAPIES

CAPD	Dialysed. Dose as in GFR<10 mL/min.
HD	Dialysed. Dose as in GFR<10 mL/min.
HDF/High flux	Dialysed. Dose as in GFR<10 mL/min.
CAV/VVHD	Not dialysed. Does as in GFR=10–20 mL/min.

IMPORTANT DRUG INTERACTIONS

Potentially hazardous interactions with other drugs
- Antidepressants: possible CNS excitation or depression (hypotension or hypertension) if administered with MAOIs or moclobemide – avoid concomitant use; sedative effects possibly increased when given with tricyclics.
- Antifungals: metabolism inhibited by ketoconazole – reduce buprenorphine dose.
- Antihistamines: sedative effects possibly increased with sedating antihistamines.
- Antipsychotics: enhanced hypotensive and sedative effects.
- Antivirals: concentration possibly increased by ritonavir; possibly reduced tipranavir concentration.
- Dopaminergics: avoid with selegiline.
- Sodium oxybate: avoid concomitant use.

ADMINISTRATION

RECONSTITUTION
–
ROUTE
- Sublingual, IM, IV, transdermal
RATE OF ADMINISTRATION
–
COMMENTS
–

OTHER INFORMATION

- It may take up to 30 hours for plasma buprenorphine concentration to decrease by 50% after the Transtec or Butrans patch has been removed.
- Do not give another opiate for 24 hours after the Transtec or Butrans patch has been removed.
- Naloxone 5–12 mg may reverse the effects of Transtec or Butrans but the effect may be delayed by 30 minutes.
- Patches are not suitable for acute pain.

Bupropion hydrochloride (amfebutamone HCL)

CLINICAL USE

Adjunct to smoking cessation

DOSE IN NORMAL RENAL FUNCTION

150 mg once daily for 6 days, then twice daily.

PHARMACOKINETICS

Molecular weight (daltons)	276.2
% Protein binding	84
% Excreted unchanged in urine	0.5
Volume of distribution (L/kg)	2000 litres
Half-life – normal/ ESRF (hrs)	14–20/–

METABOLISM

Several metabolites of bupropion are pharmacologically active and have longer half-lives, and achieve higher plasma concentrations than the parent compound. Hydroxybupropion is the major metabolite, produced by the metabolism of bupropion by the cytochrome P450 isoenzyme CYP2B6; in animal studies hydroxybupropion was one-half as potent as bupropion. Threohydrobupropion and erythrohydrobupropion are produced by reduction and are about one-fifth the potency of the parent compound. The metabolites of bupropion are excreted mainly in the urine; less than 1% of the parent drug is excreted unchanged.

DOSE IN RENAL IMPAIRMENT GFR (mL/MIN)

20–50	150 mg daily
10–20	150 mg daily
<10	150 mg daily

DOSE IN PATIENTS UNDERGOING RENAL REPLACEMENT THERAPIES

CAPD	Not dialysed. Dose as in GFR<10 mL/min.
HD	Not dialysed. Dose as in GFR<10 mL/min.
HDF/High flux	Not dialysed. Dose as in GFR<10 mL/min.
CAV/ VVHD	Unlikely to be dialysed. Dose as in GFR=10–20 mL/min.

IMPORTANT DRUG INTERACTIONS

Potentially hazardous interactions with other drugs

- Antidepressants: avoid MAOIs and linezolid with and for 2 weeks before starting treatment; avoid concomitant treatment with moclobemide; possibly increased citalopram concentration; possibly increased tricyclics concentration, increased risk of convulsions.
- Ciclosporin: may reduce ciclosporin levels.
- Hormone antagonists: possibly inhibits metabolism of tamoxifen to active metabolites – avoid.
- Methylthioninium: possible increased risk of CNS toxicity – avoid if possible.

ADMINISTRATION

RECONSTITUTION

–

ROUTE

- Oral

RATE OF ADMINISTRATION

–

COMMENTS

–

OTHER INFORMATION

- Bupropion and metabolites may accumulate in renal failure.

Buserelin

CLINICAL USE

- Treatment of advanced prostate cancer and endometriosis
- Pituitary desensitisation in preparation for ovulation induction regimens using gonadotrophins

DOSE IN NORMAL RENAL FUNCTION

- Prostate cancer: 500 mcg every 8 hours for 7 days SC then intranasally 1 spray into each nostril 6 times daily
- Endometriosis: 150 mcg is sprayed into each nostril three times daily
- Pituitary desensitisation in preparation for ovulation induction regimens using gonadotrophins: Intranasally: 600 mcg daily in 4 divided doses
- SC: 200–500 mcg daily as a single injection

PHARMACOKINETICS

Molecular weight (daltons)	1239.4 (1299.5 as acetate)
% Protein binding	15^1
% Excreted unchanged in urine	30 (SC), 0.73 (intranasal)[2]
Volume of distribution (L/kg)	No data
Half-life – normal/ ESRF (hrs)	80 minutes/–

METABOLISM

Metabolic inactivation by peptides occurs in the liver and kidney. The drug is also inactivated by pituitary membrane enzymes.

Excreted in the urine and bile as unchanged drug and metabolites.

DOSE IN RENAL IMPAIRMENT GFR (mL/MIN)

20–50	Dose as in normal renal function.
10–20	Dose as in normal renal function.
<10	Dose as in normal renal function. Monitor closely.

DOSE IN PATIENTS UNDERGOING RENAL REPLACEMENT THERAPIES

CAPD	Unlikely to be dialysed. Dose as in normal renal function.
HD	Unlikely to be dialysed. Dose as in normal renal function.
HDF/High flux	Unknown dialysability. Dose as in normal renal function.
CAV/ VVHD	Unlikely to be dialysed. Dose as in normal renal function.

IMPORTANT DRUG INTERACTIONS

Potentially hazardous interactions with other drugs
- None known

ADMINISTRATION

RECONSTITUTION
–
ROUTE
- Intranasal, SC
RATE OF ADMINISTRATION
–
COMMENTS
–

OTHER INFORMATION

- Buserelin accumulates in the liver and kidneys as well as in the anterior pituitary.

References:
1. DRUGDEX Evaluations [database on the Internet]. Buserelin. Thomson MICROMEDEX®, 2007. Available at: www. micromedex.com/ (accessed 2 April 2007).
2. Holland FJ, Fishman L, Costigan DC, et al. Pharmacokinetic characteristics of the gonadotropin-releasing hormone analog D-Ser(TBU)-6EA-10Luteinizing hormone-releasing hormone (Buserelin) after subcutaneous and intranasal administration in children with central precocious puberty. JCEM. 1986; 63(5): 1065.

Buspirone hydrochloride

CLINICAL USE

Anxiolytic

DOSE IN NORMAL RENAL FUNCTION

Initially 5 mg 2–3 times daily. Usual range 15–30 mg daily in divided doses (maximum 45 mg daily).

PHARMACOKINETICS

Molecular weight (daltons)	422
% Protein binding	95
% Excreted unchanged in urine	0
Volume of distribution (L/kg)	2.69–7.91
Half-life – normal/ESRF (hrs)	2–11/4–13[1]

METABOLISM

Systemic bioavailability of buspirone is low because of extensive first-pass metabolism. Metabolism in the liver is extensive via the cytochrome P450 isoenzyme CYP3A4; hydroxylation yields several inactive metabolites and oxidative dealkylation produces 1-(2-pyrimidinyl)-piperazine, which is reported to be about 25% as potent as the parent drug in one model of anxiolytic activity. Buspirone is excreted mainly as metabolites in the urine, and also the faeces.

DOSE IN RENAL IMPAIRMENT GFR (mL/MIN)

20–50	Start at a low dose and give twice daily.
10–20	Start at a low dose and give twice daily.
<10	Reduce by 25–50% if patient is anuric.[2]

DOSE IN PATIENTS UNDERGOING RENAL REPLACEMENT THERAPIES

CAPD	Not dialysed. Dose as in GFR<10 mL/min.
HD	Not dialysed. Dose as in GFR<10 mL/min.
HDF/High flux	Not dialysed. Dose as in GFR<10 mL/min.
CAV/ VVHD	Not dialysed. Does as in GFR=10–20 mL/min.

IMPORTANT DRUG INTERACTIONS

Potentially hazardous interactions with other drugs

- Antibacterials: concentration increased by erythromycin – reduce dose; concentration reduced by rifampicin.
- Antidepressants: risk of severe hypertension with MAOIs – avoid concomitant use.
- Antifungals: concentration increased by itraconazole – reduce dose.
- Antipsychotics: enhanced sedative effects; haloperidol concentration increased.
- Antivirals: concentration increased by ritonavir, increased risk of toxicity.
- Calcium-channel blockers: concentration increased by diltiazem and verapamil – reduce dose.
- Grapefruit juice: concentration increased by grapefruit juice – reduce dose.

ADMINISTRATION

RECONSTITUTION

–

ROUTE

- Oral

RATE OF ADMINISTRATION

–

COMMENTS

–

OTHER INFORMATION

- *Drug Prescribing in Renal Failure*, 5th edition, by Aronoff *et al.* advises no reduction in renal impairment.
- Peak plasma levels occur 60–90 minutes after dosing.
- Steady state plasma concentrations achieved within 2 days, although response to treatment may take 2 weeks.
- Non-sedative.
- Do not use in patients with severe hepatic disease.
- Use in severe renal impairment not recommended; risk of accumulation of active metabolites.

References:
1. Mahmood I, Sahajwalla C. Clinical pharmacokinetics and pharmacodynamics of buspirone. *Clin Pharmacokinet.* 1999; **36**(4): 277–87.
2. Caccia S, Vigano GL, Mingardi G, *et al.* Clinical pharmacokinetics of oral buspirone in patients with impaired renal function. *Clin Pharmacokinet.* 1988; **14**: 171–7.

Busulfan

CLINICAL USE

- Chronic myeloid leukaemia
- Remission of polycythaemia vera
- Essential thrombocythaemia and myelofibrosis
- Conditioning before bone marrow transplantation

DOSE IN NORMAL RENAL FUNCTION

Oral:
- Chronic myeloid leukaemia: 60 mcg/kg daily (maximum 4 mg daily); maintenance: 0.5–2 mg daily
- Polycythaemia vera: 4–6 mg daily; maintenance: 2–3 mg daily
- Myelofibrosis: 2–4 mg daily
IV infusion:
- Conditioning before bone marrow transplantation: 0.8 mg/kg every 6 hours over 4 days for 16 doses

PHARMACOKINETICS

Molecular weight (daltons)	246.3
% Protein binding	7–32
% Excreted unchanged in urine	1–2
Volume of distribution (L/kg)	0.62–0.85
Half-life – normal/ ESRF (hrs)	3/–

METABOLISM

Busulfan is extensively metabolised in the liver, mainly by conjugation with glutathione, either spontaneously or mediated by the enzyme glutathione-S-transferase. About 12 inactive metabolites have been identified, which are excreted in the urine. About 1% of busulfan is excreted unchanged. Elimination in the faeces is considered to be negligible.

DOSE IN RENAL IMPAIRMENT GFR (mL/MIN)

20–50	Dose as in normal renal function.
10–20	Dose as in normal renal function.
<10	Dose as in normal renal function.

DOSE IN PATIENTS UNDERGOING RENAL REPLACEMENT THERAPIES

CAPD	Unknown dialysability. Dose as in normal renal function.
HD	Dialysed. Dose as in normal renal function.
HDF/High flux	Dialysed. Dose as in normal renal function.
CAV/ VVHD	Unknown dialysability. Dose as in normal renal function.

IMPORTANT DRUG INTERACTIONS

Potentially hazardous interactions with other drugs
- Antibacterials: concentration increased by metronidazole.
- Antipsychotics: avoid concomitant use with clozapine, increased risk of agranulocytosis.
- Antifungals: metabolism inhibited by itraconazole, monitor for signs of busulfan toxicity.

ADMINISTRATION

RECONSTITUTION
–
ROUTE
- Oral, IV infusion
RATE OF ADMINISTRATION
- Over 2 hours
COMMENTS
- Dilute the solution to 500 mcg/mL with sodium chloride or glucose 5%.
- Give via a central venous catheter.

OTHER INFORMATION

- Can cause haemorrhagic cystitis.
- Can cause an increase in creatinine and haematuria.

Cabazitaxel

CLINICAL USE

Mitotic inhibitor:
- Used in combination with prednisolone for the treatment of patients with hormone refractory metastatic prostate cancer previously treated with a docetaxel-containing regimen

DOSE IN NORMAL RENAL FUNCTION

$25 \, mg/m^2$ every 3 weeks

PHARMACOKINETICS

Molecular weight (daltons)	835.9
% Protein binding	89–92
% Excreted unchanged in urine	2.3
Volume of distribution (L/kg)	4870 litres
Half-life – normal/ ESRF (hrs)	α, β, and γ half-lives of 4 minutes, 2 hours, and 95 hours, respectively.

METABOLISM

Extensively metabolised in the liver (>95%), mainly by the CYP3A4 isoenzyme (80–90%). Cabazitaxel is the main circulating compound in human plasma. Seven metabolites were detected in plasma (including 3 active metabolites issued form O-demethylations), with the main one accounting for 5% of parent exposure.

Excreted as metabolites into the urine (4%) and faeces (76%).

DOSE IN RENAL IMPAIRMENT GFR (mL/MIN)

30–50	Dose as in normal renal function.
10–30	Dose as in normal renal function. Use with caution.
<10	Dose as in normal renal function. Use with caution.

DOSE IN PATIENTS UNDERGOING RENAL REPLACEMENT THERAPIES

CAPD	Unlikely to be dialysed. Dose as in GFR<10mL/min.
HD	Unlikely to be dialysed. Dose as in GFR<10mL/min.
HDF/High flux	Unlikely to be dialysed. Dose as in GFR<10mL/min.
CAV/ VVHD	Unlikely to be dialysed. Dose as in GFR=10–30mL/min.

IMPORTANT DRUG INTERACTIONS

Potentially hazardous interactions with other drugs
- Antibacterials: avoid concomitant use with clarithromycin, rifabutin, rifampicin & telithromycin.
- Antidepressants: avoid concomitant use with St John's wort.
- Antiepileptics: avoid concomitant use with carbamazepine, phenobarbital & phenytoin.
- Antifungals: avoid concomitant use with itraconazole, ketoconazole & voriconazole.
- Antipsychotics: avoid concomitant use with clozapine (increased risk of agranulocytosis).
- Antivirals: avoid concomitant use with atazanavir, indinavir, ritonavir & saquinavir.

ADMINISTRATION

RECONSTITUTION
- Dilute with solvent provided

ROUTE
- IV infusion

RATE OF ADMINISTRATION
- 60 minutes

COMMENTS
- Dilute in sodium chloride 0.9% or glucose 5% to give a final concentration of 0.1–0.26 mg/mL
- Administer via a 0.22 micron in-line filter.
- PVC containers and polyurethane infusion sets should not be used.

OTHER INFORMATION

- Premedication should be administered at least 30 minutes prior to each administration.
- Throughout the treatment, adequate hydration of the patient needs to be ensured, in order to prevent renal failure.
- No studies have been done in renal impairment so the company advises to monitor closely and use with caution.
- BC Cancer Agency *Cancer Drug Manual* advises to use normal dose (accessed 1 November 2013).

Cabergoline

CLINICAL USE

- Endocrine disorders
- Adjunct to levodopa (with a decarboxylase inhibitor) in Parkinson's disease
- Inhibition/suppression of lactation

DOSE IN NORMAL RENAL FUNCTION

- Parkinson's disease: 1–3 mg daily
- Hyperprolactinaemic disorders: 0.25–2 mg weekly
- Inhibition of lactation: single 1 mg dose during first day post partum
- Suppression of lactation: 0.25 mg twice a day for 2 days

PHARMACOKINETICS

Molecular weight (daltons)	451.6
% Protein binding	41–42
% Excreted unchanged in urine	2–3
Volume of distribution (L/kg)	No data
Half-life – normal/ ESRF (hrs)	63–68 (healthy individuals), 79–115 (hyperprolactinaemic individuals)/ Unchanged

METABOLISM

Cabergoline is subject to first-pass metabolism and is extensively metabolised to several metabolites that do not appear to contribute to its pharmacological activity. Cabergoline is mainly eliminated via the faeces (72%); a small proportion is excreted in the urine (18%).

DOSE IN RENAL IMPAIRMENT GFR (mL/MIN)

20–50	Dose as in normal renal function.
10–20	Dose as in normal renal function.
<10	Dose as in normal renal function.

DOSE IN PATIENTS UNDERGOING RENAL REPLACEMENT THERAPIES

CAPD	Dialysed. Dose as in normal renal function.
HD	Dialysed. Dose as in normal renal function.
HDF/High flux	Dialysed. Dose as in normal renal function.
CAV/ VVHD	Dialysed. Dose as in normal renal function.

IMPORTANT DRUG INTERACTIONS

Potentially hazardous interactions with other drugs
- None known

ADMINISTRATION

RECONSTITUTION
–
ROUTE
- Oral
RATE OF ADMINISTRATION
–
COMMENTS
–

Calcitonin (salmon)/salcatonin

CLINICAL USE

- Hypercalcaemia of malignancy
- Paget's disease of bone
- Postmenopausal osteoporosis
- Prevention of acute bone loss due to sudden immobility

DOSE IN NORMAL RENAL FUNCTION

- Hypercalcaemia of malignancy: 100–400 units every 6–8 hours (SC/IM); in severe or emergency situation, up to 10 units/kg by IV infusion.
- Paget's disease of bone: 50 units 3 times a week to 100 units daily (SC/IM).
- Prevention of acute bone loss due to sudden immobility: 100 units daily in 1–2 divided doses for 2–4 weeks then reduce to 50 units daily until fully mobile (SC/IM).

PHARMACOKINETICS

Molecular weight (daltons)	3431.9
% Protein binding	30–40
% Excreted unchanged in urine	Minimal
Volume of distribution (L/kg)	9.9 litres
Half-life – normal/ ESRF (hrs)	50–90 minutes (parenteral); 16–43 minutes (intranasal)/Increased

METABOLISM

Animal studies have shown that calcitonin is primarily metabolised via proteolysis in the kidney following parenteral administration. The metabolites lack the specific biological activity of calcitonin.

Salmon calcitonin is primarily and almost exclusively degraded in the kidneys, forming pharmacologically inactive fragments of the molecule. Therefore, the metabolic clearance is much lower in patients with end-stage renal failure than in healthy subjects. However, the clinical relevance of this finding is not known.

DOSE IN RENAL IMPAIRMENT GFR (mL/MIN)

20–50	Dose as in normal renal function.
10–20	Dose as in normal renal function.
<10	Dose as in normal renal function.

DOSE IN PATIENTS UNDERGOING RENAL REPLACEMENT THERAPIES

CAPD	Unlikely to be dialysed. Dose as in normal renal function.
HD	Unlikely to be dialysed. Dose as in normal renal function.
HDF/High flux	Unlikely to be dialysed. Dose as in normal renal function.
CAV/ VVHD	Unlikely to be dialysed. Dose as in normal renal function.

IMPORTANT DRUG INTERACTIONS

Potentially hazardous interactions with other drugs
- None known

ADMINISTRATION

RECONSTITUTION
–
ROUTE
- IM, IV, SC
RATE OF ADMINISTRATION
- Over at least 6 hours
COMMENTS
- Dilute in 500 mL sodium chloride 0.9% and administer immediately; dilution may result in a loss of potency.

OTHER INFORMATION

- Peak plasma concentration occurs 15–25 minutes after parenteral administration.
- Mainly GI side effects.

Calcitriol

CLINICAL USE

Vitamin D analogue:
- Promotes intestinal calcium absorption
- Suppresses PTH production and release

DOSE IN NORMAL RENAL FUNCTION

- Orally: 250 nanograms daily or on alternate days, increased if necessary in steps of 250 nanograms at intervals of 2–4 weeks. Usual dose 0.5–1 micrograms daily.
- IV (unlicensed): treatment of hyperparathyroidism in haemodialysis patients: initially 500 nanograms (10 nanograms/kg) 3 times a week, increased if necessary in steps of 250–500 nanograms at intervals of 2–4 weeks. Usual dose 0.5–3 micrograms 3 times a week after dialysis.

PHARMACOKINETICS

Molecular weight (daltons)	416.6
% Protein binding	99.9
% Excreted unchanged in urine	7–10
Volume of distribution (L/kg)	No data
Half-life – normal/ ESRF (hrs)	9–10/18–20

METABOLISM

During transport in the blood at physiological concentrations, calcitriol is mostly bound to a specific vitamin D binding protein (DBP), but also, to a lesser degree, to lipoproteins and albumin. At higher blood calcitriol concentrations, DBP appears to become saturated, and increased binding to lipoproteins and albumin occurs.

Calcitriol is inactivated in both the kidney and the intestine, through the formation of a number of intermediates including the formation of the 1,24,25-trihydroxy derivatives. It is excreted in the bile and faeces and is subject to enterohepatic circulation.

DOSE IN RENAL IMPAIRMENT GFR (mL/MIN)

20–50	Dose as in normal renal function. Titrate to response.
10–20	Dose as in normal renal function. Titrate to response.
<10	Dose as in normal renal function. Titrate to response.

DOSE IN PATIENTS UNDERGOING RENAL REPLACEMENT THERAPIES

CAPD	Unlikely to be dialysed. Dose as in normal renal function.
HD	Unlikely to be dialysed. Dose as in normal renal function.
HDF/High flux	Unlikely to be dialysed. Dose as in normal renal function.
CAV/ VVHD	Unknown dialysability. Dose as in normal renal function.

IMPORTANT DRUG INTERACTIONS

Potentially hazardous interactions with other drugs
- Anti-epileptics: the effects of vitamin D may be reduced in patients taking barbiturates or anticonvulsants.
- Diuretics: increased risk of hypercalcaemia with thiazides.
- Sevelamer: absorption may be impaired by sevelamer.

ADMINISTRATION

RECONSTITUTION
–
ROUTE
- Oral, IV
RATE OF ADMINISTRATION
- Bolus
COMMENTS
–

OTHER INFORMATION

- IV preparation available from IDIS.
- Check plasma calcium concentrations at regular intervals (initially weekly).
- Dose of phosphate-binding agent may need to be modified as phosphate transport in the gut and bone may be affected.
- Hypercalcaemia and hypercalciuria are the major side effects, and indicate excessive dosage.

Calcium acetate

CLINICAL USE

Phosphate binding agent

DOSE IN NORMAL RENAL FUNCTION

1–4 tablets, 3 times daily

PHARMACOKINETICS

Molecular weight (daltons)	158.2
% Protein binding	–
% Excreted unchanged in urine	–
Volume of distribution (L/kg)	–
Half-life – normal/ ESRF (hrs)	–

METABOLISM

The residual acetate will be metabolised through bicarbonate, which will be further excreted via normal metabolic routes.

Any unbound calcium not involved in the binding of phosphate will be variable and may be absorbed. Calcium is absorbed mainly from the small intestine by active transport and passive diffusion. About one-third of ingested calcium is absorbed although this can vary depending upon dietary factors and the state of the small intestine. 1,25-Dihydroxycholecalciferol (calcitriol), a metabolite of vitamin D, enhances the active phase of absorption.

Excess calcium is mainly excreted renally. Unabsorbed calcium is eliminated in the faeces, together with that secreted in the bile and pancreatic juice. Minor amounts are lost in the sweat, skin, hair, and nails.

DOSE IN RENAL IMPAIRMENT GFR (mL/MIN)

20–50	Dose as in normal renal function. Titrate to response.
10–20	Dose as in normal renal function. Titrate to response.
<10	Dose as in normal renal function. Titrate to response.

DOSE IN PATIENTS UNDERGOING RENAL REPLACEMENT THERAPIES

CAPD	Unknown dialysability. Dose as in normal renal function.
HD	Unknown dialysability. Dose as in normal renal function.
HDF/High flux	Unknown dialysability. Dose as in normal renal function.
CAV/ VVHD	Unknown dialysability. Dose as in normal renal function.

IMPORTANT DRUG INTERACTIONS

Potentially hazardous interactions with other drugs
- Can impair absorption of some drugs, e.g. iron, ciprofloxacin.

ADMINISTRATION

RECONSTITUTION

–

ROUTE
- Oral

RATE OF ADMINISTRATION

–

COMMENTS
- Take tablets with meals.

OTHER INFORMATION

- Phosex: calcium content per tablet = 250 mg (6.2 mmol).
- PhosLo: calcium content per tablet = 169 mg (4.2 mmol).
- Renacet: calcium content per tablet = 120.25 mg (3 mmol).

Calcium carbonate

CLINICAL USE

- Phosphate binding agent
- Calcium supplement

DOSE IN NORMAL RENAL FUNCTION

Dose adjusted according to serum phosphate and calcium levels.

PHARMACOKINETICS

Molecular weight (daltons)	100.1
% Protein binding	40
% Excreted unchanged in urine	–
Volume of distribution (L/kg)	–
Half-life – normal/ ESRF (hrs)	–

METABOLISM

Under the influence of gastric acid, any residual carbonate will be converted to carbon dioxide and water.

Any unbound calcium not involved in the binding of phosphate will be variable and may be absorbed. Calcium is absorbed mainly from the small intestine by active transport and passive diffusion. About one-third of ingested calcium is absorbed although this can vary depending upon dietary factors and the state of the small intestine. 1,25-Dihydroxycholecalciferol (calcitriol), a metabolite of vitamin D, enhances the active phase of absorption.

Excess calcium is mainly excreted renally. Unabsorbed calcium is eliminated in the faeces, together with that secreted in the bile and pancreatic juice. Minor amounts are lost in the sweat, skin, hair, and nails.

DOSE IN RENAL IMPAIRMENT GFR (mL/MIN)

20–50	Dose as in normal renal function. Titrate to response.
10–20	Dose as in normal renal function. Titrate to response.
<10	Dose as in normal renal function. Titrate to response.

DOSE IN PATIENTS UNDERGOING RENAL REPLACEMENT THERAPIES

CAPD	Unknown dialysability. Dose as in normal renal function.
HD	Unknown dialysability. Dose as in normal renal function.
HDF/High flux	Unknown dialysability. Dose as in normal renal function.
CAV/ VVHD	Unknown dialysability. Dose as in normal renal function.

IMPORTANT DRUG INTERACTIONS

Potentially hazardous interactions with other drugs

- Can impair absorption of some drugs, e.g. iron, ciprofloxacin.

ADMINISTRATION

RECONSTITUTION

–

ROUTE

- Oral

COMMENTS

- Take with or immediately before meals.

OTHER INFORMATION

- Monitor for hypercalcaemia particularly if patient is also taking alfacalcidol.
- Calcichew contains 1250 mg calcium carbonate (500 mg elemental calcium).
- Calcium 500 contains 1250 mg calcium carbonate (500 mg elemental calcium).
- Cacit contains 1250 mg calcium carbonate (500 mg elemental calcium).
- Adcal contains 1500 mg calcium carbonate (600 mg elemental calcium).

Calcium gluconate

CLINICAL USE

Hypocalcaemia

DOSE IN NORMAL RENAL FUNCTION

Depending on indication
Acute hypocalcaemia: 10–20 mL calcium
gluconate 10% (2.25–4.5 mmol calcium) slow
IV injection over 3–10 minutes.
Oral: Dose varies depending on
requirements.

PHARMACOKINETICS

Molecular weight (daltons)	448.4
% Protein binding	–
% Excreted unchanged in urine	–
Volume of distribution (L/kg)	–
Half-life – normal/ ESRF (hrs)	–

METABOLISM

Calcium is absorbed mainly from the
small intestine by active transport and
passive diffusion. About one-third of
ingested calcium is absorbed although
this can vary depending upon dietary
factors and the state of the small intestine.
1,25-Dihydroxycholecalciferol (calcitriol), a
metabolite of vitamin D, enhances the active
phase of absorption.
   Excess calcium is mainly excreted renally.
Unabsorbed calcium is eliminated in the
faeces, together with that secreted in the bile
and pancreatic juice. Minor amounts are lost
in the sweat, skin, hair, and nails.

DOSE IN RENAL IMPAIRMENT GFR (mL/MIN)

20–50	Dose as in normal renal function. Titrate to response.
10–20	Dose as in normal renal function. Titrate to response.
<10	Dose as in normal renal function. Titrate to response.

DOSE IN PATIENTS UNDERGOING RENAL REPLACEMENT THERAPIES

CAPD	Dialysed. Dose as in normal renal function.
HD	Dialysed. Dose as in normal renal function.
HDF/High flux	Dialysed. Dose as in normal renal function.
CAV/ VVHD	Dialysed. Dose as in normal renal function.

IMPORTANT DRUG INTERACTIONS

Potentially hazardous interactions with other
drugs
● Can impair absorption of some drugs, e.g.
iron, ciprofloxacin.

ADMINISTRATION

RECONSTITUTION
–
ROUTE
● Oral, IV, IM
RATE OF ADMINISTRATION
● IV: slow 3–4 minutes for each 10 mL
(2.25 mmol calcium); not greater than
20 mmol/hour for continuous infusions
COMMENTS
● Can be added to glucose 5% or sodium
chloride 0.9%.
● IV: Can be used undiluted for continuous
and intermittent infusions (UK Critical
Care Group, *Minimum Infusion Volumes
for Fluid Restricted Critically Ill Patients*,
3rd edition, 2006).

OTHER INFORMATION

● Check patient's magnesium levels.
● Monitor calcium and PO_4 serum levels.
● Sandocal 1000: 25 mmol calcium per tablet
● Calcium Sandoz syrup: 2.7 mmol/5 mL.
● Calcium levels cannot be corrected until
magnesium levels are normal.

Calcium resonium

CLINICAL USE

Hyperkalaemia (not for emergency treatment)

DOSE IN NORMAL RENAL FUNCTION

Oral: 15 g 3–4 times daily in water
PR: 30 g in methylcellulose solution retained for 9 hours
Sorbisterit: Oral: 20 g 1–3 times daily in 150 mL of water
PR: 40 g in 150 mL of glucose 5% 1–3 times daily retained for 6 hours

PHARMACOKINETICS

Molecular weight (daltons)	–
% Protein binding	–
% Excreted unchanged in urine	0
Volume of distribution (L/kg)	–
Half-life – normal/ ESRF (hrs)	–

METABOLISM

Not applicable as calcium resonium is not systemically absorbed.

DOSE IN RENAL IMPAIRMENT GFR (mL/MIN)

20–50	Dose as in normal renal function. Titrate to response.
10–20	Dose as in normal renal function. Titrate to response.
<10	Dose as in normal renal function. Titrate to response.

DOSE IN PATIENTS UNDERGOING RENAL REPLACEMENT THERAPIES

CAPD	Not dialysed. Dose as in normal renal function.
HD	Not dialysed. Dose as in normal renal function.
HDF/High flux	Not dialysed. Dose as in normal renal function.
CAV/ VVHD	Not dialysed. Dose as in normal renal function.

IMPORTANT DRUG INTERACTIONS

Potentially hazardous interactions with other drugs
- None known

ADMINISTRATION

RECONSTITUTION
- PR: Mix with methylcellulose solution 2%.
- Oral: Mix with a little water, sweetened if preferred.

ROUTE
- Oral, PR

RATE OF ADMINISTRATION
–

COMMENTS
–

OTHER INFORMATION

- Ensure a regular laxative is prescribed – can mix calcium resonium powder with lactulose to be taken orally.
- Some units mix dose with a little water and give PR 4 times/day. Not retained for so long, but still effective.

Candesartan cilexetil

CLINICAL USE

Angiotensin-II antagonist:
- Hypertension
- Heart failure

DOSE IN NORMAL RENAL FUNCTION

2–32 mg daily

PHARMACOKINETICS

Molecular weight (daltons)	610.7
% Protein binding	>99
% Excreted unchanged in urine	26
Volume of distribution (L/kg)	0.1
Half-life – normal/ESRF (hrs)	9/18

METABOLISM

Candesartan is mainly eliminated unchanged via urine and bile and only to a minor extent eliminated by hepatic metabolism (CYP2C9).

The renal elimination of candesartan is both by glomerular filtration and active tubular secretion. Following an oral dose of ^{14}C-labelled candesartan cilexetil, approximately 26% of the dose is excreted in the urine as candesartan and 7% as an inactive metabolite while approximately 56% of the dose is recovered in the faeces as candesartan and 10% as the inactive metabolite.

DOSE IN RENAL IMPAIRMENT GFR (mL/MIN)

20–50	Dose as in normal renal function.
10–20	Initial dose 2 mg and increase according to response.
<10	Initial dose 2 mg and increase according to response.

DOSE IN PATIENTS UNDERGOING RENAL REPLACEMENT THERAPIES

CAPD	Unlikely to be dialysed. Dose as in GFR<10 mL/min.
HD	Not dialysed. Dose as in GFR<10 mL/min.
HDF/High flux	Not dialysed. Dose as in GFR<10 mL/min.
CAV/ VVHD	Unlikely to be dialysed. Dose as in GFR=10–20 mL/min.

IMPORTANT DRUG INTERACTIONS

Potentially hazardous interactions with other drugs
- Anaesthetics: enhanced hypotensive effect.
- Analgesics: antagonism of hypotensive effect and increased risk of renal impairment with NSAIDs; hyperkalaemia with ketorolac and other NSAIDs.
- Ciclosporin: increased risk of hyperkalaemia and nephrotoxicity.
- Diuretics: enhanced hypotensive effect; hyperkalaemia with potassium-sparing diuretics.
- ESAs: increased risk of hyperkalaemia; antagonism of hypotensive effect.
- Lithium: reduced excretion, possibility of enhanced lithium toxicity.
- Potassium salts: increased risk of hyperkalaemia.
- Tacrolimus: increased risk of hyperkalaemia and nephrotoxicity.

ADMINISTRATION

RECONSTITUTION
–
ROUTE
- Oral
RATE OF ADMINISTRATION
–
COMMENTS
–

OTHER INFORMATION

- In patients with mild–moderate renal impairment C_{max} and AUC are increased by 50% and 70% respectively. Corresponding changes in patients with severe renal impairment are 50% and 110% respectively.
- Adverse reactions, especially hyperkalaemia, are more common in patients with renal impairment.
- Renal failure has been reported in association with angiotensin-II antagonists in patients with renal artery stenosis, post renal transplant, and in those with congestive heart failure.
- Close monitoring of renal function during therapy is necessary in those with renal insufficiency.

Capecitabine

CLINICAL USE

Antineoplastic agent (antimetabolite):
- Colorectal, colon, advanced gastric and breast cancer

DOSE IN NORMAL RENAL FUNCTION

- Monotherapy, also combination therapy in breast cancer: $1.25\,g/m^2$ twice daily for 14 days, repeated after 7 days.
- Combination therapy for colon, rectal or gastric cancer: $800-1000\,mg/m^2$ twice daily for 14 days, repeated after 7 days
- Or $625\,mg/m^2$ twice daily continuously

PHARMACOKINETICS

Molecular weight (daltons)	359.4
% Protein binding	54
% Excreted unchanged in urine	3
Volume of distribution (L/kg)	No data
Half-life – normal/ ESRF (hrs)	0.85/Increased

METABOLISM

Capecitabine is a prodrug. It is hydrolysed in the liver to 5'-deoxy-5-fluorocytidine (5'-DFCR), which is then converted to 5'-deoxy-5-fluorouridine (5'-DFUR) and subsequently to the active 5-fluorouracil in body tissues, via the enzyme thymidine phosphorylase. 5-Fluorouracil is further metabolised to 5-fluorouridine monophosphate and 5-fluorodeoxyuridine monophosphate. About 15% of 5-fluorouracil is excreted unchanged in the urine within 6 hours. The remainder is inactivated mainly in the liver and is catabolised via dihydropyrimidine dehydrogenase. A large amount is excreted as respiratory carbon dioxide; urea and other metabolites are also produced. About 3% of a dose of capecitabine is excreted in the urine unchanged.

DOSE IN RENAL IMPAIRMENT GFR (mL/MIN)

30–50	75% of $1.2\,g/m^2$ dose ($950\,mg/m^2$ twice daily), use with care.
10–30	Avoid.
<10	Avoid.

DOSE IN PATIENTS UNDERGOING RENAL REPLACEMENT THERAPIES

CAPD	Unknown dialysability. Dose as in GFR<10 mL/min.
HD	Unlikely to be dialysed. Dose as in GFR<10 mL/min.
HDF/High flux	Unknown dialysability. Dose as in GFR<10 mL/min.
CAV/ VVHD	Unknown dialysability. Dose as in GFR=10–30 mL/min.

IMPORTANT DRUG INTERACTIONS

Potentially hazardous interactions with other drugs
- Allopurinol: avoid concomitant use.
- Anticoagulants: possibly enhances effect of coumarins.
- Anti-epileptics: reported toxicity with phenytoin, due to increased phenytoin levels.
- Antipsychotics: avoid concomitant use with clozapine – increased risk of agranulocytosis.

ADMINISTRATION

RECONSTITUTION
–
ROUTE
- Oral
RATE OF ADMINISTRATION
–
COMMENTS
- Give after food.

OTHER INFORMATION

- Contraindicated in severe renal impairment due to increased incidence of grade 3 or 4 adverse reactions in patients with a GFR of 30–50 mL/min.

Capreomycin

CLINICAL USE

Antibacterial agent in combination with other drugs:
- Tuberculosis that is resistant to first-line drugs

DOSE IN NORMAL RENAL FUNCTION

Deep IM injection: 1 g daily (not more than 20 mg/kg) for 2–4 months, then 1 g 2–3 times each week

PHARMACOKINETICS

Molecular weight (daltons)	668.7
% Protein binding	No data
% Excreted unchanged in urine	50
Volume of distribution (L/kg)	0.37–0.42
Half-life – normal/ ESRF (hrs)	2/55.5

METABOLISM

Approximately 50% of a dose is excreted unchanged in the urine by glomerular filtration within 12 hours.

DOSE IN RENAL IMPAIRMENT GFR (mL/MIN)

20–50	Dose as in normal renal function.
10–20	Dose as in normal renal function.
<10	1 g every 48 hours.

DOSE IN PATIENTS UNDERGOING RENAL REPLACEMENT THERAPIES

CAPD	Not dialysed. Dose as in GFR<10 mL/min.
HD	Dialysed. Dose as in GFR<10 mL/min.
HDF/High flux	Dialysed. Dose as in GFR<10 mL/min.
CAV/ VVHD	Not dialysed. Dose as in normal renal function.

IMPORTANT DRUG INTERACTIONS

Potentially hazardous interactions with other drugs
- Increased risk of nephrotoxicity and ototoxicity with aminoglycosides and vancomycin.

ADMINISTRATION

RECONSTITUTION
- Dissolve in 2 mL of sodium chloride 0.9% or water for injection. Allow 2–3 minutes for complete dissolution.

ROUTE
- Deep IM injection

RATE OF ADMINISTRATION
–

COMMENTS
–

OTHER INFORMATION

- Nephrotoxic.
- Check potassium levels as hypokalaemia may occur.
- Desired steady state serum capreomycin level is 10 micrograms/mL.
- Dose should not exceed 1 g/day in renal failure.
- Doses in renal impairment from *Drug Prescribing in Renal Failure*, 5th edition, by Aronoff *et al.*
- Capreomycin sulphate 1 000 000 Units is approximately equivalent to capreomycin base 1 g.
  Manufacturer has a table based on mg/kg:

Creatinine Clearance (mL/min)	Dose for these dosing intervals (mg/kg)		
	24 h	48 h	72 h
0	1.29	2.58	3.87
10	2.43	4.87	7.30
20	3.58	7.16	10.70
30	4.72	9.45	14.20
40	5.87	11.70	
50	7.01	14.00	
60	8.16		
80	10.40		
100	12.70		
110	13.90		

Captopril

CLINICAL USE

Angiotensin-converting enzyme inhibitor:
- Hypertension
- Heart failure
- Post myocardial infarction
- Diabetic nephropathy

DOSE IN NORMAL RENAL FUNCTION

6.25–50 mg 2–3 times daily
Diabetic nephropathy: 75–100 mg daily in
divided doses

PHARMACOKINETICS

Molecular weight (daltons)	217.3
% Protein binding	25–30
% Excreted unchanged in urine	40–50
Volume of distribution (L/kg)	2
Half-life – normal/ ESRF (hrs)	2–3/21–32

METABOLISM

About half the absorbed dose of captopril
is rapidly metabolised, mainly to captopril-
cysteine disulfide and the disulfide dimer
of captopril. *In vitro* studies suggest that
captopril and its metabolites may undergo
reversible interconversions. It has been
suggested that the drug may be more
extensively metabolised in patients with renal
impairment than in patients with normal
renal function.

Captopril and its metabolites are excreted
in urine. Renal excretion of unchanged
captopril occurs principally via tubular
secretion. In patients with normal renal
function, more than 95% of an absorbed
dose is excreted in urine in 24 hours; about
40–50% of the drug excreted in urine is
unchanged captopril and the remainder is
mainly the disulfide dimer of captopril and
captopril-cysteine disulfide. In one study in
healthy individuals, about 20% of a single
dose of captopril was recovered in faeces in
5 days, apparently representing unabsorbed
drug.

DOSE IN RENAL IMPAIRMENT GFR (mL/MIN)

20–50	Start low – adjust according to response.
10–20	Start low – adjust according to response.
<10	Start low – adjust according to response.

DOSE IN PATIENTS UNDERGOING RENAL REPLACEMENT THERAPIES

CAPD	Not dialysed. Dose as in GFR<10 mL/min.
HD	Dialysed. Dose as in GFR<10 mL/ min.
HDF/High flux	Dialysed. Dose as in GFR<10 mL/ min.
CAV/ VVHD	Dialysed. Dose as in GFR=10– 20 mL/min.

IMPORTANT DRUG INTERACTIONS

Potentially hazardous interactions with other
drugs
- Anaesthetics: enhanced hypotensive effect.
- Analgesics: antagonism of hypotensive effect and increased risk of renal impairment with NSAIDs; hyperkalaemia with ketorolac and other NSAIDs.
- Ciclosporin: increased risk of hyperkalaemia and nephrotoxicity.
- Diuretics: enhanced hypotensive effect; hyperkalaemia with potassium-sparing diuretics.
- ESAs: increased risk of hyperkalaemia; antagonism of hypotensive effect.
- Gold: flushing and hypotension with sodium aurothiomalate.
- Lithium: reduced excretion, possibility of enhanced lithium toxicity.
- Potassium salts: increased risk of hyperkalaemia.
- Tacrolimus: increased risk of hyperkalaemia and nephrotoxicity.

ADMINISTRATION

RECONSTITUTION
–
ROUTE
- Oral
RATE OF ADMINISTRATION
–
COMMENTS
- Tablets may be dispersed in water.

OTHER INFORMATION

- Adverse reactions, especially hyperkalaemia, are more common in patients with renal impairment.
- Effective sublingually in emergencies.
- As renal function declines a hepatic elimination route for captopril becomes increasingly more significant.
- Renal failure has been reported in association with ACE inhibitors in patients with renal artery stenosis, post renal transplant, or in those with congestive heart failure.
- A high incidence of anaphylactoid reactions has been reported in patients dialysed with high-flux polyacrylonitrile membranes and treated concomitantly with an ACE inhibitor – this combination should therefore be avoided.
- Close monitoring of renal function during therapy is necessary in those with renal insufficiency.

Carbamazepine

CLINICAL USE

- All forms of epilepsy except absence seizures
- Trigeminal neuralgia
- Prophylaxis in manic depressive illness
- Unlicensed: alcohol withdrawal and diabetic neuropathy

DOSE IN NORMAL RENAL FUNCTION

- Epilepsy: initially 100–200 mg 1–2 times daily, increased to maintenance of 0.4–1.2 g daily in divided doses; maximum 1.6–2 g daily.
- Rectal: maximum 1 g daily in 4 divided doses for up to 7 days use.
- Trigeminal neuralgia: Initially 100 mg 1–2 times daily; usual dose 200 mg 3–4 times daily; maximum 1.6 g/day; reduce dose gradually as pain goes into remission.
- Prophylaxis in manic-depressive illness: 400–600 mg daily in divided doses, maximum 1.6 g/day.
- Alcohol withdrawal: 800 mg daily in divided doses reducing to 200 mg daily over 5 days
- Diabetic neuropathy: 100 mg 1–2 times daily increasing according to response, usual dose 200 mg 3–4 times daily, max 1.6 g daily

PHARMACOKINETICS

Molecular weight (daltons)	236.3
% Protein binding	70–80
% Excreted unchanged in urine	2
Volume of distribution (L/kg)	0.8–1.9
Half-life – normal/ ESRF (hrs)	5–26/Unchanged

METABOLISM

Carbamazepine is metabolised in the liver by cytochrome P450 3A4, where the epoxide pathway of biotransformation yields the 10, 11-transdiol derivative and its glucuronide as the main metabolites.

9-hydroxymethyl-10-carbamoyl-acridan is a minor metabolite related to this pathway.

Other important biotransformation pathways for carbamazepine lead to various monohydroxylated compounds, as well as to the N-glucuronide of carbamazepine produced by UGT2B7.

After administration of a single oral dose of 400 mg carbamazepine, 72% is excreted in the urine and 28% in the faeces. In the urine, about 2% of the dose is recovered as unchanged drug and about 1% as the pharmacologically active 10, 11-epoxide metabolite.

DOSE IN RENAL IMPAIRMENT GFR (mL/MIN)

20–50	Dose as in normal renal function.
10–20	Dose as in normal renal function.
<10	Dose as in normal renal function.

DOSE IN PATIENTS UNDERGOING RENAL REPLACEMENT THERAPIES

CAPD	Not dialysed. Dose as in normal renal function.
HD	Not dialysed. Dose as in normal renal function.
HDF/High flux	Unknown dialysability. Dose as in normal renal function.
CAV/ VVHD	Not dialysed. Dose as in normal renal function.

IMPORTANT DRUG INTERACTIONS

Potentially hazardous interactions with other drugs

- Analgesics: effect enhanced by dextropropoxyphene; decreased effect of tramadol and methadone; possibly increases paracetamol metabolism, also reports of hepatotoxicity.
- Anti-arrhythmics: possibly reduces dronedarone concentration – avoid.
- Antibacterials: reduced effect of doxycycline; concentration increased by clarithromycin, erythromycin and isoniazid; increased risk of isoniazid hepatotoxicity; concentration reduced by rifabutin; concentration of telithromycin reduced – avoid concomitant use.
- Anticoagulants: metabolism of coumarins accelerated (reduced anticoagulant effect); concentration of dabigatran possibly reduced – avoid.
- Antidepressants: antagonism of anticonvulsant effect; concentration increased by fluoxetine and fluvoxamine; concentration of mianserin, mirtazapine, paroxetine, reboxetine, trazodone and tricyclics reduced; avoid concomitant use

with MAOIs; concentration reduced by St John's wort – avoid concomitant use.

- Anti-epileptics: concentration of eslicarbazepine possibly reduced but risk of side effects increased; concentration of ethosuximide, phenobarbital, retigabine, topiramate and valproate possibly reduced, concentration of active carbamazepine metabolite increased by valproate; concentration of lamotrigine, perampanel, tiagabine and zonisamide reduced; increased risk of carbamazepine toxicity with levetiracetam; concentration sometimes reduced by oxcarbazepine but active metabolite of carbamazepine may be increased and oxcarbazepine metabolite reduced; concentration of both drugs reduced with phenytoin and rufinamide, phenytoin concentration may also be increased; concentration increased by stiripentol.
- Antifungals: concentration possibly increased by fluconazole, ketoconazole and miconazole; concentration of itraconazole, caspofungin, posaconazole and voriconazole possibly reduced, avoid with voriconazole, consider increasing caspofungin dose.
- Antimalarials: avoid with piperaquine with artenimol; chloroquine, hydroxychloroquine and mefloquine antagonise anticonvulsant effect.
- Antipsychotics: antagonism of anticonvulsant effect; reduced concentration of aripiprazole (increase aripiprazole dose), haloperidol, clozapine, olanzapine, paliperidone, quetiapine and risperidone; avoid concomitant use with other drugs that can cause agranulocytosis.
- Antivirals: concentration of boceprevir and rilpivirine reduced – avoid; possibly reduced concentration of darunavir, fosamprenavir, indinavir, lopinavir, nevirapine, saquinavir and tipranavir; concentration possibly increased by indinavir and ritonavir; concentration of both drugs reduced in combination with efavirenz; avoid with etravirine and telaprevir.
- Calcium-channel blockers: effects enhanced by diltiazem and verapamil; reduced effect of felodipine, isradipine and probably dihydropyridines, nicardipine, nifedipine and nimodipine – avoid with nimodipine.
- Ciclosporin: metabolism accelerated (reduced ciclosporin concentration).
- Clopidogrel: possibly reduced anti-platelet effect.
- Corticosteroids: reduced effect of corticosteroids.
- Cytotoxics: possibly reduced concentration of axitinib, increase axitinib dose; possibly reduced concentration of crizotinib, imatinib, lapatinib and vandetanib – avoid; avoid with cabazitaxel, gefitinib and vemurafenib; concentration of irinotecan and its active metabolite and possibly eribulin reduced.
- Diuretics: increased risk of hyponatraemia; concentration increased by acetazolamide; reduced eplerenone concentration – avoid concomitant use.
- Hormone antagonists: metabolism inhibited by danazol; possibly accelerated metabolism of toremifene.
- Lipid-regulating drugs: concentration of simvastatin reduced.
- Oestrogens and progestogens: reduced contraceptive effect.
- Orlistat: possibly increased risk of convulsions.
- Ulcer-healing drugs: concentration increased by cimetidine.
- Ulipristal: contraceptive effect possibly reduced – avoid.

ADMINISTRATION

RECONSTITUTION

–

ROUTE
- Oral, rectal

RATE OF ADMINISTRATION

–

COMMENTS
- When switching a patient from tablets to liquid the same total dose may be used, but given in smaller more frequent doses.
- 125 mg suppository is equivalent 100 mg of tablets.
- Important to initiate carbamazepine therapy at a low dose and build this up over 1–2 weeks, as it autoinduces its metabolism.
- May cause inappropriate antidiuretic hormone secretion.
- Therapeutic plasma concentration range: 4–12 micrograms/mL (20–50 micromol/L at steady state).

Carbimazole

CLINICAL USE

Treatment of hyperthyroidism

DOSE IN NORMAL RENAL FUNCTION

5–60 mg daily

PHARMACOKINETICS

Molecular weight (daltons)	186.2
% Protein binding	Unbound (methimazole is 5%)
% Excreted unchanged in urine	<12 (methimazole)
Volume of distribution (L/kg)	0.5 (methimazole)
Half-life – normal/ ESRF (hrs)	3–6.4 (methimazole)/ Increased

METABOLISM

Carbimazole is rapidly metabolised to thiamazole, which is concentrated in the thyroid gland. Over 90% of orally administered carbimazole is excreted in the urine as thiamazole or its metabolites. The remainder appears in faeces. There is 10% enterohepatic circulation. Thiamazole is metabolised, probably by the liver, and excreted in the urine. Less than 12% of a dose of thiamazole may be excreted as unchanged drug.

DOSE IN RENAL IMPAIRMENT GFR (mL/MIN)

20–50	Dose as in normal renal function.
10–20	Dose as in normal renal function.
<10	Dose as in normal renal function.

DOSE IN PATIENTS UNDERGOING RENAL REPLACEMENT THERAPIES

CAPD	Not dialysed. Dose as in normal renal function.
HD	Not dialysed. Dose as in normal renal function.
HDF/High flux	Unknown dialysability. Dose as in normal renal function.
CAV/ VVHD	Unknown dialysability. Dose as in normal renal function.

IMPORTANT DRUG INTERACTIONS

Potentially hazardous interactions with other drugs
- None known

ADMINISTRATION

RECONSTITUTION
–
ROUTE
- Oral
RATE OF ADMINISTRATION
–
COMMENTS
–

OTHER INFORMATION

- There have been reports of glomerulonephritis associated with the development of antineutrophil cytoplasmic antibodies in patients receiving thiourea anti-thyroid drugs.

Carboplatin

CLINICAL USE

Antineoplastic platinum agent:
- Ovarian carcinoma of epithelial origin
- Small cell carcinoma of the lung

DOSE IN NORMAL RENAL FUNCTION

$400\,mg/m^2$
Or dose = Target AUC × [GFR (mL/min) + 25]
where AUC is commonly 5 or 7 depending
on protocol used (Calvert equation)

PHARMACOKINETICS

Molecular weight (daltons)	371.2
% Protein binding	29–89
% Excreted unchanged in urine	32–70
Volume of distribution (L/kg)	0.23–0.28
Half-life – normal/ESRF (hrs)	1.5–6/Increased

METABOLISM

There is little, if any, true metabolism of
carboplatin. Excretion is primarily by
glomerular filtration in the urine, with 70% of
the drug excreted within 24 hours, most of it
in the first 6 hours. Approximately 32% of the
dose is excreted unchanged.

Platinum from carboplatin slowly becomes
protein bound, and is subsequently excreted
with a terminal half-life of 5 days or more.

DOSE IN RENAL IMPAIRMENT GFR (mL/MIN)

20–50	Dose as in normal renal function. See 'Other information'.
10–20	Dose as in normal renal function. See 'Other information'.
<10	Dose as in normal renal function. See 'Other information'.

DOSE IN PATIENTS UNDERGOING RENAL REPLACEMENT THERAPIES

CAPD	Unknown dialysability. Dose as in GFR<10 mL/min.
HD	Dialysed. Dose as in GFR<10 mL/min.
HDF/High flux	Dialysed. Dose as in GFR<10 mL/min.
CAV/ VVHD	Unknown dialysability. Dose as in GFR=10–20 mL/min.

IMPORTANT DRUG INTERACTIONS

Potentially hazardous interactions with other
drugs
- Aminoglycosides: increased risk of
  nephrotoxicity and possibly ototoxicity
  with aminoglycosides, capreomycin,
  polymyxins or vancomycin.
- Antipsychotics: avoid concomitant
  use with clozapine, increased risk of
  agranulocytosis.

ADMINISTRATION

RECONSTITUTION
–
ROUTE
- IV
RATE OF ADMINISTRATION
- IV infusion over 15–60 minutes.
COMMENTS
- Therapy should not be repeated until
  4 weeks after the previous carboplatin
  course.
- May be diluted with glucose 5%, or sodium
  chloride 0.9% to concentrations as low as
  0.5 mg/mL.

OTHER INFORMATION

- Patients with abnormal kidney function
  or receiving concomitant therapy with
  nephrotoxic drugs are likely to experience
  more severe and prolonged myelotoxicity.
- Blood counts and renal function should be
  monitored closely.
- Contraindicated by manufacturer if
  GFR<20 mL/min.
- *Drug Prescribing in Renal Failure*, 5th
  edition, by Aronoff *et al.* recommend 50%
  of dose if GFR=10–50 mL/min and 25% of
  dose if GFR<10 mL/min.
- Some units still use a dose in normal renal
  function of $400\,mg/m^2$. In this instance, the
  dose should be reduced to 50% of normal
  dose for a GFR of 10–20 mL/min, and to
  25% of normal dose for a GFR<10 mL/min.

Carmustine

CLINICAL USE

Alkylating agent:
- Myeloma, lymphoma and brain tumours

DOSE IN NORMAL RENAL FUNCTION

150–200 mg/m^2 as a single dose or
75–100 mg/m^2 on 2 consecutive days every
6 weeks
Implants: 7.7 mg, maximum 8 implants

PHARMACOKINETICS

Molecular weight (daltons)	214.1
% Protein binding	77
% Excreted unchanged in urine	77
Volume of distribution (L/kg)	3.25
Half-life – normal/ ESRF (hrs)	22 minutes/–

METABOLISM

Intravenous carmustine is rapidly
metabolised, and no intact drug is detectable
after 15 minutes. It is partially metabolised
to active metabolites by liver microsomal
enzymes, which have a long half-life. It is
thought that the antineoplastic activity may
be due to metabolites. Approximately 30% of
a dose is excreted in the urine after 24 hours,
and 60–70% of the total dose after 96 hours.
About 10% is excreted as respiratory CO_2.
Terminal half-life of the metabolites is about
1 hour.

DOSE IN RENAL IMPAIRMENT GFR (mL/MIN)

45–60	Implant: Dose as in normal renal function. IV: 80% of dose.[1]
30–45	Implant: Dose as in normal renal function. IV: 75% of dose.[1]
<30	Implant: Dose as in normal renal function. IV: Avoid.[1]

DOSE IN PATIENTS UNDERGOING RENAL REPLACEMENT THERAPIES

CAPD	Not dialysed. Dose as in GFR<30 mL/min.
HD	Not dialysed. Dose as in GFR<30 mL/min. See 'Other information'.
HDF/High flux	Unknown dialysability. Dose as in GFR<30 mL/min. See 'Other information'.
CAV/ VVHD	Not dialysed. Dose as in GFR=30–45 mL/min.

IMPORTANT DRUG INTERACTIONS

Potentially hazardous interactions with other
drugs
- Antipsychotics: avoid concomitant use with clozapine (increased risk of agranulocytosis).

ADMINISTRATION

RECONSTITUTION
- 3 mL of the supplied diluent (absolute ethanol) then add 27 mL of sterile water for injection.

ROUTE
- IV

RATE OF ADMINISTRATION
- Administer by IV drip over a period of 1–2 hours.

COMMENTS
- Therapy should not be repeated before 6 weeks.
- Can further dilute the reconstituted solution with 500 mL of sodium chloride 0.9% or glucose 5%.

OTHER INFORMATION

- Renal abnormalities, e.g. a decrease in kidney size: progressive azotaemia and renal failure have been reported in patients receiving large cumulative doses after prolonged therapy.
- Carmustine has been used at normal dose in a haemodialysis patient without any problems.[2]

References:
1. Kintzel PE, Dorr RT. Anticancer drug renal toxicity and elimination: dosing guidelines for altered renal function. *Cancer Treat Rev.* 1995; **21**: 33–64.
2. Boesler B, Czock D, Keller F, *et al.* Clinical course of haemodialysis patients with malignancies and dose-adjusted chemotherapy. *Nephrol Dial Transplant.* 2005; **20**: 1187–91.

Carvedilol

CLINICAL USE

Beta-adrenoceptor blocker with alpha$_1$-blocking action:
- Hypertension
- Angina
- Heart failure

DOSE IN NORMAL RENAL FUNCTION

- Hypertension: 12.5–50 mg daily in single or divided doses
- Angina: 12.5–25 mg twice daily
- Heart failure: 3.125–25 mg twice daily (50 mg twice daily if wt>85 kg)

PHARMACOKINETICS

Molecular weight (daltons)	406.5
% Protein binding	>98
% Excreted unchanged in urine	<2
Volume of distribution (L/kg)	2
Half-life – normal/ ESRF (hrs)	6–10/Unchanged

METABOLISM

Carvedilol is subject to considerable first-pass metabolism in the liver; the absolute bioavailability is about 25%. It is extensively metabolised in the liver, primarily by the cytochrome P450 isoenzymes CYP2D6 and CYP2C9, and the metabolites are excreted mainly in the bile.

DOSE IN RENAL IMPAIRMENT GFR (mL/MIN)

20–50	Dose as in normal renal function.
10–20	Dose as in normal renal function.
<10	Dose as in normal renal function.

DOSE IN PATIENTS UNDERGOING RENAL REPLACEMENT THERAPIES

CAPD	Unlikely dialysability. Dose as in normal renal function. Start with low doses and titrate according to response.
HD	Not dialysed. Dose as in normal renal function. Start with low doses and titrate according to response.
HDF/High flux	Unknown dialysability. Dose as in normal renal function. Start with low doses and titrate according to response.
CAV/VVHD	Unlikely dialysability. Dose as in normal renal function. Start with low doses and titrate according to response.

IMPORTANT DRUG INTERACTIONS

Potentially hazardous interactions with other drugs
- Anaesthetics: enhanced hypotensive effect.
- Analgesics: NSAIDs antagonise hypotensive effect.
- Anti-arrhythmics: increased risk of myocardial depression and bradycardia; increased risk of bradycardia, myocardial depression and AV block with amiodarone; increased risk of myocardial depression and bradycardia with flecainide.
- Antibacterials: concentration reduced by rifampicin.
- Antidepressants: enhanced hypotensive effect with MAOIs.
- Antihypertensives; enhanced hypotensive effect; increased risk of withdrawal hypertension with clonidine; increased risk of first dose hypotensive effect with post-synaptic alpha-blockers such as prazosin.
- Antimalarials: increased risk of bradycardia with mefloquine.
- Antipsychotics enhanced hypotensive effect with phenothiazines.
- Calcium-channel blockers: increased risk of bradycardia and AV block with diltiazem; hypotension and heart failure possible with nifedipine and nisoldipine; asystole, severe hypotension and heart failure with verapamil.
- Ciclosporin: increased trough concentration, reduce dose by 20% in affected patients.
- Cytotoxics: possible increased risk of bradycardia with crizotinib.
- Diuretics: enhanced hypotensive effect.
- Fingolimod: possibly increased risk of bradycardia.
- Moxisylyte: possible severe postural hypotension.
- Sympathomimetics: severe hypertension with adrenaline and noradrenaline and possibly with dobutamine.

ADMINISTRATION

RECONSTITUTION
–

ROUTE
● Oral

RATE OF ADMINISTRATION
–

COMMENTS
–

Caspofungin

CLINICAL USE

- Invasive aspergillosis in adult patients who are refractory to or intolerant of amphotericin B and/or itraconazole
- Invasive candidiasis
- Empirical treatment of systemic fungal infections in patients with neutropenia.

DOSE IN NORMAL RENAL FUNCTION

70 mg loading dose on day 1 followed by 50 mg daily, thereafter.
If patient weighs >80 kg use 70 mg daily

PHARMACOKINETICS

Molecular weight (daltons)	1213.4 (as acetate)
% Protein binding	97
% Excreted unchanged in urine	1.4
Volume of distribution (L/kg)	No data
Half-life – normal/ ESRF (hrs)	12–15 days/Increased but not significantly. See 'Other information'.

METABOLISM

Plasma concentrations of caspofungin decline in a polyphasic manner after intravenous infusion. The initial short α-phase occurs immediately post-infusion and is followed by a β-phase with a half-life of 9 to 11 hours; an additional longer γ-phase also occurs with a half-life of 40 to 50 hours. Plasma clearance is dependent on distribution rather than on biotransformation or excretion. Caspofungin undergoes spontaneous degradation to an open ring compound. There is further slow metabolism of caspofungin by hydrolysis and N-acetylation and excretion in faeces and urine.

DOSE IN RENAL IMPAIRMENT GFR (mL/MIN)

20–50	Dose as in normal renal function.
10–20	Dose as in normal renal function.
<10	Dose as in normal renal function.

DOSE IN PATIENTS UNDERGOING RENAL REPLACEMENT THERAPIES

CAPD	Not dialysed. Dose as in normal renal function.
HD	Not dialysed. Dose as in normal renal function.
HDF/High flux	Unlikely to be dialysed. Dose as in normal renal function.
CAV/ VVHD	Not dialysed. Dose as in normal renal function.

IMPORTANT DRUG INTERACTIONS

Potentially hazardous interactions with other drugs
- Ciclosporin: monitor liver enzymes as transient increases in ALT and AST have been reported with concomitant administration. Avoid co-administration if possible. Increases AUC of caspofungin by 35%.
- Tacrolimus: reduces tacrolimus trough concentration by 26%.

ADMINISTRATION

RECONSTITUTION
- 10.5 mL water for injection
ROUTE
- IV infusion
RATE OF ADMINISTRATION
- Approximately 1 hour
COMMENTS
- Caspofungin is unstable in fluids containing glucose; add to 250 mL sodium chloride 0.9% or lactated Ringer's solution.
- If patient is fluid restricted, doses of 35 or 50 mg may be added to 100 mL infusion fluid.

OTHER INFORMATION

- In established renal failure the AUC is increased by 30–49% but a change in dosage schedule is not required.
- Caspofungin has been used at a dose of 50 mg daily in combination with IV amphotericin B to successfully treat fungal peritonitis in 1 case study; the catheter was removed. (Fourtounas C, Marangos M, Kalliakmani P, et al. Treatment of peritoneal dialysis related fungal peritonitis with caspofungin plus amphotericin B combination therapy. Nephrol Dial Transplant. 2006; 21: 236.)

Cefaclor

CLINICAL USE

Antibacterial agent

DOSE IN NORMAL RENAL FUNCTION

250 mg every 8 hours (dose may be doubled for more severe infections – maximum 4 g daily)

PHARMACOKINETICS

Molecular weight (daltons)	385.8
% Protein binding	25
% Excreted unchanged in urine	60–85
Volume of distribution (L/kg)	0.24–0.35
Half-life – normal/ ESRF (hrs)	0.5–0.9/2.3–2.8

METABOLISM

Cefaclor is rapidly excreted by the kidneys; up to 85% of a dose appears unchanged in the urine within 8 hours, the greater part within 2 hours. Probenecid delays excretion.

DOSE IN RENAL IMPAIRMENT GFR (mL/MIN)

20–50	Dose as in normal renal function.
10–20	Dose as in normal renal function.
<10	Dose as in normal renal function.

DOSE IN PATIENTS UNDERGOING RENAL REPLACEMENT THERAPIES

CAPD	Dialysed. 250–500 mg every 8 hours.
HD	Dialysed. 250–500 mg every 6–8 hours.
HDF/High flux	Dialysed. 250–500 mg every 6–8 hours.
CAV/ VVHD	Dialysed. Dose as in normal renal function.

IMPORTANT DRUG INTERACTIONS

Potentially hazardous interactions with other drugs

● Anticoagulants: effects of coumarins may be enhanced.

ADMINISTRATION

RECONSTITUTION
–
ROUTE
● Oral
RATE OF ADMINISTRATION
–
COMMENTS
–

OTHER INFORMATION

● Cefaclor is associated with protracted skin reactions.

Cefadroxil

CLINICAL USE

Antibacterial agent

DOSE IN NORMAL RENAL FUNCTION

500 mg – 1 g every 12–24 hours

PHARMACOKINETICS

Molecular weight (daltons)	381.4
% Protein binding	20
% Excreted unchanged in urine	>90
Volume of distribution (L/kg)	0.31
Half-life – normal/ ESRF (hrs)	1.3–2/22

METABOLISM

More than 90% of a dose of cefadroxil may be excreted unchanged in the urine within 24 hours by glomerular filtration and tubular secretion.

DOSE IN RENAL IMPAIRMENT GFR (mL/MIN)

25–50	1 g stat then 500–1000 mg every 12 hours.
10–25	1 g stat then 500–1000 mg every 24 hours.
<10	1 g stat then 500–1000 mg every 36 hours.

DOSE IN PATIENTS UNDERGOING RENAL REPLACEMENT THERAPIES

CAPD	Not dialysed. Dose as in GFR<10 mL/min.
HD	Dialysed. Dose as in GFR<10 mL/ min.
HDF/High flux	Dialysed. Dose as in GFR<10 mL/ min.
CAV/ VVHD	Unknown dialysability. Dose as in GFR=10–25 mL/min.

IMPORTANT DRUG INTERACTIONS

Potentially hazardous interactions with other drugs
- Anticoagulants: effects of coumarins may be enhanced.

ADMINISTRATION

RECONSTITUTION
–
ROUTE
- Oral
RATE OF ADMINISTRATION
–
COMMENTS
–

OTHER INFORMATION

- 63% of a 1 g dose is removed after 6–8 hours of haemodialysis.

Cefalexin

CLINICAL USE

Antibacterial agent

DOSE IN NORMAL RENAL FUNCTION

250 mg every 6 hours or 500 mg every
8–12 hours; maximum 6 g daily.
Recurrent UTI prophylaxis: 125 mg at night

PHARMACOKINETICS

Molecular weight (daltons)	365.4
% Protein binding	15
% Excreted unchanged in urine	80–90
Volume of distribution (L/kg)	0.35
Half-life – normal/ ESRF (hrs)	1/16

METABOLISM

Cefalexin is not metabolised. About 80%
or more of a dose is excreted unchanged in
the urine in the first 6 hours by glomerular
filtration and tubular secretion. Probenecid
delays urinary excretion. Therapeutically
effective concentrations may be found in the
bile and some may be excreted by this route.

DOSE IN RENAL IMPAIRMENT GFR (mL/MIN)

20–50	Dose as in normal renal function.
10–20	250–500 mg every 8–12 hours.[1,2]
<10	250–500 mg every 8–12 hours.[2]

DOSE IN PATIENTS UNDERGOING RENAL REPLACEMENT THERAPIES

CAPD	Dialysed. Dose as in GFR<10 mL/min.
HD	Dialysed. Dose as in GFR<10 mL/min.
HDF/High flux	Dialysed. Dose as in GFR<10 mL/min.
CAV/ VVHD	Dialysed. Dose as in GFR=10–20 mL/min.

IMPORTANT DRUG INTERACTIONS

Potentially hazardous interactions with other
drugs
- Anticoagulants: effects of coumarins may
  be enhanced.

ADMINISTRATION

RECONSTITUTION
–

ROUTE
- Oral

RATE OF ADMINISTRATION
–

COMMENTS
–

OTHER INFORMATION

- Use dose for normal renal function to treat
  urinary tract infection in ERF.
- High doses, together with the
  use of nephrotoxic drugs such as
  aminoglycosides or potent diuretics, may
  adversely affect renal function.

References:
1. Vaziri S. *Guidelines for Prescribing Drugs
in Adults with Impaired Renal Function.*
Renal dosing protocols. Detroit VA Medical
Centre.
2. www.uphs.upenn.edu/bugdrug/antibiotic_
manual/renal.htm.

Cefixime

Antibacterial agent

DOSE IN NORMAL RENAL FUNCTION

200–400 mg/day (given as a single dose or in 2 divided doses).

PHARMACOKINETICS

Molecular weight (daltons)	507.5
% Protein binding	65
% Excreted unchanged in urine	20 (50% of absorbed dose)
Volume of distribution (L/kg)	0.11–0.6
Half-life – normal/ ESRF (hrs)	3–4/11.5

METABOLISM

About 20% of an oral dose (or 50% of an absorbed dose) is excreted unchanged in the urine via glomerular filtration within 24 hours. Up to 60% may be eliminated by non-renal mechanisms; there is no evidence of metabolism but some drug is probably excreted into the faeces from bile.

DOSE IN RENAL IMPAIRMENT GFR (mL/MIN)

20–50	Dose as in normal renal function.
10–20	Dose as in normal renal function.[1]
<10	200 mg/day

DOSE IN PATIENTS UNDERGOING RENAL REPLACEMENT THERAPIES

CAPD	Not dialysed. Dose as in GFR<10 mL/min.
HD	Not dialysed. Dose as in GFR<10 mL/min.
HDF/High flux	Unknown dialysability. Dose as in GFR<10 mL/min.
CAV/ VVHD	Dialysed. Dose as in normal renal function.

IMPORTANT DRUG INTERACTIONS

Potentially hazardous interactions with other drugs
- Anticoagulants: effects of coumarins may be enhanced.

ADMINISTRATION

RECONSTITUTION
–
ROUTE
- Oral
RATE OF ADMINISTRATION
–
COMMENTS
–

OTHER INFORMATION

- Manufacturer recommends that patients with a GFR<20 mL/min or having regular APD or HD should not have a dose greater than 200 mg/day.

Reference:
1. Fillastre JP, Singlas E. Pharmacokinetics of newer drugs in patients with renal impairment (part I). *Clin Pharmacokinet.* 1991, **20**(4): 293–310.

Cefotaxime

CLINICAL USE

Antibacterial agent

DOSE IN NORMAL RENAL FUNCTION

- Mild infection: 1 g every 12 hours
- Moderate infection: 1 g every 8 hours
- Severe infection: 2 g every 6 hours
- Life-threatening infection: up to 12 g daily in 3–4 divided doses.

PHARMACOKINETICS

Molecular weight (daltons)	477.4 (as sodium salt)
% Protein binding	40
% Excreted unchanged in urine	40–60
Volume of distribution (L/kg)	0.15–0.55
Half-life – normal/ ESRF (hrs)	0.9–1.14/2.5 (10 hours for the metabolite)

METABOLISM

After partial metabolism in the liver to desacetyl-cefotaxime and inactive metabolites, elimination is mainly by the kidneys and about 40–60% of a dose has been recovered unchanged in the urine within 24 hours; a further 20% is excreted as the desacetyl metabolite. Relatively high concentrations of cefotaxime and desacetyl-cefotaxime occur in bile and about 20% of a dose has been recovered in the faeces.

Probenecid competes for renal tubular secretion with cefotaxime resulting in higher and prolonged plasma concentrations of cefotaxime and its desacetyl metabolite.

DOSE IN RENAL IMPAIRMENT GFR (mL/MIN)

20–50	Dose as in normal renal function.
5–20	Dose as in normal renal function.
<5	Reduce dose by 50% and keep frequency the same.

DOSE IN PATIENTS UNDERGOING RENAL REPLACEMENT THERAPIES

CAPD	Not dialysed. Dose as in GFR<5 mL/min.
HD	Dialysed. Dose as in GFR<5 mL/min.
HDF/High flux	Dialysed. Dose as in GFR<5 mL/min.
CAV/ VVHD	Dialysed. 1–2 g every 12 hours.[1]
CVVHD/ HDF	Dialysed. 2 g every 12 hours.[1]

IMPORTANT DRUG INTERACTIONS

Potentially hazardous interactions with other drugs
- Anticoagulants: effects of coumarins may be enhanced.

ADMINISTRATION

RECONSTITUTION
- IV Bolus/IM: 4 mL water for injection to 1 g
- IV Infusion: 1 g in 50 mL sodium chloride 0.9%

ROUTE
- IV, IM

RATE OF ADMINISTRATION
- Bolus over 3–4 minutes; infusion over 20–60 minutes

OTHER INFORMATION

- 1 g contains 2.09 mmol sodium.
- Reduce dose further if concurrent hepatic and renal failure.

Reference:
1. Trotman RL, Williamson JC, Shoemaker DM, *et al.* Antibiotic dosing in critically ill adult patients receiving continuous renal replacement therapy. *Clin Infect Dis.* 2005 Oct 15; **41**: 1159–66.

Cefpodoxime

Antibacterial agent

DOSE IN NORMAL RENAL FUNCTION

100–200 mg every 12 hours

PHARMACOKINETICS

Molecular weight (daltons)	557.6 (as proxetil)
% Protein binding	20–40
% Excreted unchanged in urine	80
Volume of distribution (L/kg)	0.6–1.2
Half-life – normal/ ESRF (hrs)	2.4/26

METABOLISM

Cefpodoxime proxetil is taken up in the intestine and is hydrolysed to the active metabolite cefpodoxime. It is excreted unchanged in the urine.

DOSE IN RENAL IMPAIRMENT GFR (mL/MIN)

30–50	Dose as in normal renal function.
10–30	100–200 mg every 24 hours.[1]
<10	100–200 mg every 24 hours.[1]

DOSE IN PATIENTS UNDERGOING RENAL REPLACEMENT THERAPIES

CAPD	Not dialysed. Dose as in GFR<10 mL/min.
HD	Dialysed. Dose as in GFR<10 mL/min.
HDF/High flux	Dialysed. Dose as in GFR<10 mL/min.
CAV/ VVHD	Dialysed. Dose as in GFR=10–30 mL/min.

IMPORTANT DRUG INTERACTIONS

Potentially hazardous interactions with other drugs

- Anticoagulants: effects of coumarins may be enhanced.

ADMINISTRATION

RECONSTITUTION

–

ROUTE

- Oral

RATE OF ADMINISTRATION

–

COMMENTS

- Take with food.
- Antacids and H_2-blockers should be taken 2–3 hours after administration of cefpodoxime.

OTHER INFORMATION

Reference:
1. www.thedrugmonitor.com/rdosing.html

Cefradine

CLINICAL USE

Antibacterial agent

DOSE IN NORMAL RENAL FUNCTION

- Oral: 250–500 mg every 6 hours (or 500 mg – 1 g every 12 hours)
- Severe infections: 1 g every 6 hours

PHARMACOKINETICS

Molecular weight (daltons)	349.4
% Protein binding	8–12
% Excreted unchanged in urine	>90
Volume of distribution (L/kg)	0.25–0.46
Half-life – normal/ ESRF (hrs)	1/6–15

METABOLISM

Cefradine is excreted unchanged in the urine by glomerular filtration and tubular secretion, over 90% of an oral dose or 60–80% of an intramuscular dose being recovered within 6 hours. Probenecid delays excretion.

DOSE IN RENAL IMPAIRMENT GFR (mL/MIN)

20–50	Dose as in normal renal function.
10–20	Dose as in normal renal function.
<10	250–500 mg every 6 hours.

DOSE IN PATIENTS UNDERGOING RENAL REPLACEMENT THERAPIES

CAPD	Dialysed. Dose as in GFR<10 mL/ min.
HD	Dialysed. Dose as in GFR<10 mL/ min.
HDF/High flux	Dialysed. Dose as in GFR<10 mL/ min.
CAV/ VVHD	Dialysed. Dose as in normal renal function.

IMPORTANT DRUG INTERACTIONS

Potentially hazardous interactions with other drugs

- Anticoagulants: effects of coumarins may be enhanced.

ADMINISTRATION

RECONSTITUTION

–

ROUTE

- Oral

RATE OF ADMINISTRATION

–

COMMENTS

–

OTHER INFORMATION

- Dose in severe renal impairment estimated from evaluation of pharmacokinetics.

Ceftaroline

CLINICAL USE

Antibacterial agent

DOSE IN NORMAL RENAL FUNCTION

600 mg every 12 hours

PHARMACOKINETICS

Molecular weight (daltons)	762.75 (as fosamil)
% Protein binding	20
% Excreted unchanged in urine	88
Volume of distribution (L/kg)	20.3 litres
Half-life – normal/ ESRF (hrs)	2.5/Increased

METABOLISM

Ceftaroline fosamil (prodrug) is converted into the active ceftaroline in plasma by phosphatase enzymes. Hydrolysis of the beta-lactam ring of ceftaroline occurs to form the microbiologically inactive, open-ring metabolite, ceftaroline M-1.

Ceftaroline is mainly eliminated by the kidneys. Renal clearance is approximately equal to, or slightly lower than, the glomerular filtration rate in the kidney, and *in vitro* transporter studies indicate that active secretion does not contribute to the renal elimination of ceftaroline.

DOSE IN RENAL IMPAIRMENT GFR (mL/MIN)

30–50	400 mg every 12 hours.
15–30	300 mg every 12 hours.
<15	200 mg every 12 hours.

DOSE IN PATIENTS UNDERGOING RENAL REPLACEMENT THERAPIES

CAPD	Dialysed. Dose as in GFR<15 mL/min.
HD	Dialysed. Dose as in GFR<15 mL/min.
HDF/High flux	Dialysed. Dose as in GFR<15 mL/min.
CAV/ VVHD	Dialysed. Dose as in GFR=15–30 mL/min.

IMPORTANT DRUG INTERACTIONS

Potentially hazardous interactions with other drugs
- Anticoagulants: effects of coumarins may be enhanced.

ADMINISTRATION

RECONSTITUTION
- 20 mL water for injection

ROUTE
- IV infusion

RATE OF ADMINISTRATION
- Over 60 minutes

COMMENTS
- Normally added to 250 mL of infusion fluid but in cases of fluid restriction can be added to 50–100 mL.
- Can be added to sodium chloride 0.9%, glucose 5% or Lactated Ringer's solution.

OTHER INFORMATION

- Administer within 6 hours of preparation.
- Side effects are more likely in patients with renal impairment.
- Doses in severe renal impairment are taken from the American data sheet.

Ceftazidime

CLINICAL USE

Antibacterial agent

DOSE IN NORMAL RENAL FUNCTION

- 0.5–2 g every 8–12 hours
- Severe infections: 3 g every 12 hours
- Pseudomonal lung infections in cystic fibrosis: 100–150 mg/kg in 3 divided doses
- Surgical prophylaxis: 1 g at induction

PHARMACOKINETICS

Molecular weight (daltons)	637.7
% Protein binding	<10
% Excreted unchanged in urine	80–90
Volume of distribution (L/kg)	0.28–0.4
Half-life – normal/ ESRF (hrs)	2/13–25

METABOLISM

Ceftazidime is passively excreted in bile, although only a small proportion (1%) is eliminated by this route. It is mainly excreted by the kidneys, almost exclusively by glomerular filtration; probenecid has little effect on the excretion. About 80–90% of a dose appears unchanged in the urine within 24 hours.

DOSE IN RENAL IMPAIRMENT GFR (mL/MIN)

31–50	1–2 g every 12 hours
16–30	1–2 g every 24 hours
6–15	500 mg – 1 g every 24 hours
<5	500 mg – 1 g every 48 hours

DOSE IN PATIENTS UNDERGOING RENAL REPLACEMENT THERAPIES

CAPD	Dialysed. 500 mg – 1 g every 24 hours.
HD	Dialysed. 500 mg – 1 g every every 48 hours or post dialysis.
HDF/High flux	Dialysed. 500 mg – 2 g every 48 hours or post dialysis.
CAV/ VVHD	Dialysed. 2 g every 8 hours[1] or 1–2 g every 12 hours.[1,2,3]
CVVHD/ HDF	Dialysed. 2 g every 12 hours.[3]

IMPORTANT DRUG INTERACTIONS

Potentially hazardous interactions with other drugs
- Anticoagulants: effects of coumarins may be enhanced.
- Ciclosporin: may cause increased ciclosporin levels.

ADMINISTRATION

RECONSTITUTION
- Water for injection:
  - 1.5 mL to 500 mg vial for IM administration
  - 5 mL to 500 mg vial for IV injection
  - 3 mL to 1 g vial for IM administration
  - 10 mL to 1 g vial for IV injection

ROUTE
- IV/IM rarely

RATE OF ADMINISTRATION
- Bolus: 3–4 minutes
- Infusion: over 30 minutes

COMMENTS
- May be given IP in CAPD fluid 125–250 mg/2L.
- Reconstituted solutions vary in colour, but this is quite normal.
- Compatible with most IV fluids, e.g. sodium chloride 0.9%, glucose-saline, glucose 5%.

OTHER INFORMATION

- Volume of distribution increases with infection.
- In exceptional circumstances, patients on haemodialysis may be given a dose of 2 g, 3 times a week post HD.

References:
1. Traunmüller F, Schenk P, Mittermeyer C, et al. Clearance of ceftazidime during continuous veno-venous haemofiltration in critically ill patients. J Antimicrob Chemother. 2002; 49: 129–34. (Assumes that polysulphone membranes are used.)
2. CVVH Initial Drug Dosing Guidelines on www.thedrugmonitor.com.
3. Trotman RL, Williamson JC, Shoemaker DM, et al. Antibiotic dosing in critically ill adult patients receiving continuous renal replacement therapy. Clin Infect Dis. 2005 Oct 15; 41: 1159–66.

Ceftriaxone

CLINICAL USE

Antibacterial agent

DOSE IN NORMAL RENAL FUNCTION

1 g daily (severe infections: 2–4 g daily)
Gonorrhoea: single dose 250 mg IM

PHARMACOKINETICS

Molecular weight (daltons)	661.6 (as sodium salt)
% Protein binding	85–95
% Excreted unchanged in urine	40–60
Volume of distribution (L/kg)	0.12–0.18
Half-life – normal/ ESRF (hrs)	6–9/14.7

METABOLISM

About 40–65% of a dose of ceftriaxone is
excreted unchanged in the urine, principally
by glomerular filtration; the remainder
is excreted in the bile and is ultimately
found in the faeces as unchanged drug and
microbiologically inactive compounds.

DOSE IN RENAL IMPAIRMENT GFR (mL/MIN)

20–50	Dose as in normal renal function.
10–20	Dose as in normal renal function.
<10	Dose as in normal renal function. Maximum 2 g daily.

DOSE IN PATIENTS UNDERGOING RENAL REPLACEMENT THERAPIES

CAPD	Not dialysed. Dose as in GFR<10 mL/min.
HD	Not dialysed. Dose as in GFR<10 mL/min.
HDF/High flux	Unknown dialysability. Dose as in GFR<10 mL/min.
CAV/ VVHD	Unknown dialysability. 2 g every 12–24 hours.[1]
CVVHD/ HDF	Likely dialysability. 2 g every 12–24 hours.[1]

IMPORTANT DRUG INTERACTIONS

Potentially hazardous interactions with other
drugs
- Anticoagulants: effects of coumarins may
  be enhanced.
- Ciclosporin: may cause increased
  ciclosporin levels.

ADMINISTRATION

RECONSTITUTION
- 250 mg: IV – 5 mL water for injection; IM
  – 1 mL 1% lidocaine hydrochloride.
- 1 g: IV – 10 mL water for injection; IM –
  3.5 mL 1% lidocaine hydrochloride.
- Infusion: 2 g in 40 mL of calcium-free
  solution, e.g. sodium chloride 0.9%,
  glucose 5%.
- Incompatible with calcium containing
  solutions, e.g. Hartmann's, Ringer's.
ROUTE
- IV, IM, SC
RATE OF ADMINISTRATION
- Bolus: over 2–4 minutes.
- Infusion: over at least 30 minutes.
COMMENTS
- For IM injection: doses greater than 1 g
  should be divided and injected at more
  than one site.

OTHER INFORMATION

- Calcium ceftriaxone has appeared as a
  precipitate in urine, or been mistaken as
  gallstones in patients receiving higher than
  recommended doses.
- Contains 3.6 mmol sodium per gram of
  ceftriaxone.
- Information from the company shows that
  the bioavailability of SC administration is
  equivalent to IV. The maximum amount
  able to be given in a single SC injection
  is 500 mg dissolved in 2 mL lidocaine 1%.
  Administration was said to be tolerable.

Reference:
1. Trotman RL, Williamson JC, Shoemaker
DM, *et al.* Antibiotic dosing in critically ill
adult patients receiving continuous renal
replacement therapy. *Clin Infect Dis.* 2005
Oct 15; **41**: 1159–66.

Cefuroxime (oral)

CLINICAL USE

Antibacterial agent

DOSE IN NORMAL RENAL FUNCTION

125–500 mg every 12 hours
Gonorrhoea: single dose of 1 g

PHARMACOKINETICS

Molecular weight (daltons)	510.5 (as axetil)
% Protein binding	50
% Excreted unchanged in urine	85–90
Volume of distribution (L/kg)	0.13–1.8
Half-life – normal/ ESRF (hrs)	1.2/17

METABOLISM

After oral administration cefuroxime axetil
is rapidly hydrolysed in the intestinal mucosa
and blood to release active cefuroxime.
Cefuroxime is excreted unchanged in the
urine, 50% by glomerular filtration and
50% by renal tubular secretion. Probenecid
competes for renal tubular secretion
with cefuroxime resulting in higher and
more prolonged plasma concentrations of
cefuroxime. Small amounts of cefuroxime are
excreted in bile.

DOSE IN RENAL IMPAIRMENT GFR (mL/MIN)

20–50	Dose as in normal renal function.
10–20	Dose as in normal renal function.
<10	Dose as in normal renal function.

DOSE IN PATIENTS UNDERGOING RENAL REPLACEMENT THERAPIES

CAPD	Dialysed. Dose as in normal renal function.
HD	Dialysed. Dose as in normal renal function.
HDF/High flux	Dialysed. Dose as in normal renal function.
CAV/ VVHD	Dialysed. Dose as in normal renal function.

IMPORTANT DRUG INTERACTIONS

Potentially hazardous interactions with other
drugs
- Anticoagulants: effects of coumarins may
  be enhanced.

ADMINISTRATION

RECONSTITUTION
–
ROUTE
- Oral
RATE OF ADMINISTRATION
–
COMMENTS
- Take with or after food

OTHER INFORMATION

- Doses in renal impairment are taken from
  Drug Prescribing in Renal Failure, 5th
  edition, by Aronoff *et al.*

Cefuroxime (parenteral)

CLINICAL USE

Antibacterial agent

DOSE IN NORMAL RENAL FUNCTION

750 mg – 1.5 g every 6–8 hours
Meningitis: 3 g every 8 hours

PHARMACOKINETICS

Molecular weight (daltons)	446.4 (as sodium salt)
% Protein binding	50
% Excreted unchanged in urine	85–90
Volume of distribution (L/kg)	0.13–1.8
Half-life – normal/ ESRF (hrs)	1.2/17

METABOLISM

Cefuroxime is excreted unchanged in the urine, 50% by glomerular filtration and 50% by renal tubular secretion. On injection, most of a dose of cefuroxime is excreted within 24 hours, the majority within 6 hours. Probenecid competes for renal tubular secretion with cefuroxime resulting in higher and more prolonged plasma concentrations of cefuroxime. Small amounts of cefuroxime are excreted in bile.

DOSE IN RENAL IMPAIRMENT GFR (mL/MIN)

20–50	Dose as in normal renal function.
10–20	750 mg – 1.5 g every 12 hours
<10	750 mg – 1.5 g every 24 hours

DOSE IN PATIENTS UNDERGOING RENAL REPLACEMENT THERAPIES

CAPD	Dialysed. Dose as in GFR<10 mL/min.
HD	Dialysed. Dose as in GFR<10 mL/min.
HDF/High flux	Dialysed. Dose as in GFR<10 mL/min.
CAV/VVHD	Dialysed. Dose as in GFR=10–20 mL/min.

IMPORTANT DRUG INTERACTIONS

Potentially hazardous interactions with other drugs
- Anticoagulants: effects of coumarins may be enhanced.

ADMINISTRATION

RECONSTITUTION
- IM: 1 mL of water for injection to each 250 mg
- IV bolus: 2 mL of water for injection to each 250 mg, but 15 mL of water for injection to 1.5 g
- IV infusion: 1.5 g in 50 mL of water for injection

ROUTE
- IM, IV

RATE OF ADMINISTRATION
- IV bolus: over 3–5 minutes
- IV infusion: over 30 minutes

COMMENTS
- Do not mix in syringe with aminoglycoside antibiotics.
- Injection may also be reconstituted with: sodium chloride 0.9%, glucose 5%, glucose saline, Hartmann's solution.
- Cefuroxime and metronidazole can be mixed (see manufacturer's guidelines).

OTHER INFORMATION

- At high doses, take care in patients receiving concurrent treatment with potent diuretics such as furosemide, or aminoglycosides, as combination can adversely affect renal function.
- Each 750 mg vial ≡ 1.8 mmol sodium.

Celecoxib

CLINICAL USE

Cox 2 inhibitor and analgesic

DOSE IN NORMAL RENAL FUNCTION

100–200 mg once or twice daily

PHARMACOKINETICS

Molecular weight (daltons)	381.4
% Protein binding	97
% Excreted unchanged in urine	<3
Volume of distribution (L/kg)	400 litres
Half-life – normal/ ESRF (hrs)	8–12/Unchanged

METABOLISM

Celecoxib is metabolised in the liver mainly by the cytochrome P450 isoenzyme CYP2C9, which shows genetic polymorphism; the three identified metabolites are inactive as inhibitors of cyclo-oxygenase-1 (COX-1) or COX-2 enzymes. It is eliminated mainly as metabolites in the faeces and urine; less than 3% is recovered as unchanged drug.

DOSE IN RENAL IMPAIRMENT GFR (mL/MIN)

30–50	Dose as in normal renal function. Use with caution.
10–30	Dose as in normal renal function, but avoid if possible.
<10	Dose as in normal renal function, but only use if on dialysis.

DOSE IN PATIENTS UNDERGOING RENAL REPLACEMENT THERAPIES

CAPD	Unlikely to be dialysed. Dose as in normal renal function. See 'Other information'.
HD	Unlikely to be dialysed. Dose as in normal renal function. See 'Other information'.
HDF/High flux	Unknown dialysability. Dose as in normal renal function. See 'Other information'.
CAV/ VVHD	Unknown dialysability. Dose as in GFR=10–20 mL/min.

IMPORTANT DRUG INTERACTIONS

Potentially hazardous interactions with other drugs

- ACE inhibitors and angiotensin-II antagonists: antagonism of hypotensive effect; increased risk of nephrotoxicity and hyperkalaemia.
- Analgesics: avoid concomitant use of 2 or more NSAIDs, including aspirin (increased side effects); avoid with ketorolac (increased risk of side effects and haemorrhage).
- Antibacterials: possibly increased risk of convulsions with quinolones; concentration reduced by rifampicin.
- Anticoagulants: effects of coumarins and phenindione enhanced; possibly increased risk of bleeding with heparins and dabigatran.
- Antidepressants: increased risk of bleeding with SSRIs and venlafaxine.
- Antidiabetic agents: effects of sulphonylureas enhanced.
- Anti-epileptics: possibly increased phenytoin concentration.
- Antifungals: if used with fluconazole, halve the dose of celecoxib.
- Antivirals: increased risk of haematological toxicity with zidovudine; concentration possibly increased by ritonavir.
- Ciclosporin: may potentiate nephrotoxicity.
- Cytotoxic agents: reduced excretion of methotrexate; increased risk of bleeding with erlotinib.
- Diuretics: increased risk of nephrotoxicity; antagonism of diuretic effect; hyperkalaemia with potassium-sparing diuretics.
- Lithium: excretion decreased.
- Pentoxifylline: possibly increased risk of bleeding.
- Tacrolimus: increased risk of nephrotoxicity.

ADMINISTRATION

RECONSTITUTION

–

ROUTE

- Oral

RATE OF ADMINISTRATION

–

COMMENTS

–

OTHER INFORMATION

- Clinical trials have shown renal effects similar to those observed with comparative NSAIDs. Monitor patient for deterioration in renal function and fluid retention.
- Inhibition of renal prostaglandin synthesis by NSAIDs may interfere with renal function, especially in the presence of existing renal disease. Avoid if possible; if not, check serum creatinine 48–72 hours after starting NSAID. If raised, discontinue NSAID therapy.
- Use normal doses in patients with ERF on dialysis if they do not pass any urine.
- Use with caution in renal transplant recipients – can reduce intrarenal autocoid synthesis.
- Celecoxib should be used with caution in uraemic patients predisposed to gastrointestinal bleeding or uraemic coagulopathies.
- Contraindicated in patients with ischaemic heart disease or cerebrovascular disease and class II–IV NYHA congestive heart failure.

Celiprolol hydrochloride

CLINICAL USE

Beta-adrenoceptor blocker:
- Mild to moderate hypertension

DOSE IN NORMAL RENAL FUNCTION

200–400 mg daily

PHARMACOKINETICS

Molecular weight (daltons)	416
% Protein binding	25
% Excreted unchanged in urine	12–18
Volume of distribution (L/kg)	4.5
Half-life – normal/ ESRF (hrs)	5–6/Unchanged

METABOLISM

Metabolism of celiprolol is minimal and it is mainly excreted unchanged in the urine (50%) and faeces (50%).

DOSE IN RENAL IMPAIRMENT GFR (mL/MIN)

20–50	Dose as in normal renal function.
10–20	Dose as in normal renal function.
<10	Start low – adjust according to response.

DOSE IN PATIENTS UNDERGOING RENAL REPLACEMENT THERAPIES

CAPD	Unknown dialysability. Dose as in GFR<10 mL/min.
HD	Unknown dialysability. Dose as in GFR<10 mL/min.
HDF/High flux	Unknown dialysability. Dose as in GFR<10 mL/min.
CAV/ VVHD	Unknown dialysability. Dose as in normal renal function.

IMPORTANT DRUG INTERACTIONS

Potentially hazardous interactions with other drugs
- Anaesthetics: enhanced hypotensive effect.
- Analgesics: NSAIDs antagonise hypotensive effect.
- Anti-arrhythmics: increased risk of myocardial depression and bradycardia; increased risk of bradycardia, myocardial depression and AV block with amiodarone; increased risk of myocardial depression and bradycardia with flecainide.
- Antidepressants: enhanced hypotensive effect with MAOIs.
- Antihypertensives; enhanced hypotensive effect; increased risk of withdrawal hypertension with clonidine; increased risk of first dose hypotensive effect with post-synaptic alpha-blockers such as prazosin.
- Antimalarials: increased risk of bradycardia with mefloquine.
- Antipsychotics: enhanced hypotensive effect with phenothiazines.
- Calcium-channel blockers: increased risk of bradycardia and AV block with diltiazem; hypotension and heart failure possible with nifedipine and nisoldipine; asystole, severe hypotension and heart failure with verapamil.
- Cytotoxics: possible increased risk of bradycardia with crizotinib.
- Diuretics: enhanced hypotensive effect.
- Fingolimod: possibly increased risk of bradycardia.
- Moxisylyte: possible severe postural hypotension.
- Sympathomimetics: severe hypertension with adrenaline and noradrenaline and possibly with dobutamine.

ADMINISTRATION

RECONSTITUTION

–

ROUTE
- Oral

RATE OF ADMINISTRATION

–

COMMENTS
- Take half to one hour before food.

Certolizumab pegol

CLINICAL USE

Tumour necrosis factor alpha inhibitor:
- Treatment of moderate to severe rheumatoid arthritis in combination with methotrexate
- Treatment of ankylosing spondylitis

DOSE IN NORMAL RENAL FUNCTION

200 mg in 2 separate injections at weeks 0, 2, and 4 then maintenance of 200 mg every 2 weeks

PHARMACOKINETICS

Molecular weight (daltons)	91 000
% Protein binding	No data
% Excreted unchanged in urine	Mainly FAB
Volume of distribution (L/kg)	8.01 litres
Half-life – normal/ ESRF (hrs)	14 days/–

METABOLISM

The Fab fragment comprises protein compounds and is expected to be degraded to peptides and amino acids by proteolysis. The de-conjugated PEG component is rapidly eliminated from plasma and is to an unknown extent excreted renally.

DOSE IN RENAL IMPAIRMENT GFR (mL/MIN)

20–50	Dose as in normal renal function.
10–20	Use with caution.
<10	Use with caution.

DOSE IN PATIENTS UNDERGOING RENAL REPLACEMENT THERAPIES

CAPD	Unlikely to be dialysed. Dose as in GFR<10 mL/min.
HD	Unlikely to be dialysed. Dose as in GFR<10 mL/min.
HDF/High flux	Unlikely to be dialysed. Dose as in GFR<10 mL/min.
CAV/ VVHD	Unlikely to be dialysed. Dose as in GFR=10–20 mL/min.

IMPORTANT DRUG INTERACTIONS

Potentially hazardous interactions with other drugs
- Live vaccines: avoid concomitant use.
- Anakinra & abatacept: avoid concomitant use.

ADMINISTRATION

RECONSTITUTION
–
ROUTE
- SC
RATE OF ADMINISTRATION
–
COMMENTS
- Suitable injection sites are the thigh and abdomen.

OTHER INFORMATION

- Manufacturer is unable to provide a dose in moderate to severe renal impairment due to lack of studies.
- Contraindicated in patients with severe infections and moderate to severe heart failure.
- Bioavailability is 76–88%.
- Clearance following subcutaneous dosing was estimated to be 21 mL/h in a rheumatoid arthritis population pharmacokinetic analysis, with an inter-subject variability of 30.8% and an inter-occasion variability of 22%. The presence of antibodies to certolizumab pegol resulted in an approximately 3-fold increase in clearance. Compared with a 70 kg person, clearance is 29% lower and 38% higher, respectively, in individual RA patients weighing 40 kg and 120 kg.

Cetirizine hydrochloride

CLINICAL USE

Antihistamine:
- Symptomatic relief of allergy such as hay fever, urticaria

DOSE IN NORMAL RENAL FUNCTION

10 mg daily

PHARMACOKINETICS

Molecular weight (daltons)	461.8
% Protein binding	93
% Excreted unchanged in urine	50–60
Volume of distribution (L/kg)	0.45
Half-life – normal/ ESRF (hrs)	8–10/20

METABOLISM

Cetirizine does not undergo extensive first pass metabolism. About two thirds of the dose is excreted unchanged in urine.

DOSE IN RENAL IMPAIRMENT GFR (mL/MIN)

20–50	Dose as in normal renal function.
10–20	Dose as in normal renal function.
<10	5–10 mg daily

DOSE IN PATIENTS UNDERGOING RENAL REPLACEMENT THERAPIES

CAPD	Unlikely dialysability. Dose as in GFR<10 mL/min.
HD	Not dialysed. Dose as in GFR<10 mL/min.
HDF/High flux	Not dialysed. Dose as in GFR<10 mL/min.
CAV/ VVHD	Unknown dialysability. Dose as in normal renal function.

IMPORTANT DRUG INTERACTIONS

Potentially hazardous interactions with other drugs
- Antivirals: concentration possibly increased by ritonavir.

ADMINISTRATION

RECONSTITUTION
–
ROUTE
- Oral
RATE OF ADMINISTRATION
–
COMMENTS
- Available as tablets and solution

OTHER INFORMATION

- Manufacturers recommend halving dose in renal impairment.
- Dose may be titrated up but may result in increased sedation.
- Less than 10% of a dose is removed by haemodialysis.

Cetuximab

CLINICAL USE

Monoclonal antibody:
- Treatment of EGFR-expressing metastatic colorectal cancer in combination with irinotecan after failure of irinotecan-including cytotoxic therapy
- Treatment of head and neck cancer

DOSE IN NORMAL RENAL FUNCTION

Initial dose 400 mg/m^2 then 250 mg/m^2 weekly.

PHARMACOKINETICS

Molecular weight (daltons)	152 000
% Protein binding	No data
% Excreted unchanged in urine	minimal
Volume of distribution (L/kg)	1.5–6.2 L/m^2
Half-life – normal/ ESRF (hrs)	70–100/Unchanged

METABOLISM

Several pathways have been described that may contribute to the metabolism of antibodies. All of these pathways involve the biodegradation of the antibody to smaller molecules, i.e. small peptides or amino acids.

DOSE IN RENAL IMPAIRMENT GFR (mL/MIN)

20–50	Dose as in normal renal function. Use with caution.
10–20	Dose as in normal renal function. Use with caution.
<10	Dose as in normal renal function. Use with caution.

DOSE IN PATIENTS UNDERGOING RENAL REPLACEMENT THERAPIES

CAPD	Not dialysed. Dose as in GFR<10 mL/min.
HD	Not dialysed. Dose as in GFR<10 mL/min. See 'Other information'.
HDF/High flux	Not dialysed. Dose as in GFR<10 mL/min.
CAV/ VVHD	Not dialysed. Dose as in GFR=10–20 mL/min.

IMPORTANT DRUG INTERACTIONS

Potentially hazardous interactions with other drugs
- None known

ADMINISTRATION

RECONSTITUTION
–
ROUTE
- IV infusion.

RATE OF ADMINISTRATION
- 1st dose: 120 minutes
- Further doses: 60 minutes
- Maximum infusion rate must not exceed 5 mL/min

COMMENTS
- Administer via a 0.2 micrometer in-line filter
- The filter may clog and need to be replaced during the infusion

OTHER INFORMATION

- Delayed hypersensitivity reactions may occur and patients should be warned to contact their doctor if this occurs.
- Premedication with an antihistamine is recommended.
- 2% of patients receiving cetuximab developed renal failure.
- Give irinotecan at least 1 hour after the end of cetuximab infusion.
- Manufacturer has no information in renal impairment.
- There have been some case studies using cetuximab in haemodialysis patients successfully at normal doses. (Thariat J, Azzopardi N, Peyrade F, *et al.* Cetuximab pharmacokinetics in end-stage kidney disease under hemodialysis. *J Clin Oncol.* 2008 Sep 1; **26**(25): 4223–4.)

Chloral hydrate

CLINICAL USE

Insomnia (short term use)

DOSE IN NORMAL RENAL FUNCTION

- Mixture: 5–20 mL at night
- Welldorm (707 mg): 1–2 tablets at night; maximum 2 g (5 tablets/day)
- Syrup: 15–45 mL at night

PHARMACOKINETICS

Molecular weight (daltons)	165.4
% Protein binding	70–80
% Excreted unchanged in urine	<1
Volume of distribution (L/kg)	0.6
Half-life – normal/ ESRF (hrs)	7–11/–

METABOLISM

Chloral hydrate is rapidly metabolised to trichloroethanol (the active metabolite) and trichloroacetic acid in the erythrocytes, liver, and other tissues. It is excreted partly in the urine as trichloroethanol and its glucuronide (urochloralic acid) and as trichloroacetic acid. Some is also excreted in the bile.

DOSE IN RENAL IMPAIRMENT GFR (mL/MIN)

20–50	Dose as in normal renal function.
10–20	1 tablet at night.
<10	Avoid

DOSE IN PATIENTS UNDERGOING RENAL REPLACEMENT THERAPIES

CAPD	Unknown dialysability. Avoid.
HD	Dialysed. Avoid.
HDF/High flux	Dialysed. Avoid.
CAV/ VVHD	Dialysed. Dose as in GFR=10–20 mL/min.

IMPORTANT DRUG INTERACTIONS

Potentially hazardous interactions with other drugs

- Anticoagulants: may transiently enhance effect of coumarins.
- Antipsychotics: enhanced sedative effects.
- Antivirals: concentration possibly increased by ritonavir.

ADMINISTRATION

RECONSTITUTION

–

ROUTE

- Oral

RATE OF ADMINISTRATION

–

COMMENTS

- Take with water (or milk) 15–30 minutes before bedtime.

OTHER INFORMATION

- Manufacturer advises to avoid in patients with marked hepatic or renal impairment, severe cardiac disease, marked gastritis and those susceptible to acute attacks of porphyria.
- Chloral hydrate followed by intravenous furosemide may result in sweating, hot flushes, and variable blood pressure including hypertension.

Chlorambucil

CLINICAL USE

Alkylating agent:
- Hodgkin's disease
- Non-Hodgkin's lymphoma (NHL)
- Chronic lymphocytic leukaemia (CLL)
- Waldenström's macroglobulinaemia (WM)

DOSE IN NORMAL RENAL FUNCTION

- Hodgkin's disease: 200 mcg/kg/day (4–8 weeks)
- NHL: 100–200 mcg/kg/day (4–8 weeks) then reduce dose or give intermittently
- CLL: initially 150 mcg/kg/day, then 4 weeks after 1st course ended 100 mcg/kg/day
- WM = initially 6–12 mg daily, then reduce to 2–8 mg daily

PHARMACOKINETICS

Molecular weight (daltons)	304.2
% Protein binding	99
% Excreted unchanged in urine	<1
Volume of distribution (L/kg)	0.86
Half-life – normal/ ESRF (hrs)	1.5/–

METABOLISM

Chlorambucil is extensively metabolised in the liver via the hepatic microsomal enzyme oxidation system, principally to phenylacetic acid mustard, which is pharmacologically active, and which also undergoes some spontaneous degradation to further derivatives. Chlorambucil is excreted in the urine, almost exclusively as metabolites with less than 1% unchanged.

DOSE IN RENAL IMPAIRMENT GFR (mL/MIN)

20–50	Dose as in normal renal function. See 'Other information'.
10–20	Dose as in normal renal function. See 'Other information'.
<10	Dose as in normal renal function. See 'Other information'.

DOSE IN PATIENTS UNDERGOING RENAL REPLACEMENT THERAPIES

CAPD	Not dialysed. Dose as in normal renal function.
HD	Not dialysed. Dose as in normal renal function.
HDF/High flux	Unknown dialysability. Dose as in normal renal function.
CAV/ VVHD	Not dialysed. Dose as in normal renal function.

IMPORTANT DRUG INTERACTIONS

Potentially hazardous interactions with other drugs
- Ciclosporin: ciclosporin concentration possibly reduced.
- Patients who receive phenylbutazone may require reduced doses of chlorambucil.

ADMINISTRATION

RECONSTITUTION
–
ROUTE
- Oral
RATE OF ADMINISTRATION
–
COMMENTS
–

OTHER INFORMATION

- Monitor patients with renal impairment closely as they are at increased risk of myelosuppression associated with azotaemia.
- Oral absorption slowed and decreased by 10–20% if ingested with food.

Chloramphenicol

CLINICAL USE

Antibacterial agent

DOSE IN NORMAL RENAL FUNCTION

Oral/IV: 12.5 mg/kg every 6 hours (maximum 100 mg/kg/day)

PHARMACOKINETICS

Molecular weight (daltons)	323.1
% Protein binding	60
% Excreted unchanged in urine	5–10
Volume of distribution (L/kg)	0.5–1
Half-life – normal/ ESRF (hrs)	1.5–4/Unchanged

METABOLISM

Chloramphenicol is excreted mainly in the urine but only 5–10% of an oral dose appears unchanged; the remainder is inactivated in the liver, mostly by conjugation with glucuronic acid to inactive metabolites. About 3% is excreted in the bile. However, most is reabsorbed and only about 1%, mainly in the inactive form, is excreted in the faeces.

DOSE IN RENAL IMPAIRMENT GFR (mL/MIN)

20–50	Dose as in normal renal function.
10–20	Dose as in normal renal function.
<10	Dose as in normal renal function.

DOSE IN PATIENTS UNDERGOING RENAL REPLACEMENT THERAPIES

CAPD	Not dialysed. Dose as in normal renal function.
HD	Dialysed. Dose as in normal renal function.
HDF/High flux	Dialysed. Dose as in normal renal function.
CAV/ VVHD	Not dialysed. Dose as in normal renal function.

IMPORTANT DRUG INTERACTIONS

Potentially hazardous interactions with other drugs
- Anticoagulants: effect of coumarins enhanced.
- Antidiabetics: effect of sulphonylureas enhanced.
- Anti-epileptics: metabolism accelerated by phenobarbital (reduced concentration of chloramphenicol); increased concentration of phenytoin (risk of toxicity).
- Antipsychotics: avoid concomitant use with clozapine (increased risk of agranulocytosis).
- Ciclosporin: possibly increases ciclosporin concentration.
- Clopidogrel: possibly reduces anti-platelet effect.
- Tacrolimus: possibly increases tacrolimus concentration.

ADMINISTRATION

RECONSTITUTION
- Kemicetine: 1 g vial – reconstitute with water for injection, sodium chloride 0.9% or glucose 5%.
- 1.7 mL = 400 mg/mL solution
- 3.2 mL = 250 mg/mL solution
- 4.2 mL = 200 mg/mL solution
ROUTE
- Oral, IV, IM (Kemicetine only).
RATE OF ADMINISTRATION
- over at least 1 minute
COMMENTS
–

OTHER INFORMATION

- Manufacturers recommend monitoring serum levels in patients with renal impairment – Micromedex therapeutic range 10–25 micrograms/mL.
- Levels should be taken 1 hour after IV administration, aim for 15–25 mg/L, trough <15 mg/L.
- Kemicetine 1 g vial = 3.14 mmol sodium.

Chlordiazepoxide hydrochloride

CLINICAL USE

- Anxiety (short term use)
- Alcohol withdrawal

DOSE IN NORMAL RENAL FUNCTION

- Anxiety: 30–100 mg daily in divided doses.
- Alcohol withdrawal: 10–50 mg 4 times a day, reducing gradually.

PHARMACOKINETICS

Molecular weight (daltons)	336.2
% Protein binding	96
% Excreted unchanged in urine	1–2
Volume of distribution (L/kg)	0.3–0.5
Half-life – normal/ ESRF (hrs)	6–30/Unchanged

METABOLISM

Chlordiazepoxide is extensively metabolised in the liver. The elimination half-life of chlordiazepoxide ranges from about 6 to 30 hours, but its main active metabolite desmethyldiazepam (nordazepam) has a half-life of several days. Other pharmacologically active metabolites of chlordiazepoxide include desmethylchlordiazepoxide, demoxepam, and oxazepam. Unchanged drug and metabolites are excreted in the urine, mainly as conjugated metabolites.

DOSE IN RENAL IMPAIRMENT GFR (mL/MIN)

20–50	Dose as in normal renal function.
10–20	Dose as in normal renal function.
<10	50% of normal dose.

DOSE IN PATIENTS UNDERGOING RENAL REPLACEMENT THERAPIES

CAPD	Unlikely to be dialysed. Dose as in GFR<10 mL/min.
HD	Not dialysed. Dose as in GFR<10 mL/min.
HDF/High flux	Unknown dialysability. Dose as in GFR<10 mL/min.
CAV/ VVHD	Unknown dialysability. Dose as in normal renal function.

IMPORTANT DRUG INTERACTIONS

Potentially hazardous interactions with other drugs
- Antibacterials: metabolism possibly increased by rifampicin.
- Antipsychotics: enhanced sedative effects.
- Antivirals: concentration possibly increased by ritonavir.
- Sodium oxybate: enhanced effects of sodium oxybate – avoid.
- Ulcer-healing drugs: metabolism inhibited by cimetidine.

ADMINISTRATION

RECONSTITUTION
–
ROUTE
- Oral
RATE OF ADMINISTRATION
–
COMMENTS
–

Chloroquine

CLINICAL USE

- Treatment and prophylaxis of malaria
- Discoid and systemic lupus erythematosus
- Rheumatoid arthritis

DOSE IN NORMAL RENAL FUNCTION

- Orally.
- Malaria treatment: 600 mg, followed by 300 mg 6–8 hours later, then 300 mg/day for 2 days.
- Malaria prophylaxis: 300 mg once a week on the same day each week (start 1 week before exposure to risk and continue until 4 weeks after leaving the malarial area).
- SLE: 150 mg daily.
- Rheumatoid arthritis: 150 mg daily; maximum 2.5 mg/kg.

PHARMACOKINETICS

Molecular weight (daltons)	319.9 (515.9 as phosphate), (436 as sulphate)
% Protein binding	50–70
% Excreted unchanged in urine	42–47
Volume of distribution (L/kg)	>100
Half-life – normal/ ESRF (hrs)	10–60 days/5–50 days

METABOLISM

Chloroquine is extensively metabolised in the liver, mainly to monodesethylchloroquine with smaller amounts of bisdesethylchloroquine (didesethylchloroquinine) and other metabolites being formed. Monodesethylchloroquine has been reported to have some activity against *Plasmodium falciparum*. Chloroquine and its metabolites are excreted in the urine, with about half of a dose appearing as unchanged drug and about 10% as the monodesethyl metabolite. Chloroquine may be detected in urine for several months.

DOSE IN RENAL IMPAIRMENT GFR (mL/MIN)

20–50	Dose as in normal renal function.
10–20	Dose as in normal renal function.
<10	50% of normal dose.

DOSE IN PATIENTS UNDERGOING RENAL REPLACEMENT THERAPIES

CAPD	Not dialysed. Dose as in GFR<10 mL/min.
HD	Not dialysed. Dose as in GFR<10 mL/min.
HDF/High flux	Unknown dialysability. Dose as in GFR<10 mL/min.
CAV/ VVHD	Not dialysed. Dose as in normal renal function.

IMPORTANT DRUG INTERACTIONS

Potentially hazardous interactions with other drugs

- Anti-arrhythmics: increased risk of ventricular arrhythmias with amiodarone – avoid concomitant use.
- Antibacterials: increased risk of ventricular arrhythmias with moxifloxacin – avoid concomitant use.
- Anti-epileptics: antagonism of anticonvulsant effect.
- Antimalarials: increased risk of convulsions with mefloquine; avoid concomitant use with artemether/ lumefantrine.
- Antipsychotics: increased risk of ventricular arrhythmias with droperidol – avoid.
- Ciclosporin: increases ciclosporin concentration – increased risk of toxicity.
- Digoxin: possibly increased concentration of digoxin.
- Lanthanum: absorption possibly reduced by lanthanum, give at least 2 hours apart.

ADMINISTRATION

RECONSTITUTION
–
ROUTE
- Oral, IV, IM/SC in rare cases
RATE OF ADMINISTRATION
- IV infusion: Administer dose of 10 mg/kg of chloroquine base in sodium chloride 0.9% by slow IV infusion over 8 hours followed by 3 further 8 hour infusions containing 5 mg base/kg (total dose 25 mg base/kg over 32 hours)
COMMENTS
- Oral: Do not take indigestion remedies at the same time of day as this medicine.
- Chloroquine sulphate inj. is available: 5.45% w/v (equivalent to 40 mg chloroquine base per mL).

OTHER INFORMATION

- Excretion is increased in alkaline urine.
- Manufacturer advises to use with caution in patients with renal or hepatic disease.
- Dose in severe renal impairment is from *Drug Prescribing in Renal Failure*, 5th edition, by Aronoff *et al.*
- Bone marrow suppression may occur with extended treatment.
- 150 mg chloroquine base is equivalent to 200 mg of sulphate and 250 mg of phosphate.

Chlorphenamine maleate (chlorpheniramine)

CLINICAL USE

Antihistamine:
- Relief of allergy, pruritus
- Treatment/prophylaxis of anaphylaxis

DOSE IN NORMAL RENAL FUNCTION

- Oral: 4 mg 4–6 times a day (maximum 24 mg/day)
- IV/IM/SC: 10–20 mg (maximum 40 mg/day)

PHARMACOKINETICS

Molecular weight (daltons)	390.9
% Protein binding	Approx 70
% Excreted unchanged in urine	Approx 22
Volume of distribution (L/kg)	3
Half-life – normal/ESRF (hrs)	12–43/–

METABOLISM

Chlorphenamine appears to undergo extensive first-pass metabolism. Chlorphenamine maleate is extensively metabolised in the liver. Metabolites include desmethyl- and didesmethylchlorphenamine. Unchanged drug and metabolites are excreted mainly in the urine; excretion is dependent on urinary pH and flow rate. Only trace amounts have been found in the faeces.

DOSE IN RENAL IMPAIRMENT GFR (mL/MIN)

20–50	Dose as in normal renal function.
10–20	Dose as in normal renal function.
<10	Dose as in normal renal function. See 'Other information'.

DOSE IN PATIENTS UNDERGOING RENAL REPLACEMENT THERAPIES

CAPD	Not dialysed. Dose as in normal renal function.
HD	Dialysed. Dose as in normal renal function.
HDF/High flux	Dialysed. Dose as in normal renal function.
CAV/VVHD	Dialysed. Dose as in normal renal function.

IMPORTANT DRUG INTERACTIONS

Potentially hazardous interactions with other drugs
- Analgesics: sedative effects possibly increased with opioid analgesics.
- Antivirals: concentration possibly increased by lopinavir.
- Inhibits phenytoin metabolism and can lead to phenytoin toxicity.

ADMINISTRATION

RECONSTITUTION
–
ROUTE
- Oral, IV
RATE OF ADMINISTRATION
- Bolus over 1 minute
COMMENTS
- Injection reported to cause stinging or burning sensation at site of injection.

OTHER INFORMATION

- Increased cerebral sensitivity in patients with renal impairment.

Chlorpromazine hydrochloride

CLINICAL USE

- Anti-emetic
- Anxiolytic
- Antipsychotic
- Hiccups

DOSE IN NORMAL RENAL FUNCTION

- Anti-emetic:
  - Oral: 10–25 mg every 4–6 hours
  - IM: 25–50 mg every 3–4 hours
- Antipsychotic, anxiolytic:
  - Oral: 25 mg every 8 hours (or 75 mg at night) initially; increase as necessary; usual maintenance dose 75–300 mg daily (up to 1 g daily)
  - IM: 25–50 mg every 6–8 hours
- Induction of hypothermia: 25–50 mg every 6–8 hours
- Hiccups: Oral: 25–50 mg every 6–8 hours
- PR (unlicensed): 100 mg every 6–8 hours

PHARMACOKINETICS

Molecular weight (daltons)	355.3
% Protein binding	95–98
% Excreted unchanged in urine	<1
Volume of distribution (L/kg)	7–20[1]
Half-life – normal/ ESRF (hrs)	23–37/Unchanged

METABOLISM

Chlorpromazine is subject to considerable first-pass metabolism in the gut wall and is also extensively metabolised in the liver. Paths of metabolism of chlorpromazine include hydroxylation and conjugation with glucuronic acid, N-oxidation, oxidation of a sulfur atom, and dealkylation. Chlorpromazine is excreted in the urine and bile in the form of both active and inactive metabolites; there is some evidence of enterohepatic recycling.

DOSE IN RENAL IMPAIRMENT GFR (mL/MIN)

20–50	Dose as in normal renal function.
10–20	Dose as in normal renal function.
<10	Start with small dose and increase according to response.

DOSE IN PATIENTS UNDERGOING RENAL REPLACEMENT THERAPIES

CAPD	Not dialysed. Dose as in GFR<10 mL/min.
HD	Not dialysed. Dose as in GFR<10 mL/min.
HDF/High flux	Unknown dialysability. Dose as in GFR<10 mL/min.
CAV/ VVHD	Unknown dialysability. Dose as in normal renal function.

IMPORTANT DRUG INTERACTIONS

Potentially hazardous interactions with other drugs

- Anaesthetics: enhanced hypotensive effect.
- Analgesics: increased risk of convulsions with tramadol; enhanced hypotensive and sedative effects with opioids; increased risk of ventricular arrhythmias with methadone.
- Anti-arrhythmics: increased risk of ventricular arrhythmias with anti-arrhythmics that prolong the QT interval and disopyramide; avoid concomitant use with amiodarone and dronedarone.
- Antibacterials: increased risk of ventricular arrhythmias with moxifloxacin and telithromycin – avoid with moxifloxacin.
- Antidepressants: increased level of tricyclics, possibly increased risk of ventricular arrhythmias and antimuscarinic side effects.
- Anticonvulsant: antagonises anticonvulsant effect; concentration of phenytoin possibly increased or decreased; concentration of both drugs reduced with phenobarbital.
- Antimalarials: avoid concomitant use with artemether/lumefantrine and piperaquine with artenimol.
- Antipsychotics: increased risk of ventricular arrhythmias with droperidol and pimozide – avoid concomitant use; concentration of haloperidol possibly increased.
- Antivirals: concentration possibly increased with ritonavir.
- Anxiolytics and hypnotics: increased sedative effects.
- Atomoxetine: increased risk of ventricular arrhythmias.

- Beta-blockers: enhanced hypotensive effect; concentration of both drugs may increase with propranolol; increased risk of ventricular arrhythmias with sotalol.
- Cytotoxics: increased risk of ventricular arrhythmias with vandetanib – avoid; increased risk of ventricular arrhythmias with arsenic trioxide.
- Diuretics: enhanced hypotensive effect.
- Lithium: increased risk of extrapyramidal side effects and possibly neurotoxicity.
- Pentamidine: increased risk of ventricular arrhythmias.
- Ulcer-healing drugs: effects enhanced by cimetidine.

ADMINISTRATION

RECONSTITUTION

–

ROUTE
- Oral, deep IM, PR (unlicensed)

RATE OF ADMINISTRATION

–

COMMENTS

–

OTHER INFORMATION

- Start with small doses in severe renal impairment due to increased cerebral sensitivity.
- Manufacturer advises to use with caution due to risk of accumulation.

Reference:
1. Ereshefsky L. Pharmacokinetics and drug interactions: update for new antipsychotics. *J Clin Psychiatry.* 1996; **57**(Suppl. 11): 12–25.

Chlortalidone (chlorthalidone)

CLINICAL USE

Thiazide-like diuretic:
- Hypertension
- Ascites
- Oedema
- Diabetes insipidus
- Mild to moderate heart failure

DOSE IN NORMAL RENAL FUNCTION

- Hypertension: 25–50 mg daily.
- Oedema: 50 mg daily initially.
- Diabetes insipidus: 100 mg every 12 hours initially, reducing to 50 mg daily where possible.
- Heart failure: 25–50 mg daily increasing to 100–200 mg daily.

PHARMACOKINETICS

Molecular weight (daltons)	338.8
% Protein binding	76
% Excreted unchanged in urine	50
Volume of distribution (L/kg)	3.9
Half-life – normal/ ESRF (hrs)	40–60/Unchanged

METABOLISM

Chlortalidone is highly bound to red blood cells; the receptor to which it is bound has been identified as carbonic anhydrase. It is much less strongly bound to plasma proteins. Chlortalidone is mainly excreted unchanged in the urine.

DOSE IN RENAL IMPAIRMENT GFR (mL/MIN)

30–50	Dose as in normal renal function.
<30	Avoid. See 'Other information'.

DOSE IN PATIENTS UNDERGOING RENAL REPLACEMENT THERAPIES

CAPD	Unlikely to be dialysed. Avoid.
HD	Not dialysed. Avoid.
HDF/High flux	Unknown dialysability. Avoid.
CAV/ VVHD	Unknown dialysability. Dose as in normal renal function.

IMPORTANT DRUG INTERACTIONS

Potentially hazardous interactions with other drugs
- Analgesics: increased risk of nephrotoxicity with NSAIDs; antagonism of diuretic effect.
- Anti-arrhythmics: hypokalaemia leads to increased cardiac toxicity; effects of lidocaine and mexiletine antagonised.
- Antibacterials: avoid administration with lymecycline.
- Antidepressants: increased risk of hypokalaemia with reboxetine; enhanced hypotensive effect with MAOIs; increased risk of postural hypotension with tricyclics.
- Anti-epileptics: increased risk of hyponatraemia with carbamazepine.
- Antifungals: increased risk of hypokalaemia with amphotericin.
- Antihypertensives: enhanced hypotensive effect; increased risk of first dose hypotension with post-synaptic alpha-blockers like prazosin; hypokalaemia increases risk of ventricular arrhythmias with sotalol.
- Antipsychotics: hypokalaemia increases risk of ventricular arrhythmias with amisulpride; enhanced hypotensive effect with phenothiazines; hypokalaemia increases risk of ventricular arrhythmias with pimozide – avoid concomitant use.
- Atomoxetine: hypokalaemia increases risk of ventricular arrhythmias.
- Cardiac glycosides: increased toxicity if hypokalaemia occurs.
- Ciclosporin: increased risk of nephrotoxicity and hypomagnesaemia.
- Cytotoxics: increased risk of ventricular arrhythmias due to hypokalaemia with arsenic trioxide; increased risk of nephrotoxicity and ototoxicity with platinum compounds.
- Lithium excretion reduced, increased toxicity.

ADMINISTRATION

RECONSTITUTION

–

ROUTE
- Oral

RATE OF ADMINISTRATION

–

COMMENTS
- A single dose at breakfast time is preferable.

OTHER INFORMATION

- Can precipitate diabetes mellitus and gout, and cause severe electrolyte disturbances and an increase in serum lipids.
- Thiazide diuretics are unlikely to be of use once GFR<30 mL/min.

Ciclosporin

CLINICAL USE

Immunosuppressant:
- Prophylaxis of solid organ transplant rejection
- Nephrotic syndrome
- Atopic dermatitis
- Psoriasis
- Rheumatoid arthritis
- Ulcerative colitis

DOSE IN NORMAL RENAL FUNCTION

- Organ transplantation:
  — Oral: 2–15 mg/kg/day based on levels. (See local protocol.)
  — IV: One-third to one-half of oral dose. (See local protocol.)
- Bone marrow transplantation:
  — Oral: 12.5–15 mg/kg daily
  — IV: 3–5 mg/kg daily
- Nephrotic syndrome: 5 mg/kg orally in 2 divided doses
- Atopic dermatitis/psoriasis: 2.5–5 mg/kg orally in 2 divided doses
- Rheumatoid arthritis: Oral: 2.5–4 mg/kg in 2 divided doses
- Ulcerative colitis: IV infusion: 2 mg/kg daily over 24 hours

PHARMACOKINETICS

Molecular weight (daltons)	1202.6
% Protein binding	Approx 90
% Excreted unchanged in urine	0.1
Volume of distribution (L/kg)	3–5
Half-life – normal/ESRF (hrs)	5–20/ Unchanged

METABOLISM

Ciclosporin is widely distributed throughout the body. Distribution in the blood is concentration-dependent, with 41–58% in erythrocytes and 10–20% in leucocytes; the remainder is found in plasma, about 90% protein-bound, mostly to lipoprotein. Clearance from the blood is biphasic. Ciclosporin is extensively metabolised in the liver and mainly excreted in faeces via the bile. About 6% of a dose is reported to be excreted in the urine, less than 0.1% unchanged.

DOSE IN RENAL IMPAIRMENT GFR (mL/MIN)

20–50	Dose as in normal renal function.
10–20	Dose as in normal renal function.
<10	Dose as in normal renal function.

DOSE IN PATIENTS UNDERGOING RENAL REPLACEMENT THERAPIES

CAPD	Not dialysed. Dose as in normal renal function; adjust according to levels.
HD	Not dialysed. Dose as in normal renal function; adjust according to levels.
HDF/High flux	Unknown dialysability. Dose as in normal renal function; adjust according to levels.
CAV/ VVHD	Not dialysed. Dose as in normal renal function; adjust according to levels.

IMPORTANT DRUG INTERACTIONS

Potentially hazardous interactions with other drugs
- Increased risk of hyperkalaemia with ACE inhibitors, angiotensin-II antagonists, potassium-sparing diuretics, potassium salts.
- Increased risk of nephrotoxicity with acetazolamide, aminoglycosides, amphotericin, co-trimoxazole, disopyramide, foscarnet, melphalan, NSAIDs, polymyxins, quinolones, sulphonamides, thiazide diuretics, trimethoprim and vancomycin.
- Increased ciclosporin levels with aciclovir, amiodarone, atazanavir, boceprevir, carvedilol, chloramphenicol, chloroquine, cimetidine, clarithromycin, colchicine, danazol, diltiazem, doxycycline, erythromycin, famotidine, fluconazole, fluoxetine, fluvoxamine, fosamprenavir, glibenclamide, glipizide, grapefruit juice, hydroxychloroquine, imatinib, indinavir, itraconazole, ketoconazole, lercanidipine (concentration of both drugs increased – avoid), macrolides, micafungin, miconazole, high-dose methylprednisolone, metoclopramide, metronidazole, muromonab-CD3, nicardipine, posaconazole, progestogens, propafenone, ritonavir, saquinavir and telaprevir (concentration of both drugs increased), tacrolimus, telithromycin, verapamil and voriconazole.

- Decreased ciclosporin levels with barbiturates, bupropion, carbamazepine, efavirenz, griseofulvin, lanreotide, modafinil, octreotide, oxcarbazepine, pasireotide, phenytoin, primidone, quinine, red wine, rifampicin, St John's wort, sulfadiazine, IV sulfadimidine, sulfasalazine, sulfinpyrazone, terbinafine, ticlopidine and IV trimethoprim and possibly by oxcarbazepine.
- Aliskiren: concentration of aliskiren increased – avoid.
- Ambrisentan: concentration of ambrisentan increased.
- Antibacterials: increased risk of myopathy with daptomycin – try to avoid concomitant use.
- Anticoagulants: concentration of dabigatran increased – avoid.
- Antidiabetics: may increase repaglinide concentration, risk of hypoglycaemia.
- Antimuscarinics: avoid with darifenacin.
- Basiliximab: may alter ciclosporin levels.
- Bosentan: co-administration of ciclosporin and bosentan is contraindicated. When ciclosporin and bosentan are co-administered, initial trough concentrations of bosentan are 30 times higher than normal. At steady state, trough levels are 3–4 times higher than normal. Blood concentrations of ciclosporin decreased by 50%.
- Calcium-channel blockers: increased nifedipine concentration and toxicity.
- Cardiac glycosides: increased digoxin concentration and toxicity.
- Caspofungin: caspofungin concentration increased – monitor LFTs.
- Colchicine: risk of myopathy or rhabdomyolysis; also increased blood-ciclosporin concentrations and nephrotoxicity.
- Cytotoxics: increased risk of neurotoxicity with doxorubicin; concentration of epirubicin, everolimus and idarubicin increased; reduced excretion of mitoxantrone; increased toxicity with methotrexate; seizures have been reported in bone marrow transplant patients taking busulfan and cyclophosphamide; use crizotinib with caution; concentration of etoposide possibly increased (increased risk of toxicity); possible interaction with docetaxel.
- Fidaxomicin: avoid concomitant use.

- Lipid-lowering agents: absorption reduced by colesevelam, increased risk of myopathy with statins (avoid concomitant use with simvastatin, max dose of atorvastatin should be 10 mg[1]); avoid with rosuvastatin; increased risk of nephrotoxicity with fenofibrate; bezafibrate may increase creatinine and reduce ciclosporin levels; concentration of both drugs may be increased with ezetimibe.
- Mycophenolate mofetil: some studies show that ciclosporin decreases plasma MPA AUC levels – no dose change required.
- NSAIDs: diclofenac concentration increased – reduce diclofenac dose.
- Omeprazole: may alter ciclosporin concentration.
- Orlistat: absorption of ciclosporin possibly reduced.
- Prednisolone: increased prednisolone concentration.
- Sirolimus: increased absorption of sirolimus – give sirolimus 4 hours after ciclosporin; sirolimus concentration increased; long term concomitant administration may be associated with deterioration in renal function.
- Tacrolimus: increased ciclosporin concentration and toxicity – avoid concomitant use.
- Ursodeoxycholic acid: unpredictably increased absorption and raised ciclosporin levels in some patients.

ADMINISTRATION

RECONSTITUTION
–
ROUTE
- Oral, IV peripherally or centrally.
RATE OF ADMINISTRATION
- Over 2–6 hours peripherally or 1 hour centrally
COMMENTS
- Dilute 50 mg in 20–100 mL with sodium chloride 0.9% or glucose 5%.

OTHER INFORMATION

- To convert from IV to oral multiply by 2–3 (usually 2.5)
- Dose and monitor blood levels in accordance with local protocol.

Reference:
1. MHRA. *Drug Safety Update*. Statins: interactions and updated advice. August 2012; **6**(1): 2–4.

Cidofovir

CLINICAL USE

- Treatment of CMV retinitis in patients with AIDS, if other agents are unsuitable
- Treatment of BK polyoma virus in transplant patients (unlicensed)

DOSE IN NORMAL RENAL FUNCTION

5 mg/kg weekly for 2 weeks then once every 2 weeks.
(See further information for BK polyoma virus treatment.)

PHARMACOKINETICS

Molecular weight (daltons)	279.2
% Protein binding	<6
% Excreted unchanged in urine	80–100
Volume of distribution (L/kg)	0.3–0.8
Half-life – normal/ESRF (hrs)	1.7–2.7/16–25[1]

METABOLISM

After IV doses of cidofovir, serum concentrations decline with a reported terminal half-life of about 2.2 hours (the intracellular half-life of the active diphosphate may be up to 65 hours). Cidofovir is eliminated mainly by renal excretion, both by glomerular filtration and tubular secretion. About 80–100% of a dose is recovered unchanged from the urine within 24 hours. Use with probenecid may reduce the excretion of cidofovir to some extent by blocking tubular secretion, although 70–85% has still been reported to be excreted unchanged in the urine within 24 hours.

DOSE IN RENAL IMPAIRMENT GFR (mL/MIN)

>55	Dose as in normal renal function.
<55	Avoid. See 'Other information'.

DOSE IN PATIENTS UNDERGOING RENAL REPLACEMENT THERAPIES

CAPD	Not dialysed. 0.5 mg/kg/dose
HD	Dialysed. 0.5 mg/kg/dose
HDF/High flux	Dialysed. 0.5 mg/kg/dose
CAV/VVHD	Unknown dialysability. 0.5 mg/kg/dose

IMPORTANT DRUG INTERACTIONS

Potentially hazardous interactions with other drugs
- Antivirals: avoid concomitant use with tenofovir.

ADMINISTRATION

RECONSTITUTION
–
ROUTE
- IV infusion
RATE OF ADMINISTRATION
- Over 60 minutes
COMMENTS
- Dilute in 100 mL sodium chloride 0.9%.

OTHER INFORMATION

- Always administer with oral probenecid and intravenous sodium chloride 0.9%.
- Administer 2 hours before dialysis session to benefit from peak concentration without having delayed clearance.
- 52–75% of dose dialysed out with high-flux haemodialysis.
- Information for the treatment of BK polyoma virus in transplant patients is from Pittsburgh. Starting dose was 0.25 mg/kg (if GFR<30 mL/min) in 100 mL sodium chloride 0.9% administered over 1 hour, given every 10–14 days. Hydration pre- and post-dose with 1 litre of sodium chloride 0.9% if tolerated. If no change within 10–14 days increase to 0.3–0.5 mg/kg; dose can be increased up to 1 mg/kg depending on response and side effects. Most patients would need a cumulative dose of 1–1.5 mg/kg. Initially use without probenecid. Monitor blood and urine samples for PCR measurement of viral load.
- The manufacturer advises to avoid in renal failure but theoretical doses, based on a 70 kg person, are suggested in the following paper:

Reference:
1. Brody SR, Humphreys MH, Gambertoglio JG, *et al.* Pharmacokinetics of cidofovir in renal insufficiency and in continuous ambulatory peritoneal dialysis or high-flux haemodialysis. *Clin Pharmacol Ther.* 1999; **65**: 21–8.

CL$_{CR}$ (mL/min/kg)	Dose (mg/kg)
1.3–1.8	5
1–1.2	4
0.8–0.9	3
0.7	2.5
0.5–0.6	2
0.4	1.5
0.2–0.3	1
0.1	0.5

Cilazapril

CLINICAL USE

Angiotensin-converting enzyme inhibitor:
- Hypertension
- Heart failure

DOSE IN NORMAL RENAL FUNCTION

0.5–5 mg daily

PHARMACOKINETICS

Molecular weight (daltons)	435.5
% Protein binding	No data
% Excreted unchanged in urine	80–90
Volume of distribution (L/kg)	0.5–0.8
Half-life – normal/ ESRF (hrs)	9/Increased

METABOLISM

Cilazapril acts as a prodrug of the diacid cilazaprilat, its active metabolite. After oral absorption cilazapril is rapidly metabolised in the liver to cilazaprilat, the bioavailability of which is about 60%. Peak plasma concentrations of cilazaprilat occur within 2 hours of an oral dose of cilazapril. Cilazaprilat is eliminated unchanged in the urine.

DOSE IN RENAL IMPAIRMENT GFR (mL/MIN)

40–50	Start at low dose and adjust according to response.
10–40	Start at low dose and adjust according to response.
<10	Start at low dose and adjust according to response.

DOSE IN PATIENTS UNDERGOING RENAL REPLACEMENT THERAPIES

CAPD	Unknown dialysability. Dose as in GFR<10 mL/min.
HD	Dialysed. Dose as in GFR<10 mL/min.
HDF/High flux	Dialysed. Dose as in GFR<10 mL/min.
CAV/ VVHD	Unknown dialysability. Dose as in GFR=10–40 mL/min.

IMPORTANT DRUG INTERACTIONS

Potentially hazardous interactions with other drugs
- Anaesthetics: enhanced hypotensive effect.
- Ciclosporin: decreased renal function and increased risk of hyperkalaemia.
- NSAIDs: antagonism of hypotensive effect and increased risk of renal failure; hyperkalaemia.
- Diuretics: enhanced hypotensive effect; hyperkalaemia with potassium-sparing diuretics.
- ESAs: increased risk of hyperkalaemia.
- Gold: flushing and hypotension with sodium aurothiomalate.
- Lithium: ACE inhibitors reduce excretion of lithium (increased plasma lithium concentration).
- Potassium salts: hyperkalaemia.
- Tacrolimus: decreased renal function and increased risk of hyperkalaemia.

ADMINISTRATION

RECONSTITUTION
–
ROUTE
- Oral
RATE OF ADMINISTRATION
–
COMMENTS
- Take dose about the same time each day.

OTHER INFORMATION

- Data refer to active drug – cilazaprilat.
- Symptomatic hypotension reported in patients with sodium or volume depletion, i.e. sickness, diarrhoea, on diuretics, low sodium diet or post dialysis.
- Renal failure has been associated with ACE inhibitors in patients with renal artery stenosis, post renal transplant, and congestive heart failure.
- A high incidence of anaphylactoid reactions has been reported in patients dialysed with high-flux polyacrylonitrile membranes and treated concomitantly with an ACE inhibitor – this combination should therefore be avoided.
- Hyperkalaemia and other side effects are more common in patients with impaired renal function.
- Close monitoring of renal function during therapy is necessary in those with renal insufficiency.

Cilostazol

CLINICAL USE

Intermittent claudication

DOSE IN NORMAL RENAL FUNCTION

100 mg twice daily, 30 minutes before or
2 hours after food

PHARMACOKINETICS

Molecular weight (daltons)	369.5
% Protein binding	95–98
% Excreted unchanged in urine	<2 as dehydro-cilostazol (74% as metabolites)
Volume of distribution (L/kg)	No data
Half-life – normal/ESRF (hrs)	10.5–13/Unchanged

METABOLISM

Cilostazol is extensively metabolised in the
liver by cytochrome P450 isoenzymes, mainly
CYP3A4 and to a lesser extent CYP2C19, to
both active and inactive metabolites; these
are mainly excreted in the urine (74%) with
the remainder in the faeces (20%). The active
metabolites have apparent elimination half-
lives of 11 to 13 hours.

DOSE IN RENAL IMPAIRMENT
GFR (mL/MIN)

25–50	Dose as in normal renal function.
10–25	Dose as in normal renal function. Use with caution. See 'Other information'.
<10	Dose as in normal renal function. Use with caution. See 'Other information'.

DOSE IN PATIENTS UNDERGOING
RENAL REPLACEMENT THERAPIES

CAPD	Not dialysed. Dose as in GFR<10 mL/min.
HD	Not dialysed. Dose as in GFR<10 mL/min.
HDF/High flux	Unknown dialysability. Dose as in GFR<10 mL/min.
CAV/VVHD	Unlikely to be dialysed. Dose as in GFR=10–25 mL/min.

IMPORTANT DRUG INTERACTIONS

Potentially hazardous interactions with other
drugs
- Anagrelide: avoid concomitant use.
- Antibacterials: concentration increased
  by erythromycin – consider reducing
  cilostazol dose.
- Antifungals: concentration possibly
  increased by ketoconazole – consider
  reducing cilostazol dose.
- Calcium-channel blockers: concentration
  increased by diltiazem – consider reducing
  cilostazol dose.
- Ulcer-healing drugs: concentration
  increased by omeprazole – consider
  reducing cilostazol dose.

ADMINISTRATION

RECONSTITUTION
–
ROUTE
- Oral
RATE OF ADMINISTRATION
–
COMMENTS
–

OTHER INFORMATION

- There are two major metabolites, a
  dehydro-cilostazol and a 4'-trans-
  hydroxy cilostazol, both of which have
  similar apparent half-lives. The dehydro
  metabolite is 4–7 times as active a platelet
  anti-aggregant as the parent compound,
  and the 4'-trans-hydroxy metabolite is one
  fifth as active.
- In subjects with severe renal impairment,
  the free fraction of cilostazol was 27%
  higher and both C_{max} and AUC were
  29% and 39% lower respectively than in
  subjects with normal renal function. The
  C_{max} and AUC of the dehydro metabolite
  were 41% and 47% lower respectively in
  the severely renally impaired subjects
  compared to subjects with normal renal
  function. The C_{max} and AUC of 4'-trans-
  hydroxy cilostazol were 173% and 209%
  greater in subjects with severe renal
  impairment. The drug should be used with
  great caution if administered to patients
  with a creatinine clearance <25 mL/min.
- Contraindicated in patients with heart
  failure.
- Contraindicated by manufacturer if GFR
  <25 mL/min in the UK but only use with
  caution in the USA SPC.

- Cilostazol is under investigation for its antiplatelet effect after coronary stent implantation.
- Dose can also be reduced to 50 mg twice daily if used with drugs which affect its clearance.

Cimetidine

CLINICAL USE

H_2 antagonist:
- Conditions associated with hyperacidity
- Refractory uraemic pruritus (unlicensed use)

DOSE IN NORMAL RENAL FUNCTION

- Oral: duodenal and gastric ulceration treatment: 800 mg at night, or 400 mg twice daily; rarely, up to 1.6 g daily. Prophylaxis: 400 mg at night or 400 mg twice daily. Prophylaxis of stress ulceration: 200–400 mg every 4–6 hours.
- Reflux oesophagitis: 400 mg every 6 hours.
- Zollinger-Ellison syndrome: 400 mg every 4–6 hours.

PHARMACOKINETICS

Molecular weight (daltons)	252.3
% Protein binding	20
% Excreted unchanged in urine	50–75
Volume of distribution (L/kg)	1–1.3
Half-life – normal/ ESRF (hrs)	2–3/5

METABOLISM

The bioavailability of cimetidine after oral doses is about 60–70%, due to hepatic first-pass metabolism. Cimetidine is partially metabolised in the liver to the sulfoxide and to hydroxymethyl cimetidine. About 50% of an oral dose, and 75% of an intravenous dose, is excreted unchanged in the urine in 24 hours. After an oral or parenteral dose of 300 mg, blood concentrations remain above that required to provide 80% inhibition of basal gastric acid secretion for 4 to 5 hours.

DOSE IN RENAL IMPAIRMENT GFR (mL/MIN)

30–50	200 mg four times daily.
15–30	200 mg three times daily.
<15	200 mg twice daily.

DOSE IN PATIENTS UNDERGOING RENAL REPLACEMENT THERAPIES

CAPD	Not dialysed. Dose as in GFR<15 mL/min.
HD	Dialysed. Dose as in GFR<15 mL/min.
HDF/High flux	Dialysed. Dose as in GFR<15 mL/min.
CAV/ VVHD	Not dialysed. 300 mg every 8 hours.[1]

IMPORTANT DRUG INTERACTIONS

Potentially hazardous interactions with other drugs
- Alpha-blockers: effects of tolazoline antagonised.
- Anti-arrhythmics: increased concentration of amiodarone, flecainide, lidocaine procainamide and propafenone.
- Anticoagulants: enhanced effect of coumarins.
- Anti-epileptics: metabolism of carbamazepine, phenytoin and valproate inhibited.
- Antifungals: absorption of itraconazole and ketoconazole reduced; posaconazole concentration reduced – avoid; terbinafine concentration increased.
- Antimalarials: avoid concomitant use with artemether/lumefantrine; metabolism of chloroquine, hydroxychloroquine and quinine inhibited.
- Antipsychotics: possibly enhanced effect of antipsychotics, chlorpromazine and clozapine.
- Antivirals: concentration of atazanavir reduced; concentration of raltegravir and saquinavir possibly increased – avoid; avoid for 12 hours before and 4 hours after rilpivirine.
- Ciclosporin: possibly increased ciclosporin levels.
- Clopidogrel: possibly reduces anti-platelet effect.
- Cytotoxics: possibly enhances myelosuppressive effects of carmustine and lomustine; concentration of epirubicin and fluorouracil increased; avoid with erlotinib; possibly reduced absorption of lapatinib; possibly reduced absorption of pazopanib – give at least 2 hours before or 10 hours after cimetidine.
- Ergot alkaloids: increased risk of ergotism – avoid concomitant use.
- Fampridine: avoid concomitant use.
- Theophylline: metabolism of theophylline inhibited.
- Ulipristal: contraceptive effect possibly reduced – avoid with high dose ulipristal.

ADMINISTRATION

RECONSTITUTION

–

ROUTE

- Oral

OTHER INFORMATION

- Inhibits tubular secretion of creatinine.
- Uraemic patients susceptible to mental confusion.

Reference:
1. Dose from CVVH Initial Drug Dosing Guidelines on www.thedrugmonitor.com.

Cinacalcet

CLINICAL USE

Calcimimetic agent:
- Treatment of secondary hyperparathyroidism in patients with CKD 5 on dialysis
- Treatment of primary hyperparathyroidism
- Treatment of hypercalcaemia in patients with parathyroid carcinoma

DOSE IN NORMAL RENAL FUNCTION

- Secondary hyperparathyroidism: 30–180 mg once daily.
- Parathyroid carcinoma and primary hyperparathyroidism: 30 mg twice daily increasing to a maximum of 90 mg 4 times a day.

PHARMACOKINETICS

Molecular weight (daltons)	393.9 as Hydrochloride
% Protein binding	93–97
% Excreted unchanged in urine	80
Volume of distribution (L/kg)	1000 litres
Half-life – normal/ ESRF (hrs)	30–40/Unchanged

METABOLISM

Cinacalcet is rapidly and extensively metabolised by cytochrome P450 isoenzymes CYP3A4 and CYP1A2, by oxidation followed by conjugation. The major circulating metabolites are inactive, and are renally excreted, with 80% of the dose recovered in the urine, and 15% in the faeces.

DOSE IN RENAL IMPAIRMENT GFR (mL/MIN)

20–50	Dose as in normal renal function.
10–20	Dose as in normal renal function.
<10	Dose as in normal renal function.

DOSE IN PATIENTS UNDERGOING RENAL REPLACEMENT THERAPIES

CAPD	Not dialysed. Dose as in normal renal function.
HD	Not dialysed. Dose as in normal renal function.
HDF/High flux	Unlikely to be dialysed. Dose as normal renal function.
CAV/ VVHD	Not Dialysed. Dose as in normal renal function.

IMPORTANT DRUG INTERACTIONS

Potentially hazardous interactions with other drugs
- Antifungals: metabolism inhibited by ketoconazole.
- Hormone antagonists: metabolism of tamoxifen to active metabolite inhibited – avoid.
- Tobacco: metabolism increased by tobacco.

ADMINISTRATION

RECONSTITUTION
–
ROUTE
- Oral
RATE OF ADMINISTRATION
–
COMMENTS
- Take with food or shortly after a meal

OTHER INFORMATION

- Adjust dose according to response.
- Monitor calcium levels to prevent hypocalcaemia.
- Can be used in combination with vitamin D analogues and phosphate binders.
- Steady state is achieved after 7 days.

Cinnarizine

- Vestibular disorders
- Motion sickness

DOSE IN NORMAL RENAL FUNCTION

- Vestibular disorders: 30 mg 3 times a day
- Motion sickness: 30 mg 2 hours before travel then 15 mg every 8 hours when required.

PHARMACOKINETICS

Molecular weight (daltons)	368.5
% Protein binding	80
% Excreted unchanged in urine	<20
Volume of distribution (L/kg)	No data
Half-life – normal/ ESRF (hrs)	3–6/–

METABOLISM

Cinnarizine is extensively metabolised mainly via CYP2D6, but there is considerable inter-individual variation in the extent of metabolism.

The elimination of metabolites occurs as follows: one third in the urine (unchanged as metabolites and glucuronide conjugates) and two thirds in the faeces.

DOSE IN RENAL IMPAIRMENT GFR (mL/MIN)

20–50	Dose as in normal renal function.
10–20	Dose as in normal renal function.
<10	Dose as in normal renal function.

DOSE IN PATIENTS UNDERGOING RENAL REPLACEMENT THERAPIES

CAPD	Unlikely to be dialysed. Dose as in normal renal function.
HD	Unlikely to be dialysed. Dose as in normal renal function.
HDF/High flux	Unknown dialysability. Dose as in normal renal function.
CAV/ VVHD	Unlikely to be dialysed. Dose as in normal renal function.

IMPORTANT DRUG INTERACTIONS

Potentially hazardous interactions with other drugs
- None known

ADMINISTRATION

RECONSTITUTION
–
ROUTE
- Oral
RATE OF ADMINISTRATION
–

Ciprofibrate

CLINICAL USE
Hyperlipidaemia

DOSE IN NORMAL RENAL FUNCTION
100 mg daily

PHARMACOKINETICS

Molecular weight (daltons)	289.2
% Protein binding	95–99
% Excreted unchanged in urine	20–25
Volume of distribution (L/kg)	12 litres
Half-life – normal/ ESRF (hrs)	38–86/171.9

METABOLISM
Approximately 30–75% of a single dose administered to volunteers was excreted in the urine in 72 hours, either as unchanged ciprofibrate (20–25% of the total excreted) or as a glucuronide conjugate. Subjects with moderate renal impairment excreted on average 7% of a single dose as unchanged ciprofibrate over 96 hours, compared with 6.9% in normal subjects. In subjects with severe insufficiency this was reduced to 4.7%.

DOSE IN RENAL IMPAIRMENT GFR (mL/MIN)

20–50	Dose as in normal renal function.
10–20	100 mg every 48 hours.
<10	Avoid. See 'Other information'.

DOSE IN PATIENTS UNDERGOING RENAL REPLACEMENT THERAPIES

CAPD	Not dialysed. Avoid.
HD	Not dialysed. Avoid.
HDF/High flux	Unknown dialysability. Avoid.
CAV/ VVHD	Unknown dialysability. Dose as in GFR=10–20 mL/min

IMPORTANT DRUG INTERACTIONS
Potentially hazardous interactions with other drugs
- Antibacterials: increased risk of myopathy with daptomycin – try to avoid concomitant use.
- Anticoagulants: enhances effect of coumarins and phenindione. Dose of anticoagulant should be reduced by up to 50% and readjusted by monitoring INR.
- Antidiabetics: may improve glucose tolerance and have an additive effect with insulin or sulphonylureas.
- Colchicine: possible increased risk of myopathy.
- Lipid-regulating drugs: increased risk of myopathy in combination with statins and ezetimibe (do not exceed 10 mg of simvastatin and 20 mg of rosuvastatin[1]) – avoid concomitant use with ezetimibe.

ADMINISTRATION
RECONSTITUTION
–
ROUTE
- Oral
RATE OF ADMINISTRATION
–
COMMENTS
–

OTHER INFORMATION
- Increased risk of rhabdomyolysis in doses of 200 mg or greater.

Reference:
1. MHRA. *Drug Safety Update*. Statins: interactions and updated advice. August 2012; **6**(1): 2–4.

Ciprofloxacin

CLINICAL USE

Antibacterial agent

DOSE IN NORMAL RENAL FUNCTION

Oral: 250–750 mg every 12 hours
IV: 100–400 mg every 8–12 hours

PHARMACOKINETICS

Molecular weight (daltons)	331.3
% Protein binding	20–40
% Excreted unchanged in urine	40–70
Volume of distribution (L/kg)	2.5
Half-life – normal/ ESRF (hrs)	3–5/8

METABOLISM

Ciprofloxacin is eliminated principally by urinary excretion, but non-renal clearance may account for about one-third of elimination and includes hepatic metabolism, biliary excretion, and possibly transluminal secretion across the intestinal mucosa. At least 4 active metabolites have been identified. Oxociprofloxacin appears to be the major urinary metabolite and sulfociprofloxacin the primary faecal metabolite.

Urinary excretion is by active tubular secretion as well as glomerular filtration and is reduced by probenecid; it is virtually complete within 24 hours. About 40–50% of an oral dose is excreted unchanged in the urine and about 15% as metabolites. Up to 70% of a parenteral dose may be excreted unchanged within 24 hours and 10% as metabolites. Faecal excretion over 5 days has accounted for 20–35% of an oral dose and 15% of an intravenous dose.

DOSE IN RENAL IMPAIRMENT GFR (mL/MIN)

30–50	Dose as in normal renal function.
10–30	50–100% of normal dose.
<10	50% of normal dose. (100% dose may be given for short periods under exceptional circumstances.)

DOSE IN PATIENTS UNDERGOING RENAL REPLACEMENT THERAPIES

CAPD	Not dialysed. Oral: 250 mg every 8–12 hours. IV: 200 mg every 12 hours.
HD	Not dialysed. Oral: 250–500 mg every 12 hours. IV: 200 mg every 12 hours.
HDF/High flux	Unknown dialysability. Oral: 250–500 mg every 12 hours. IV: 200 mg every 12 hours.
CAV/ VVHD	Dialysed. Oral: 500–750 mg every 12 hours. IV: 200–400 mg every 12 hours.[1]

IMPORTANT DRUG INTERACTIONS

Potentially hazardous interactions with other drugs

- Analgesics: increased risk of convulsions with NSAIDs.
- Anticoagulants: anticoagulant effect of coumarins enhanced.
- Antidepressants: metabolism of duloxetine inhibited – avoid; avoid with agomelatine.
- Antimalarials: manufacturer of artemether with lumefantrine advises avoid concomitant use.
- Antipsychotics: possibly increased concentration of olanzapine and clozapine.
- Ciclosporin: variable response; no interaction seen locally; some reports of increased nephrotoxicity.
- Clopidogrel: possibly reduced anti-platelet effect.
- Cytotoxics: possibly reduced excretion of methotrexate; concentration of erlotinib increased.
- Muscle relaxants: tizanidine concentration increased – avoid concomitant use.
- Tacrolimus: increased levels (anecdotally).
- Theophylline: possibly increased risk of convulsions; increased levels of theophylline.

ADMINISTRATION

RECONSTITUTION

–

ROUTE

- Oral, IV

RATE OF ADMINISTRATION

- Infusion: over 30–60 minutes

COMMENTS

- Swallow tablets whole, do not chew.
- Do not take milk, iron preparations, indigestion remedies or phosphate binders at the same time as ciprofloxacin orally.

OTHER INFORMATION

- Intraperitoneal ciprofloxacin in CAPD, dose range from 25 mg/L to 100 mg/L.
- In CAPD peritonitis oral ciprofloxacin up to 500 mg twice daily may be administered.
- Long term use in severe renal impairment can lead to the patients becoming nauseous.
- Oral bioavailability is 70–80%.
- Only very small amounts removed by dialysis.

Reference:

1. Trotman RL, Williamson JC, Shoemaker DM, *et al.* Antibiotic dosing in critically ill adult patients receiving continuous renal replacement therapy. *Clinical Practice.* 2005; **42**(15 0ctober): 1159–66.

Cisplatin

CLINICAL USE

Antineoplastic platinum agent:
- Testicular and metastatic ovarian tumours
- Cervical tumours
- Lung carcinoma
- Bladder cancer
- Squamous cell cancer of head and neck

DOSE IN NORMAL RENAL FUNCTION

- Single agent therapy: 50–120 mg/m^2 as a single dose every 3–4 weeks or 15–20 mg/m^2 daily for 5 days every 3–4 weeks.
- Combination therapy: 20 mg/m^2 and upward, every 3–4 weeks.
- Cervical cancer in combination with radiotherapy: 40 mg/m^2 weekly for 6 weeks.

PHARMACOKINETICS

Molecular weight (daltons)	300
% Protein binding	>90
% Excreted unchanged in urine	27–45
Volume of distribution (L/kg)	0.5
Half-life – normal/ ESRF (hrs)	0.3–1 (terminal T$_{1/2}$ 2–5 days)/–

METABOLISM

Cisplatin is non-enzymatically transformed into multiple metabolites. More than 90% of the platinum from a dose is protein bound within 2 to 4 hours; only the unbound fraction has significant antineoplastic activity. There is good uptake of cisplatin in the kidneys, liver and intestine. It also distributes into third spaces such as ascites and pleural fluid. Excretion of intact drug and metabolites is mainly in the urine but is incomplete and prolonged: up to about 50% of a dose has been reported to be excreted in urine over 5 days, and platinum may be detected in tissue for several months afterwards. The unbound fraction, which is more rapidly cleared (20–80% within 24 hours), may be actively secreted by the renal tubules.

DOSE IN RENAL IMPAIRMENT GFR (mL/MIN)

20–50	See 'Other information'.
10–20	See 'Other information'.
<10	See 'Other information'.

DOSE IN PATIENTS UNDERGOING RENAL REPLACEMENT THERAPIES

CAPD	Not dialysed. Dose as in GFR<10 mL/min.
HD	Not dialysed. Dose as in GFR<10 mL/min.
HDF/High flux	Dialysed. Dose as in GFR<10 mL/min.
CAV/ VVHD	Unknown dialysability. Dose as in GFR=10–20 mL/min.

IMPORTANT DRUG INTERACTIONS

Potentially hazardous interactions with other drugs
- Aldesleukin: avoid concomitant use.
- Aminoglycosides: increased risk of nephrotoxicity and possibly ototoxicity with aminoglycosides, capreomycin, polymyxins or vancomycin.
- Antipsychotics: avoid concomitant use with clozapine, increased risk of agranulocytosis.
- Cytotoxics: increased risk of ototoxicity with ifosfamide; increased pulmonary toxicity with bleomycin and methotrexate.

ADMINISTRATION

RECONSTITUTION
- Water for injection to form a 1 mg/mL solution

ROUTE
- IV infusion

RATE OF ADMINISTRATION
- Over 6–8 hours

COMMENTS
- Pre-treatment hydration, with 1–2 litres of fluid infused for 8–12 hours prior to cisplatin dose, is recommended in order to initiate diuresis. The drug is then well diluted in 2 litres sodium chloride 0.9% or glucose-saline solutions to ensure hydration and maintain urine output. Adequate hydration must be maintained during the following 24 hours, with potassium and magnesium supplementation given as necessary.
- Cisplatin solutions react with aluminium – do not use equipment containing aluminium.

OTHER INFORMATION

- Contraindicated by manufacturer.
- Dose modification depends not only on the degree of renal dysfunction, but also on the intended dose and the therapeutic end-point. In general, any patient with a GFR<70 mL/min should be highlighted as 'at risk' from cisplatin renal toxicity.
- Kintzel PE, Dorr RT. Anticancer drug renal toxicity and elimination: dosing guidelines for altered renal function. *Cancer Treat Rev.* 1995; **21**: 33–64.

GFR (mL/min)	Dose
>60	100%
50–60	75%
40–50	50%
<40	Avoid

- Bennett

GFR (mL/min)	Dose
>50	100%
10–50	75%
<10 and HD	50%

- An alternative approach is to consider changing to carboplatin, which can be dosed specifically according to GFR.
- Ototoxicity, nephrotoxicity and myelosuppression reported. Check hearing, renal function and haematology before treatment and before each subsequent course.
- Toxicity is also associated with cumulative doses of cisplatin.
- Hypomagnesaemia, hypocalcaemia and hyperuricaemia observed.
- The addition of mannitol to the infusion may aid diuresis and protect the kidneys.

Citalopram

CLINICAL USE

SSRI antidepressant:
- Depressive illness
- Panic disorder

DOSE IN NORMAL RENAL FUNCTION

10–40 mg daily
Oral drops: 8–32 mg (4 drops = 8 mg liquid = 10 mg tablet)

PHARMACOKINETICS

Molecular weight (daltons)	324.4
% Protein binding	<80
% Excreted unchanged in urine	12
Volume of distribution (L/kg)	12.3
Half-life – normal/ESRF (hrs)	36/49.5

METABOLISM

Citalopram is metabolised by demethylation, deamination, and oxidation to active and inactive metabolites. The demethylation of citalopram to one of its active metabolites, demethylcitalopram, involves the cytochrome P450 isoenzymes CYP3A4 and CYP2C19; the metabolism of citalopram is also partly dependent on CYP2D6. Didemethylcitalopram has also been identified as a metabolite of citalopram. It is excreted mainly via the liver (85%) with the remainder via the kidneys. About 12% is excreted in the urine as unchanged drug.

DOSE IN RENAL IMPAIRMENT GFR (mL/MIN)

20–50	Dose as in normal renal function.
10–20	Dose as in normal renal function.
<10	Dose as in normal renal function. Use with caution.

DOSE IN PATIENTS UNDERGOING RENAL REPLACEMENT THERAPIES

CAPD	Unlikely to be dialysed. Dose as in GFR<10 mL/min.
HD	Not dialysed. Dose as in GFR<10 mL/min.
HDF/High flux	Not dialysed. Dose as in GFR<10 mL/min.
CAV/ VVHD	Unlikely to be dialysed. Dose as in normal renal function.

IMPORTANT DRUG INTERACTIONS

Potentially hazardous interactions with other drugs
- Analgesics: increased risk of bleeding with aspirin and NSAIDs; risk of CNS toxicity increased with tramadol.
- Antibacterials: possibly increased risk of ventricular arrhythmias with telithromycin.
- Anticoagulants: effect of coumarins possibly enhanced; possibly increased risk of bleeding with dabigatran.
- Antidepressants: avoid concomitant use with MAOIs and moclobemide, increased risk of toxicity; avoid concomitant use with St John's wort; possibly enhanced serotonergic effects with duloxetine; can increase tricyclics' antidepressant concentration; increased agitation and nausea with tryptophan.
- Anti-epileptics: convulsive threshold lowered.
- Antimalarials: avoid concomitant use with artemether/lumefantrine and piperaquine with artenimol.
- Antipsychotics: possibly increased clozapine concentration; avoid concomitant administration with pimozide due to prolongation of QT interval.
- Antivirals: concentration possibly increased by ritonavir.
- Dopaminergics: avoid with selegiline; increased risk of CNS toxicity with rasagiline.
- $5HT_1$ agonist: increased risk of CNS toxicity – avoid; possibly increased risk of serotonergic effects with naratriptan.
- Linezolid: use with care, possibly increased risk of side effects.
- Lithium: increased risk of CNS effects.
- Methylthioninium: risk of CNS toxicity – avoid if possible.

ADMINISTRATION

RECONSTITUTION
–
ROUTE
- Oral
RATE OF ADMINISTRATION
–

OTHER INFORMATION

- Only 1% of drug is removed by haemodialysis.
- There is reduced clearance of citalopram in severe renal failure.
- Use with caution due to lack of information from manufacturer.
- Risk of QT prolongation and ventricular arrhythmias. Maximum dose in elderly, poor metabolisers of CYP2C19 and patients with hepatic failure is 20 mg.

Cladribine

CLINICAL USE

Antineoplastic agent:
- Hairy cell leukaemia (HCL)
- Chronic lymphocytic leukaemia (CLL) in patients who have failed to respond to standard regimens.

DOSE IN NORMAL RENAL FUNCTION

Leustat
- HCL: 0.09 mg/kg (3.6 mg/m^2) daily for 7 days
- CLL: 0.12 mg/kg (4.8 mg/m^2) daily for 2 hours on days 1 to 5 of a 28 day cycle

Litak
- HCL: 0.14 mg/kg/day for 5 days by subcutaneous injection
- or according to local protocol

PHARMACOKINETICS

Molecular weight (daltons)	285.7
% Protein binding	20
% Excreted unchanged in urine	18
Volume of distribution (L/kg)	9
Half-life – normal/ESRF (hrs)	3–22/No data

METABOLISM

Cladribine is extensively distributed and penetrates into the CNS. Cladribine is phosphorylated within cells by deoxycytidine kinase to form 2-chlorodeoxyadenosine-5'-monophosphate which is further phosphorylated to the diphosphate by nucleoside monophosphate kinase and to the active metabolite 2-chlorodeoxyadenosine-5'-triphosphate (CdATP) by nucleoside diphosphate kinase. CdATP inhibits DNA synthesis and repair, particularly in lymphocytes and monocytes.

There is little information available on the route of excretion of cladribine in man. An average of 18% of the administered dose has been reported to be excreted in urine of patients with solid tumours during a 5-day continuous intravenous infusion.

DOSE IN RENAL IMPAIRMENT GFR (mL/MIN)

20–50	75% of dose. Use with caution. See 'Other information'.
10–20	75% of dose. Use with caution. See 'Other information'.
<10	50% of dose. Use with caution. See 'Other information'.

DOSE IN PATIENTS UNDERGOING RENAL REPLACEMENT THERAPIES

CAPD	Unknown dialysability. Dose as in GFR<10 mL/min.
HD	Unknown dialysability. Dose as in GFR<10 mL/min.
HDF/High flux	Unknown dialysability. Dose as in GFR<10 mL/min.
CAV/VVHD	Unknown dialysability. Dose as in GFR=10–20 mL/min.

IMPORTANT DRUG INTERACTIONS

Potentially hazardous interactions with other drugs
- Caution when administering with any other immunosuppressive or myelosuppressive therapy.

ADMINISTRATION

RECONSTITUTION
–

ROUTE
- SC, IV infusion

RATE OF ADMINISTRATION
- 24 hours or 2 hours depending on condition being treated.

COMMENTS
- Add to 100–500 mL of sodium chloride 0.9%

OTHER INFORMATION

- Prodrug – activated by intracellular phosphorylation. The nucleotide that is formed accumulates in the cell and is incorporated into the DNA.
- Regular monitoring is recommended in renal failure.
- Acute renal insufficiency has developed in some patients receiving high-dose cladribine.
- Use with caution advised by manufacturer due to inadequate data on dosing of patients with renal insufficiency therefore use according to clinical need.
- Dosing in renal impairment is from *Drug Prescribing in Renal Failure*, 5th edition, by Aronoff *et al.*
- A study showed that <10% of dose is excreted in urine as metabolites and <20% as parent drug.

Clarithromycin

CLINICAL USE

Antibacterial agent:
- Also adjunct in treatment of duodenal ulcers by eradication of *H. pylori*.

DOSE IN NORMAL RENAL FUNCTION

- Oral: 250–500 mg every 12 hours
- XL: 500–1000 mg once daily
- IV: 500 mg every 12 hours

PHARMACOKINETICS

Molecular weight (daltons)	748
% Protein binding	80
% Excreted unchanged in urine	15–40
Volume of distribution (L/kg)	2–4
Half-life – normal/ ESRF (hrs)	3–7/Prolonged

METABOLISM

The microbiologically active metabolite 14-hydroxyclarithromycin is formed by first pass metabolism. The pharmacokinetics of clarithromycin are non linear. At 250 mg bd, 15–20% of unchanged drug is excreted in the urine. With 500 mg bd dosing urinary excretion is approximately 36%. The 14-hydroxyclarithromycin is the major urinary metabolite and accounts for 10–15% of the dose. Most of the remainder of the dose is eliminated in the faeces, primarily via the bile. Five to 10 per cent of the parent drug is recovered from the faeces.

DOSE IN RENAL IMPAIRMENT GFR (mL/MIN)

30–50	Dose as in normal renal function.
10–30	Oral: 250–500 mg every 12 hours. IV: 250–500 mg every 12 hours.
<10	Oral: 250–500 mg every 12 hours. IV: 250–500 mg every 12 hours. See 'Other information'.

DOSE IN PATIENTS UNDERGOING RENAL REPLACEMENT THERAPIES

CAPD	Unknown dialysability. Dose as in GFR<10 mL/min.
HD	Dialysed. Dose as in GFR<10 mL/min.
HDF/High flux	Dialysed. Dose as in GFR<10 mL/min.
CAV/ VVHD	Unknown dialysability. Dose as in GFR=10–30 mL/min.

IMPORTANT DRUG INTERACTIONS

Potentially hazardous interactions with other drugs
- Anti-arrhythmics: possibly increased disopyramide concentration; increased risk of ventricular arrhythmias with dronedarone – avoid.
- Antibacterials: increased rifabutin concentration – reduce rifabutin dose; clarithromycin concentration reduced by rifamycins.
- Anticoagulants: effect of coumarins enhanced.
- Antidepressants: avoid concomitant use with reboxetine; concentration of trazodone possibly enhanced.
- Anti-epileptics: increased carbamazepine and phenytoin concentration.
- Antihistamines: metabolism of mizolastine inhibited – avoid concomitant use.
- Antimalarials: avoid concomitant administration with artemether/ lumefantrine; increased risk of ventricular arrhythmias with piperaquine with artenimol – avoid.
- Antimuscarinics: avoid concomitant use with tolterodine.
- Antipsychotics: increased risk of ventricular arrhythmias with droperidol and pimozide – avoid concomitant use; possibly increased quetiapine concentration – avoid.
- Antivirals: concentration of both drugs increased with atazanavir and telaprevir; increased risk of rash with efavirenz; concentration of etravirine increased and clarithromycin concentration reduced; concentration of maraviroc possibly increased – consider reducing maraviroc dose; concentration reduced by nevirapine but active metabolite increased also nevirapine concentration increased; concentration of rilpivirine possibly increased – avoid; increased risk of

ventricular arrhythmisa with saquinavir –
avoid; oral clarithromycin reduces
absorption of zidovudine; concentration
increased by ritonavir and tipranavir, also
concentration of tipranavir increased –
reduce dose of clarithromycin in renal
impairment.

- Anxiolytics: metabolism of midazolam
  inhibited.
- Calcium-channel blockers: possibly
  inhibits metabolism of calcium-channel
  blockers.
- Ciclosporin: increased ciclosporin
  concentration (although may take ≅
  5 days after starting clarithromycin before
  increase in ciclosporin levels is seen).
- Colchicine: treatment with both agents has
  been shown in a study to increase the risk
  of fatal colchicine toxicity, especially in
  patients with renal impairment – avoid.[1]
- Cytotoxics: concentration of axitinib
  increased – reduce axitinib dose;
  concentration of crizotinib and everolimus
  possibly increased – avoid; avoid with
  cabazitaxel, nilotinib and pazopanib;
  reduce dose of ruxolitinib; increased risk
  of neutropenia with vinorelbine.
- Diuretics: increased eplerenone
  concentration – avoid concomitant use.
- Ergot alkaloids: increase risk of ergotism –
  avoid concomitant use.
- 5HT$_1$ agonists: increased eletriptan
  concentration – avoid concomitant use.
- Ivabradine: increased ivabradine
  concentration – avoid concomitant use.
- Lipid-lowering drugs: concentration
  of pravastatin increased; increased
  risk of myopathy with atorvastatin and
  simvastatin, avoid with simvastatin and
  max dose of atorvastatin 20 mg.[2]
- Ranolazine: concentration of ranolazine
  possibly increased – avoid.
- Sirolimus: possibly increased sirolimus
  concentration – avoid concomitant use.
- Tacrolimus: increased tacrolimus levels.
- Theophylline: possibly increased
  theophylline concentration.
- Ticagrelor: concentration of ticagrelor
  possibly increased – avoid.

ADMINISTRATION

RECONSTITUTION
- Add 10 mL water for injection to vial
  (500 mg). Add reconstituted product to
  250 mL glucose 5% or sodium chloride
  0.9%. (Stable in 100 mL, but more likely to
  cause phlebitis, pain and inflammation at
  the injection site.)

ROUTE
- IV infusion into one of the larger proximal
  veins.
- Not to be administered by bolus or IM
  injection.

RATE OF ADMINISTRATION
- Over 60 minutes.

OTHER INFORMATION

- Use with caution in renal or hepatic
  failure.
- Oral bioavailability is 55%.
- Patients with GFR<10 mL/min, vomiting
  may be a problem with high doses.

References:
1. Ladva S. Colchicine toxicity reported with
concurrent colchicine and clarithromycin.
Clin Infect Dis. 2005; **41**: 291–300.
2. MHRA. *Drug Safety Update.* Statins:
interactions and updated advice. August
2012; **6**(1): 2–4.

Clemastine

CLINICAL USE

Antihistamine:
- Symptomatic relief of allergy such as hay fever, urticaria

DOSE IN NORMAL RENAL FUNCTION

1–3 mg twice daily

PHARMACOKINETICS

Molecular weight (daltons)	460 (as fumarate)
% Protein binding	95–98[1]
% Excreted unchanged in urine	<1
Volume of distribution (L/kg)	7–15
Half-life – normal/ ESRF (hrs)	21/–

METABOLISM

Extensively metabolised in the liver mainly by mono- and didemethylation and glucuronide conjugation. The metabolites are mainly excreted in the urine.

DOSE IN RENAL IMPAIRMENT GFR (mL/MIN)

20–50	Dose as in normal renal function.
10–20	Dose as in normal renal function.
<10	Dose as in normal renal function.

DOSE IN PATIENTS UNDERGOING RENAL REPLACEMENT THERAPIES

CAPD	Unlikely to be dialysed. Dose as in normal renal function.
HD	Unlikely to be dialysed. Dose as in normal renal function.
HDF/High flux	Probably dialysed. Dose as in normal renal function.
CAV/ VVHD	Probably dialysed. Dose as in normal renal function.

IMPORTANT DRUG INTERACTIONS

Potentially hazardous interactions with other drugs
- Analgesics: sedative properties increased with opioid analgesics.

ADMINISTRATION

RECONSTITUTION

–

ROUTE
- Oral

RATE OF ADMINISTRATION

–

OTHER INFORMATION

Reference:
1. Hansson H, Bergvall K, Bondesson U, *et al*. Clinical pharmacology of clemastine in healthy dogs. *Vet Dermatol*. 2004 Jun; **15**(3): 152–8.

Clindamycin

CLINICAL USE

Antibacterial agent

DOSE IN NORMAL RENAL FUNCTION

- Oral: 150–450 mg every 6 hours.
- Endocarditis prophylaxis: 600 mg 1 hour before procedure.
- IV/IM: 0.6–4.8 g daily in 2–4 divided doses.
- Prophylaxis: 300 mg 15 minutes before procedure then 150 mg 6 hours later.

PHARMACOKINETICS

Molecular weight (daltons)	461.4 (as hydrochloride); 505 (as phosphate)
% Protein binding	>90
% Excreted unchanged in urine	10
Volume of distribution (L/kg)	0.6–1.2
Half-life – normal/ESRF (hrs)	2–3/3–5

METABOLISM

Clindamycin undergoes metabolism, presumably in the liver, to the active N-demethyl and sulfoxide metabolites, and also to some inactive metabolites. About 10% of a dose is excreted in the urine as active drug or metabolites and about 4% in the faeces; the remainder is excreted as inactive metabolites. Excretion is slow, and takes place over several days.

DOSE IN RENAL IMPAIRMENT GFR (mL/MIN)

20–50	Dose as in normal renal function.
10–20	Dose as in normal renal function.
<10	Dose as in normal renal function. See 'Other information'.

DOSE IN PATIENTS UNDERGOING RENAL REPLACEMENT THERAPIES

CAPD	Not dialysed. Dose as in normal renal function.
HD	Not dialysed. Dose as in normal renal function.
HDF/High flux	Unknown dialysability. Dose as in normal renal function.
CAV/VVHD	Not dialysed. Dose as in normal renal function.

IMPORTANT DRUG INTERACTIONS

Potentially hazardous interactions with other drugs

- Ciclosporin: may cause reduced ciclosporin levels.
- Erythromycin: antagonism demonstrated *in vitro*; manufacturers recommend that the two drugs should not be administered concurrently.
- Muscle relaxants: enhanced neuromuscular blockade.

ADMINISTRATION

RECONSTITUTION

–

ROUTE

- Oral, IV, IM

RATE OF ADMINISTRATION

- 10–60 minutes.

COMMENTS

- Dilute prior to IV administration: up to 900 mg, in at least 50 mL of diluent; over 900 mg, in 100 mL of diluent. Compatible with sodium chloride 0.9% or glucose 5%.
- Administration of more than 1200 mg in a single 1 hour infusion is not recommended.
- Doses greater than 600 mg should be given as IV infusions.

OTHER INFORMATION

- Capsules should be swallowed whole with a glass of water.
- Pseudomembranous colitis may occur.
- Periodic kidney and liver function tests should be carried out during prolonged therapy.
- Dosage may require reduction in patients with severe renal impairment due to prolonged half-life.

Clobazam

CLINICAL USE

Benzodiazepine:
- Anticonvulsant
- Anxiolytic

DOSE IN NORMAL RENAL FUNCTION

20–30 mg daily; maximum 60 mg daily

PHARMACOKINETICS

Molecular weight (daltons)	300.7
% Protein binding	85
% Excreted unchanged in urine	87 (unchanged drug and metabolite)
Volume of distribution (L/kg)	0.87–1.83
Half-life – normal/ ESRF (hrs)	11–77 (42 hours for metabolite)/–

METABOLISM

Clobazam is metabolised in the liver by demethylation and hydroxylation; the cytochrome P450 isoenzyme CYP2C19 plays a role in its metabolism. Unlike the 1,4-benzodiazepines such as diazepam, clobazam, a 1,5-benzodiazepine, is hydroxylated at the 4-position rather than the 3-position. Clobazam is excreted unchanged and as its main active metabolite, N-desmethylclobazam, mainly in the urine.

DOSE IN RENAL IMPAIRMENT GFR (mL/MIN)

20–50	Dose as in normal renal function.
10–20	Dose as in normal renal function.
<10	Dose as in normal renal function. Start with low doses.

DOSE IN PATIENTS UNDERGOING RENAL REPLACEMENT THERAPIES

CAPD	Unlikely to be dialysed. Dose as in GFR<10mL/min.
HD	Not dialysed. Dose as in GFR<10mL/min.
HDF/High flux	Unlikely to be dialysed. Dose as in GFR<10mL/min.
CAV/ VVHD	Unknown dialysability. Dose as in normal renal function.

IMPORTANT DRUG INTERACTIONS

Potentially hazardous interactions with other drugs
- Antibacterials: metabolism possibly increased by rifampicin.
- Antipsychotics: increased sedative effects.
- Antivirals: concentration possibly increased by ritonavir.
- Disulfiram: metabolism of clobazam inhibited; increased sedative effects.
- Sodium oxybate: enhanced effects of sodium oxybate – avoid.

ADMINISTRATION

RECONSTITUTION
–
ROUTE
- Oral
RATE OF ADMINISTRATION
–
COMMENTS
–

OTHER INFORMATION

- Syrup is available.
- Causes less sedation than clonazepam.
- There is a case report of clobazam being used to treat phantom limb pain at a dose of 10 mg 3 times a day. (Rice-Oxley CP. The limited list: clobazam for phantom limb pain. BMJ. 1986; 293: 1309.)

Clofazimine

CLINICAL USE

Treatment of leprosy

DOSE IN NORMAL RENAL FUNCTION

- Multibacillary leprosy: 300 mg once monthly (supervised) and 50 mg daily or 100 mg alternate days (unsupervised)
- *Lepromatous lepra* reactions: 300 mg daily

PHARMACOKINETICS

Molecular weight (daltons)	473.4
% Protein binding	Low[1]
% Excreted unchanged in urine	<1
Volume of distribution (L/kg)	High[1]
Half-life – normal/ ESRF (hrs)	10–70 days/ Unchanged[1]

METABOLISM

Because of its lipophilic nature, clofazimine is mainly distributed to fatty tissue and reticuloendothelial cells, including macrophages. Clofazimine accumulates in the body and is largely excreted unchanged in the faeces, both as unabsorbed drug and via biliary excretion. About 1% of the dose is excreted in 24 hours in the urine as unchanged clofazimine and metabolites. A small amount of clofazimine is also excreted through sebaceous and sweat glands, and in sputum.

DOSE IN RENAL IMPAIRMENT GFR (mL/MIN)

20–50	Dose as in normal renal function.
10–20	Dose as in normal renal function.
<10	Dose as in normal renal function.

DOSE IN PATIENTS UNDERGOING RENAL REPLACEMENT THERAPIES

CAPD	Not dialysed. Dose as in normal renal function.
HD	Not dialysed. Dose as in normal renal function.
HDF/High flux	Unknown dialysability. Dose as in normal renal function.
CAV/ VVHD	Unknown dialysability. Dose as in normal renal function.

IMPORTANT DRUG INTERACTIONS

Potentially hazardous interactions with other drugs
- None known

ADMINISTRATION

RECONSTITUTION
–
ROUTE
- Oral
RATE OF ADMINISTRATION
–

OTHER INFORMATION

- In the sunlight a red/brown discolouration may appear on the skin.
- Secretions may also become a red/brown colour.
- Available on a named patient basis.

Reference:
1. Swan SK, Bennett WM. Drug dosing guidelines in patients with renal failure. *West J Med.* 1992 Jun; **156**(6): 633–8.

Clomethiazole (chlormethiazole)

CLINICAL USE

- Alcohol withdrawal
- Insomnia
- Restlessness and agitation.

DOSE IN NORMAL RENAL FUNCTION

- Alcohol withdrawal: 2–4 capsules stat, then:
  — Day 1: 3 capsules 3 or 4 times daily
  — Day 2: 2 capsules 3 or 4 times daily
  — Day 3: 1 capsule 4 times daily
  — Reduce over a further 4–6 days; give a total treatment of not more than 9 days.
- Insomnia: 1–2 capsules at night.
- Restlessness and agitation: 1 capsule 3 times daily.

PHARMACOKINETICS

Molecular weight (daltons)	161.7
% Protein binding	65
% Excreted unchanged in urine	0.1–5
Volume of distribution (L/kg)	4–16
Half-life – normal/ ESRF (hrs)	4/Unchanged

METABOLISM

Clomethiazole is extensively metabolised, probably by first-pass metabolism in the liver with only small amounts appearing unchanged in the urine. The rate of elimination is decreased by about 30% in liver cirrhosis.

DOSE IN RENAL IMPAIRMENT GFR (mL/MIN)

20–50	Dose as in normal renal function.
10–20	Dose as in normal renal function.
<10	Dose as in normal renal function. See 'Other information'.

DOSE IN PATIENTS UNDERGOING RENAL REPLACEMENT THERAPIES

CAPD	Unknown dialysability. Dose as in GFR<10mL/min.
HD	Dialysed. Dose as in GFR<10mL/min.
HDF/High flux	Dialysed. Dose as in GFR<10mL/min.
CAV/ VVHD	Dialysed. Dose as in normal renal function.

IMPORTANT DRUG INTERACTIONS

Potentially hazardous interactions with other drugs
- Antipsychotics: enhanced sedative effects.
- Antivirals: concentration possibly increased by ritonavir.
- Cimetidine: inhibits metabolism of clomethiazole

ADMINISTRATION

RECONSTITUTION
–
ROUTE
- Oral
RATE OF ADMINISTRATION
–
COMMENTS
- Syrup should be stored in a fridge.

OTHER INFORMATION

- Clomethiazole has a high hepatic extraction ratio.
- Increased cerebral sensitivity in renal impairment.
- Manufacturers recommend caution should be observed in patients with chronic renal disease.

Clomipramine hydrochloride

CLINICAL USE

- Depressive illness
- Phobic and obsessional states
- Adjunctive treatment of cataplexy associated with narcolepsy.

DOSE IN NORMAL RENAL FUNCTION

10–250 mg daily
Cataplexy: 10–75 mg daily

PHARMACOKINETICS

Molecular weight (daltons)	351.3
% Protein binding	97.6
% Excreted unchanged in urine	2
Volume of distribution (L/kg)	12–17
Half-life – normal/ ESRF (hrs)	12–36/–

METABOLISM

Clomipramine is extensively demethylated during first-pass metabolism in the liver to its primary active metabolite, desmethylclomipramine.

Clomipramine has been estimated to have a plasma elimination half-life of about 21 hours; that of desmethylclomipramine is longer (about 36 hours).

Paths of metabolism of both clomipramine and desmethylclomipramine include hydroxylation and N-oxidation. About two-thirds of a single dose of clomipramine is excreted in the urine, mainly in the form of its metabolites, either free or in conjugated form; the remainder of the dose appears in the faeces.

DOSE IN RENAL IMPAIRMENT GFR (mL/MIN)

20–50	Dose as in normal renal function.
10–20	Start at lower doses and increase according to response.
<10	Start at lower doses and increase according to response.

DOSE IN PATIENTS UNDERGOING RENAL REPLACEMENT THERAPIES

CAPD	Not dialysed. Dose as in GFR<10 mL/min.
HD	Not dialysed. Dose as in GFR<10 mL/min.
HDF/High flux	Unknown dialysability. Dose as in GFR<10 mL/min.
CAV/ VVHD	Not dialysed. Dose as in GFR=10–20 mL/min.

IMPORTANT DRUG INTERACTIONS

Potentially hazardous interactions with other drugs

- Alcohol: increased sedative effect.
- Analgesics: increased risk of CNS toxicity with tramadol; possibly increased risk of side effects with nefopam; possibly increased sedative effects with opioids.
- Anti-arrhythmics: increased risk of ventricular arrhythmias with amiodarone – avoid concomitant use; increased risk of ventricular arrhythmias with disopyramide, flecainide or propafenone; avoid with dronedarone.
- Antibacterials: increased risk of ventricular arrhythmias with moxifloxacin and possibly telithromycin – avoid concomitant use with moxifloxacin.
- Anticoagulants: may alter anticoagulant effect of coumarins.
- Antidepressants: possibly increased serotonergic effects with duloxetine; enhanced CNS excitation and hypertension with MAOIs and moclobemide; concentration possibly increased with SSRIs.
- Anti-epileptics: convulsive threshold lowered; concentration reduced by carbamazepine, phenobarbital and possibly phenytoin.
- Antimalarials: avoid concomitant use with artemether/lumefantrine and piperaquine with artenimol.
- Antipsychotics: increased risk of ventricular arrhythmias especially with droperidol and pimozide – avoid; increased antimuscarinic effects with clozapine and phenothiazines; concentration increased by antipsychotics.
- Antivirals: increased risk of ventricular arrhythmias with saquinavir – avoid;

concentration possibly increased with ritonavir.

- Atomoxetine: increased risk of ventricular arrhythmias and possibly convulsions.
- Beta-blockers: increased risk of ventricular arrhythmias with sotalol.
- Clonidine: tricyclics antagonise hypotensive effect; increased risk of hypertension on clonidine withdrawal.
- Cytotoxics: increased risk of ventricular arrhythmias with arsenic trioxide.
- Dopaminergics: avoid use with entacapone; CNS toxicity reported with selegiline and rasagiline.
- Methylthioninium: risk of CNS toxicity – avoid if possible.
- Pentamidine: increased risk of ventricular arrhythmias.
- Sympathomimetics: increased risk of hypertension and arrhythmias with adrenaline and noradrenaline; metabolism possibly inhibited by methylphenidate.

ADMINISTRATION

RECONSTITUTION

–

ROUTE

- Oral

OTHER INFORMATION

- Normal doses have been used in dialysis patients long term, but caution as parent drug and active metabolites may accumulate.

Clonazepam

CLINICAL USE

Benzodiazepine:
- Anticonvulsant
- Anxiolytic
- Restless legs syndrome

DOSE IN NORMAL RENAL FUNCTION

- Oral: 0.5–20 mg daily in 3–4 divided doses or as a single dose at night once on maintenance therapy; normal maintenance dose: 4–8 mg daily.
- IV: 1 mg, repeated if necessary.
- Restless legs syndrome: 0.5–4 mg at night.

PHARMACOKINETICS

Molecular weight (daltons)	315.7
% Protein binding	86
% Excreted unchanged in urine	<0.5
Volume of distribution (L/kg)	3
Half-life – normal/ ESRF (hrs)	20–60/–

METABOLISM

Clonazepam is extensively metabolised in the liver, its principal metabolite being 7-aminoclonazepam, which has no antiepileptic activity; minor metabolites are the 7-acetamido- and 3-hydroxy-derivatives. It is excreted mainly in the urine almost entirely as its metabolites in free or conjugated form.

DOSE IN RENAL IMPAIRMENT GFR (mL/MIN)

20–50	Start at low dose and increase according to response.
10–20	Start at low dose and increase according to response.
<10	Start at low dose and increase according to response.

DOSE IN PATIENTS UNDERGOING RENAL REPLACEMENT THERAPIES

CAPD	Unlikely to be dialysed. Dose as in GFR<10 mL/min.
HD	Not dialysed. Dose as in GFR<10 mL/min.
HDF/High flux	Unknown dialysability. Dose as GFR<10 mL/min.
CAV/ VVHD	Not dialysed. Dose as in GFR=10–20 mL/min.

IMPORTANT DRUG INTERACTIONS

Potentially hazardous interactions with other drugs
- Antibacterials: metabolism possibly increased by rifampicin.
- Antipsychotics: increased sedative effects.
- Antivirals: concentration possibly increased by ritonavir.
- Disulfiram: metabolism inhibited, increased sedative effects.
- Sodium oxybate: enhanced effects of sodium oxybate – avoid.

ADMINISTRATION

RECONSTITUTION
- IV bolus: Reconstitute with 1 mL diluent (water for injection) to give 1 mg in 1 mL solution.
- IV infusion: up to 3 mg (3 amps) added to 250 mL sodium chloride 0.9% or glucose 5%.

ROUTE
- Oral, IV bolus or infusion.

RATE OF ADMINISTRATION
- IV bolus: 0.25–0.5 mg over 1 minute.

COMMENTS
- IV infusion of clonazepam is potentially hazardous (especially if prolonged), calling for close and constant observation; best carried out in specialist centres with ICU facilities. Risks include apnoea, hypotension and deep unconsciousness.

OTHER INFORMATION

- In long term administration, active metabolites may accumulate and lower doses should be used.
- Clonazepam is one of several agents that are used in restless legs syndrome, and has also been tried in the management of intractable hiccup where chlorpromazine has failed.

Clonidine hydrochloride

CLINICAL USE

- Hypertension
- Migraine
- Gilles de la Tourette syndrome
- Menopausal flushing.

DOSE IN NORMAL RENAL FUNCTION

- Hypertension: 50–100 mcg 3 times a day, increasing gradually to 1.2 mg daily.
- Slow IV: 150–300 micrograms; maximum 750 mcg in 24 hours.
- Migraine, menopausal flushing, Gilles de la Tourette syndrome: 50–75 mcg twice daily.

PHARMACOKINETICS

Molecular weight (daltons)	266.6
% Protein binding	30–40
% Excreted unchanged in urine	40–60
Volume of distribution (L/kg)	3–6
Half-life – normal/ ESRF (hrs)	10–20/41

METABOLISM

About 50% of a clonidine dose is metabolised in the liver. It is excreted in the urine as unchanged drug and metabolites, 40–60% of an oral dose being excreted in 24 hours as unchanged drug; about 20% of a dose is excreted in the faeces, probably via enterohepatic circulation.

DOSE IN RENAL IMPAIRMENT GFR (mL/MIN)

20–50	Dose as in normal renal function.
10–20	Dose as in normal renal function.
<10	Dose as in normal renal function.

DOSE IN PATIENTS UNDERGOING RENAL REPLACEMENT THERAPIES

CAPD	Not dialysed. Dose as in normal renal function.
HD	Not dialysed. Dose as in normal renal function.
HDF/High flux	Unknown dialysability. Dose as in normal renal function.
CAV/ VVHD	Unknown dialysability. Dose as in normal renal function.

IMPORTANT DRUG INTERACTIONS

Potentially hazardous interactions with other drugs

- Antidepressants: tricyclics antagonise hypotensive effect and also increase risk of hypertension on clonidine withdrawal; increased hypotensive effect with MAOIs; hypotensive effect possibly antagonised by mirtazapine.
- Beta-adrenoreceptor antagonists: increased risk of hypertension on withdrawal.
- Ciclosporin: may increase ciclosporin levels.
- Sympathomimetics: possibly increased risk of hypertension with adrenaline and noradrenaline; serious adverse effects reported with methylphenidate.

ADMINISTRATION

RECONSTITUTION

–

ROUTE

- Oral, IV

RATE OF ADMINISTRATION

- Slow IV injection

COMMENTS

- Minimum volume for infusion 6–50 mcg/ mL in sodium chloride 0.9% or glucose 5%, (UK Critical Care Group, *Minimum Infusion Volumes for Fluid Restricted Critically Ill Patients*, 3rd edition, 2006)

OTHER INFORMATION

- Use in renal impairment: clonidine plasma concentrations for a given dose are 2–3 times higher in patients with severe renal impairment; however, blood pressure control appears satisfactory and adverse effects are not increased.
- Clonidine withdrawal: rebound hypertension if drug is abruptly withdrawn.
- Tricyclic antidepressants may decrease efficacy.

Clopidogrel

CLINICAL USE

Antiplatelet agent

DOSE IN NORMAL RENAL FUNCTION

75 mg daily
Acute coronary syndrome and post-MI:
300 mg loading dose then 75 mg daily (with
aspirin 75–325 mg daily)

PHARMACOKINETICS

Molecular weight (daltons)	419.9 (as hydrogen sulphate)
% Protein binding	98
% Excreted unchanged in urine	50
Volume of distribution (L/kg)	No data
Half-life – normal/ ESRF (hrs)	8 (active metabolite)/–

METABOLISM

Clopidogrel is a prodrug and is extensively
metabolised in the liver, mainly to the
inactive carboxylic acid derivative;
metabolism is mediated by cytochrome P450
isoenzymes including CYP3A4 and CYP2B6,
CYP1A2, CYP1A1, and CYP2C19. The active
metabolite appears to be a thiol derivative.
Clopidogrel and its metabolites are excreted
in urine and in faeces; about 50% of an oral
dose is recovered from the urine and about
46% from the faeces.

DOSE IN RENAL IMPAIRMENT GFR (mL/MIN)

20–50	Dose as in normal renal function.
10–20	Dose as in normal renal function.
<10	Dose as in normal renal function.

DOSE IN PATIENTS UNDERGOING RENAL REPLACEMENT THERAPIES

CAPD	Unlikely to be dialysed. Dose as in normal renal function.
HD	Unlikely to be dialysed. Dose as in normal renal function.
HDF/High flux	Unknown dialysability. Dose as in normal renal function.
CAV/ VVHD	Unlikely to be dialysed. Dose as in normal renal function.

IMPORTANT DRUG INTERACTIONS

Potentially hazardous interactions with other
drugs

- Antibacterials: antiplatelet effect possibly reduced by chloramphenicol, ciprofloxacin and erythromycin.
- Anticoagulants: enhanced anticoagulant effect with coumarins and phenindione; manufacturer advises to avoid concomitant use with warfarin.
- Heparin: increased risk of bleeding.
- Antidepressants: antiplatelet effect possibly reduced by fluoxetine, fluvoxamine and moclobemide.
- Antiepileptics: antiplatelet effect possibly reduced by carbamazepine and oxcarbazepine.
- Antifungals: antiplatelet effect possibly reduced by fluconazole, itraconazole, ketoconazole and voriconazole.
- Antivirals: antiplatelet effect possibly reduced by etravirine.
- Ulcer healing drugs: avoid concomitant use with PPIs and cimetidine if possible due to reduced efficacy of clopidogrel.

ADMINISTRATION

RECONSTITUTION
–

ROUTE
- Oral
RATE OF ADMINISTRATION
–

OTHER INFORMATION
–

Clozapine

CLINICAL USE

Atypical antipsychotic:
- Schizophrenia
- Psychosis in Parkinson's disease

DOSE IN NORMAL RENAL FUNCTION

- Schizophrenia: 200–450 mg daily in divided doses, maximum 900 mg daily
- Psychosis in Parkinson's disease: 25–37.5 mg daily at night, maximum 100 mg daily in 1–2 divided doses

PHARMACOKINETICS

Molecular weight (daltons)	326.8
% Protein binding	95–97
% Excreted unchanged in urine	Minimal (50% as metabolites)
Volume of distribution (L/kg)	1.6–6
Half-life – normal/ ESRF (hrs)	6–26/–

METABOLISM

Clozapine undergoes extensive first-pass metabolism. The systemic drug is almost completely metabolised and routes of metabolism include N-demethylation, hydroxylation, and N-oxidation; the desmethyl metabolite (norclozapine) has limited activity. The metabolism of clozapine is mediated mainly by the cytochrome P450 isoenzyme CYP1A2. Metabolites and trace amounts of unchanged drug are excreted mainly in the urine and also in the faeces.

DOSE IN RENAL IMPAIRMENT GFR (mL/MIN)

20–50	Dose as in normal renal function; use with caution.
10–20	Dose as in normal renal function; use with caution.
<10	Start with a low dose and titrate slowly.

DOSE IN PATIENTS UNDERGOING RENAL REPLACEMENT THERAPIES

CAPD	Unlikely to be dialysed. Dose as in GFR<10 mL/min.
HD	Unlikely to be dialysed. Dose as in GFR<10 mL/min.
HDF/High flux	Unknown dialysability. Dose as in GFR<10 mL/min.
CAV/ VVHD	Unknown dialysability. Dose as in GFR=10–20 mL/min.

IMPORTANT DRUG INTERACTIONS

Potentially hazardous interactions with other drugs
- Anaesthetics: enhanced hypotensive effect.
- Analgesics: increased risk of convulsions with tramadol; enhanced hypotensive and sedative effects with opioids; increased risk of ventricular arrhythmias with methadone.
- Anti-arrhythmics: increased risk of ventricular arrhythmias with anti-arrhythmics that prolong the QT interval; increased risk of arrhythmias with flecainide.
- Antibacterials: concentration possibly increased by erythromycin (possible increased risk of convulsions); concentration increased by ciprofloxacin; concentration possibly reduced by rifampicin; avoid concomitant use with chloramphenicol and sulphonamides (increased risk of agranulocytosis).
- Antidepressants: concentration possibly increased by citalopram, fluoxetine, fluvoxamine, paroxetine, sertraline and venlafaxine (increased risk of toxicity); possibly increased CNS effects of MAOIs; possibly increased antimuscarinic effects with tricyclics; increased concentration of tricyclics.
- Anti-epileptics: antagonises anticonvulsant effect; metabolism accelerated by carbamazepine, phenytoin and possibly phenobarbital; avoid concomitant use with drugs known to cause agranulocytosis; concentration possibly increased or decreased by valproate.
- Antimalarials: avoid concomitant use with artemether/lumefantrine.
- Antipsychotics: avoid concomitant use with depot formulations (cannot be withdrawn quickly if neutropenia occurs).
- Antivirals: concentration increased by ritonavir – avoid concomitant use; increased risk of ventricular arrhythmias with saquinavir – avoid.
- Anxiolytics and hypnotics: increased sedative effects; adverse reports with clozapine and benzodiazepines.
- Atomoxetine: increased risk of ventricular arrhythmias.

- Cytotoxics: increased risk of agranulocytosis – avoid concomitant use; increased risk of ventricular arrhythmias with arsenic trioxide.
- Lithium: increased risk of extrapyramidal side effects and possibly neurotoxicity.
- Penicillamine: increased risk of agranulocytosis – avoid concomitant use.
- Ulcer-healing drugs: effects possibly enhanced by cimetidine; concentration possibly reduced by omeprazole.

ADMINISTRATION

RECONSTITUTION
–

ROUTE
- Oral

RATE OF ADMINISTRATION
–

OTHER INFORMATION

- Contraindicated by manufacturer in severe renal impairment.
- Patient must be registered with appropriate company monitoring scheme.
- Associated with myocarditis (increased risk in the first 2 months) and cardiomyopathy.
- Potentially fatal agranulocytosis and neutropenia have been reported. WCC has to be monitored at least weekly for the first 18 weeks then 2 weekly for weeks 18–52 and then at least 4 weekly.
- Increased risk of side effects especially seizures in doses above 450 mg daily.
- Rarely interstitial nephritis has been reported with clozapine.
- Dose in severe renal impairment taken from personal experience.
- Clozapine can cause severe constipation so patients must be monitored closely especially PD patients.

Co-amoxiclav (amoxicillin/clavulanic acid)

CLINICAL USE

Antibacterial agent

DOSE IN NORMAL RENAL FUNCTION

- IV: 1.2 g every 8 hours (increasing to every 6 hours in severe infections)
- Oral: 375–625 mg 3 times daily

PHARMACOKINETICS

Molecular weight (daltons)	Amoxicillin: 365.4; Clavulanic acid: 199.2
% Protein binding	Amoxicillin: 20; Clavulanic acid: 25
% Excreted unchanged in urine	Amoxicillin: 60; Clavulanic acid: 40
Volume of distribution (L/kg)	Amoxicillin: 0.3; Clavulanic acid: 0.3
Half-life – normal/ ESRF (hrs)	Amoxicillin: 1–1.5/7–20; Clavulanic acid: 1/3–4

METABOLISM

Amoxicillin is metabolised to a limited extent to penicilloic acid which is excreted in the urine. About 60% of an oral dose of amoxicillin is excreted unchanged in the urine by glomerular filtration and tubular secretion. High concentrations have been reported in bile; some may be excreted in the faeces.

Clavulanic acid is mainly excreted in urine (73%). Elimination also occurs via expired air (17%) and in the faeces (8%).

DOSE IN RENAL IMPAIRMENT GFR (mL/MIN)

30–50	Dose as in normal renal function.
10–30	IV: 1.2 g every 12 hours Oral: Dose as in normal renal function.
<10	IV: 1.2 g stat followed by 600 mg every 8 hours or 1.2 g every 12 hours Oral: Dose as in normal renal function.

DOSE IN PATIENTS UNDERGOING RENAL REPLACEMENT THERAPIES

CAPD	Dialysed. Dose as in GFR<10 mL/min.
HD	Dialysed. Dose as in GFR<10 mL/min.
HDF/High flux	Dialysed. Dose as in GFR<10 mL/min.
CAV/ VVHD	Dialysed. Dose as in GFR=10–30 mL/min.

IMPORTANT DRUG INTERACTIONS

Potentially hazardous interactions with other drugs

- Anticoagulants: effects of coumarins are potentially enhanced.
- Oral contraceptives: potentially reduced efficacy.
- Methotrexate: reduced excretion thereby increasing risk of toxicity.
- See 'Other information'.

ADMINISTRATION

RECONSTITUTION
- 600 mg with 10 mL water for injection; 1.2 g with 20 mL water for injection.

ROUTE
- Oral, IV

RATE OF ADMINISTRATION
- IV bolus: over 3–4 minutes.
- Infusion: infuse over 30–40 minutes in 50–100 mL sodium chloride 0.9%.

COMMENTS
- IV preparation is less stable in infusion solutions containing glucose, dextran or bicarbonate. May be injected into drip tubing over period of 3–4 minutes.
- Do not mix with aminoglycosides.

OTHER INFORMATION

- CSM has advised that cholestatic jaundice may occur if treatment exceeds a period of 14 days or up to 6 weeks after treatment has been stopped. The incidence of cholestatic jaundice occurring with co-amoxiclav is higher in males than in females, and prevalent particularly in men over the age of 65 years.
- The probability of co-amoxiclav associated cholestatic jaundice is 6 times more

common than with amoxicillin, and with higher doses of clavulanic acid.
- Doses in renal impairment are taken from personal experience.
- Each 1.2 g vial contains: sodium 2.7 mmol, potassium 1 mmol.
- In patients receiving mycophenolate mofetil, reduction in pre-dose concentration of the active metabolite mycophenolic acid (MPA) of approximately 50% has been reported after starting oral co-amoxiclav. The change in pre-dose level may not accurately represent changes in overall MPA exposure. Therefore, a change in the dose of mycophenolate mofetil should not normally be necessary in the absence of clinical evidence of graft dysfunction. However, close clinical monitoring should be performed during the combination and shortly after antibiotic treatment.

Co-beneldopa (Madopar)

CLINICAL USE
Treatment of Parkinsonism

DOSE IN NORMAL RENAL FUNCTION
150–800 mg daily in divided doses after meals (expressed as levodopa)
MR: Initially 1–2 capsules 3 times daily

PHARMACOKINETICS

Molecular weight (daltons)	Benserazide: 293.7 (as HCl), Levodopa: 197.2
% Protein binding	Benserazide: 0, Levodopa: 10–30
% Excreted unchanged in urine	Benserazide: 0 (64 as metabs), Levodopa: <1
Volume of distribution (L/kg)	Benserazide: No Data, Levodopa: 0.36–1.6
Half-life – normal/ ESRF (hrs)	Benserazide: 1.5/ Increased, Levodopa: 1.5/Increased by 25%

METABOLISM
Levodopa is rapidly decarboxylated by the enzyme aromatic l-amino acid decarboxylase, mostly in the gut, liver, and kidney, to dopamine, which is metabolised in turn, principally to dihydroxyphenylacetic acid (DOPAC) and homovanillic acid (HVA). Other routes of metabolism include O-methylation, transamination, and oxidation, producing a variety of minor metabolites including noradrenaline and 3-O-methyldopa; the latter may accumulate in the CNS due to its relatively long half-life. About 80% of an oral dose of levodopa is excreted in the urine within 24 hours, mainly as dihydroxyphenylacetic and homovanillic acids. Only small amounts of levodopa are excreted unchanged in the faeces.

Benserazide is rapidly excreted in the urine in the form of metabolites, mostly within the first 6 hours; 85% of urinary excretion occurs within 12 hours. It is mainly metabolised in the gut and appears to protect levodopa against decarboxylation primarily in the gut, but also in the rest of the body, mainly by way of its metabolite trihydroxybenzylhydrazine.

DOSE IN RENAL IMPAIRMENT GFR (mL/MIN)

20–50	Dose as in normal renal function.
10–20	Dose as in normal renal function.
<10	Dose as in normal renal function.

DOSE IN PATIENTS UNDERGOING RENAL REPLACEMENT THERAPIES

CAPD	Unlikely to be dialysed. Dose as in normal renal function.
HD	Unlikely to be dialysed. Dose as in normal renal function.
HDF/High flux	Dialysed. Dose as in normal renal function.
CAV/ VVHD	Unknown dialysability. Dose as in normal renal function.

IMPORTANT DRUG INTERACTIONS
Potentially hazardous interactions with other drugs
- Anaesthetics: risk of arrhythmias with volatile liquid anaesthetics such as halothane.
- Antidepressants: hypertensive crisis with MAOIs and linezolid (including moclobemide) – avoid for at least 2 weeks after stopping MAOI.
- Bupropion: increased risk of side effects of levodopa
- Ferrous sulphate: reduces AUC of levodopa by 30–50%, clinically significant in some but not all patients.

ADMINISTRATION
RECONSTITUTION
–
ROUTE
- Oral
RATE OF ADMINISTRATION
–

OTHER INFORMATION
- Can be used to treat restless legs syndrome at a dose of 62.5–125 mg.
- Urine may be red-tinged and turn dark on standing, due to metabolites.
- Serum uric acid and blood urea nitrogen levels are occasionally elevated.

Co-careldopa (Sinemet)

CLINICAL USE

Treatment of Parkinsonism

DOSE IN NORMAL RENAL FUNCTION

150–800 mg carbidopa daily in divided doses after meals
MR: initially 1 tablet twice daily

PHARMACOKINETICS

Molecular weight (daltons)	Carbidopa: 244.2, Levodopa: 197.2
% Protein binding	Carbidopa: 36, Levodopa: 10–30
% Excreted unchanged in urine	Carbidopa: 30, Levodopa: <1
Volume of distribution (L/kg)	Carbidopa: No data, Levodopa: 0.36–1.6
Half-life – normal/ ESRF (hrs)	Carbidopa: 2–3, Levodopa: 0.6–1.3/ Unknown

METABOLISM

Levodopa is rapidly decarboxylated by the enzyme aromatic l-amino acid decarboxylase, mostly in the gut, liver, and kidney, to dopamine, which is metabolised in turn, principally to dihydroxyphenylacetic acid (DOPAC) and homovanillic acid (HVA). Other routes of metabolism include O-methylation, transamination, and oxidation, producing a variety of minor metabolites including noradrenaline and 3-O-methyldopa; the latter may accumulate in the CNS due to its relatively long half-life. About 80% of an oral dose of levodopa is excreted in the urine within 24 hours, mainly as dihydroxyphenylacetic and homovanillic acids. Only small amounts of levodopa are excreted unchanged in the faeces.

Carbidopa inhibits the peripheral decarboxylation of levodopa to dopamine. It is rapidly excreted in the urine both unchanged and in the form of metabolites.

DOSE IN RENAL IMPAIRMENT GFR (mL/MIN)

20–50	Dose as in normal renal function.
10–20	Dose as in normal renal function.
<10	Dose as in normal renal function.

DOSE IN PATIENTS UNDERGOING RENAL REPLACEMENT THERAPIES

CAPD	Unlikely to be dialysed. Dose as in normal renal function.
HD	Unlikely to be dialysed. Dose as in normal renal function.
HDF/High flux	Dialysed. Dose as in normal renal function.
CAV/ VVHD	Unknown dialysability. Dose as in normal renal function.

IMPORTANT DRUG INTERACTIONS

Potentially hazardous interactions with other drugs
- Anaesthetics: risk of arrhythmias with volatile liquid anaesthetics such as halothane.
- Antidepressants: hypertensive crisis with MAOIs and linezolid (including moclobemide) – avoid for at least 2 weeks after stopping MAOI.
- Bupropion: increased risk of side effects of levodopa
- Ferrous sulphate: reduces AUC of levodopa by 30–50%, clinically significant in some but not all patients.

ADMINISTRATION

RECONSTITUTION

–

ROUTE
- Oral

RATE OF ADMINISTRATION

–

OTHER INFORMATION

- Can be used to treat restless legs syndrome.
- May cause dark urine.

Co-codamol (paracetamol and codeine phosphate)

CLINICAL USE
Analgesic

DOSE IN NORMAL RENAL FUNCTION
1–2 tablets up to 4 times a day.

PHARMACOKINETICS

Molecular weight (daltons)	Paracetamol: 151.2; Codeine: 317.4 (Codeine phosphate 406.4)
% Protein binding	Paracetamol: 20–30; Codeine: 7
% Excreted unchanged in urine	Paracetamol: <5; Codeine: 0
Volume of distribution (L/kg)	Paracetamol: 1–1.2; Codeine: 3–4
Half-life – normal/ ESRF (hrs)	Paracetamol: 1–4/ Unchanged; Codeine: 2.5–4/13

METABOLISM
Paracetamol is metabolised mainly in the liver and excreted in the urine mainly as the glucuronide and sulfate conjugates. Less than 5% is excreted as unchanged paracetamol. A minor hydroxylated metabolite (N-acetyl-p-benzoquinoneimine) is usually produced in very small amounts by cytochrome P450 isoenzymes (mainly CYP2E1 and CYP3A4) in the liver and kidney. It is usually detoxified by conjugation with glutathione but may accumulate after paracetamol overdosage and cause tissue damage.

Codeine is metabolised by O- and N-demethylation in the liver to morphine, norcodeine, and other metabolites including normorphine and hydrocodone. Metabolism to morphine is mediated by the cytochrome P450 isoenzyme CYP2D6, which shows genetic polymorphism. Codeine and its metabolites are excreted almost entirely by the kidney, mainly as conjugates with glucuronic acid.

DOSE IN RENAL IMPAIRMENT GFR (mL/MIN)

20–50	Dose as in normal renal function.
10–20	Dose as in normal renal function.
<10	Dose as in normal renal function.

DOSE IN PATIENTS UNDERGOING RENAL REPLACEMENT THERAPIES

CAPD	Unlikely to be dialysed. Dose as in normal renal function.
HD	Not dialysed. Dose as in normal renal function.
HDF/High flux	Unknown dialysability. Dose as in normal renal function.
CAV/ VVHD	Not dialysed. Dose as in normal renal function.

IMPORTANT DRUG INTERACTIONS
Potentially hazardous interactions with other drugs
- Antibacterials: metabolism increased by rifampicin.
- Antidepressants: possible CNS excitation or depression with MAOIs – avoid concomitant use, and for 2 weeks after stopping MAOI; possible CNS excitation or depression with moclobemide; increased sedative effects with tricyclics.
- Antihistamines: increased sedative effects with sedating antihistamines.
- Antipsychotics: enhanced hypotensive and sedative effects.
- Dopaminergics: avoid with selegiline.
- Sodium oxybate: enhanced effect of sodium oxybate – avoid concomitant use.

ADMINISTRATION
RECONSTITUTION
–
ROUTE
- Oral
RATE OF ADMINISTRATION
–

OTHER INFORMATION

- Available in 3 strengths: (1) 8/500; 8 mg codeine phosphate/500 mg paracetamol, (2) 15/500; 15 mg codeine phosphate/500 mg paracetamol; (3) 30/500; 30 mg codeine phosphate/500 mg paracetamol.
- 30/500 formulation: may cause drowsiness, due to increased cerebral sensitivity in patients with renal failure and put patients at risk of constipation.

- Effervescent formulations of Solpadol and Tylex (30/500) should be avoided in renal impairment. They contain 16.9 mmol and 13.6 mmol sodium per tablet respectively.

Codeine phosphate

CLINICAL USE

- Analgesic
- Antidiarrhoeal
- Cough suppressant.

DOSE IN NORMAL RENAL FUNCTION

30–60 mg up to every 4 hours.

PHARMACOKINETICS

Molecular weight (daltons)	406.4
% Protein binding	7
% Excreted unchanged in urine	0
Volume of distribution (L/kg)	3–4
Half-life – normal/ ESRF (hrs)	2.5–4/13

METABOLISM

Codeine is metabolised by O- and N-demethylation in the liver to morphine, norcodeine, and other metabolites including normorphine and hydrocodone. Metabolism to morphine is mediated by the cytochrome P450 isoenzyme CYP2D6, which shows genetic polymorphism. Codeine and its metabolites are excreted almost entirely by the kidney, mainly as conjugates with glucuronic acid.

DOSE IN RENAL IMPAIRMENT GFR (mL/MIN)

20–50	Dose as in normal renal function.
10–20	30 mg up to every 4 hours. Increase if tolerated.
<10	30 mg up to every 6 hours. Increase if tolerated.

DOSE IN PATIENTS UNDERGOING RENAL REPLACEMENT THERAPIES

CAPD	Unlikely to be dialysed. Dose as in GFR<10 mL/min.
HD	Not dialysed. Dose as in GFR<10 mL/min.
HDF/High flux	Unknown dialysability. Dose as in GFR<10 mL/min.
CAV/ VVHD	Not dialysed. Dose as in GFR=10–20 mL/min.

IMPORTANT DRUG INTERACTIONS

Potentially hazardous interactions with other drugs

- Antibacterials: metabolism increased by rifampicin.
- Antidepressants: possible CNS excitation or depression with MAOIs – avoid concomitant use, and for 2 weeks after stopping MAOI; possible CNS excitation or depression with moclobemide; increased sedative effects with tricyclics.
- Antihistamines: increased sedative effects with sedating antihistamines.
- Antipsychotics: enhanced hypotensive and sedative effects.
- Dopaminergics: avoid with selegiline.
- Sodium oxybate: enhanced effect of sodium oxybate – avoid concomitant use.

ADMINISTRATION

RECONSTITUTION
–
ROUTE
- Oral, IV, IM, SC
RATE OF ADMINISTRATION
- IV bolus
COMMENTS
–

OTHER INFORMATION

- Increased risk of drowsiness due to increased cerebral sensitivity in patients with renal failure.
- Increased risk of constipation – caution in patients on peritoneal dialysis.

Co-dydramol (paracetamol and dihydrocodeine)

CLINICAL USE

Analgesic

DOSE IN NORMAL RENAL FUNCTION

1–2 tablets up to 4 times a day.

PHARMACOKINETICS

Molecular weight (daltons)	Paracetamol: 151.2; Dihydrocodeine: 451.5 (as tartrate)
% Protein binding	Paracetamol: 20–30; Dihydrocodeine: –
% Excreted unchanged in urine	Paracetamol: <5; Dihydrocodeine: 13–22
Volume of distribution (L/kg)	Paracetamol: 1–2; Dihydrocodeine: 1.1
Half-life – normal/ ESRF (hrs)	Paracetamol: 1–4/Unchanged; Dihydrocodeine: 3.5–5/6+

METABOLISM

Paracetamol is metabolised mainly in the liver and excreted in the urine mainly as the glucuronide and sulfate conjugates. Less than 5% is excreted as unchanged paracetamol. A minor hydroxylated metabolite (N-acetyl-p-benzoquinoneimine) is usually produced in very small amounts by cytochrome P450 isoenzymes (mainly CYP2E1 and CYP3A4) in the liver and kidney. It is usually detoxified by conjugation with glutathione but may accumulate after paracetamol overdosage and cause tissue damage.

Dihydrocodeine is metabolised in the liver via the cytochrome P450 isoenzyme CYP2D6, to dihydromorphine, which has potent analgesic activity, although the analgesic effect of dihydrocodeine appears to be mainly due to the parent compound; some is also converted via CYP3A4 to nordihydrocodeine. Dihydrocodeine is excreted in urine as unchanged drug and metabolites, including glucuronide conjugates.

DOSE IN RENAL IMPAIRMENT GFR (mL/MIN)

20–50	Dose as in normal renal function.
10–20	50–100% of dose every 6 hours.
<10	50–100% of dose every 6–8 hours.

DOSE IN PATIENTS UNDERGOING RENAL REPLACEMENT THERAPIES

CAPD	Not dialysed. Dose as in GFR<10 mL/min.
HD	Not dialysed. Dose as in GFR<10 mL/min.
HDF/High flux	Unknown dialysability. Dose as in GFR<10 mL/min.
CAV/ VVHD	Unknown dialysability. Dose as in GFR=10–20 mL/min.

IMPORTANT DRUG INTERACTIONS

Potentially hazardous interactions with other drugs
- Antidepressants: possible CNS excitation or depression with MAOIs – avoid concomitant use, and for 2 weeks after stopping MAOI; possible CNS excitation or depression with moclobemide; increased sedative effects with tricyclics.
- Antihistamines: increased sedative effects with sedating antihistamines.
- Antipsychotics: enhanced hypotensive and sedative effects.
- Dopaminergics: avoid with selegiline.
- Sodium oxybate: enhanced effect of sodium oxybate – avoid concomitant use.

ADMINISTRATION

RECONSTITUTION
–

ROUTE
- Oral

RATE OF ADMINISTRATION
–

COMMENTS
–

OTHER INFORMATION

- Active metabolites of dihydrocodeine accumulate in renal impairment (drowsiness/lightheadedness/constipation). Increased cerebral sensitivity in patients with renal failure.

Colchicine

CLINICAL USE

- Acute gout
- Short term prophylaxis during initial therapy with allopurinol and uricosuric drugs
- Prophylaxis of familial Mediterranean fever (unlicensed).

DOSE IN NORMAL RENAL FUNCTION

- Acute: 500 micrograms 2–4 times daily until pain relieved or vomiting/diarrhoea occurs. Maximum of 6 mg per course. Do not repeat course within 3 days.
- Short term prophylaxis: 500 micrograms 2 times per day.
- Prophylaxis of familial Mediterranean fever: 0.5–2 mg daily.

PHARMACOKINETICS

Molecular weight (daltons)	399.4
% Protein binding	30–50
% Excreted unchanged in urine	5–20
Volume of distribution (L/kg)	1–2
Half-life – normal/ ESRF (hrs)	4.4/18.8

METABOLISM

The absorption of colchicine from the gastrointestinal tract is thought to be limited by its expulsion by P-glycoprotein, for which colchicine is a substrate. It is demethylated in the liver via the cytochrome P450 isoenzyme CYP3A4 to 2 primary metabolites, 2-O-demethylcolchicine and 3-O-demethylcolchicine (2-DMC and 3-DMC, respectively), and 1 minor metabolite, 10-O-demethylcolchicine (also known as colchiceine). Enterohepatic recycling occurs. The main route of elimination is hepatobiliary excretion in the faeces. Renal excretion accounts for 10–20% of colchicine elimination in patients with normal renal function.

DOSE IN RENAL IMPAIRMENT GFR (mL/MIN)

20–50	Reduce dose or dosage interval by 50%.
10–20	Reduce dose or dosage interval by 50%
<10	500 mcg 3–4 times a day; maximum total dose of 3 mg.

DOSE IN PATIENTS UNDERGOING RENAL REPLACEMENT THERAPIES

CAPD	Not dialysed. Dose as in GFR<10 mL/min.
HD	Not dialysed. Dose as in GFR<10 mL/min.
HDF/High flux	Unknown dialysability. Dose as in GFR<10 mL/min.
CAV/ VVHD	Unknown dialysability. Dose as in GFR=10–20 mL/min.

IMPORTANT DRUG INTERACTIONS

Potentially hazardous interactions with other drugs

- Anti-arrhythmics: possible increased risk of toxicity with amiodarone.
- Antibacterials: possible increased risk of toxicity with azithromycin, clarithromycin, erythromycin and telithromycin – suspend or reduce dose of colchicine, avoid concomitant use in renal or hepatic failure.
- Antifungals: possible increased risk of toxicity with itraconazole and ketoconazole – suspend or reduce dose of colchicine, avoid concomitant use in renal or hepatic failure.
- Antivirals: possible increased risk of toxicity with atazanavir, indinavir, ritonavir and telaprevir – suspend or reduce dose of colchicine, avoid concomitant use in renal or hepatic failure.
- Calcium-channel blockers: possible increased risk of toxicity with diltiazem and verapamil – suspend or reduce dose of colchicine, avoid concomitant use in renal or hepatic failure.
- Cardiac glycosides: possible increased risk of myopathy with digoxin.
- Ciclosporin: risk of myopathy or rhabdomyolysis, also increased blood-ciclosporin concentrations and nephrotoxicity – suspend or reduce dose of colchicine, avoid concomitant use in renal or hepatic failure.
- Grapefruit juice: possible increased risk of toxicity.

- Lipid-regulating drugs: possible increased risk of myopathy with fibrates and statins.

ADMINISTRATION

RECONSTITUTION

–

ROUTE

- Oral

RATE OF ADMINISTRATION

–

COMMENTS

–

OTHER INFORMATION

- Colchicine has a narrow therapeutic window and is extremely toxic and may be fatal in overdose. Patients at particular risk of toxicity are those with renal or hepatic impairment, gastrointestinal or cardiac disease, and patients at extremes of age.
- The signs of overdose may be delayed.
- If nausea, vomiting or diarrhoea occurs, stop therapy.
- Manufacturer contraindicates colchicine in GFR<10 mL/min but in practice is used routinely at low doses to treat gout in patients with severe renal impairment.
- Dose in renal impairment is from *Drug Prescribing in Renal Failure*, 5th edition, by Aronoff *et al.*, and *Drug Dosage in Renal Insufficiency* by Seyffart G.
- In CKD 5, colchicine can be administered concurrently with allopurinol, but seek specialist advice.

Colesevelam hydrochloride

CLINICAL USE

- Hyperlipidaemias

DOSE IN NORMAL RENAL FUNCTION

- Monotherapy: 3.75 g daily (in 1–2 divided doses). Maximum 4.375 g daily.
- Combination therapy: 2.5–3.75 g daily in 1–2 divided doses.

PHARMACOKINETICS

Molecular weight (daltons)	Small
% Protein binding	0
% Excreted unchanged in urine	0.05
Volume of distribution (L/kg)	Not absorbed.
Half-life – normal/ ESRF (hrs)	Not absorbed.

METABOLISM

Not absorbed.

DOSE IN RENAL IMPAIRMENT GFR (mL/MIN)

20–50	Dose as in normal renal function.
10–20	Dose as in normal renal function.
<10	Dose as in normal renal function.

DOSE IN PATIENTS UNDERGOING RENAL REPLACEMENT THERAPIES

CAPD	Not dialysed. Dose as in normal renal function.
HD	Not dialysed. Dose as in normal renal function.
HDF/High flux	Not dialysed. Dose as in normal renal function.
CAV/ VVHD	Not dialysed. Dose as in normal renal function.

IMPORTANT DRUG INTERACTIONS

Potentially hazardous interactions with other drugs

- Ciclosporin: may reduce absorption of ciclosporin.

ADMINISTRATION

RECONSTITUTION

–

ROUTE

- Oral

RATE OF ADMINISTRATION

–

COMMENTS

- Administer other drugs at least 4 hours before or after colesevelam.

Colestipol hydrochloride

CLINICAL USE

Hyperlipidaemias, particularly type IIa

DOSE IN NORMAL RENAL FUNCTION

5 g once or twice daily, increased if necessary at intervals of 1–2 months, to a maximum of 30 g daily.

PHARMACOKINETICS

Molecular weight (daltons)	–
% Protein binding	0
% Excreted unchanged in urine	0
Volume of distribution (L/kg)	Not absorbed.
Half-life – normal/ ESRF (hrs)	Not absorbed.

METABOLISM

Not applicable as colestipol is not systemically absorbed.

DOSE IN RENAL IMPAIRMENT GFR (mL/MIN)

20–50	Dose as in normal renal function.
10–20	Dose as in normal renal function.
<10	Dose as in normal renal function.

DOSE IN PATIENTS UNDERGOING RENAL REPLACEMENT THERAPIES

CAPD	Not dialysed. Dose as in normal renal function.
HD	Not dialysed. Dose as in normal renal function.
HDF/High flux	Not dialysed. Dose as in normal renal function.
CAV/ VVHD	Not dialysed. Dose as in normal renal function.

IMPORTANT DRUG INTERACTIONS

Potentially hazardous interactions with other drugs

- Anticoagulants: may enhance or reduce effects of coumarins and phenindione.
- Ciclosporin: No reports of an interaction; however, ciclosporin levels should be carefully monitored if colestipol and ciclosporin are prescribed concurrently, as colestipol may interfere with ciclosporin absorption.

ADMINISTRATION

RECONSTITUTION

–

ROUTE

- Oral

RATE OF ADMINISTRATION

–

COMMENTS

- Other drugs should be taken at least 1 hour before or 4–6 hours after colestipol to reduce possible interference with absorption.
- Colestipol granules may be administered as a suspension in water or a flavoured vehicle.
- Colestipol orange contains 32.5 mg aspartame (18.2 mg phenylalanine) per sachet.

OTHER INFORMATION

- Colestipol may interfere with the absorption of fat soluble vitamins.

Colestyramine (cholestyramine)

CLINICAL USE

- Hyperlipidaemias
- Pruritis associated with partial biliary obstruction and primary biliary cirrhosis
- Diarrhoeal disorders.

DOSE IN NORMAL RENAL FUNCTION

- Lipid reduction: 12–24 g daily (in single or up to 4 divided doses). Maximum 36 g daily.
- Pruritis: 4–8 g daily.
- Diarrhoeal disorders: 12–24 g daily. Maximum 36 g daily.

PHARMACOKINETICS

Molecular weight (daltons)	–
% Protein binding	0
% Excreted unchanged in urine	0
Volume of distribution (L/kg)	Not absorbed.
Half-life – normal/ ESRF (hrs)	Not absorbed.

METABOLISM

Not applicable as colestyramine resin is not absorbed from the digestive tract.

DOSE IN RENAL IMPAIRMENT GFR (mL/MIN)

20–50	Dose as in normal renal function.
10–20	Dose as in normal renal function.
<10	Dose as in normal renal function.

DOSE IN PATIENTS UNDERGOING RENAL REPLACEMENT THERAPIES

CAPD	Not dialysed. Dose as in normal renal function.
HD	Not dialysed. Dose as in normal renal function.
HDF/High flux	Not dialysed. Dose as in normal renal function.
CAV/ VVHD	Not dialysed. Dose as in normal renal function.

IMPORTANT DRUG INTERACTIONS

Potentially hazardous interactions with other drugs

- Anticoagulants: effect of coumarins and phenindione may be enhanced or reduced.
- Ciclosporin: may interact unpredictably with ciclosporin. Take ciclosporin at least 1 hour before or 4–6 hours after to prevent problems with absorption.
- Leflunomide: avoid concomitant use.
- Raloxifene, thyroid hormones, bile acids, valproate, cardiac glycosides and mycophenolate mofetil: absorption reduced.

ADMINISTRATION

RECONSTITUTION
- Mix with water, or a suitable liquid such as fruit juice, and stir to a uniform consistency.
- May also be mixed with skimmed milk, thin soups, apple sauce, etc.

ROUTE
- Oral

RATE OF ADMINISTRATION
–

COMMENTS
- Do not take in dry form.
- Administer other drugs at least 1 hour before or 4–6 hours after colestyramine.
- Prepare powder immediately prior to administration.

OTHER INFORMATION

- Hyperchloraemic acidosis occasionally reported on prolonged use of colestyramine.
- On chronic use, an increased bleeding tendency may occur associated with vitamin K deficiency.

Colistimethate sodium (Colistin)

CLINICAL USE

Polymyxins:
- Antibacterial agent

DOSE IN NORMAL RENAL FUNCTION

- IV: <60 kg: 50 000–75 000 units/kg in 3 divided doses
- >60 kg 1–2 million units every 8 hours
- Nebulised solution: 1–2 million units every 12 hours

PHARMACOKINETICS

Molecular weight (daltons)	Approximately 1748
% Protein binding	55[1]
% Excreted unchanged in urine	80
Volume of distribution (L/kg)	0.09–0.34[1]
Half-life – normal/ESRF (hrs)	1.5–8/13–20 (IV), 6.8–14 (Nebulised)

METABOLISM

Studies on the gastrointestinal absorption of colistin have shown no significant systemic absorption following oral administration.

Colistimethate sodium is converted to the colistin base by hydrolysis *in vivo*. As 80% of the dose can be recovered unchanged in the urine, and there is no biliary excretion, it can be assumed that the remaining drug is inactivated in the tissues. The mechanism is unknown.

DOSE IN RENAL IMPAIRMENT GFR (mL/MIN)

See 'other information'. Weight assumed to be >60 kg.

20–50	IV: 1–2 million units every 8 hours.
10–20	IV: 1 million units every 12–18 hours.
<10	IV: 1 million units every 18–24 hours.

DOSE IN PATIENTS UNDERGOING RENAL REPLACEMENT THERAPIES

CAPD	Dialysed. Dose as in GFR<10 mL/min.
HD	Not dialysed. Dose as in GFR<10 mL/min.
HDF/High flux	Dialysed. Dose as in GFR<10 mL/min.
CAV/VVHD	Not dialysed. 2 million units every 48 hours.[1]

IMPORTANT DRUG INTERACTIONS

Potentially hazardous interactions with other drugs
- Antibacterials: increased risk of nephrotoxicity with aminoglycosides and capreomycin; increased risk of nephrotoxicity and ototoxicity with vancomycin.
- Ciclosporin: increased risk of nephrotoxicity.
- Cytotoxics: increased risk of nephrotoxicity and possibly ototoxicity with platinum agents.
- Diuretics: increased risk of ototoxicity with loop diuretics.
- Muscle relaxants: polymyxins enhance the effect of non-depolarising muscle relaxants and suxamethonium.
- Parasympathomimetics: polymyxins antagonise the effect of neostigmine and pyridostigmine.

ADMINISTRATION

RECONSTITUTION
- Sodium chloride 0.9% or water for injection

ROUTE
- IV, Nebulised, Topical

RATE OF ADMINISTRATION
- Infusion: over 30 minutes
- Bolus: over 5 minutes (only if patient has a totally implantable venous access device, TIVAD)

COMMENTS
- IV: Give in 10–50 mL sodium chloride 0.9% or water for injection.
- Inhalation: Dissolve in 2–4 mL sodium chloride 0.9% or water for injection.

OTHER INFORMATION

- Less than 0.5 mmol/L sodium per 0.5–2 million unit vial (before reconstitution).
- Pharmacokinetic data: (Lee CS, Marbury TC. Drug therapy in patients undergoing haemodialysis: clinical pharmacokinetic considerations. *Clin Pharmacokinet*. 1984; **9**: 42–66.)

- Can cause renal failure, muscle weakness and apnoea in overdose. Risk factors are usually the IV route, high doses, concomitant use with other nephrotoxic agents, and if the dose is not reduced appropriately in renal failure.
- In renal impairment, neonates, and cystic fibrosis patients, plasma concentrations of 10–15 mg/L (125–200 units/mL) are usually adequate.
- Dosage schedules in renal impairment vary according to which preparation is being used. Doses in the following table are from Colomycin SPC.
- Promixin SPC (IV):
  GFR:
  40–75 mL/min: 1–1.5 MIU twice daily
  25–40 mL/min: 1 MIU once or twice daily
  <25 mL/min: 1–1.5 MIU every 36 hours

Reference:

1. Trotman RL, Williamson JC, Shoemaker DM, *et al.* Antibiotic dosing in critically ill adult patients receiving continuous renal replacement therapy. *Clin Infect Dis.* 2005 Oct 15; **41**: 1159–66.

Co-trimoxazole (trimethoprim + sulfamethoxazole)

CLINICAL USE

Antibacterial agent:
- Treatment and prophylaxis of *Pneumocystis jiroveci* pneumonia (PCP)
- Acute exacerbations of chronic bronchitis
- Urinary tract infections, on microbiological advice

DOSE IN NORMAL RENAL FUNCTION

- PCP: 120 mg/kg/day in 2–4 divided doses. Oral prophylaxis: 480–960 mg daily or 960 mg on alternate days.
- Acute exacerbations of chronic bronchitis and urinary tract infections on microbiological advice:
  — IV: 960 mg – 1.44 g twice a day
  — Oral: 960 mg twice a day.

PHARMACOKINETICS

Molecular weight (daltons)	Sulfamethoxazole: 253.3; Trimethoprim: 290.3
% Protein binding	Sulfamethoxazole: 70; Trimethoprim: 45
% Excreted unchanged in urine	Sulfamethoxazole: 15–30; Trimethoprim: 40–60
Volume of distribution (L/kg)	Sulfamethoxazole: 0.28–0.38; Trimethoprim: 1–2.2
Half-life – normal/ ESRF (hrs)	Sulfamethoxazole: 6–12/20–50; Trimethoprim: 8–10/20–49

METABOLISM

Sulfamethoxazole undergoes conjugation mainly in the liver, chiefly to the inactive N^{4}-acetyl derivative; this metabolite represents about 15% of the total amount of sulfamethoxazole in the blood. Metabolism is increased in patients with renal impairment and decreased in those with hepatic impairment. Elimination in the urine is dependent on pH. About 80 to 100% of a dose is excreted in the urine, of which about 60% is in the form of the acetyl derivative, with the remainder as unchanged drug and glucuronide.

Trimethoprim is excreted mainly by the kidneys through glomerular filtration and tubular secretion. About 10–20% of trimethoprim is metabolised in the liver and small amounts are excreted in the faeces via the bile, but most, about 40–60% of a dose, is excreted in urine, mainly as unchanged drug, within 24 hours.

DOSE IN RENAL IMPAIRMENT GFR (mL/MIN)

GFR	
30–50	Dose as in normal renal function.
15–30	50% of dose; PCP: 60 mg/kg twice daily for 3 days then 30 mg/kg twice daily.
<15	50% of dose; PCP: 30 mg/kg twice daily. (This should only be given if haemodialysis facilities are available.)

DOSE IN PATIENTS UNDERGOING RENAL REPLACEMENT THERAPIES

CAPD	Not dialysed. Dose as in GFR<15 mL/min.
HD	Dialysed. Dose as in GFR<15 mL/ min.
HDF/High flux	Dialysed. Dose as in GFR<15 mL/ min.
CAV/ VVHD	Dialysed. Dose as in GFR=15– 30 mL/min.

IMPORTANT DRUG INTERACTIONS

Potentially hazardous interactions with other drugs
- Anti-arrhythmics: increased risk of ventricular arrhythmias with amiodarone – avoid concomitant use; concentration of procainamide increased.
- Antibacterials: increased risk of crystalluria with methenamine.
- Anticoagulants: effect of coumarins enhanced; metabolism of phenindione possibly inhibited.
- Anti-epileptics: antifolate effect and concentration of phenytoin increased.
- Antimalarials: increased risk of antifolate effect with pyrimethamine.
- Antipsychotics: avoid concomitant use with clozapine, increased risk of agranulocytosis.

- Ciclosporin: increased risk of nephrotoxicity; possibly reduced ciclosporin levels.
- Cytotoxics: increased risk of haematological toxicity with azathioprine, methotrexate and mercaptopurine. Antifolate effect of methotrexate increased.

ADMINISTRATION

RECONSTITUTION

–

ROUTE

- IV, oral

RATE OF ADMINISTRATION

- Over 60–90 minutes
- Alternatively: 2–3 hours for high doses as undiluted solution via central line (unlicensed)

COMMENTS

- For an IV infusion dilute each 5 mL co-trimoxazole strong solution with 125 mL sodium chloride 0.9% or glucose 5%.
- Glaxo Smith Kline: dilute 5 mL to 75 mL glucose 5% and administer over 1 hour if fluid restricted.

OTHER INFORMATION

- Alternative dosing (for acute exacerbations of chronic bronchitis and urinary tract infections) on microbiological advice only; not PCP.
- After 2–3 days, plasma samples collected 12 hours post dose should have levels of sulfamethoxazole not higher than 150 micrograms/mL. If higher, stop treatment until levels fall below 120 micrograms/mL.
- Plasma levels of trimethoprim should be 5 micrograms/mL or higher, for optimum efficacy for PCP.
- Folic acid supplementation may be necessary during chronic therapy.
- Monthly blood counts advisable.

Crisantaspase

CLINICAL USE

Antineoplastic agent:
- Treatment of acute lymphoblastic leukaemia and other neoplastic conditions

DOSE IN NORMAL RENAL FUNCTION

6000 units/m^2 (200 Units/kg), three times a week for 3 weeks.
Or according to local protocol

PHARMACOKINETICS

Molecular weight (daltons)	31 732
% Protein binding	No data
% Excreted unchanged in urine	Minimal
Volume of distribution (L/kg)	5 L/m^2
Half-life – normal/ ESRF (hrs)	7–13/–

METABOLISM

No data

DOSE IN RENAL IMPAIRMENT GFR (mL/MIN)

20–50	Dose as in normal renal function.
10–20	Dose as in normal renal function.
<10	Dose as in normal renal function.

DOSE IN PATIENTS UNDERGOING RENAL REPLACEMENT THERAPIES

CAPD	Unlikely to be dialysed. Dose as in normal renal function.
HD	Unlikely to be dialysed. Dose as in normal renal function.
HDF/High flux	Unlikely to be dialysed. Dose as in normal renal function.
CAV/ VVHD	Unlikely to be dialysed. Dose as in normal renal function.

IMPORTANT DRUG INTERACTIONS

Potentially hazardous interactions with other drugs
- None known

ADMINISTRATION

RECONSTITUTION
- 1–2 mL sodium chloride 0.9%

ROUTE
- IM, IV, SC

RATE OF ADMINISTRATION
–

COMMENTS
- Use within 15 minutes of preparation

Crizotinib

CLINICAL USE

Antineoplastic tyrosine kinase inhibitor:
- Treatment of ALK-positive non-small cell lung cancer

DOSE IN NORMAL RENAL FUNCTION

250 mg twice daily (reduce dose if side effects occur)

PHARMACOKINETICS

Molecular weight (daltons)	450.3
% Protein binding	91
% Excreted unchanged in urine	2.3
Volume of distribution (L/kg)	1772 litres
Half-life – normal/ ESRF (hrs)	42/–

METABOLISM

Mainly metabolised in the liver by CYP3A4/5. The main metabolic pathways are oxidation (to crizotinib lactam) and O-dealkylation.

Excreted 53% via faeces (53% unchanged) and 22% via urine (2% unchanged).

DOSE IN RENAL IMPAIRMENT GFR (mL/MIN)

30–50	Dose as in normal renal function.
10–30	Start with a dose of 250 mg once daily. Use with caution.
<10	Start with a dose of 250 mg once daily. Use with caution.

DOSE IN PATIENTS UNDERGOING RENAL REPLACEMENT THERAPIES

CAPD	Unlikely dialysability. Dose as in GFR<10 mL/min.
HD	Unlikely dialysability. Dose as in GFR<10 mL/min.
HDF/High flux	Unlikely dialysability. Dose as in GFR<10 mL/min.
CAV/ VVHD	Unlikely dialysability Dose as in GFR=10–30 mL/min.

IMPORTANT DRUG INTERACTIONS

Potentially hazardous interactions with other drugs
- Analgesics: use alfentanil and fentanyl with caution.
- Antibacterials: concentration reduced by rifabutin and rifampicin – avoid; concentration increased by clarithromycin and telithromycin – avoid.
- Antidepressants: St John's wort may reduce concentration of crizotinib – avoid concomitant use.
- Antiepileptics: concentration possibly reduced by carbamazepine, phenobarbital and phenytoin – avoid concomitant use.
- Antifungals: concentration increased by ketoconazole and possibly with itraconazole and voriconazole – avoid concomitant use.
- Antipsychotics: avoid concomitant use with clozapine (increased risk of agranulocytosis); avoid concomitant use with pimozide.
- Antivirals: concentration possibly increased by atazanavir, indinavir, ritonavir and saquinavir – avoid concomitant use.
- Anxiolytics and hypnotics: increases concentration of midazolam.
- Ciclosporin: use with caution.
- Ergot alkaloids: use with caution.
- Grapefruit juice: may increase concentration of crizotinib, avoid concomitant use.
- Oestrogens & progestogens: contraceptive effect possibly reduced – avoid.
- Sirolimus: use with caution.
- Tacrolimus: use with caution.

ADMINISTRATION

RECONSTITUTION
–
ROUTE
- Oral
RATE OF ADMINISTRATION
–

OTHER INFORMATION

- Manufacturer in UK SPC has no data in severe renal impairment so advises to use with caution.
- Dose in renal impairment from US data sheet.
- Clearances were similar in studies down to 30 mL/min.
- The mean AUC for crizotinib increased by 79% and mean C_{max} increased by 34%

in patients with severe renal impairment compared to those with normal renal function.

- May cause QT prolongation.
- Crizotinib has also been associated with fatal hepatotoxicity.
- Bioavailability is 43%.

Cyclizine

CLINICAL USE

- Nausea and vomiting
- Vertigo
- Motion sickness
- Labyrinthine disorders

DOSE IN NORMAL RENAL FUNCTION

50 mg up to 3 times daily

PHARMACOKINETICS

Molecular weight (daltons)	266.4
% Protein binding	No data
% Excreted unchanged in urine	<1
Volume of distribution (L/kg)	No data
Half-life – normal/ ESRF (hrs)	20/–

METABOLISM

Cyclizine is metabolised in the liver to the relatively inactive N-demethylated metabolite, norcyclizine. Both cyclizine and norcyclizine have plasma elimination half-lives of 20 hours. Less than 1% of the total oral dose is eliminated in the urine in 24 hours.

DOSE IN RENAL IMPAIRMENT GFR (mL/MIN)

20–50	Dose as in normal renal function.
10–20	Dose as in normal renal function.
<10	Dose as in normal renal function.

DOSE IN PATIENTS UNDERGOING RENAL REPLACEMENT THERAPIES

CAPD	Unknown dialysability. Dose as in normal renal function.
HD	Unknown dialysability. Dose as in normal renal function.
HDF/High flux	Unknown dialysability. Dose as in normal renal function.
CAV/ VVHD	Unknown dialysability. Dose as in normal renal function.

IMPORTANT DRUG INTERACTIONS

Potentially hazardous interactions with other drugs
- None known

ADMINISTRATION

RECONSTITUTION
–
ROUTE
- IV, IM, Oral
RATE OF ADMINISTRATION
- Slow IV
COMMENTS
- Increased cerebral sensitivity in patients with renal failure

Cyclopenthiazide

CLINICAL USE

Thiazide diuretic:
- Hypertension
- Heart failure
- Oedema

DOSE IN NORMAL RENAL FUNCTION

- Hypertension: 250–500 mcg once daily
- Heart failure: 250 mcg – 1 mg once daily
- Oedema: up to 500 mcg once daily

PHARMACOKINETICS

Molecular weight (daltons)	379.9
% Protein binding	No data
% Excreted unchanged in urine	100
Volume of distribution (L/kg)	No data
Half-life – normal/ ESRF (hrs)	12/Increased

METABOLISM

Cyclopenthiazide appears to be entirely excreted unchanged in the urine.

DOSE IN RENAL IMPAIRMENT GFR (mL/MIN)

20–50	Dose as in normal renal function.
10–30	Unlikely to work.
<10	Unlikely to work.

DOSE IN PATIENTS UNDERGOING RENAL REPLACEMENT THERAPIES

CAPD	Unknown dialysability. Unlikely to work.
HD	Unknown dialysability. Unlikely to work.
HDF/High flux	Unknown dialysability. Unlikely to work.
CAV/ VVHD	Unknown dialysability. Unlikely to work.

IMPORTANT DRUG INTERACTIONS

Potentially hazardous interactions with other drugs
- Analgesics: increased risk of nephrotoxicity with NSAIDs; antagonism of diuretic effect.
- Anti-arrhythmics: hypokalaemia leads to increased cardiac toxicity; effects of lidocaine and mexiletine antagonised.
- Antibacterials: avoid administration with lymecycline.
- Antidepressants: increased risk of hypokalaemia with reboxetine; enhanced hypotensive effect with MAOIs; increased risk of postural hypotension with tricyclics.
- Anti-epileptics: increased risk of hyponatraemia with carbamazepine.
- Antifungals: increased risk of hypokalaemia with amphotericin.
- Antihypertensives: enhanced hypotensive effect; increased risk of first dose hypotension with post-synaptic alpha-blockers like prazosin; hypokalaemia increases risk of ventricular arrhythmias with sotalol.
- Antipsychotics: hypokalaemia increases risk of ventricular arrhythmias with amisulpride; enhanced hypotensive effect with phenothiazines; hypokalaemia increases risk of ventricular arrhythmias with pimozide – avoid concomitant use.
- Atomoxetine: hypokalaemia increases risk of ventricular arrhythmias.
- Cardiac glycosides: increased toxicity if hypokalaemia occurs.
- Ciclosporin: increased risk of nephrotoxicity and possibly hypomagnesaemia.
- Cytotoxics: increased risk of ventricular arrhythmias due to hypokalaemia with arsenic trioxide; increased risk of nephrotoxicity and ototoxicity with platinum compounds.
- Lithium: excretion reduced, increased toxicity.

ADMINISTRATION

RECONSTITUTION
–
ROUTE
- Oral
RATE OF ADMINISTRATION
–

COMMENTS
–

OTHER INFORMATION

- Monitor for hypokalaemia.
- Acts within 1–3 hours, peaks in 4–8 hours and lasts up to 12 hours.

Cyclophosphamide

CLINICAL USE

Alkylating agent:
- Immunosuppression of autoimmune diseases including rheumatoid arthritis
- Treatment of malignant disease

DOSE IN NORMAL RENAL FUNCTION

- Autoimmune disease:
  - Oral: 1–2.5 mg/kg/day
  - IV: Usually 0.5–1 g/m² or 10–15 mg/kg repeated at intervals, e.g. monthly (pulse therapy)
- Malignant disease:
  - Oral: 50–250 mg/m² daily or according to local protocol.

PHARMACOKINETICS

Molecular weight (daltons)	279.1
% Protein binding	Parent drug 0–10: alkylating metabolites >60
% Excreted unchanged in urine	5–25
Volume of distribution (L/kg)	0.78
Half-life – normal/ ESRF (hrs)	3–12/10

METABOLISM

Cyclophosphamide is a prodrug and undergoes activation by various cytochrome P450 isoenzymes (notably CYP2B6) in the liver (great inter-patient variability in metabolism). The initial metabolites are 4-hydroxycyclophosphamide and its acyclic tautomer, aldophosphamide, which both undergo further metabolism; aldophosphamide may undergo non-enzymatic conversion to active phosphoramide mustard. Acrolein is also produced and may be responsible for bladder toxicity. Cyclophosphamide is excreted principally in urine, as metabolites and some unchanged drug.

DOSE IN RENAL IMPAIRMENT GFR (mL/MIN)

20–50	Dose as in normal renal function.
10–20	75–100%[1] of normal dose depending on clinical indication and local protocol.
<10	50–100%[1] of normal dose depending on clinical indication and local protocol.

DOSE IN PATIENTS UNDERGOING RENAL REPLACEMENT THERAPIES

CAPD	Dialysed. Dose as in GFR<10 mL/min. Following dose, do not perform CAPD exchange for 12 hours.
HD	Dialysed. Dose as in GFR<10 mL/min. Dose at minimum of 12 hours before HD session.
HDF/High flux	Dialysed. Dose as in GFR<10 mL/min. Dose at minimum of 12 hours before HDF session.
CAV/VVHD	Dialysed. Dose as in GFR=10–20 mL/min.

IMPORTANT DRUG INTERACTIONS

Potentially hazardous interactions with other drugs
- Antipsychotics: avoid concomitant use with clozapine, increased risk of agranulocytosis.
- Cytotoxics: increased toxicity with high-dose cyclophosphamide and pentostatin – avoid concomitant use.

ADMINISTRATION

RECONSTITUTION
- Add 5 mL water for injection to each 100 mg
- (sodium chloride 0.9% for Endoxana).

ROUTE
- Oral, IV

RATE OF ADMINISTRATION
- Directly into vein over 2–3 minutes, OR directly into tubing of fast running IV infusion with patient supine.

COMMENTS
- IV route occasionally used for pulse therapy. Can be administered as an IV infusion.
- Injection can be administered orally down a NG tube.

OTHER INFORMATION

- Reduce IV dose to 75% of oral dose, bioavailability is 75%.
- Cyclophosphamide and its alkylating metabolites can be eliminated by dialysis.
- Patients receiving chronic indefinite therapy may be at increased risk of developing urothelial carcinoma.
- If patient is anuric and on dialysis, neither cyclophosphamide nor its metabolites, nor Mesna, should appear in the urinary tract. The use of Mesna may therefore be unnecessary, although this would be a clinical decision.
- If the patient is still passing urine, Mesna should be given to prevent urothelial toxicity.

Reference:
1. Kintzel PE, Dorr RT. Anticancer drug renal toxicity and elimination: dosing guidelines for altered renal function. *Cancer Treat Rev.* 1995; **21**: 33–64.

Cycloserine

CLINICAL USE

Antibacterial agent:
● Tuberculosis

DOSE IN NORMAL RENAL FUNCTION

Initially 250 mg every 12 hours for
2 weeks; then increased according to blood
concentration and response to maximum
500 mg every 12 hours.

PHARMACOKINETICS

Molecular weight (daltons)	102.1
% Protein binding	<20
% Excreted unchanged in urine	50–70
Volume of distribution (L/kg)	0.11–0.26
Half-life – normal/ ESRF (hrs)	8–12/Increased

METABOLISM

Cycloserine is excreted largely unchanged
by glomerular filtration. About 50% of a
single 250-mg dose is excreted unchanged
in the urine within 12 hours and about 70%
is excreted within 72 hours. As negligible
amounts of cycloserine appear in the faeces,
it is assumed that the remainder of a dose is
metabolised to unidentified metabolites.

DOSE IN RENAL IMPAIRMENT GFR (mL/MIN)

20–50	250–500 mg every 24 hours. Monitor blood levels weekly.
10–20	250–500 mg every 24 hours. Monitor blood levels weekly.
<10	250–500 mg every 36–48 hours. Monitor blood levels weekly.

DOSE IN PATIENTS UNDERGOING RENAL REPLACEMENT THERAPIES

CAPD	Unknown dialysability. Dose as in GFR<10 mL/min.
HD	Dialysed. Dose as in GFR<10 mL/min.
HDF/High flux	Dialysed. Dose as in GFR<10 mL/min.
CAV/ VVHD	Likely dialysability. Dose as in GFR=10–20 mL/min.

IMPORTANT DRUG INTERACTIONS

Potentially hazardous interactions with other
drugs
● Alcohol: Increased risk of seizures.

ADMINISTRATION

RECONSTITUTION
–
ROUTE
● Oral
RATE OF ADMINISTRATION
–
COMMENTS
–

OTHER INFORMATION

● May cause drowsiness – increased
  cerebral sensitivity in patients with renal
  impairment.
● Blood concentration monitoring is
  required, especially in renal impairment,
  if dose exceeds 500 mg daily, or if signs of
  toxicity. Blood concentration should not
  exceed 30 mg/L.
● Contraindicated by manufacturer in severe
  renal insufficiency.
● Doses in renal impairment from *Drug
  Prescribing in Renal Failure*, 5th edition, by
  Aronoff *et al.*
● Can cause CNS toxicity.
● Pyridoxine has been used in an attempt to
  treat or prevent neurological reactions, but
  its value is unproven.

Cyproheptadine hydrochloride

CLINICAL USE

Antihistamine:
- Symptomatic relief of allergy such as hay fever, urticaria

DOSE IN NORMAL RENAL FUNCTION

4–20 mg daily in divided doses. Maximum dose 32 mg daily

PHARMACOKINETICS

Molecular weight (daltons)	350.9
% Protein binding	96–99
% Excreted unchanged in urine	<2
Volume of distribution (L/kg)	Large
Half-life – normal/ ESRF (hrs)	1–4/Increased

METABOLISM

Undergoes almost complete metabolism in the liver. The main metabolite found in humans is a quaternary ammonium glucuronide conjugate of cyproheptadine.

Forty per cent is excreted in the urine mainly as metabolites and 2–20% via the faeces.

DOSE IN RENAL IMPAIRMENT GFR (mL/MIN)

20–50	Dose as in normal renal function.
10–20	Dose as in normal renal function.
<10	Dose as in normal renal function.

DOSE IN PATIENTS UNDERGOING RENAL REPLACEMENT THERAPIES

CAPD	Unlikely to be dialysed. Dose as in normal renal function.
HD	Unlikely to be dialysed. Dose as in normal renal function.
HDF/High flux	Unlikely to be dialysed. Dose as in normal renal function.
CAV/VVHD	Unlikely to be dialysed. Dose as in normal renal function.

IMPORTANT DRUG INTERACTIONS

Potentially hazardous interactions with other drugs
- Analgesics: sedative properties increased with opioid analgesics.

ADMINISTRATION

RECONSTITUTION
–
ROUTE
- Oral
RATE OF ADMINISTRATION
–

OTHER INFORMATION

- May cause excessive drowsiness in renal patients. Start with a low dose and gradually increase.

Cyproterone acetate

CLINICAL USE

- Control of libido in severe hypersexuality and sexual deviation in adult male
- Management of patients with prostatic cancer (LHRH 'flare', palliative treatment)
- Hot flushes post orchidectomy

DOSE IN NORMAL RENAL FUNCTION

- Control of hypersexuality: 50 mg twice daily
- Prostatic cancer: 200–300 mg/day in 2–3 divided doses
- Hot flushes: 50–150 mg daily in 1–3 divided doses

PHARMACOKINETICS

Molecular weight (daltons)	416.9
% Protein binding	Approx 96
% Excreted unchanged in urine	<1
Volume of distribution (L/kg)	10–30
Half-life – normal/ ESRF (hrs)	32.1–56.7/–

METABOLISM

Cyproterone is metabolised by various pathways including hydroxylation and conjugation; about 35% of a dose is excreted in urine, the remainder being excreted in the bile. The principal metabolite, 15β-hydroxycyproterone, has anti-androgenic activity.

DOSE IN RENAL IMPAIRMENT GFR (mL/MIN)

20–50	Dose as in normal renal function.
10–20	Dose as in normal renal function.
<10	Dose as in normal renal function.

DOSE IN PATIENTS UNDERGOING RENAL REPLACEMENT THERAPIES

CAPD	Unknown dialysability. Dose as in normal renal function.
HD	Unknown dialysability. Dose as in normal renal function.
HDF/High flux	Unknown dialysability. Dose as in normal renal function.
CAV/ VVHD	Unknown dialysability. Dose as in normal renal function.

IMPORTANT DRUG INTERACTIONS

Potentially hazardous interactions with other drugs
- None known

ADMINISTRATION

RECONSTITUTION
–
ROUTE
- Oral
RATE OF ADMINISTRATION
–
COMMENTS
–

OTHER INFORMATION

- May cause drowsiness – increased CNS sensitivity in patients with renal impairment.
- CSM has advised that in view of the hepatotoxicity associated with long-term doses of 300 mg daily, the use of cyproterone acetate in prostatic cancer should be restricted to short courses, to cover testosterone 'flare' associated with gonadorelin analogues, treatment of hot flushes after orchidectomy or gonadorelin analogues, and for patients who have not responded to (or are intolerant of) other treatments.
- Direct hepatic toxicity including jaundice, hepatitis and hepatic failure have been reported. Liver function tests should be performed before treatment and whenever symptoms suggestive of hepatotoxicity occur.

Cytarabine

CLINICAL USE

Antineoplastic agent:
- Acute leukaemias and lymphomas
- Meningeal neoplasms

DOSE IN NORMAL RENAL FUNCTION

- Continuous: 0.5–2 mg/kg/day
- Intermittent: 3–5 mg/kg/day
- Single agent in acute leukaemia: up to 200 mg/m^2
- Maintenance: 1–1.5 mg/kg once or twice a week
- Lymphomatous meningitis: 50 mg (Intrathecal) every 14–28 days. See SPC for more information, depends on place in treatment
- Or according to local policy

PHARMACOKINETICS

Molecular weight (daltons)	243.2
% Protein binding	13
% Excreted unchanged in urine	5.8–10
Volume of distribution (L/kg)	2.6
Half-life – normal/ ESRF (hrs)	1–3 (Intrathecal liposomal: 100–263)/ Unchanged

METABOLISM

Cytarabine is converted by phosphorylation to an active form, which is rapidly deaminated, mainly in the liver and the kidneys, by cytidine deaminase to inactive 1-β-d-arabinofuranosyluracil (uracil arabinoside, ara-U). Approximately 80% of an intravenous dose is excreted in the urine within 24 hours, mostly as the inactive metabolite with about 10% as unchanged cytarabine. A small amount is excreted in the bile.

DOSE IN RENAL IMPAIRMENT GFR (mL/MIN)

20–50	100% of conventional low dose regime. For high dose, see 'Other information'.
10–20	100% of conventional low dose regime. For high dose, see 'Other information'.
<10	100% of conventional low dose regime. For high dose, see 'Other information'.

DOSE IN PATIENTS UNDERGOING RENAL REPLACEMENT THERAPIES

CAPD	Not dialysed. Dose as in GFR<10 mL/min.
HD	Not dialysed. Dose as in GFR<10 mL/min.
HDF/High flux	Dialysed. Dose as in GFR<10 mL/min.
CAV/ VVHD	Unknown dialysability. Dose as in GFR=10–20 mL/min.

IMPORTANT DRUG INTERACTIONS

Potentially hazardous interactions with other drugs
- Antipsychotics: avoid concomitant use with clozapine, increased risk of agranulocytosis.

ADMINISTRATION

RECONSTITUTION
–
ROUTE
- IV infusion, IV injection, SC, Intrathecal
RATE OF ADMINISTRATION
- IV injection: rapid
- IV infusion: 1–24 hours
COMMENTS
- Patients generally tolerate higher doses when medication given by rapid IV injection (compared with slow infusion), due to the rapid metabolism of cytarabine and the consequent short duration of action of the high dose.

OTHER INFORMATION

- Elevated baseline serum creatinine (>1.2 mg/dl) is an independent risk factor for the development of neurotoxicity during treatment with high-dose cytarabine.
- Retrospective analysis implicates impaired renal function as an independent risk factor for high-dose cytarabine-induced cerebral and cerebellar toxicity.
- The incidence of neurotoxicity was 86–100% following administration of high-dose cytarabine to patients with CRCL <40 mL/min and 60–76% following administration to patients with CRCL <60 mL/min. In contrast, when patients with CRCL >60 mL/min received

high-dose cytarabine, the incidence of neurotoxicity was found to be 8%, which correlates with the overall incidence of this adverse effect.

- Accordingly, it has been suggested that high-dose cytarabine should be used with caution in patients with impaired renal function (Kintzel PE, Dorr RT. Anticancer drug renal toxicity and elimination: dosing guidelines for altered renal function. *Cancer Treat Rev.* 1995; **21**: 33–64).

GFR (mL/min)	Dose
45–60	60%
30–45	50%
<30	Avoid

- Anecdotally, an initial dose of 25% of the normal dose has been given to patients with a GFR<20 mL/min, with subsequent doses escalated according to tolerance.

Cytomegalovirus (CMV) human immunoglobulin (unlicensed product)

CLINICAL USE

- Prophylaxis for renal transplant recipients at risk of primary cytomegalovirus (CMV) disease
- Treatment of CMV disease (usually with ganciclovir)

DOSE IN NORMAL RENAL FUNCTION

See local protocols.

PHARMACOKINETICS

Molecular weight (daltons)	150
% Protein binding	N/A
% Excreted unchanged in urine	0
Volume of distribution (L/kg)	1
Half-life – normal/ ESRF (hrs)	50

METABOLISM

The metabolism and elimination of CMV human immunoglobulin is similar to endogenous IgG, i.e. primarily via proteolytic catabolism throughout the body, including endothelial cells, and does not rely primarily on elimination through the kidneys and liver.

DOSE IN RENAL IMPAIRMENT GFR (mL/MIN)

20–50	Dose as in normal renal function.
10–20	Dose as in normal renal function.
<10	Dose as in normal renal function.

DOSE IN PATIENTS UNDERGOING RENAL REPLACEMENT THERAPIES

CAPD	Not dialysed. Dose as in normal renal function.
HD	Not dialysed. Dose as in normal renal function.
HDF/High flux	Unknown dialysability. Dose as in normal renal function.
CAV/ VVHD	Not dialysed. Dose as in normal renal function.

IMPORTANT DRUG INTERACTIONS

Potentially hazardous interactions with other drugs
- Ciclosporin: no effect on efficacy of CMV immunoglobulin.

ADMINISTRATION

RECONSTITUTION
–

ROUTE
- IV peripherally or centrally

RATE OF ADMINISTRATION
–

COMMENTS
- Follow guidelines supplied by company.

OTHER INFORMATION

- Can give 10 mg IV chlorphenamine 1 hour before administration.
- Monitor for anaphylaxis, have epinephrine available.
- Do not mix with any other drugs or infusion fluids.

Dabigatran etexilate

CLINICAL USE

Direct thrombin inhibitor:
- Prevention of venous thromboembolism in adult patients undergoing elective hip or knee replacement surgery (VTE)
- Prevention of stroke and systemic embolism in AF (AF)

DOSE IN NORMAL RENAL FUNCTION

- VTE: 110 mg within 1–4 hours of completed surgery and thereafter 220 mg once daily (length of course depends on type of surgery)
- Elderly or on amiodarone or verapamil: 75 mg once daily then 150 mg daily
- AF: 150 mg twice daily
- Elderly or high risk of bleeding: 110 mg twice daily

PHARMACOKINETICS

Molecular weight (daltons)	627.7
% Protein binding	34–35
% Excreted unchanged in urine	85
Volume of distribution (L/kg)	60–70 litres
Half-life – normal/ESRF (hrs)	12–14 (14–17 after major orthopaedic surgery)/24–28

METABOLISM

Dabigatran etexilate is a prodrug which does not exhibit any pharmacological activity. After oral administration, dabigatran etexilate is rapidly absorbed and converted to dabigatran by esterase-catalysed hydrolysis in plasma and in the liver. Dabigatran is a potent, competitive, reversible direct thrombin inhibitor and is the main active principle in plasma.

Mainly excreted in the urine (85%) and 6% via the faeces.

DOSE IN RENAL IMPAIRMENT GFR (mL/MIN)

30–50	VTE: 75 mg within 1–4 hours of completed surgery and thereafter 150 mg once daily; 75 mg if also on CYP450 inhibitor. AF: Dose as in normal renal function.
10–30	Avoid. See 'Other information'.
<10	Avoid. See 'Other information'.

DOSE IN PATIENTS UNDERGOING RENAL REPLACEMENT THERAPIES

CAPD	Dialysed. Dose as in GFR<10 mL/min.
HD	Dialysed. Dose as in GFR<10 mL/min.
HDF/High flux	Dialysed. Dose as in GFR<10 mL/min.
CAV/VVHD	Dialysed. Dose as in GFR=10–30 mL/min.

IMPORTANT DRUG INTERACTIONS

Potentially hazardous interactions with other drugs
- Analgesics: possible increased risk of bleeding with NSAIDs; increased risk of haemorrhage with ketorolac or IV diclofenac – avoid concomitant use.
- Anti-arrhythmics: concentration increased by amiodarone, reduce dose of dabigatran; concentration increased by dronedarone – avoid.
- Antibacterials: concentration reduced by rifampicin – avoid.
- Anticoagulants: increased risk haemorrhage with other anticoagulants – avoid.
- Antidepressants: possible increased risk of bleeding with SSRIs; concentration possibly reduced by St John's wort – avoid.
- Antifungals: concentration increased by ketoconazole and possibly itraconazole – avoid
- Verapamil: reduce dose of dabigatran to 150 mg daily, 75 mg in GFR=30–50 mL/min.
- Ciclosporin: concentration possibly increased by ciclosporin – avoid.
- Sulfinpyrazone: possible increased risk of bleeding.
- Tacrolimus: concentration possibly increased by tacrolimus – avoid.

ADMINISTRATION

RECONSTITUTION
–

ROUTE
- Oral

RATE OF ADMINISTRATION
–

OTHER INFORMATION

- Oral bioavailability is 6.5%.
- Haemodialysis removes approximately 50–60% of dabigatran over 4 hours with a 700 mL/min dialysate flow rate and a blood flow rate of 200 mL/min or 350–390 mL/min respectively.
- Contraindicated by manufacturer in renal failure due to increased risk of bleeding.
- Information from US data sheet for AF:

GFR (mL/min)	Dose
>30	Dose as in normal renal function
15–30	75 mg twice daily. Avoid if also on a CYP450 inhibitor

- In people with GFR=30–50 mL/min and 10–30 mL/min, the AUC was approximately 2.7 and 6 times higher respectively compared to people with normal renal function.
- It is recommended to wait 12 hours after the last dose before switching from dabigatran to a parenteral anticoagulant.

Dacarbazine

CLINICAL USE

Antineoplastic agent:
- Metastatic melanoma
- Hodgkin's disease
- Soft tissue sarcomas

DOSE IN NORMAL RENAL FUNCTION

- Single agent: 200–250 mg/m^2 daily for 5 days, repeated every 3 weeks or 850 mg/m^2 on day 1 then once every 3 weeks.
- Hodgkin's disease: 375 mg/m^2 every 15 days in combination.

PHARMACOKINETICS

Molecular weight (daltons)	182.2
% Protein binding	0–5
% Excreted unchanged in urine	20–50
Volume of distribution (L/kg)	1.49
Half-life – normal/ ESRF (hrs)	0.5–5/Increased

METABOLISM

Dacarbazine (DTIC) is assumed to be inactive. Dacarbazine is extensively metabolised in the liver by the cytochrome P450 isoenzymes CYP1A2 and CYP2E1 (and possibly in the tissues by CYP1A1) to its active metabolite 5-(3-methyl-triazen-1-yl)-imidazole-4-carboxamide (MTIC), which spontaneously decomposes to the major metabolite 5-amino-imidazole-4-carboxamide (AIC). About half of a dose is excreted in the urine by tubular secretion; 50% as unchanged DTIC and approximately 50% as AIC.

DOSE IN RENAL IMPAIRMENT GFR (mL/MIN)

45–60	80% of dose
30–45	75% of dose
<30	70% of dose, use with caution

DOSE IN PATIENTS UNDERGOING RENAL REPLACEMENT THERAPIES

CAPD	Likely dialysability. Dose as in GFR<30 mL/min.
HD	Likely dialysability. Dose as in GFR<30 mL/min.
HDF/High flux	Likely dialysability. Dose as in GFR<30 mL/min.
CAV/ VVHD	Likely dialysability. Dose as in GFR<30 mL/min.

IMPORTANT DRUG INTERACTIONS

Potentially hazardous interactions with other drugs
- Aldesleukin: avoid concomitant use.
- Antipsychotics: avoid with clozapine, increased risk of agranulocytosis.

ADMINISTRATION

RECONSTITUTION
- 10 mL water for injection per 100 mg vial (50 mL for 1 g vial)
ROUTE
- IV
RATE OF ADMINISTRATION
- Bolus: 1–2 minutes
- Infusion: 15–30 minutes
COMMENTS
- For infusion can be diluted with up to 125–300 mL glucose 5% or sodium chloride 0.9%.
- Avoid contact with skin and mucous membranes.
- Protect from light.
- Doses above 200 mg/m^2 should be given as infusions.

OTHER INFORMATION

- Nadir for white cell count usually occurs 21–25 days after a dose.
- Contraindicated by manufacturer in severe renal impairment due to lack of data.
- Doses from Kintzel PE, Dorr RT. Anticancer drug renal toxicity and elimination: dosing guidelines for altered renal function. *Cancer Treat Rev.* 1995; **21**: 33–64.

Dactinomycin

CLINICAL USE

Antineoplastic antibiotic

DOSE IN NORMAL RENAL FUNCTION

Dose varies according to patient tolerance, size and location of neoplasm.
Maximum dose: 15 mcg/kg or 400–600 mcg/m^2 daily for 5 days per 2 week cycle.

PHARMACOKINETICS

Molecular weight (daltons)	1255.4
% Protein binding	5
% Excreted unchanged in urine	30
Volume of distribution (L/kg)	>12.1
Half-life – normal/ ESRF (hrs)	36/–

METABOLISM

Intravenous doses of dactinomycin are rapidly distributed with high concentrations in bone marrow and nucleated cells. It undergoes only minimal metabolism and is slowly excreted in urine and bile. Fifteen per cent is eliminated by hepatic metabolism. Approximately 30% of the dose was recovered in the urine and faeces in 1 week.

DOSE IN RENAL IMPAIRMENT GFR (mL/MIN)

20–50	Dose as in normal renal function.
10–20	Use with caution. Dose as in normal renal function.
<10	Use with caution. Dose as in normal renal function.

DOSE IN PATIENTS UNDERGOING RENAL REPLACEMENT THERAPIES

CAPD	Unlikely to be dialysed. Dose as in GFR<10 mL/min
HD	Unlikely to be dialysed. Dose as in GFR<10 mL/min
HDF/High flux	Unknown dialysability. Dose as in GFR<10 mL/min
CAV/ VVHD	Unknown dialysability. Dose as in GFR=10–20 mL/min

IMPORTANT DRUG INTERACTIONS

Potentially hazardous interactions with other drugs
● None known

ADMINISTRATION

RECONSTITUTION
● 1.1 mL water for injection without preservative
ROUTE
● IV
RATE OF ADMINISTRATION
● 15 minutes
COMMENTS
● Add to 50 mL glucose 5% or sodium chloride 0.9% (maximum concentration 10 mg/mL) or to a fast running IV infusion.
● Avoid direct contact with the skin.

OTHER INFORMATION

● Nadir for platelet and white cell count usually occurs after 14–21 days, with recovery in 21–25 days.
● Can cause renal abnormalities.

Dalteparin sodium (LMWH)

CLINICAL USE

1. Peri- and postoperative surgical and medical thromboprophylaxis
2. Prevention of clotting in extracorporeal circuits
3. Treatment of DVT
4. Acute coronary syndrome

DOSE IN NORMAL RENAL FUNCTION

1. Dose according to risk of thrombosis:
   Moderate risk: 2500 IU daily.
   High risk and medical: 5000 IU daily.
2. Dose for >4 hour session: IV bolus of 30–40 IU/kg, followed by infusion of 10–15 IU/kg/hour.
   Dose for <4 hour session: as above or single IV bolus injection of 5000 IU.
   If at increased risk of bleeding IV bolus of 5–10 IU/kg, followed by infusion of 4–5 IU/kg/hour. See 'Other information'.
3. 200 IU/kg daily (maximum 18 000 units as a single dose) or 100 IU/kg twice daily.
4. 120 IU/kg every 12 hours maximum 10 000 IU twice daily for 5–8 days.

PHARMACOKINETICS

Molecular weight (daltons)	Average 6000
% Protein binding	No data
% Excreted unchanged in urine	No data
Volume of distribution (L/kg)	0.04–0.06
Half-life – normal/ ESRF (hrs)	IV: 2; SC: 3.5–4/ Prolonged

METABOLISM

Liver and the reticuloendothelial system are the sites of biotransformation of dalteparin. It is partially metabolised by desulphation and depolymerisation. The kidneys are the major site of dalteparin excretion (approximately 70% based on animal studies).

DOSE IN RENAL IMPAIRMENT GFR (mL/MIN)

20–50	Dose as in normal renal function.
10–20	Dose as in normal renal function only for prophylaxis doses. See 'Other information'.
<10	Dose as in normal renal function only for prophylaxis doses. See 'Other information'.

DOSE IN PATIENTS UNDERGOING RENAL REPLACEMENT THERAPIES

CAPD	Not dialysed. Dose as in GFR<10 mL/min.
HD	Not dialysed. Dose as in GFR<10 mL/min.
HDF/High flux	Dialysed. Dose as in GFR<10 mL/min.
CAV/ VVHD	Not dialysed. Dose as in GFR=10–20 mL/min.

IMPORTANT DRUG INTERACTIONS

Potentially hazardous interactions with other drugs
- Analgesics: increased risk of bleeding with NSAIDs, avoid concomitant use with IV diclofenac; increased risk of haemorrhage with ketorolac – avoid concomitant use.
- Nitrates: anticoagulant effect reduced by infusions of glyceryl trinitrate.
- Use with care in patients receiving oral anticoagulants, platelet aggregation inhibitors, aspirin or dextran.

ADMINISTRATION

RECONSTITUTION
–
ROUTE
- SC injection into abdominal wall (pre-filled syringes)
- IV bolus/infusion (ampoules)
RATE OF ADMINISTRATION
–
COMMENTS
- Dalteparin solution for injection (ampoules) is compatible with sodium chloride 0.9% and glucose 5%.

OTHER INFORMATION

- Low molecular weight heparins are renally excreted and hence accumulate in severe renal impairment. While the doses recommended for prophylaxis against DVT and prevention of thrombus formation in extracorporeal circuits are well tolerated in patients with ERF, the doses recommended for treatment of DVT and PE have been associated with severe, sometimes fatal, bleeding episodes in such patients. Hence the use of unfractionated heparin would be preferable in these instances.

- In patients with GFR ≤ 30 mL/min, monitoring for anti-Xa levels is recommended to determine the appropriate dalteparin dose. Target anti-Xa range is 0.5–1.5 IU/mL. When monitoring anti-Xa in these patients, sampling should be performed 4–6 hours after dosing and only after the patient has received 3–4 doses.

- Antifactor-Xa levels should be regularly monitored in new patients on haemodialysis, during the first weeks; later, less frequent monitoring is generally required. Consult manufacturer's literature.

- Additional doses may be required if using LMWHs for anticoagulation in HDF.

- Bleeding may occur especially at high doses corresponding with antifactor-Xa levels greater than 1.5 IU/mL.

- The prolongation of the APTT induced by dalteparin is fully neutralised by protamine, but the anti-Xa activity is only neutralised to about 25–50%.

- 1 mg of protamine inhibits the effect of 100 IU (antifactor-Xa) of dalteparin.

- Heparin can suppress adrenal secretion of aldosterone leading to hypercalcaemia, particularly in patients with chronic renal impairment and diabetes mellitus.

- Alternative dosing for haemodialysis is 70 IU/kg as a single bolus into the arterial line at the start of dialysis; the dose may need to be greatly reduced in people on warfarin. An anti-Xa level >0.4 IU/mL after 4 hours of dialysis inhibits significant clotting during haemodialysis. (Sagedal S, Hartmann A, Sundstrom K, *et al.* A single dose of dalteparin effectively prevents clotting during haemodialysis. *Nephrol Dial Transplant.* 1999; **14**: 1943–7.)

Danaparoid sodium

CLINICAL USE

- Prophylaxis of DVT and PE
- Thromboembolic disease requiring parenteral anticoagulation in patients with heparin induced thrombocytopenia (HIT)
- Anticoagulation for haemodialysis

DOSE IN NORMAL RENAL FUNCTION

- Prophylaxis, DVT and PE: 750 units twice daily for 7–10 days (SC).
- HIT: 2500 units IV bolus (Wt<55 kg: 1250 units; >90 kg: 3750 units) then an IV infusion of 400 units/hour for 2 hours, 300 units/hour for 2 hours, then 200 units/hour for 5 days.
- Haemodialysis: see 'Other information'.

PHARMACOKINETICS

Molecular weight (daltons)	Approx 6500
% Protein binding	No data
% Excreted unchanged in urine	40–50
Volume of distribution (L/kg)	8–9
Half-life – normal/ESRF (hrs)	25/>31

METABOLISM

Danaparoid sodium is mainly eliminated by renal excretion and animal experiments indicate that the liver is not involved in its metabolism.

DOSE IN RENAL IMPAIRMENT GFR (mL/MIN)

20–50	Dose as in normal renal function.
10–20	Use with caution.
<10	Use with caution. Reduce second and subsequent doses for thromboembolism prophylaxis.

DOSE IN PATIENTS UNDERGOING RENAL REPLACEMENT THERAPIES

CAPD	Not dialysed. Dose as in GFR<10 mL/min.
HD	Not dialysed. Dose as in GFR<10 mL/min.
HDF/High flux	Unknown dialysability. Dose as in GFR<10 mL/min.
CAV/VVHD	Not dialysed. Dose as in GFR=10–20 mL/min.

IMPORTANT DRUG INTERACTIONS

Potentially hazardous interactions with other drugs
- Enhances effects of oral anticoagulants.
- Interferes with laboratory monitoring of prothrombin time – monitor anticoagulation closely.

ADMINISTRATION

RECONSTITUTION
- Glucose 5% or sodium chloride 0.9%
ROUTE
- SC, IV
RATE OF ADMINISTRATION
- See dose.
COMMENTS
–

OTHER INFORMATION

- Contraindicated by manufacturer in severe renal impairment unless patient has HIT and there is no other alternative.
- Pharmacokinetic information is from *Pharmacy Update*. 1997 Nov/Dec; www.cc.nih.gov/phar/updates/97novdec.html
- Monitor anti-Xa activity in patients >90 kg and with renal impairment.
Can also be used for haemodialysis anticoagulation:
- 2–3 times a week dialysis:
  — 1st and 2nd dialysis: 3750 units IV bolus prior to dialysis. (If patient weighs <55 kg then give 2500 unit IV bolus.)
  — Subsequent dialysis: 3000 units by IV bolus prior to dialysis, provided there are no fibrin threads in the bubble chamber. (If patient weighs <55 kg then give 2000 unit IV bolus.)
- Daily dialysis:
  — 1st dialysis: 3750 units IV bolus prior to dialysis; if patient <55 kg give 2500 units.
  — 2nd dialysis: 2500 units IV bolus prior to dialysis; if patient <55 kg give 2000 units.
  — Prior to the second and subsequent dialysis a specimen should be drawn for plasma anti-Xa levels (to be used for dosing a third and subsequent dialysis).
- Expected pre-dialysis ranges of anti-Xa levels:

— If plasma anti-Xa levels are <0.3 U/mL, then 3rd or subsequent dialysis dose should be 3000 units. For patients weighing <55 kg use 2000 units.
— If plasma anti-Xa levels are 0.3–0.35 U/mL, then 3rd or subsequent dialysis dose should be 2500 units. For patients weighing <55 kg use 1500 units.
— If plasma anti-Xa levels are 0.35–0.4 U/mL, then 3rd or subsequent dialysis dose should be 2000 units. For patients weighing <55 kg use 1500 units.
— If plasma anti-Xa levels are >0.4 U/mL, then do not give any danaparoid before dialysis. However, if fibrin threads form in the bubble chamber, then the patient may be given 1500 units IV bolus (irrespective of the patient's weight).
- During dialysis the plasma anti-Xa level should be 0.5–0.8 U/mL.
- If needed take a blood sample prior to every dialysis and during dialysis (at 30 minutes and at 4 hours).
- Protamine is no use as an antidote for bleeding complications. If no anti-Xa monitoring is available then the first 4 dialysis sessions should have pre-dialysis IV bolus of 3750, 3750, 3000 and 2500 units respectively, then 2500 units thereafter. Take blood sample prior to 4th and 7th dialysis to ensure there is no accumulation.
- Oozing from puncture sites has been noted 24–36 hours post dose.
- Haemofiltration: 55–90 kg: 2500 units bolus followed by 600 units/hr for 4 hours then 400 units/hr for 4 hours then 200–600 units/hr to maintain adequate anti-Xa levels. If patient <55 kg reduce bolus to 2000 units followed by 400 units/hr for 4 hours then 150–400 units/hr to maintain adequate anti-Xa levels. (*Drug Information Handbook*, 22nd edition. American Pharmacists Association. Lexicomp.)
- For CVVH, an initial bolus of 750 units followed by an infusion of 0.7–2 units/kg/hr can be given. (Wester JPJ. Guidelines for anticoagulation with danaparoid sodium and lepirudin in continuous venovenous hemofiltration. *Neth J Crit Care*. 2004; **8**(4): 293–301). Although there are many different regimes this one uses the least amount of danaparoid.

Dapagliflozin

CLINICAL USE

Selective and reversible inhibitor of sodium-glucose co-transporter 2
- Treatment of type 2 diabetes

DOSE IN NORMAL RENAL FUNCTION

10 mg once daily

PHARMACOKINETICS

Molecular weight (daltons)	408.9
% Protein binding	91
% Excreted unchanged in urine	<2
Volume of distribution (L/kg)	118 litres
Half-life – normal/ ESRF (hrs)	12.9/–

METABOLISM

Dapagliflozin is extensively metabolised, primarily to dapagliflozin 3-O-glucuronide, which is an inactive metabolite. The formation of dapagliflozin 3-O-glucuronide is mediated by UGT1A9, an enzyme present in the liver and kidney, and CYP-mediated metabolism was a minor clearance pathway in humans. About 75% of the dose is excreted in the urine and 21% in the faeces.

DOSE IN RENAL IMPAIRMENT GFR (mL/MIN)

20–60	Avoid
10–20	Avoid
<10	Avoid

DOSE IN PATIENTS UNDERGOING RENAL REPLACEMENT THERAPIES

CAPD	Avoid
HD	Avoid
HDF/High flux	Avoid
CAV/ VVHD	Avoid

IMPORTANT DRUG INTERACTIONS

Potentially hazardous interactions with other drugs
- None known

ADMINISTRATION

RECONSTITUTION
–
ROUTE
- Oral
RATE OF ADMINISTRATION
–

OTHER INFORMATION

- Not recommended by manufacturer if GFR<60 mL/min due to increased side effects and lack of efficacy.
- In subjects with moderate renal impairment (patients with CRCL <60 mL/min or eGFR<60 mL/min/1.73 m^2), a higher proportion of subjects treated with dapagliflozin had an increase in creatinine, phosphate, parathyroid hormone and hypotension, compared with placebo.
- Oral bioavailability is 78%.
- Efficacy is reduced with reducing renal function.

Dapsone

CLINICAL USE

- Treatment and prophylaxis of leprosy
- Dermatitis herpetiformis
- *Pneumocystis jiroveci* pneumonia (PCP)
- Malaria prophylaxis

DOSE IN NORMAL RENAL FUNCTION

- Leprosy: 1–2 mg/kg or 100 mg daily
- PCP (with trimethoprim): 50–100 mg daily, 100 mg twice weekly or 200 mg once weekly
- Dermatitis herpetiformis: 50–300 mg daily
- Malaria prophylaxis: 100 mg weekly in combination with pyrimethamine 12.5 mg weekly

PHARMACOKINETICS

Molecular weight (daltons)	248.3
% Protein binding	50–80
% Excreted unchanged in urine	20
Volume of distribution (L/kg)	1–1.5
Half-life – normal/ ESRF (hrs)	10–80/–

METABOLISM

Dapsone undergoes enterohepatic recycling. Dapsone is acetylated to monoacetyldapsone, the major metabolite, and other mono and diacetyl derivatives. Acetylation shows genetic polymorphism. Hydroxylation is the other major metabolic pathway resulting in hydroxylamine dapsone, which may be responsible for dapsone-associated methaemoglobinaemia and haemolysis.

Dapsone is mainly excreted in the urine, only 20% of a dose as unchanged drug.

DOSE IN RENAL IMPAIRMENT GFR (mL/MIN)

20–50	Dose as in normal renal function.
10–20	Dose as in normal renal function, use with caution.
<10	50–100 mg daily, use with caution. No dose reduction is required for malaria prophylaxis. See 'Other information'.

DOSE IN PATIENTS UNDERGOING RENAL REPLACEMENT THERAPIES

CAPD	Likely dialysability. Dose as in GFR<10 mL/min.
HD	Dialysed. Dose as in GFR<10 mL/min.
HDF/High flux	Dialysed. Dose as in GFR<10 mL/min.
CAV/ VVHD	Likely dialysability. Dose as in GFR=10–20 mL/min.

IMPORTANT DRUG INTERACTIONS

Potentially hazardous interactions with other drugs

- Antivirals: increased risk of ventricular arrhythmias with saquinavir – avoid concomitant use.

ADMINISTRATION

RECONSTITUTION
–
ROUTE
- Oral
RATE OF ADMINISTRATION
–
COMMENTS
–

OTHER INFORMATION

- Greater risk of haemolytic side effects in patients with glucose-6-phosphate-dehydrogenase deficiency.
- Regular blood counts are recommended in patients with severe anaemia or renal impairment: weekly for the 1st month, then monthly for 6 months, then semi-annually.
- Almost all patients lose 1–2 g of haemoglobin.
- The dose for herpetiformis can be reduced if the patient is on a gluten free diet.
- One study used dapsone in a haemodialysis patient for bullous dermatosis: therapy was initiated at 100 mg but the dose had to be reduced to 50 mg due to haemolytic effects. (Serwin AB, Mysliwiec H, Laudanska H, *et al.* Linear IgA bullous dermatosis in a diabetic patient with chronic renal failure. *Int J Dermatol.* 2002 Nov; **41**(11): 778–80).

Daptomycin

CLINICAL USE

Antibacterial agent

DOSE IN NORMAL RENAL FUNCTION

4–6 mg/kg once daily for 7 to 14 days depending on indication

PHARMACOKINETICS

Molecular weight (daltons)	1620.7
% Protein binding	90–92
% Excreted unchanged in urine	Approximately 50%
Volume of distribution (L/kg)	0.092–0.104
Half-life – normal/ ESRF (hrs)	8.1–9/29.4[1]

METABOLISM

In vitro studies indicate that daptomycin is not metabolised by, and does not affect, the cytochrome P450 isoenzyme system. Little or no metabolism is thought to take place although 4 minor metabolites have been detected in the urine.

Daptomycin is excreted mainly via renal filtration with about 78% and 6% of a dose recovered in the urine and faeces, respectively.

DOSE IN RENAL IMPAIRMENT GFR (mL/MIN)

30–50	Dose as in normal renal function.
<30	4–6 mg/kg every 48 hours.

DOSE IN PATIENTS UNDERGOING RENAL REPLACEMENT THERAPIES

CAPD	Not dialysed. Dose as in GFR<30 mL/min.
HD	Not dialysed. Dose as in GFR<30 mL/min.
HDF/High flux	Dialysed. Dose as in GFR<30 mL/min.
CAV/ VVHD	Slightly dialysed. 4–6 mg/kg every 48 hours.[2]

IMPORTANT DRUG INTERACTIONS

Potentially hazardous interactions with other drugs
- Warfarin: monitor INR when on daptomycin.
- Ciclosporin: increased risk of myopathy – try to avoid concomitant use.
- Lipid-regulating drugs: increased risk of myopathy with fibrates and statins – try to avoid concomitant use.

ADMINISTRATION

RECONSTITUTION
- Infusion: 7 mL sodium chloride 0.9% to give a solution of 50 mg/mL
- Bolus: 10 mL sodium chloride 0.9%.
ROUTE
- IV infusion, IV Bolus
RATE OF ADMINISTRATION
- Infusion: over 30 minutes
- Bolus: over 2 minutes
COMMENTS
- Once reconstituted, stable for 12 hours at room temperature and 48 hours refrigerated.
- Add to 50 mL sodium chloride 0.9% before administration. Stable for 12 hours at room temperature or 24 hours refrigerated.
- Incompatible with dextrose solutions.
- Compatible with solutions containing aztreonam, ceftazidime, ceftriaxone, gentamicin, fluconazole, levofloxacin, dopamine, heparin and lidocaine.

OTHER INFORMATION

- May cause renal impairment.
- Vials do not contain any bacteriostatic or fungiostatic agents.
- Company advises to administer post dialysis.
- Monitor creatinine phosphokinase levels, muscle pain or weakness.
- Increased risk of myopathy in severe renal failure due to increased daptomycin levels.
- 15% of dose is removed by 4 hours of haemodialysis and 11% over 48 hours by peritoneal dialysis.
- Therapeutic concentrations of daptomycin are unlikely due to low PD clearance of drug therefore systemic use for peritonitis is unlikely to work.[3]
- There is a case study using IP daptomycin for VRE peritonitis at a dose of 100 mg/L. (Huen SC, Hall I & Topal J *et al.* Successful

use of intraperitoneal daptomycin in the treatment of vancomycin-resistant enterococcus. peritonitis. *Am J Kidney Dis.* 2009 Sep; **54**(3): 538–41.)

References:
1. Fenton C, Keating GM, Curran MP. Daptomycin. *Drugs.* 2004; **64**(4): 445–55.
2. Trotman RL, Williamson JC, Shoemaker DM, *et al.* Antibiotic dosing in critically ill adult patients receiving continuous renal replacement therapy. *Clin Infect Dis.* 2005 Oct 15; **41**: 1159–66.
3. Salzer W. Antimicrobial-resistant gram-positive bacteria in PD peritonitis and the newer antibiotics used to treat them. *Perit Dial Int.* 2005; **25**: 313–19.

Darbepoetin alfa

CLINICAL USE

Treatment of anaemia associated with chronic renal failure, and with non-haematological malignancies in adult cancer patients receiving chemotherapy

DOSE IN NORMAL RENAL FUNCTION

- Renal failure: 0.45 micrograms/kg once a week; dose is adjusted by 25% every 4 weeks according to response; maintenance every 1–2 weeks.
- Patients not on dialysis: 0.75 mcg/kg every 2 weeks; maintenance may be every 1–4 weeks.
- Chemotherapy related anaemia: 2.25 mcg/kg once a week, or 6.75 mcg/kg every 3 weeks; adjust doses by 50% every 4 weeks according to response.

PHARMACOKINETICS

Molecular weight (daltons)	30 000–37 000
% Protein binding	No data
% Excreted unchanged in urine	No data
Volume of distribution (L/kg)	0.05
Half-life – normal/ ESRF (hrs)	21 (IV), 73 (SC)/ Unchanged

METABOLISM

The metabolic fate of both endogenous and recombinant erythropoietin is poorly understood. Current evidence from studies in animals suggests that hepatic metabolism contributes only minimally to elimination of the intact hormone, but desialylated epoetin (i.e. terminal sialic acid groups removed) appears to undergo substantial hepatic clearance via metabolic pathways and/or binding. Desialylation and/or removal of the oligosaccharide side chains of erythropoietin appear to occur principally in the liver; bone marrow also may have a role in catabolism of the hormone. Elimination of desialylated drug by the kidneys, bone marrow, and spleen also may occur; results of animal studies suggest that proximal renal tubular secretion may be involved in renal elimination. In preclinical studies it has been shown that renal clearance of darbepoetin is minimal (up to 2% of total clearance).

DOSE IN RENAL IMPAIRMENT GFR (mL/MIN)

20–50	Dose as in normal renal function.
10–20	Dose as in normal renal function.
<10	Dose as in normal renal function.

DOSE IN PATIENTS UNDERGOING RENAL REPLACEMENT THERAPIES

CAPD	Not dialysed. Dose as in normal renal function.
HD	Not dialysed. Dose as in normal renal function.
HDF/High flux	Not dialysed. Dose as in normal renal function.
CAV/ VVHD	Not dialysed. Dose as in normal renal function.

IMPORTANT DRUG INTERACTIONS

Potentially hazardous interactions with other drugs

- Ciclosporin and tacrolimus: monitor ciclosporin and tacrolimus levels; since these drugs are bound to red blood cells there is a potential risk of a drug interaction as haemoglobin concentration increases.
- ACE inhibitors and angiotensin-II antagonists: increased risk of hyperkalaemia.

ADMINISTRATION

RECONSTITUTION
–
ROUTE
- SC, IV
RATE OF ADMINISTRATION
–
COMMENTS
–

OTHER INFORMATION

- To convert to darbepoetin from epoetin, divide total weekly epoetin dose by 200 although that may slightly overestimate the darbepoetin dose.
- Same dose may be given either SC or IV – monitor response.
- Use with caution in patients with a history of epilepsy as convulsions have been reported in patients with CKD.
- Once a pre-filled pen has been removed from the fridge and brought to room temperature it must be used within 7 days.
- Pre-treatment checks and appropriate correction/treatment needed for iron,

folate and B12 deficiency, infection, inflammation or aluminium toxicity to produce optimum response to therapy.

- Concomitant iron therapy (200–300 mg elemental oral iron) needed daily. IV iron may be needed for patients with very low serum ferritin (<100 nanograms/mL).
- May increase heparin requirement during HD.

- Reported association of pure red cell aplasia (PRCA) with epoetin therapy. This is a very rare condition; due to failed production of red blood cell precursors in the bone marrow, resulting in profound anaemia. Possibly due to an immune response to the protein backbone of R-HuEPO. Resulting antibodies render the patient unresponsive to the therapeutic effects of all epoetins and darbepoetin.

Darifenacin

CLINICAL USE

Symptomatic treatment of urinary
incontinence, frequency or urgency

DOSE IN NORMAL RENAL FUNCTION

7.5–15mg once daily

PHARMACOKINETICS

Molecular weight (daltons)	426.6 (507.5 as hydrobromide)
% Protein binding	98
% Excreted unchanged in urine	3
Volume of distribution (L/kg)	163 litres
Half-life – normal/ ESRF (hrs)	13–19/Unchanged

METABOLISM

After an oral dose, darifenacin is subject to
extensive first-pass metabolism and has a
bioavailability of about 15–19%. Darifenacin
is metabolised in the liver by the cytochrome
P450 isoenzymes CYP2D6 and CYP3A4.
Most of a dose is excreted as metabolites in
the urine and faeces.

DOSE IN RENAL IMPAIRMENT GFR (mL/MIN)

20–50	Dose as in normal renal function.
10–20	Dose as in normal renal function.
<10	Dose as in normal renal function.

DOSE IN PATIENTS UNDERGOING RENAL REPLACEMENT THERAPIES

CAPD	Unlikely to be dialysed. Dose as in normal renal function.
HD	Unlikely to be dialysed. Dose as in normal renal function.
HDF/High flux	Unlikely to be dialysed. Dose as in normal renal function.
CAV/ VVHD	Unlikely to be dialysed. Dose as in normal renal function.

IMPORTANT DRUG INTERACTIONS

Potentially hazardous interactions with other
drugs
- Anti-arrhythmics: increased risk
  of antimuscarinic side effects with
  disopyramide.
- Antifungals: concentration increased by
  ketoconazole – avoid concomitant use;
  avoid with itraconazole.
- Antivirals: avoid concomitant use with
  fosamprenavir, atazanavir, indinavir,
  lopinavir, ritonavir, saquinavir and
  tipranavir.
- Calcium-channel blockers: avoid
  concomitant use with verapamil.
- Ciclosporin: avoid concomitant use.

ADMINISTRATION

RECONSTITUTION

–

ROUTE

- Oral

RATE OF ADMINISTRATION

–

COMMENTS

–

Darunavir

CLINICAL USE

Protease inhibitor:
- Treatment of HIV infection with 100 mg of ritonavir, in combination with other antiretroviral medication

DOSE IN NORMAL RENAL FUNCTION

- Previously treated with antiretrovirals: 600 mg twice daily
- Not previously treated with antiretrovirals: 800 mg once daily

PHARMACOKINETICS

Molecular weight (daltons)	593.7 (as ethanolate)
% Protein binding	95
% Excreted unchanged in urine	7.7
Volume of distribution (L/kg)	29.1–147.1 litres (81.1–180.9 litres with ritonavir)
Half-life – normal/ ESRF (hrs)	15 (with ritonavir)/ Unchanged

METABOLISM

Darunavir is metabolised by oxidation by the cytochrome P450 system (mainly the isoenzyme CYP3A4), with at least 3 metabolites showing some antiretroviral activity. About 80% of a dose is excreted in the faeces, with 41.2% of this as unchanged drug; 14% is excreted in the urine, with 7.7% being unchanged drug.

DOSE IN RENAL IMPAIRMENT GFR (mL/MIN)

20–50	Dose as in normal renal function.
10–20	Dose as in normal renal function.
<10	Dose as in normal renal function.

DOSE IN PATIENTS UNDERGOING RENAL REPLACEMENT THERAPIES

CAPD	Unlikely to be dialysed. Dose as in normal renal function.
HD	Unlikely to be dialysed. Dose as in normal renal function.
HDF/High flux	Unlikely to be dialysed. Dose as in normal renal function.
CAV/ VVHD	Unlikely to be dialysed. Dose as in normal renal function.

IMPORTANT DRUG INTERACTIONS

Potentially hazardous interactions with other drugs
- Antibacterials: rifabutin concentration increased – reduce dose of rifabutin; darunavir concentration reduced by rifampicin – avoid concomitant use.
- Antidepressants: possibly reduced concentration of paroxetine and sertraline; darunavir concentration reduced by St John's wort – avoid concomitant use.
- Antimalarials: concentration of lumefantrine increased; possibly increases concentration of quinine.
- Antipsychotics: possibly increases quetiapine concentration – avoid.
- Antivirals: avoid with boceprevir or telaprevir; concentration reduced by efavirenz – adjust dose; concentration of both drugs increased with indinavir; concentration reduced by lopinavir, also concentration of lopinavir increased – avoid; concentration of maraviroc increased, consider reducing dose of maraviroc; concentration reduced by saquinavir.
- Cytotoxics: possibly increases everolimus concentration – avoid.
- Lipid-lowering drugs: possibly increased risk of myopathy with atorvastatin and rosuvastatin, avoid with rosuvastatin; possibly increases pravastatin concentration; avoid concomitant use with simvastatin.[1]
- Ranolazine: possibly increases ranolazine concentration – avoid.

ADMINISTRATION

RECONSTITUTION
–

ROUTE
- Oral

RATE OF ADMINISTRATION
–

COMMENTS
–

Reference:
1. MHRA. *Drug Safety Update*. Statins: interactions and updated advice. August 2012; **6**(1): 2–4.

Dasatinib

CLINICAL USE

- Chronic myeloid leukaemia (CML) in patients who have resistance or intolerance to previous therapy, including imatinib
- Philadelphia chromosome-positive acute lymphoblastic leukaemia in adults who are resistant to or intolerant of prior therapy

DOSE IN NORMAL RENAL FUNCTION

- Chronic CML: 100 mg once daily
- All other indications: 140 mg daily; Maximum: 180 mg once daily

PHARMACOKINETICS

Molecular weight (daltons)	488
% Protein binding	96
% Excreted unchanged in urine	0.1
Volume of distribution (L/kg)	2505 litres
Half-life – normal/ ESRF (hrs)	5–6/–

METABOLISM

Dasatinib is extensively metabolised, mainly via the cytochrome P450 isoenzyme CYP3A4, forming an active metabolite. Elimination is predominantly in the faeces, mostly as metabolites. Following a single oral dose of $[^{14}C]$-labelled dasatinib, approximately 89% of the dose was eliminated within 10 days, with 4% and 85% of the radioactivity recovered in the urine and faeces, respectively. Unchanged dasatinib accounted for 0.1% and 19% of the dose in urine and faeces, respectively, with the remainder of the dose as metabolites.

DOSE IN RENAL IMPAIRMENT GFR (mL/MIN)

20–50	Dose as in normal renal function.
10–20	Dose as in normal renal function.
<10	Dose as in normal renal function. Use with caution.

DOSE IN PATIENTS UNDERGOING RENAL REPLACEMENT THERAPIES

CAPD	Unlikely to be dialysed. Dose as in GFR<10 mL/min.
HD	Unlikely to be dialysed. Dose as in GFR<10 mL/min.
HDF/High flux	Unlikely to be dialysed. Dose as in GFR<10 mL/min.
CAV/ VVHD	Unlikely to be dialysed. Dose as in normal renal function.

IMPORTANT DRUG INTERACTIONS

Potentially hazardous interactions with other drugs

- Antibacterials: metabolism accelerated by rifampicin – avoid concomitant use.
- Antipsychotics: avoid concomitant use with clozapine, increased risk of agranulocytosis.
- Antivirals: avoid with boceprevir.

ADMINISTRATION

RECONSTITUTION
–
ROUTE
- Oral
RATE OF ADMINISTRATION
–
COMMENTS
–

OTHER INFORMATION

- No studies have been done with dasatinib in renal impairment but due to the low renal excretion there is unlikely to be a reduction in clearance.
- Most common adverse effects of dasatinib include fluid retention, gastrointestinal disturbances, and bleeding. Fluid retention may be severe, and can result in pleural and pericardial effusion, pulmonary oedema and ascites.

Daunorubicin

CLINICAL USE

Antineoplastic agent:
- Acute leukaemias
- HIV-related Kaposi's sarcoma

DOSE IN NORMAL RENAL FUNCTION

40–60 mg/m^2 frequency varies according to indication
Dose depends on indication or as for local protocol.

PHARMACOKINETICS

Molecular weight (daltons)	564 (as hydrochloride)
% Protein binding	50–90
% Excreted unchanged in urine	5–18
Volume of distribution (L/kg)	39.2
Half-life – normal/ ESRF (hrs)	18.5; Liposomal: 4–5.2/–

METABOLISM

Daunorubicin is rapidly taken up by the tissues, especially by the kidneys, liver, spleen and heart. Subsequent release of drug and metabolites is slow (t½ ~ 55 hours). It is rapidly metabolised in the liver and the major metabolite, daunorubicinol, is also active. It is excreted slowly in the urine, mainly as metabolites with 25% excreted within 5 days. Biliary excretion accounts for 40–50% elimination.

DOSE IN RENAL IMPAIRMENT GFR (mL/MIN)

20–50	Dose as in normal renal function. See 'Other information'.
10–20	Dose as in normal renal function. See 'Other information'.
<10	Dose as in normal renal function. See 'Other information'.

DOSE IN PATIENTS UNDERGOING RENAL REPLACEMENT THERAPIES

CAPD	Unlikely to be dialysed. Dose as GFR<10 mL/min.
HD	Unlikely to be dialysed. Dose as GFR<10 mL/min.
HDF/High flux	Unknown dialysability. Dose as GFR<10 mL/min.
CAV/ VVHD	Unlikely to be dialysed. Dose as GFR=10–20 mL/min.

IMPORTANT DRUG INTERACTIONS

Potentially hazardous interactions with other drugs
- None known

ADMINISTRATION

RECONSTITUTION
- Reconstitute 20 mg vial with 4 mL water for injection giving a concentration of 5 mg/mL. Dilute calculated dose of daunorubicin further in sodium chloride 0.9% to give a final concentration of 1 mg/mL.

ROUTE
- IV

RATE OF ADMINISTRATION
- Acute leukaemia: 1 mg/mL solution should be infused over 20 minutes into the tubing or a side arm of a rapidly flowing IV infusion of sodium chloride 0.9%.
- HIV-related Kaposi's sarcoma: 30–60 minutes.

OTHER INFORMATION

- Potentially cardiotoxic.
- Monitor blood uric acid and urea levels.
- Manufacturer's literature suggests that in patients with a serum creatinine of 105–265 µmol/L the dose should be reduced to 75% of normal; if the creatinine is >265 µmol/L, the dose should be 50% of normal.
- Dose in renal impairment is from *Drug Prescribing in Renal Failure*, 5th edition, by Aronoff *et al.*
- A liposomal formulation of daunorubicin is now available (DaunoXome®). Dilute to 0.2–1 mg/mL with glucose 5% and administer over 30–60 minutes.

Decitabine

CLINICAL USE

Antineoplastic antimetabolite agent:
- Treatment of acute myeloid leukaemia

DOSE IN NORMAL RENAL FUNCTION

$20 \, mg/m^2$ daily for 5 days repeated every 4 weeks

PHARMACOKINETICS

Molecular weight (daltons)	228.2
% Protein binding	<1
% Excreted unchanged in urine	Approx 4
Volume of distribution (L/kg)	69.1 litres[1]
Half-life – normal/ ESRF (hrs)	30–35 minutes/–

METABOLISM

The exact route of metabolism and elimination is unknown but thought to be through deamination by cytidine deaminase in the liver, kidney, intestinal epithelium and blood to form inactive metabolites.

DOSE IN RENAL IMPAIRMENT GFR (mL/MIN)

20–50	Dose as in normal renal function. Use with caution.
10–20	Dose as in normal renal function. Use with caution.
<10	Dose as in normal renal function. Use with caution.

DOSE IN PATIENTS UNDERGOING RENAL REPLACEMENT THERAPIES

CAPD	Possibly dialysed. Dose as in GFR<10 mL/min.
HD	Probably dialysed. Dose as in GFR<10 mL/min.
HDF/High flux	Dialysed. Dose as in GFR<10 mL/min.
CAV/ VVHD	Dialysed. Dose as in GFR=10–20 mL/min.

IMPORTANT DRUG INTERACTIONS

Potentially hazardous interactions with other drugs
- Antipsychotics: avoid with clozapine, increased risk of agranulocytosis.

ADMINISTRATION

RECONSTITUTION
- 10 mL water for injection

ROUTE
- IV infusion

RATE OF ADMINISTRATION
- 1 hour

COMMENTS
- After reconstitution dilute to 0.1–1 mg/mL with sodium chloride 0.9%, glucose 5% or lactated Ringer's solution.

OTHER INFORMATION

- Manufacturer has not done any studies in renal failure but because of low renal clearance use doses as for normal renal function.

Reference:
1. Mistry B, Gibiansky L, Hussein Z. Pharmacokinetic modelling of decitabine in patients with myelodysplastic syndromes (MDS) and acute myeloid leukemia (AML). *J Clin Oncol.* **29**: 2011 (suppl; abstr 6551).

Deferasirox

CLINICAL USE

Treatment of iron overload

DOSE IN NORMAL RENAL FUNCTION

10–30 mg/kg once daily rounded to the nearest whole tablet
Maximum 40 mg/kg daily

PHARMACOKINETICS

Molecular weight (daltons)	373.4
% Protein binding	99
% Excreted unchanged in urine	8
Volume of distribution (L/kg)	14 litres
Half-life – normal/ESRF (hrs)	8–16/–

METABOLISM

Metabolism of deferasirox is mainly glucuronidation by uridine diphosphate glucuronosyltransferase (UGT) enzymes. Cytochrome P450 isoenzyme-mediated metabolism appears to be minor. Deconjugation of the glucuronidates in the intestine and subsequent enterohepatic recycling are likely to occur. It is excreted mainly in the faeces via bile, as metabolites and as unchanged drug. About 8% of a dose is excreted in the urine.

DOSE IN RENAL IMPAIRMENT GFR (mL/MIN)

20–50	Avoid. See 'Other information'.
10–20	Avoid. See 'Other information'.
<10	Avoid. See 'Other information'.

DOSE IN PATIENTS UNDERGOING RENAL REPLACEMENT THERAPIES

CAPD	Unlikely to be dialysed. Avoid.
HD	Dialysed. Avoid.
HDF/High flux	Dialysed. Avoid.
CAV/VVHD	Dialysed. Avoid.

IMPORTANT DRUG INTERACTIONS

Potentially hazardous interactions with other drugs
- Aluminium-containing antacids: avoid concomitant use.
- Theophylline: concentration of theophylline increased, consider reducing theophylline dose.
- Other nephrotoxic agents: avoid concomitant therapy.

ADMINISTRATION

RECONSTITUTION
–
ROUTE
- Oral
RATE OF ADMINISTRATION
–
COMMENTS
- Take on an empty stomach.
- Disperse in a glass of water, orange or apple juice.

OTHER INFORMATION

- UK manufacturer advises to avoid in moderate to severe renal impairment due to lack of data. New Zealand data sheet advises to use normal dose with caution if GFR=40–60 mL/min. US data sheet advises to use 50% of dose if GFR=40–60 mL/min.
- Increased risk of potentially fatal renal failure and cytopenias in patients with other comorbidities who also had an advanced haematological condition. www.medscape.com/viewarticle/557118.
- During clinical trials, increases in serum creatinine of >33% on 2 consecutive occasions (sometimes above the upper limit of the normal range) occurred in about 36% of patients. These were dose-dependent. Cases of acute renal failure have been reported following post-marketing use of deferasirox.
- Patients with pre-existing renal conditions and patients who are receiving medicinal products that depress renal function may be more at risk of complications.
- Tests for proteinuria should be performed monthly. Other markers of renal tubular function may also be monitored (e.g. glycosuria in non-diabetics and low levels of serum potassium, phosphate, magnesium or urate, phosphaturia, aminoaciduria).
- If, despite dose reduction and interruption, the serum creatinine remains significantly elevated and there is also persistent abnormality in another marker of renal function (e.g. proteinuria, Fanconi's syndrome), the patient should be referred to a renal specialist, and further specialised investigations (such as renal biopsy) may be considered.
- Closely monitor patients who are taking other agents which may cause ulceration, e.g. NSAIDs.

Deferiprone

CLINICAL USE

Orally administered chelator:
* Treatment of transfusional iron overload

DOSE IN NORMAL RENAL FUNCTION

25 mg/kg 3 times daily.
Maximum 100 mg/kg daily.

PHARMACOKINETICS

Molecular weight (daltons)	139.2
% Protein binding	No data
% Excreted unchanged in urine	15 – See 'Other information'
Volume of distribution (L/kg)	1.55–1.73
Half-life – normal/ ESRF (hrs)	2–3/Unknown

METABOLISM

Deferiprone is hepatically metabolised to an inactive glucuronide metabolite and is excreted mainly in the urine as the metabolite and the iron-deferiprone complex, with a small amount of unchanged drug.

DOSE IN RENAL IMPAIRMENT GFR (mL/MIN)

20–50	Dose as in normal renal function.
10–20	Use with caution.
<10	Use with caution.

DOSE IN PATIENTS UNDERGOING RENAL REPLACEMENT THERAPIES

CAPD	Unknown dialysability. Dose as in GFR<10 mL/min.
HD	Dialysed. Dose as in GFR<10 mL/min.
HDF/High flux	Dialysed. Dose as in GFR<10 mL/min.
CAV/ VVHD	Dialysed. Dose as in GFR=10–20 mL/min.

IMPORTANT DRUG INTERACTIONS

Potentially hazardous interactions with other drugs
* None known

ADMINISTRATION

RECONSTITUTION

–

ROUTE
* Oral

RATE OF ADMINISTRATION

–

COMMENTS

–

OTHER INFORMATION

* Manufacturer advises to use with caution due to lack of studies. Since deferiprone is eliminated mainly via the kidneys, there may be an increased risk of complications in patients with impaired renal function.
* Side effects include reversible neutropenia, agranulocytosis, musculoskeletal and joint pain, subclinical ototoxicity, plus case reports of systemic vasculitis and fatal SLE.
* Can cause subnormal serum zinc levels.
* Reddish-brown discolouration of the urine reported in 40% of thalassaemia patients undergoing deferiprone therapy.
* Deferiprone removed aluminium *in vitro* from blood samples of 46 patients undergoing chronic haemodialysis. Only patients with serum aluminium concentrations >80 mcg/mL were included. Deferiprone removed the aluminium faster and more effectively from higher molecular weight proteins than desferrioxamine. (Canteros-Piccotto MA, Fernández-Martin JL, Cannata-Ortiz MJ, *et al.* Effectiveness of deferiprone (L1) releasing the aluminium bound to plasma proteins in chronic renal failure. *Nephrol Dial Transplant.* 1996; **11**(7): 1488–9).

Deflazacort

CLINICAL USE

Glucocorticoid:
- Suppression of inflammatory and allergic disorders

DOSE IN NORMAL RENAL FUNCTION

3–18 mg daily
(Acute disorders up to 120 mg daily initially)

PHARMACOKINETICS

Molecular weight (daltons)	441.5
% Protein binding	40
% Excreted unchanged in urine	70
Volume of distribution (L/kg)	1.2
Half-life – normal/ ESRF (hrs)	1.1–1.9/Unchanged

METABOLISM

Deflazacort is immediately converted by plasma esterases to the pharmacologically active metabolite (D 21-OH). It is 40% protein-bound and has no affinity for corticosteroid-binding-globulin (transcortin). Elimination takes place primarily through the kidneys; 70% of the administered dose is excreted in the urine. The remaining 30% is eliminated in the faeces. Metabolism of D 21-OH is extensive; only 18% of urinary excretion represents D 21-OH. The metabolite of D 21-OH, deflazacort 6-beta-OH, represents one third of the urinary elimination.

DOSE IN RENAL IMPAIRMENT GFR (mL/MIN)

20–50	Dose as in normal renal function.
10–20	Dose as in normal renal function.
<10	Dose as in normal renal function.

DOSE IN PATIENTS UNDERGOING RENAL REPLACEMENT THERAPIES

CAPD	Unlikely to be dialysed. Dose as in normal renal function.
HD	Not dialysed. Dose as in normal renal function.
HDF/High flux	Unknown dialysability. Dose as in normal renal function.
CAV/ VVHD	Unlikely to be dialysed. Dose as in normal renal function.

IMPORTANT DRUG INTERACTIONS

Potentially hazardous interactions with other drugs
- Aldesleukin: avoid concomitant use.
- Antibacterials: metabolism accelerated by rifampicin; metabolism possibly inhibited by erythromycin; concentration of isoniazid possibly reduced.
- Anticoagulants: efficacy of coumarins and phenindione may be altered.
- Anti-epileptics: metabolism accelerated by carbamazepine, phenobarbital and phenytoin.
- Antifungals: increased risk of hypokalaemia with amphotericin – avoid concomitant use; metabolism possibly inhibited by itraconazole and ketoconazole.
- Antivirals: concentration possibly increased by ritonavir.
- Ciclosporin: rare reports of convulsions in patients on ciclosporin and high-dose corticosteroids; increased half-life of deflazacort.
- Diuretics: enhanced hypokalaemic effects of acetazolamide, loop diuretics and thiazide diuretics.
- Vaccines: high dose corticosteroids can impair immune response to vaccines; avoid concomitant use with live vaccines.

ADMINISTRATION

RECONSTITUTION

–

ROUTE
- Oral

RATE OF ADMINISTRATION

–

COMMENTS

–

OTHER INFORMATION

- 6 mg of deflazacort is equivalent to 5 mg prednisolone.

Degarelix

CLINICAL USE

Gonadotrophin releasing hormone antagonist:
- Treatment of advanced prostate cancer

DOSE IN NORMAL RENAL FUNCTION

240 mg starting dose (administered as 2 separate injections of 120 mg) followed by 80 mg every 28 days

PHARMACOKINETICS

Molecular weight (daltons)	1632.3
% Protein binding	90
% Excreted unchanged in urine	20–30
Volume of distribution (L/kg)	1
Half-life – normal/ ESRF (hrs)	43–53 days (28 after 80 mg maintenance dose)/–

METABOLISM

Undergoes peptide hydrolysis in the hepato-biliary system, and is mainly (70–80%) excreted as peptide fragments in the faeces.

DOSE IN RENAL IMPAIRMENT GFR (mL/MIN)

20–50	Dose as in normal renal function.
10–20	Dose as in normal renal function.
<10	Dose as in normal renal function. Use with caution.

DOSE IN PATIENTS UNDERGOING RENAL REPLACEMENT THERAPIES

CAPD	Unlikely to be dialysed. Dose as in GFR<10 mL/min. Use with caution.
HD	Unlikely to be dialysed. Dose as in GFR<10 mL/min. Use with caution.
HDF/High flux	Unlikely to be dialysed. Dose as in GFR<10 mL/min. Use with caution.
CAV/ VVHD	Unlikely to be dialysed. Dose as in normal renal function.

IMPORTANT DRUG INTERACTIONS

Potentially hazardous interactions with other drugs
- None known

ADMINISTRATION

RECONSTITUTION
- 3 mL solvent provided

ROUTE
- SC

RATE OF ADMINISTRATION
–

OTHER INFORMATION

- Use with caution in severe renal impairment due to lack of experience.
- May prolong QT interval.
- Degarelix is injected to form a subcutaneous depot, and the pharmacokinetics of the drug is strongly influenced by the concentration of the injected solution.
- A phase III study has demonstrated that the clearance of degarelix in patients with mild to moderate renal impairment is reduced by approximately 23% so no dose adjustment is required.

Demeclocycline hydrochloride

CLINICAL USE

Antibacterial agent:
- Treatment of syndrome of inappropriate antidiuretic hormone secretion

DOSE IN NORMAL RENAL FUNCTION

- 150 mg 4 times a day or 300 mg twice daily
- Syndrome of inappropriate antidiuretic hormone: 900–1200 mg daily in divided doses
- Maintenance: 600–900 mg daily in divided doses

PHARMACOKINETICS

Molecular weight (daltons)	501.3
% Protein binding	41–90
% Excreted unchanged in urine	42
Volume of distribution (L/kg)	1.7
Half-life – normal/ ESRF (hrs)	10–15/42–68

METABOLISM

Demeclocycline hydrochloride, like other tetracyclines, is concentrated in the liver, where it is metabolised and excreted into the bile. It is found in much higher concentrations in the bile compared with the blood. Following a single 150 mg dose of demeclocycline hydrochloride in normal volunteers, 44% (n = 8) was excreted in urine and 13% and 46%, respectively, were excreted in faeces in two patients within 96 hours as active drug.

DOSE IN RENAL IMPAIRMENT GFR (mL/MIN)

20–50	Dose as in normal renal function.
10–20	600 mg every 24–48 hours.
<10	600 mg every 24–48 hours.

DOSE IN PATIENTS UNDERGOING RENAL REPLACEMENT THERAPIES

CAPD	Not dialysed. 600 mg every 48 hours.
HD	Dialysed. 600 mg post dialysis.
HDF/High flux	Dialysed. 600 mg post dialysis.
CAV/ VVHD	Unknown dialysability. Dose as in GFR=10–20 mL/min.

IMPORTANT DRUG INTERACTIONS

Potentially hazardous interactions with other drugs
- Anticoagulants: possibly enhanced anticoagulant effect of coumarins and phenindione.
- Oestrogens: possibly reduced contraceptive effects of oestrogens (risk probably small).
- Retinoids: possible increased risk of benign intracranial hypertension, avoid concomitant use.

ADMINISTRATION

RECONSTITUTION

–

ROUTE
- Oral

RATE OF ADMINISTRATION

–

COMMENTS

–

OTHER INFORMATION

- Avoid if possible in renal impairment due to its potential nephrotoxicity.
- May be administered to anuric patients every 3–4 days.
- Dose in renal impairment is from *Drug Dosage in Renal Insufficiency* by Seyffart G.

Denosumab

CLINICAL USE

Human monoclonal antibody (IgG2):
- Osteoporosis in postmenopausal women and men with prostate cancer after hormone ablation at risk of fractures
- Reduction of bone damage in patients with bone metastases from solid tumours

DOSE IN NORMAL RENAL FUNCTION

- Osteoporosis: 60 mg every 6 months
- Reduction of bone damage: 120 mg every 4 weeks

PHARMACOKINETICS

Molecular weight (daltons)	144 700
% Protein binding	No data
% Excreted unchanged in urine	No data
Volume of distribution (L/kg)	No data
Half-life – normal/ ESRF (hrs)	14–55 days/ Unchanged

METABOLISM

Metabolism and elimination are expected to follow the immunoglobulin clearance pathways, resulting in degradation to small peptides and individual amino acids.

DOSE IN RENAL IMPAIRMENT GFR (mL/MIN)

30–50	Dose as in normal renal function.
10–30	Dose as in normal renal function. See 'Other information'.
<10	Dose as in normal renal function. See 'Other information'.

DOSE IN PATIENTS UNDERGOING RENAL REPLACEMENT THERAPIES

CAPD	Unlikely to be dialysed. Dose as in GFR<10 mL/min.
HD	Unlikely to be dialysed. Dose as in GFR<10 mL/min.
HDF/High flux	Unlikely to be dialysed. Dose as in GFR<10 mL/min.
CAV/ VVHD	Unlikely to be dialysed. Dose as in GFR=10–30 mL/min.

IMPORTANT DRUG INTERACTIONS

Potentially hazardous interactions with other drugs
- None known

ADMINISTRATION

RECONSTITUTION
–
ROUTE
- SC
RATE OF ADMINISTRATION
–

OTHER INFORMATION

- There is limited data from the manufacturer for monthly administration therefore use with caution.
- Hypocalcaemia is a major risk if GFR<30 mL/min.
- Calcium and vitamin D supplements must be taken.
- Osteonecrosis of the jaw has occurred although rarely.

Desferrioxamine mesilate

CLINICAL USE

Chelating agent:
- Acute iron poisoning
- Chronic iron or aluminium overload

DOSE IN NORMAL RENAL FUNCTION

- SC/IV: Initially 500 mg then 20–60 mg/kg/day 3–7 times a week. Exact dosages should be determined for each individual.
- IM: 0.5–2 g daily as stat, maintenance dose as per response.
- Oral: acute iron poisoning: 5–10 g should be dissolved in 50–100 mL water.
- Aluminium overload in HD: (IV) 5 mg/kg weekly over last hour of dialysis.
- PD: (SC, IM, IV, IP) 5 mg/kg weekly before the final exchange of the day.

PHARMACOKINETICS

Molecular weight (daltons)	656.8
% Protein binding	<10
% Excreted unchanged in urine	22
Volume of distribution (L/kg)	2–2.5
Half-life – normal/ ESRF (hrs)	6/–

METABOLISM

When given parenterally desferrioxamine forms chelates with iron and aluminium ions to form ferrioxamine and aluminoxamine, respectively. The chelates are excreted in the urine and faeces via the bile. Desferrioxamine is metabolised, mainly in the plasma. Four metabolites of desferrioxamine were isolated from urine of patients with iron overload. The following biotransformation reactions were found to occur with desferrioxamine: transamination and oxidation yielding an acid metabolite, beta-oxidation also yielding an acid metabolite, decarboxylation and N-hydroxylation yielding neutral metabolites.

DOSE IN RENAL IMPAIRMENT GFR (mL/MIN)

20–50	Dose as in normal renal function. See 'Other information'.
10–20	See 'Other information'.
<10	See 'Other information'.

DOSE IN PATIENTS UNDERGOING RENAL REPLACEMENT THERAPIES

CAPD	Dialysed. Treatment of aluminium overload: 1 g once or twice each week prior to final exchange of the day by slow IV infusion, IM, SC or IP.
HD	Dialysed. Treatment of aluminium overload: 1 g once each week administered during the last hour of dialysis as a slow IV infusion.
HDF/High flux	Dialysed. Treatment of aluminium overload: 1 g once each week administered during the last hour of dialysis as a slow IV infusion.
CAV/ VVHD	Dialysed. Dose schedule unknown. Metal chelates will be removed by dialysis.

IMPORTANT DRUG INTERACTIONS

Potentially hazardous interactions with other drugs
- Avoid prochlorperazine, levomepromazine and methotrimeprazine (prolonged unconsciousness).
- Do not administer with blood.

ADMINISTRATION

RECONSTITUTION
- Dissolve contents of one vial (500 mg) in 5 mL of water for injection =10% solution. If for IV administration, the 10% solution can be diluted with sodium chloride 0.9%, glucose 5% or glucose/sodium chloride.

ROUTE
- IV, SC (bolus or continuous infusion), IM, IP, oral

RATE OF ADMINISTRATION
- IV (acute overdose): Maximum 15 mg/kg/ hour. Reduce after 4–6 hours so that total dose does not exceed 80 mg/kg/24 hours.
- SC: Infuse over 8–24 hours. Local irritation may occur.

COMMENTS
- The urine may appear orange/red in patients treated with desferrioxamine for severe iron intoxication.
- SC infusion is about 90% as effective as IV administration, which is now the route of choice in transfusion-related iron overload.
- IM injection is less effective than SC.

OTHER INFORMATION

- Studies suggest that during HD only a small amount of plasma desferrioxamine crosses the dialysis membrane.
- Manufacturer advises to use with caution in renal impairment except those on dialysis as the metal complexes are excreted via the kidney.
- *Drug Prescribing in Renal Failure*, 5th edition, by Aronoff *et al.* advises to use 25–50% of dose if GFR=10–50 mL/min and to avoid if GFR<10 mL/min.
- 100 mg desferrioxamine mesilate can bind 4.1 mg Al^{3+}.

- Desferrioxamine may predispose to development of infection with *Yersinia* species.
- In haemodialysis patients treated with desferrioxamine post dialysis, the half-life has been found to be extended to 19 hours between dialysis sessions.
- Anecdotally, escalating doses of up to 2 g, 3 times a week have been successfully used for iron overload in patients on haemodialysis.
- In treatment of acute iron poisoning, effectiveness of treatment is dependent on an adequate urine output. If oliguria or anuria develop, PD or HD may be necessary.

Desirudin (unlicensed product)

CLINICAL USE

Prophylaxis of DVT in patients undergoing orthopaedic surgery

DOSE IN NORMAL RENAL FUNCTION

15 mg 5–15 minutes before surgery then 15 mg twice daily for 9–12 days or until mobile

PHARMACOKINETICS

Molecular weight (daltons)	6963.4
% Protein binding	No data
% Excreted unchanged in urine	40–50
Volume of distribution (L/kg)	0.25
Half-life – normal/ ESRF (hrs)	2–3/–

METABOLISM

Desirudin is metabolised and excreted by the kidney, and 40 to 50% of a dose is excreted unchanged in the urine.

DOSE IN RENAL IMPAIRMENT GFR (mL/MIN)

31–60	Initially 5 mg twice daily. Aim for APTT <0.85 seconds.
<31	Initially 1.7 mg twice daily and monitor APTT.

DOSE IN PATIENTS UNDERGOING RENAL REPLACEMENT THERAPIES

CAPD	Not dialysed. Dose as in GFR<31 mL/min.
HD	Not dialysed. Dose as in GFR<31 mL/min.
HDF/High flux	Unknown dialysability. Dose as in GFR<31 mL/min.
CAV/ VVHD	Not dialysed. Dose as in GFR<31 mL/min.

IMPORTANT DRUG INTERACTIONS

Potentially hazardous interactions with other drugs
- Anticoagulants, antiplatelets, fondaparinux, NSAIDs, heparin and dextran – increased risk of bleeding.

ADMINISTRATION

RECONSTITUTION
- With diluent supplied

ROUTE
- SC

RATE OF ADMINISTRATION
–

COMMENTS
–

OTHER INFORMATION

- Doses from *Drug Information Handbook*, 22nd edition. American Pharmacists Association. Lexicomp.
- The effect is poorly reversible.
- APTT levels can be reduced by IV DDAVP.
- Available on a named patient basis from Aventis Pharma.
- 7% of dose is metabolised by the kidneys.

Desloratadine

CLINICAL USE

Antihistamine:
- Symptomatic relief of allergy such as hay fever, urticaria

DOSE IN NORMAL RENAL FUNCTION

5 mg daily

PHARMACOKINETICS

Molecular weight (daltons)	310.8
% Protein binding	83–87
% Excreted unchanged in urine	40.6 (as active metabolites)
Volume of distribution (L/kg)	No data
Half-life – normal/ ESRF (hrs)	27/Increased

METABOLISM

Desloratadine is the primary active metabolite of loratadine. Approximately 40% of the dose is excreted in the urine and 42% in the faeces over a 10 day period and mainly in the form of conjugated metabolites. Approximately 27% of the dose is eliminated in the urine during the first 24 hours. Less than 1% of the active substance is excreted unchanged in the active form, as desloratadine.

DOSE IN RENAL IMPAIRMENT GFR (mL/MIN)

20–50	Dose as in normal renal function.
10–20	Dose as in normal renal function.
<10	Dose as in normal renal function. Use with caution.

DOSE IN PATIENTS UNDERGOING RENAL REPLACEMENT THERAPIES

CAPD	Not dialysed. Dose as in normal renal function.
HD	Not dialysed. Dose as in normal renal function.
HDF/High flux	Unknown dialysability. Dose as in normal renal function.
CAV/ VVHD	Unlikely to be dialysed. Dose as in normal renal function.

IMPORTANT DRUG INTERACTIONS

Potentially hazardous interactions with other drugs
- Antivirals: concentration possibly increased by ritonavir.

ADMINISTRATION

RECONSTITUTION
–
ROUTE
- Oral
RATE OF ADMINISTRATION
–
COMMENTS
–

OTHER INFORMATION

Full dose may result in increased sedation in patients with GFR<10 mL/min.

Desmopressin (DDAVP)

CLINICAL USE

- Diabetes insipidus
- Nocturnal enuresis
- Post-biopsy bleeding (unlicensed indication)
- Pre-biopsy prophylaxis (unlicensed indication)

DOSE IN NORMAL RENAL FUNCTION

- Diabetes insipidus: Oral: 0.2–1.2 mg daily in 3 divided doses. IV: 1–4 mcg daily. Inhaled: 10–40 mcg in 1 or 2 divided doses. Sub-lingual: 120–720 mcg daily.
- Nocturnal enuresis: Oral: 200–400 mcg at bedtime.
- Biopsy: Males – 16 mcg; Females – 12 mcg or 300–400 nanograms/kg.
- Pre-biopsy prophylaxis in uraemic patients: 20 mcg (IV) over 30 minutes.

PHARMACOKINETICS

Molecular weight (daltons)	1069.20
% Protein binding	0
% Excreted unchanged in urine	45
Volume of distribution (L/kg)	0.2–0.41
Half-life – normal/ ESRF (hrs)	Inhaled: 55 minutes; Oral: 2.8 hours; IV: 51–158 minutes/–

METABOLISM

Metabolic fate of desmopressin is unknown. It is not affected by liver microsomal cytochrome P450 enzymes. As a peptide, desmopressin is expected to undergo catabolism to its constituent amino acids, with subsequent recycling of the amino acid in the body pool.

DOSE IN RENAL IMPAIRMENT GFR (mL/MIN)

20–50	Dose as in normal renal function.
10–20	Dose as in normal renal function.
<10	Dose as in normal renal function.

DOSE IN PATIENTS UNDERGOING RENAL REPLACEMENT THERAPIES

CAPD	Unlikely to be dialysed. Dose as in normal renal function.
HD	Unlikely to be dialysed. Dose as in normal renal function.
HDF/High flux	Unknown dialysability. Dose as in normal renal function.
CAV/ VVHD	Unlikely to be dialysed. Dose as in normal renal function.

IMPORTANT DRUG INTERACTIONS

Potentially hazardous interactions with other drugs
- None known

ADMINISTRATION

RECONSTITUTION
–

ROUTE
- IV, intranasally, oral, SC, IM, SL
RATE OF ADMINISTRATION
- Over 20–60 minutes
COMMENTS
- Dilute dose to 50 mL with sodium chloride 0.9%.
- Do not inject at a faster rate – greater risk of tachyphylaxis.
- In patients with ischaemic heart disease, infuse more slowly – increased risk of acute ischaemic event.

OTHER INFORMATION

- Emergency treatment of more generalised bleeding unresponsive to normal treatments: 0.1–0.5 micrograms/kg 4 times a day + IV conjugated oestrogens (premarin) 0.6 mg/kg/day for up to 5 days.
- DDAVP works as a haemostatic by stimulating factor VIII production.
- Onset of action less than 1 hour. Duration of effect 4–8 hours.

Dexamethasone

CLINICAL USE

Corticosteroid:
- Cerebral oedema
- Bacterial meningitis (unlicensed indication)
- Suppression of inflammatory and allergic disorders
- Rheumatic disease
- Congenital adrenal hyperplasia
- Anti-emetic (unlicensed indication)

DOSE IN NORMAL RENAL FUNCTION

- Cerebral oedema, bacterial meningitis: depends on preparation.
- Rheumatic disease:
  — intra-articular, intrasynovial: according to preparation and size of joint
  — soft tissue infiltration: 1.7–5 mg
- Oral: 0.5–10 mg daily, IV/IM: 0.4–20 mg

PHARMACOKINETICS

Molecular weight (daltons)	392.5 (472.4 as phosphate)
% Protein binding	77
% Excreted unchanged in urine	65
Volume of distribution (L/kg)	0.8–1
Half-life – normal/ ESRF (hrs)	3.5–4.5/–

METABOLISM

Corticosteroids are metabolised mainly in the liver but also in other tissues, and are excreted in the urine. The slower metabolism of the synthetic corticosteroids with their lower protein-binding affinity may account for their increased potency compared with the natural corticosteroids. Up to 65% of a dose of dexamethasone is excreted in urine within 24 hours.

DOSE IN RENAL IMPAIRMENT GFR (mL/MIN)

20–50	Dose as in normal renal function.
10–20	Dose as in normal renal function.
<10	Dose as in normal renal function.

DOSE IN PATIENTS UNDERGOING RENAL REPLACEMENT THERAPIES

CAPD	Not dialysed. Dose as in normal renal function.
HD	Not dialysed. Dose as in normal renal function.
HDF/High flux	Unknown dialysability. Dose as in normal renal function.
CAV/ VVHD	Removal unlikely. Dose as in normal renal function.

IMPORTANT DRUG INTERACTIONS

Potentially hazardous interactions with other drugs
- Aldesleukin: avoid concomitant use.
- Antibacterials: metabolism accelerated by rifampicin; metabolism possibly inhibited by erythromycin; concentration of isoniazid possibly reduced.
- Anticoagulants: efficacy of coumarins and phenindione may be altered.
- Anti-epileptics: metabolism accelerated by carbamazepine, phenobarbital and phenytoin.
- Antifungals: increased risk of hypokalaemia with amphotericin – avoid concomitant use; metabolism possibly inhibited by itraconazole and ketoconazole; caspofungin concentration possibly reduced (may need to increase dose).
- Antivirals: concentration of indinavir, lopinavir, saquinavir and telaprevir possibly reduced; avoid with rilpivirine; concentration possibly increased by ritonavir.
- Ciclosporin: rare reports of convulsions in patients on ciclosporin and high-dose corticosteroids.
- Cytotoxics: possibly decreases axitinib concentration, increase dose of axitinib.
- Diuretics: enhanced hypokalaemic effects of acetazolamide, loop diuretics and thiazide diuretics.
- Vaccines: high dose corticosteroids can impair immune response to vaccines; avoid concomitant use with live vaccines.

ADMINISTRATION

RECONSTITUTION

–

ROUTE

- Oral, IV, IM, intra-articular, intrasynovial

RATE OF ADMINISTRATION

- IV slowly over not less than 5 minutes. If underlying cardiac pathology, infusion over 20–30 minutes advised.

COMMENTS

- Dexamethasone sodium phosphate 1.3 mg = dexamethasone 1 mg.
- 750 mcg of dexamethasone is equivalent to 5 mg prednisolone.
- Injection solution can be administered orally or via nasogastric tube.
- Tablets will disperse in water.

Dexibuprofen

CLINICAL USE

NSAID and analgesic

DOSE IN NORMAL RENAL FUNCTION

- Initially: 600–900 mg daily in divided doses, after food
- Maximum 1.2 g daily (900 mg daily for dysmenorrhoea)
- Maximum single dose: 400 mg (300 mg for dysmenorrhoea)

PHARMACOKINETICS

Molecular weight (daltons)	206.3
% Protein binding	>99
% Excreted unchanged in urine	82 (mainly as inactive metabolites)
Volume of distribution (L/kg)	10–11 litres
Half-life – normal/ ESRF (hrs)	1.6–1.9/Unchanged

METABOLISM

Dexibuprofen is the $S(+)$-enantiomer of ibuprofen. After metabolic transformation in the liver (hydroxylation and carboxylation), the pharmacologically inactive metabolites are completely excreted, mainly by the kidneys (90%), but also in the bile.

DOSE IN RENAL IMPAIRMENT GFR (mL/MIN)

20–50	Dose as in normal renal function, but avoid if possible.
10–20	Dose as in normal renal function, but avoid if possible.
<10	Dose as in normal renal function, but only use if on dialysis.

DOSE IN PATIENTS UNDERGOING RENAL REPLACEMENT THERAPIES

CAPD	Not dialysed. Dose as in GFR<10 mL/min.
HD	Not dialysed. Dose as in GFR<10 mL/min.
HDF/High flux	Unknown dialysability. Dose as in GFR<10 mL/min.
CAV/ VVHD	Not dialysed. Dose as in GFR=10–20 mL/min.

IMPORTANT DRUG INTERACTIONS

Potentially hazardous interactions with other drugs
- ACE inhibitors and angiotensin-II antagonists: antagonism of hypotensive effect, increased risk of nephrotoxicity and hyperkalaemia.
- Analgesics: avoid concomitant use of 2 or more NSAIDs, including aspirin (increased side effects); avoid with ketorolac (increased risk of side effects and haemorrhage).
- Antibacterials: possibly increased risk of convulsions with quinolones.
- Anticoagulants: effects of coumarins and phenindione enhanced; possibly increased risk of bleeding with heparins and dabigatran.
- Antidepressants: increased risk of bleeding with SSRIs and venlafaxine.
- Antidiabetic agents: effects of sulphonylureas enhanced.
- Anti-epileptics: possibly increased phenytoin concentration.
- Antivirals: increased risk of haematological toxicity with zidovudine; concentration possibly increased by ritonavir.
- Ciclosporin: may potentiate nephrotoxicity.
- Cytotoxic agents: reduced excretion of methotrexate; increased risk of bleeding with erlotinib.
- Diuretics: increased risk of nephrotoxicity; antagonism of diuretic effect; hyperkalaemia with potassium-sparing diuretics.
- Lithium: excretion decreased.
- Pentoxifylline: increased risk of bleeding.
- Tacrolimus: increased risk of nephrotoxicity.

ADMINISTRATION

RECONSTITUTION
–
ROUTE
- Oral
RATE OF ADMINISTRATION
–
COMMENTS
–

OTHER INFORMATION

- Inhibition of renal prostaglandin synthesis by NSAIDs may interfere with renal function, especially in the presence of existing renal disease – avoid if possible; if not, check serum creatinine 48–72 hours after starting NSAID – if raised, discontinue NSAID therapy.

- Use normal doses in patients with CKD 5 on dialysis.
- Use with caution in renal transplant recipients – can reduce intrarenal autocoid synthesis.

Dexketoprofen

CLINICAL USE

NSAID and analgesic

DOSE IN NORMAL RENAL FUNCTION

12.5 mg every 4–6 hours
or 25 mg every 8 hours

PHARMACOKINETICS

Molecular weight (daltons)	254.3
% Protein binding	99
% Excreted unchanged in urine	<10
Volume of distribution (L/kg)	0.24
Half-life – normal/ ESRF (hrs)	1.65/Increased

METABOLISM

Dexketoprofen is the *S*-enantiomer of ketoprofen. The main elimination route for dexketoprofen is glucuronide conjugation in the liver followed by renal excretion.

DOSE IN RENAL IMPAIRMENT GFR (mL/MIN)

20–50	Dose as in normal renal function but use with caution.
10–20	Dose as in normal renal function but avoid if possible.
<10	Dose as in normal renal function but only if on dialysis.

DOSE IN PATIENTS UNDERGOING RENAL REPLACEMENT THERAPIES

CAPD	Dialysed. Dose as in normal renal function. See 'Other information'.
HD	Dialysed. Dose as in normal renal function. See 'Other information'.
HDF/High flux	Dialysed. Dose as in normal renal function. See 'Other information'.
CAV/ VVHD	Dialysed. Dose as for GFR=10–20 mL/min.

IMPORTANT DRUG INTERACTIONS

Potentially hazardous interactions with other drugs

- ACE inhibitors and angiotensin-II antagonists: antagonism of hypotensive effect; increased risk of nephrotoxicity and hyperkalaemia.
- Analgesics: avoid concomitant use of 2 or more NSAIDs, including aspirin (increased side effects); avoid with ketorolac (increased risk of side effects and haemorrhage).
- Antibacterials: possibly increased risk of convulsions with quinolones.
- Anticoagulants: effects of coumarins and phenindione enhanced; possibly increased risk of bleeding with heparins and dabigatran.
- Antidepressants: increased risk of bleeding with SSRIs and venlafaxine.
- Antidiabetic agents: effects of sulphonylureas enhanced.
- Anti-epileptics: possibly increased phenytoin concentration.
- Antivirals: increased risk of haematological toxicity with zidovudine; concentration possibly increased by ritonavir.
- Ciclosporin: may potentiate nephrotoxicity.
- Cytotoxic agents: reduced excretion of methotrexate; increased risk of bleeding with erlotinib.
- Diuretics: increased risk of nephrotoxicity; antagonism of diuretic effect, hyperkalaemia with potassium-sparing diuretics.
- Lithium: excretion decreased.
- Pentoxifylline: increased risk of bleeding.
- Probenecid: excretion reduced by probenecid.
- Tacrolimus: increased risk of nephrotoxicity.

ADMINISTRATION

RECONSTITUTION

–

ROUTE

- Oral

RATE OF ADMINISTRATION

–

COMMENTS

–

OTHER INFORMATION

- Inhibition of renal prostaglandin synthesis by NSAIDs may interfere with renal function, especially in the presence of existing renal disease – avoid if possible; if not, check serum creatinine 48–72 hours after starting NSAID – if raised, discontinue NSAID therapy.

- Use normal doses in patients with ERF on dialysis if they do not pass any urine.
- Use with caution in renal transplant recipients – can reduce intrarenal autocoid synthesis.

- Dexketoprofen should be used with caution in uraemic patients predisposed to gastrointestinal bleeding or uraemic coagulopathies.

Diamorphine hydrochloride

CLINICAL USE

Opiate analgesic:
- Control of severe pain
- Pain relief in myocardial infarction (MI)
- Acute pulmonary oedema

DOSE IN NORMAL RENAL FUNCTION

- Severe pain: Oral/SC/IM: 5–10 mg
  4 hourly, increasing dose as necessary.
- MI, acute pulmonary oedema: IV:
  2.5–5 mg. Elderly patients – reduce dose
  by half.

PHARMACOKINETICS

Molecular weight (daltons)	423.9
% Protein binding	35
% Excreted unchanged in urine	0.1
Volume of distribution (L/kg)	40–50 litres
Half-life – normal/ESRF (hrs)	1.7–5.3 minutes/–

METABOLISM

Diamorphine is rapidly hydrolysed to the
active metabolite 6-O-monoacetylmorphine
(6-acetylmorphine) in the blood and then
to morphine. Oral doses are subject to
extensive first-pass metabolism to morphine;
neither diamorphine nor 6-acetylmorphine
has been detected in the blood after giving
diamorphine by this route. The majority
of the drug is excreted via the kidney as
glucuronides and to a much lesser extent as
morphine. About 7–10% is eliminated via the
biliary system into the faeces.

DOSE IN RENAL IMPAIRMENT GFR (mL/MIN)

20–50	Dose as in normal renal function.
10–20	Use small doses, e.g. 2.5 mg SC/IM approx 6 hourly and titrate to response.
<10	Use small doses, e.g. 2.5 mg SC/IM approx 8 hourly and titrate to response.

DOSE IN PATIENTS UNDERGOING RENAL REPLACEMENT THERAPIES

CAPD	Not dialysed. Dose as in GFR<10 mL/min.
HD	Dialysed. Dose as in GFR<10 mL/min.
HDF/High flux	Dialysed. Dose as in GFR<10 mL/min.
CAV/VVHD	Unknown dialysability. Dose as in GFR=10–20 mL/min.

IMPORTANT DRUG INTERACTIONS

Potentially hazardous interactions with other
drugs
- Anti-arrhythmics: delayed absorption of
  mexiletine.
- Antidepressants: possible CNS excitation
  or depression with MAOIs – avoid
  concomitant use and for 2 weeks after
  stopping MAOI; possible CNS excitation
  or depression with moclobemide;
  increased sedative effects with tricyclics.
- Antihistamines: increased sedative effects
  with sedating antihistamines.
- Antipsychotics: enhanced sedative and
  hypotensive effect.
- Dopaminergics: avoid with selegiline.
- Sodium oxybate: enhanced effect of
  sodium oxybate – avoid concomitant use.

ADMINISTRATION

RECONSTITUTION
- 1 mL water for injection or sodium
  chloride 0.9% (less may be used, e.g. for SC
  injection use 0.1 mL for 10 mg)

ROUTE
- IV, IM, SC, oral

RATE OF ADMINISTRATION
- IV: 1 mg/minute

COMMENTS
- Monitor BP and respiratory rates.

OTHER INFORMATION

- Increased cerebral sensitivity in renal
  impairment which can result in excessive
  sedation and serious respiratory
  depression necessitating ventilation.
- More rapid onset and shorter duration of
  action than morphine.
- Extreme caution with regular dosing –
  accumulation of active metabolites may
  occur.
- Naloxone must be readily available for
  reversal if required.

Diazepam

CLINICAL USE

Benzodiazepine:
- Perioperative sedation (IV)
- Anxiolytic
- Muscle relaxant
- Status epilepticus

DOSE IN NORMAL RENAL FUNCTION

- Pre-med: Oral: 5 mg, IV: 10–20 mg or 100–200 mcg/kg; PR: 500 mcg/kg repeated after 12 hours as rectal solution
- Anxiety: Oral: 2 mg 3 times a day, increasing if necessary to 15–30 mg daily in divided doses; PR: 10–30 mg daily in divided doses
- IM/IV: 5–10 mg repeated after not less than 4 hours
- Insomnia: 5–15 mg at night
- Status epilepticus: IV: 10 mg, repeated after 10 minutes if required; PR: 10–20 mg

PHARMACOKINETICS

Molecular weight (daltons)	284.7
% Protein binding	95–99
% Excreted unchanged in urine	<1
Volume of distribution (L/kg)	0.95–2
Half-life – normal/ ESRF (hrs)	24–48/Increased

METABOLISM

Diazepam has a biphasic half-life with an initial rapid distribution phase and a prolonged terminal elimination phase of 1 or 2 days; its action is further prolonged by the even longer half-life of 2 to 5 days of its principal active metabolite, desmethyldiazepam. Diazepam is extensively metabolised in the liver, notably via the cytochrome P450 isoenzymes CYP2C19 and CYP3A4; in addition to desmethyldiazepam, its active metabolites include oxazepam and temazepam. It is excreted in the urine, mainly in the form of free or conjugated metabolites.

DOSE IN RENAL IMPAIRMENT GFR (mL/MIN)

20–50	Dose as in normal renal function.
10–20	Use small doses and titrate to response.
<10	Use small doses and titrate to response.

DOSE IN PATIENTS UNDERGOING RENAL REPLACEMENT THERAPIES

CAPD	Not dialysed. Dose as in GFR<10 mL/min.
HD	Not dialysed. Dose as in GFR<10 mL/min.
HDF/High flux	Unknown dialysability. Dose as in GFR<10 mL/min.
CAV/ VVHD	Not dialysed. Dose as in GFR=10–20 mL/min.

IMPORTANT DRUG INTERACTIONS

Potentially hazardous interactions with other drugs
- Antibacterials: metabolism enhanced by rifampicin; metabolism inhibited by isoniazid.
- Antifungals: concentration increased by fluconazole and voriconazole – risk of prolonged sedation.
- Antipsychotics: increased sedative effects; increased risk of hypotension, bradycardia and respiratory depression with parenteral diazepam and IM olanzapine; risk serious adverse effects in combination with clozapine.
- Antivirals: concentration possibly increased by ritonavir.
- Sodium oxybate: enhanced effects of sodium oxybate – avoid.

ADMINISTRATION

RECONSTITUTION
–
ROUTE
- IV injection, infusion, oral, PR
RATE OF ADMINISTRATION
- 5 mg (1 mL)/minute
COMMENTS
- Injection can be mixed with sodium chloride 0.9% or glucose 5% to 40 mg in 500 mL

OTHER INFORMATION

- Increased cerebral sensitivity in renal impairment which may result in excessive sedation and encephalopathy.
- Always have flumazenil available to reverse effect.
- Protein binding decreased in ERF
- Volume of distribution increased in ERF.
- IV emulsion formulation (Diazemuls) less likely to cause thrombophlebitis.

Diazoxide

CLINICAL USE

- Treatment of hypertensive emergencies including severe hypertension associated with renal disease
- Hypoglycaemia

DOSE IN NORMAL RENAL FUNCTION

- Hypertension: IV: 1–3 mg/kg; maximum single dose: 150 mg, repeat after 5–15 minutes.
- Hypoglycaemia: Oral: 3–5 mg/kg in 2–3 divided doses; adjust according to response, usually 3–8 mg/kg; total doses up to 1 g have been used.

PHARMACOKINETICS

Molecular weight (daltons)	230.7
% Protein binding	>90
% Excreted unchanged in urine	50
Volume of distribution (L/kg)	0.2–0.3
Half-life – normal/ ESRF (hrs)	20–45/30–60

METABOLISM

Diazoxide is partly metabolised in the liver and is excreted in the urine both unchanged and in the form of metabolites; only small amounts are recovered from the faeces.

The plasma half-life of diazoxide greatly exceeds the duration of vascular activity.

DOSE IN RENAL IMPAIRMENT GFR (mL/MIN)

20–50	Dose as in normal renal function.
10–20	Dose as in normal renal function.
<10	Start with a lower dose and increase gradually according to response. Use with caution.

DOSE IN PATIENTS UNDERGOING RENAL REPLACEMENT THERAPIES

CAPD	Dialysed. Dose as in GFR<10 mL/min.
HD	Dialysed. Dose as in GFR<10 mL/min.
HDF/High flux	Dialysed. Dose as in GFR<10 mL/min.
CAV/VVHD	Unknown dialysability. Dose as in normal renal function.

IMPORTANT DRUG INTERACTIONS

Potentially hazardous interactions with other drugs
- Antihypertensives and vasodilators: enhanced hypotensive effect.
- MAOIs: withdraw at least 14 days before starting diazoxide.
- Phenytoin: may reduce phenytoin levels.

ADMINISTRATION

RECONSTITUTION
–
ROUTE
- IV bolus, oral
RATE OF ADMINISTRATION
- <30 seconds
COMMENTS
–

OTHER INFORMATION

- Single doses above 300 mg have been associated with angina and myocardial and cerebral infarction.
- Can cause sodium and water retention.

Diclofenac sodium

CLINICAL USE

NSAID and analgesic

DOSE IN NORMAL RENAL FUNCTION

75–150 mg daily in divided doses.

PHARMACOKINETICS

Molecular weight (daltons)	318.1
% Protein binding	99.7
% Excreted unchanged in urine	<1
Volume of distribution (L/kg)	0.12–0.17
Half-life – normal/ESRF (hrs)	1–2/Unchanged

METABOLISM

Diclofenac undergoes first-pass metabolism and is then extensively metabolised to 4'-hydroxydiclofenac, 5-hydroxydiclofenac, 3'-hydroxydiclofenac, and 4',5-dihydroxydiclofenac by glucuronidation of the intact molecule or more commonly by single and multiple hydroxylation followed by glucuronidation. It is then excreted in the form of glucuronide and sulfate conjugates, mainly in the urine (about 60%) but also in the bile (about 35%); less than 1% is excreted as unchanged diclofenac.

DOSE IN RENAL IMPAIRMENT GFR (mL/MIN)

20–50	Dose as in normal renal function.
10–20	Dose as in normal renal function, but avoid if possible.
<10	Dose as in normal renal function, but only use if on dialysis.

DOSE IN PATIENTS UNDERGOING RENAL REPLACEMENT THERAPIES

CAPD	Not dialysed. Dose as in normal renal function. See 'Other information'.
HD	Not dialysed. Dose as in normal renal function. See 'Other information'.
HDF/High flux	Not dialysed. Dose as in normal renal function. See 'Other information'.
CAV/VVHD	Not dialysed. Dose as in GFR=10–20 mL/min.

IMPORTANT DRUG INTERACTIONS

Potentially hazardous interactions with other drugs

- ACE inhibitors and angiotensin-II antagonists: antagonism of hypotensive effect; increased risk of nephrotoxicity and hyperkalaemia.
- Analgesics: avoid concomitant use of 2 or more NSAIDs, including aspirin (increased side effects); avoid with ketorolac (increased risk of side effects and haemorrhage).
- Antibacterials: possibly increased risk of convulsions with quinolones; concentration reduced by rifampicin.
- Anticoagulants: effects of coumarins and phenindione enhanced; possibly increased risk of bleeding with heparins and dabigatran; increased risk of haemorrhage with IV diclofenac – avoid concomitant use.
- Antidepressants: increased risk of bleeding with SSRIs and venlafaxine.
- Antidiabetic agents: effects of sulphonylureas enhanced.
- Anti-epileptics: possibly increased phenytoin concentration.
- Antivirals: increased risk of haematological toxicity with zidovudine; concentration possibly increased by ritonavir.
- Ciclosporin: may potentiate nephrotoxicity; concentration increased by ciclosporin.
- Cytotoxic agents: reduced excretion of methotrexate; increased risk of bleeding with erlotinib.
- Diuretics: increased risk of nephrotoxicity; antagonism of diuretic effect; hyperkalaemia with potassium-sparing diuretics.
- Lithium: excretion decreased.
- Pentoxifylline: increased risk of bleeding.
- Tacrolimus: increased risk of nephrotoxicity.

ADMINISTRATION

RECONSTITUTION
–
ROUTE
- Oral, IV, IM, PR

RATE OF ADMINISTRATION
- 25–50 mg over 15–60 minutes; 75 mg over 30–120 minutes.
- Continuous infusion of 5 mg/hour.

COMMENTS
- Dilute 75 mg in 100–500 mL of sodium chloride 0.9% or glucose 5% buffered with 0.5 mL sodium bicarbonate 8.4%.

OTHER INFORMATION

- Diclofenac should be used with caution in uraemic patients predisposed to gastrointestinal bleeding or uraemic coagulopathies.
- Inhibition of renal prostaglandin synthesis by NSAIDs may interfere with renal function, especially in the presence of existing renal disease – avoid if possible; if not, check serum creatinine 48–72 hours after starting NSAID – if raised, discontinue NSAID therapy.
- Use normal doses in patients with ERF on dialysis if they do not pass any urine.
- Use with great caution in renal transplant recipients – can reduce intrarenal autocoid synthesis.

Didanosine

CLINICAL USE

Nucleoside reverse transcriptase inhibitor:
- Treatment of HIV in combination with other antiretroviral drugs

DOSE IN NORMAL RENAL FUNCTION

>60 kg: 400 mg daily in 1–2 divided doses
<60 kg: 250 mg daily in 1–2 divided doses

PHARMACOKINETICS

Molecular weight (daltons)	236.2
% Protein binding	<5
% Excreted unchanged in urine	20
Volume of distribution (L/kg)	1
Half-life – normal/ESRF (hrs)	1.4/4.1

METABOLISM

Didanosine is metabolised intracellularly to the active antiviral metabolite dideoxyadenosine triphosphate. The terminal metabolism of didanosine in man has not been evaluated. However, based on animal studies, it is presumed that it follows the same pathways responsible for the elimination of endogenous purines. Renal clearance is by glomerular filtration and active tubular secretion; about 20% of an oral dose is recovered in the urine.

DOSE IN RENAL IMPAIRMENT GFR (mL/MIN)

30–59	<60 kg: 150 mg daily in 1 or 2 divided doses >60 kg: 200 mg daily in 1 or 2 divided doses
10–29	<60 kg: 100 mg daily >60 kg: 150 mg daily
<10	<60 kg: 75 mg daily >60 kg: 100 mg daily

DOSE IN PATIENTS UNDERGOING RENAL REPLACEMENT THERAPIES

CAPD	Not dialysed. Dose as in GFR<10 mL/min.
HD	Dialysed. Dose as in GFR<10 mL/min.
HDF/High flux	Dialysed. Dose as in GFR<10 mL/min.
CAV/VVHD	Dialysed. Dose as in GFR=10–29 mL/min.

IMPORTANT DRUG INTERACTIONS

Potentially hazardous interactions with other drugs
- Allopurinol: concentration of didanosine increased – avoid.
- Antibacterials: ciprofloxacin, tetracyclines, and other antibiotics affected by indigestion remedies – do not administer within 2 hours of didanosine.
- Antivirals: concentration possibly increased by ganciclovir and tenofovir – avoid with tenofovir; increased risk of side effects with ribavirin and stavudine – avoid with ribavirin; concentration reduced by tipranavir; give didanosine 2 hours before or 4 hours after rilpivirine.
- Cytotoxics: increased risk of toxicity with hydroxycarbamide – avoid concomitant use.

ADMINISTRATION

RECONSTITUTION
–

ROUTE
- Oral

RATE OF ADMINISTRATION
–

COMMENTS
- Give dose after dialysis on dialysis days, and at the same time on non-dialysis days.

OTHER INFORMATION

- Haemodialysis removes 20–35% of the dose.
- Administer 30 minutes to 2 hours before meals (depends on formulation).
- Magnesium content of tablets 8.6 mEq.
- Chew, crush tablet or disperse in at least 30 mL of water.
- Can be diluted in apple juice.
- Ingestion with food decreases absorption by 55%.

Digoxin

CLINICAL USE

- Supraventricular arrhythmias
- Heart failure

DOSE IN NORMAL RENAL FUNCTION

- Digitalisation: 0.75–1.5 mg in divided doses over 24 hours, followed by 62.5–500 mcg daily, adjusted according to response.
- Emergency loading (IV): 0.75–1 mg over at least 2 hours

PHARMACOKINETICS

Molecular weight (daltons)	780.9
% Protein binding	25
% Excreted unchanged in urine	50–75
Volume of distribution (L/kg)	5–8
Half-life – normal/ ESRF (hrs)	30–40/100

METABOLISM

Digoxin is mainly excreted unchanged in the urine by glomerular filtration and tubular secretion; reabsorption also occurs. Extensive metabolism has been reported in a minority of patients. Metabolites that have been detected in the urine include digoxigenin, dihydrodigoxigenin, the mono- and bisdigitoxosides of digoxigenin, and dihydrodigoxin. Digoxigenin mono- and bisdigitoxosides are known to be cardioactive whereas dihydrodigoxin is probably much less active than digoxin.

In about 10% of patients there is considerable reduction to cardio-inactive metabolites, chiefly dihydrodigoxin, and 40% or more of a dose may be excreted in the urine as dihydrodigoxin. Bacterial flora in the gastrointestinal tract appear to be responsible for this metabolism and antibacterials can reduce the process.

Excretion of digoxin is proportional to the glomerular filtration rate. After intravenous injection 50–70% of the dose is excreted unchanged.

DOSE IN RENAL IMPAIRMENT GFR (mL/MIN)

20–50	125–250 micrograms per day.
10–20	125–250 micrograms per day. Monitor levels.
<10	Dose commonly 62.5 micrograms alternate days, or 62.5 micrograms daily. Monitor levels.

DOSE IN PATIENTS UNDERGOING RENAL REPLACEMENT THERAPIES

CAPD	Not dialysed. Dose as in GFR<10 mL/min.
HD	Not dialysed. Dose as in GFR<10 mL/min.
HDF/High flux	Not dialysed. Dose as in GFR<10 mL/min.
CAV/ VVHD	Not dialysed. Dose as in GFR=10–20 mL/min.

IMPORTANT DRUG INTERACTIONS

Potentially hazardous interactions with other drugs

- Angiotensin-II antagonists: concentration increased by telmisartan.
- Anti-arrhythmics: concentration increased by amiodarone, dronedarone and propafenone (half maintenance dose of digoxin).
- Antidepressants: concentration reduced by St John's wort – avoid concomitant use.
- Antifungals: increased toxicity if hypokalaemia occurs with amphotericin; concentration increased by itraconazole.
- Antimalarials: concentration possibly increased by quinine, hydroxychloroquine and chloroquine; increased risk of bradycardia with mefloquine.
- Calcium-channel blockers: concentration increased by diltiazem, lercanidipine, nicardipine, verapamil and possibly nifedipine; increased risk of AV block and bradycardia with verapamil.
- Ciclosporin: concentration increased by ciclosporin.
- Colchicine: possibly increased risk of myopathy.
- Diuretics: increased toxicity if hypokalaemia occurs; concentration increased by spironolactone and possibly potassium canrenoate.
- Ticagrelor: concentration of digoxin increased.

ADMINISTRATION

RECONSTITUTION

–

ROUTE

- Oral, IV

RATE OF ADMINISTRATION

- Loading dose: infuse over 10–20 minutes.

COMMENTS

- IV administration: dilute dose to 4 times volume with sodium chloride 0.9% or glucose 5%.
- IV dosing may be used for very rapid control.

OTHER INFORMATION

- Complex kinetics in renal impairment: Volume of distribution and total body clearance reduced in CKD 5.
- Steady-state plasma monitoring advisable: normal range 0.8–2 nanograms/mL; take at least 8 hours post-dose, ideally before dose in the morning.
- If changing from oral to IV reduce dose by a third.
- Hypokalaemia, hypomagnesaemia, marked hypercalcaemia and hypothyroidism increase toxicity.
- Increases uraemic gastrointestinal symptoms.
- Only 3% of dose is removed after a 5 hour HD session.
- Concomitant administration of phosphate binders reduces GI absorption by up to 25%.

Dihydrocodeine tartrate

CLINICAL USE

Analgesia

DOSE IN NORMAL RENAL FUNCTION

Oral: 30 mg every 4–6 hours
SC/IM: up to 50 mg every 4–6 hours

PHARMACOKINETICS

Molecular weight (daltons)	451.5
% Protein binding	No data
% Excreted unchanged in urine	13–22
Volume of distribution (L/kg)	1.1
Half-life – normal/ ESRF (hrs)	3.5–5/>6

METABOLISM

Dihydrocodeine is metabolised in the liver via the cytochrome P450 isoenzyme CYP2D6, to dihydromorphine, which has potent analgesic activity, although the analgesic effect of dihydrocodeine appears to be mainly due to the parent compound; some is also converted via CYP3A4 to nordihydrocodeine. Dihydrocodeine is excreted in urine as unchanged drug and metabolites, including glucuronide conjugates.

DOSE IN RENAL IMPAIRMENT GFR (mL/MIN)

20–50	Dose as in normal renal function.
10–20	Use small doses and titrate to response.
<10	Use small doses and titrate to response.

DOSE IN PATIENTS UNDERGOING RENAL REPLACEMENT THERAPIES

CAPD	Unknown dialysability. Dose as in GFR<10 mL/min.
HD	Unknown dialysability. Dose as in GFR<10 mL/min.
HDF/High flux	Unknown dialysability. Dose as in GFR<10 mL/min.
CAV/ VVHD	Unknown dialysability. Dose as in GFR=10–20 mL/min.

IMPORTANT DRUG INTERACTIONS

Potentially hazardous interactions with other drugs
- Antidepressants: possible CNS excitation or depression with MAOIs – avoid concomitant use, and for 2 weeks after stopping MAOI; possible CNS excitation or depression with moclobemide; increased sedative effects with tricyclics.
- Antihistamines: increased sedative effects with sedating antihistamines.
- Antipsychotics: enhanced hypotensive and sedative effects.
- Dopaminergics: avoid with selegiline.
- Sodium oxybate: enhanced effect of sodium oxybate – avoid concomitant use.

ADMINISTRATION

RECONSTITUTION
–
ROUTE
- Oral, IM, SC
RATE OF ADMINISTRATION
–
COMMENTS
–

OTHER INFORMATION

- Increased and prolonged effect in renal impairment, enhancing respiratory depression and constipation.
- Increased CNS sensitivity in renal impairment.
- Accumulation of active metabolites can occur – caution.
- Effects can be reversed by naloxone.

Diltiazem hydrochloride

CLINICAL USE

Calcium-channel blocker:
- Prophylaxis and treatment of angina
- Hypertension

DOSE IN NORMAL RENAL FUNCTION

180–500 mg in up to 3 divided doses

PHARMACOKINETICS

Molecular weight (daltons)	451
% Protein binding	80–85
% Excreted unchanged in urine	5
Volume of distribution (L/kg)	3–8
Half-life – normal/ ESRF (hrs)	2–11; SR: 5–8/ Unchanged

METABOLISM

Diltiazem is almost completely absorbed from the gastrointestinal tract after oral doses, but undergoes extensive first-pass hepatic metabolism resulting in a bioavailability of about 40%. It is extensively metabolised in the liver, mainly by the cytochrome P450 isoenzyme CYP3A4; one of the metabolites, desacetyldiltiazem, has been reported to have 25–50% of the activity of the parent compound. About 2–4% of a dose is excreted in urine as unchanged diltiazem with the remainder excreted as metabolites in bile and urine.

DOSE IN RENAL IMPAIRMENT GFR (mL/MIN)

20–50	Dose as in normal renal function.
10–20	Dose as in normal renal function.
<10	Start with a low dose and gradually increase as tolerated.

DOSE IN PATIENTS UNDERGOING RENAL REPLACEMENT THERAPIES

CAPD	Not dialysed. Dose as in GFR<10 mL/min.
HD	Not dialysed. Dose as in GFR<10 mL/min.
HDF/High flux	Not dialysed. Dose as in GFR<10 mL/min.
CAV/ VVHD	Not dialysed. Dose as in normal renal function.

IMPORTANT DRUG INTERACTIONS

Potentially hazardous interactions with other drugs
- Anaesthetics: enhanced hypotensive effect.
- Anti-arrhythmics: increased risk of bradycardia, AV block and myocardial depression with amiodarone; increased risk of bradycardia and myocardial depression with dronedarone.
- Antibacterials: metabolism increased by rifampicin; metabolism possibly inhibited by clarithromycin, erythromycin and telithromycin.
- Antidepressants: enhanced hypotensive effect with MAOIs; concentration of imipramine and possibly other tricyclics increased.
- Anti-epileptics: effect probably reduced by barbiturates, phenytoin, and primidone; enhanced effect of carbamazepine; increased levels of phenytoin.
- Antifungals: negative inotropic effect possibly increased with itraconazole.
- Antihypertensives: enhanced hypotensive effect; increased risk of first dose hypotensive effect of post-synaptic alpha-blockers.
- Antivirals: concentration increased by atazanavir and ritonavir – reduce dose of diltiazem with atazanavir; concentration reduced by efavirenz; use telaprevir with caution.
- Beta-blockers: risk of bradycardia and AV block if co-prescribed with beta-blockers.
- Cardiac glycosides: increased digoxin concentration.
- Ciclosporin: increased ciclosporin concentrations.
- Cilostazol: increased cilostazol concentration – avoid concomitant use.
- Colchicine: possibly increased risk of colchicine toxicity – suspend or reduce colchicine, avoid concomitant use in renal or hepatic failure.
- Cytotoxics: possibly increased risk of bradycardia with crizotinib.
- Fingolimod: increased risk of bradycardia.
- Ivabradine: concentration of ivabradine increased – avoid concomitant use.
- Sirolimus: sirolimus concentration increased.
- Statins: increased atorvastatin concentration and possibly myopathy;

increased myopathy with simvastatin. Do not exceed 20 mg of simvastatin with diltiazem.[1]
- Tacrolimus: increased tacrolimus concentration.
- Theophylline: enhanced effect of theophylline.

ADMINISTRATION

RECONSTITUTION
–
ROUTE
- Oral
RATE OF ADMINISTRATION
–
COMMENTS
–

OTHER INFORMATION

- Active metabolites.
- Monitor heart rate early on in therapy. If falls below 50 beats/minute, do not increase dose.
- Maintain patient on same brand.

Reference:
1. MHRA. *Drug Safety Update.* Statins: interactions and updated advice. August 2012; **6**(1): 2–4.

Dipyridamole

CLINICAL USE

Oral: Antiplatelet agent
IV: Myocardial imaging

DOSE IN NORMAL RENAL FUNCTION

Oral: 100–200 mg 3 times daily.
Modified release: 200 mg twice daily.
IV: 0.142 mg/kg/minute (0.567 mg/kg total)
infused over 4 minutes.

PHARMACOKINETICS

Molecular weight (daltons)	504.6
% Protein binding	97–99
% Excreted unchanged in urine	1–5
Volume of distribution (L/kg)	1.33–3.53
Half-life – normal/ ESRF (hrs)	9–12/Unchanged

METABOLISM

Dipyridamole is metabolised in the liver.
Renal excretion of the parent compound
is negligible (<0.5%). Urinary excretion of
the glucuronide metabolite is low (5%), the
metabolites are mostly (about 95%) excreted
via the bile into the faeces, with some
evidence of enterohepatic recirculation.

DOSE IN RENAL IMPAIRMENT GFR (mL/MIN)

20–50	Dose as in normal renal function.
10–20	Dose as in normal renal function.
<10	Dose as in normal renal function.

DOSE IN PATIENTS UNDERGOING RENAL REPLACEMENT THERAPIES

CAPD	Not dialysed. Dose as in normal renal function.
HD	Not dialysed. Dose as in normal renal function.
HDF/High flux	Not dialysed. Dose as in normal renal function.
CAV/ VVHD	Not dialysed. Dose as in normal renal function.

IMPORTANT DRUG INTERACTIONS

Potentially hazardous interactions with other
drugs
• Anti-arrhythmics: effects of adenosine
  enhanced and extended.
• Anticoagulants: anticoagulant effect of
  coumarins, phenindione and heparin
  enhanced.

ADMINISTRATION

RECONSTITUTION
–
ROUTE
• Oral, IV infusion
RATE OF ADMINISTRATION
• Over 4 minutes
COMMENTS
–

Disodium etidronate

CLINICAL USE

Bisphosphonate:
- Paget's disease of bone
- Vertebral osteoporosis (Didronel PMO)

DOSE IN NORMAL RENAL FUNCTION

- Paget's disease: 5–20 mg/kg daily for 3–6 months
- Vertebral osteoporosis: 400 mg daily for 14 days followed by 76 days of calcium carbonate 1.25 g (= 500 mg calcium)

PHARMACOKINETICS

Molecular weight (daltons)	250
% Protein binding	Depends on calcium concentration and pH.
% Excreted unchanged in urine	50
Volume of distribution (L/kg)	0.3–1.3
Half-life – normal/ ESRF (hrs)	1–6/–

METABOLISM

Etidronate is not metabolised. Absorption averages about 1% of an oral dose of 5 mg/kg/day, increasing to 6% at 20 mg/kg/day. Most of the drug is cleared from the blood within 6 hours. Within 24 hours about half of the absorbed dose is excreted in the urine. The remainder is sequestered into bone, especially to areas of elevated osteogenesis, and is slowly eliminated. Unabsorbed drug is excreted in the faeces.

DOSE IN RENAL IMPAIRMENT GFR (mL/MIN)

20–50	Maximum dose = 5 mg/kg/day
10–20	Maximum dose = 5 mg/kg/day – use with caution. (May also use Didronel PMO for osteoporosis.)
<10	Maximum dose = 5 mg/kg/day – use with caution. (May also use Didronel PMO for osteoporosis.)

DOSE IN PATIENTS UNDERGOING RENAL REPLACEMENT THERAPIES

CAPD	Unknown dialysability. Dose as in GFR<10 mL/min.
HD	Unknown dialysability. Dose as in GFR<10 mL/min.
HDF/High flux	Unknown dialysability. Dose as in GFR<10 mL/min.
CAV/ VVHD	Unknown dialysability. Dose as in GFR=10–20 mL/min.

IMPORTANT DRUG INTERACTIONS

Potentially hazardous interactions with other drugs
- Do not give iron and mineral supplements, antacids or phosphate binders within 2 hours of an etidronate.

ADMINISTRATION

RECONSTITUTION
–
ROUTE
- Oral
RATE OF ADMINISTRATION
–
COMMENTS
- Take on an empty stomach. Recommended that patients take with water at the midpoint of a 4 hour fast (i.e. 2 hours before and 2 hours after food).
- Oral bioavailability is very low; only about 4% of dose is absorbed.

OTHER INFORMATION

- Manufacturer advises to use with caution in severe renal impairment due to lack of data and renal excretion.
- Renal clearance of etidronate is 1.2 mL/minute/kg, while the total body clearance is 2.2 mL/minute/kg.
- Elimination is likely to be reduced in patients with renal impairment and elderly with reduced renal function necessitating caution. Uptake of etidronate by bone represents non-renal clearance.

Disodium pamidronate

CLINICAL USE

Bisphosphonate:
- Hypercalcaemia
- Bone pain
- Paget's disease

DOSE IN NORMAL RENAL FUNCTION

- Hypercalcaemia: depends on serum calcium – 15–90 mg in single or divided doses
- Bone pain: 90 mg every 4 weeks
- Paget's disease: 30 mg weekly for 6 weeks, or 30 mg first dose then 60 mg every other week

PHARMACOKINETICS

Molecular weight (daltons)	369.1
% Protein binding	54
% Excreted unchanged in urine	20–55
Volume of distribution (L/kg)	0.5–0.6
Half-life – normal/ ESRF (hrs)	0.8–27/Unchanged

METABOLISM

Pamidronate is not metabolised, and about 20–55% of the dose is excreted in the urine unchanged within 72 hours; the remainder is mainly sequestered to bone and only very slowly eliminated.

DOSE IN RENAL IMPAIRMENT GFR (mL/MIN)

20–50	Dose as in normal renal function.
10–20	Dose as in normal renal function.
<10	Serum calcium >4.0, give 60 mg. Serum calcium <4.0, give 30 mg.

DOSE IN PATIENTS UNDERGOING RENAL REPLACEMENT THERAPIES

CAPD	Unknown dialysability. Dose as in GFR<10 mL/min.
HD	Dialysed. Dose as in GFR<10 mL/min.
HDF/High flux	Dialysed. Dose as in GFR<10 mL/min.
CAV/ VVHD	Unknown dialysability. Dose as in normal renal function.

IMPORTANT DRUG INTERACTIONS

Potentially hazardous interactions with other drugs
- None known

ADMINISTRATION

RECONSTITUTION
- 15 mg in 5 mL water for injection
- 30 or 90 mg in 10 mL water for injection
- Final concentration should not exceed 30 mg per 125 mL sodium chloride 0.9%

ROUTE
- IV

RATE OF ADMINISTRATION
–

COMMENTS
–

OTHER INFORMATION

- Rate of acute renal failure is 9.3%, can cause focal segmental glomerulosclerosis, especially at higher doses. (Markowitz GS, Appel GB, Fine PL, et al. Collapsing focal segmental glomerulosclerosis following treatment with high-dose pamidronate. *J Am Soc Nephrol.* 2001; **12**(6): 1164–72.)
- If pamidronate is not excreted adequately, kidney stones may be formed. In dialysis patients there is increased risk of asymptomatic hypocalcaemia with 90 mg doses (anecdotal).

Disopyramide

CLINICAL USE

Ventricular and supraventricular arrhythmias

DOSE IN NORMAL RENAL FUNCTION

- Oral: 300–800 mg daily in divided doses.
- IV: 2 mg/kg over 5 minutes to a maximum of 150 mg.
- Infusion: 400 mcg/kg/hour, maximum 300 mg in 1st hour and 800 mg daily

PHARMACOKINETICS

Molecular weight (daltons)	339.5
% Protein binding	50–65
% Excreted unchanged in urine	50–75
Volume of distribution (L/kg)	0.8–2.6
Half-life – normal/ESRF (hrs)	5–8/12–22

METABOLISM

Disopyramide is partially metabolised in the liver by the cytochrome P450 isoenzyme CYP3A4. The major metabolite is mono-N-dealkylated disopyramide which retains some antiarrhythmic and antimuscarinic activity.

The major route of excretion is through the kidney, about 50–60% as the unchanged drug, 20% as the N-dealkylated metabolite, and 10% as other metabolites. Sixty-four per cent of the N-dealkylated metabolite is excreted via the faeces.

DOSE IN RENAL IMPAIRMENT GFR (mL/MIN)

30–40	Oral: 100 mg every 8 hours. IV: Reduce dose
15–30	Oral: 100 mg every 12 hours. IV: Reduce dose.
<15	Oral: 100 mg every 24 hours (monitor levels). IV: Reduce dose.

DOSE IN PATIENTS UNDERGOING RENAL REPLACEMENT THERAPIES

CAPD	Not dialysed. Dose as in GFR<15 mL/min.
HD	Not dialysed. Dose as in GFR<15 mL/min.
HDF/High flux	Unlikely to be dialysed. Dose as in GFR<15 mL/min.
CAV/ VVHD	Unknown dialysability. Dose as in GFR=15–30 mL/min.

IMPORTANT DRUG INTERACTIONS

Potentially hazardous interactions with other drugs

- Anti-arrhythmics: increased myocardial depression with other anti-arrhythmics; amiodarone and dronedarone increase risk of ventricular arrhythmias – avoid concomitant use.
- Antibacterials: concentration possibly increased by azithromycin, clarithromycin and erythromycin (risk of toxicity); increased risk of ventricular arrhythmias with moxifloxacin – avoid concomitant use; possibly increased risk of ventricular arrhythmias with telithromycin; concentration reduced by rifamycins.
- Antidepressants: increased risk of ventricular arrhythmias with tricyclics.
- Antifungals: increased risk of ventricular arrhythmias with ketoconazole – avoid concomitant use; avoid with itraconazole.
- Antihistamines: increased risk of ventricular arrhythmias with mizolastine.
- Antihypertensives: increased myocardial depression and asystole with beta-blockers or verapamil; increased risk of ventricular arrhythmias with sotalol – avoid.
- Antimalarials: avoid concomitant use with artemether/lumefantrine and piperaquine with artenimol.
- Antimuscarinics: increased risk of antimuscarinic side effects; increased risk of ventricular arrhythmias with tolterodine.
- Antipsychotics: increased risk of ventricular arrhythmias with antipsychotics that prolong the QT interval and phenothiazines and sulpiride; increased risk of ventricular arrhythmias with amisulpride, droperidol, pimozide and zuclopenthixol and possibly haloperidol – avoid concomitant use.
- Antivirals: concentration possibly increased by ritonavir, increased risk of toxicity; increased risk of ventricular arrhythmias with saquinavir and telaprevir – avoid.
- Atomoxetine: increased risk of ventricular arrhythmias.
- Beta-blockers: increased myocardial depression; increased risk of ventricular arrhythmias with sotalol.
- Calcium-channel blockers: increased risk of myocardial depression and asystole with verapamil.

- Ciclosporin: may increase risk of nephrotoxicity with ciclosporin.
- Cytotoxics: possibly increased risk of ventricular arrhythmias with vandetanib – avoid; increased risk of ventricular arrhythmias with arsenic trioxide.
- Diuretics: increased cardiac toxicity if hypokalaemia occurs.
- Fingolimod: possible increased risk of bradycardia.
- Ivabradine: increased risk of ventricular arrhythmias.
- Pentamidine: possibly increased risk of ventricular arrhythmias.
- Ranolazine: avoid concomitant use.

ADMINISTRATION

RECONSTITUTION
–

ROUTE
- Oral, IV

RATE OF ADMINISTRATION
- 20–30 mg/hour (0.4 mg/kg/hour)

COMMENTS
- May be given by peripheral IV infusion in glucose 5%, sodium chloride 0.9% or compound sodium lactate.

OTHER INFORMATION

- Use with caution in patients with impaired renal function.
- Doses in renal impairment taken from American data sheet.
- Do not give renally impaired patients sustained release preparations.
- Optimum therapeutic plasma level 2–6 mg/L.
- Haemoperfusion can be used in cases of severe poisoning.

Disulfiram

CLINICAL USE

Adjunct in the treatment of chronic alcohol dependence

DOSE IN NORMAL RENAL FUNCTION

800 mg on day 1 reducing over 5 days to 100–200 mg daily.

PHARMACOKINETICS

Molecular weight (daltons)	296.5
% Protein binding	96
% Excreted unchanged in urine	70–76 (as metabolites)
Volume of distribution (L/kg)	No data
Half-life – normal/ ESRF (hrs)	12/–

METABOLISM

Disulfiram is rapidly reduced to diethyldithiocarbamate, mainly by the glutathione reductase system in erythrocytes; reduction may also occur in the liver. Diethyldithiocarbamate is metabolised in the liver to its glucuronide and methyl ester and to diethylamine, carbon disulfide, and sulfate ions. Metabolites are excreted mainly in the urine; carbon disulfide is exhaled in the breath.

DOSE IN RENAL IMPAIRMENT GFR (mL/MIN)

20–50	Dose as in normal renal function.
10–20	Use with caution.
<10	Avoid.

DOSE IN PATIENTS UNDERGOING RENAL REPLACEMENT THERAPIES

CAPD	Unlikely to be dialysed. Avoid.
HD	Unlikely to be dialysed. Avoid.
HDF/High flux	Unlikely to be dialysed. Avoid.
CAV/ VVHD	Unlikely to be dialysed. Dose as in GFR=10–20 mL/min.

IMPORTANT DRUG INTERACTIONS

Potentially hazardous interactions with other drugs
- Alcohol: risk of severe disulfiram reaction
- Anticoagulants: enhanced anticoagulant effect with coumarins.
- Anti-epileptics: inhibition of metabolism of phenytoin (increased risk of toxicity).
- Paraldehyde: increased risk of toxicity with paraldehyde.

ADMINISTRATION

RECONSTITUTION
–
ROUTE
- Oral
RATE OF ADMINISTRATION
–
COMMENTS
–

OTHER INFORMATION

- Review after 6 months.
- Patients should be warned about severe nature of alcohol and disulfiram reaction.
- Contraindicated in cardiovascular disease, psychoses or severe personality disorders.
- Disulfiram blocks the metabolism of alcohol and leads to an accumulation of acetaldehyde in the blood stream. Use with caution in diabetics.

Dobutamine

CLINICAL USE

Inotropic agent

DOSE IN NORMAL RENAL FUNCTION

2.5–10 micrograms/kg/minute, increasing up to 40 micrograms/kg/minute according to response.

PHARMACOKINETICS

Molecular weight (daltons)	301.4; 337.8 (as hydrochloride)
% Protein binding	No data
% Excreted unchanged in urine	<10
Volume of distribution (L/kg)	0.12–0.28
Half-life – normal/ ESRF (hrs)	2–4 minutes/–

METABOLISM

Dobutamine is metabolised in the liver and other tissues by catechol-o-methyltransferase to an inactive compound, 3–0-methyldobutamine and by conjugation with glucuronic acid. Conjugates of dobutamine and 3–0-methyldobutamine are excreted mainly in urine and to a minor extent in faeces.

DOSE IN RENAL IMPAIRMENT GFR (mL/MIN)

20–50	Dose as in normal renal function.
10–20	Dose as in normal renal function.
<10	Dose as in normal renal function.

DOSE IN PATIENTS UNDERGOING RENAL REPLACEMENT THERAPIES

CAPD	Not dialysed. Dose as in normal renal function.
HD	Not dialysed. Dose as in normal renal function.
HDF/High flux	Not dialysed. Dose as in normal renal function.
CAV/ VVHD	Not dialysed. Dose as in normal renal function.

IMPORTANT DRUG INTERACTIONS

Potentially hazardous interactions with other drugs
- Antidepressants: risk of hypertensive crisis with MAOIs and moclobemide.
- Beta-blockers: possibly severe hypotension with beta-blockers.
- Dopaminergics: effects possibly enhanced by entacapone; avoid concomitant use with rasagiline.

ADMINISTRATION

RECONSTITUTION
–
ROUTE
- Continuous IV infusion centrally via CRIP (or peripherally via a large vein)
RATE OF ADMINISTRATION
- Varies with dose
COMMENTS
- Dilute to at least 50 mL with sodium chloride 0.9% or glucose 5% (less than 5 mg/mL, ideally 0.5–1 mg/mL).
- 250 mg may be diluted in as little as 50 mL diluent.
- Minimum volume 10 mg/mL or even undiluted; give strong solution via central line, (UK Critical Care Group, *Minimum Infusion Volumes for Fluid Restricted Critically Ill Patients*, 3rd edition, 2006).

OTHER INFORMATION

- Cardiac and BP monitoring advised.
- Sodium bicarbonate rapidly inactivates dobutamine.
- Solution may turn pink, but potency is unaffected.
- Can cause hypokalaemia.

Docetaxel

CLINICAL USE

Antineoplastic agent:
- Treatment of breast cancer, prostate cancer and non-small cell lung cancer unresponsive to alternative therapies, also gastric adenocarcinoma, squamous cell carcinoma of head and neck

DOSE IN NORMAL RENAL FUNCTION

75–100 mg/m^2 every 3 weeks.

PHARMACOKINETICS

Molecular weight (daltons)	807.9
% Protein binding	>95
% Excreted unchanged in urine	6
Volume of distribution (L/kg)	113 litres
Half-life – normal/ ESRF (hrs)	4 min(α)/36 min(β)/11.1 hr(γ)

METABOLISM

A study of ^{14}C-docetaxel has been conducted in three cancer patients. Docetaxel was eliminated in both the urine and faeces following cytochrome P450 3A4-mediated oxidative metabolism of the tert-butyl ester group, within 7 days, the urinary and faecal excretion accounted for about 6% and 75% of the administered radioactivity, respectively. About 80% of the radioactivity recovered in faeces is excreted during the first 48 hours as one major inactive metabolite and three minor inactive metabolites and very low amounts of unchanged medicinal product.

DOSE IN RENAL IMPAIRMENT GFR (mL/MIN)

20–50	Dose as in normal renal function.
10–20	Dose as in normal renal function.
<10	Dose as in normal renal function.

DOSE IN PATIENTS UNDERGOING RENAL REPLACEMENT THERAPIES

CAPD	Unlikely to be dialysed. Dose as in normal renal function.
HD	Unlikely to be dialysed. Dose as in normal renal function.
HDF/High flux	Unlikely to be dialysed. Dose as in normal renal function.
CAV/ VVHD	Unlikely to be dialysed. Dose as in normal renal function.

IMPORTANT DRUG INTERACTIONS

Potentially hazardous interactions with other drugs
- Antipsychotics: avoid concomitant use with clozapine – increased risk of agranulocytosis.
- Antivirals: concentration possibly increased by ritonavir, increased risk of toxicity.
- Ciclosporin: possibly inhibits metabolism of ciclosporin; bioavailability of docetaxel increased by ciclosporin.

ADMINISTRATION

RECONSTITUTION
- With diluent provided
ROUTE
- IV
RATE OF ADMINISTRATION
- Over 1 hour
COMMENTS
- Allow vials to come to room temperature for 5 minutes.
- Doses of up to 200 mg can be added to 250 mL infusion bags of glucose 5% or sodium chloride 0.9%.
- Doses greater than 200 mg should be diluted to a concentration of 0.74 mg/mL.
- Administer within 4 hours of dilution.

OTHER INFORMATION

- Give premedication with oral dexamethasone 16 mg daily for 3 days, starting 1 day before commencing chemotherapy.

Domperidone

CLINICAL USE

- Acute nausea and vomiting (including that caused by levodopa and bromocriptine)
- Gastro-oesophageal reflux
- Dyspepsia

DOSE IN NORMAL RENAL FUNCTION

Nausea and vomiting: Adults 10–20 mg orally 3–4 times daily, maximum 80 mg daily.
PR: 60 mg twice daily.

PHARMACOKINETICS

Molecular weight (daltons)	425.9
% Protein binding	>90
% Excreted unchanged in urine	<1
Volume of distribution (L/kg)	5.7
Half-life – normal/ ESRF (hrs)	7–9/20.8

METABOLISM

Domperidone undergoes extensive first-pass hepatic and intestinal metabolism. It undergoes rapid and extensive hepatic metabolism. The main metabolic pathways are N-dealkylation by cytochrome P450 isoenzyme CYP3A4, and aromatic hydroxylation by CYP3A4, CYP1A2, and CYP2E1. About 30% of an oral dose is excreted in urine within 24 hours, almost entirely as metabolites; the remainder of a dose is excreted in faeces over several days, about 10% as unchanged drug.

DOSE IN RENAL IMPAIRMENT GFR (mL/MIN)

20–50	Dose as in normal renal function.
10–20	Dose as in normal renal function.
<10	Dose as in normal renal function.

DOSE IN PATIENTS UNDERGOING RENAL REPLACEMENT THERAPIES

CAPD	Unlikely to be dialysed. Dose as in normal renal function.
HD	Unlikely to be dialysed. Dose as in normal renal function.
HDF/High flux	Unlikely to be dialysed. Dose as in normal renal function.
CAV/ VVHD	Unknown dialysability. Dose as in normal renal function.

IMPORTANT DRUG INTERACTIONS

Potentially hazardous interactions with other drugs

- Antibacterials: possible increased risk of ventricular arrhythmias with erythromycin.
- Antifungals: possibly increased risk of ventricular arrhythmias with ketoconazole – avoid.
- Antimalarials: possible increased risk of ventricular arrhythmias with piperaquine with artenimol – avoid.
- Antivirals: concentration increased by telaprevir – avoid.

ADMINISTRATION

RECONSTITUTION

–

ROUTE

- Oral, PR

RATE OF ADMINISTRATION

–

COMMENTS

- Treatment of acute nausea and vomiting: maximum period of treatment is 12 weeks.
- Treatment of dyspepsia: administer before food; maximum period of treatment is 12 weeks.

OTHER INFORMATION

- Domperidone has the advantage over metoclopramide and phenothiazines of being less likely to cause CNS effects, such as sedation and dystonic reactions, as it does not readily cross the blood-brain barrier.
- Due to minimal renal excretion no dose change is recommended although with prolonged administration the frequency in severe renal impairment may need to be reduced to once or twice daily.
- The European Medicines Agency (7/3/2014) recommends that domperidone should only be used short-term for nausea and vomiting with a maximum dose of 30 mg daily for weight >35 kg. It also should not be used in patients with liver impairment or heart arrhythmias due to the risk of QT prolongation.

Donepezil hydrochloride

CLINICAL USE

Treatment of dementia in mild to moderate Alzheimer's disease

DOSE IN NORMAL RENAL FUNCTION

5–10 mg daily

PHARMACOKINETICS

Molecular weight (daltons)	416
% Protein binding	95
% Excreted unchanged in urine	17
Volume of distribution (L/kg)	12
Half-life – normal/ ESRF (hrs)	70/Unchanged

METABOLISM

Donepezil hydrochloride is both excreted in the urine intact and metabolised by the cytochrome P450 system to multiple metabolites, not all of which have been identified. Following administration of a single 5 mg dose of ^{14}C-labelled donepezil hydrochloride, plasma radioactivity, expressed as a percentage of the administered dose, was present primarily as intact donepezil hydrochloride (30%), 6-O-desmethyl donepezil (11% – only metabolite that exhibits activity similar to donepezil hydrochloride), donepezil-cis-N-oxide (9%), 5-O-desmethyl donepezil (7%) and the glucuronide conjugate of 5-O-desmethyl donepezil (3%). Approximately 57% of the total administered radioactivity was recovered from the urine (17% as unchanged donepezil), and 14.5% was recovered from the faeces, suggesting biotransformation and urinary excretion as the primary routes of elimination. There is no evidence to suggest enterohepatic recirculation of donepezil hydrochloride and/or any of its metabolites.

DOSE IN RENAL IMPAIRMENT GFR (mL/MIN)

20–50	Dose as in normal renal function.
10–20	Dose as in normal renal function.
<10	Dose as in normal renal function.

DOSE IN PATIENTS UNDERGOING RENAL REPLACEMENT THERAPIES

CAPD	Unlikely to be dialysed. Dose as in normal renal function.
HD	Unlikely to be dialysed. Dose as in normal renal function.
HDF/High flux	Unknown dialysability. Dose as in normal renal function.
CAV/ VVHD	Unlikely to be dialysed. Dose as in normal renal function.

IMPORTANT DRUG INTERACTIONS

Potentially hazardous interactions with other drugs
● None known

ADMINISTRATION

RECONSTITUTION
–
ROUTE
● Oral
RATE OF ADMINISTRATION
–
COMMENTS
–

OTHER INFORMATION

Metabolised via CYP450 3A4 and 2D6 so may interact with other drugs metabolised by these pathways.

Dopamine hydrochloride

CLINICAL USE
Cardiogenic shock in infarction or cardiac surgery

DOSE IN NORMAL RENAL FUNCTION
Initially 2–5 mcg/kg/minute

PHARMACOKINETICS

Molecular weight (daltons)	189.6
% Protein binding	No data
% Excreted unchanged in urine	Minimal
Volume of distribution (L/kg)	No data
Half-life – normal/ ESRF (hrs)	2 min/–

METABOLISM
Dopamine is a metabolic precursor of noradrenaline and, whereas a proportion is excreted as the metabolic products of noradrenaline, the majority is mainly metabolised into 3,4,-dihydroxyphenylacetic acid (DOPAC) and 3-methoxy-4-hydroxyphenylacetic (HVA) which are rapidly excreted in the urine.

DOSE IN RENAL IMPAIRMENT GFR (mL/MIN)

20–50	Dose as in normal renal function.
10–20	Dose as in normal renal function.
<10	Dose as in normal renal function.

DOSE IN PATIENTS UNDERGOING RENAL REPLACEMENT THERAPIES

CAPD	Not dialysed. Dose as in normal renal function.
HD	Not dialysed. Dose as in normal renal function.
HDF/High flux	Not dialysed. Dose as in normal renal function.
CAV/ VVHD	Not dialysed. Dose as in normal renal function.

IMPORTANT DRUG INTERACTIONS
Potentially hazardous interactions with other drugs
- Alpha-blockers: avoid concomitant use with tolazoline.
- Antidepressants: risk of hypertensive crisis with MAOIs and moclobemide.
- Ciclosporin: may reduce risk of ciclosporin nephrotoxicity.
- Dopaminergics: effects possibly enhanced by entacapone; avoid concomitant use with rasagiline; risk of hypertensive crisis with selegiline.

ADMINISTRATION
RECONSTITUTION
–
ROUTE
- IV peripherally into large vein (centrally for inotropic dose). Central route always preferable.
RATE OF ADMINISTRATION
- Via CRIP as indicated below.
COMMENTS
- Minimum dilution 200 mg in 50 mL.
- Not compatible with sodium bicarbonate – rapid deactivation of dopamine.

OTHER INFORMATION
- Renal dose is 2–5 mcg/kg/min but little evidence that it can improve renal function.
- Causes renal vasoconstriction at inotropic dose.
- Cardiac and BP monitoring advised.
- Very severe tissue damage caused by extravasation.

Dopexamine hydrochloride

CLINICAL USE

Inotropic support in exacerbations of heart failure and heart failure associated with cardiac surgery

DOSE IN NORMAL RENAL FUNCTION

IV infusion: 0.5 –1 mcg/kg/minute and then in increments (0.5–1 micrograms/kg/minute) up to 6 micrograms/kg/minute at not less than 15 minute intervals.

PHARMACOKINETICS

Molecular weight (daltons)	429.4
% Protein binding	No data
% Excreted unchanged in urine	10
Volume of distribution (L/kg)	0.45
Half-life – normal/ ESRF (hrs)	6–11 minutes/–

METABOLISM

Dopexamine is rapidly eliminated from blood with a half-life of approximately 6–7 minutes in healthy volunteers and around 11 minutes in patients with cardiac failure. Subsequent elimination of the metabolites is by urinary and biliary excretion.

DOSE IN RENAL IMPAIRMENT GFR (mL/MIN)

20–50	Dose as in normal renal function and adjust to response.
10–20	Dose as in normal renal function and adjust to response.
<10	Dose as in normal renal function and adjust to response.

DOSE IN PATIENTS UNDERGOING RENAL REPLACEMENT THERAPIES

CAPD	Unknown dialysability. Dose as in normal renal function.
HD	Unknown dialysability. Dose as in normal renal function.
HDF/High flux	Unknown dialysability. Dose as in normal renal function.
CAV/ VVHD	Unknown dialysability. Dose as in normal renal function.

IMPORTANT DRUG INTERACTIONS

Potentially hazardous interactions with other drugs
- Antidepressants: risk of hypertensive crisis with MAOIs and moclobemide.
- Beta-blockers: risk of severe hypertension.
- Dopaminergics: avoid concomitant use with rasagiline.
- Sympathomimetics: effects of adrenaline and noradrenaline possibly enhanced.

ADMINISTRATION

RECONSTITUTION
–
ROUTE
- By intravenous infusion into a central or large peripheral vein.
RATE OF ADMINISTRATION
- See dosage instructions.
COMMENTS
- IV infusion of 400 or 800 micrograms/mL in glucose 5% or sodium chloride 0.9%.
- Peripheral administration: concentration of infusion solution must not exceed 1 mg/mL.
- Central administration: concentration not >4 mg/mL.
- Rate of administration and duration of therapy should be adjusted according to the patient's response as determined by heart rate and rhythm, blood pressure, urine flow and measurement of cardiac output.

OTHER INFORMATION

Avoid abrupt withdrawal.

Doripenem

CLINICAL USE

Carbapenem antibacterial agent

DOSE IN NORMAL RENAL FUNCTION

500–1000 mg every 8 hours

PHARMACOKINETICS

Molecular weight (daltons)	438.5
% Protein binding	8.1
% Excreted unchanged in urine	71
Volume of distribution (L/kg)	16.8 litres
Half-life – normal/ ESRF (hrs)	1/Increased

METABOLISM

Metabolised via hydrolysis of its beta-lactam ring by dehydropeptidase I to an open-ringed inactive metabolite (doripenem-M1).

Mainly excreted in the urine by tubular secretion and glomerular filtration. About 70% and 15% of a dose is recovered as unchanged drug and metabolite, respectively, in the urine within 48 hours. Less than 1% is excreted in faeces.

DOSE IN RENAL IMPAIRMENT GFR (mL/MIN)

30–50	250–500 mg every 8 hours
10–30	250–500 mg every 12 hours
<10	250–500 mg every 12 hours, use with caution.

DOSE IN PATIENTS UNDERGOING RENAL REPLACEMENT THERAPIES

CAPD	Dialysed. Dose as in GFR<10 mL/min.
HD	Dialysed. Dose as in GFR<10 mL/min.
HDF/High flux	Dialysed. Dose as in GFR<10 mL/min.
CAV/VVHD	Dialysed. 500 mg every 12 hours.

IMPORTANT DRUG INTERACTIONS

Potentially hazardous interactions with other drugs
- Anti-epileptics: reduced valproic acid concentration – avoid concomitant use.

ADMINISTRATION

RECONSTITUTION
- 10 mL water for injection or sodium chloride 0.9%

ROUTE
- IV

RATE OF ADMINISTRATION
- 60 minutes (4 hours for VAP)

COMMENTS
- Add to 100 mL of sodium chloride 0.9% or glucose 5%.
- Do not use glucose 5% for infusions lasting >1 hour.

OTHER INFORMATION

- SPC recommends using with caution in severe renal impairment due to limited clinical data and increased exposure to doripenem and its metabolite.
- Following a single 500 mg dose, doripenem AUC increased 1.6-fold, 2.8-fold, and 5.1-fold in subjects with GFR=51–79 mL/min, 31–50 mL/min and ≤ 30 mL/min respectively, compared to people with normal renal function. AUC of the microbiologically inactive metabolite is expected to be considerably increased in patients with severe renal impairment compared with healthy subjects.
- AUCs of doripenem and its metabolite are substantially increased in patients who require haemodialysis compared with healthy subjects. In a study where six subjects on haemodialysis received a single dose of 500 mg doripenem, the amount of doripenem removed during the 4 hour haemodialysis session was 231 mg (46% of the dose).

Dornase alfa

CLINICAL USE

To improve pulmonary function in cystic fibrosis

DOSE IN NORMAL RENAL FUNCTION

2.5 mg (2500 u) daily via nebuliser can be increased to twice daily if over 21 years of age.

PHARMACOKINETICS

Molecular weight (daltons)	29 249.6
% Protein binding	No data
% Excreted unchanged in urine	No data
Volume of distribution (L/kg)	No data
Half-life – normal/ ESRF (hrs)	11 (from lungs in rats)

METABOLISM

Dornase alfa acts as a mucolytic by hydrolysing DNA that has accumulated in sputum from decaying neutrophils. It is expected to be metabolised by proteases present in biological fluids.

DOSE IN RENAL IMPAIRMENT GFR (mL/MIN)

20–50	Dose as in normal renal function.
10–20	Dose as in normal renal function.
<10	Dose as in normal renal function.

DOSE IN PATIENTS UNDERGOING RENAL REPLACEMENT THERAPIES

CAPD	Unlikely to be dialysed. Dose as in normal renal function.
HD	Unlikely to be dialysed. Dose as in normal renal function.
HDF/High flux	Unlikely to be dialysed. Dose as in normal renal function.
CAV/ VVHD	Unlikely to be dialysed. Dose as in normal renal function.

IMPORTANT DRUG INTERACTIONS

Potentially hazardous interactions with other drugs
● None known

ADMINISTRATION

RECONSTITUTION
–
ROUTE
● Nebulised
RATE OF ADMINISTRATION
–

COMMENTS
● <15% of dose is systemically absorbed.

OTHER INFORMATION

● No pharmacokinetic data available; little systemic absorption therefore little accumulation expected.
● Use undiluted, using recommended jet nebuliser/compressor system. Refer to data sheet.

Dosulepin hydrochloride (dothiepin)

CLINICAL USE

Tricyclic antidepressant

DOSE IN NORMAL RENAL FUNCTION

50–225 mg daily

PHARMACOKINETICS

Molecular weight (daltons)	331.9
% Protein binding	84
% Excreted unchanged in urine	56 (mainly as metabolites)
Volume of distribution (L/kg)	45
Half-life – normal/ ESRF (hrs)	14–24/–

METABOLISM

Dosulepin hydrochloride is readily absorbed from the gastrointestinal tract, and extensively demethylated by first-pass metabolism in the liver to its primary active metabolite, desmethyldothiepin (also termed northiaden). Paths of metabolism also include S-oxidation.

Dosulepin is excreted in the urine, mainly in the form of its metabolites; small amounts are also excreted in the faeces. Elimination half-lives of about 14 to 24 and 23 to 46 hours have been reported for dosulepin and its metabolites, respectively.

DOSE IN RENAL IMPAIRMENT GFR (mL/MIN)

20–50	Dose as in normal renal function.
10–20	Start with small dose, and titrate according to response.
<10	Start with small dose, and titrate according to response.

DOSE IN PATIENTS UNDERGOING RENAL REPLACEMENT THERAPIES

CAPD	Not dialysed. Dose as in GFR<10 mL/min.
HD	Not dialysed. Dose as in GFR<10 mL/min.
HDF/High flux	Unknown dialysability. Dose as in GFR<10 mL/min.
CAV/ VVHD	Unknown dialysability. Dose as in GFR=10–20 mL/min.

IMPORTANT DRUG INTERACTIONS

Potentially hazardous interactions with other drugs

- Alcohol: increased sedative effect.
- Analgesics: increased risk of CNS toxicity with tramadol; possibly increased risk of side effects with nefopam; possibly increased sedative effects with opioids.
- Anti-arrhythmics: increased risk of ventricular arrhythmias with amiodarone – avoid concomitant use; increased risk of ventricular arrhythmias with disopyramide, flecainide or propafenone; avoid with dronedarone.
- Antibacterials: increased risk of ventricular arrhythmias with moxifloxacin and possibly telithromycin – avoid concomitant use with moxifloxacin.
- Anticoagulants: may alter anticoagulant effect of coumarins.
- Antidepressants: enhanced CNS excitation and hypertension with MAOIs and moclobemide – avoid concomitant use; concentration possibly increased with SSRIs.
- Anti-epileptics: convulsive threshold lowered; concentration reduced by carbamazepine, phenobarbital and possibly phenytoin.
- Antimalarials: avoid concomitant use with artemether/lumefantrine and piperaquine with artenimol.
- Antipsychotics: increased risk of ventricular arrhythmias especially with droperidol and pimozide – avoid; increased antimuscarinic effects with clozapine and phenothiazines; concentration increased by antipsychotics.
- Antivirals: increased risk of ventricular arrhythmias with saquinavir – avoid; concentration possibly increased with ritonavir.
- Atomoxetine: increased risk of ventricular arrhythmias and possibly convulsions.
- Beta-blockers: increased risk of ventricular arrhythmias with sotalol.
- Clonidine: Tricyclics antagonise hypotensive effect; increased risk of hypertension on clonidine withdrawal.
- Dopaminergics: avoid use with entacapone; CNS toxicity reported with selegiline and rasagiline.

- Pentamidine: increased risk of ventricular arrhythmias.
- Sympathomimetics: increased risk of hypertension and arrhythmias with adrenaline and noradrenaline; metabolism possibly inhibited by methylphenidate.

ADMINISTRATION

RECONSTITUTION

–

ROUTE

- Oral

RATE OF ADMINISTRATION

–

COMMENTS

–

OTHER INFORMATION

- Metabolites are active and partly renally excreted.
- Metabolites accumulate and cause excessive sedation.
- 25–50 mg usually effective without too much sedation.

Doxapram hydrochloride

CLINICAL USE

- Postoperative respiratory depression
- Acute respiratory failure

DOSE IN NORMAL RENAL FUNCTION

- Postoperative respiratory depression: IV injection 1–1.5 mg/kg repeated at hourly intervals, or IV infusion 2–3 mg/minute, adjusted according to response.
- Acute respiratory failure: 1.5–4 mg/minute as an IV infusion, adjusted according to response.

PHARMACOKINETICS

Molecular weight (daltons)	433
% Protein binding	No data
% Excreted unchanged in urine	<5
Volume of distribution (L/kg)	0.58–2.74
Half-life – normal/ ESRF (hrs)	2.4–4.1/–

METABOLISM

Doxapram is extensively metabolised in the liver, and the major route of excretion of metabolites and a small amount of unchanged drug is thought to be via bile to the faeces. Less than 5% of an IV dose is excreted unchanged in the urine in 24 hours.

DOSE IN RENAL IMPAIRMENT GFR (mL/MIN)

20–50	Dose as in normal renal function.
10–20	Dose as in normal renal function.
<10	Dose as in normal renal function.

DOSE IN PATIENTS UNDERGOING RENAL REPLACEMENT THERAPIES

CAPD	Unknown dialysability. Dose as in normal renal function.
HD	Unknown dialysability. Dose as in normal renal function.
HDF/High flux	Unknown dialysability. Dose as in normal renal function.
CAV/ VVHD	Unknown dialysability. Dose as in normal renal function.

IMPORTANT DRUG INTERACTIONS

Potentially hazardous interactions with other drugs
- Anaesthetics: increased risk of arrhythmias with volatile liquid general anaesthetics – avoid for at least 10 minutes after volatile liquid general anaesthetics.

ADMINISTRATION

RECONSTITUTION
–
ROUTE
- IV bolus, IV infusion
RATE OF ADMINISTRATION
- IV injection: over at least 30 seconds
- IV infusion as indication
COMMENTS
- Doxapram has a narrow margin of safety; the minimum effective dosage should be used and maximum recommended dosages should not be exceeded.

OTHER INFORMATION

Unlike naloxone, doxapram does not reverse the other effects of opioid analgesics (i.e. analgesia).

Doxazosin

CLINICAL USE

Alpha-adrenoceptor blocker:
- Hypertension
- Benign prostatic hyperplasia (BPH)

DOSE IN NORMAL RENAL FUNCTION

- Hypertension: 1–16 mg daily
- XL preparation: 4–8 mg once daily
- BPH: 1–8 mg daily

PHARMACOKINETICS

Molecular weight (daltons)	547.6 (as mesilate)
% Protein binding	98
% Excreted unchanged in urine	<5
Volume of distribution (L/kg)	1–1.7
Half-life – normal/ ESRF (hrs)	22/Unchanged

METABOLISM

Doxazosin is extensively metabolised in the liver, and excreted in faeces as inactive metabolites (6-hydroxydoxazosin) and a small amount of unchanged drug.

DOSE IN RENAL IMPAIRMENT GFR (mL/MIN)

20–50	Dose as in normal renal function.
10–20	Dose as in normal renal function.
<10	Dose as in normal renal function.

DOSE IN PATIENTS UNDERGOING RENAL REPLACEMENT THERAPIES

CAPD	Not dialysed. Dose as in normal renal function.
HD	Not dialysed. Dose as in normal renal function.
HDF/High flux	Unknown dialysability. Dose as in normal renal function.
CAV/ VVHD	Not dialysed. Dose as in normal renal function.

IMPORTANT DRUG INTERACTIONS

Potentially hazardous interactions with other drugs
- Anaesthetics: enhanced hypotensive effect.
- Antidepressants: enhanced hypotensive effect with MAOIs.
- Beta-blockers: enhanced hypotensive effect; increased risk of first dose hypotensive effect.
- Calcium-channel blockers: enhanced hypotensive effect, increased risk of first dose hypotensive effect.
- Diuretics: enhanced hypotensive effect, increased risk of first dose hypotensive effect.
- Moxisylyte: possibly severe postural hypotension when used in combination.
- Vardenafil, sildenafil and tadalafil: enhanced hypotensive effect, avoid concomitant use.

ADMINISTRATION

RECONSTITUTION
–
ROUTE
- Oral
RATE OF ADMINISTRATION
–
COMMENTS
–

OTHER INFORMATION

–

Doxepin

CLINICAL USE

Tricyclic antidepressant

DOSE IN NORMAL RENAL FUNCTION

25–300 mg daily, doses above 100 mg given in 3 divided doses

PHARMACOKINETICS

Molecular weight (daltons)	315.8 (as hydrochloride)
% Protein binding	76
% Excreted unchanged in urine	<3
Volume of distribution (L/kg)	20
Half-life – normal/ ESRF (hrs)	8–24/10–30

METABOLISM

Approximately 55%-87% of doxepin undergoes first pass metabolism in the liver, forming the primary active metabolite desmethyldoxepin. Doxepin is excreted in the urine, mainly in the form of its metabolites, either free or in conjugated form.

DOSE IN RENAL IMPAIRMENT GFR (mL/MIN)

20–50	Dose as in normal renal function.
10–20	Start with small dose, and titrate according to response.
<10	Start with small dose, and titrate according to response.

DOSE IN PATIENTS UNDERGOING RENAL REPLACEMENT THERAPIES

CAPD	Not dialysed. Dose as in GFR<10 mL/min.
HD	Not dialysed. Dose as in GFR<10 mL/min.
HDF/High flux	Unknown dialysability. Dose as in GFR<10 mL/min.
CAV/ VVHD	Unknown dialysability. Dose as in GFR=10–20 mL/min.

IMPORTANT DRUG INTERACTIONS

Potentially hazardous interactions with other drugs

- Alcohol: increased sedative effect.
- Analgesics: increased risk of CNS toxicity with tramadol; possibly increased risk of side effects with nefopam; possibly increased sedative effects with opioids.
- Anti-arrhythmics: increased risk of ventricular arrhythmias with amiodarone – avoid concomitant use; increased risk of ventricular arrhythmias with disopyramide, flecainide or propafenone; avoid with dronedarone.
- Antibacterials: increased risk of ventricular arrhythmias with moxifloxacin and possibly telithromycin – avoid concomitant use with moxifloxacin.
- Anticoagulants: may alter anticoagulant effect of coumarins.
- Antidepressants: enhanced CNS excitation and hypertension with MAOIs and moclobemide – avoid concomitant use; concentration possibly increased with SSRIs.
- Anti-epileptics: convulsive threshold lowered; concentration reduced by carbamazepine, phenobarbital and possibly phenytoin.
- Antimalarials: avoid concomitant use with artemether/lumefantrine and piperaquine with artenimol.
- Antipsychotics: increased risk of ventricular arrhythmias especially with droperidol and pimozide – avoid; increased antimuscarinic effects with clozapine and phenothiazines; concentration increased by antipsychotics.
- Antivirals: increased risk of ventricular arrhythmias with saquinavir – avoid; concentration possibly increased with ritonavir.
- Atomoxetine: increased risk of ventricular arrhythmias and possibly convulsions.
- Beta-blockers: increased risk of ventricular arrhythmias with sotalol.
- Clonidine: tricyclics antagonise hypotensive effect; increased risk of hypertension on clonidine withdrawal.
- Dopaminergics: avoid use with entacapone; CNS toxicity reported with selegiline and rasagiline.
- Pentamidine: increased risk of ventricular arrhythmias.
- Sympathomimetics: increased risk of hypertension and arrhythmias with

adrenaline and noradrenaline; metabolism possibly inhibited by methylphenidate.

ADMINISTRATION

RECONSTITUTION

–

ROUTE

● Oral

RATE OF ADMINISTRATION

–

COMMENTS

–

OTHER INFORMATION

● The half-life of desmethyldoxepin (active metabolite) ranged from 33–80 hours (mean 51 hours).

Doxorubicin hydrochloride

CLINICAL USE

Antineoplastic agent:
- Acute leukaemias
- Lymphomas
- Sarcomas
- Various solid tumours

DOSE IN NORMAL RENAL FUNCTION

Varies according to local protocol

PHARMACOKINETICS

Molecular weight (daltons)	580
% Protein binding	50–85
% Excreted unchanged in urine	<15
Volume of distribution (L/kg)	>20–30
Half-life – normal/ ESRF (hrs)	30; (Liposomal: 55–75; Pegylated: 24–231)/Unchanged

METABOLISM

The elimination of doxorubicin from the blood is triphasic with mean half-lives of 12 minutes (distribution), 3.3 hours and about 30 hours. Doxorubicin undergoes rapid metabolism in the liver. The main metabolite is the pharmacologically active doxorubicinol. Other metabolites are deoxyrubicin aglycone, glucuronide and sulphate conjugate. About 40–50% of a dose is excreted in bile within 7 days, of which about half is excreted as unchanged drug and the rest as metabolites. Only 5–15% of the administered dose is eliminated in urine.

DOSE IN RENAL IMPAIRMENT GFR (mL/MIN)

20–50	Dose as in normal renal function.
10–20	Dose as in normal renal function.
<10	75–100% of dose. Caelyx: No data.

DOSE IN PATIENTS UNDERGOING RENAL REPLACEMENT THERAPIES

CAPD	Not dialysed. Dose as in GFR<10mL/min.
HD	Not dialysed. Dose as in GFR<10mL/min.
HDF/High flux	Unknown dialysability. Dose as in GFR<10mL/min.
CAV/ VVHD	Unknown dialysability. Dose as in normal renal function.

IMPORTANT DRUG INTERACTIONS

Potentially hazardous interactions with other drugs
- Antipsychotics: avoid concomitant use with clozapine, increased risk of agranulocytosis.
- Ciclosporin: increased risk of neurotoxicity.

ADMINISTRATION

RECONSTITUTION
- Reconstitute with water for injection or sodium chloride 0.9%, 10mg in 5mL, 50mg in 25mL

ROUTE
- IV, intra-arterial, intravesical (bladder instillation)

RATE OF ADMINISTRATION
- Via the tubing of a fast running intravenous infusion of sodium chloride 0.9% or glucose 5%
- Injection: over 3–5 minutes
- Continuous infusion: over 24 hours
- Caelyx: initially 1 mg/min, if no reactions further doses over 60 minutes
- AIDS-related Kaposi's sarcoma: dilute in 250mL glucose 5% over 30 minutes

COMMENTS
- For bladder instillation, concentration of doxorubicin in bladder should be 50mg per 50mL. To avoid undue dilution in urine, the patient should be instructed not to drink any fluid in the 12 hours prior to instillation. This should limit urine production to approximately 50mL per hour.

OTHER INFORMATION

- Manufacturer of Caelyx® has no information in GFR<30 mL/min.
- *Drug Prescribing in Renal Failure*, 5th edition, by Aronoff *et al.* suggests using 100% of the dose for conventional doxorubicin.
- A cumulative dose of 450–550 mg/m² should only be exceeded with extreme caution. Above this level, the risk of irreversible congestive cardiac failure increases greatly.
- Patients with impaired hepatic function have prolonged and elevated plasma concentrations of both the drug and its metabolites. Dose reduction is required.
- Liposomal preparations available: up to 90 mg in 250 mL glucose 5%; if greater than 90 mg dilute in 500 mL glucose 5%.

Doxycycline

CLINICAL USE

Antibacterial agent
- Also prophylaxis/treatment of malaria

DOSE IN NORMAL RENAL FUNCTION

- 200 mg on day 1, then 100 mg daily; severe infections 200 mg daily.
- Syphilis: 100–200 mg twice daily.
- Malaria: treatment: 200 mg once daily; prophylaxis: 100 mg daily.

PHARMACOKINETICS

Molecular weight (daltons)	462.4
% Protein binding	>90
% Excreted unchanged in urine	33–45
Volume of distribution (L/kg)	0.7
Half-life – normal/ ESRF (hrs)	18/Unchanged

METABOLISM

Doxycycline is concentrated in the bile. About 40% of the administered dose is eliminated in 3 days in active form in the urine. However, the majority of a dose of doxycycline is excreted in the faeces after chelation in the intestines. Urinary concentrations are roughly 10 times higher than plasma concentrations at the same time.

In the presence of impaired renal function, urinary elimination decreases, faecal elimination increases and the half-life remains unchanged.

DOSE IN RENAL IMPAIRMENT GFR (mL/MIN)

20–50	Dose as in normal renal function.
10–20	Dose as in normal renal function.
<10	Dose as in normal renal function.

DOSE IN PATIENTS UNDERGOING RENAL REPLACEMENT THERAPIES

CAPD	Not dialysed. Dose as in normal renal function.
HD	Not dialysed. Dose as in normal renal function.
HDF/High flux	Unknown dialysability. Dose as in normal renal function.
CAV/ VVHD	Not dialysed. Dose as in normal renal function.

IMPORTANT DRUG INTERACTIONS

Potentially hazardous interactions with other drugs
- Anticoagulants: possibly enhanced anticoagulant effect of coumarins and phenindione.
- Ciclosporin: possibly increases plasma-ciclosporin concentration.
- Oestrogens: possibly reduced contraceptive effects of oestrogens (risk probably small).
- Retinoids: possible increased risk of benign intracranial hypertension – avoid concomitant use.

ADMINISTRATION

RECONSTITUTION

–

ROUTE
- Oral

RATE OF ADMINISTRATION

–

COMMENTS
- Do not take iron preparations, indigestion remedies or phosphate binders at the same time of day as doxycycline.

Dronedarone

CLINICAL USE

Anti-arrhythmic:
- Maintenance of sinus rhythm after successful cardioversion in adult clinically stable patients with paroxysmal or persistent atrial fibrillation

DOSE IN NORMAL RENAL FUNCTION

400 mg twice daily

PHARMACOKINETICS

Molecular weight (daltons)	556.8 (593.2 as hydrochloride)
% Protein binding	99.7
% Excreted unchanged in urine	0 (6% as metabolites)
Volume of distribution (L/kg)	1200–1400 litres
Half-life – normal/ ESRF (hrs)	25–30/Unchanged

METABOLISM

Dronedarone is extensively metabolised in the liver, mainly by the cytochrome P450 isoenzyme CYP3A4 to a less active N-debutyl metabolite, and several inactive metabolites.

About 6% of an oral dose is excreted in the urine (entirely metabolites) and 84% in the faeces (metabolites and unchanged drug).

DOSE IN RENAL IMPAIRMENT GFR (mL/MIN)

30–50	Dose as in normal renal function.
10–30	Dose as in normal renal function. See 'Other information'.
<10	Dose as in normal renal function. See 'Other information'.

DOSE IN PATIENTS UNDERGOING RENAL REPLACEMENT THERAPIES

CAPD	Not dialysed. Dose as GFR<10 mL/min.
HD	Not dialysed. Dose as GFR<10 mL/min.
HDF/High flux	Unknown dialysability. Dose as GFR<10 mL/min.
CAV/ VVHD	Not dialysed. Dose as in GFR=10–30 mL/min.

IMPORTANT DRUG INTERACTIONS

Potentially hazardous interactions with other drugs
- Anti-arrhythmics: increased risk of myocardial depression with other anti-arrhythmics; increased risk of ventricular arrhythmias with amiodarone or disopyramide – avoid concomitant use.
- Antibacterials: increased risk of ventricular arrhythmias with clarithromycin, telithromycin & erythromycin; concentration reduced by rifampicin – avoid concomitant use.
- Anticoagulants: increased anticoagulant effect with coumarins & phenindione; increased dabigatran concentration – avoid concomitant use; avoid concomitant use with rivaroxaban.
- Antidepressants: concentration possibly reduced by St John's wort – avoid concomitant use; increased risk of ventricular arrhythmias with tricyclic antidepressants – avoid concomitant use.
- Anti-epileptics: concentration possibly reduced by phenytoin, carbamazepine and phenobarbital – avoid concomitant use.
- Antifungals: concentration increased by ketoconazole – avoid concomitant use; avoid concomitant use with itraconazole, posaconazole & voriconazole.
- Antipsychotics: increased risk of ventricular arrhythmias with antipsychotics that prolong the QT interval; increased risk of ventricular arrhythmias with phenothiazines – avoid concomitant use.
- Antivirals: avoid concomitant use with ritonavir; increased risk of ventricular arrhythmias with saquinavir – avoid concomitant use.
- Beta-blockers: increased risk of myocardial depression; concentration of metoprolol & propranolol possibly increased; increased risk of ventricular arrhythmias with sotalol – avoid concomitant use.
- Calcium-channel blockers: concentration increased by nifedipine; increased risk of bradycardia & myocardial depression with diltiazem & verapamil.
- Digoxin: increased concentration (halve digoxin maintenance dose).
- Fingolimod: possibly increased risk of bradycardia.
- Grapefruit juice: concentration of dronedarone increased – avoid concomitant use.

- Lipid-lowering drugs: concentration of atorvastatin & rosuvastatin possibly increased; increased risk of myopathy with simvastatin.
- Sirolimus: manufacturer advises use with caution.
- Tacrolimus: manufacturer advises use with caution.

ADMINISTRATION

RECONSTITUTION

–

ROUTE

- Oral

RATE OF ADMINISTRATION

–

OTHER INFORMATION

- Contraindicated by manufacturer in the UK but no dose alteration in the USA for severe renal impairment.
- Cases of life-threatening acute liver injury have been reported. Monitor LFTs before and during treatment.
- Cases of new-onset or worsening heart failure have been reported.
- An increase in plasma creatinine (mean increase 10 µmol/l) has been observed in healthy subjects and in patients. In most patients this increase occurs early after treatment initiation and reaches a plateau after 7 days. It is recommended to measure plasma creatinine values prior to and 7 days after initiation of dronedarone. If an increase in creatininemia is observed, serum creatinine should be remeasured after a further 7 days. If no further increase in creatinine is observed, this value should be used as the new reference baseline taking into account that this may be expected with dronedarone. If serum creatinine continues to rise then consideration should be given to further investigation and discontinuing treatment.
- Oral bioavailability is 4% (15% with food).

Droperidol

CLINICAL USE

- Treatment of postoperative nausea and vomiting (PONV)

DOSE IN NORMAL RENAL FUNCTION

PONV: 0.625–125 mg every 6 hours
Prevention of PONV due to opioids in PCA:
15–50 mcg of droperidol for every 1 mg of
morphine, maximum 5 mg

PHARMACOKINETICS

Molecular weight (daltons)	379.4
% Protein binding	85–90
% Excreted unchanged in urine	1
Volume of distribution (L/kg)	1.5
Half-life – normal/ ESRF (hrs)	121–147 minutes/–

METABOLISM

Extensively metabolised in the liver,
and undergoes oxidation, dealkylation,
demethylation and hydroxylation by
cytochrome P450 isoenzymes 1A2 and
3A4, and to a lesser extent by 2C19. The
metabolites are inactive.

About 75% of a dose is excreted in the
urine, with 1% being excreted unchanged;
11% appears in the faeces.

DOSE IN RENAL IMPAIRMENT GFR (mL/MIN)

20–50	Dose as in normal renal function.
10–20	625 mcg every 6 hours. Reduce dose of infusion.
<10	625 mcg every 6 hours. Reduce dose of infusion.

DOSE IN PATIENTS UNDERGOING RENAL REPLACEMENT THERAPIES

CAPD	Unlikely to be dialysed. Dose as in GFR<10 mL/min.
HD	Unlikely to be dialysed. Dose as in GFR<10 mL/min.
HDF/High flux	Unknown dialysability. Dose as in GFR<10 mL/min.
CAV/ VVHD	Unlikely to be dialysed. Dose as in GFR=10–20 mL/min.

IMPORTANT DRUG INTERACTIONS

Potentially hazardous interactions with
other drugs

- Anaesthetics: enhanced hypotensive effect; effects of thiopental enhanced.
- Analgesics: increased risk of ventricular arrhythmias with methadone; increased risk of convulsions with tramadol; enhanced hypotensive and sedative effects with opioids.
- Anti-arrhythmics increased risk of ventricular arrhythmias with anti-arrhythmics that prolong the QT interval, e.g. procainamide, disopyramide, dronedarone and amiodarone – avoid concomitant use with amiodarone and dronedarone.
- Antibacterials: increased risk of ventricular arrhythmias with moxifloxacin and macrolides – avoid concomitant use.
- Antidepressants: increased risk of ventricular arrhythmias with fluoxetine, fluvoxamine, sertraline or tricyclics – avoid.
- Anti-epileptics: antagonised (convulsive threshold lowered).
- Antimalarials: avoid concomitant use with artemether/lumefantrine and piperaquine with artenimol; increased risk of ventricular arrhythmias with chloroquine, hydroxychloroquine or quinine – avoid.
- Antipsychotics: increased risk of ventricular arrhythmias with amisulpride, pimozide, sulpiride, phenothiazines that prolong QT interval or haloperidol – avoid concomitant use.
- Antivirals: concentration possibly increased with ritonavir.
- Anxiolytics and hypnotics: increased sedative effects.
- Atomoxetine: increased risk of ventricular arrhythmias.
- Beta-blockers: enhanced hypotensive effect; increased risk of ventricular arrhythmias with sotalol – avoid.
- Cytotoxics: increased risk of ventricular arrhythmias with arsenic trioxide.
- Desferrioxamine: avoid concomitant use.
- Diuretics: enhanced hypotensive effect.
- Hormone antagonists: increased risk of ventricular arrhythmias with tamoxifen – avoid.
- Lithium: increased risk of extrapyramidal side effects and possibly neurotoxicity.
- Pentamidine: increased risk of ventricular arrhythmias.

- Tacrolimus: increased risk of ventricular arrhythmias – avoid.

ADMINISTRATION

RECONSTITUTION

–

ROUTE

- IV

RATE OF ADMINISTRATION

- Bolus or continuous infusion

OTHER INFORMATION

- Increased CNS sensitivity in severe renal impairment.
- Droperidol has been associated with QT prolongation, serious ventricular arrhythmias and sudden death. Withdrawn by Janssen-Cilag in 2001 but is still available in the UK and USA from other suppliers.

Duloxetine

CLINICAL USE

- Moderate to severe stress urinary incontinence
- Depression
- Diabetic peripheral neuropathy
- Generalised anxiety disorder

DOSE IN NORMAL RENAL FUNCTION

- Incontinence: 20–40 mg twice daily
- Depression and diabetic peripheral neuropathy: 60 mg daily
- Anxiety: 30–120 mg daily

PHARMACOKINETICS

Molecular weight (daltons)	333.9 (as hydrochloride)
% Protein binding	95–96
% Excreted unchanged in urine	<1 (77% as metabolites)
Volume of distribution (L/kg)	1640 litres
Half-life – normal/ ESRF (hrs)	8–17/Unchanged

METABOLISM

Duloxetine is extensively metabolised and the metabolites are excreted principally in urine. Both cytochromes P450–2D6 and 1A2 catalyse the formation of the two major metabolites, glucuronide conjugate of 4-hydroxy duloxetine and sulphate conjugate of 5-hydroxy, 6-methoxy duloxetine.

Based upon *in vitro* studies, the circulating metabolites of duloxetine are considered pharmacologically inactive.

DOSE IN RENAL IMPAIRMENT GFR (mL/MIN)

30–50	Dose as in normal renal function; start with a low dose.
10–30	Start at low dose and increase according to response.
<10	Start at very low dose and increase according to response.

DOSE IN PATIENTS UNDERGOING RENAL REPLACEMENT THERAPIES

CAPD	Not dialysed. Dose as in GFR <10 mL/min.
HD	Not dialysed. Dose as in GFR <10 mL/min.
HDF/High flux	Unlikely to be dialysed. Dose as in GFR <10 mL/min.
CAV/ VVHD	Not dialysed. Dose as in GFR =10–30 mL/min.

IMPORTANT DRUG INTERACTIONS

Potentially hazardous interactions with other drugs

- Antibacterials: metabolism inhibited by ciprofloxacin – avoid concomitant use.
- Anticoagulants: possibly increased risk of bleeding with dabigatran.
- Other CNS medication: enhanced effect.
- Antidepressants: avoid concomitant use with MAOIs, moclobemide, St John's wort, tryptophan, venlafaxine, amitriptyline, clomipramine and SSRIs due to increased risk of serotonin syndrome; increased risk of side effects with tricyclic antidepressants; fluvoxamine decreases the clearance of duloxetine by 77% – avoid concomitant use.
- Antimalarials: avoid concomitant use with artemether/lumefantrine and piperaquine with artenimol.
- Methylthioninium: risk of CNS toxicity – avoid if possible.

ADMINISTRATION

RECONSTITUTION
–
ROUTE
- Oral
RATE OF ADMINISTRATION
–
COMMENTS
–

OTHER INFORMATION

- In CKD 5 there is a 2-fold increase in C_{max} and AUC. The renally excreted metabolites 4-hydroxy duloxetine glucuronide and 5-hydroxy, 6-methoxy duloxetine sulphate were 7–9 times higher than in people with normal renal function.
- Contraindicated in uncontrolled hypertension due to potential risk of hypertensive crisis.
- Contraindicated by manufacturer if GFR<30 mL/min due to increased plasma concentration and limited data. New Zealand data sheet advises to start at a low dose, e.g. 30 mg, and gradually increase in severe renal impairment.

Dutasteride

CLINICAL USE

Testosterone-5-alpha-reductase inhibitor:
- Benign prostatic hyperplasia

DOSE IN NORMAL RENAL FUNCTION

500 mcg daily

PHARMACOKINETICS

Molecular weight (daltons)	528.5
% Protein binding	>99.5
% Excreted unchanged in urine	0.1
Volume of distribution (L/kg)	300–500 litres
Half-life – normal/ ESRF (hrs)	3–5 weeks/ Unchanged

METABOLISM

Dutasteride is metabolised by the cytochrome P450 isoenzymes CYP3A4 and CYP3A5, and most of a dose is excreted as metabolites in the faeces.

DOSE IN RENAL IMPAIRMENT GFR (mL/MIN)

20–50	Dose as in normal renal function.
10–20	Dose as in normal renal function.
<10	Dose as in normal renal function.

DOSE IN PATIENTS UNDERGOING RENAL REPLACEMENT THERAPIES

CAPD	Unlikely to be dialysed. Dose as in normal renal function.
HD	Unlikely to be dialysed. Dose as in normal renal function.
HDF/High flux	Unlikely to be dialysed. Dose as in normal renal function.
CAV/ VVHD	Unlikely to be dialysed. Dose as in normal renal function.

IMPORTANT DRUG INTERACTIONS

Potentially hazardous interactions with other drugs
- None known

ADMINISTRATION

RECONSTITUTION
–
ROUTE
- Oral
RATE OF ADMINISTRATION
–

OTHER INFORMATION

- Oral bioavailability is approximately 60%.

Eculizumab

CLINICAL USE

Recombinant monoclonal antibody:
- Paroxysmal nocturnal haemoglobinuria (PNH)
- Atypical haemolytic uraemic syndrome (aHUS)

DOSE IN NORMAL RENAL FUNCTION

- PNH: 600 mg once a week for 4 weeks then 900 mg every 12–16 days
- aHUS: 900 mg once a week for 4 weeks then 1200 mg every 12–16 days

PHARMACOKINETICS

Molecular weight (daltons)	148 000
% Protein binding	No data
% Excreted unchanged in urine	No data
Volume of distribution (L/kg)	7.7 litres
Half-life – normal/ ESRF (hrs)	11–12 days/–

METABOLISM

Human antibodies undergo endocytotic digestion in the cells of the reticuloendothelial system. Eculizumab contains only naturally occurring amino acids and has no known active metabolites. Human antibodies are predominately catabolised by lysosomal enzymes to small peptides and amino acids.

DOSE IN RENAL IMPAIRMENT GFR (mL/MIN)

20–50	Dose as in normal renal function.
10–20	Dose as in normal renal function.
<10	Dose as in normal renal function.

DOSE IN PATIENTS UNDERGOING RENAL REPLACEMENT THERAPIES

CAPD	Unlikely to be dialysed. Dose as in normal renal function.
HD	Unlikely to be dialysed. Dose as in normal renal function.
HDF/High flux	Unlikely to be dialysed. Dose as in normal renal function.
CAV/ VVHD	Unlikely to be dialysed. Dose as in normal renal function.

IMPORTANT DRUG INTERACTIONS

Potentially hazardous interactions with other drugs
- None known

ADMINISTRATION

RECONSTITUTION
–
ROUTE
- IV infusion
RATE OF ADMINISTRATION
- 25–45 minutes

OTHER INFORMATION

- A 1 hour session of plasma exchange causes a 50% decline in concentration of eculizumab.

Efavirenz

CLINICAL USE

Non-nucleoside reverse transcriptase inhibitor:
- HIV infection in combination with other antiretroviral drugs

DOSE IN NORMAL RENAL FUNCTION

600 mg once daily (tablets and capsules should be taken on an empty stomach to minimise side effects)
Oral solution: 720 mg once daily

PHARMACOKINETICS

Molecular weight (daltons)	315.7
% Protein binding	99.5–99.75
% Excreted unchanged in urine	<1
Volume of distribution (L/kg)	2–4
Half-life – normal/ ESRF (hrs)	40–55 (multiple dosing); 52–76 (single dosing)/Unchanged

METABOLISM

Studies in humans and *in vitro* studies using human liver microsomes have demonstrated that efavirenz is principally metabolised by the cytochrome P450 system to hydroxylated metabolites with subsequent glucuronidation of these hydroxylated metabolites. These metabolites are essentially inactive against HIV-1. The *in vitro* studies suggest that CYP3A4 and CYP2B6 are the major isozymes responsible for efavirenz metabolism and that it inhibited P450 isozymes 2C9, 2C19, and 3A4. In *in vitro* studies efavirenz did not inhibit CYP2E1 and inhibited CYP2D6 and CYP1A2 only at concentrations well above those achieved clinically.

Approximately 14–34% of a radiolabelled dose of efavirenz was recovered in the urine and less than 1% of the dose was excreted in urine as unchanged efavirenz.

DOSE IN RENAL IMPAIRMENT GFR (mL/MIN)

20–50	Dose as in normal renal function.
10–20	Dose as in normal renal function.
<10	Dose as in normal renal function.

DOSE IN PATIENTS UNDERGOING RENAL REPLACEMENT THERAPIES

CAPD	Not dialysed. Dose as in normal renal function.
HD	Not dialysed. Dose as in normal renal function.
HDF/High flux	Not dialysed. Dose as in normal renal function.
CAV/ VVHD	Not dialysed. Dose as in normal renal function.

IMPORTANT DRUG INTERACTIONS

Potentially hazardous interactions with other drugs
- Antibacterials: concentration of rifabutin reduced.
- Anticoagulants: possibly affects concentration of coumarins.
- Antidepressants: concentration reduced by St John's wort – avoid concomitant use.
- Antifungals: itraconazole, posaconazole and voriconazole concentration reduced; voriconazole increases efavirenz concentration – reduce dose of efavirenz by 50% and increase dose of voriconazole to 400 mg twice daily; possibly reduces caspofungin concentration – may possibly need to increase caspofungin dose.
- Antipsychotics: possibly increased risk of ventricular arrhythmias with pimozide – avoid concomitant use; possibly reduces aripiprazole concentration – increase aripiprazole dose.
- Antivirals: concentration of atazanavir and boceprevir reduced – avoid; saquinavir concentration significantly reduced; concentration of darunavir, indinavir, lopinavir, telaprevir and possibly etravirine and maraviroc reduced – adjust darunavir, lopinavir, maraviroc and telaprevir dose, avoid with etravirine; concentration reduced by nevirapine; monitor LFTs when used in combination with ritonavir.
- Anxiolytics and hypnotics: risk of prolonged sedation with midazolam – avoid concomitant use.
- Atovaquone: concentration of atovaquone reduced – avoid.
- Ciclosporin: concentration of ciclosporin possibly reduced.
- Ergot alkaloids: risk of ergotism – avoid concomitant use.
- Grapefruit juice: concentration possibly increased.

- Progestogens: possibly reduced contraceptive effect.
- Tacrolimus: possibly affects tacrolimus concentration.

ADMINISTRATION

RECONSTITUTION
–
ROUTE
- Oral
RATE OF ADMINISTRATION
–
COMMENTS
–

OTHER INFORMATION

- Induces its own metabolism.
- Monitor cholesterol levels as increases of 10–20% in total cholesterol have been reported.
- Half-life of 10 hours in haemodialysis patients has been reported.
- Bioavailability of oral solution is less than that for capsules or tablets – therefore not interchangeable.

Eletriptan

CLINICAL USE

5HT$_1$ receptor agonist:
- Acute relief of migraine

DOSE IN NORMAL RENAL FUNCTION

40–80 mg repeated after 2 hours if migraine recurs (do not take 2nd dose for the same attack).
Maximum 80 mg in 24 hours.

PHARMACOKINETICS

Molecular weight (daltons)	463.4 (as hydrobromide)
% Protein binding	85
% Excreted unchanged in urine	9
Volume of distribution (L/kg)	2–2.5
Half-life – normal/ ESRF (hrs)	4/Unchanged

METABOLISM

In vitro studies indicate that eletriptan is primarily metabolised by hepatic cytochrome P-450 enzyme CYP3A4. This finding is substantiated by increased plasma concentrations of eletriptan following co-administration with erythromycin and ketoconazole, known selective and potent CYP3A4 inhibitors. *In vitro* studies also indicate a small involvement of CYP2D6 although clinical studies do not indicate any evidence of polymorphism with this enzyme.
There are two major circulating metabolites identified that significantly contribute to plasma radioactivity following administration of ^{14}C-labelled eletriptan. The metabolite formed by N-oxidation has demonstrated no activity in animal *in vitro* models. The metabolite formed by N-demethylation has been demonstrated to have similar activity to eletriptan in animal *in vitro* models. A third area of radioactivity in plasma has not been formally identified, but is most likely to be a mixture of hydroxylated metabolites which have also been observed excreted in urine and faeces.
The plasma concentrations of the N-demethylated active metabolite are only 10–20% of those of the parent, so would not be expected to significantly contribute to the therapeutic action of eletriptan. Non-renal clearance accounts for approximately 90% of the total clearance indicating that eletriptan is eliminated primarily by metabolism.

DOSE IN RENAL IMPAIRMENT GFR (mL/MIN)

30–50	20 mg; maximum daily dose 40 mg.
10–30	20 mg; maximum daily dose 40 mg, use with caution.
<10	20 mg; maximum daily dose 40 mg, use with caution.

DOSE IN PATIENTS UNDERGOING RENAL REPLACEMENT THERAPIES

CAPD	Unknown dialysability. Dose as in GFR<10 mL/min.
HD	Unknown dialysability. Dose as in GFR<10 mL/min.
HDF/High flux	Unknown dialysability. Dose as in GFR<10 mL/min.
CAV/VVHD	Unknown dialysability. Dose as in GFR=10–30 mL/min.

IMPORTANT DRUG INTERACTIONS

Potentially hazardous interactions with other drugs
- Antibacterials: concentration increased by clarithromycin and erythromycin – avoid concomitant use.
- Antidepressants: increased risk of CNS toxicity with citalopram – avoid; possibly increased serotonergic effects with duloxetine and venlafaxine; increased serotonergic effects with St John's wort – avoid concomitant use.
- Antifungals: concentration increased by itraconazole and ketoconazole – avoid concomitant use.
- Antivirals: concentration increased by indinavir and ritonavir – avoid concomitant use.
- Ergot alkaloids: increased risk of vasospasm – avoid.

ADMINISTRATION

RECONSTITUTION
–
ROUTE
- Oral
RATE OF ADMINISTRATION
–
COMMENTS
–

OTHER INFORMATION

- Manufacturer in UK SPC advises to avoid in severe renal impairment due to enhanced hypertensive effect but no contraindication in US data sheet.
- Contraindicated in uncontrolled hypertension.

Eltrombopag

CLINICAL USE

Thrombopoetin receptor agonist:
- Treatment of chronic immune idiopathic thrombocytopenic purpura (ITP)
- Chronic hepatitis C associated thrombocytopenia (HCV)

DOSE IN NORMAL RENAL FUNCTION

ITP: 25–75 mg daily
HCV: 25–100 mg daily

PHARMACOKINETICS

Molecular weight (daltons)	442.5 (564.6 as olamine)
% Protein binding	>99.9
% Excreted unchanged in urine	0 (31% as metabolites)
Volume of distribution (L/kg)	8.72 litres[1]
Half-life – normal/ ESRF (hrs)	21–32/–

METABOLISM

Mainly hepatically metabolised through cleavage, oxidation by cytochrome P450 isoenzymes CYP1A2 and CYP 2C8 and conjugation with glucuronic acid, glutathione, or cysteine.

Approximately 31% of a dose is eliminated in the urine as metabolites, and about 59% in the faeces (20% unchanged).

DOSE IN RENAL IMPAIRMENT GFR (mL/MIN)

20–50	Dose as in normal renal function.
10–20	Dose as in normal renal function.
<10	Dose as in normal renal function. Use with caution.

DOSE IN PATIENTS UNDERGOING RENAL REPLACEMENT THERAPIES

CAPD	Not dialysed. Dose as in GFR<10 mL/min.
HD	Not dialysed. Dose as in GFR<10 mL/min.
HDF/High flux	Not dialysed. Dose as in GFR<10 mL/min.
CAV/ VVHD	Not dialysed. Dose as in normal renal function.

IMPORTANT DRUG INTERACTIONS

Potentially hazardous interactions with other drugs
- Statins: increased rosuvastatin concentration, may need to reduce rosuvastatin dose.

ADMINISTRATION

RECONSTITUTION
–
ROUTE
- Oral
RATE OF ADMINISTRATION
–

COMMENTS
- Take at least 4 hours before or after antacids, dairy products (or other calcium containing food products), or mineral supplements containing polyvalent cations (e.g. iron, calcium, magnesium, aluminium, selenium and zinc).

OTHER INFORMATION

- Patients with impaired renal function should use eltrombopag with caution and close monitoring, for example by measuring creatinine and/or urine analysis.
- LFTs should be measured before treatment and then every 2 weeks while the dose is adjusted; once the dose is established, monthly monitoring is recommended. Tests should be repeated within 3 to 5 days if found to be abnormal, liver function should be monitored every week. If alanine aminotransferase levels increase to 3 times the upper limit of normal or above, and these are progressive or persist for 4 weeks or longer or are accompanied by increased bilirubin or by signs of hepatic injury or decompensation, eltrombopag should be stopped.
- The most common serious adverse effect of eltrombopag is haemorrhage.
- Following administration of a single 50 mg-dose, the $AUC_{0-\infty}$ of eltrombopag was 32–36% lower in patients with mild to moderate renal impairment, and 60% lower in severe renal impairment compared with healthy volunteers.
- Plasma-eltrombopag exposure is about 70% higher in some patients of East Asian origin (e.g. Japanese, Chinese, Taiwanese, and Korean), compared with Caucasian patients so a lower starting dose is recommended.

Reference:
1. Page 18 (2009) Abstr 1494 [www.page-meeting.org/?abstract=1494] – poster presentation, Abstracts of the Annual Meeting of the Population Approach Group in Europe.

Emtricitabine

CLINICAL USE

Nucleoside reverse transcriptase inhibitor:
- Treatment of HIV-1 in combination with other antiretroviral agents

DOSE IN NORMAL RENAL FUNCTION

200 mg once daily (if weight >33 kg)
Oral solution: 240 mg once daily, (6 mg/kg if weight <33 kg)

PHARMACOKINETICS

Molecular weight (daltons)	247.2
% Protein binding	<4
% Excreted unchanged in urine	86
Volume of distribution (L/kg)	1.1–1.7
Half-life – normal/ESRF (hrs)	10/Increased

METABOLISM

There is limited metabolism of emtricitabine. The biotransformation of emtricitabine includes oxidation of the thiol moiety to form the 3'-sulphoxide diastereomers (approximately 9% of dose) and conjugation with glucuronic acid to form 2'-O-glucuronide (approximately 4% of dose). Emtricitabine is primarily excreted by the kidneys with complete recovery of the dose achieved in urine (approximately 86%) and faeces (approximately 14%). Thirteen per cent of the emtricitabine dose was recovered in urine as three metabolites.

Pharmacokinetic parameters were determined following administration of a single dose of 200 mg emtricitabine hard capsules to 30 non-HIV infected subjects with varying degrees of renal insufficiency. Subjects were grouped according to baseline creatinine clearance (>80 mL/min as normal function; 50–80 mL/min as mild impairment; 30–49 mL/min as moderate impairment; <30 mL/min as severe impairment; <15 mL/min as functionally anephric requiring haemodialysis). The systemic emtricitabine exposure (mean ± standard deviation) increased from 11.8±2.9 μg·h/mL in subjects with normal renal function to 19.9±1.1, 25±5.7 and 34±2.1 μg·h/mL, in patients with mild, moderate and severe renal impairment, respectively.

DOSE IN RENAL IMPAIRMENT GFR (mL/MIN)

30–50	Tablets: 200 mg every 48 hours; Oral solution: 120 mg daily.
15–30	Tablets: 200 mg every 72 hours; Oral solution: 80 mg daily.
<15	Tablets: 200 mg every 96 hours; Oral Solution: 60 mg daily

DOSE IN PATIENTS UNDERGOING RENAL REPLACEMENT THERAPIES

CAPD	Unknown dialysability. Dose as in GFR<15 mL/min.
HD	Dialysed. Dose as in GFR<15 mL/min.
HDF/High flux	Dialysed. Dose as in GFR<15 mL/min.
CAV/VVHD	Dialysed. Dose as in GFR=15–30 mL/min.

IMPORTANT DRUG INTERACTIONS

Potentially hazardous interactions with other drugs
- Antivirals: avoid concomitant use with lamivudine.

ADMINISTRATION

RECONSTITUTION
–
ROUTE
- Oral
RATE OF ADMINISTRATION
–
COMMENTS
–

OTHER INFORMATION

- Haemodialysis should be started at least 12 hours after the last dose of emtricitabine.
- In patients with ESRD on haemodialysis, approximately 30% of the emtricitabine dose was recovered in dialysate over a 3 hour dialysis period which had been started within 1.5 hours of emtricitabine dosing (blood flow rate of 400 mL/min and dialysate flow rate of approximately 600 mL/min).
- 200 mg of the hard capsules is equivalent to 240 mg of the oral solution.
- Dose may be reduced instead of increasing dosage interval.
- Up to 30% of dose is removed by a 3 hour haemodialysis session.

Enalapril maleate

CLINICAL USE

Angiotensin converting enzyme inhibitor:
- Hypertension
- Heart failure

DOSE IN NORMAL RENAL FUNCTION

2.5–40 mg daily

PHARMACOKINETICS

Molecular weight (daltons)	492.5
% Protein binding	50–60
% Excreted unchanged in urine	20
Volume of distribution (L/kg)	0.17[1]
Half-life – normal/ ESRF (hrs)	11/34–60

METABOLISM

Following absorption, oral enalapril is rapidly and extensively hydrolysed to enalaprilat, a potent angiotensin converting enzyme inhibitor. Peak serum concentrations of enalaprilat occur about 4 hours after an oral dose of enalapril tablet, and the effective half-life is 11 hours.

Excretion of enalaprilat is primarily renal. The principal components in urine are enalaprilat, accounting for about 40% of the dose, and intact enalapril (about 20%).

DOSE IN RENAL IMPAIRMENT GFR (mL/MIN)

20–50	Dose as in normal renal function.
10–20	Start with 2.5 mg per day and increase according to response.
<10	Start with 2.5 mg per day and increase according to response.

DOSE IN PATIENTS UNDERGOING RENAL REPLACEMENT THERAPIES

CAPD	Dialysed. Dose as in GFR<10 mL/ min.
HD	Dialysed. Dose as in GFR<10 mL/ min.
HDF/High flux	Dialysed. Dose as in GFR<10 mL/ min.
CAV/ VVHD	Dialysed. Dose as in GFR=10– 20 mL/min.

IMPORTANT DRUG INTERACTIONS

Potentially hazardous interactions with other drugs
- Anaesthetics: enhanced hypotensive effect.
- Analgesics: antagonism of hypotensive effect and increased risk of renal impairment with NSAIDs; hyperkalaemia with ketorolac and other NSAIDs.
- Ciclosporin: increased risk of hyperkalaemia and nephrotoxicity.
- Diuretics: enhanced hypotensive effect; hyperkalaemia with potassium-sparing diuretics.
- ESAs: increased risk of hyperkalaemia; antagonism of hypotensive effect.
- Gold: flushing and hypotension with sodium aurothiomalate.
- Lithium: reduced excretion, possibility of enhanced lithium toxicity.
- Potassium salts: increased risk of hyperkalaemia.
- Tacrolimus: increased risk of hyperkalaemia and nephrotoxicity.

ADMINISTRATION

RECONSTITUTION
–
ROUTE
- Oral
RATE OF ADMINISTRATION
–
COMMENTS
–

OTHER INFORMATION

- Side effects (e.g. hyperkalaemia, metabolic acidosis) are more common in patients with impaired renal function.
- Close monitoring of renal function during therapy is necessary in those with renal insufficiency.
- Renal failure has been reported in association with ACE inhibitors in patients with renal artery stenosis, post renal transplant, and in those with severe congestive heart failure.
- High incidence of anaphylactoid reactions has been reported in patients dialysed with high-flux polyacrylonitrile membranes and treated concomitantly with an ACE inhibitor – this combination should therefore be avoided.
- ACE inhibitor cough may be helped by sodium cromoglycate inhalers.
- Enalaprilat injection available on a named patient basis.

Reference:
1. Oberg KC, Just VL, Bauman JL, *et al.*
Reduced bioavailability of enalapril in
patients with severe heart failure. *J Am Coll
Cardiol.* 1994 Feb; **23**(special issue): 381 A.

Enfuvirtide

CLINICAL USE

Treatment of HIV-1 in combination with other antiretroviral agents

DOSE IN NORMAL RENAL FUNCTION

90 mg twice daily

PHARMACOKINETICS

Molecular weight (daltons)	4491.9
% Protein binding	92
% Excreted unchanged in urine	No data
Volume of distribution (L/kg)	4.4–6.6 litres
Half-life – normal/ ESRF (hrs)	3.2–4.4/Probably unchanged

METABOLISM

As a peptide, enfuvirtide is expected to undergo catabolism to its constituent amino acids, with subsequent recycling of the amino acids in the body pool. *In vitro* human microsomal studies and *in vivo* studies indicate that enfuvirtide is not an inhibitor of CYP450 enzymes. In *in vitro* human microsomal and hepatocyte studies, hydrolysis of the amide group of the C-terminus amino acid, phenylalanine, results in a deamidated metabolite. Mass balance studies to determine elimination pathway(s) of enfuvirtide have not been performed in humans.

DOSE IN RENAL IMPAIRMENT GFR (mL/MIN)

35–50	Dose as in normal renal function.
10–35	Dose as in normal renal function.[1]
<10	Dose as in normal renal function.[1]

DOSE IN PATIENTS UNDERGOING RENAL REPLACEMENT THERAPIES

CAPD	Unlikely to be dialysed. Dose as in GFR<10 mL/min.
HD	13% dialysed.[1] Dose as in GFR<10 mL/min.
HDF/High flux	Unlikely to be dialysed. Dose as in GFR<10 mL/min.
CAV/ VVHD	Unlikely to be dialysed. Dose as in GFR=10–35 mL/min.

IMPORTANT DRUG INTERACTIONS

Potentially hazardous interactions with other drugs
- None known

ADMINISTRATION

RECONSTITUTION
- 1.1 mL water for injection

ROUTE
- SC

RATE OF ADMINISTRATION

–

COMMENTS
- Do not shake vial or turn it upside down as this causes foaming.
- The powder may take up to 45 minutes to dissolve.
- Use within 24 hours if kept in refrigerator. Allow to reach room temperature before injecting.

OTHER INFORMATION

- Renal calculi have been reported with enfuvirtide therapy.
- C_{max} and AUC are increased in CKD 5 patients.[2]

References:
1. Tebas P, Bellos N, Lucasti C, *et al.* Enfuvirtide does not require dose-adjustment in patients with chronic renal failure: the results of a pharmacokinetic study of enfuvirtide in HIV-1 infected patients with impaired renal function. *14th Conference on Retroviruses and Opportunistic Infections*; 2007 Feb 25–28; Los Angeles.
2. www.centerwatch.com/patient/trialresults/stur11.html

Enoxaparin sodium (LMWH)

CLINICAL USE

- Prophylaxis of thromboembolic disorders of venous origin
- Treatment of deep vein thrombosis and pulmonary embolism
- Anticoagulation of the extracorporeal circulation during haemodialysis
- Acute coronary syndrome

DOSE IN NORMAL RENAL FUNCTION

- Prophylaxis DVT:
  — Moderate risk surgery: 20 mg once daily
  — High risk surgery/medical prophylaxis: 40 mg once daily
- Treatment DVT and PE: 1.5 mg/kg every 24 hours.
- Anticoagulation of extracorporeal circuits – see 'Other information'.
- Acute coronary syndrome: 1 mg/kg every 12 hours

PHARMACOKINETICS

Molecular weight (daltons)	Mean = 4500
% Protein binding	No data
% Excreted unchanged in urine	10
Volume of distribution (L/kg)	5 litres
Half-life – normal/ ESRF (hrs)	4–5/Increased

METABOLISM

A linear relationship between anti-Xa plasma clearance and creatinine clearance at steady-state has been observed, which indicates decreased clearance of enoxaparin sodium in patients with reduced renal function.
In patients with severe renal impairment (creatinine clearance <30 mL/min), the AUC at steady state is significantly increased by an average of 65% after repeated, once daily subcutaneous doses of 40 mg.
   Hepatic metabolism by desulphation and depolymerisation also contributes to elimination.

DOSE IN RENAL IMPAIRMENT GFR (mL/MIN)

50–80	Dose as in normal renal function.
30–50	Dose as in normal renal function. Monitor carefully.
<30	Treatment: 1 mg/kg daily. Initial stat dose of 30 mg for patients who have had a STEMI & are <75 years. Prophylaxis: 20 mg daily. See 'Other information'.

DOSE IN PATIENTS UNDERGOING RENAL REPLACEMENT THERAPIES

CAPD	Not dialysed. Dose as in GFR<30 mL/min.
HD	Not dialysed. Dose as in GFR<30 mL/min.
HDF/High flux	Dialysed. Dose as in GFR<30 mL/min.
CAV/ VVHD	Not dialysed. Dose as in GFR=30–50 mL/min

IMPORTANT DRUG INTERACTIONS

Potentially hazardous interactions with other drugs

- Analgesics: increased risk of bleeding with NSAIDs – avoid concomitant use with IV diclofenac; increased risk of haemorrhage with ketorolac – avoid concomitant use.
- Nitrates: anticoagulant effect reduced by infusions of glyceryl trinitrate.
- Use with care in patients receiving oral anticoagulants, platelet aggregation inhibitors, aspirin or dextran.

ADMINISTRATION

RECONSTITUTION
–
ROUTE
- SC
RATE OF ADMINISTRATION
–
COMMENTS
–

OTHER INFORMATION

- In extracorporeal circulation during haemodialysis, 1 mg/kg enoxaparin is introduced into the arterial line of the circuit at the beginning of the session. The effect of this dose is usually sufficient for a 4 hour session. If fibrin rings are found, a further dose of 0.5–1 mg/kg may be given.
- For patients with a high risk of haemorrhage, the dose should be reduced

to 0.5 mg/kg for double vascular access or 0.75 mg/kg for single vascular access.

- The dose of protamine to neutralise the effect of enoxaparin should equal the dose of enoxaparin: 50 anti-heparin units of protamine should neutralise the anti-factor-Xa activity generated by 1 mg of enoxaparin. If prothrombin time is still raised 2–4 hours later give 0.5 mg/kg infusion of protamine. (Hovanessian H. Letter. *Ann Emerg Med.* 2006; **36**(3): 278.)

- Manufacturer advises monitoring of the anti-factor-Xa activity, whatever the severity of the renal impairment, when treatment doses are being employed. They also advise monitoring patients if given prolonged treatment with prophylactic doses.

- Low molecular weight heparins are renally excreted and hence accumulate in severe renal impairment. While the doses recommended for prophylaxis against DVT and prevention of thrombus formation in extracorporeal circuits are well tolerated in patients with ESRF, the doses recommended for treatment of DVT and PE have been associated with severe, sometimes fatal, bleeding episodes in such patients. Hence the use of unfractionated heparin would be preferable in these instances.

- Additional doses may be required if using LMWHs for anticoagulation in HDF.

Entacapone

CLINICAL USE

Catechol-O-methyltransferase inhibitor:
- Treatment of Parkinson's disease

DOSE IN NORMAL RENAL FUNCTION

200 mg with each dose of levodopa with dopadecarboxylase inhibitor
Max 2 g daily

PHARMACOKINETICS

Molecular weight (daltons)	305.3
% Protein binding	98 (mainly albumin)
% Excreted unchanged in urine	Traces (10–20% as unchanged drug and metabolites)
Volume of distribution (L/kg)	20 litres
Half-life – normal/ ESRF (hrs)	1–6-3.4/Unchanged

METABOLISM

Entacapone undergoes extensive first-pass metabolism to form glucuronide metabolites.
   It is eliminated mainly in the faeces with about 10–20% being excreted in the urine, mainly as glucuronide conjugates.

DOSE IN RENAL IMPAIRMENT GFR (mL/MIN)

20–50	Dose as in normal renal function.
10–20	Dose as in normal renal function.
<10	Dose as in normal renal function.

DOSE IN PATIENTS UNDERGOING RENAL REPLACEMENT THERAPIES

CAPD	Unlikely to be dialysed. Dose as in normal renal function.
HD	Unlikely to be dialysed. Dose as in normal renal function.
HDF/High flux	Unlikely to be dialysed. Dose as in normal renal function.
CAV/ VVHD	Unlikely to be dialysed. Dose as in normal renal function.

IMPORTANT DRUG INTERACTIONS

Potentially hazardous interactions with other drugs
- Anticoagulants: enhances anticoagulant effect of warfarin.
- Antidepressants: use with caution in combination with moclobemide, tricyclics and venlafaxine; avoid with MAOIs.
- Dopaminergics: possibly enhances effects of apomorphine; possibly reduces concentration of rasagiline; max dose of selegiline is 10 mg in combination.

ADMINISTRATION

ROUTE
- Oral
RATE OF ADMINISTRATION
–

OTHER INFORMATION

- Manufacturer suggests that a longer dosing interval may be required in dialysis patients.
- Bioavailability is 35%.

Entecavir

CLINICAL USE

Treatment of chronic hepatitis B infection

DOSE IN NORMAL RENAL FUNCTION

500 mcg daily; 1000 mcg daily in lamivudine-refractory patients.

PHARMACOKINETICS

Molecular weight (daltons)	295.3
% Protein binding	13
% Excreted unchanged in urine	75
Volume of distribution (L/kg)	Large
Half-life – normal/ ESRF (hrs)	128–149/–

METABOLISM

Entecavir is not a substrate, inhibitor or inducer of the CYP450 enzyme system. Following administration of ^{14}C-entecavir, no oxidative or acetylated metabolites and minor amounts of the phase II metabolites, glucuronide and sulfate conjugates, were observed.

Entecavir is predominantly eliminated by the kidney: renal clearance is independent of dose and ranges between 360 mL/min and 471 mL/min suggesting that entecavir undergoes both glomerular filtration and net tubular secretion.

DOSE IN RENAL IMPAIRMENT GFR (mL/MIN)

30–50	250 mcg daily or 500 mcg every 48 hours; 500 mcg daily in lamivudine-refractory patients.
10–30	150 mcg daily or 500 mcg every 72 hours; 300 mcg daily or 500 mcg every 48 hours in lamivudine-refractory patients.
<10	50 mcg daily or 500 mcg every 5–7 days; 100 mcg daily or 500 mcg every 72 hours in lamivudine-refractory patients.

DOSE IN PATIENTS UNDERGOING RENAL REPLACEMENT THERAPIES

CAPD	0.3% dialysed. Dose as in GFR<10 mL/min.
HD	13% dialysed. Dose as in GFR<10 mL/min.
HDF/High flux	Dialysed. Dose as in GFR<10 mL/min.
CAV/VVHD	Likely to be dialysed. Dose as in GFR=10–30 mL/min.

IMPORTANT DRUG INTERACTIONS

Potentially hazardous interactions with other drugs
• None known

ADMINISTRATION

RECONSTITUTION
–
ROUTE
• Oral
RATE OF ADMINISTRATION
–
COMMENTS
–

OTHER INFORMATION

Entecavir clearance decreases with decreasing creatinine clearance. A 4 hour period of haemodialysis removed ≈13% of the dose, and 0.3% was removed by CAPD.

Epirubicin hydrochloride

CLINICAL USE

Antineoplastic agent:
- Leukaemias
- Malignant lymphomas
- Multiple myeloma
- Various solid tumours

DOSE IN NORMAL RENAL FUNCTION

- 60–90 mg/m^2 every 3 weeks.
- High dose: 60–135 mg/m^2 every 3–4 weeks, or 45 mg/m^2 on days 1, 2, and 3, every 3 weeks.
- Dose and frequency depend on condition and whether monotherapy or combination therapy
- Or according to local protocol.

PHARMACOKINETICS

Molecular weight (daltons)	580
% Protein binding	77
% Excreted unchanged in urine	9–10
Volume of distribution (L/kg)	14–38
Half-life – normal/ ESRF (hrs)	30–40/Unchanged

METABOLISM

Epirubicin is extensively and rapidly metabolised in the liver; 27–40% eliminated by biliary excretion. Slow elimination through the liver is due to extensive tissue distribution. Also is metabolised in other organs and cells, including red blood cells. Four main metabolic pathways have been identified. Only the metabolite epirubicinol (13-OH epirubicin) appears to have cytotoxic activity; however, epirubicinol is unlikely to reach *in vivo* concentrations sufficient to produce cytotoxic effects. Epirubicin and its major metabolites are eliminated in faeces via biliary excretion (40% of the administered dose being recovered in the bile in 72 hours) and to a lesser extent in urine (10% of a dose in 48 hours).

DOSE IN RENAL IMPAIRMENT GFR (mL/MIN)

20–50	Dose as in normal renal function.
10–20	Dose as in normal renal function.
<10	Dose as in normal renal function, but use lower dose.

DOSE IN PATIENTS UNDERGOING RENAL REPLACEMENT THERAPIES

CAPD	Unlikely to be dialysed. Dose as in GFR<10 mL/min.
HD	Unlikely to be dialysed. Dose as in GFR<10 mL/min.
HDF/High flux	Unknown dialysability. Dose as in GFR<10 mL/min
CAV/ VVHD	Unknown dialysability. Dose as in GFR<10 mL/min.

IMPORTANT DRUG INTERACTIONS

Potentially hazardous interactions with other drugs
- Antipsychotics: avoid concomitant use with clozapine – increased risk of agranulocytosis.
- Ciclosporin: increased risk of neurotoxicity.
- Ulcer-healing drugs: concentration increased by cimetidine.

ADMINISTRATION

RECONSTITUTION
- Reconstitute with water for injection or sodium chloride 0.9% (rapid dissolution only)

ROUTE
- IV, intravesical (bladder instillation), intrathecal

RATE OF ADMINISTRATION
- IV: give via the tubing of a fast running intravenous infusion of sodium chloride 0.9% or glucose 5%, taking 3–5 minutes over the injection.
- IV infusion: 30 minutes

COMMENTS
- For bladder instillation: concentration of epirubicin in bladder should be 50–80 mg per 50 mL once a week.
- To avoid undue dilution in urine, the patient should be instructed not to drink any fluid in the 12 hours prior to instillation.
- In the case of local toxicity dose is reduced to 30 mg per 50 mL.

OTHER INFORMATION

- A cumulative dose of 900–1000 mg/m^2 should only be exceeded with extreme caution. Above this level, the risk of irreversible congestive cardiac failure increases greatly.
- Patients with impaired hepatic function have prolonged and elevated plasma concentrations of epirubicin – dose reduction is required.
- Epirubicin may make the urine red for 1–2 days after administration.

Eplerenone

CLINICAL USE

Aldosterone antagonist:
- Left ventricular dysfunction and heart failure

DOSE IN NORMAL RENAL FUNCTION

25–50 mg daily

PHARMACOKINETICS

Molecular weight (daltons)	414.5
% Protein binding	50
% Excreted unchanged in urine	<5
Volume of distribution (L/kg)	43–57 litres
Half-life – normal/ ESRF (hrs)	3–6/–

METABOLISM

Eplerenone metabolism is primarily mediated via CYP3A4. No active metabolites of eplerenone have been identified in human plasma. Less than 5% of an eplerenone dose is recovered as unchanged drug in the urine and faeces. Following a single oral dose of radiolabelled drug, approximately 32% of the dose was excreted in the faeces and approximately 67% was excreted in the urine.

DOSE IN RENAL IMPAIRMENT GFR (mL/MIN)

20–50	Dose as in normal renal function.[1]
10–20	Dose as in normal renal function.[1]
<10	Dose as in normal renal function.[1]

DOSE IN PATIENTS UNDERGOING RENAL REPLACEMENT THERAPIES

CAPD	Unknown dialysability. Dose as in GFR<10 mL/min.
HD	10% dialysed.[1] Dose as in GFR<10 mL/min.
HDF/High flux	Unknown dialysability. Dose as in GFR<10 mL/min.
CAV/ VVHD	Unknown dialysability. Dose as in GFR=10–20 mL/min.

IMPORTANT DRUG INTERACTIONS

Potentially hazardous interactions with other drugs
- ACE inhibitors or AT-II antagonists: enhanced hypotensive effect; risk of severe hyperkalaemia.
- Anti-arrhythmics: concentration increased by amiodarone – reduce eplerenone dose.
- Antibacterials: concentration increased by clarithromycin and telithromycin – avoid concomitant use; concentration increased by erythromycin – reduce eplerenone dose; concentration reduced by rifampicin – avoid concomitant use; avoid concomitant use with lymecycline; increased risk of hyperkalaemia with trimethoprim.
- Antidepressants: concentration reduced by St John's wort – avoid concomitant use; increased risk of postural hypotension with tricyclics; enhanced hypotensive effect with MAOIs.
- Anti-epileptics: concentration reduced by carbamazepine, phenytoin and phenobarbital – avoid concomitant use.
- Antifungals: concentration increased by itraconazole and ketoconazole – avoid concomitant use; concentration increased by fluconazole – reduce eplerenone dose.
- Antihypertensives: enhanced hypotensive effect, increased risk of first dose hypotensive effect with post-synaptic alpha-blockers.
- Antivirals: concentration increased by ritonavir – avoid concomitant use; concentration increased by saquinavir – reduce eplerenone dose.
- Ciclosporin: increased risk of hyperkalaemia and nephrotoxicity.
- Cytotoxics: increased risk of nephrotoxicity and ototoxicity with platinum compounds.
- NSAIDs: increased risk of hyperkalaemia (especially with indomethacin); increased risk of nephrotoxicity; antagonism of diuretic effect.
- Potassium salts: increased risk of hyperkalaemia.
- Lithium: reduced lithium excretion – avoid concomitant use.
- Tacrolimus: increased risk of hyperkalaemia and nephrotoxicity.
- CYP3A4 inhibitors: Do not exceed a dose of 25 mg daily for eplerenone.
- CYP3A4 inducers: reduced eplerenone concentration – avoid concomitant use.

ADMINISTRATION

RECONSTITUTION

–

ROUTE

• Oral

RATE OF ADMINISTRATION

–

COMMENTS

–

OTHER INFORMATION

• Monitor potassium levels regularly in people with renal impairment.
• Contraindicated by manufacturer due to risk of hyperkalaemia in severe renal impairment.

• From personal experience can be used safely in severe renal impairment with close monitoring.

Reference:

1. Ravis WR, Reid S, Sica DA, *et al.* Pharmacokinetics of eplerenone after single and multiple dosing in subjects with and without renal impairment. *J Clin Pharmacol.* 2005; **45**: 810–21.

Epoetin alfa (Eprex)

CLINICAL USE

- Anaemia associated with renal impairment in pre-dialysis and dialysis patients, and in patients receiving cancer chemotherapy
- Increased yield of autologous blood

DOSE IN NORMAL RENAL FUNCTION

- Renal:
  - CORRECTION PHASE: (To raise haemoglobin to target level) 50 u/kg 2–3 times weekly; increase, according to response, by 25 u/kg 3 times weekly at intervals of 4 weeks. Rise in haemoglobin should not exceed 2 g/100 mL/month (optimum rise in haemoglobin up to 1 g/100 mL/month to avoid hypertension). Target haemoglobin usually 10–12 g/100 mL.
  - MAINTENANCE PHASE: Adjust dose to maintain required haemoglobin level; usual dose needed is 75–300 u/kg weekly in 1–3 divided doses.
- Cancer: Initially 150 u/kg 3 times a week and adjust according to response.
- Autologous blood harvest: 600 u/kg IV once or twice a week for 3 weeks prior to surgery.

PHARMACOKINETICS

Molecular weight (daltons)	30 400
% Protein binding	No data
% Excreted unchanged in urine	No data
Volume of distribution (L/kg)	0.03–0.05
Half-life – normal/ESRF (hrs)	IV: 4/5 SC: ≅24/Unchanged

METABOLISM

The metabolic fate of both endogenous and recombinant erythropoietin is poorly understood. Current evidence from studies in animals suggests that hepatic metabolism contributes only minimally to elimination of the *intact* hormone, but desialylated epoetin (i.e. terminal sialic acid groups removed) appears to undergo substantial hepatic clearance via metabolic pathways and/or binding. Desialylation and/or removal of the oligosaccharide side chains of erythropoietin appear to occur principally in the liver; bone marrow also may have a role in catabolism of the hormone. Elimination of desialylated drug by the kidneys, bone marrow, and spleen also may occur; results of animal studies suggest that proximal renal tubular secretion may be involved in renal elimination.

DOSE IN RENAL IMPAIRMENT GFR (mL/MIN)

20–50	Dose as in normal renal function.
10–20	Dose as in normal renal function.
<10	Dose as in normal renal function.

DOSE IN PATIENTS UNDERGOING RENAL REPLACEMENT THERAPIES

CAPD	Not dialysed. Dose as in normal renal function.
HD	Not dialysed. Dose as in normal renal function.
HDF/High flux	Not dialysed. Dose as in normal renal function.
CAV/ VVHD	Not dialysed. Dose as in normal renal function.

IMPORTANT DRUG INTERACTIONS

Potentially hazardous interactions with other drugs
- Hyperkalaemia with ACE inhibitors and angiotensin-II antagonists.

ADMINISTRATION

RECONSTITUTION
–
ROUTE
- IV/SC (maximum 1 mL per injection site)
RATE OF ADMINISTRATION
- 1–5 minutes
COMMENTS
- When given IV, higher doses normally needed to produce required response

OTHER INFORMATION

- Reported association of pure red cell aplasia (PRCA) with epoetin therapy. This is a very rare condition; due to failed production of red blood cell precursors in the bone marrow, resulting in profound anaemia. Possibly due to an immune response to the protein backbone of R-HuEPO. Resulting antibodies render the patient unresponsive to the therapeutic effects of all epoetins and darbepoetin.

- Pre-treatment checks and appropriate correction/treatment needed for iron, folate and B12 deficiency, infection, inflammation or aluminium toxicity, to produce optimum response to therapy.

- Concomitant iron therapy (200–300 mg elemental oral iron) needed daily. IV iron may be needed for patients with very low serum ferritin (<100 nanograms/mL).
- May increase heparin requirement during HD.

Epoetin beta (Neorecormon)

CLINICAL USE

Anaemia associated with renal impairment in pre-dialysis and dialysis patients, and in patients receiving cancer chemotherapy

DOSE IN NORMAL RENAL FUNCTION

- Renal:
  - CORRECTION PHASE: (To raise haemoglobin to target level) 60 u/kg SC or 40 u/kg IV 3 times weekly for 4 weeks; increase, according to response, in steps of 20 u/kg 3 times weekly at monthly intervals. Maximum dose 720 u/kg weekly. Target haemoglobin usually 10–12 g/100 mL.
  - MAINTENANCE DOSE: (To maintain haemoglobin at target level) Half correction phase dose, then adjust according to response at intervals of 1–2 weeks.
- Cancer: Initially 450 u/kg weekly in 3–7 divided doses and adjust according to response.

PHARMACOKINETICS

Molecular weight (daltons)	30 400
% Protein binding	No data
% Excreted unchanged in urine	No data
Volume of distribution (L/kg)	0.03–0.05
Half-life – normal/ ESRF (hrs)	IV: 4–12/Unchanged SC: 13–28/Unchanged

METABOLISM

The metabolic fate of both endogenous and recombinant erythropoietin is poorly understood. Current evidence from studies in animals suggests that hepatic metabolism contributes only minimally to elimination of the *intact* hormone, but desialylated epoetin (i.e. terminal sialic acid groups removed) appears to undergo substantial hepatic clearance via metabolic pathways and/or binding. Desialylation and/or removal of the oligosaccharide side chains of erythropoietin appear to occur principally in the liver; bone marrow also may have a role in catabolism of the hormone. Elimination of desialylated drug by the kidneys, bone marrow, and spleen also may occur; results of animal studies suggest that proximal renal tubular secretion may be involved in renal elimination.

DOSE IN RENAL IMPAIRMENT GFR (mL/MIN)

20–50	Dose as in normal renal function.
10–20	Dose as in normal renal function.
<10	Dose as in normal renal function.

DOSE IN PATIENTS UNDERGOING RENAL REPLACEMENT THERAPIES

CAPD	Not dialysed. Dose as in normal renal function.
HD	Not dialysed. Dose as in normal renal function.
HDF/High flux	Not dialysed. Dose as in normal renal function.
CAV/VVHD	Not dialysed. Dose as in normal renal function.

IMPORTANT DRUG INTERACTIONS

Potentially hazardous interactions with other drugs
- Risk of hyperkalaemia with ACE inhibitors and angiotensin-II antagonists.

ADMINISTRATION

RECONSTITUTION
- Reconstitute using diluent provided only for multidose vial and penfill cartridges.

ROUTE
- SC, IV

RATE OF ADMINISTRATION
- 2 minutes

COMMENTS
- May also be given IV, but higher doses are needed to produce required response.

OTHER INFORMATION

- Pre-treatment checks and appropriate correction/treatment needed for iron, folate and B12 deficiencies, infection, inflammation or aluminium toxicity to produce optimum response to therapy.
- Concomitant iron therapy (200–300 mg elemental oral iron) needed daily. IV iron may be needed for patients with very low serum ferritin (<100 nanograms/mL).
- May increase heparin requirement during HD.

- Reported association of pure red cell aplasia (PRCA) with epoetin therapy. This is a very rare condition; due to failed production of red blood cell precursors in the bone marrow, resulting in profound anaemia. Possibly due to an immune response to the protein backbone of R-HuEPO. Resulting antibodies render the patient unresponsive to the therapeutic effects of all epoetins and darbepoetin.

Epoprostenol (prostacyclin)

CLINICAL USE

- Vasodilation and inhibition of platelet aggregation without prolonging bleeding time
- Alternative to heparin in haemodialysis
- Treatment of peripheral vascular disease and pulmonary hypertension

DOSE IN NORMAL RENAL FUNCTION

- 2–50 ng/kg/minute, adjusted according to response.
- Dialysis anticoagulation: 4 ng/kg/minute starting 10–15 minutes before and continuing during dialysis via the arterial line, adjusted according to response (range: 0.5–12 ng/kg/minute).

PHARMACOKINETICS

Molecular weight (daltons)	352.5
% Protein binding	No data
% Excreted unchanged in urine	<5 (40–90 as drug + metabolites)
Volume of distribution (L/kg)	0.357–1.015
Half-life – normal/ ESRF (hrs)	2–6 minutes/–

METABOLISM

On intravenous infusion epoprostenol is hydrolysed rapidly to the more stable but much less active 6-keto-prostaglandin $F_{1\alpha}$ (6-oxo-prostaglandin $F_{1\alpha}$). A second metabolite, 6,15-diketo-13,14-dihydro-prostaglandin $F_{1\alpha}$, is formed by enzymatic degradation.

Following the administration of radiolabelled epoprostenol to humans, at least 16 metabolites were found, 10 of which were structurally identified.

Unlike many other prostaglandins, epoprostenol is not metabolised during passage through the pulmonary circulation. The urinary and faecal recoveries of radioactivity were 82% and 4%, respectively.

DOSE IN RENAL IMPAIRMENT GFR (mL/MIN)

20–50	Dose as in normal renal function.
10–20	Dose as in normal renal function.
<10	Dose as in normal renal function.

DOSE IN PATIENTS UNDERGOING RENAL REPLACEMENT THERAPIES

CAPD	Unknown dialysability. Dose as in normal renal function.
HD	Unknown dialysability. Dose as in normal renal function.
HDF/High flux	Unknown dialysability. Dose as in normal renal function.
CAV/ VVHD	Unknown dialysability. Dose as in normal renal function.

IMPORTANT DRUG INTERACTIONS

Potentially hazardous interactions with other drugs
- Increased hypotensive effect with 'acetate' dialysis

ADMINISTRATION

RECONSTITUTION
- 500 microgram vial with diluent provided gives solution of 10 micrograms/mL. Can be diluted further.

ROUTE
- IV or into blood supplying dialyser.

RATE OF ADMINISTRATION
- Via CRIP

COMMENTS
- Complicated dosing schedule – check calculations carefully.
- Infusion rate may be calculated by the following formula:

Dose rate (mL/hr) =

$$\frac{\text{Dosage (ng/kg/min)} \times \text{body wt (kg)} \times 60}{\text{Concentration of infusion (ng/mL)}}$$

(usually 10 000 ng/mL)

OTHER INFORMATION

- Monitor BP and heart rate. Reduce dose if patient becomes hypotensive. Cardiovascular effects cease 30 minutes after stopping the infusion.
- Some patients may exhibit allergic reaction to buffer solution used to reconstitute epoprostenol.
- Solution retains 90% potency for 12 hours after dilution.
- The concentrated solution should be filtered using the filter provided in the pack.

Eprosartan

CLINICAL USE

Angiotensin-II antagonist:
• Hypertension

DOSE IN NORMAL RENAL FUNCTION

300–800 mg daily

PHARMACOKINETICS

Molecular weight (daltons)	520.6 (as mesilate)
% Protein binding	98
% Excreted unchanged in urine	<2 (as metabolites)
Volume of distribution (L/kg)	13 litres
Half-life – normal/ ESRF (hrs)	5–9/Unchanged

METABOLISM

Following oral and intravenous dosing with [^{14}C] eprosartan in human subjects, eprosartan was the only drug-related compound found in the plasma and faeces. In the urine, approximately 20% of the radioactivity excreted was an acyl glucuronide of eprosartan with the remaining 80% being unchanged eprosartan. Eprosartan is eliminated by both biliary and renal excretion. Following intravenous [^{14}C] eprosartan, about 61% of radioactivity is recovered in the faeces and about 37% in the urine. Following an oral dose of [^{14}C] eprosartan, about 90% of radioactivity is recovered in the faeces and about 7% in the urine.

DOSE IN RENAL IMPAIRMENT GFR (mL/MIN)

20–50	Dose as in normal renal function.
10–20	Dose as in normal renal function.
<10	Dose as in normal renal function. Initially 300 mg daily and increase according to response.

DOSE IN PATIENTS UNDERGOING RENAL REPLACEMENT THERAPIES

CAPD	Unlikely to be dialysed. Dose as in normal renal function.
HD	Not dialysed. Dose as in normal renal function.
HDF/High flux	Not dialysed. Dose as in normal renal function.
CAV/ VVHD	Not dialysed. Dose as in normal renal function.

IMPORTANT DRUG INTERACTIONS

Potentially hazardous interactions with other drugs
• Anaesthetics: enhanced hypotensive effect.
• Analgesics: antagonism of hypotensive effect and increased risk of renal impairment with NSAIDs; hyperkalaemia with ketorolac and other NSAIDs.
• Ciclosporin: increased risk of hyperkalaemia and nephrotoxicity.
• Diuretics: enhanced hypotensive effect; hyperkalaemia with potassium-sparing diuretics.
• Epoetin: increased risk of hyperkalaemia; antagonism of hypotensive effect.
• Lithium: reduced excretion, possibility of enhanced lithium toxicity.
• Potassium salts: increased risk of hyperkalaemia.
• Tacrolimus: increased risk of hyperkalaemia and nephrotoxicity.

ADMINISTRATION

RECONSTITUTION
–
ROUTE
• Oral
RATE OF ADMINISTRATION
–
COMMENTS
–

OTHER INFORMATION

• Side effects (e.g. hyperkalaemia, metabolic acidosis) are more common in patients with impaired renal function.
• Close monitoring of renal function during therapy is necessary in those with renal insufficiency.
• Renal failure has been reported in association with AT-II antagonists in patients with renal artery stenosis, post renal transplant, and in those with severe congestive heart failure.

Eptifibatide

CLINICAL USE

Antiplatelet agent:
- Prevention of early myocardial infarction in patients with unstable angina or non-ST segment-elevation myocardial infarction and with last episode of chest pain within 24 hours

DOSE IN NORMAL RENAL FUNCTION

IV bolus of 180 mcg/kg then by IV infusion at a rate of 2 mcg/kg/minute for up to 72–96 hours.

PHARMACOKINETICS

Molecular weight (daltons)	832
% Protein binding	25
% Excreted unchanged in urine	50
Volume of distribution (L/kg)	0.185–0.26
Half-life – normal/ ESRF (hrs)	2.5/Increased

METABOLISM

Renal excretion accounts for approximately 50% of total body clearance of eptifibatide; approximately 50% of the amount cleared is excreted unchanged in the urine.

DOSE IN RENAL IMPAIRMENT GFR (mL/MIN)

30–50	Normal bolus dose. Reduce infusion to 1 mcg/kg/minute and use with caution due to limited experience.
10–30	Normal bolus dose. Reduce infusion to 1 mcg/kg/minute and use with caution due to limited experience.
<10	Normal bolus dose. Reduce infusion to 1 mcg/kg/minute and use with caution due to limited experience.

DOSE IN PATIENTS UNDERGOING RENAL REPLACEMENT THERAPIES

CAPD	Unknown dialysability. Dose as in GFR<10 mL/min.
HD	Dialysed. Dose as in GFR<10 mL/min.
HDF/High flux	Dialysed. Dose as in GFR<10 mL/min.
CAV/ VVHD	Unknown dialysability. Dose as in GFR=10–30 mL/min.

IMPORTANT DRUG INTERACTIONS

Potentially hazardous interactions with other drugs
- Iloprost: increased risk of bleeding.

ADMINISTRATION

RECONSTITUTION
–
ROUTE
- IV bolus, IV infusion
RATE OF ADMINISTRATION
- 1–2 mcg/kg/minute depending on renal function.
COMMENTS
–

OTHER INFORMATION

- Antiplatelet effect lasts for about 4 hours after stopping infusion.
- Main side effect is bleeding.
- In patients with a GFR<50 mL/min, clearance is halved and plasma concentration doubled.
- Contraindicated by UK SPC if GFR<30 mL/min but not in US data sheet. Although contraindicated in dialysis dependent patients in US data sheet.

Eribulin

CLINICAL USE

Antineoplastic agent
- Treatment of metastatic breast cancer

DOSE IN NORMAL RENAL FUNCTION

$1.23 \, mg/m^2$ (as base) on Days 1 and 8 of every
21-day cycle
Consult relevant local protocol.

PHARMACOKINETICS

Molecular weight (daltons)	729.9 (826 as mesilate)
% Protein binding	49–65
% Excreted unchanged in urine	9
Volume of distribution (L/kg)	$43–114 \, litres/m^2$
Half-life – normal/ ESRF (hrs)	40/–

METABOLISM

Minimal metabolism.
    Eribulin is eliminated primarily by biliary
excretion. The transport protein involved
in the excretion is presently unknown.
Preclinical studies indicate that eribulin is
transported by Pgp. However, it is unknown
whether Pgp is contributing to the biliary
excretion of eribulin.

DOSE IN RENAL IMPAIRMENT GFR (mL/MIN)

40–50	Dose as in normal renal function.
40–30	$1.1 \, mg/m^2/dose.$
<30	Reduce dose.

DOSE IN PATIENTS UNDERGOING RENAL REPLACEMENT THERAPIES

CAPD	Not dialysed. Dose as in GFR<30 mL/min.
HD	Not dialysed. Dose as in GFR<30 mL/min.
HDF/High flux	Not dialysed. Dose as in GFR<30 mL/min.
CAV/ VVHD	Not dialysed. Dose as in GFR=30–40 mL/min.

IMPORTANT DRUG INTERACTIONS

Potentially hazardous interactions with other
drugs
- Antipsychotics: avoid concomitant use with clozapine (increased risk of agranulocytosis).

ADMINISTRATION

RECONSTITUTION
–
ROUTE
- IV
RATE OF ADMINISTRATION
- Over 2–5 minutes
COMMENTS
- May be diluted in 100 mL of sodium chloride 0.9%

OTHER INFORMATION

- Due to lack of data the manufacturer cannot recommend a dose if GFR<40 mL/ min.
- Information in GFR=30–40 mL/min from US data sheet.
- A study in patients with different degrees of impaired renal function showed that the exposure of eribulin in patients with creatinine clearance ≥ 40 to 59 mL/min, n=6) was similar to patients with normal renal function while the exposure in patients with creatinine clearance <40 mL/ min was increased by 75%, n=4.

Erlotinib

CLINICAL USE

Tyrosine kinase inhibitor, antineoplastic agent:
- Treatment of locally advanced or metastatic non-small cell lung cancer after failure of at least 1 other regime
- Pancreatic cancer

DOSE IN NORMAL RENAL FUNCTION

- Non-small cell lung cancer: 150 mg once daily at least 1 hour before or 2 hours after food.
- Pancreatic cancer: 100 mg once daily. Or see local protocol.

PHARMACOKINETICS

Molecular weight (daltons)	429.9 (as hydrochloride)
% Protein binding	93–95
% Excreted unchanged in urine	9 (<2% as unchanged drug)
Volume of distribution (L/kg)	232 litres
Half-life – normal/ESRF (hrs)	36/–

METABOLISM

Erlotinib is metabolised mainly by the cytochrome P450 isoenzyme CYP3A4, and to a lesser extent by CYP1A2. Extrahepatic metabolism by CYP3A4 in intestine, CYP1A1 in lung, and 1B1 in tumour tissue potentially contribute to the metabolic clearance of erlotinib.

Metabolic pathways include demethylation, to metabolites OSI-420 and OSI-413, oxidation, and aromatic hydroxylation. The metabolites OSI-420 and OSI-413 have comparable potency to erlotinib in non-clinical *in vitro* assays and *in vivo* tumour models. They are present in plasma at levels that are <10% of erlotinib and display similar pharmacokinetics as erlotinib. Erlotinib is excreted predominantly as metabolites via the faeces (>90%) with renal elimination accounting for only a small amount (approximately 9%) of an oral dose. Less than 2% of the orally administered dose is excreted as parent substance.

DOSE IN RENAL IMPAIRMENT GFR (mL/MIN)

20–50	Dose as in normal renal function.
15–20	Dose as in normal renal function.
<15	Use with caution.

DOSE IN PATIENTS UNDERGOING RENAL REPLACEMENT THERAPIES

CAPD	Unlikely to be dialysed. Dose as in GFR<15 mL/min
HD	Unlikely to be dialysed. Dose as in GFR<15 mL/min
HDF/High flux	Unlikely to be dialysed. Dose as in GFR<15 mL/min
CAV/VVHD	Unlikely to be dialysed. Dose as in normal renal function.

IMPORTANT DRUG INTERACTIONS

Potentially hazardous interactions with other drugs
- Analgesics: increased risk of bleeding with NSAIDs.
- Antacids: concentration possibly reduced by antacids, give at least 4 hours before or 2 hours after erlotinib.
- Anticoagulants: increased risk of bleeding with coumarins.
- Antipsychotics: avoid concomitant use with clozapine, increased risk of agranulocytosis.
- Antivirals: avoid with boceprevir.
- Ulcer-healing drugs: avoid with cimetidine, esomeprazole, famotidine, lansoprazole, nizatidine, pantoprazole and rabeprazole; concentration reduced by ranitidine, give at least 2 hours before or 10 hours after ranitidine; concentration reduced by omeprazole – avoid.

ADMINISTRATION

RECONSTITUTION
–

ROUTE
- Oral

RATE OF ADMINISTRATION
–

COMMENTS
–

OTHER INFORMATION

- Has not been studied in patients with a GFR<15 mL/min; therefore use with caution, but drug has limited renal excretion.
- Major side effects are rash and diarrhoea.
- Can cause interstitial lung disease and abnormal liver function tests.
- Smoking may reduce erlotinib concentration by increasing clearance.

Ertapenem

CLINICAL USE

Antibacterial agent

DOSE IN NORMAL RENAL FUNCTION

1 g daily

PHARMACOKINETICS

Molecular weight (daltons)	497.5 (as sodium)
% Protein binding	85–95
% Excreted unchanged in urine	38
Volume of distribution (L/kg)	0.1
Half-life – normal/ ESRF (hrs)	4/14

METABOLISM

After intravenous infusion of radiolabelled 1 g ertapenem, the plasma radioactivity consists predominantly (94%) of ertapenem. The major metabolite of ertapenem is the ring-opened derivative formed by dehydropeptidase-I-mediated hydrolysis of the beta-lactam ring. Approximately 80% of a dose is recovered in urine and 10% in faeces. Of the 80% recovered in urine, approximately 38% is excreted as unchanged ertapenem and approximately 37% as the ring-opened metabolite.

DOSE IN RENAL IMPAIRMENT GFR (mL/MIN)

30–50	Dose as in normal renal function.
10–30	Use 50–100% of dose.
<10	Use 50% of dose, or 1 g 3 times a week. See 'Other information'.

DOSE IN PATIENTS UNDERGOING RENAL REPLACEMENT THERAPIES

CAPD	Dialysed. Dose as in GFR<10 mL/min.
HD	Dialysed. Dose as in GFR<10 mL/min.
HDF/High flux	Dialysed. Dose as in GFR<10 mL/min.
CAV/VVHD	Dialysed. Dose as in GFR=10–30 mL/min.

IMPORTANT DRUG INTERACTIONS

Potentially hazardous interactions with other drugs
- Anti-epileptics: concentration of valproate reduced – avoid concomitant use.

ADMINISTRATION

RECONSTITUTION
- 10 mL water for injection or sodium chloride 0.9%.

ROUTE
- IV, (IM – not licensed)

RATE OF ADMINISTRATION
- IV Infusion: 30 minutes.

COMMENTS
- Dilute in sodium chloride 0.9% only.
- Incompatible with glucose.
- Dilute solutions are stable for 6 hours at room temperature or 24 hours in a refrigerator. Use within 4 hours of removal from refrigerator.

OTHER INFORMATION

- Not recommended by UK manufacturer due to lack of data in GFR<30 mL/min but a dose of 50% is recommended in US data sheet.
- Doses in renal impairment are from *Drug Prescribing in Renal Failure*, 5th edition, by Aronoff *et al.*
- Approximately 30% of dose is dialysed after a 4 hour haemodialysis session.
- Anecdotally ertapenem has been used at a dose of 1 g 3 times a week in haemodialysis patients.
- Give at least 6 hours before haemodialysis session if unable to give post dialysis.

Erythromycin

CLINICAL USE

Antibacterial agent

DOSE IN NORMAL RENAL FUNCTION

- IV: 6.25–12.5 mg/kg every 6 hours
- Oral: 250–500 mg every 6 hours or 0.5–1 g every 12 hours
- Maximum 4 g daily

PHARMACOKINETICS

Molecular weight (daltons)	733.9
% Protein binding	70–95
% Excreted unchanged in urine	2–15
Volume of distribution (L/kg)	0.6–1.2 (increased in CKD 5)
Half-life – normal/ ESRF (hrs)	1.5–2/4–7

METABOLISM

Erythromycin is partly metabolised in the liver by the cytochrome P450 isoenzyme CYP3A4 via N-demethylation to inactive, unidentified metabolites. It is excreted in high concentrations in the bile and undergoes intestinal reabsorption. About 2–5% of an oral dose is excreted unchanged in the urine and as much as 12–15% of an intravenous dose may be excreted unchanged by the urinary route.

DOSE IN RENAL IMPAIRMENT GFR (mL/MIN)

20–50	Dose as in normal renal function.
10–20	Dose as in normal renal function.
<10	Dose as in normal renal function. See 'Other information'.

DOSE IN PATIENTS UNDERGOING RENAL REPLACEMENT THERAPIES

CAPD	Not dialysed. Dose as in normal renal function.
HD	Not dialysed. Dose as in normal renal function.
HDF/High flux	Unknown dialysability. Dose as in normal renal function.
CAV/ VVHD	Unknown dialysability. Dose as in normal renal function.

IMPORTANT DRUG INTERACTIONS

Potentially hazardous interactions with other drugs

- Anti-arrhythmics: increased risk of ventricular arrhythmias with IV erythromycin and amiodarone – avoid concomitant use; increased toxicity with disopyramide; increased risk of ventricular arrhythmias with dronedarone – avoid.
- Antibacterials: increased risk of ventricular arrhythmias with moxifloxacin and IV erythromycin – avoid concomitant use; increased rifabutin concentration.
- Anticoagulants: enhanced effect of coumarins.
- Antidepressants: avoid concomitant use with reboxetine.
- Anti-epileptics: increased carbamazepine concentration and possibly valproate.
- Antihistamines: possibly increases loratadine concentration; inhibits mizolastine metabolism – avoid concomitant use; concentration of rupatadine increased.
- Antimalarials: avoid concomitant administration with artemether/ lumefantrine; increased risk of ventricular arrhythmias with piperaquine with artenimol – avoid.
- Antimuscarinics: avoid concomitant use with tolterodine.
- Antipsychotics: increased risk of ventricular arrhythmias with sulpiride and zuclopenthixol and IV erythromycin avoid concomitant use; possibly increases clozapine concentration leading to increased risk of convulsions; possibly increased risk of ventricular arrhythmias with amisulpride, droperidol and pimozide – avoid concomitant use; possibly increased quetiapine concentration.
- Antivirals: concentration of both drugs increased with telaprevir; concentration increased by ritonavir; avoid with rilpivirine, concentration increased; increased risk of ventricular arrhythmias with saquinavir – avoid.
- Anxiolytics and hypnotics: inhibits midazolam and zopiclone metabolism; increases buspirone concentration.
- Atomoxetine: increased risk of ventricular arrhythmias with parenteral erythromycin.
- Calcium-channel blockers: possibly inhibit metabolism of calcium-channel blockers; avoid concomitant use with lercanidipine.

- Ciclosporin: markedly elevated ciclosporin blood levels – decreased levels on withdrawing drug. Monitor blood levels of ciclosporin carefully and adjust dose promptly as necessary.
- Clopidogrel: possibly reduced anti-platelet effect.
- Colchicine: increased risk of colchicine toxicity – suspend or reduce dose of colchicine, avoid in hepatic or renal impairment.
- Cytotoxics: concentration of axitinib increased – reduce axitinib dose; concentration of everolimus possibly increased; increased risk of ventricular arrhythmias with IV erythromycin and vandetanib – avoid; possible interaction with docetaxel; increased risk of ventricular arrhythmias with arsenic trioxide; increases vinblastine toxicity – avoid concomitant use.
- Diuretics: increased eplerenone concentration – reduce eplerenone dose.
- Domperidone: possible increased risk of ventricular arrhythmias.
- Ergot alkaloids: increase risk of ergotism – avoid concomitant use.
- 5HT$_1$ agonists: increased eletriptan concentration – avoid concomitant use.
- Ivabradine: increased risk of ventricular arrhythmias – avoid concomitant use.
- Lipid-lowering drugs: increased risk of myopathy; concentration of rosuvastatin reduced; avoid concomitant use with simvastatin.[1]
- Pentamidine: increased risk of ventricular arrhythmias with IV erythromycin.
- Sirolimus: concentration of both drugs increased.
- Tacrolimus: markedly elevated tacrolimus blood levels – decreased levels on withdrawing drug. Monitor blood levels of tacrolimus carefully and adjust dose promptly as necessary.
- Theophylline: inhibits theophylline metabolism; if erythromycin given orally decreased erythromycin concentration.
- Ticagrelor: concentration of ticagrelor possibly increased.

ADMINISTRATION

RECONSTITUTION
- 1 g with 20 mL water for injection, then dilute resultant solution further to 1–5 mg/mL.

ROUTE
- IV, oral

RATE OF ADMINISTRATION
- 20–60 minutes using constant rate infusion pump

COMMENTS
- Use central line if concentration greater than 5 mg/mL; if >10 mg/mL monitor carefully (some units use 1 g in 100 mL of sodium chloride 0.9%). (UK Critical Care Group, *Minimum Infusion Volumes for Fluid Restricted Critically Ill Patients*, 3rd edition, 2006)

OTHER INFORMATION

- May also give one third of daily dose by infusion over 8 hours peripherally at concentration of 1 g/250 mL (4 mg/mL). Repeat 8 hourly, i.e. continuously.
- Increased risk of ototoxicity in renal impairment especially at high doses.
- Avoid peaks produced by oral twice-daily dosing, i.e. dose 4 times daily.
- Monitor closely for thrombophlebitic reactions at site of infusion.

Reference:
1. MHRA. *Drug Safety Update*. Statins: interactions and updated advice. August 2012; **6**(1): 2–4.

Escitalopram

CLINICAL USE

SSRI antidepressant:
- Depressive illness
- Panic and social anxiety disorder

DOSE IN NORMAL RENAL FUNCTION

- Antidepressant: 10–20 mg daily
- Panic and social anxiety disorder: 5–20 mg
- Patients >65 years: maximum 10 mg daily

PHARMACOKINETICS

Molecular weight (daltons)	414.4 (as Oxalate)
% Protein binding	<80
% Excreted unchanged in urine	8
Volume of distribution (L/kg)	12–26
Half-life – normal/ ESRF (hrs)	22–32/Slightly increased

METABOLISM

Escitalopram is metabolised in the liver to the demethylated and didemethylated metabolites. Both of these are pharmacologically active. Alternatively, the nitrogen may be oxidised to form the N-oxide metabolite. Both parent substance and metabolites are partly excreted as glucuronides. After multiple dosing the mean concentrations of the demethyl and didemethyl metabolites are usually 28–31% and <5%, respectively, of the escitalopram concentration. Biotransformation of escitalopram to the demethylated metabolite is mediated primarily by CYP2C19. Some contribution by the enzymes CYP3A4 and CYP2D6 is possible. The major metabolites have a significantly longer half-life than the parent drug.

Escitalopram and major metabolites are assumed to be eliminated by both hepatic and renal routes, with the major part of the dose excreted as metabolites in the urine.

DOSE IN RENAL IMPAIRMENT GFR (mL/MIN)

30–50	Dose as in normal renal function.
10–30	Dose as in normal renal function. Start with a low dose and titrate slowly.
<10	Dose as in normal renal function. Start with a low dose and titrate slowly.

DOSE IN PATIENTS UNDERGOING RENAL REPLACEMENT THERAPIES

CAPD	Unlikely to be dialysed. Dose as in GFR<10 mL/min.
HD	Not dialysed. Dose as in GFR<10 mL/min.
HDF/High flux	Not dialysed. Dose as in GFR<10 mL/min.
CAV/ VVHD	Unlikely to be dialysed. Dose as in GFR=10–30 mL/min.

IMPORTANT DRUG INTERACTIONS

Potentially hazardous interactions with other drugs
- Analgesics: increased risk of bleeding with aspirin and NSAIDs; risk of CNS toxicity increased with tramadol.
- Anticoagulants: effect of coumarins possibly enhanced; possibly increased risk of bleeding with dabigatran.
- Antidepressants: avoid concomitant use with MAOI, increased risk of toxicity; increased risk of CNS toxicity with moclobemide – avoid concomitant use; avoid concomitant use with St John's wort; possibly enhanced serotonergic effects with duloxetine; can increase concentration of tricyclics; increased agitation and nausea with tryptophan.
- Anti-epileptics: convulsive threshold lowered.
- Antimalarials: avoid concomitant use with artemether/lumefantrine and piperaquine with artenimol.
- Antipsychotics: possibly increased risk of ventricular arrhythmias with pimozide – avoid.
- Antivirals: concentration possibly increased by ritonavir.
- Dopaminergics: avoid with selegiline; increased risk of CNS toxicity with rasagiline.
- $5HT_1$ agonist: increased risk of CNS toxicity with sumatriptan; possibly increased risk of serotonergic effects with naratriptan.
- Linezolid: use with care, possibly increased risk of side effects.
- Lithium: increased risk of CNS effects.
- Methylthioninium: risk of CNS toxicity – avoid if possible.

ADMINISTRATION

RECONSTITUTION

–

ROUTE

- Oral

RATE OF ADMINISTRATION

–

COMMENTS

- Oral drops: 20 drops = 10 mg

OTHER INFORMATION

- Escitalopram is an isomer of citalopram.
- Risk of QT prolongation and ventricular arrhythmias.

Eslicarbazepine acetate

CLINICAL USE

Anti-epileptic

DOSE IN NORMAL RENAL FUNCTION

400–1200 mg once daily

PHARMACOKINETICS

Molecular weight (daltons)	296.3
% Protein binding	<40
% Excreted unchanged in urine	<1[1] (90 plus metabolites)
Volume of distribution (L/kg)	2.7[1]
Half-life – normal/ ESRF (hrs)	10–20/Increased

METABOLISM

Eslicarbazepine acetate is rapidly and extensively biotransformed to its major active metabolite eslicarbazepine by hydrolytic first-pass metabolism. Minor metabolites in plasma are R-licarbazepine and oxcarbazepine, which were shown to be active, and the glucuronic acid conjugates of eslicarbazepine acetate, eslicarbazepine, R-licarbazepine and oxcarbazepine.

Eslicarbazepine acetate and its metabolites are mainly excreted in the urine unchanged.

DOSE IN RENAL IMPAIRMENT GFR (mL/MIN)

30–60	Initially 400 mg every 48 hours or 200 mg once daily increased to 400 mg daily. Dose may be increased as required.
10–30	400 mg alternate days for 2 weeks, increasing to 400 mg once daily, max dose 600 mg daily.[2]
<10	400 mg alternate days for 2 weeks, increasing to 400 mg once daily, max dose 600 mg daily.[2]

DOSE IN PATIENTS UNDERGOING RENAL REPLACEMENT THERAPIES

CAPD	Probably dialysed. Dose as in GFR<10 mL/min.
HD	Dialysed. 400–600 mg post dialysis.
HDF/High flux	Dialysed. 400–600 mg post dialysis.
CAV/ VVHD	Dialysed. Dose as in GFR=10–30 mL/min.

IMPORTANT DRUG INTERACTIONS

Potentially hazardous interactions with other drugs

- Antidepressants: anticonvulsant effect possibly antagonised by MAOIs, SSRIs and TADs; avoid with St John's wort
- Antiepileptics: avoid concomitant use with carbamazepine, oxcarbazepine; concentration reduced by phenytoin and concentration of phenytoin increased.
- Antimalarials: anticonvulsant effect antagonised by mefloquine.
- Antipsychotics: antagonism of anticonvulsant effect.
- Oestrogens & progestogens: reduced contraceptive effect.
- Orlistat: possibly increased risk of convulsions.

ADMINISTRATION

RECONSTITUTION

–

ROUTE

- Oral

RATE OF ADMINISTRATION

–

OTHER INFORMATION

- Not recommended by manufacturer in GFR<30 mL/min due to lack of data.
- May prolong PR interval.
- High bioavailability.
- Metabolites are effectively cleared by haemodialysis.

References:
1. Patsalos, PN, editor. *Antiepileptic Drug Interactions: a clinical guide*. p. 36.
2. Diaz A, Deliz B, Benbadis SR. The use of newer antiepileptic drugs in patients with renal failure. *Expert Rev Neurother*. 2012; **12**(1): 99–105.

Esmolol hydrochloride

CLINICAL USE

Beta-adrenoceptor blocker:
- Short-term treatment of supraventricular arrhythmias (including AF, atrial flutter, sinus tachycardia)
- Tachycardia and hypertension in the perioperative period

DOSE IN NORMAL RENAL FUNCTION

50–200 micrograms/kg/minute; see product literature for titration schedule.

PHARMACOKINETICS

Molecular weight (daltons)	331.8
% Protein binding	55
% Excreted unchanged in urine	<2
Volume of distribution (L/kg)	1.9
Half-life – normal/ESRF (hrs)	9 minutes/ Unchanged

METABOLISM

Esmolol hydrochloride is metabolised by esterases into an acid metabolite (ASL-8123) and methanol. This occurs through hydrolysis of the ester group by esterases in the red blood cells. Esmolol hydrochloride is excreted by the kidneys, partly unchanged (less than 2% of the administered amount), partly as acid metabolite that has a weak (less than 0.1% of esmolol) beta-blocking activity. The acid metabolite is also excreted in the urine.

DOSE IN RENAL IMPAIRMENT GFR (mL/MIN)

20–50	Dose as in normal renal function.
10–20	Dose as in normal renal function.
<10	Dose as in normal renal function.

DOSE IN PATIENTS UNDERGOING RENAL REPLACEMENT THERAPIES

CAPD	Dialysed. Dose as in normal renal function.
HD	Dialysed. Dose as in normal renal function.
HDF/High flux	Dialysed. Dose as in normal renal function.
CAV/ VVHD	Unknown dialysability. Dose as in normal renal function.

IMPORTANT DRUG INTERACTIONS

Potentially hazardous interactions with other drugs
- Anaesthetics: enhanced hypotensive effect.
- Analgesics: NSAIDs antagonise hypotensive effect.
- Anti-arrhythmics: increased risk of myocardial depression and bradycardia; with amiodarone, increased risk of bradycardia and AV block and myocardial depression; increased risk of myocardial depression and bradycardia with flecainide.
- Antidepressants: enhanced hypotensive effect with MAOIs.
- Antimalarials: increased risk of bradycardia with mefloquine.
- Antipsychotics: enhanced hypotensive effect with phenothiazines.
- Calcium-channel blockers: increased risk of bradycardia and AV block with diltiazem; severe hypotension and heart failure occasionally with nifedipine and possibly other dihydropyridines; asystole, severe hypotension and heart failure with verapamil – avoid concomitant verapamil use.
- Antihypertensives: enhanced hypotensive effect; increased risk of withdrawal hypertension with clonidine; increased risk of first dose hypotensive effect with post-synaptic alpha-blockers.
- Cytotoxics: possible increased risk of bradycardia with crizotinib.
- Diuretics: enhanced hypotensive effect.
- Fingolimod: possibly increased risk of bradycardia.
- Moxisylyte: possible severe postural hypotension.
- Sympathomimetics: severe hypertension with adrenaline and noradrenaline and possibly dobutamine.

ADMINISTRATION

RECONSTITUTION
–
ROUTE
- IV infusion
RATE OF ADMINISTRATION
- 50–200 mcg/kg/minute
COMMENTS
- Incompatible with sodium bicarbonate solutions.

- Dilute to a concentration of 10 mg/mL with sodium chloride 0.9% or glucose 5%.
- Local irritation has occurred with infusions of 20 mg/mL.

OTHER INFORMATION

- Hyperkalaemia can occur in CKD 5.
- Titrate dose according to blood pressure response.

Esomeprazole

CLINICAL USE

Gastric acid suppression

DOSE IN NORMAL RENAL FUNCTION

- Oral: 20–40 mg daily
- Zollinger-Ellison syndrome: 80–160 mg daily (doses >80 mg given in divided doses)
- IV: 20–40 mg daily
- Severe peptic ulcer bleeding: 80 mg over 30 minutes then 8 mg/hour for 72 hours

PHARMACOKINETICS

Molecular weight (daltons)	345.4
% Protein binding	97
% Excreted unchanged in urine	<1
Volume of distribution (L/kg)	0.22
Half-life – normal/ ESRF (hrs)	1.3/Unchanged

METABOLISM

Esomeprazole is completely metabolised by the cytochrome P450 system (CYP). The major part of the metabolism of esomeprazole is dependent on the polymorphic CYP2C19, responsible for the formation of the hydroxy- and desmethyl metabolites of esomeprazole. The remaining part is dependent on another specific isoform, CYP3A4, responsible for the formation of esomeprazole sulphone, the main metabolite in plasma. The major metabolites of esomeprazole have no effect on gastric acid secretion.

Almost 80% of an oral dose of esomeprazole is excreted as metabolites in the urine, the remainder in the faeces. Less than 1% of the parent drug is found in urine.

DOSE IN RENAL IMPAIRMENT GFR (mL/MIN)

20–50	Dose as in normal renal function.
10–20	Dose as in normal renal function.
<10	Dose as in normal renal function.

DOSE IN PATIENTS UNDERGOING RENAL REPLACEMENT THERAPIES

CAPD	Unlikely to be dialysed. Dose as in normal renal function.
HD	Not dialysed. Dose as in normal renal function.
HDF/High flux	Unlikely to be dialysed. Dose as in normal renal function.
CAV/ VVHD	Unlikely to be dialysed. Dose as in normal renal function.

IMPORTANT DRUG INTERACTIONS

Potentially hazardous interactions with other drugs
- Anticoagulants: effect of coumarins possibly enhanced.
- Anti-epileptics: effects of phenytoin enhanced.
- Antifungals: absorption of itraconazole and ketoconazole reduced; avoid with posaconazole; concentration possibly increased by voriconazole.
- Antivirals: concentration of atazanavir and rilpivirine reduced – avoid concomitant use; concentration of raltegravir and saquinavir possibly increased – avoid; concentration of esomeprazole reduced by tipranavir.
- Clopidogrel: reduced anti-platelet effect.
- Cytotoxics: possibly reduced excretion of methotrexate; avoid with erlotinib and vandetanib; possibly reduced lapatinib absorption; possibly reduced absorption of pazopanib.
- Ulipristal: reduced contraceptive effect, avoid with high dose ulipristal.

ADMINISTRATION

RECONSTITUTION
- 5 mL sodium chloride 0.9%
ROUTE
- Oral, IV
RATE OF ADMINISTRATION
- Bolus: over 3 minutes
- Infusion: 10–30 minutes
COMMENTS
- Dilute with up to 100 mL sodium chloride 0.9%.

OTHER INFORMATION

- Can be dispersed in half a glass of non-carbonated water. Stir well until it disintegrates; the liquid with pellets should be drunk immediately or within 30 minutes of preparation. The glass should then be rinsed with water which should also be drunk.
- Do not crush or chew.
- Manufacturer advises to use with caution due to lack of data.

Estramustine phosphate

CLINICAL USE

Alkylating agent:
Prostate cancer

DOSE IN NORMAL RENAL FUNCTION

0.14–1.4 g daily in divided doses (usual initial
dose 560–840 mg daily)

PHARMACOKINETICS

Molecular weight (daltons)	564.3 (as sodium phosphate)
% Protein binding	No data
% Excreted unchanged in urine	22–36
Volume of distribution (L/kg)	0.43[1]
Half-life – normal/ ESRF (hrs)	10 (estromustine: 20)/–

METABOLISM

Estramustine sodium phosphate is absorbed
from the gastrointestinal tract and rapidly
dephosphorylated in the intestine and
prostate to estramustine and its oxidised
isomer estromustine. Some hydrolysis
of the carbamate linkage occurs in the
liver, releasing estradiol, estrone, and
the normustine group. Estramustine
and estromustine are excreted with their
metabolites mainly in the faeces.

DOSE IN RENAL IMPAIRMENT GFR (mL/MIN)

20–50	Dose as in normal renal function.
10–20	Dose as in normal renal function.
<10	Dose as in normal renal function.

DOSE IN PATIENTS UNDERGOING RENAL REPLACEMENT THERAPIES

CAPD	Unknown dialysability. Dose as in normal renal function.
HD	Unknown dialysability. Dose as in normal renal function.
HDF/High flux	Unknown dialysability. Dose as in normal renal function.
CAV/ VVHD	Unknown dialysability. Dose as in normal renal function.

IMPORTANT DRUG INTERACTIONS

Potentially hazardous interactions with
other drugs
- Antipsychotics: avoid concomitant
  use with clozapine (increased risk of
  agranulocytosis).
- Bisphosphonates: concentration increased
  by sodium clodronate.

ADMINISTRATION

RECONSTITUTION
–
ROUTE
- Oral
RATE OF ADMINISTRATION
–
COMMENTS
- Don't give less than 1 hour before or
  2 hours after meals.

OTHER INFORMATION

- Can cause fluid retention so use with
  caution in renal impairment.

Reference:
1. Gunnarsson PO, Andersson SB, Johansson
SÅ, et al. Pharmacokinetics of estramustine
phosphate (Estracyt) in prostatic cancer
patients. *Eur J Clin Pharmacol*. 1984 Jan;
26(1): 113–19.

Etamsylate

CLINICAL USE

- Short-term treatment of blood loss in menorrhagia
- Prophylaxis of surgical bleeding (unlicensed)

DOSE IN NORMAL RENAL FUNCTION

- Menorrhagia: 500 mg 4 times a day during menstruation
- Surgical bleeding: 1–1.5 g daily or 250–500 mg every 4–6 hours

PHARMACOKINETICS

Molecular weight (daltons)	263.3
% Protein binding	>90
% Excreted unchanged in urine	72–80
Volume of distribution (L/kg)	No data
Half-life – normal/ESRF (hrs)	3.7–8/–

METABOLISM

Etamsylate is excreted unchanged, mainly in the urine.

DOSE IN RENAL IMPAIRMENT GFR (mL/MIN)

20–50 Dose as in normal renal function.
10–20 Dose as in normal renal function.
<10 Dose as in normal renal function.

DOSE IN PATIENTS UNDERGOING RENAL REPLACEMENT THERAPIES

CAPD	Unlikely to be dialysed. Dose as in normal renal function.
HD	Unlikely to be dialysed. Dose as in normal renal function.
HDF/High flux	Unknown dialysability. Dose as in normal renal function.
CAV/ VVHD	Unlikely to be dialysed. Dose as in normal renal function.

IMPORTANT DRUG INTERACTIONS

Potentially hazardous interactions with other drugs
- None known

ADMINISTRATION

RECONSTITUTION
–
ROUTE
- Oral
RATE OF ADMINISTRATION
–
COMMENTS
–

Etanercept

CLINICAL USE

Tumour necrosis factor alpha inhibitor
- Treatment of moderate to severe rheumatoid arthritis in combination with methotrexate
- Psoriatic arthritis
- Ankylosing spondylitis

DOSE IN NORMAL RENAL FUNCTION

25 mg twice weekly or 50 mg weekly

PHARMACOKINETICS

Molecular weight (daltons)	150 000
% Protein binding	No data
% Excreted unchanged in urine	No data
Volume of distribution (L/kg)	10.4 litres
Half-life – normal/ ESRF (hrs)	72–132/Unchanged

METABOLISM

Since etanercept is a fusion glycoprotein, consisting entirely of human protein components, it is expected to undergo proteolysis.

DOSE IN RENAL IMPAIRMENT GFR (mL/MIN)

20–50	Dose as in normal renal function.
10–20	Dose as in normal renal function.
<10	Dose as in normal renal function.

DOSE IN PATIENTS UNDERGOING RENAL REPLACEMENT THERAPIES

CAPD	Unlikely to be dialysed. Dose as in normal renal function.
HD	Unlikely to be dialysed. Dose as in normal renal function.
HDF/High flux	Unlikely to be dialysed. Dose as in normal renal function.
CAV/ VVHD	Unlikely to be dialysed. Dose as in normal renal function.

IMPORTANT DRUG INTERACTIONS

Potentially hazardous interactions with other drugs
- Live vaccines: avoid concomitant use.
- Anakinra & abatacept: avoid concomitant use.

ADMINISTRATION

RECONSTITUTION
- 1 mL water for injection (solvent provided)
ROUTE
- SC
RATE OF ADMINISTRATION
–

OTHER INFORMATION

- Contraindicated in patients with severe infections and moderate to severe heart failure.
- Bioavailability is 76%.
- Case reports of glomerulonephritis have been reported with etanercept.[1]

Reference:
1. Stokes MB, Foster K, Markowitz GS, *et al.* Development of glomerulonephritis during anti-TNF-α therapy for rheumatoid arthritis. *Nephrol Dial Transplant.* **20**(7): 1400–6.

Ethambutol hydrochloride

CLINICAL USE

Antibacterial agent:
- Tuberculosis

DOSE IN NORMAL RENAL FUNCTION

15 mg/kg/day or 30 mg/kg 3 times a week
(supervised dosing)

PHARMACOKINETICS

Molecular weight (daltons)	277.2
% Protein binding	20–30
% Excreted unchanged in urine	50
Volume of distribution (L/kg)	1.6–3.2
Half-life – normal/ ESRF (hrs)	3–4/5–15

METABOLISM

Ethambutol is partially metabolised in the
liver to the aldehyde and dicarboxylic acid
derivatives, which are inactive. Up to 80% of
a dose appears in the urine within 24 hours,
50% as unchanged drug and 8–15% as the
inactive metabolites. About 20% of the dose
is excreted unchanged in the faeces.

DOSE IN RENAL IMPAIRMENT GFR (mL/MIN)

20–50	Dose as in normal renal function.
10–20	15 mg/kg every 24–36 hours, or 7.5–15 mg/kg/day
<10	15 mg/kg every 48 hours, or 5–7.5 mg/kg/day

DOSE IN PATIENTS UNDERGOING RENAL REPLACEMENT THERAPIES

CAPD	Not dialysed. Dose as in GFR<10 mL/min.
HD	Dialysed. Dose as in GFR<10 mL/min, or on dialysis days only give 25 mg/kg 4–6 hours before dialysis.
HDF/High flux	Dialysed. Dose as in GFR<10 mL/min, or on dialysis days only give 25 mg/kg 4–6 hours before dialysis.
CAV/ VVHD	Dialysed. Dose as in GFR=10–20 mL/min.

IMPORTANT DRUG INTERACTIONS

Potentially hazardous interactions with
other drugs
- None known

ADMINISTRATION

RECONSTITUTION

–

ROUTE
- Oral

RATE OF ADMINISTRATION

–

COMMENTS

–

OTHER INFORMATION

- Monitor plasma levels. Dosages should be individually determined and adjusted according to measured levels and renal replacement therapy.
- Peak levels are taken 2–2.5 hours post dose (2–6 mg/L or 7–22 micromol/L); trough is taken pre dose (<1 mg/L or <4 micromol/L).
- Baseline visual acuity tests should be performed prior to initiating ethambutol.
- Daily dosing is preferred by some specialists to aid compliance and ensure maximum therapeutic effect.
- Dose in renal impairment is from *Drug Prescribing in Renal Failure*, 5th edition, by Aronoff *et al.*

Ethosuximide

CLINICAL USE

Epilepsy

DOSE IN NORMAL RENAL FUNCTION

500 mg – 2 g daily in divided doses.

PHARMACOKINETICS

Molecular weight (daltons)	141.2
% Protein binding	0[1]
% Excreted unchanged in urine	12–20
Volume of distribution (L/kg)	0.6–0.9
Half-life – normal/ ESRF (hrs)	40–60/Unchanged

METABOLISM

Ethosuximide is extensively hydroxylated in the liver to its principal metabolite which is reported to be inactive.

Ethosuximide is excreted in the urine mainly in the form of its metabolites, either free or conjugated, but about 12–20% is also excreted unchanged.

DOSE IN RENAL IMPAIRMENT GFR (mL/MIN)

20–50	Dose as in normal renal function.
10–20	Dose as in normal renal function.
<10	Dose as in normal renal function.

DOSE IN PATIENTS UNDERGOING RENAL REPLACEMENT THERAPIES

CAPD	Dialysed. Dose as in normal renal function.
HD	Dialysed. Dose as in normal renal function.
HDF/High flux	Dialysed. Dose as in normal renal function.
CAV/ VVHD	Dialysed. Dose as in normal renal function.

IMPORTANT DRUG INTERACTIONS

Potentially hazardous interactions with other drugs

- Antibacterials: concentration increased by isoniazid.
- Antidepressants: lower convulsive threshold; avoid with St John's wort.
- Anti-epileptics: concentration possibly reduced by carbamazepine, phenytoin and phenobarbital; concentration of phenytoin possibly increased; concentration increased by valproate.
- Antimalarials: anticonvulsant effect antagonised by mefloquine.
- Antipsychotics: lower convulsive threshold.
- Orlistat: possible increased risk of convulsions.

ADMINISTRATION

RECONSTITUTION
–
ROUTE
- Oral
RATE OF ADMINISTRATION
–
COMMENTS
–

OTHER INFORMATION

Reference:
1. Browne T. Pharmacokinetics of anti-epileptic drugs. *Neurology*. 1998; **51**(Suppl. 4): S2–7.

Etodolac

CLINICAL USE

NSAID and analgesic

DOSE IN NORMAL RENAL FUNCTION

300–600 mg daily in 1–2 divided doses
XL: 600 mg once daily

PHARMACOKINETICS

Molecular weight (daltons)	287.4
% Protein binding	>99
% Excreted unchanged in urine	1
Volume of distribution (L/kg)	0.4
Half-life – normal/ ESRF (hrs)	6–7.4/Unchanged

METABOLISM

Excretion of etodolac is mainly in the urine as hydroxylated metabolites and glucuronide conjugates; some may be excreted in the bile.

DOSE IN RENAL IMPAIRMENT GFR (mL/MIN)

20–50	Dose as in normal renal function, but avoid if possible.
10–20	Dose as in normal renal function, but avoid if possible.
<10	Dose as in normal renal function, but only use if on dialysis.

DOSE IN PATIENTS UNDERGOING RENAL REPLACEMENT THERAPIES

CAPD	Not dialysed. Dose as in normal renal function. See 'Other information'.
HD	Not dialysed. Dose as in normal renal function. See 'Other information'.
HDF/High flux	Unknown dialysability. Dose as in normal renal function. See 'Other information'.
CAV/ VVHD	Unlikely to be dialysed. Use lowest possible dose.

IMPORTANT DRUG INTERACTIONS

Potentially hazardous interactions with other drugs
- ACE inhibitors and angiotensin-II antagonists: antagonism of hypotensive effect, increased risk of nephrotoxicity and hyperkalaemia.
- Analgesics: avoid concomitant use of 2 or more NSAIDs, including aspirin (increased side effects); avoid with ketorolac, increased risk of side effects and haemorrhage.
- Antibacterials: possibly increased risk of convulsions with quinolones.
- Anticoagulants: effects of coumarins and phenindione enhanced; possibly increased risk of bleeding with heparins and dabigatran.
- Antidepressants: increased risk of bleeding with SSRIs and venlafaxine.
- Antidiabetic agents: effects of sulphonylureas enhanced.
- Anti-epileptics: possibly increased phenytoin concentration.
- Antivirals: increased risk of haematological toxicity with zidovudine; concentration possibly increased by ritonavir.
- Ciclosporin: may potentiate nephrotoxicity.
- Cytotoxic agents: reduced excretion of methotrexate; increased risk of bleeding with erlotinib.
- Diuretics: increased risk of nephrotoxicity; antagonism of diuretic effect; hyperkalaemia with potassium-sparing diuretics.
- Lithium: excretion decreased.
- Pentoxifylline: increased risk of bleeding.
- Tacrolimus: increased risk of nephrotoxicity.

ADMINISTRATION

RECONSTITUTION

–

ROUTE
- Oral

RATE OF ADMINISTRATION

–

COMMENTS
- Take with or after food.

OTHER INFORMATION

- Inhibition of renal prostaglandin synthesis by NSAIDs may interfere with renal function, especially in the presence of existing renal disease – avoid if possible; if not, check serum creatinine 48–72 hours after starting NSAID – if increased, discontinue therapy.
- In patients with renal, cardiac or hepatic impairment, especially those taking diuretics, caution is required since the use of NSAIDs may result in deterioration of renal function. The dose should be kept as low as possible and renal function should be monitored.
- Use normal doses in patients with ERF on dialysis if they do not pass any urine.
- Use with caution in renal transplant recipients – can reduce intrarenal autocoid synthesis.
- Accumulation of etodolac is unlikely in AKI, CKD or dialysis patients as it is metabolised in the liver.

Etomidate

CLINICAL USE

Induction of anaesthesia

DOSE IN NORMAL RENAL FUNCTION

150–300 mcg/kg, maximum total dose 60 mg with Hypnomidate®

PHARMACOKINETICS

Molecular weight (daltons)	244.3
% Protein binding	76
% Excreted unchanged in urine	2
Volume of distribution (L/kg)	2–4.5
Half-life – normal/ ESRF (hrs)	4–5/Unchanged

METABOLISM

Etomidate is rapidly redistributed from the CNS to other body tissues, and undergoes rapid metabolism in the liver and plasma. Pharmacokinetics are complex and have been described by both 2- and 3-compartment models. Etomidate is about 76% bound to plasma proteins. Etomidate is metabolised in the liver. After 24 hours, 75% of the administered dose of etomidate has been eliminated in the urine primarily as metabolites, although some is excreted in the bile. Only 2% of etomidate is excreted unchanged via the urine.

DOSE IN RENAL IMPAIRMENT GFR (mL/MIN)

20–50	Dose as in normal renal function.
10–20	Dose as in normal renal function.
<10	Dose as in normal renal function.

DOSE IN PATIENTS UNDERGOING RENAL REPLACEMENT THERAPIES

CAPD	Unknown dialysability. Dose as in normal renal function.
HD	Unknown dialysability. Dose as in normal renal function.
HDF/High flux	Unknown dialysability. Dose as in normal renal function.
CAV/ VVHD	Unknown dialysability. Dose as in normal renal function.

IMPORTANT DRUG INTERACTIONS

Potentially hazardous interactions with other drugs

- Adrenergic neurone blockers: enhanced hypotensive effect.
- Antihypertensives: enhanced hypotensive effect.
- Antidepressants: avoid MAOIs for 2 weeks before surgery; increased risk of arrhythmias and hypotension with tricyclics.
- Antipsychotics: enhanced hypotensive effect.

ADMINISTRATION

ROUTE
- Intravenous injection only

RATE OF ADMINISTRATION
–

COMMENTS
–

OTHER INFORMATION

- In cases of adrenocortical gland dysfunction and during very long surgical procedures, a prophylactic cortisol supplement may be required (e.g. 50–100 mg hydrocortisone).

Etoposide

CLINICAL USE

Antineoplastic agent

DOSE IN NORMAL RENAL FUNCTION

- IV: 50–120 mg/m^2 daily according to local protocol.
- Oral: 120–240 mg/m^2 daily.
  Or according to local protocol.

PHARMACOKINETICS

Molecular weight (daltons)	588.6
% Protein binding	74–94
% Excreted unchanged in urine	29
Volume of distribution (L/kg)	0.17–0.5
Half-life – normal/ ESRF (hrs)	4–11/19

METABOLISM

Etoposide is metabolised by the cytochrome P450 isoenzyme CYP3A4, yielding inactive metabolites.

Etoposide is excreted in urine and faeces as unchanged drug and metabolites: Approximately 45% of an administered dose is excreted in the urine, 29% being excreted unchanged in 72 hours. Up to 16% is recovered in the faeces.

DOSE IN RENAL IMPAIRMENT GFR (mL/MIN)

30–50	IV: 75% of dose and see 'Other information'. Oral: Dose as in normal renal function.
15–30	IV: 75% of dose and see 'Other information'. Oral: Dose as in normal renal function.
<15	IV: 50% of dose, based on clinical response and see 'Other information'. Oral: Dose as in normal renal function.

DOSE IN PATIENTS UNDERGOING RENAL REPLACEMENT THERAPIES

CAPD	Not dialysed. Dose as in GFR<15 mL/min.
HD	Not dialysed. Dose as in GFR<15 mL/min.
HDF/High flux	Not dialysed. Dose as in GFR<15 mL/min.
CAV/ VVHD	Unknown dialysability. Dose as in GFR=15–30 mL/min.

IMPORTANT DRUG INTERACTIONS

Potentially hazardous interactions with other drugs
- Anticoagulants: possibly enhanced anticoagulant effect with coumarins.
- Antipsychotics: avoid concomitant use with clozapine, increased risk of agranulocytosis.
- Ciclosporin: 50% reduction in etoposide clearance.

ADMINISTRATION

RECONSTITUTION
- 5–10 mL of infusion fluid or water for injection
ROUTE
- Oral, IV
RATE OF ADMINISTRATION
- IV infusion: 5 minutes – 3.5 hours
COMMENTS
- Dilute with sodium chloride 0.9% or glucose 5% to give a solution concentration as low as 100 mcg/mL of etoposide.

OTHER INFORMATION

- Avoid skin contact.
- One study suggested that patients with serum creatinine >130 μmol/L require a 30% dose reduction (Joel S, Clark P, Slevin M. Renal function and etoposide pharmacokinetics: is dose modification necessary? *Am Soc Clin Oncol.* 1991; **10**: 103). This dose adjustment was calculated to result in equivalent total dose exposure in patients with reduced renal function.
- Patients with a raised bilirubin and/or decreased albumin may have an increase in free etoposide and hence greater myelosuppression.
- Reaches high concentration in kidney: possible accumulation in renal impairment.
- Plasma clearance is reduced and volume of distribution increased in renal impairment.
- Kintzel PE, Dorr RT. Anticancer drug renal toxicity and elimination: dosing guidelines for altered renal function. *Cancer Treat Rev.* 1995; **21**: 33–64. – suggest 85% of dose for GFR 60 mL/min, 80% for 45 mL/min and 75% for 30 mL/min.

- Dose in severe renal impairment is from *Drug Prescribing in Renal Failure*, 5th edition, by Aronoff *et al.*
- Has been used without any problems in a haemodialysis patient, using a dose that increased gradually to 250 mg per treatment. (Holthius JJM, Van de Vyver FL, Van Oort WJ, *et al.* Pharmacokinetic evaluation of increased dosages of etoposide in a chronic haemodialysis patient. *Cancer Treat Rev.* 1985; **69**(11): 1279–82.)
- Bristol-Myers Squibb advise giving 75% of dose if GFR is 15–50 mL/min.

Etoricoxib

CLINICAL USE

Cox-2 inhibitor and analgesic

DOSE IN NORMAL RENAL FUNCTION

- RA: 90 mg once daily
- OA and other indications: 60 mg once daily
- Acute gout: 120 mg once daily

PHARMACOKINETICS

Molecular weight (daltons)	358.8
% Protein binding	92
% Excreted unchanged in urine	<1
Volume of distribution (L/kg)	120 litres
Half-life – normal/ ESRF (hrs)	22/Unchanged

METABOLISM

Etoricoxib is extensively metabolised with <1% of a dose recovered in urine as the parent drug. The major route of metabolism to form the 6'-hydroxymethyl derivative is catalysed by CYP enzymes. CYP3A4 appears to contribute to the metabolism of etoricoxib *in vivo*. Five metabolites have been identified in man. The principal metabolite is the 6'-carboxylic acid derivative of etoricoxib formed by further oxidation of the 6'-hydroxymethyl derivative. These principal metabolites either demonstrate no measurable activity or are only weakly active as COX-2 inhibitors. None of these metabolites inhibit COX-1.

Elimination of etoricoxib occurs almost exclusively through metabolism followed by renal excretion.

Following administration of a single 25-mg radiolabelled intravenous dose of etoricoxib to healthy subjects, 70% of radioactivity was recovered in urine and 20% in faeces, mostly as metabolites. Less than 2% was recovered as unchanged drug.

DOSE IN RENAL IMPAIRMENT GFR (mL/MIN)

20–50	Dose as in normal renal function, but avoid if possible.
10–20	Dose as in normal renal function, but avoid if possible.
<10	Dose as in normal renal function, but only use if on dialysis.

DOSE IN PATIENTS UNDERGOING RENAL REPLACEMENT THERAPIES

CAPD	Unknown dialysability. Dose as in normal renal function.
HD	Not dialysed. Dose as in normal renal function.
HDF/High flux	Unknown dialysability. Dose as in normal renal function.
CAV/VVHD	Unknown dialysability. Use lowest possible dose.

IMPORTANT DRUG INTERACTIONS

Potentially hazardous interactions with other drugs

- ACE inhibitors and angiotensin-II antagonists: antagonism of hypotensive effect; increased risk of nephrotoxicity and hyperkalaemia.
- Analgesics: avoid concomitant use of 2 or more NSAIDs, including aspirin (increased side effects); avoid with ketorolac, increased risk of side effects and haemorrhage.
- Antibacterials: possibly increased risk of convulsions with quinolones; concentration reduced by rifampicin.
- Anticoagulants: effects of coumarins and phenindione enhanced; possibly increased risk of bleeding with heparins and dabigatran.
- Antidepressants: increased risk of bleeding with SSRIs and venlafaxine.
- Antidiabetic agents: effects of sulphonylureas enhanced.
- Anti-epileptics: possibly increased phenytoin concentration.
- Antivirals: increased risk of haematological toxicity with zidovudine; concentration possibly increased by ritonavir.
- Ciclosporin: may potentiate nephrotoxicity.
- Cytotoxic agents: reduced excretion of methotrexate; increased risk of bleeding with erlotinib.

- Diuretics: increased risk of nephrotoxicity; antagonism of diuretic effect; hyperkalaemia with potassium-sparing diuretics.
- Lithium: excretion decreased.
- Pentoxifylline: increased risk of bleeding.
- Tacrolimus: increased risk of nephrotoxicity.

ADMINISTRATION

RECONSTITUTION

–

ROUTE

- Oral

RATE OF ADMINISTRATION

–

COMMENTS

- Take with or without food but onset of action is faster without food.

OTHER INFORMATION

- Clinical trials have shown renal effects similar to those observed with comparative NSAIDs. Monitor patient for deterioration in renal function and fluid retention.
- Inhibition of renal prostaglandin synthesis by NSAIDs may interfere with renal function, especially in the presence of existing renal disease – avoid if possible; if not, check serum creatinine 48–72 hours after starting NSAID – if raised, discontinue NSAID therapy.
- Use normal doses in patients with ERF on dialysis if they do not pass any urine.
- Use with caution in renal transplant recipients – can reduce intrarenal autocoid synthesis.
- Etoricoxib should be used with caution in uraemic patients predisposed to gastrointestinal bleeding or uraemic coagulopathies.

Etravirine

CLINICAL USE

Non-nucleoside reverse transcriptase
inhibitor:
- Treatment of HIV infection in
  combination with other antiretrovirals

DOSE IN NORMAL RENAL FUNCTION

200 mg twice daily

PHARMACOKINETICS

Molecular weight (daltons)	435.3
% Protein binding	99.9
% Excreted unchanged in urine	0 (1.2% as metabolites)
Volume of distribution (L/kg)	No data
Half-life – normal/ ESRF (hrs)	30–40/Probably unchanged

METABOLISM

Etravirine is extensively metabolised by
hepatic microsomal enzymes, mainly by
the cytochrome P450 isoenzymes CYP3A4,
CYP2C9, and CYP2C19, to substantially less
active metabolites.

Unchanged etravirine accounted for 81.2
to 86.4% of the administered dose in faeces.
Unchanged etravirine was not detected in
urine.

DOSE IN RENAL IMPAIRMENT GFR (mL/MIN)

20–50	Dose as in normal renal function.
10–20	Dose as in normal renal function.
<10	Dose as in normal renal function.

DOSE IN PATIENTS UNDERGOING RENAL REPLACEMENT THERAPIES

CAPD	Not dialysed. Dose as in normal renal function.
HD	Not dialysed. Dose as in normal renal function.
HDF/High flux	Not dialysed. Dose as in normal renal function.
CAV/ VVHD	Unknown dialysability. Dose as in normal renal function.

IMPORTANT DRUG INTERACTIONS

Potentially hazardous interactions with other
drugs
- Antibacterials: concentration increased
  by clarithromycin, also concentration of
  clarithromycin reduced; concentration of
  both drugs reduced with rifabutin; avoid
  concomitant use with rifampicin.
- Antivirals: concentration possibly
  reduced by efavirenz and nevirapine –
  avoid concomitant use; concentration
  of fosamprenavir increased, consider
  reducing fosamprenavir dose; possibly
  reduces indinavir concentration – avoid
  concomitant use; possibly reduces
  concentration of maraviroc; concentration
  reduced by tipranavir and tipranavir
  concentration increased – avoid
  concomitant use.
- Clopidogrel: possibly reduced antiplatelet
  effect.

ADMINISTRATION

RECONSTITUTION
–
ROUTE
- Oral
RATE OF ADMINISTRATION
–
COMMENTS
- Give after food

OTHER INFORMATION

- Etravirine is readily absorbed after oral
  doses and peak plasma concentrations
  occur after about 2.5 to 4 hours;
  absorption is increased by food.

Everolimus

CLINICAL USE

Protein kinase inhibitor:
1. Treatment of advanced renal cell carcinoma, breast cancer and neuroendocrine tumours
2. Renal angiomyolipoma associated with tuberous sclerosis complex
3. Prophylaxis of acute rejection in allogenic renal and cardiac transplants, in combination with ciclosporin and prednisolone – Unlicensed

DOSE IN NORMAL RENAL FUNCTION

1. Oral: 10 mg daily
2. Intravenous 0.75 mg twice daily
(Titrate according to levels – see 'Other information'.)

PHARMACOKINETICS

Molecular weight (daltons)	958.2
% Protein binding	74
% Excreted unchanged in urine	<5
Volume of distribution (L/kg)	235–449 litres
Half-life – normal/ESRF (hrs)	18–35/ Unchanged

METABOLISM

Everolimus is metabolised in the liver and to some extent in the gastrointestinal wall, and is a substrate of P-glycoprotein and the cytochrome P450 isoenzyme CYP3A4. Six main metabolites of everolimus have been detected in human blood, including three monohydroxylated metabolites, two hydrolytic ring-opened products, and a phosphatidylcholine conjugate of everolimus. These metabolites were shown to have approximately 100 times less activity than everolimus itself. Following the administration of a single dose of radiolabelled everolimus, 80% of the radioactivity was recovered from the faeces, while 5% was excreted in the urine. The parent substance was not detected in urine or faeces.

DOSE IN RENAL IMPAIRMENT GFR (mL/MIN)

20–50	Dose as in normal renal function.
10–20	Dose as in normal renal function.
<10	Dose as in normal renal function.

DOSE IN PATIENTS UNDERGOING RENAL REPLACEMENT THERAPIES

CAPD	Unknown dialysability. Dose as in normal renal function.
HD	Unknown dialysability. Dose as in normal renal function.
HDF/High flux	Unknown dialysability. Dose as in normal renal function.
CAV/ VVHD	Unknown dialysability. Dose as in normal renal function.

IMPORTANT DRUG INTERACTIONS

Potentially hazardous interactions with other drugs
- Ciclosporin: increases everolimus AUC by 168% and C_{max} by 82%.
- Antibacterials: erythromycin, clarithromycin and telithromycin increase everolimus levels – avoid with clarithromycin & telithromycin; rifampicin decreases everolimus levels by factor of 3.
- Antifungals: concentration increased by ketoconazole and possibly itraconazole, posaconazole and voriconazole – avoid.
- Antipsychotics: increased risk of agranulocytosis with clozapine – avoid.
- Antivirals: concentration possibly increased by atazanavir, darunavir, indinavir, ritonavir and saquinavir – avoid.
- Calcium-channel blockers: concentration of both drugs increased with verapamil.
- St John's wort: decreases everolimus levels.
- Grapefruit juice: increases everolimus levels.

ADMINISTRATION

RECONSTITUTION
–
ROUTE
- Oral
RATE OF ADMINISTRATION
–
COMMENTS
–

OTHER INFORMATION

- C_{max} and AUC are reduced by 60% and 16% respectively when everolimus is taken with a high fat meal. Take doses consistently either with or without food to achieve consistent blood levels.
- Patients achieving whole-blood trough levels of ≥3 ng/mL have been found to have a lower incidence of biopsy-proven acute rejection.

Exemestane

CLINICAL USE

Irreversible, steroidal aromatase inhibitor:
- Treatment of breast cancer

DOSE IN NORMAL RENAL FUNCTION

25 mg daily

PHARMACOKINETICS

Molecular weight (daltons)	296.4
% Protein binding	90
% Excreted unchanged in urine	<1
Volume of distribution (L/kg)	20 000 litres
Half-life – normal/ ESRF (hrs)	24/–

METABOLISM

Metabolised via oxidation by the cytochrome P450 isoenzyme CYP3A4, and via reduction by aldoketoreductase.

Metabolites are excreted in the urine (39–45%) and faeces (36–48%).

DOSE IN RENAL IMPAIRMENT GFR (mL/MIN)

20–50	Dose as in normal renal function.
10–20	Dose as in normal renal function.
<10	Dose as in normal renal function.

DOSE IN PATIENTS UNDERGOING RENAL REPLACEMENT THERAPIES

CAPD	Unlikely to be dialysed. Dose as in normal renal function.
HD	Unlikely to be dialysed. Dose as in normal renal function.
HDF/High flux	Unlikely to be dialysed. Dose as in normal renal function.
CAV/ VVHD	Unlikely to be dialysed. Dose as in normal renal function.

IMPORTANT DRUG INTERACTIONS

Potentially hazardous interactions with other drugs
- None known

ADMINISTRATION

RECONSTITUTION
–
ROUTE
- Oral
RATE OF ADMINISTRATION
–

OTHER INFORMATION

- In patients with severe renal impairment (CRCL <30 mL/min) the systemic exposure to exemestane was 2 times higher compared with healthy volunteers but due to the safety profile no dose alteration is required.

Exenatide

CLINICAL USE

Adjunctive therapy in type 2 diabetes
mellitus

DOSE IN NORMAL RENAL FUNCTION

5–10 mcg twice daily within 60 minutes
before the morning and evening meal
MR: 2 mg once weekly

PHARMACOKINETICS

Molecular weight (daltons)	4186.6
% Protein binding	No data
% Excreted unchanged in urine	Majority
Volume of distribution (L/kg)	28 litres
Half-life – normal/ ESRF (hrs)	2.4/5.95[1]

METABOLISM

Exenatide is eliminated through the
kidneys by glomerular filtration followed by
proteolytic degradation.

DOSE IN RENAL IMPAIRMENT GFR (mL/MIN)

30–50	Increase dose to 10 mcg with caution. Avoid MR.
10–30	Avoid. See 'Other information'.
<10	Avoid. See 'Other information'.

DOSE IN PATIENTS UNDERGOING RENAL REPLACEMENT THERAPIES

CAPD	Unknown dialysability. Dose as in GFR<10 mL/min.
HD	Unknown dialysability. Dose as in GFR<10 mL/min.
HDF/High flux	Unknown dialysability. Dose as in GFR<10 mL/min.
CAV/ VVHD	Unknown dialysability. Dose as in GFR=10–30 mL/min.

IMPORTANT DRUG INTERACTIONS

Potentially hazardous interactions with
other drugs
- Anticoagulants: possibly enhances
  anticoagulant effect of warfarin.
- Other nephrotoxins: avoid concomitant
  use.

ADMINISTRATION

RECONSTITUTION
–
ROUTE
- SC
RATE OF ADMINISTRATION
–
COMMENTS
–

OTHER INFORMATION

- Clearance is reduced by 84% in patients
  with established renal failure.
- US data sheet: Increased gastrointestinal
  side effects in patients with severe renal
  impairment and on dialysis.
- May cause renal failure including
  proteinuria. Avoid in patients with pre-
  existing renal impairment.

Reference:
1. www.medscape.com/viewarticle/521830_4

Ezetimibe

CLINICAL USE

Hypercholesterolaemia either in combination with a statin or as monotherapy

DOSE IN NORMAL RENAL FUNCTION

10 mg daily

PHARMACOKINETICS

Molecular weight (daltons)	409.4
% Protein binding	99.7
% Excreted unchanged in urine	11
Volume of distribution (L/kg)	No data
Half-life – normal/ ESRF (hrs)	22/–

METABOLISM

Ezetimibe is rapidly absorbed and extensively conjugated to a pharmacologically active phenolic glucuronide (ezetimibe-glucuronide). Ezetimibe is metabolised primarily in the small intestine and liver via glucuronide conjugation (a phase II reaction) with subsequent biliary excretion. Ezetimibe and ezetimibe-glucuronide are the major drug-derived compounds detected in plasma, constituting approximately 10–20% and 80–90% of the total drug in plasma, respectively. Both ezetimibe and ezetimibe-glucuronide are slowly eliminated from plasma with evidence of significant enterohepatic recycling. Following oral administration of ^{14}C-ezetimibe (20 mg) to human subjects, total ezetimibe accounted for approximately 93% of the total radioactivity in plasma. Approximately 78% and 11% of the administered radioactivity were recovered in the faeces and urine, respectively, over a 10-day collection period. After 48 hours, there were no detectable levels of radioactivity in the plasma.

DOSE IN RENAL IMPAIRMENT GFR (mL/MIN)

20–50	Dose as in normal renal function.
10–20	Dose as in normal renal function.
<10	Dose as in normal renal function.

DOSE IN PATIENTS UNDERGOING RENAL REPLACEMENT THERAPIES

CAPD	Unlikely to be dialysed. Dose as in normal renal function.
HD	Unlikely to be dialysed. Dose as in normal renal function.
HDF/High flux	Unlikely to be dialysed. Dose as in normal renal function.
CAV/ VVHD	Unlikely to be dialysed. Dose as in normal renal function.

IMPORTANT DRUG INTERACTIONS

Potentially hazardous interactions with other drugs
- Ciclosporin: concentration of both drugs possibly increased.
- Fibrates: avoid concomitant administration.

ADMINISTRATION

RECONSTITUTION
–
ROUTE
- Oral
RATE OF ADMINISTRATION
–
COMMENTS
–

OTHER INFORMATION

- When used with a statin LFTs should be monitored before initiation of therapy and then at regular intervals.
- If GFR<30 mL/min there is a 1.5 increase in the AUC of ezetimibe but no dose adjustment is required.
- Very rarely, cases of rhabdomyolysis have occurred – discontinue if myopathy is suspected.

Famciclovir

CLINICAL USE

Antiviral agent

DOSE IN NORMAL RENAL FUNCTION

- Zoster: 250 mg 3 times a day or 750 mg once daily.
- (Immunocompromised: 500 mg 3 times daily or 750 mg twice daily)
- First genital herpes infection: 250 mg 3 times a day.
- Acute recurrent genital herpes: 250 mg twice a day.
- (Immunocompromised: 500 mg twice a day)
- Suppression: 250 mg twice daily (HIV patients: 500 mg twice daily)
- Herpes simplex (Immunocompromised): 500 mg twice daily

PHARMACOKINETICS

Molecular weight (daltons)	321.3
% Protein binding	<20 as penciclovir
% Excreted unchanged in urine	0
Volume of distribution (L/kg)	0.91–1.25
Half-life – normal/ ESRF (hrs)	2 (penciclovir)/3.2–23.6 (3.8–25: penciclovir)

METABOLISM

Famciclovir is a pro-drug; it is rapidly converted to penciclovir; virtually no famciclovir is detectable in the plasma or urine. Bioavailability of penciclovir is reported to be 77%. Famciclovir is mainly excreted in the urine (partly by renal tubular secretion) as penciclovir and its 6-deoxy precursor. No unchanged famciclovir has been detected in urine.

DOSE IN RENAL IMPAIRMENT GFR (mL/MIN)

For immunocompromised patients, see 'Other information'.

30–59	Zoster, and first episode genital herpes: 250 mg once daily. Recurrent genital herpes: 250 mg once daily. Suppression: Dose as in normal renal function.
10–29	Zoster, and first episode genital herpes: 125 mg once daily. Recurrent genital herpes: 125 mg once daily. Suppression: 125 mg twice daily
<10	Zoster, and first episode genital herpes: 250 mg 3 times a week. Recurrent genital herpes: 125 mg 3 times a week.

DOSE IN PATIENTS UNDERGOING RENAL REPLACEMENT THERAPIES

CAPD	Moderate dialysability likely. Dose as in GFR<10 mL/min.
HD	Dialysed. Dose as in GFR<10 mL/min post dialysis on dialysis days.
HDF/High flux	Dialysed. Dose as in GFR<10 mL/min post dialysis on dialysis days.
CAV/ VVHD	Likely dialysability. Dose as in GFR=10–29 mL/min.

IMPORTANT DRUG INTERACTIONS

Potentially hazardous interactions with other drugs

- Probenecid: decreased excretion of famciclovir.
- Increased famciclovir levels reported with mycophenolate mofetil.

ADMINISTRATION

RECONSTITUTION

–

ROUTE

- Oral

RATE OF ADMINISTRATION

–

COMMENTS

–

OTHER INFORMATION

- Treatment of herpes infections in immunocompromised patients

GFR (mL/min)	Dose	
	Zoster	Simplex
30–59	250 mg 2×/day	250 mg 2×/day
10–29	125 mg 1×/day	125 mg 2×/day

- Four hours' haemodialysis results in approximately 75% reduction in plasma concentration of penciclovir.

Famotidine

CLINICAL USE

H_2-blocker:
- Conditions associated with hyperacidity

DOSE IN NORMAL RENAL FUNCTION

20–80 mg daily
- Zollinger-Ellison syndrome: 80–800 mg daily in divided doses.

PHARMACOKINETICS

Molecular weight (daltons)	337.4
% Protein binding	15–20
% Excreted unchanged in urine	25–30
Volume of distribution (L/kg)	1.1–1.4
Half-life – normal/ ESRF (hrs)	3/>20

METABOLISM

Metabolism of famotidine occurs in the liver, with formation of an inactive metabolite, the sulfoxide. Following oral administration, the mean urinary excretion of famotidine is 65–70% of the absorbed dose, 25–30% as unchanged compound. Renal clearance is 250 to 450 mL/min, indicating some tubular excretion. A small amount may be excreted as the sulfoxide.

DOSE IN RENAL IMPAIRMENT GFR (mL/MIN)

20–50	50% of normal dose or increase dose to every 36–48 hours.
10–20	50% of normal dose or increase dose to every 36–48 hours.
<10	20 mg at night (maximum or increase dose to every 36–48 hours).

DOSE IN PATIENTS UNDERGOING RENAL REPLACEMENT THERAPIES

CAPD	Not dialysed. Dose as in GFR<10 mL/min.
HD	Not dialysed. Dose as in GFR<10 mL/min.
HDF/High flux	Not dialysed. Dose as in GFR<10 mL/min.
CAV/VVHD	Not dialysed. Dose as in GFR=10–20 mL/min.

IMPORTANT DRUG INTERACTIONS

Potentially hazardous interactions with other drugs
- Antifungals: absorption of itraconazole and ketoconazole reduced; concentration of posaconazole possibly reduced – avoid.
- Antivirals: concentration of atazanavir reduced; concentration of raltegravir possibly increased – avoid; avoid for 12 hours before and 4 hours after rilpivirine.
- Ciclosporin: possibly increased ciclosporin levels.
- Cytotoxics: possibly reduced dasatinib concentration; avoid with erlotinib; possibly reduced absorption of pazopanib – give at least 2 hours before or 10 hours after famotidine; possibly reduced absorption of lapatinib.
- Ulipristal: contraceptive effect possibly reduced – avoid with high dose ulipristal.

ADMINISTRATION

RECONSTITUTION
–
ROUTE
- Oral
RATE OF ADMINISTRATION
–

COMMENTS
–

OTHER INFORMATION

- CNS effects have been seen in patients with moderate to severe renal impairment.
- Contraindicated in UK SPC in moderate to severe renal impairment but doses in monograph are from US data sheet.

Febuxostat

CLINICAL USE

Xanthine oxidase inhibitor
● Treatment of chronic gout

DOSE IN NORMAL RENAL FUNCTION

80–120 mg daily

PHARMACOKINETICS

Molecular weight (daltons)	316.4
% Protein binding	99.2
% Excreted unchanged in urine	3 (49% as metabolites)
Volume of distribution (L/kg)	29–75 litres
Half-life – normal/ ESRF (hrs)	5–8/Increased

METABOLISM

Extensively metabolised by conjugation via the uridine diphosphate glucuronosyltransferase (UDPGT) enzyme system, and by oxidation via the cytochrome P450 isoenzyme system to form active metabolites.

About 49% of a dose is excreted via the urine, and 45% via the faeces (12% as unchanged drug).

DOSE IN RENAL IMPAIRMENT GFR (mL/MIN)

30–50	Dose as in normal renal function.
10–30	Start with 40 mg and monitor closely. See 'Other information'.
<10	Start with 40 mg and monitor closely. See 'Other information'.

DOSE IN PATIENTS UNDERGOING RENAL REPLACEMENT THERAPIES

CAPD	Unlikely to be dialysed. Dose as in GFR<10 mL/min.
HD	Unlikely to be dialysed. Dose as in GFR<10 mL/min.
HDF/High flux	Unlikely to be dialysed. Dose as in GFR<10 mL/min.
CAV/ VVHD	Unlikely to be dialysed. Dose as in GFR=10–30 mL/min.

IMPORTANT DRUG INTERACTIONS

Potentially hazardous interactions with other drugs
● Azathioprine: avoid concomitant use, increased risk of neutropenia.
● Cytotoxics: avoid concomitant use with mercaptopurine.
● Theophylline: use with caution.

ADMINISTRATION

RECONSTITUTION
–
ROUTE
● Oral
RATE OF ADMINISTRATION
–

OTHER INFORMATION

● Not recommended in UK SPC in severe renal impairment due to lack of data.
● Advise to use with caution in severe renal impairment in US data sheet, starting with a dose of 40 mg in moderate renal impairment.
● In patients with severe renal impairment (GFR=10–29), peak plasma concentrations of febuxostat did not alter compared to those with normal renal function; although the mean AUC was increased by 1.8.
● A study found that although exposure to febuxostat and its metabolites was generally higher in subjects with increasing degrees of renal impairment, decreases in uric acid were comparable regardless of renal function.[1]
● Treatment in patients with ischaemic heart disease or congestive heart failure is not recommended.
● There have been 2 case reports of febuxostat causing neutropenia in 2 haemodialysis patients.[2]
● There is a series of cases from Japan using febuxostat in haemodialysis patients at a dose of 10–20 mg daily with good effect.[3]

References:
1. Mayer MD, et al. Pharmacokinetics and pharmacodynamics of febuxostat, a new non-purine selective inhibitor of xanthine oxidase in subjects with renal impairment. Am J Ther. 2005; 12: 22–34.

2. Kobayashi S, Ogura M, Hosoya T. Acute neutropenia associated with initiation of febuxostat therapy for hyperuricaemia in patients with chronic kidney disease. *J Clin Pharm Ther.* 2013 Jun; **38**(3): 258–61.

3. Horikoshi R, Akimoto T, Inoue M, *et al.* Febuxostat for hyperuricemia: experience with patients on chronic hemodialysis treatment. *Clin Exp Nephrol.* February 2013; **17**(1): 149–50.

Felodipine

CLINICAL USE

Calcium-channel blocker:
- Hypertension
- Angina

DOSE IN NORMAL RENAL FUNCTION

Hypertension: 5–20 mg once daily
Angina: 5–10 mg daily

PHARMACOKINETICS

Molecular weight (daltons)	384.3
% Protein binding	99
% Excreted unchanged in urine	<0.5
Volume of distribution (L/kg)	10
Half-life – normal/ ESRF (hrs)	24/Unchanged

METABOLISM

Felodipine is metabolised in the liver and all identified metabolites are devoid of vasodilating properties.

Approximately 70% of a given dose is excreted as metabolites in the urine and about 10% with the faeces. Less than 0.5% of the dose is excreted unchanged in the urine.

DOSE IN RENAL IMPAIRMENT GFR (mL/MIN)

20–50	Dose as in normal renal function.
10–20	Dose as in normal renal function.
<10	Dose as in normal renal function.

DOSE IN PATIENTS UNDERGOING RENAL REPLACEMENT THERAPIES

CAPD	Not dialysed. Dose as in normal renal function.
HD	Not dialysed. Dose as in normal renal function.
HDF/High flux	Not dialysed. Dose as in normal renal function.
CAV/ VVHD	Not dialysed. Dose as in normal renal function.

IMPORTANT DRUG INTERACTIONS

Potentially hazardous interactions with other drugs
- Anaesthetics: enhanced hypotensive effect.
- Antibacterials metabolism possibly inhibited by clarithromycin, erythromycin & telithromycin.
- Antidepressants: enhanced hypotensive effect with MAOIs.
- Anti-epileptics: effect reduced by carbamazepine, barbiturates, phenytoin and primidone.
- Antifungals: metabolism inhibited by itraconazole and ketoconazole; negative inotropic effect possibly increased with itraconazole.
- Antihypertensives: enhanced hypotensive effect, increased risk of first dose hypotensive effect of post-synaptic alpha-blockers.
- Antivirals: concentration possibly increased by ritonavir; use with caution with telaprevir.
- Grapefruit juice: concentration increased – avoid concomitant use.
- Tacrolimus: possibly increased tacrolimus concentration.
- Theophylline: possibly increased theophylline concentration.

ADMINISTRATION

RECONSTITUTION
-

ROUTE
- Oral

RATE OF ADMINISTRATION
-

COMMENTS
-

Fenofibrate

CLINICAL USE

Treatment of hyperlipidaemias types IIa, IIb, III, IV and V

DOSE IN NORMAL RENAL FUNCTION

Depends on preparation

PHARMACOKINETICS

Molecular weight (daltons)	360.8
% Protein binding	99
% Excreted unchanged in urine	0
Volume of distribution (L/kg)	0.89
Half-life – normal/ ESRF (hrs)	20/140–360

METABOLISM

After oral administration, fenofibrate is rapidly hydrolysed by esterases to the active metabolite fenofibric acid.

No unchanged fenofibrate can be detected in the plasma. Fenofibric acid is excreted mainly in the urine, mainly as the glucuronide conjugate, but also as a reduced form of fenofibric acid and its glucuronide; practically all the drug is eliminated from the body within 6 days.

DOSE IN RENAL IMPAIRMENT GFR (mL/MIN)

20–60	134 mg daily
10–20	67 mg daily
<10	Avoid.

DOSE IN PATIENTS UNDERGOING RENAL REPLACEMENT THERAPIES

CAPD	Unlikely to be dialysed. Avoid.
HD	Not dialysed. Avoid.
HDF/High flux	Unlikely to be dialysed. Avoid.
CAV/ VVHD	Unlikely to be dialysed. Dose as in GFR=10–20 mL/min.

IMPORTANT DRUG INTERACTIONS

Potentially hazardous interactions with other drugs

- Antibacterials: increased risk of myopathy with daptomycin – try to avoid concomitant use.
- Anticoagulants: enhances effect of coumarins and phenindione; dose of anticoagulant should be reduced by up to 50% and readjusted by monitoring INR.
- Antidiabetics: may improve glucose tolerance and have an additive effect with insulin or sulphonylureas.
- Ciclosporin: ciclosporin levels appear to be unaffected; however, it is recommended that concomitant therapy should be avoided because of the possibility of elevated serum creatinine levels.
- Colchicine: possible increased risk of myopathy.
- Lipid-regulating drugs: increased risk of myopathy in combination with statins and ezetimibe (maximum 20 mg of rosuvastatin); increased risk of cholelithiasis and gallbladder disease with ezetimibe – avoid with ezetimibe.

ADMINISTRATION

RECONSTITUTION

–

ROUTE

- Oral

RATE OF ADMINISTRATION

–

COMMENTS

–

OTHER INFORMATION

- A few studies have noted that use of second-generation fibrates in transplant recipients is hampered by frequent rises in serum creatinine.
- Avoid use in patients with GFR<10 mL/ min due to increased risk of rhabdomyolysis.
- Contraindicated by manufacturer if GFR<20 mL/min.

Fenoprofen

CLINICAL USE

NSAID and analgesic

DOSE IN NORMAL RENAL FUNCTION

300–600 mg 3–4 times a day; maximum 3 g daily.

PHARMACOKINETICS

Molecular weight (daltons)	558.6 (as calcium salt)
% Protein binding	>99
% Excreted unchanged in urine	2–5
Volume of distribution (L/kg)	0.10
Half-life – normal/ ESRF (hrs)	3/Unchanged

METABOLISM

Approximately 90% of a dose is excreted in the urine in 24 hours, chiefly as the glucuronide and the glucuronide of hydroxylated fenoprofen.

DOSE IN RENAL IMPAIRMENT GFR (mL/MIN)

20–50	Start with low dose, but avoid if possible.
10–20	Start with low dose, but avoid if possible.
<10	Start with low dose, but only use if on dialysis.

DOSE IN PATIENTS UNDERGOING RENAL REPLACEMENT THERAPIES

CAPD	Unlikely to be dialysed. Start with low doses and increase according to response. See 'Other information'.
HD	Not dialysed. Start with low doses and increase according to response. See 'Other information'.
HDF/High flux	Not dialysed. Start with low doses and increase according to response. See 'Other information'.
CAV/ VVHD	Not dialysed. Dose as in GFR=10–20 mL/min. See 'Other information'.

IMPORTANT DRUG INTERACTIONS

Potentially hazardous interactions with other drugs

- ACE inhibitors and angiotensin-II antagonists: increased risk of hyperkalaemia and nephrotoxicity; reduced hypotensive effect.
- Analgesics: avoid concomitant use with other NSAIDs or aspirin; avoid concomitant use with ketorolac (increased side effects and haemorrhage).
- Antibacterials: possibly increased risk of convulsions with quinolones.
- Anticoagulants: effects of coumarins and phenindione enhanced; possibly increased risk of bleeding with heparins and dabigatran.
- Antidepressants: increased risk of bleeding with SSRIs or venlafaxine.
- Antidiabetic agents: effects of sulphonylureas enhanced.
- Anti-epileptics: possibly enhanced effect of phenytoin.
- Antivirals: concentration possibly increased by ritonavir; increased risk of haematological toxicity with zidovudine.
- Ciclosporin: may potentiate nephrotoxicity.
- Cytotoxic agents: reduced excretion of methotrexate; increased risk of bleeding with erlotinib.
- Lithium: excretion reduced.
- Diuretics: increased risk of nephrotoxicity; antagonism of diuretic effect; hyperkalaemia with potassium-sparing diuretics.
- Pentoxifylline: increased risk of bleeding.
- Tacrolimus: increased risk of nephrotoxicity.

ADMINISTRATION

RECONSTITUTION

–

ROUTE
- Oral

RATE OF ADMINISTRATION

–

COMMENTS

–

OTHER INFORMATION

- Contraindicated in patients with history of significantly impaired renal function.
- Inhibition of renal prostaglandin synthesis by NSAIDs may interfere with renal function, especially in the presence

of existing renal disease – avoid use if possible; if not, check serum creatinine 48–72 hours after starting NSAID – if it has increased, discontinue therapy.
- Possibility of decreased platelet aggregation.
- Can use normal doses in patients with ERF on dialysis.
- Use with caution in renal transplant recipients – can reduce intrarenal autocoid synthesis.
- Associated with nephrotic syndrome, interstitial nephritis, hyperkalaemia, sodium retention.

Fentanyl

CLINICAL USE

Opioid analgesic:
- Short surgical procedures
- Ventilated patients
- Chronic intractable pain

DOSE IN NORMAL RENAL FUNCTION

- IV injection:
  - with spontaneous respiration: 50–200 mcg, then 25–50 mcg as required.
  - with assisted ventilation: 0.3–3.5 mg, then 100–200 mcg as required.
- IV infusion:
  - with spontaneous respiration: 3–4.8 micrograms/kg/hour adjusted according to response.
  - with assisted ventilation: 10 mcg/kg over 10 minutes, then 6 mcg/kg/hour, may require up to 180 mcg/kg/hr during cardiac surgery.
- Topical (chronic pain): Initially 12–25 mcg/hour, patches changed every 72 hours increased according to response.
- Oral: varies according to preparation, see SPC for more information.
- Nasal spray: varies according to preparation, see SPC for more information.

PHARMACOKINETICS

Molecular weight (daltons)	336.5
% Protein binding	80–85
% Excreted unchanged in urine	<7
Volume of distribution (L/kg)	4
Half-life – normal/ESRF (hrs)	2–7/Possibly increased

METABOLISM

Fentanyl is metabolised in the liver by N-dealkylation and hydroxylation via the cytochrome P450 isoenzyme CYP3A4. Metabolites and some unchanged drug are excreted mainly in the urine. The short duration of action is probably due to rapid redistribution into the tissues rather than metabolism and excretion. The relatively longer elimination half-life reflects slower release from tissue depots.

The main metabolites of fentanyl, which are excreted in the urine, have been identified as 4-N-(N-propionylanilino) piperidine and 4-N-(N-hydroxypropionylanilino) piperidine; 1-(2-phenethyl)-4-N-(N-hydroxypropionylanilino) piperidine is a minor metabolite. Fentanyl has no active or toxic metabolites.

DOSE IN RENAL IMPAIRMENT GFR (mL/MIN)

20–50	75% of normal dose. Titrate according to response.
10–20	75% of normal dose. Titrate according to response.
<10	50% of normal dose. Titrate according to response.

DOSE IN PATIENTS UNDERGOING RENAL REPLACEMENT THERAPIES

CAPD	Not dialysed. Dose as in GFR<10 mL/min.
HD	Not dialysed. Dose as in GFR<10 mL/min.
HDF/High flux	Not dialysed. Dose as in GFR<10 mL/min.
CAV/VVHD	Not dialysed. Dose as in GFR=10–20 mL/min.

IMPORTANT DRUG INTERACTIONS

Potentially hazardous interactions with other drugs
- Antibacterials: metabolism increased by rifampicin.
- Antidepressants: possible CNS excitation or depression (hypertension or hypotension) in patients also receiving MAOIs (including moclobemide) – avoid concomitant use; possibly increased sedative effects with tricyclics.
- Antifungals: concentration increased by triazoles.
- Antihistamines: increased sedative effects with sedating antihistamines.
- Antipsychotics: enhanced hypotensive and sedative effects.
- Antivirals: concentration increased by ritonavir; increased risk of ventricular arrhythmias with saquinavir – avoid.
- Cytotoxics: use crizotinib with caution.
- Dopaminergics: avoid with selegiline.
- Sodium oxybate: enhanced effect of sodium oxybate – avoid concomitant use.

ADMINISTRATION

RECONSTITUTION

–

ROUTE

- IV, IM, topically buccal, sublingual, intranasal

RATE OF ADMINISTRATION

–

COMMENTS

- Compatible with sodium chloride 0.9% and glucose 5%.

OTHER INFORMATION

- For short surgical procedures the degree of renal impairment is irrelevant.
- For other indications, renal impairment may have a moderate effect on the elimination of the drug; however, as fentanyl is titrated to response the usual dose and method of administration remain valid.
- Doses in renal impairment are from *Drug Prescribing in Renal Failure*, 5th edition, by Aronoff *et al.*
- Like other opiates, start with a low dose and titrate as tolerated.

Ferric carboxymaltose

CLINICAL USE

Ferric carboxymaltose complex:
- Treatment of iron deficiency anaemia (when oral treatment is ineffective or contraindicated)

DOSE IN NORMAL RENAL FUNCTION

Dose calculated according to weight.

PHARMACOKINETICS

Molecular weight (daltons)	Approx 150 000
% Protein binding	No data
% Excreted unchanged in urine	0.0005[1]
Volume of distribution (L/kg)	3 litres
Half-life – normal/ ESRF (hrs)	7–12/–

METABOLISM

Most absorbed iron is bound to transferrin and transported to the bone marrow where it is incorporated into haemoglobin; the remainder is contained within the storage forms, ferritin or haemosiderin, or as myoglobin, with smaller amounts occurring in haem-containing enzymes or in plasma bound to transferrin. Only very small amounts of iron are excreted as the majority released after the destruction of the haemoglobin molecule is reused.

DOSE IN RENAL IMPAIRMENT GFR (mL/MIN)

20–50	Dose as in normal renal function.
10–20	Dose as in normal renal function.
<10	Dose as in normal renal function.

DOSE IN PATIENTS UNDERGOING RENAL REPLACEMENT THERAPIES

CAPD	Not dialysed. Dose as in normal renal function.
HD	Not dialysed. Dose as in normal renal function.
HDF/High flux	Not dialysed. Dose as in normal renal function.
CAV/ VVHD	Not dialysed. Dose as in normal renal function.

IMPORTANT DRUG INTERACTIONS

Potentially hazardous interactions with other drugs
- Dimercaprol: avoid concomitant use.
- Oral iron: reduced absorption.

ADMINISTRATION

RECONSTITUTION
–
ROUTE
- IV

RATE OF ADMINISTRATION
- Bolus (undiluted): 200–500 mg at a rate of 100 mg/min
- Doses >500 mg over 15 minutes

COMMENTS
- Doses 100–200 mg can be added to a maximum of 50 mL sodium chloride 0.9%
- Doses 200–500 mg can be added to a maximum of 100 mL sodium chloride 0.9%
- Doses >500 mg can be added to a maximum of 250 mL sodium chloride 0.9%
- Patients should be monitored during and for 30 minutes after administration.

OTHER INFORMATION

- After a single 100 mg IV iron dose of ferric carboxymaltose (n=6) injected over 1 min, serum iron concentration peaked at a mean of 15 min. After 500, 800 or 1000 mg iron in 250 mL normal saline infused over 15 min (n=6 for each dose), serum iron concentration peaked at means of 20 min, 1 hour and 1.2 hours, respectively. (www.medsafe.govt.nz/profs/datasheet/f/ferinjectinj.pdf).

Reference:
1. Geisser P, Banké-Bochita J. Pharmacokinetics, safety and tolerability of intravenous ferric carboxymaltose: a dose-escalation study in volunteers with mild iron-deficiency anaemia. *Arzneimittelforschung*. 2010; **60**(6a): 362–72.

Ferrous fumarate

CLINICAL USE

Iron deficiency anaemia

DOSE IN NORMAL RENAL FUNCTION

Dose varies according to preparation

PHARMACOKINETICS

Molecular weight (daltons)	169.9
% Protein binding	–
% Excreted unchanged in urine	–
Volume of distribution (L/kg)	–
Half-life – normal/ ESRF (hrs)	–

METABOLISM

Following absorption, the majority of iron is bound to transferrin and transported to the bone marrow where it is incorporated into haemoglobin. The remainder is stored within ferritin or haemosiderin or is incorporated into myoglobin with smaller amounts occurring in haem-containing enzymes or in plasma bound to transferrin. Only very small amounts are excreted as the body reabsorbs the iron after the haemoglobin has broken down.

DOSE IN RENAL IMPAIRMENT GFR (mL/MIN)

20–50	Dose as in normal renal function.
10–20	Dose as in normal renal function.
<10	Dose as in normal renal function.

DOSE IN PATIENTS UNDERGOING RENAL REPLACEMENT THERAPIES

CAPD	Not dialysed. Dose as in normal renal function.
HD	Not dialysed. Dose as in normal renal function.
HDF/High flux	Not dialysed. Dose as in normal renal function.
CAV/ VVHD	Not dialysed. Dose as in normal renal function.

IMPORTANT DRUG INTERACTIONS

Potentially hazardous interactions with other drugs
- Antibacterials: reduced absorption of 4-quinolones and tetracyclines.
- Dimercaprol: avoid concomitant use.
- Mycophenolate: may significantly reduce absorption of mycophenolate.

ADMINISTRATION

RECONSTITUTION
–
ROUTE
- Oral
RATE OF ADMINISTRATION
–
COMMENTS
–

OTHER INFORMATION

- Absorption of iron may be enhanced with concurrent administration of ascorbic acid.
- Phosphate binding agents, e.g. calcium carbonate or magnesium carbonate, reduce absorption of iron from the gut.
- Absorption may be impaired in patients with CKD due to upregulation of hepcidin – consider using IV iron.
- Monitor: serum iron, transferrin saturation and ferritin levels (in line with local policy).

Ferrous gluconate

CLINICAL USE

Iron deficiency anaemia

DOSE IN NORMAL RENAL FUNCTION

- Prophylaxis: 2 tablets daily
- Therapeutic: 4–6 tablets daily in divided doses

PHARMACOKINETICS

Molecular weight (daltons)	482.2
% Protein binding	–
% Excreted unchanged in urine	–
Volume of distribution (L/kg)	–
Half-life – normal/ ESRF (hrs)	–

METABOLISM

Following absorption, the majority of iron is bound to transferrin and transported to the bone marrow where it is incorporated into haemoglobin. The remainder is stored within ferritin or haemosiderin or is incorporated into myoglobin with smaller amounts occurring in haem-containing enzymes or in plasma bound to transferrin. Only very small amounts are excreted as the body reabsorbs the iron after the haemoglobin has broken down.

DOSE IN RENAL IMPAIRMENT GFR (mL/MIN)

20–50	Dose as in normal renal function.
10–20	Dose as in normal renal function.
<10	Dose as in normal renal function.

DOSE IN PATIENTS UNDERGOING RENAL REPLACEMENT THERAPIES

CAPD	Not dialysed. Dose as in normal renal function.
HD	Not dialysed. Dose as in normal renal function.
HDF/High flux	Not dialysed. Dose as in normal renal function.
CAV/ VVHD	Not dialysed. Dose as in normal renal function.

IMPORTANT DRUG INTERACTIONS

Potentially hazardous interactions with other drugs
- Antibacterials: reduced absorption of 4-quinolones and tetracyclines.
- Dimercaprol: avoid concomitant use.
- Mycophenolate: may significantly reduce absorption of mycophenolate.

ADMINISTRATION

RECONSTITUTION

–

ROUTE
- Oral

RATE OF ADMINISTRATION

–

COMMENTS

–

OTHER INFORMATION

- One 300 mg ferrous gluconate tablet contains 35 mg elemental iron.
- Best taken before food to aid absorption.
- Phosphate binding agents, e.g. calcium carbonate or magnesium carbonate, reduce absorption of iron from the gut.
- Absorption may be impaired in patients with CKD due to upregulation of hepcidin – consider using IV iron.
- Monitor serum iron, transferrin saturation and ferritin levels (in line with local policy).

Ferrous sulphate

CLINICAL USE

Iron deficiency anaemia

DOSE IN NORMAL RENAL FUNCTION

- Prophylaxis: 200 mg daily
- Therapeutic: 200 mg 2–3 times daily
- M/R: 1–2 tablets/capsules daily

PHARMACOKINETICS

Molecular weight (daltons)	278
% Protein binding	–
% Excreted unchanged in urine	–
Volume of distribution (L/kg)	–
Half-life – normal/ ESRF (hrs)	–

METABOLISM

Following absorption, the majority of iron is bound to transferrin and transported to the bone marrow where it is incorporated into haemoglobin. The remainder is stored within ferritin or haemosiderin or is incorporated into myoglobin with smaller amounts occurring in haem-containing enzymes or in plasma bound to transferrin. Only very small amounts are excreted as the body reabsorbs the iron after the haemoglobin has broken down.

DOSE IN RENAL IMPAIRMENT GFR (mL/MIN)

20–50	Dose as in normal renal function
10–20	Dose as in normal renal function.
<10	Dose as in normal renal function.

DOSE IN PATIENTS UNDERGOING RENAL REPLACEMENT THERAPIES

CAPD	Not dialysed. Dose as in normal renal function.
HD	Not dialysed. Dose as in normal renal function.
HDF/High flux	Not dialysed. Dose as in normal renal function.
CAV/ VVHD	Not dialysed. Dose as in normal renal function.

IMPORTANT DRUG INTERACTIONS

Potentially hazardous interactions with other drugs

- Antibacterials: reduced absorption of 4-quinolones and tetracyclines.
- Dimercaprol: avoid concomitant use.
- Mycophenolate: may significantly reduce absorption of mycophenolate.

ADMINISTRATION

RECONSTITUTION

–

ROUTE

- Oral

RATE OF ADMINISTRATION

–

COMMENTS

–

OTHER INFORMATION

- One 200 mg ferrous sulphate tablet contains 65 mg elemental iron.
- Absorption of iron may be enhanced with concurrent administration of ascorbic acid.
- Phosphate binding agents, e.g. calcium carbonate or magnesium carbonate, reduce absorption of iron from the gut.
- Absorption may be impaired in patients with CKD due to upregulation of hepcidin – consider using IV iron.
- Monitor: serum iron, transferrin saturation and ferritin levels (in line with local policy).

Ferumoxytol

CLINICAL USE

Colloidal iron-carbohydrate complex:
- Prophylaxis of iron deficiency anaemia in CKD (when oral treatment is ineffective or contraindicated)

DOSE IN NORMAL RENAL FUNCTION

- Weight <50 kg & Hb >10–12 g/dL: 510 mg
- Weight >50 kg or Hb <10 g/dL: 1020 mg in 2 divided doses, 2nd dose should be 2–8 days later.

PHARMACOKINETICS

Molecular weight (daltons)	750 000
% Protein binding	No data
% Excreted unchanged in urine	No data
Volume of distribution (L/kg)	2.71 litres[1]
Half-life – normal/ ESRF (hrs)	16/Unchanged

METABOLISM

Most absorbed iron is bound to transferrin and transported to the bone marrow where it is incorporated into haemoglobin; the remainder is contained within the storage forms, ferritin or haemosiderin, or as myoglobin, with smaller amounts occurring in haem-containing enzymes or in plasma bound to transferrin. Only very small amounts of iron are excreted as the majority released after the destruction of the haemoglobin molecule is reused.

DOSE IN RENAL IMPAIRMENT GFR (mL/MIN)

20–50	Dose as in normal renal function.
10–20	Dose as in normal renal function.
<10	Dose as in normal renal function.

DOSE IN PATIENTS UNDERGOING RENAL REPLACEMENT THERAPIES

CAPD	Not dialysed. Dose as in normal renal function.
HD	Not dialysed. Dose as in normal renal function.
HDF/High flux	Not dialysed. Dose as in normal renal function.
CAV/ VVHD	Not dialysed. Dose as in normal renal function.

IMPORTANT DRUG INTERACTIONS

Potentially hazardous interactions with other drugs
- Dimercaprol: avoid concomitant use.
- Oral iron: reduced absorption.

ADMINISTRATION

RECONSTITUTION
–
ROUTE
- IV
RATE OF ADMINISTRATION
- 30 mg/second (1 mL/second)
COMMENTS
- Patients should be monitored during and for 30 minutes after administration.

OTHER INFORMATION

- Do not give if Hb >12 g/dL.
- Peak plasma concentrations of ferumoxytol occur about 20 minutes after intravenous injection.

Reference:
1. Pai AB, Nielsen JC, Kausz A, *et al.* Plasma pharmacokinetics of two consecutive doses of ferumoxytol in healthy subjects. *Clin Pharmacol Ther.* 2010 Aug; **88**(2): 237–42.

Fesoterodine fumarate

CLINICAL USE

Antimuscarinic:
- Symptomatic treatment of urinary incontinence, frequency or urgency

DOSE IN NORMAL RENAL FUNCTION

4–8 mg once daily

PHARMACOKINETICS

Molecular weight (daltons)	527.7
% Protein binding	50 (metabolite)
% Excreted unchanged in urine	70 (as metabolites)
Volume of distribution (L/kg)	169 litres
Half-life – normal/ ESRF (hrs)	7/–

METABOLISM

Rapidly and extensively hydrolysed to its active metabolite. The active metabolite is further metabolised in the liver to its carboxy, carboxy-N-desisopropyl, and N-desisopropyl metabolites via two major pathways involving CYP2D6 and CYP3A4. None of these metabolites contribute significantly to the antimuscarinic activity of fesoterodine.

Approximately 70% of an oral dose of fesoterodine is recovered in the urine as metabolites, and a smaller amount in the faeces.

DOSE IN RENAL IMPAIRMENT GFR (mL/MIN)

50–80	Dose as in normal renal function.
30–50	Dose as in normal renal function. See 'Other information'.
<30	4 mg daily. See 'Other information'.

DOSE IN PATIENTS UNDERGOING RENAL REPLACEMENT THERAPIES

CAPD	Probably dialysed. Dose as in GFR<30 mL/min.
HD	Probably dialysed. Dose as in GFR<30 mL/min.
HDF/High flux	Probably dialysed. Dose as in GFR<30 mL/min.
CAV/ VVHD	Probably dialysed. Dose as in GFR=30–50 mL/min.

IMPORTANT DRUG INTERACTIONS

Potentially hazardous interactions with other drugs
- Anti-arrhythmics: increased risk of antimuscarinic side effects with disopyramide.
- Antifungals: dose reduction advised with itraconazole and ketoconazole.
- Antivirals: dose reduction advised with atazanavir, indinavir, ritonavir and saquinavir.
- Induction of CYP3A4 may lead to subtherapeutic plasma levels. Concomitant use with CYP3A4 inducers (e.g. carbamazepine, rifampicin, phenobarbital, phenytoin, St John's wort) is not recommended.
- Co-administration of a potent CYP2D6 inhibitor may result in increased exposure and adverse events. A dose reduction to 4 mg may be needed
- See 'Other information'.

ADMINISTRATION

RECONSTITUTION
–
ROUTE
- Oral
RATE OF ADMINISTRATION
–

OTHER INFORMATION

- Bioavailability of active metabolite is 52%.
- UK licensed product information for fesoterodine fumarate states that patients with GFR=30–80 mL/min should increase their dose with caution; those also receiving moderate CYP3A4 inhibitors should not exceed an oral dose of fesoterodine fumarate of 4 mg once daily, and concomitant potent CYP3A4 inhibitors are not recommended. Patients with GFR<30 mL/min and concomitant moderate or potent CYP3A4 inhibitors are advised not to take fesoterodine.
- In patients with GFR=30–80 mL/min, C_{max} and AUC of the active metabolite increased up to 1.5 and 1.8-fold, respectively, as compared to healthy subjects. In patients with GFR<30 mL/min, C_{max} and AUC are increased 2 and 2.3-fold, respectively.

Fexofenadine hydrochloride

CLINICAL USE

Antihistamine:
- Symptomatic relief of rhinitis and urticaria

DOSE IN NORMAL RENAL FUNCTION

120–180 mg daily depending on condition

PHARMACOKINETICS

Molecular weight (daltons)	538.1
% Protein binding	60–70
% Excreted unchanged in urine	10
Volume of distribution (L/kg)	5–6
Half-life – normal/ ESRF (hrs)	11–15/19–25

METABOLISM

Fexofenadine undergoes negligible metabolism (hepatic or non-hepatic); about 5% of the total dose is metabolised, mostly by the intestinal mucosa, with 0.5–1.5% of the dose undergoing hepatic biotransformation by the cytochrome P450 system. The major route of elimination is believed to be via biliary excretion while up to 10% of ingested dose is excreted unchanged through the urine.

DOSE IN RENAL IMPAIRMENT GFR (mL/MIN)

20–50	Dose as in normal renal function. Use with care.
10–20	Dose as in normal renal function. Use with care. See 'Other information'.
<10	Dose as in normal renal function. Use with care. See 'Other information'.

DOSE IN PATIENTS UNDERGOING RENAL REPLACEMENT THERAPIES

CAPD	Unlikely dialysability. Dose as in GFR<10 mL/min.
HD	Not dialysed. Dose as in GFR<10 mL/min.
HDF/High flux	Unknown dialysability. Dose as in GFR<10 mL/min.
CAV/ VVHD	Unlikely to be dialysed. Dose as in GFR=10–20 mL/min.

IMPORTANT DRUG INTERACTIONS

Potentially hazardous interactions with other drugs
- Antibacterials: effects possibly reduced by rifampicin.
- Antivirals: concentration possibly increased by ritonavir.
- Aluminium/magnesium containing antacids: reduced absorption – avoid for 2 hours.

ADMINISTRATION

RECONSTITUTION
–
ROUTE
- Oral
RATE OF ADMINISTRATION
–
COMMENTS
- Taken before food.

OTHER INFORMATION

- Larger doses may be used in patients with renal impairment, but increase carefully as can result in increased sedation.

Fidaxomicin

CLINICAL USE

Macrolide antibacterial agent:
- Treatment of *Clostridium difficile* infection

DOSE IN NORMAL RENAL FUNCTION

200 mg twice daily for 10 days

PHARMACOKINETICS

Molecular weight (daltons)	1058
% Protein binding	No data
% Excreted unchanged in urine	<1
Volume of distribution (L/kg)	Unknown
Half-life – normal/ ESRF (hrs)	8–10/Unchanged

METABOLISM

Mainly metabolised by hydrolysis in the gut at the isobutyryl ester to form its main and microbiologically active metabolite, OP-1118.

Over 92% of a dose is excreted in the faeces as either fidaxomicin or OP-118, although very small amounts of OP-118 have been recovered in the urine.

DOSE IN RENAL IMPAIRMENT GFR (mL/MIN)

20–50	Dose as in normal renal function.
10–20	Dose as in normal renal function.
<10	Dose as in normal renal function. Use with caution.

DOSE IN PATIENTS UNDERGOING RENAL REPLACEMENT THERAPIES

CAPD	Unlikely to be dialysed. Dose as in normal renal function.
HD	Unlikely to be dialysed. Dose as in normal renal function.
HDF/High flux	Unlikely to be dialysed. Dose as in normal renal function.
CAV/ VVHD	Unlikely to be dialysed. Dose as in normal renal function.

IMPORTANT DRUG INTERACTIONS

Potentially hazardous interactions with other drugs
- Anti-arrhythmics: avoid concomitant use with amiodarone and dronedarone.
- Antibacterials: avoid concomitant use with clarithromycin and erythromycin.
- Antifungals: avoid concomitant use with ketoconazole.
- Calcium-channel blockers: avoid concomitant use with verapamil.
- Ciclosporin: increased fidaxomicin levels, avoid concomitant use.

ADMINISTRATION

RECONSTITUTION
–
ROUTE
- Oral
RATE OF ADMINISTRATION
–

OTHER INFORMATION

- UK data sheet advises to use with caution if GFR<30 mL/min due to lack of data.
- Dose in renal impairment is taken from the American data sheet.
- Volume of distribution is unknown due to minimal systemic absorption.
- Limited data suggests that there is no major difference in plasma concentration of fidaxomicin or its metabolite OP-1118 between patients with reduced renal function (creatinine clearance <50 mL/min) and patients with normal renal function (creatinine clearance ≥50 mL/min).

Filgrastim

CLINICAL USE

Recombinant human granulocyte-colony stimulating factor (rhG-CSF):
- Treatment of neutropenia

DOSE IN NORMAL RENAL FUNCTION

0.5–1.2 MU/kg/day according to indication and patient response.

PHARMACOKINETICS

Molecular weight (daltons)	18 800
% Protein binding	Very High
% Excreted unchanged in urine	0
Volume of distribution (L/kg)	0.15
Half-life – normal/ ESRF (hrs)	3.5/–

METABOLISM

Filgrastim is primarily eliminated by the kidney and neutrophils/neutrophil precursors; the latter presumably involves binding of the growth factor to the G-CSF receptor on the cell surface, internalisation of the growth factor-receptor complexes via endocytosis, and subsequent degradation inside the cells.

DOSE IN RENAL IMPAIRMENT GFR (mL/MIN)

20–50	Dose as in normal renal function and titrate dose to response.
10–20	Dose as in normal renal function and titrate dose to response.
<10	Dose as in normal renal function and titrate dose to response.

DOSE IN PATIENTS UNDERGOING RENAL REPLACEMENT THERAPIES

CAPD	Not dialysed. Dose as in GFR<10 mL/min.
HD	Not dialysed. Dose as in GFR<10 mL/min.
HDF/High flux	Not dialysed. Dose as in GFR<10 mL/min.
CAV/ VVHD	Not dialysed. Dose as in GFR=10–20 mL/min.

IMPORTANT DRUG INTERACTIONS

Potentially hazardous interactions with other drugs
- Cytotoxics: neutropenia possibly exacerbated with fluorouracil.

ADMINISTRATION

RECONSTITUTION
–
ROUTE
- IV, SC
RATE OF ADMINISTRATION
- IV: Over 30 minutes or continuous IV infusion over 24 hours.
- SC: Can give as continuous SC infusion over 24 hours.
COMMENTS
- IV: Dilute with glucose 5% ONLY; minimum concentration 0.2 MU per mL – add Human Serum Albumin if concentration is less than 1.5 MU per mL.
- SC: Continuous infusion – dilute with 20 mL of glucose 5%.
- Dilute Neupogen may be adsorbed to glass and plastic materials – follow recommendations for dilution.

OTHER INFORMATION

- One very small study (2–3 patients) concluded that body clearance of filgrastim was not affected by any degree of renal impairment.

Finasteride

CLINICAL USE

- Benign prostatic hypertrophy
- Male pattern baldness

DOSE IN NORMAL RENAL FUNCTION

- BPH: 5 mg daily
- Male pattern baldness: 1 mg daily

PHARMACOKINETICS

Molecular weight (daltons)	372.5
% Protein binding	≈93
% Excreted unchanged in urine	<0.05
Volume of distribution (L/kg)	1.07
Half-life – normal/ ESRF (hrs)	6–8/Unchanged

METABOLISM

Finasteride is metabolised primarily via the cytochrome P450 3A4 enzyme subfamily. Following an oral dose of ^{14}C-finasteride in man, two metabolites of the drug were identified that possess only a small fraction of the 5α-reductase inhibitory activity of finasteride. Thirty-nine per cent of the dose was excreted in the urine in the form of metabolites (virtually no unchanged drug was excreted in the urine) and 57% of total dose was excreted in the faeces.

DOSE IN RENAL IMPAIRMENT GFR (mL/MIN)

20–50	Dose as in normal renal function.
10–20	Dose as in normal renal function.
<10	Dose as in normal renal function.

DOSE IN PATIENTS UNDERGOING RENAL REPLACEMENT THERAPIES

CAPD	Unlikely to be dialysed. Dose as in normal renal function.
HD	Unlikely to be dialysed. Dose as in normal renal function.
HDF/High flux	Unknown dialysability. Dose as in normal renal function.
CAV/ VVHD	Unlikely to be dialysed. Dose as in normal renal function.

IMPORTANT DRUG INTERACTIONS

Potentially hazardous interactions with other drugs
- None known

ADMINISTRATION

RECONSTITUTION

–

ROUTE
- Oral

RATE OF ADMINISTRATION

–

COMMENTS

–

OTHER INFORMATION

Data sheet states that no dosage adjustment is required in renally impaired patients whose creatinine clearance is as low as 9 mL/min. No studies have been done in patients with creatinine clearance of less than 9 mL/min.

Fingolimod

CLINICAL USE

Sphingosine 1-phosphate receptor modulator
- Treatment of highly active relapsing-remitting multiple sclerosis.

DOSE IN NORMAL RENAL FUNCTION

500 micrograms once daily

PHARMACOKINETICS

Molecular weight (daltons)	307.5 (343.9 as hydrochloride)
% Protein binding	>99
% Excreted unchanged in urine	0
Volume of distribution (L/kg)	940–1460 litres
Half-life – normal/ ESRF (hrs)	6–9 days/Unchanged

METABOLISM

Transformed by reversible stereoselective phosphorylation to the pharmacologically active (S)-enantiomer of fingolimod phosphate. It is eliminated by oxidative biotransformation mainly via the cytochrome P450 4F2 isoenzyme and subsequent fatty acid-like degradation to inactive metabolites, and by formation of pharmacologically inactive non-polar ceramide analogues of fingolimod. The main enzyme involved in the metabolism of fingolimod is partially identified and may be either CYP4F2 or CYP3A4.

Eighty-one per cent excreted as inactive metabolites in the urine and <2.5% in the faeces as metabolites and unchanged drug.

DOSE IN RENAL IMPAIRMENT GFR (mL/MIN)

20–50	Dose as in normal renal function.
10–20	Dose as in normal renal function.
<10	Dose as in normal renal function.

DOSE IN PATIENTS UNDERGOING RENAL REPLACEMENT THERAPIES

CAPD	Not dialysed. Dose as in normal renal function.
HD	Not dialysed. Dose as in normal renal function.
HDF/High flux	Not dialysed. Dose as in normal renal function.
CAV/ VVHD	Not dialysed. Dose as in normal renal function.

IMPORTANT DRUG INTERACTIONS

Potentially hazardous interactions with other drugs
- Anti-arrhythmics: possible increased risk of bradycardia with amiodarone, disopyramide & dronedarone.
- Antifungals: concentration increased by ketoconazole.
- Beta-blockers: possibly increased risk of bradycardia.
- Calcium-channel blockers: possible increased risk of bradycardia with diltiazem & verapamil.

ADMINISTRATION

RECONSTITUTION
–
ROUTE
- Oral
RATE OF ADMINISTRATION
–

OTHER INFORMATION

- Oral bioavailability is 93%.
- In patients with severe renal impairment, fingolimod C_{max} and AUC are increased by 32% and 43%, respectively, and fingolimod-phosphate C_{max} and AUC are increased by 25% and 14%, respectively, with no change in apparent elimination half-life. Based on these findings, no dose change is required in patients with renal impairment. The systemic exposure of two metabolites (M2 and M3) is increased by 3- and 13-fold, respectively. The toxicity of these metabolites is not known.

Flecainide acetate

CLINICAL USE

Class Ic anti-arrhythmic agent:
- Ventricular arrhythmias and tachycardias

DOSE IN NORMAL RENAL FUNCTION

- Oral: Supraventricular arrhythmias: 100–300 mg daily in 2 divided doses.
- Oral: Ventricular arrhythmias: 200–400 mg daily in 2 divided doses.
- IV bolus: 2 mg/kg over 10–30 minutes (maximum 150 mg), then IV infusion of 1.5 mg/kg/hour for 1 hour, subsequently 0.1–0.25 mg/kg/hour; maximum 600 mg in 24 hours.

PHARMACOKINETICS

Molecular weight (daltons)	474.4
% Protein binding	32–58
% Excreted unchanged in urine	42
Volume of distribution (L/kg)	8.31
Half-life – normal/ ESRF (hrs)	12–27/19–26

METABOLISM

Flecainide is extensively metabolised (subject to genetic polymorphism), the two major metabolites being m-O-dealkylated flecainide and m-O-dealkylated lactam of flecainide, both of which may have some activity. Its metabolism appears to involve the cytochrome P450 isoenzyme CYP2D6, which shows genetic polymorphism.

Flecainide is excreted mainly in the urine, approximately 30% as unchanged drug and the remainder as metabolites. About 5% is excreted in the faeces. Haemodialysis removes only about 1% of unchanged flecainide.

DOSE IN RENAL IMPAIRMENT GFR (mL/MIN)

35–50	Dose as in normal renal function.
10–35	Oral: Initially 100 mg daily (or 50 mg twice daily). IV: Reduce dose by 50%. See 'Other information'.
<10	Oral: Initially 100 mg daily (or 50 mg twice daily). IV: Reduce dose by 50%. See 'Other information'.

DOSE IN PATIENTS UNDERGOING RENAL REPLACEMENT THERAPIES

CAPD	≈1% dialysed.[1] Dose as in GFR<10 mL/min.
HD	≈1% dialysed.[1] Dose as in GFR<10 mL/min.
HDF/High flux	Unknown dialysability. Dose as in GFR<10 mL/min.
CAV/ VVHD	Minimal removal. Dose as in GFR=10–35 mL/min.

IMPORTANT DRUG INTERACTIONS

Potentially hazardous interactions with other drugs
- Anti-arrhythmics: concentration increased by amiodarone – halve dose of flecainide; increased myocardial depression with other anti-arrhythmics.
- Antidepressants: concentration increased by fluoxetine; increased risk of ventricular arrhythmias with tricyclics.
- Antihistamines: increased risk of ventricular arrhythmias with mizolastine.
- Antihypertensives: increased myocardial depression and bradycardia with beta-blockers; increased myocardial depression and asystole with verapamil.
- Antimalarials: concentration increased by quinine; avoid concomitant use with artemether/lumefantrine.
- Antimuscarinics: increased risk of ventricular arrhythmias with tolterodine.
- Antipsychotics: increased risk of ventricular arrhythmias with antipsychotics that prolong the QT interval and phenothiazines; increased risk of arrhythmias with clozapine.
- Antivirals: concentration possibly increased by fosamprenavir, indinavir, lopinavir, ritonavir and saquinavir, increased risk of ventricular arrhythmias – avoid concomitant use; use telaprevir with caution.
- Diuretics: increased cardiac toxicity if hypokalaemia occurs.

ADMINISTRATION

RECONSTITUTION
–
ROUTE
- Oral, IV bolus, IV infusion

RATE OF ADMINISTRATION
- See 'Other information'.

COMMENTS
- Infusion: Dilute with 5% glucose infusion; if chloride containing solutions are used the injection should be added to a volume of not less than 500 mL, otherwise a precipitate will form.
- Trough plasma levels of 200–1000 nanograms/mL may be needed to obtain the maximum therapeutic effect. Plasma levels above 700–1000 nanograms/mL are associated with increased likelihood of adverse events.

OTHER INFORMATION

- Manufacturer recommends frequent plasma level monitoring in severe renal impairment.
- Electrolyte disturbances should be corrected before using flecainide.

Reference:
1. Singlas E, Fillastre JP. Pharmacokinetics of newer drugs in patients with renal impairment (part II). *Clin Pharmacokinet.* 1991; **20**(5): 389–410.

Flucloxacillin

CLINICAL USE

Antibacterial agent

DOSE IN NORMAL RENAL FUNCTION

- Oral: 250–500 mg every 6 hours
- IV: 250 mg – 2 g every 6 hours
- IM: 250–500 mg every 6 hours
- Endocarditis: maximum 2 g every 4 hours if >85 kg
- Osteomyelitis: maximum 8 g daily in divided doses

PHARMACOKINETICS

Molecular weight (daltons)	453.9
% Protein binding	95
% Excreted unchanged in urine	66–76
Volume of distribution (L/kg)	0.13
Half-life – normal/ ESRF (hrs)	53–60 minutes/ 135–173 minutes

METABOLISM

In normal subjects approximately 10% of the flucloxacillin administered is metabolised to penicilloic acid. Excretion occurs mainly through the kidney. Between 65.5% (oral route) and 76.1% (parenteral route) of the dose administered is recovered in unaltered active form in the urine within 8 hours. A small portion of the dose administered is excreted in the bile.

DOSE IN RENAL IMPAIRMENT GFR (mL/MIN)

20–50	Dose as in normal renal function.
10–20	Dose as in normal renal function.
<10	Dose as in normal renal function up to a total daily dose of 4 g.

DOSE IN PATIENTS UNDERGOING RENAL REPLACEMENT THERAPIES

CAPD	Not dialysed. Dose as in GFR<10 mL/min.
HD	Not dialysed. Dose as in GFR<10 mL/min.
HDF/High flux	Not dialysed. Dose as in GFR<10 mL/min.
CAV/ VVHD	Not dialysed. Dose as in normal renal function.

IMPORTANT DRUG INTERACTIONS

Potentially hazardous interactions with other drugs
- Reduces excretion of methotrexate.

ADMINISTRATION

RECONSTITUTION
- IV: 250 mg and 500 mg in 5–10 mL water for injection; 1 g in 15–20 mL water for injection.
- IM: 250 mg in 1.5 mL water for injection; 500 mg in 2 mL water for injection

ROUTE
- IV, IM, Oral

RATE OF ADMINISTRATION
- Bolus: 3–4 minutes
- Infusion: 30–60 minutes

COMMENTS
- Compatible with various infusion fluids.

OTHER INFORMATION

- Monitor urine for protein at high doses.
- Sodium content of injection: 2.26 mmol/g.
- Monitor liver function tests in hypoalbuminaemic patients receiving high doses of flucloxacillin (e.g. CAPD patients).

Fluconazole

CLINICAL USE

Antifungal agent

DOSE IN NORMAL RENAL FUNCTION

50–400 mg daily, maximum 800 mg daily
(unlicensed dose)

PHARMACOKINETICS

Molecular weight (daltons)	306.3
% Protein binding	11–12
% Excreted unchanged in urine	80
Volume of distribution (L/kg)	0.65–0.7
Half-life – normal/ESRF (hrs)	30/98

METABOLISM

Fluconazole is metabolised only to a minor
extent. Of a radioactive dose, only 11% is
excreted as metabolites in the urine. The
major route of excretion is renal, with
approximately 80% of the administered
dose appearing in the urine as unchanged
medicinal product. Fluconazole clearance is
proportional to creatinine clearance. There is
no evidence of circulating metabolites.

DOSE IN RENAL IMPAIRMENT GFR (mL/MIN)

20–50	50–100% of normal dose.[1] See 'Other information'.
10–20	50–100% of normal dose.[1] See 'Other information'.
<10	50% of normal dose. See 'Other information'.

DOSE IN PATIENTS UNDERGOING RENAL REPLACEMENT THERAPIES

CAPD	Dialysed. Dose as in GFR<10 mL/min.
HD	Dialysed. 50% of normal dose daily, or 100% of normal dose 3 times a week after dialysis.
HDF/High flux	Dialysed. 50% of normal dose daily, or 100% of normal dose 3 times a week after dialysis.
CAV/VVH	Dialysed. Dose as in normal renal function.
CVVHD/HDF	Dialysed. 400–800 mg every 24 hours.[2]

IMPORTANT DRUG INTERACTIONS

Potentially hazardous interactions with
other drugs

- Analgesics: increases concentration of celecoxib – halve celecoxib dose; concentration of flurbiprofen, ibuprofen and methadone increased; increases concentration of parecoxib – reduce parecoxib dose; inhibits metabolism of alfentanil; concentration of fentanyl possibly increased.
- Antibacterials: avoid with erythromycin; increases rifabutin levels – reduce dose; metabolism accelerated by rifampicin.
- Anticoagulants: potentiates effect of coumarins.
- Antidepressants: avoid concomitant use with reboxetine; concentration of amitriptyline and nortriptyline increased.
- Antidiabetics: possibly enhances hypoglycaemic effect of nateglinide; increases concentration of sulphonylureas.
- Anti-epileptics: increases phenytoin levels; possibly increased carbamazepine concentration.
- Antimalarials: avoid concomitant administration with artemether/lumefantrine and piperaquine with artenimol.
- Antipsychotics: increased risk of ventricular arrhythmias with pimozide – avoid concomitant use; possibly increased quetiapine levels – reduce dose of quetiapine.
- Antivirals: increases nevirapine, ritonavir, tipranavir and zidovudine levels, and possibly saquinavir.
- Anxiolytics and hypnotics: increases diazepam and midazolam levels.
- Bosentan: increased bosentan levels – avoid concomitant use.
- Ciclosporin: increases blood/serum ciclosporin levels.
- Clopidogrel: possibly reduced anti-platelet effect.
- Cytotoxics: possibly increased side effects of cyclophosphamide; reduce dose of ruxolitinib.
- Diuretics: increased eplerenone levels – avoid concomitant use; concentration of fluconazole increased by hydrochlorothiazide.
- Ergot alkaloids: increased risk of ergotism – avoid concomitant use.
- Ivabradine: increased ivabradine levels – reduce initial dose.

- Lipid-lowering drugs: possibly increased risk of myopathy with atorvastatin or simvastatin; concentration of fluvastatin increased, possibly increased risk of myopathy.
- Retinoids: possibly increased risk of tretinoin toxicity.
- Sirolimus: may increase sirolimus concentration.
- Tacrolimus: increases blood/serum tacrolimus levels.
- Theophylline: possibly increases theophylline levels.

ADMINISTRATION

RECONSTITUTION

–

ROUTE
- Oral, IV

RATE OF ADMINISTRATION
- IV: 5–10 mL/minute peripherally

COMMENTS
- Oral≡IV dose. Very high bioavailability.

OTHER INFORMATION

- Oral bioavailability is 90%.
- Approximately 50% is removed during a 3 hour haemodialysis session.
- Has been used as adjunct to IV amphotericin and IP flucytosine in CAPD peritonitis.
- No dose adjustment is required for single dose therapy.
- Recurrent yeast peritonitis: Flucytosine 2000 mg orally stat, then 1000 mg daily in addition to fluconazole 150 mg IP or 200 mg orally on alternate days. Remove Tenckhoff if no response.
- Dose of 800 mg is appropriate in CRRT as long as dialysate flow rate is 2 L/hour and treating a relatively resistant organism.[2]

References:
1. Mojgan S. *Section 1: Clinical Pharmacology in the ICU* (1994): p. 61.
2. Trotman RL, Williamson JC, Shoemaker DM, *et al.* Antibiotic dosing in critically ill adult patients receiving continuous renal replacement therapy. *Clin Infect Dis.* 2005; **41**: 1159–66.

Flucytosine

CLINICAL USE

Antifungal agent

DOSE IN NORMAL RENAL FUNCTION

100–200 mg/kg per day in 4 divided doses

PHARMACOKINETICS

Molecular weight (daltons)	129.1
% Protein binding	2–4
% Excreted unchanged in urine	90
Volume of distribution (L/kg)	0.65–0.91
Half-life – normal/ ESRF (hrs)	3–6/75–200

METABOLISM

About 90% of a dose of flucytosine is excreted unchanged in the urine. A small amount of flucytosine may be metabolised to 5-flurouracil.

DOSE IN RENAL IMPAIRMENT GFR (mL/MIN)

20–40	50 mg/kg 12 hourly
10–20	50 mg/kg 24 hourly
<10	50 mg/kg then dose according to levels. Dose of 0.5–1 g daily is usually adequate.

DOSE IN PATIENTS UNDERGOING RENAL REPLACEMENT THERAPIES

CAPD	Dialysed. Give 50 mg/kg daily in 4 divided doses. Monitor levels.
HD	Dialysed. Dose as in GFR<10 mL/ min, given post dialysis. Monitor trough level pre dialysis, and reduce post-dialysis dose accordingly.
HDF/High flux	Dialysed. Dose as in GFR<10 mL/ min, given post dialysis. Monitor trough level pre dialysis, and reduce post-dialysis dose accordingly.
CAV/ VVHD	Dialysed. Give dose as in GFR=10–20 mL/min and monitor blood levels, pre dose.

IMPORTANT DRUG INTERACTIONS

Potentially hazardous interactions with other drugs
- Cytarabine: concentration of flucytosine possibly reduced.

ADMINISTRATION

RECONSTITUTION

–

ROUTE
- Oral, IV peripherally through a blood filter

RATE OF ADMINISTRATION
- 20–40 minutes

COMMENTS

–

OTHER INFORMATION

- Monitor blood levels 24 hours after therapy commences. Pre-dose level 25–50 mg/L is usually adequate. Do not exceed 80 mg/L.
- 250 mL intravenous flucytosine infusion contains 34.5 mmol sodium.
- Bone marrow suppression more common in patients with renal impairment.
- Tablets available on named patient basis only.
- Can be given IP at a dose of 50 mg/L.

Fludarabine phosphate

CLINICAL USE

B-cell chronic lymphocytic leukaemia

DOSE IN NORMAL RENAL FUNCTION

- IV: 25 mg/m^2 daily for 5 days, repeated every 28 days.
- Oral: 40 mg/m^2 for 5 days every 28 days.

PHARMACOKINETICS

Molecular weight (daltons)	365.2
% Protein binding	19–29
% Excreted unchanged in urine	40–60
Volume of distribution (L/kg)	0.8–4
Half-life – normal/ ESRF (hrs)	20/24

METABOLISM

Intravenous fludarabine phosphate is rapidly dephosphorylated to fludarabine which is taken up by lymphocytes and rephosphorylated via the enzyme deoxycytidine kinase to the active triphosphate nucleotide. Clearance of fludarabine from the plasma is triphasic; elimination is mostly via renal excretion: 40–60% of an intravenous dose is excreted in the urine. The pharmacokinetics of fludarabine show considerable inter-individual variation.

DOSE IN RENAL IMPAIRMENT GFR (mL/MIN)

30–70	50–75% of normal dose.
10–30	50–75% of normal dose. Use with care.
<10	50% of normal dose. Use with care.

DOSE IN PATIENTS UNDERGOING RENAL REPLACEMENT THERAPIES

CAPD	Unknown dialysability. Dose as in GFR<10 mL/min.
HD	Unknown dialysability. Dose as in GFR<10 mL/min.
HDF/High flux	Unknown dialysability. Dose as in GFR<10 mL/min.
CAV/ VVHD	Unknown dialysability. Dose as in GFR=10–30 mL/min.

IMPORTANT DRUG INTERACTIONS

Potentially hazardous interactions with other drugs
- Antipsychotics: avoid concomitant use with clozapine, increased risk of agranulocytosis.
- Cytotoxics: increased pulmonary toxicity with pentostatin (unacceptably high incidence of fatalities); increases intracellular concentration of cytarabine.

ADMINISTRATION

RECONSTITUTION
- Reconstitute each vial with 2 mL of water to give a concentration of 25 mg/mL.
ROUTE
- IV, oral
RATE OF ADMINISTRATION
- Infusion should be administered over 30 minutes.
COMMENTS
- IV bolus in 10 mL of sodium chloride 0.9%.
- IV infusion in 100 mL of sodium chloride 0.9%.

OTHER INFORMATION

- Rapidly dephosphorylated in plasma to (2-F-9-ß-D-arabinofuranosyladenine) 2-F-ara-ATP, which is necessary for cellular uptake.
- Approximately 60% of an administered dose is excreted in the urine within 24 hrs.
- Administer up to achievement of clinical response (usually 6 cycles) then discontinue.
- In a study, patients with a GFR=17–41 mL/min/m^2 received 20 mg/m^2 and those with a GFR<17 mL/min/m^2 received 15 mg/m^2. The patients with a GFR=17–41 mL/min/m^2 had a similar AUC as patients with normal renal function receiving the full dose but the AUC was increased in those with a GFR<17 mL/min/m^2. (Lichtman S, Etcubanas E, Budman DR. The pharmacokinetics and pharmacodynamics of fludarabine phosphate in patients with renal impairment: a prospective dose adjustment study. *Cancer Investigation*. 2002; **20**(7&8): 904–13.)
- Dose in severe renal impairment is from *Drug Prescribing in Renal Failure*, 5th edition, by Aronoff *et al.*

Fludrocortisone acetate

CLINICAL USE

Replacement therapy in adrenal insufficiency

DOSE IN NORMAL RENAL FUNCTION

50–300 micrograms daily

PHARMACOKINETICS

Molecular weight (daltons)	422.5
% Protein binding	70–80
% Excreted unchanged in urine	80% (as metabolites)
Volume of distribution (L/kg)	Widely distributed
Half-life – normal/ ESRF (hrs)	3.5 (Biological half-life 18–36 hours)/–

METABOLISM

Fludrocortisone is hydrolysed to produce the non-esterified alcohol. In human volunteers, excretion through urine was about 80%, and it was concluded that about 20% was excreted by a different route. It is likely that, as for the metabolism of other steroids, excretion into the bile is balanced by reabsorption in the intestine and some part is excreted with the faeces.

DOSE IN RENAL IMPAIRMENT GFR (mL/MIN)

20–50	Dose as in normal renal function.
10–20	Dose as in normal renal function.
<10	Dose as in normal renal function.

DOSE IN PATIENTS UNDERGOING RENAL REPLACEMENT THERAPIES

CAPD	Unknown dialysability. Dose as in normal renal function.
HD	Unknown dialysability. Dose as in normal renal function.
HDF/High flux	Unknown dialysability. Dose as in normal renal function.
CAV/ VVHD	Unknown dialysability. Dose as in normal renal function.

IMPORTANT DRUG INTERACTIONS

Potentially hazardous interactions with other drugs
- Aldesleukin: avoid concomitant use.
- Antibacterials: metabolism accelerated by rifamycins; metabolism possibly inhibited by erythromycin; possibly reduce isoniazid concentration.
- Anticoagulants: efficacy of coumarins and phenindione may be altered.
- Anti-epileptics: metabolism accelerated by carbamazepine, phenobarbital and phenytoin.
- Antifungals: increased risk of hypokalaemia with amphotericin – avoid concomitant use; metabolism possibly inhibited by itraconazole and ketoconazole.
- Antivirals: concentration possibly increased by ritonavir.
- Vaccines: high dose corticosteroids can impair immune response to vaccines – avoid concomitant use with live vaccines.

ADMINISTRATION

RECONSTITUTION
–
ROUTE
- Oral
RATE OF ADMINISTRATION
–
COMMENTS
- Use for as short a time and as low a dose as possible.

Flumazenil

CLINICAL USE

Reversal of sedative effects of benzodiazepines in anaesthetic, intensive care, and diagnostic procedures

DOSE IN NORMAL RENAL FUNCTION

- Initially 200 micrograms over 15 seconds, then 100 micrograms at 60 second intervals if required; usual dose range 300–600 micrograms; maximum dose 1 mg, or 2 mg in intensive care situations.
- If drowsiness recurs, an IV infusion of 100–400 micrograms per hour may be given.

PHARMACOKINETICS

Molecular weight (daltons)	303.3
% Protein binding	50
% Excreted unchanged in urine	<0.1
Volume of distribution (L/kg)	0.6–1.1
Half-life – normal/ ESRF (hrs)	0.7–1.3/Unchanged

METABOLISM

Flumazenil is extensively metabolised in the liver. The carboxylic acid metabolite is the main metabolite in plasma (free form) and urine (free form and its glucuronide). This main metabolite showed no benzodiazepine agonist or antagonist activity in pharmacological tests.

Flumazenil is almost completely (99%) eliminated by non-renal routes. Practically no unchanged flumazenil is excreted in the urine, suggesting complete metabolic degradation of the drug. Elimination of radiolabelled drug is essentially complete within 72 hours, with 90–95% of the radioactivity appearing in urine and 5–10% in the faeces.

DOSE IN RENAL IMPAIRMENT GFR (mL/MIN)

20–50	Dose as in normal renal function.
10–20	Dose as in normal renal function.
<10	Dose as in normal renal function.

DOSE IN PATIENTS UNDERGOING RENAL REPLACEMENT THERAPIES

CAPD	Unknown dialysability. Dose as in normal renal function.
HD	Unknown dialysability. Dose as in normal renal function.
HDF/High flux	Unknown dialysability. Dose as in normal renal function.
CAV/ VVHD	Unknown dialysability. Dose as in normal renal function.

IMPORTANT DRUG INTERACTIONS

Potentially hazardous interactions with other drugs
- None known

ADMINISTRATION

RECONSTITUTION
–
ROUTE
- IV injection, IV infusion
RATE OF ADMINISTRATION
- See 'Dose in normal renal function'.
COMMENTS
- Infusion: suitable diluents include sodium chloride 0.9%, sodium chloride 0.45% and glucose 5%.

OTHER INFORMATION

The half-life of flumazenil is shorter than those of diazepam and midazolam – patients should be closely monitored to avoid the risk of them becoming re-sedated.

Fluorouracil

CLINICAL USE

Antineoplastic agent

DOSE IN NORMAL RENAL FUNCTION

- IV infusion: 15 mg/kg/day to a total dose of 12–15 g.
- IV bolus: 12 mg/kg/day for 3 days, then 6 mg/kg on alternate days or 15 mg/kg once a week.
- Maintenance: 5–15 mg/kg once a week.
- Intra-arterial infusion: 5–7.5 mg/kg by continuous 24–hour infusion.
- Or consult relevant local chemotherapy protocol.

PHARMACOKINETICS

Molecular weight (daltons)	130.1
% Protein binding	10
% Excreted unchanged in urine	15
Volume of distribution (L/kg)	0.25–0.5
Half-life – normal/ ESRF (hrs)	16 minutes/ Unchanged

METABOLISM

After intravenous injection fluorouracil is cleared rapidly from plasma. It is distributed throughout body tissues and fluids, and disappears from the plasma within about 3 hours. Within the target cell fluorouracil is converted to 5-fluorouridine monophosphate and floxuridine monophosphate (5-fluorodeoxyuridine monophosphate), the former undergoing conversion to the triphosphate which can be incorporated into RNA while the latter inhibits thymidylate synthetase. About 15% of an intravenous dose is excreted unchanged in the urine within 6 hours. Approximately 80% is inactivated mainly in the liver and is catabolised via dihydropyrimidine dehydrogenase (DPD) similarly to endogenous uracil, 60–80% is excreted as respiratory carbon dioxide; urea and other metabolites are also produced, and 2–3% by the biliary system.

DOSE IN RENAL IMPAIRMENT GFR (mL/MIN)

20–50	Dose as in normal renal function.
10–20	Dose as in normal renal function.
<10	Dose as in normal renal function. Use with caution.

DOSE IN PATIENTS UNDERGOING RENAL REPLACEMENT THERAPIES

CAPD	Some removal likely. Dose as in normal renal function.
HD	Dialysed. Dose as in normal renal function.
HDF/High flux	Dialysed. Dose as in normal renal function.
CAV/ VVHD	Dialysed. Dose as in normal renal function.

IMPORTANT DRUG INTERACTIONS

Potentially hazardous interactions with other drugs
- Anticoagulants: possibly enhances effect of coumarins.
- Antipsychotics: avoid concomitant use with clozapine, increased risk of agranulocytosis.
- Metronidazole and cimetidine inhibit metabolism (increased toxicity).
- Temoporfin: increased skin photosensitivity with topical fluorouracil.

ADMINISTRATION

RECONSTITUTION
- Consult relevant local protocol.
ROUTE
- IV infusion: intermittent or continuous IV injection, intra-arterial, topical
RATE OF ADMINISTRATION
- 30–60 minutes, 4 hours
- or as a continuous infusion over 24 hours
- or consult relevant local protocol.
COMMENTS
–

OTHER INFORMATION

- Use ideal body weight in patients showing obesity, ascites, and oedema.

Fluoxetine

CLINICAL USE

SSRI antidepressant:
- Depressive illness
- Bulimia nervosa
- Obsessive compulsive disorder

DOSE IN NORMAL RENAL FUNCTION

20–60 mg daily depending on indication.

PHARMACOKINETICS

Molecular weight (daltons)	345.8 (as hydrochloride)
% Protein binding	94.5
% Excreted unchanged in urine	<10
Volume of distribution (L/kg)	20–40
Half-life – normal/ ESRF (hrs)	Acute dosing: 24–72/ Unchanged Chronic dosing: 4–6 days/Increased

METABOLISM

Fluoxetine is extensively metabolised by the enzyme CYP2D6 in the liver to its primary active metabolite norfluoxetine (desmethylfluoxetine), by desmethylation.

The elimination half-life of fluoxetine is 4 to 6 days and for norfluoxetine 4 to 16 days. Excretion is mainly (about 60%) via the kidney.

DOSE IN RENAL IMPAIRMENT GFR (mL/MIN)

20–50	Dose as in normal renal function.
10–20	Dose as in normal renal function.
<10	Use low dose, or on alternate days and increase according to response.

DOSE IN PATIENTS UNDERGOING RENAL REPLACEMENT THERAPIES

CAPD	Not dialysed. Dose as in GFR<10 mL/min.
HD	Not dialysed. Dose as in GFR<10 mL/min.
HDF/High flux	Not dialysed. Dose as in GFR<10 mL/min.
CAV/ VVHD	Not dialysed. Dose as in GFR=10–20 mL/min.

IMPORTANT DRUG INTERACTIONS

Potentially hazardous interactions with other drugs
- Analgesics: increased risk of bleeding with aspirin and NSAIDs; risk of CNS toxicity increased with tramadol; concentration of methadone possibly increased.
- Anti-arrhythmics: increased flecainide concentration.
- Anticoagulants: effect of coumarins possibly enhanced; possibly increased risk of bleeding with dabigatran.
- Antidepressants: avoid concomitant use with MAOIs and moclobemide, increased risk of toxicity; avoid concomitant use with St John's wort; possibly enhanced serotonergic effects with duloxetine and mirtazapine; can increase concentration of tricyclics; increased agitation and nausea with tryptophan.
- Anti-epileptics: antagonism (lowered convulsive threshold); concentration of carbamazepine and phenytoin increased.
- Antimalarials: avoid concomitant use with artemether/lumefantrine and piperaquine with artenimol.
- Antipsychotics: concentration of haloperidol, clozapine and risperidone increased; possibly inhibits aripiprazole metabolism – reduce aripiprazole dose; increased risk of ventricular arrhythmias with droperidol and pimozide – avoid.
- Antivirals: concentration possibly increased by ritonavir.
- Anxiolytics & hypnotics: concentration of alprazolam increased.
- Ciclosporin: may increase ciclosporin concentration.
- Clopidogrel: possibly reduced antiplatelet effect.
- Dopaminergics: increased risk of hypertension and CNS excitation with selegiline – avoid concomitant use; increased risk of CNS toxicity with rasagiline – avoid concomitant use.
- Hormone antagonists: metabolism of tamoxifen to active metabolite possibly reduced – avoid.
- $5HT_1$ agonist: increased risk of CNS toxicity with sumatriptan; possibly increased risk of serotonergic effects with naratriptan.
- Lithium: increased risk of CNS effects (lithium toxicity reported).
- Methylthioninium: risk of CNS toxicity – avoid if possible.

ADMINISTRATION

RECONSTITUTION

–

ROUTE

● Oral

RATE OF ADMINISTRATION

–

COMMENTS

–

OTHER INFORMATION

● Accumulation may occur in patients with severe renal failure during chronic treatment (metabolites are excreted renally).

● Choong-Ki L, Var T, Blaine T W. Fluoxetine in depressed patients with renal failure and in depressed patients with normal kidney function. *General Hosp Psychiatry.* 1996; **18**(1): 8–13, studied 7 patients undergoing haemodialysis and concluded that the process of HD does not alter the pharmacokinetics of fluoxetine or its major metabolite. All patients received fluoxetine 20 mg per day for 8 weeks.

● Contraindicated in ESRD by some manufacturers in the UK but not the US.

● *Drug Prescribing in Renal Failure*, 5th edition, by Aronoff *et al.* advises to use 100% of dose.

Flupentixol

CLINICAL USE

Antipsychotic:
- Schizophrenia and other psychoses
- Depression

DOSE IN NORMAL RENAL FUNCTION

- Psychosis:
  — Oral: 3–9 mg twice daily, max 18 mg daily
  — Deep IM: 50 mg 4 weekly – 300 mg 2 weekly; maximum dose 400 mg weekly; 20–40 mg every 2–4 weeks may be adequate in some patients.
- Depression: 0.5–3 mg daily (doses above 2 mg should be in 2 divided doses, and 2nd dose should not be after 4 pm).

PHARMACOKINETICS

Molecular weight (daltons)	434.5 (588.8 as decanoate)
% Protein binding	>95
% Excreted unchanged in urine	Negligible
Volume of distribution (L/kg)	12–14
Half-life – normal/ ESRF (hrs)	22–36 (IM: 3–8 days)/ Increased

METABOLISM

Flupentixol is readily absorbed from the gastrointestinal tract after oral use and is probably subject to first-pass metabolism in the gut wall. It is also extensively metabolised in the liver and is excreted in the urine and faeces in the form of numerous metabolites; there is evidence of enterohepatic recycling. Paths of metabolism of flupentixol include sulfoxidation, side-chain N-dealkylation, and glucuronic acid conjugation.

DOSE IN RENAL IMPAIRMENT GFR (mL/MIN)

20–50	Dose as in normal renal function.
10–20	Dose as in normal renal function.
<10	Start with quarter to half of the dose and titrate slowly.

DOSE IN PATIENTS UNDERGOING RENAL REPLACEMENT THERAPIES

CAPD	Not dialysed. Dose as in GFR<10 mL/min.
HD	Not dialysed. Dose as in GFR<10 mL/min.
HDF/High flux	Unknown dialysability. Dose as in GFR<10 mL/min.
CAV/ VVHD	Not dialysed. Dose as in normal renal function.

IMPORTANT DRUG INTERACTIONS

Potentially hazardous interactions with other drugs
- Alcohol: enhanced effects.
- Anaesthetics: enhanced hypotensive effects.
- Analgesics: increased risk of convulsions with tramadol; enhanced hypotensive and sedative effects with opioids.
- Antidepressants: increased concentration of tricyclics.
- Anti-epileptics: anticonvulsant effect antagonised.
- Antimalarials: avoid concomitant use with artemether/lumefantrine.
- Antipsychotics: avoid concomitant use of clozapine with depot preparations in case of neutropenia.
- Antivirals: concentration possibly increased with ritonavir.
- Anxiolytics and hypnotics: increased sedative effects.
- Avoid concomitant use with drugs that prolong the QT interval.

ADMINISTRATION

RECONSTITUTION
–
ROUTE
- Oral, IM
RATE OF ADMINISTRATION
–
COMMENTS
–

OTHER INFORMATION

- May cause hypotension and sedation in renal impairment.
- Increased CNS sensitivity in renally impaired patients – start with small doses as can accumulate.
- For IM injection a 20 mg test dose should first be given.
- Oral bioavailability is 40–55%.
- Peak levels occur 7 days after IM injection and 4 hours after oral administration.

Flurbiprofen

CLINICAL USE

NSAID and analgesic

DOSE IN NORMAL RENAL FUNCTION

- 150–200 mg daily in divided doses, increased in acute conditions to 300 mg daily.
- Dysmenorrhoea: 50–100 mg every 4–6 hours; maximum 300 mg daily.

PHARMACOKINETICS

Molecular weight (daltons)	244.3
% Protein binding	99
% Excreted unchanged in urine	<3
Volume of distribution (L/kg)	0.1–0.2
Half-life – normal/ ESRF (hrs)	3–6/Unchanged

METABOLISM

Flurbiprofen is metabolised mainly by hydroxylation (via the cytochrome P450 isoenzyme CYP2C9) and conjugation in the liver and excreted in the urine. The rate of urinary excretion of flurbiprofen and its two major metabolites ([2-(2-fluoro-4'-hydroxy-4-biphenylyl) propionic acid] and [2-(2-fluoro-3'-hydroxy-4'-methoxy-4-biphenylyl) propionic acid]) in both free and conjugated states is similar for both the oral and rectal routes of administration.

DOSE IN RENAL IMPAIRMENT GFR (mL/MIN)

20–50	Dose as in normal renal function, but avoid if possible.
10–20	Dose as in normal renal function, but avoid if possible.
<10	Dose as in normal renal function, but only if on dialysis.

DOSE IN PATIENTS UNDERGOING RENAL REPLACEMENT THERAPIES

CAPD	Removal very unlikely. Dose as in GFR<10 mL/min. See 'Other information'.
HD	Removal very unlikely. Dose as in GFR<10 mL/min. See 'Other information'.
HDF/High flux	Unknown dialysability. Dose as in GFR<10 mL/min. See 'Other information'.
CAV/ VVHD	Removal very unlikely. Dose as in GFR=10–20 mL/min.

IMPORTANT DRUG INTERACTIONS

Potentially hazardous interactions with other drugs

- ACE inhibitors and angiotensin-II antagonists: antagonism of hypotensive effect; increased risk of nephrotoxicity and hyperkalaemia.
- Analgesics: avoid concomitant use with other NSAIDs or aspirin; avoid concomitant use with ketorolac (increased side effects and haemorrhage).
- Antibacterials: possibly increased risk of convulsions with quinolones.
- Anticoagulants: effects of coumarins and phenindione enhanced; possibly increased risk of bleeding with heparins and dabigatran.
- Antidepressants: increased risk of bleeding with SSRIs or venlafaxine.
- Antidiabetic agents: effects of sulphonylureas enhanced.
- Anti-epileptics: possibly enhanced effect of phenytoin.
- Antivirals: concentration possibly increased by ritonavir; increased risk of haematological toxicity with zidovudine.
- Ciclosporin: may potentiate nephrotoxicity.
- Cytotoxic agents: reduced excretion of methotrexate; increased risk of bleeding with erlotinib.
- Lithium: excretion reduced (risk of lithium toxicity).
- Diuretics: increased risk of nephrotoxicity; antagonism of diuretic effect; hyperkalaemia with potassium-sparing diuretics.
- Pentoxifylline: increased risk of bleeding.
- Tacrolimus: increased risk of nephrotoxicity.

ADMINISTRATION

RECONSTITUTION

–

ROUTE

- Oral

RATE OF ADMINISTRATION

–

COMMENTS

–

OTHER INFORMATION

- NSAIDs have been reported to cause nephrotoxicity in various forms; interstitial nephritis, nephrotic syndrome and renal failure. In patients with renal, cardiac or hepatic impairment, caution is required since the use of NSAIDs may result in deterioration of renal function.
- Inhibition of renal prostaglandin synthesis by NSAIDs may interfere with renal function, especially in the presence of existing renal disease – avoid if possible; if not, check serum creatinine 48–72 hours after starting NSAID – if creatinine has increased, discontinue therapy.
- Use normal doses in patients with ERF on dialysis if they do not pass any urine.
- Use with caution in renal transplant recipients – can reduce intrarenal autocoid synthesis.

Flutamide

CLINICAL USE

Treatment of advanced prostate cancer

DOSE IN NORMAL RENAL FUNCTION

250 mg every 8 hours; start 3 days before
LHRH agonist.

PHARMACOKINETICS

Molecular weight (daltons)	276.2
% Protein binding	>90
% Excreted unchanged in urine	45
Volume of distribution (L/kg)	No data
Half-life – normal/ ESRF (hrs)	6/Slightly increased (active metabolite)

METABOLISM

It is rapidly and extensively metabolised;
the major metabolite (2-hydroxyflutamide)
possesses anti-androgenic properties. Both
flutamide and 2-hydroxyflutamide are
more than 90% bound to plasma proteins.
Excretion is mainly in the urine with only
minor amounts appearing in the faeces.

DOSE IN RENAL IMPAIRMENT GFR (mL/MIN)

20–50	Dose as in normal renal function.
10–20	Dose as in normal renal function.
<10	Dose as in normal renal function.

DOSE IN PATIENTS UNDERGOING RENAL REPLACEMENT THERAPIES

CAPD	Not dialysed. Dose as in normal renal function.
HD	Not dialysed. Dose as in normal renal function.
HDF/High flux	Not dialysed. Dose as in normal renal function.
CAV/ VVHD	Not dialysed. Dose as in normal renal function.

IMPORTANT DRUG INTERACTIONS

Potentially hazardous interactions with
other drugs
● Anticoagulants: effects of coumarins
   enhanced.

ADMINISTRATION

RECONSTITUTION
–
ROUTE
● Oral
RATE OF ADMINISTRATION
–
COMMENTS
–

Fluvastatin

CLINICAL USE

HMG CoA reductase inhibitor:
- Primary hypercholesterolaemia
- Slowing progression of atherosclerosis
- Secondary prevention of coronary events after percutaneous coronary intervention

DOSE IN NORMAL RENAL FUNCTION

20–80 mg daily in the evening
XL: 80 mg daily

PHARMACOKINETICS

Molecular weight (daltons)	433.4 (as sodium salt)
% Protein binding	>98
% Excreted unchanged in urine	6
Volume of distribution (L/kg)	0.35
Half-life – normal/ ESRF (hrs)	1.4–3.2/Unchanged

METABOLISM

Fluvastatin is rapidly and completely absorbed from the gastrointestinal tract and undergoes extensive first-pass metabolism in the liver. Metabolism is mainly by the cytochrome P450 isoenzyme CYP2C9, with only a small amount metabolised by CYP3A4. The major components circulating in the blood are fluvastatin and the pharmacologically inactive N-desisopropyl-propionic acid metabolite. The hydroxylated metabolites have pharmacological activity but do not circulate systemically. About 93% is excreted in the faeces, mainly as metabolites, with only about 6% being excreted in the urine.

DOSE IN RENAL IMPAIRMENT GFR (mL/MIN)

30–50	Dose as in normal renal function.
10–30	Dose as in normal renal function. See 'Other information'.
<10	Dose as in normal renal function. See 'Other information'.

DOSE IN PATIENTS UNDERGOING RENAL REPLACEMENT THERAPIES

CAPD	Removal unlikely. Dose as in GFR<10 mL/min.
HD	Removal unlikely. Dose as in GFR<10 mL/min.
HDF/High flux	Removal unlikely. Dose as in GFR<10 mL/min.
CAV/ VVHD	Removal unlikely. Dose as in GFR=10–30 mL/min.

IMPORTANT DRUG INTERACTIONS

Potentially hazardous interactions with other drugs
- Antibacterials: rifampicin increases metabolism; increased risk of myopathy with daptomycin.
- Anticoagulants: anticoagulant effect enhanced.
- Anti-epileptics: concentration of either or both drugs may be increased with phenytoin.
- Antifungals: concentration increased by fluconazole – increased risk of myopathy.
- Ciclosporin: concomitant treatment with ciclosporin may lead to risk of muscle toxicity.
- Colchicine: isolated cases of myopathy have been reported.
- Lipid-lowering drugs: increased risk of myopathy with gemfibrozil, fibrates and nicotinic acid – avoid concomitant use with gemfibrozil.

ADMINISTRATION

RECONSTITUTION
–
ROUTE
- Oral
RATE OF ADMINISTRATION
–
COMMENTS
–

OTHER INFORMATION

- The Committee on Safety of Medicines has advised that rhabdomyolysis associated with lipid-lowering drugs, such as the fibrates and statins, appears to be rare (approx. 1 case in every 100 000 treatment years), but may be increased in those with renal impairment and possibly in those with hypothyroidism.
- Manufacturer advises to use doses above 40 mg in patients with GFR<30 mL/min with caution due to lack of data.
- *Drug Prescribing in Renal Failure*, 5th edition, by Aronoff *et al.* advises to use 100% of dose.

Fluvoxamine maleate

CLINICAL USE

SSRI antidepressant:
- Depression
- Obsessive compulsive disorder

DOSE IN NORMAL RENAL FUNCTION

- 50–300 mg daily (doses over 150 mg in divided doses)
- Depression: usual maintenance dose 100 mg daily
- Obsessive compulsive disorder: usual maintenance dose 100–300 mg daily

PHARMACOKINETICS

Molecular weight (daltons)	434.4
% Protein binding	80
% Excreted unchanged in urine	2
Volume of distribution (L/kg)	25
Half-life – normal/ESRF (hrs)	13–15/ Unchanged

METABOLISM

Fluvoxamine undergoes extensive hepatic transformation by CYP2D6, mainly via oxidative demethylation, into at least 9 metabolites. The two major metabolites showed negligible pharmacological activity. The other metabolites are not expected to be pharmacologically active. Excretion is mainly in the urine; about 2% of a dose is excreted as unchanged drug.

DOSE IN RENAL IMPAIRMENT GFR (mL/MIN)

30–50	Dose as in normal renal function.
10–20	Dose as in normal renal function.
<10	Dose as in normal renal function but titrate slowly.

DOSE IN PATIENTS UNDERGOING RENAL REPLACEMENT THERAPIES

CAPD	Not dialysed. Dose as in GFR<10 mL/min.
HD	Not dialysed. Dose as in GFR<10 mL/min.
HDF/High flux	Not dialysed. Dose as in GFR<10 mL/min.
CAV/ VVHD	Unknown dialysability. Dose as in normal renal function.

IMPORTANT DRUG INTERACTIONS

Potentially hazardous interactions with other drugs

- Analgesics: increased risk of bleeding with aspirin and NSAIDs; risk of CNS toxicity increased with tramadol; concentration of methadone possibly increased.
- Anti-arrhythmics: increased risk of toxicity with mexiletine.
- Anticoagulants: effect of coumarins possibly enhanced; possibly increased risk of bleeding with dabigatran.
- Antidepressants: avoid concomitant use with reboxetine, MAOIs, moclobemide and St John's wort; possibly enhanced serotonergic effects with duloxetine and mirtazapine; fluvoxamine inhibits metabolism of duloxetine – avoid concomitant use; can increase tricyclics concentration; increased agitation and nausea with tryptophan; metabolism of agomelatine reduced.
- Anti-epileptics: antagonise anticonvulsant threshold; concentration of carbamazepine and phenytoin increased.
- Antimalarials: avoid concomitant use with artemether/lumefantrine and piperaquine with artenimol.
- Antipsychotics: concentration of asenapine, haloperidol, clozapine and olanzapine increased; increased risk of ventricular arrhythmias with droperidol and possibly pimozide – avoid.
- Antivirals: concentration possibly increased by ritonavir.
- Ciclosporin: may increase ciclosporin concentration.
- Clopidogrel: possibly reduced antiplatelet effect.
- Dopaminergics: increased risk of CNS toxicity with rasagiline – avoid; hypertension and CNS excitation with selegiline – avoid concomitant use.
- $5HT_1$ agonist: risk of CNS toxicity increased with sumatriptan; possibly increased risk of serotonergic effects with naratriptan; inhibits metabolism of frovatriptan; possibly inhibits metabolism of zolmitriptan – reduce zolmitriptan dose.
- Linezolid: use with care, possibly increased risk of side effects.

- Lithium: increased risk of CNS effects – monitor levels.
- Methylthioninium: risk of CNS toxicity – avoid if possible.
- Muscle relaxants: increased risk of toxicity with tizanidine – avoid.
- Theophylline: increased theophylline concentrations – avoid concomitant use; if not possible, halve theophylline dose and monitor levels.

ADMINISTRATION

RECONSTITUTION

–

ROUTE

- Oral

RATE OF ADMINISTRATION

–

COMMENTS

–

Folic acid

CLINICAL USE

- Folate-deficient megaloblastic anaemia
- Supplement in HD patients

DOSE IN NORMAL RENAL FUNCTION

- 5 mg daily for 4 months, then weekly according to response
- Maintenance: 5 mg every 1–7 days

PHARMACOKINETICS

Molecular weight (daltons)	441.4
% Protein binding	70
% Excreted unchanged in urine	Varies with daily dose
Volume of distribution (L/kg)	No data
Half-life – normal/ ESRF (hrs)	2.5/–

METABOLISM

Folic acid given therapeutically enters the portal circulation largely unchanged, since it is a poor substrate for reduction by dihydrofolate reductase. It is converted to the metabolically active form 5-methyltetrahydrofolate in the plasma and liver. Folate undergoes enterohepatic circulation. Folate metabolites are eliminated in the urine and folate in excess of body requirements is excreted unchanged in the urine.

DOSE IN RENAL IMPAIRMENT GFR (mL/MIN)

20–50	Dose as in normal renal function.
10–20	Dose as in normal renal function.
<10	Dose as in normal renal function.

DOSE IN PATIENTS UNDERGOING RENAL REPLACEMENT THERAPIES

CAPD	Dialysed. Dose as in normal renal function.
HD	Dialysed. Dose as in normal renal function.
HDF/High flux	Dialysed. Dose as in normal renal function.
CAV/ VVHD	Dialysed. Dose as in normal renal function.

IMPORTANT DRUG INTERACTIONS

Potentially hazardous interactions with other drugs
- Anti-epileptics: reduces phenytoin, primidone and phenobarbital levels.
- Cytotoxics: avoid with raltitrexed.

ADMINISTRATION

RECONSTITUTION
–
ROUTE
- Oral
RATE OF ADMINISTRATION
–
COMMENTS
–

OTHER INFORMATION

- If seriously folate deficient, give 10 mg/day for 1 month, then 5 mg/day.
- Doses up to 15 mg daily have been used in cases of malabsorption.
- Most nutritionists recommend 0.5–1 mg folic acid daily for patients on HD or CAPD; may accumulate in uraemic patients.
- Dosage used by dialysis units varies from 5 mg daily to 5 mg once weekly.

Folinic acid (calcium folinate)

CLINICAL USE

- Folinic acid rescue
- Enhancement of 5-fluorouracil cytotoxicity in advanced colorectal cancer
- Folate deficiency

DOSE IN NORMAL RENAL FUNCTION

Varies according to indication.

PHARMACOKINETICS

Molecular weight (daltons)	511.5
% Protein binding	54
% Excreted unchanged in urine	80–90 (as inactive metabolites)
Volume of distribution (L/kg)	17.5
Half-life – normal/ ESRF (hrs)	32–35 minutes/–

METABOLISM

Folinic acid is a racemate where the L-form (L-5-formyl-tetrahydrofolate, L-5-formyl-THF) is the active enantiomer. The major metabolic product of folinic acid is 5-methyl-tetrahydrofolic acid (5-methyl-THF) which is predominantly produced in the liver and intestinal mucosa, 80–90% with the urine (5- and 10-formyl-tetrahydrofolates inactive metabolites), 5–8% with the faeces.

DOSE IN RENAL IMPAIRMENT GFR (mL/MIN)

20–50	Dose as in normal renal function.
10–20	Dose as in normal renal function.
<10	Dose as in normal renal function.

DOSE IN PATIENTS UNDERGOING RENAL REPLACEMENT THERAPIES

CAPD	Some removal likely. Dose as in normal renal function.
HD	Some removal likely. Dose as in normal renal function.
HDF/High flux	Dialysed. Dose as in normal renal function.
CAV/ VVHD	Some removal likely. Dose as in normal renal function.

IMPORTANT DRUG INTERACTIONS

Potentially hazardous interactions with other drugs

- Should not be administered simultaneously with a folic acid antagonist as this may nullify the effect of the antagonist.
- Cytotoxics: avoid with raltitrexed.

ADMINISTRATION

RECONSTITUTION
- For IV infusion, compatible with: sodium chloride 0.9%, glucose 5%, sodium lactate injection.

ROUTE
- IM, IV injection, IV infusion, oral

RATE OF ADMINISTRATION
- Because of the calcium content of leucovorin solutions, no more than 160 mg/minute should be injected IV.

COMMENTS
–

OTHER INFORMATION

–

Fondaparinux sodium

CLINICAL USE

- Prophylaxis of deep vein thrombosis
- Treatment of deep vein thrombosis, pulmonary embolism, unstable angina and after a myocardial infarction

DOSE IN NORMAL RENAL FUNCTION

- Prophylaxis DVT
  - Surgical: 2.5 mg 6 hours after surgery, then 2.5 mg daily
  - Medical: 2.5 mg daily
  - Treatment of superficial-vein thrombosis: 2.5 mg daily (if weight >50 kg)
  - Unstable angina & MI: 2.5 mg daily·
- Treatment DVT and PE:
  - <50 kg: 5 mg daily
  - 50–100 kg: 7.5 mg daily
  - >100 kg: 10 mg daily

PHARMACOKINETICS

Molecular weight (daltons)	1728
% Protein binding	97–98.6 (to anti-thrombin)
% Excreted unchanged in urine	64–77
Volume of distribution (L/kg)	0.1–0.12
Half-life – normal/ ESRF (hrs)	17–21/72

METABOLISM

Although not fully evaluated, there is no evidence of fondaparinux metabolism and in particular no evidence for the formation of active metabolites. Fondaparinux is excreted to 64–77% by the kidney as unchanged compound.

DOSE IN RENAL IMPAIRMENT GFR (mL/MIN)

20–50	1.5 mg daily. See 'Other information'.
10–20	Reduce dose. See 'Other information'.
<10	Reduce dose. See 'Other information'.

DOSE IN PATIENTS UNDERGOING RENAL REPLACEMENT THERAPIES

CAPD	Unlikely to be dialysed. Dose as in GFR<10 mL/min.
HD	Dialysed. Dose as in GFR<10 mL/min.
HDF/High flux	Dialysed. Dose as in GFR<10 mL/min.
CAV/ VVHD	Unknown dialysability. Dose as in GFR=10–20 mL/min.

IMPORTANT DRUG INTERACTIONS

Potentially hazardous interactions with other drugs
- Increased risk of bleeding in combination with any other drugs that affect coagulation.

ADMINISTRATION

RECONSTITUTION
–
ROUTE
- SC
RATE OF ADMINISTRATION
–
COMMENTS
–

OTHER INFORMATION

- In patients with a GFR of 30–50 mL/min and weight >100 kg, give an initial dose of 10 mg then reduce to 7.5 mg daily for treatment of a DVT; use with caution.
- Manufacturer advises to avoid in severe renal impairment due to increased risk of bleeding.
- Clearance of fondaparinux increases by up to 20% during haemodialysis.
- Has been used successfully at a dose of 2.5 mg for concomitant treatment of a DVT and dialysis anticoagulation every 48 hours for 10 weeks without any problems. (Haase M, Bellomo R, Rocktaeschel J, et al. Use of fondaparinux (arixtra) in a dialysis patient with symptomatic heparin-induced thrombocytopenia type II. Nephrol Dial Transplant. 2005 Feb; 20(2): 444–6.)
- It has also been used for dialysis anticoagulation at a dose of 2.5 mg daily for 4 hours of dialysis using low flux dialysers. Although anti-Xa levels were still

increased before the next dialysis session increasing the bleeding risk. (Sombolos KI, Fragia TK, Gionanlis LC, *et al.* Use of fondaparinux as an anticoagulant during hemodialysis: a preliminary study. *Int J Clin Pharmacol Ther.* 2008 Apr; **46**(4): 198–203.)

- Some units have used fondaparinux for haemodiafiltration in doses ranging from 2.5 mg to 5 mg pre dialysis.

- The following study recommends an initial dose of 0.03 mg/kg pre dialysis for dialysis anti-coagulation. Mahieu E, Claes K, Jacquemin M, *et al.* Anticoagulation with fondaparinux for hemodiafiltration in patients with heparin-induced thrombocytopenia: dose-finding study and safety evaluation. *Artif Organs.* 2013 May; **37**(5): 482–7.

Formoterol fumarate (eformoterol)

CLINICAL USE

Long acting selective beta-2 agonist

DOSE IN NORMAL RENAL FUNCTION

1–2 puffs twice daily.
Turbohaler: 6–24 mcg 1–2 times daily as
a single dose, up to 72 mcg daily may be
needed.

PHARMACOKINETICS

Molecular weight (daltons)	804.9
% Protein binding	61–64
% Excreted unchanged in urine	6.4–8
Volume of distribution (L/kg)	No data
Half-life – normal/ ESRF (hrs)	8/–

METABOLISM

Formoterol is eliminated primarily by
metabolism, direct glucuronidation being
the major pathway of biotransformation,
with O-demethylation followed by further
glucuronidation being another pathway.
Minor pathways involve sulphate conjugation
of formoterol and deformylation followed
by sulphate conjugation. After a single oral
dose of ^{3}H-formoterol, 59–62% of the dose
was recovered in the urine and 32–34%
in the faeces. Approximately 6.4–8% of
the dose was recovered in the urine as
unchanged formoterol, with the (R,R) and
(S,S)-enantiomers contributing 40% and 60%
respectively.

DOSE IN RENAL IMPAIRMENT GFR (mL/MIN)

20–50	Dose as in normal renal function.
10–20	Dose as in normal renal function.
<10	Dose as in normal renal function.

DOSE IN PATIENTS UNDERGOING RENAL REPLACEMENT THERAPIES

CAPD	Not dialysed. Dose as in normal renal function.
HD	Unlikely to be dialysed. Dose as in normal renal function.
HDF/High flux	Unlikely to be dialysed. Dose as in normal renal function.
CAV/ VVHD	Not dialysed. Dose as in normal renal function.

IMPORTANT DRUG INTERACTIONS

Potentially hazardous interactions with
other drugs
● None known

ADMINISTRATION

RECONSTITUTION
–
ROUTE
● Inhaled
RATE OF ADMINISTRATION
–
COMMENTS
–

Fosamprenavir

CLINICAL USE

Protease inhibitor:
- For HIV infection, in combination with other antiretroviral drugs

DOSE IN NORMAL RENAL FUNCTION

700 mg twice daily with ritonavir 100 mg twice daily

PHARMACOKINETICS

Molecular weight (daltons)	625.7 (as calcium salt)
% Protein binding	90 (amprenavir)
% Excreted unchanged in urine	<1 (amprenavir)
Volume of distribution (L/kg)	6 (amprenavir)
Half-life – normal/ESRF (hrs)	7.7/Unchanged (amprenavir)

METABOLISM

Fosamprenavir is rapidly and almost completely hydrolysed to amprenavir and inorganic phosphate as it is absorbed through the gut epithelium, following oral administration. The primary route of metabolism of amprenavir is via the cytochrome P450 3A4 enzyme. The primary route of elimination of amprenavir is via hepatic metabolism with less than 1% excreted unchanged in the urine and no detectable amprenavir in faeces. Metabolites account for approximately 14% of the administered amprenavir dose in the urine, and approximately 75% in the faeces.

DOSE IN RENAL IMPAIRMENT GFR (mL/MIN)

20–50	Dose as in normal renal function.
10–20	Dose as in normal renal function.
<10	Dose as in normal renal function.

DOSE IN PATIENTS UNDERGOING RENAL REPLACEMENT THERAPIES

CAPD	Unlikely to be dialysed. Dose as in normal renal function.
HD	Unlikely to be dialysed. Dose as in normal renal function.
HDF/High flux	Unlikely to be dialysed. Dose as in normal renal function.
CAV/ VVHD	Unlikely to be dialysed. Dose as in normal renal function.

IMPORTANT DRUG INTERACTIONS

Potentially hazardous interactions with other drugs
- Anti-arrhythmics: possibly increased concentration of amiodarone, flecainide, lidocaine and propafenone (increased risk of ventricular arrhythmias) – avoid concomitant use.
- Antibacterials: increases concentration of rifabutin – reduce rifabutin dose; concentration significantly reduced by rifampicin – avoid concomitant use; avoid concomitant use with telithromycin in severe renal and hepatic impairment.
- Antidepressants: concentration reduced by St John's wort – avoid concomitant use.
- Antimalarials: use artemether/ lumefantrine with caution; possibly increases quinine concentration.
- Antipsychotics: possibly inhibits aripiprazole metabolism – reduce aripiprazole dose; possibly increases quetiapine concentration – avoid; possibly increases pimozide concentration (increased risk of ventricular arrhythmias) – avoid concomitant use.
- Antivirals: avoid with boceprevir, raltegravir and telaprevir; concentration increased by etravirine, consider reducing dose of fosamprenavir; concentration reduced by lopinavir and tipranavir; effect on lopinavir unpredictable – avoid; concentration possibly reduced by nevirapine.
- Anxiolytics and hypnotics: increased risk of prolonged sedation and respiratory depression with midazolam – avoid with oral midazolam.
- Ergot alkaloids: increased risk of ergotism – avoid concomitant use.
- Immunosuppressants: monitor ciclosporin, tacrolimus and sirolimus levels.
- Ranolazine: possibly increases ranolazine concentration – avoid.
- Statins: possibly increased risk of myopathy with atorvastatin; possibly increased myopathy with simvastatin and rosuvastatin – avoid concomitant use.

ADMINISTRATION

RECONSTITUTION
–
ROUTE
- Oral

RATE OF ADMINISTRATION
–
COMMENTS
–

OTHER INFORMATION

Prodrug of amprenavir, 700 mg of fosamprenavir is equivalent to 600 mg amprenavir.

Fosaprepitant

CLINICAL USE

Prevention of acute and delayed nausea and vomiting associated with moderate and highly emetogenic cancer chemotherapy

DOSE IN NORMAL RENAL FUNCTION

150 mg 30 minutes before chemotherapy on day 1 of cycle

PHARMACOKINETICS

Molecular weight (daltons)	614.4
% Protein binding	97
% Excreted unchanged in urine	0
Volume of distribution (L/kg)	82 litres
Half-life – normal/ ESRF (hrs)	11/Unchanged

METABOLISM

Fosaprepitant is a prodrug and is rapidly metabolised to aprepitant.

Aprepitant undergoes extensive hepatic metabolism, mainly via oxidation by the cytochrome P450 isoenzyme CYP3A4; the isoenzymes CYP1A2 and CYP2C19 mediate minor metabolic pathways. The resultant metabolites have weak activity and are excreted in the urine and in the faeces. Aprepitant is not excreted unchanged in the urine.

DOSE IN RENAL IMPAIRMENT GFR (mL/MIN)

20–50	Dose as in normal renal function.
10–20	Dose as in normal renal function.
<10	Dose as in normal renal function.

DOSE IN PATIENTS UNDERGOING RENAL REPLACEMENT THERAPIES

CAPD	Not dialysed. Dose as in normal renal function.
HD	Not dialysed. Dose as in normal renal function.
HDF/High flux	Not dialysed. Dose as in normal renal function.
CAV/ VVHD	Not dialysed. Dose as in normal renal function.

IMPORTANT DRUG INTERACTIONS

Potentially hazardous interactions with other drugs
- Avoid concomitant use with pimozide or St John's wort.
- Oestrogens and progestogens: may cause contraceptive failure.

ADMINISTRATION

RECONSTITUTION
- 5 mL of sodium chloride 0.9%
ROUTE
- IV infusion
RATE OF ADMINISTRATION
- 20–30 minutes
COMMENTS
- Add to 145 mL of sodium chloride 0.9%

OTHER INFORMATION

- Less than 0.2% of the dose is dialysed.

Foscarnet sodium

CLINICAL USE

Antiviral agent:
- Treatment and maintenance therapy of cytomegalovirus retinitis (CMV)
- Mucocutaneous herpes simplex infection (HSI)

DOSE IN NORMAL RENAL FUNCTION

- CMV: 60 mg/kg every 8 hours induction dose for 2–3 weeks, then 60 mg/kg daily, increase to 90–120 mg/kg if tolerated.
- Mucocutaneous herpes simplex infection: 40 mg/kg every 8 hours.

PHARMACOKINETICS

Molecular weight (daltons)	300
% Protein binding	14–17
% Excreted unchanged in urine	85
Volume of distribution (L/kg)	0.4–0.6
Half-life – normal/ ESRF (hrs)	2–4/>100

METABOLISM

There is no metabolic conversion of foscarnet and it is eliminated by the kidneys as unchanged drug mainly through glomerular filtration, with some active tubular secretion.

DOSE IN RENAL IMPAIRMENT GFR (mL/MIN)

20–50	28 mg/kg every 8 hours.
10–20	15 mg/kg every 8 hours.
<10	6 mg/kg every 8 hours.

DOSE IN PATIENTS UNDERGOING RENAL REPLACEMENT THERAPIES

CAPD	Dialysed. Dose as in GFR<10 mL/min. See 'Other information'.
HD	Dialysed. Dose as in GFR<10 mL/min. See 'Other information'.
HDF/High flux	Dialysed. Dose as in GFR<10 mL/min. See 'Other information'.
CAV/ VVHD	Dialysed. Dose as in GFR=10–20 mL/min. See 'Other information'.

IMPORTANT DRUG INTERACTIONS

Potentially hazardous interactions with other drugs
- Ciclosporin: may cause acute renal failure in combination.
- Pentamidine: increased risk of hypocalcaemia with parenteral pentamidine.

ADMINISTRATION

RECONSTITUTION
–
ROUTE
- Centrally (undiluted); peripherally (diluted).
RATE OF ADMINISTRATION
- Continuous infusion over 24 hours,
- or intermittent infusion over at least 60 minutes.
COMMENTS
- If given peripherally dilute with glucose 5% or sodium chloride 0.9% to a concentration of 12 mg/mL or less.
- Alternatively, piggy-back the undiluted foscarnet dose to 1 litre of a glucose 5% or sodium chloride 0.9% infusion.
- If given centrally, can be administered undiluted but additional fluids should be given to reduce the risk of nephrotoxicity.

OTHER INFORMATION

- Doses in renal impairment are from *Drug Prescribing in Renal Failure*, 5th edition, by Aronoff *et al.*

Some renal units dose by creatinine clearance/weight as follows (Based on SPC):

Treatment doses for CMV and HSV

Clearance mL/min/kg	Dose for CMV: mg/kg 8 hourly	Dose for HSV: mg/kg 8 hourly
1.6–1.4	55	37
1.4–1.2	49	33
1.2–1	42	28
1–0.8	35	24
0.8–0.6	28	19
0.6–0.4	21	14
0.4–0.2	14	9
0.2–0.1	10	5

Maintenance therapy doses for CMV

Clearance mL/min/kg	Dose: mg/kg daily
1.6–1.4	55
1.4–1.2	49
1.2–1	42
1–0.8	35
0.8–0.6	28
0.6–0.4	21
0.4–0.2	14
0.2–0.1	10

- Maintain adequate hydration to prevent renal toxicity.
- Monitor serum calcium and magnesium.
- Some units use full-dose ganciclovir and half-dose foscarnet concomitantly for treatment of resistant CMV disease.

Fosfomycin (unlicensed)

CLINICAL USE

Antibacterial agent

DOSE IN NORMAL RENAL FUNCTION

- Oral: 3 g sachet as a stat dose
- IV/IM: 0.5–1 g every 6–8 hours (up to 20 g daily have been given IV in severe infections)

PHARMACOKINETICS

Molecular weight (daltons)	138.1 (259.2 as tromethamine)
% Protein binding	0
% Excreted unchanged in urine	38
Volume of distribution (L/kg)	92–180.2
Half-life – normal/ ESRF (hrs)	2.9–8.5/40

METABOLISM

Fosfomycin undergoes no biotransformation and is excreted mainly unchanged through the kidneys. This results in very high urinary concentrations (up to 3 mg/mL) within 2–4 hours of a dose. Therapeutic concentrations of 200–300 mcg/mL in urine are usually maintained for at least 36 hours, and can last 48–72 hours.

DOSE IN RENAL IMPAIRMENT GFR (mL/MIN)

20–50	Dose as in normal renal function
10–20	Dose as in normal renal function
<10	Contraindicated due to prolonged half-life. See 'Other information'.

DOSE IN PATIENTS UNDERGOING RENAL REPLACEMENT THERAPIES

CAPD	Dialysed. Dose as in GFR<10 mL/min.
HD	Dialysed. Dose as in GFR<10 mL/min.
HDF/High flux	Dialysed. Dose as in GFR<10 mL/min.
CAV/VVHD	Dialysed. Dose as in GFR=10–20 mL/min.

IMPORTANT DRUG INTERACTIONS

Potentially hazardous interactions with other drugs
- Metoclopramide: metoclopramide increases gastrointestinal motility and therefore lowers the serum concentration and urinary excretion of fosfomycin.

ADMINISTRATION

ROUTE
- IM, IV, Oral

OTHER INFORMATION

- Oral bioavailability is 30–40%.
- In 5 anuric patients undergoing haemodialysis, the t½ of fosfomycin during haemodialysis was 40 hours. In patients with varying degrees of renal impairment (creatinine clearances varying from 54 mL/min to 7 mL/min), the t½ of fosfomycin increased from 11 hours to 50 hours. The percentage of fosfomycin recovered in urine decreased from 32% to 11% indicating that renal impairment significantly decreases the excretion of fosfomycin.
- Development of bacterial resistance under therapy is a frequent occurrence and makes fosfomycin unsuitable for sustained therapy of severe infections.
- In severe renal impairment a 3 g dose can maintain therapeutic plasma levels for 7–10 days.

Fosinopril sodium

CLINICAL USE

Angiotensin-converting enzyme inhibitor:
- Hypertension
- Heart failure

DOSE IN NORMAL RENAL FUNCTION

10–40 mg once daily

PHARMACOKINETICS

Molecular weight (daltons)	585.6
% Protein binding	95
% Excreted unchanged in urine	<1
Volume of distribution (L/kg)	0.15
Half-life – normal/ ESRF (hrs)	11.5–14/14–32

METABOLISM

Fosinopril acts as a prodrug of the diacid fosinoprilat, its active metabolite. Fosinopril is rapidly and completely hydrolysed to fosinoprilat in both gastrointestinal mucosa and liver. Fosinoprilat is excreted both in urine and in the faeces via the bile.

DOSE IN RENAL IMPAIRMENT
GFR (mL/MIN)

20–50	Dose as in normal renal function.
10–20	Dose as in normal renal function. Start with low dose.
<10	Dose as in normal renal function. Start with low dose.

DOSE IN PATIENTS UNDERGOING RENAL REPLACEMENT THERAPIES

CAPD	Not dialysed. Dose as in GFR<10 mL/min.
HD	Not dialysed. Dose as in GFR<10 mL/min.
HDF/High flux	Unlikely to be dialysed. Dose as in GFR<10 mL/min.
CAV/ VVHD	Unlikely to be dialysed. Dose as in GFR=10–20 mL/min.

IMPORTANT DRUG INTERACTIONS

Potentially hazardous interactions with other drugs
- Anaesthetics: enhanced hypotensive effect.
- Analgesics: antagonism of hypotensive effect and increased risk of renal impairment with NSAIDs; hyperkalaemia with ketorolac and other NSAIDs.
- Ciclosporin: increased risk of hyperkalaemia and nephrotoxicity.
- Diuretics: enhanced hypotensive effect; hyperkalaemia with potassium-sparing diuretics.
- ESAs: increased risk of hyperkalaemia; antagonism of hypotensive effect.
- Gold: flushing and hypotension with sodium aurothiomalate.
- Lithium: reduced excretion, possibility of enhanced lithium toxicity.
- Potassium salts: increased risk of hyperkalaemia.
- Tacrolimus: increased risk of hyperkalaemia and nephrotoxicity.

ADMINISTRATION

RECONSTITUTION
–
ROUTE
- Oral
RATE OF ADMINISTRATION
–
COMMENTS
–

OTHER INFORMATION

- Hepatobiliary elimination compensates for diminished renal excretion.
- Hyperkalaemia and other side effects more common in patients with impaired renal function.
- Close monitoring of renal function during therapy necessary in those with renal insufficiency.
- Renal failure has been reported in association with ACE inhibitors in patients with renal artery stenosis, post renal transplant, and those with congestive heart failure.
- High incidence of anaphylactoid reactions has been reported in patients dialysed with high-flux polyacrylonitrile membranes and treated concomitantly with an ACE inhibitor – this combination should therefore be avoided.

Fosphenytoin sodium

CLINICAL USE

- Control of status epilepticus
- Seizures associated with neurosurgery or head injury when oral phenytoin is not possible

DOSE IN NORMAL RENAL FUNCTION

- Status epilepticus:
  - Treatment: 20 mg PE/kg (loading dose) by IV infusion
  - Maintenance: 4–5 mg PE/kg daily in 1–2 divided doses
- Prophylaxis or treatment of seizures: 10–15 mg PE/kg by IV infusion; then convert to phenytoin or 4–5 mg PE/kg daily in 1–2 divided doses

PHARMACOKINETICS

Molecular weight (daltons)	406.2
% Protein binding	95–99
% Excreted unchanged in urine	1–5
Volume of distribution (L/kg)	4.3–10.8 litres
Half-life – normal/ESRF (hrs)	18.9 (IV), 41.2 (IM)/Unchanged

METABOLISM

Fosphenytoin is rapidly and completely hydrolysed to phenytoin with a conversion half-life of about 15 minutes; 1 mmol of fosphenytoin yields 1 mmol of phenytoin. Phenytoin is hydroxylated in the liver to inactive metabolites, chiefly 5-(4-hydroxyphenyl)-5-phenylhydantoin by an enzyme system which is saturable. Phenytoin undergoes enterohepatic recycling and is excreted in the urine, mainly as its hydroxylated metabolite, in either free or conjugated form.

DOSE IN RENAL IMPAIRMENT GFR (mL/MIN)

20–50	Reduce dose or rate by 10–25% and monitor carefully (except for status epilepticus).
10–20	Reduce dose or rate by 10–25% and monitor carefully (except for status epilepticus).
<10	Reduce dose or rate by 10–25% and monitor carefully (except for status epilepticus).

DOSE IN PATIENTS UNDERGOING RENAL REPLACEMENT THERAPIES

CAPD	Unlikely to be dialysed. Dose as in GFR<10 mL/min.
HD	Not dialysed. Dose as in GFR<10 mL/min.
HDF/High flux	Unlikely to be dialysed. Dose as in GFR<10 mL/min.
CAV/ VVHD	Not dialysed. Dose as in GFR=10–20 mL/min.

IMPORTANT DRUG INTERACTIONS

Potentially hazardous interactions with other drugs

- Analgesics: enhanced effect with NSAIDs; metabolism of methadone accelerated.
- Anti-arrhythmics: increased concentration with amiodarone; concentration of disopyramide and possibly dronedarone reduced – avoid with dronedarone.
- Antibacterials: level increased by clarithromycin, chloramphenicol, isoniazid, metronidazole, sulfonamides and trimethoprim (+ antifolate effect); concentration increased or decreased by ciprofloxacin; concentration of doxycycline and telithromycin reduced – avoid with telithromycin; concentration reduced by rifamycins.
- Anticoagulants: increased metabolism of coumarins (reduced effect but also reports of enhancement); possibly reduced dabigatran concentration – avoid.
- Antidepressants: antagonise anticonvulsant effect; concentration increased by fluoxetine and fluvoxamine and possibly sertraline; concentration of mianserin, mirtazapine and paroxetine and possibly tricyclics reduced; concentration reduced by St John's wort – avoid.
- Anti-epileptics: concentration of both drugs reduced with carbamazepine, concentration may also be increased by carbamazepine, eslicarbazepine, ethosuximide, oxcarbazepine, stiripentol and topiramate; concentration of ethosuximide, active oxcarbazepine metabolite, retigabine, rufinamide (concentration of phenytoin possibly increased), topiramate and valproate possibly reduced; concentration of eslicarbazepine, ethosuximide,

lamotrigine, perampanel, tiagabine and zonisamide reduced; concentration of phenobarbital often increased; phenobarbital and valproate may alter concentration; concentration reduced by vigabatrin.
- Antifungals: concentration of ketoconazole, itraconazole, posaconazole, voriconazole and possibly caspofungin reduced – avoid with itraconazole, increase voriconazole dose and possibly caspofungin; levels increased by fluconazole, miconazole and voriconazole.
- Antimalarials: avoid with piperaquine with artenimol, mefloquine and pyrimethamine – antagonise anticonvulsant effect; increased antifolate effect with pyrimethamine.
- Antipsychotics: antagonise anticonvulsant effect; possibly reduced aripiprazole concentration – increase aripiprazole dose; metabolism of clozapine, haloperidol, quetiapine and sertindole increased; concentration increased or decreased with chlorpromazine.
- Antivirals: possibly reduced concentration of abacavir, darunavir, indinavir, lopinavir, ritonavir and saquinavir; concentration of boceprevir and rilpivirine reduced – avoid; concentration possibly increased by indinavir and ritonavir; concentration increased or decreased with zidovudine; avoid with etravirine and telaprevir.
- Calcium-channel blockers: levels increased by diltiazem; concentration of diltiazem, felodipine, isradipine, nimodipine and verapamil reduced; avoid with isradipine and nimodipine.
- Ciclosporin: reduced ciclosporin levels.
- Corticosteroids: metabolism accelerated (effect reduced).
- Cytotoxics: metabolism possibly inhibited by fluorouracil; increased antifolate effect with methotrexate; reduced phenytoin absorption; concentration of busulfan, eribulin, etoposide and imatinib reduced – avoid with imatinib; concentration possibly reduced by cisplatin; possibly reduced concentration of axitinib, increase axitinib dose; possibly reduced concentration of crizotinib – avoid; avoid with cabazitaxel, gefitinib, lapatinib and vemurafenib; concentration of irinotecan and its active metabolite reduced.
- Disulfiram: levels of phenytoin increased.
- Diuretics: concentration increased by acetazolamide; concentration of eplerenone reduced – avoid concomitant use; increased risk of osteomalacia with carbonic anhydrase inhibitors; antagonises effect of furosemide.
- Muscle relaxants: long-term use of phenytoin reduces effects of non-depolarising muscle relaxants, but acute use may enhance effects.
- Oestrogens and progestogens: metabolism increased (reduced contraceptive effect).
- Orlistat: possibly increased risk of convulsions.
- Sulfinpyrazone: concentration increased by sulfinpyrazone.
- Theophylline: concentration of both drugs reduced.
- Ulcer-healing drugs: metabolism inhibited by cimetidine; absorption reduced by sucralfate; enhanced effect with esomeprazole and omeprazole.
- Ulipristal: contraceptive effect possibly reduced – avoid.

ADMINISTRATION

RECONSTITUTION
–
ROUTE
- IV, IM
RATE OF ADMINISTRATION
- Status epilepticus: 100–150 mg PE/min
- Treatment and prophylaxis of seizures: 50–100 mg PE/min
COMMENTS
- Dilute further when using for IV infusion with sodium chloride 0.9% or glucose 5% to 1.5–25 mg PE/mL.

OTHER INFORMATION

- 75 mg of fosphenytoin sodium is equivalent to 50 mg of phenytoin.
- 0.037 mmol of phosphate/mg of fosphenytoin.
- Decreased protein binding in renal failure.
- Monitor ECG, BP and respiratory function during infusion.
- When substituting IV, IM use same dose and frequency as for oral phenytoin, administer at a rate of 50–100 mg PE/min.
- May increase blood glucose in diabetic patients.
- Some is dialysed out, as not all PE is protein-bound.
- Half-life of fosphenytoin to phenytoin is 15 minutes; more rapid in renal failure due to reduced protein binding.

Frovatriptan

CLINICAL USE

$5HT_1$ receptor agonist:
- Acute relief of migraine

DOSE IN NORMAL RENAL FUNCTION

2.5 mg; a second dose can be taken if required after at least 2 hours.
Maximum daily dose is 5 mg.

PHARMACOKINETICS

Molecular weight (daltons)	243.3
% Protein binding	15
% Excreted unchanged in urine	10–32
Volume of distribution (L/kg)	3–4.2
Half-life – normal/ ESRF (hrs)	26/Unchanged

METABOLISM

Following oral administration of radiolabelled frovatriptan, 32% of the dose was recovered in urine and 62% in faeces. Radiolabelled compounds excreted in urine were unchanged frovatriptan, hydroxy frovatriptan, N-acetyl desmethyl frovatriptan, hydroxy N-acetyl desmethyl frovatriptan, and desmethyl frovatriptan, together with several other minor metabolites formed under the action of CYP1A2. Desmethyl frovatriptan had about 3-fold lower affinity at 5-HT1 receptors than the parent compound. N-acetyl desmethyl frovatriptan had negligible affinity at 5-HT1 receptors. The activity of other metabolites has not been studied. Renal clearance accounted for 38% (82 mL/min) and 49% (65 mL/min) of total clearance in males and females, respectively.

DOSE IN RENAL IMPAIRMENT GFR (mL/MIN)

20–50	Dose as in normal renal function.
10–20	Dose as in normal renal function.
<10	Dose as in normal renal function.

DOSE IN PATIENTS UNDERGOING RENAL REPLACEMENT THERAPIES

CAPD	Likely dialysability. Dose as in normal renal function.
HD	Likely dialysability. Dose as in normal renal function.
HDF/High flux	Likely dialysability. Dose as in normal renal function.
CAV/ VVHD	Likely dialysability. Dose as in normal renal function.

IMPORTANT DRUG INTERACTIONS

Potentially hazardous interactions with other drugs
- Antidepressants: increased CNS toxicity with citalopram – avoid; blood levels of frovatriptan increased 27–49% by fluvoxamine – avoid concomitant use; possibly increased serotonergic effects with duloxetine, venlafaxine and SSRIs; increased serotonergic effects with St John's wort – avoid concomitant use.
- Ergot alkaloids: increased risk of vasospasm – avoid.

ADMINISTRATION

RECONSTITUTION
–
ROUTE
- Oral
RATE OF ADMINISTRATION
–
COMMENTS
–

Fulvestrant

CLINICAL USE

Treatment of postmenopausal women with oestrogen-receptor-positive, locally advanced or metastatic breast cancer

DOSE IN NORMAL RENAL FUNCTION

500 mg every 2 weeks for the first 3 doses then 500 mg every month

PHARMACOKINETICS

Molecular weight (daltons)	606.8
% Protein binding	99
% Excreted unchanged in urine	<1
Volume of distribution (L/kg)	3–5
Half-life – normal/ ESRF (hrs)	40 days/Unchanged

METABOLISM

The metabolism of fulvestrant has not been fully evaluated, but involves combinations of a number of possible biotransformation pathways analogous to those of endogenous steroids. Identified metabolites (includes 17-ketone, sulphone, 3-sulphate, 3- and 17-glucuronide metabolites) are either less active or exhibit similar activity to fulvestrant in anti-oestrogen models.

Fulvestrant is eliminated mainly in metabolised form. The major route of excretion is via the faeces, with less than 1% being excreted in the urine.

DOSE IN RENAL IMPAIRMENT GFR (mL/MIN)

30–50	Dose as in normal renal function.
10–30	Dose as in normal renal function.
<10	Dose as in normal renal function.

DOSE IN PATIENTS UNDERGOING RENAL REPLACEMENT THERAPIES

CAPD	Unlikely to be dialysed. Dose as in normal renal function.
HD	Unlikely to be dialysed. Dose as in normal renal function.
HDF/High flux	Unlikely to be dialysed. Dose as in normal renal function.
CAV/ VVHD	Unlikely to be dialysed. Dose as in normal renal function.

IMPORTANT DRUG INTERACTIONS

Potentially hazardous interactions with other drugs
- None known

ADMINISTRATION

RECONSTITUTION
–
ROUTE
- IM
RATE OF ADMINISTRATION
- 1–2 minutes
COMMENTS
- Administer as 2 separate injections, one in each buttock

OTHER INFORMATION

- As it is an intramuscular injection, use with caution in patients who are heparinised.
- Manufacturer in UK SPC advises to use with caution due to lack of data if GFR<30 mL/min but US data sheet has no restrictions as minimal renal excretion.

Furosemide (frusemide)

CLINICAL USE

Loop diuretic.

DOSE IN NORMAL RENAL FUNCTION

- Oral: 20 mg – 1 g daily
- IV: 20 mg – 1.5 g daily

Doses titrated to response.

PHARMACOKINETICS

Molecular weight (daltons)	330.7
% Protein binding	91–99
% Excreted unchanged in urine	80–90
Volume of distribution (L/kg)	0.07–0.2
Half-life – normal/ ESRF (hrs)	0.5–2/9.7

METABOLISM

Little biotransformation of furosemide takes place. It is mainly eliminated via the kidneys (80–90%); a small fraction of the dose undergoes biliary elimination and 10–15% of the activity can be recovered from the faeces.

DOSE IN RENAL IMPAIRMENT GFR (mL/MIN)

20–50	Dose as in normal renal function.
10–20	Dose as in normal renal function; increased doses may be required.
<10	Dose as in normal renal function; increased doses may be required.

DOSE IN PATIENTS UNDERGOING RENAL REPLACEMENT THERAPIES

CAPD	Not dialysed. Dose as in GFR<10 mL/min.
HD	Not dialysed. Dose as in GFR<10 mL/min.
HDF/High flux	Not dialysed. Dose as in GFR<10 mL/min.
CAV/ VVHD	Not dialysed. Dose as in GFR=10–20 mL/min.

IMPORTANT DRUG INTERACTIONS

Potentially hazardous interactions with other drugs

- Analgesics: increased risk of nephrotoxicity with NSAIDs; antagonism of diuretic effect with NSAIDs.
- Anti-arrhythmics: risk of cardiac toxicity with anti-arrhythmics if hypokalaemia occurs; effects of lidocaine and mexiletine antagonised.
- Antibacterials: increased risk of ototoxicity with aminoglycosides, polymyxins and vancomycin; avoid concomitant use with lymecycline.
- Antidepressants: increased risk of hypokalaemia with reboxetine; enhanced hypotensive effect with MAOIs; increased risk of postural hypotension with tricyclics.
- Anti-epileptics: increased risk of hyponatraemia with carbamazepine; effects antagonised by phenytoin.
- Antifungals: increased risk of hypokalaemia with amphotericin.
- Antihypertensives: enhanced hypotensive effect; increased risk of first dose hypotensive effect with alpha-blockers; increased risk of ventricular arrhythmias with sotalol if hypokalaemia occurs.
- Antipsychotics: increased risk of ventricular arrhythmias with amisulpride or pimozide (avoid with pimozide) if hypokalaemia occurs; enhanced hypotensive effect with phenothiazines.
- Atomoxetine: hypokalaemia increases risk of ventricular arrhythmias.
- Cardiac glycosides: increased toxicity if hypokalaemia occurs.
- Ciclosporin: variable reports of increased nephrotoxicity, ototoxicity and hepatotoxicity.
- Cytotoxics: increased risk of ventricular arrhythmias due to hypokalaemia with arsenic trioxide; increased risk of nephrotoxicity and ototoxicity with platinum compounds.
- Lithium: risk of toxicity.

ADMINISTRATION

RECONSTITUTION

–

ROUTE
- IV peripherally or centrally, IM, Oral

RATE OF ADMINISTRATION
- 1 hour; not greater than 4 mg/minute

COMMENTS
  — 250 mg to 50 mL sodium chloride 0.9% or undiluted via CRIP
  — Increased danger of ototoxicity and nephrotoxicity if infused at faster rate than approximately 4 mg/minute.
  — Protect from light

OTHER INFORMATION

- 500 mg orally ≡ 250 mg IV
- Excreted by tubular secretion, therefore in severe renal impairment (GFR=5–10 mL/min) higher doses may be required due to a reduction in the number of functioning nephrons.
- Furosemide acts within 1 hour of oral administration (after IV peak effect within 30 minutes), diuresis complete within 6 hours.

Gabapentin

CLINICAL USE

Anti-epileptic:
- Adjunctive treatment of partial seizures with or without secondary generalisation
- Neuropathic pain
- Migraine prophylaxis (unlicensed)

DOSE IN NORMAL RENAL FUNCTION

- Epilepsy: 300 mg on day 1; 300 mg twice daily on day 2; 300 mg 3 times daily on day 3.
- Usual range 0.9–3.6 g daily in 3 divided doses, max 4.8 g daily in divided doses.
- Neuropathic pain: Maximum 3.6 g in 3 divided doses.
- Migraine prophylaxis: Initially 300 mg daily increasing up to 2.4 g daily in divided doses.

PHARMACOKINETICS

Molecular weight (daltons)	171.2
% Protein binding	<3
% Excreted unchanged in urine	≈100
Volume of distribution (L/kg)	0.7
Half-life – normal/ ESRF (hrs)	5–7/52

METABOLISM

There is no evidence of gabapentin metabolism in humans. Gabapentin is eliminated unchanged solely by renal excretion.

DOSE IN RENAL IMPAIRMENT GFR (mL/MIN)

30–60	Start at low dose and increase dose according to response.
15–30	Start at low dose and increase dose according to response.
<15	300 mg on alternate days or 100 mg at night initially, increase according to tolerability.

DOSE IN PATIENTS UNDERGOING RENAL REPLACEMENT THERAPIES

CAPD	Probably dialysed. Dose as in GFR<15 mL/min. See 'Other information'.
HD	Dialysed. Loading dose of 300–400 mg in patients who have never received gabapentin. Maintenance dose of 200–300 mg after each HD session and increase according to tolerability. See 'Other information'.
HDF/High flux	Dialysed. Loading dose of 300–400 mg in patients who have never received gabapentin. Maintenance dose of 200–300 mg after each HD session and increase according to tolerability. See 'Other information'.
CAV/ VVHD	Dialysed. Dose as in GFR=15–30 mL/min.

IMPORTANT DRUG INTERACTIONS

Potentially hazardous interactions with other drugs
- Antacids: reduce absorption.
- Antidepressants: antagonism of anticonvulsive effect (convulsive threshold lowered); avoid with St John's wort.
- Antimalarials: anticonvulsant effect antagonised by mefloquine.
- Orlistat: possible increased risk of convulsions.

ADMINISTRATION

RECONSTITUTION
–
ROUTE
- Oral
RATE OF ADMINISTRATION
–
COMMENTS
–

OTHER INFORMATION

- For neuropathic pain in renal patients do not give loading dose.
- Can cause false positive readings with some urinary protein tests.
- For neuropathic pain or restless legs in patients with moderate to severe renal impairment, start with 100 mg daily and increase according to response.
- Can be used to treat dialysis itch. (Gunal AI, Ozalp G, Yoldas TK, *et al.* Gabapentin therapy for pruritus in haemodialysis patients: a randomized, placebo-controlled, double-blind trial. *Nephrol Dial Transplant.* 2004; **19**(12): 3137–9.)

Galantamine

CLINICAL USE

Mild to moderate dementia in Alzheimer's disease

DOSE IN NORMAL RENAL FUNCTION

4–12 mg twice daily
XL: 8–24 mg once daily

PHARMACOKINETICS

Molecular weight (daltons)	368.3 (as hydrobromide)
% Protein binding	18
% Excreted unchanged in urine	18–22
Volume of distribution (L/kg)	175 litres
Half-life – normal/ ESRF (hrs)	7–8 (XL: 8–10)/ Increased

METABOLISM

Galantamine is partially (up to 75%) metabolised by the cytochrome P450 isoenzymes CYP2D6 and CYP3A4; a number of active metabolites are formed. The elimination half-life is about 7 to 8 hours. After 7 days, 90–97% of a single oral dose is recovered in the urine with up to about 6% detected in the faeces; about 20–30% of the dose is excreted in the urine as unchanged galantamine. Clearance is reported to be 20% lower in females than in males and 25% lower in poor metabolisers than in extensive metabolisers.

DOSE IN RENAL IMPAIRMENT GFR (mL/MIN)

20–50	Dose as in normal renal function.
10–20	Dose as in normal renal function.
<10	Dose as in normal renal function but start with lower doses.

DOSE IN PATIENTS UNDERGOING RENAL REPLACEMENT THERAPIES

CAPD	Dialysed. Dose as in GFR<10 mL/min.
HD	Dialysed. Dose as in GFR<10 mL/min.
HDF/High flux	Dialysed. Dose as in GFR<10 mL/min.
CAV/VVHD	Dialysed. Dose as in normal renal function.

IMPORTANT DRUG INTERACTIONS

Potentially hazardous interactions with other drugs
- Antibacterials: erythromycin increases concentration of galantamine.

ADMINISTRATION

RECONSTITUTION
–
ROUTE
- Oral
RATE OF ADMINISTRATION
–
COMMENTS
–

OTHER INFORMATION

- Manufacturer advises to avoid use if GFR<9 mL/min due to lack of studies

Ganciclovir

CLINICAL USE

Antiviral agent:
- Treatment of life- or sight-threatening cytomegalovirus (CMV) in immunocompromised people
- CMV prophylaxis in immunosuppressed patients secondary to organ transplantation

DOSE IN NORMAL RENAL FUNCTION

- Induction/treatment of active CMV disease: 5 mg/kg 12 hourly for 14–21 days.
- Maintenance for CMV retinitis: 6 mg/kg per day for 5 days per week or 5 mg/kg daily until recovery of adequate immunity.

PHARMACOKINETICS

Molecular weight (daltons)	255.2
% Protein binding	<2
% Excreted unchanged in urine	84.6–94.6
Volume of distribution (L/kg)	0.54–0.87
Half-life – normal/ESRF (hrs)	2.9/28.5

METABOLISM

Renal excretion of unchanged drug by glomerular filtration and active tubular secretion is the major route of elimination of ganciclovir. In patients with normal renal function, 89.6 ± 5.0% of IV administered ganciclovir was recovered unmetabolised in the urine.

DOSE IN RENAL IMPAIRMENT GFR (mL/MIN)

20–50	See 'Other information'.
10–20	See 'Other information'.
<10	See 'Other information'.

DOSE IN PATIENTS UNDERGOING RENAL REPLACEMENT THERAPIES

CAPD	Dialysed. 1.25 mg/kg every day.
HD	Dialysed. 1.25 mg/kg every day, given post dialysis on dialysis days.
HDF/High flux	Dialysed. 1.25 mg/kg every day, given post dialysis on dialysis days.
CAV/ VVHD	Dialysed. 2.5 mg/kg per day. See 'Other information'.

IMPORTANT DRUG INTERACTIONS

Potentially hazardous interactions with other drugs
- Antibacterials: increased risk of convulsions with imipenem/cilastatin.
- Antivirals: possibly increased didanosine concentration; profound myelosuppression with zidovudine – avoid if possible.
- Increased risk of myelosuppression with other myelosuppressive drugs.
- Mycophenolate: concomitant treatment with ganciclovir and mycophenolate causes increased concentration of ganciclovir and inactive mycophenolate metabolite.

ADMINISTRATION

RECONSTITUTION
- Reconstitute 1 vial (500 mg) with 10 mL water for injection (50 mg/mL), then transfer dose to 100 mL sodium chloride 0.9%.

ROUTE
- IV peripherally in fast-flowing vein or centrally – see below.

RATE OF ADMINISTRATION
- Over 1 hour

COMMENTS
- May give 50% dose over 15 minutes after HD in washback (unlicensed).

OTHER INFORMATION

From SPC:

Creatinine Clearance (mL/min)	Dose
>70	5 mg/kg 12 hourly
50–69	2.5 mg/kg 12 hourly
25–49	2.5 mg/kg 24 hourly
10–24	1.25 mg/kg 24 hourly
<10	1.25 mg/kg 24 hourly, given after haemodialysis on dialysis days

Alternative regimen used by some units:

Creatinine Clearance (mL/min)	Dose
>50	5 mg/kg 12 hourly
25–50	2.5 mg/kg 12 hourly
10–25	2.5 mg/kg 24 hourly
<10	1.25 mg/kg 24 hourly

- Some units use 2.5 mg/kg twice daily in CAV/VVHD.

- Monitor patient for myelosuppression, particularly in patients receiving prophylactic co-trimoxazole therapy.
- Pre-dialysis therapeutic blood levels in range 5–12 mg/L.
- For intermittent haemodialysis, the fraction of ganciclovir removed in a single dialysis session varied from 50% to 63%.
- Not to be infused in concentrations over 10 mg/mL peripherally.

Gefitinib

CLINICAL USE

Tyrosine kinase inhibitor:
- Treatment of non-small cell lung cancer

DOSE IN NORMAL RENAL FUNCTION

250 mg once daily
Consult relevant local protocol

PHARMACOKINETICS

Molecular weight (daltons)	446.9
% Protein binding	90
% Excreted unchanged in urine	<4
Volume of distribution (L/kg)	1400 litres
Half-life – normal/ ESRF (hrs)	41–48/Unchanged

METABOLISM

Extensively metabolised in the liver, mainly by the cytochrome P450 isoenzymes CYP3A4 and CYP2D6; the major metabolite is O-desmethylgefitinib, which is much less potent than gefitinib, and unlikely to contribute to its clinical activity.

Gefitinib is excreted mainly as metabolites via the faeces (86%); renal elimination of gefitinib and its metabolites accounts for <4% of the dose.

DOSE IN RENAL IMPAIRMENT GFR (mL/MIN)

20–50	Dose as in normal renal function.
10–20	Dose as in normal renal function. Use with caution.
<10	Dose as in normal renal function. Use with caution.

DOSE IN PATIENTS UNDERGOING RENAL REPLACEMENT THERAPIES

CAPD	Not dialysed. Dose as in GFR<10 mL/min.
HD	Not dialysed. Dose as in GFR<10 mL/min.
HDF/High flux	Not dialysed. Dose as in GFR<10 mL/min.
CAV/ VVHD	Not dialysed. Dose as in GFR=10–20 mL/min.

IMPORTANT DRUG INTERACTIONS

Potentially hazardous interactions with other drugs
- Antibacterials: avoid concomitant use with rifampicin (reduced gefitinib concentration).
- Anticoagulants: possibly enhanced anticoagulant effect with warfarin.
- Antipsychotics: avoid concomitant use with clozapine (increased risk of agranulocytosis).
- Antivirals: avoid concomitant use with boceprevir.
- Ulcer-healing drugs: concentration reduced by ranitidine.
- Avoid concomitant use with other inhibitors or inducers of CYP3A4. Dose alterations may be required.

ADMINISTRATION

RECONSTITUTION
–
ROUTE
- Oral
RATE OF ADMINISTRATION
–

OTHER INFORMATION

- Manufacturer advises to use gefitinib with caution if GFR<20 mL/min due to lack of studies but clearance is unlikely to be affected due to low renal excretion.
- Bioavailability is 59%.
- Adverse effects are related to dose and exposure.

Gemcitabine

CLINICAL USE

Antineoplastic agent:
- Palliative treatment, or first-line treatment with cisplatin, of locally advanced or metastatic non-small cell lung cancer
- Pancreatic and breast cancer
- Bladder cancer in combination with cisplatin

DOSE IN NORMAL RENAL FUNCTION

$1-1.25 \text{ mg/m}^2$, frequency dependent on chemotherapy regimen; dose reduced according to toxicity.

PHARMACOKINETICS

Molecular weight (daltons)	299.7 (as Hydrochloride)
% Protein binding	Negligible
% Excreted unchanged in urine	<10
Volume of distribution (L/kg)	12.4 litres/m^2 (women); 17.5 litres/m^2 (men)
Half-life – normal/ ESRF (hrs)	42–94 minutes/–

METABOLISM

After intravenous doses gemcitabine is rapidly cleared from the blood and metabolised by cytidine deaminase in the liver, kidney, blood, and other tissues. Clearance is about 25% lower in women than in men. Almost all (99%) of the dose is excreted in urine as 2'-deoxy-2',2'-difluorouridine (dFdU), only about 1% being found in the faeces. Intracellular metabolism produces mono-, di-, and triphosphate metabolites, the latter two active. The active intracellular metabolites have not been detected in plasma or urine.

DOSE IN RENAL IMPAIRMENT GFR (mL/MIN)

20–50	Dose as in normal renal function.
10–20	Use with caution. See 'Other information'.
<10	Use with caution. See 'Other information'.

DOSE IN PATIENTS UNDERGOING RENAL REPLACEMENT THERAPIES

CAPD	Likely dialysability. Dose as in GFR <10 mL/min.
HD	Dialysed. Dose as in GFR <10 mL/min. Dose after dialysis, and give next dialysis after 48 hours.
HDF/High flux	Dialysed. Dose as in GFR <10 mL/min. Dose after dialysis, and give next dialysis after 48 hours.
CAV/ VVHD	Dialysed. Dose as in GFR=10–20 mL/min.

IMPORTANT DRUG INTERACTIONS

Potentially hazardous interactions with other drugs
- Antipsychotics: avoid concomitant use with clozapine, increased risk of agranulocytosis.

ADMINISTRATION

RECONSTITUTION
- Reconstitute with sodium chloride 0.9%, 5 mL to 200 mg vial and 25 mL to 1 g vial.
- Can be further diluted in sodium chloride 0.9% if required.

ROUTE
- IV

RATE OF ADMINISTRATION
- 30 minutes

OTHER INFORMATION

- Manufacturer advises to use with caution due to lack of studies.
- Causes reversible haematuria with or without proteinuria in about 50% of patients; no evidence for cumulative renal toxicity with repeated dosing of gemcitabine.
- Haemolytic uraemic syndrome (HUS) has been reported with a crude incidence rate of 0.015%.
- A study looking at the use of gemcitabine 500–1000 mg/m^2 administered IV on days 1, 8, and 15 every 28 days in patients with renal dysfunction concluded that this regimen was well tolerated in patients with a GFR as low as 30 mL/min. (Data on file from Eli Lilly)
- Another study in patients with serum creatinine in the range 130–420 μmol/L, at doses of 650–800 mg/m^2 weekly for 3 weeks out of a 4 week cycle, found dose limiting toxicities, including neutropenia, fever, raised transaminases and increased

serum creatinine. It was concluded that a reduced dose of gemcitabine might be appropriate in patients with established renal impairment. (Egorin MJ, Venook MP, Rosner G, *et al.* Phase 1 study of gemcitabine (G) in patients with organ dysfunction. *Proc Annual Meet Am Soc Clin Oncol.* 1998; **17**: A719).

- The following series of 5 cases showed that gemcitabine can be used safely at doses of 800–1000 mg as long as the patients are on haemodialysis: Matsuda M. Gemcitabine for patients with chronic renal failure on hemodialysis. *J Clin Oncol.* 2007; **25**(18S) (June 20 Supplement): 15189. 2007 ASCO Annual Meeting Proceedings.

Gemfibrozil

CLINICAL USE

Hyperlipidaemias of types IIa, IIb, III, IV and V

DOSE IN NORMAL RENAL FUNCTION

1.2 g daily, usually in 2 divided doses; range 0.9–1.2 g daily.

PHARMACOKINETICS

Molecular weight (daltons)	250.3
% Protein binding	>97
% Excreted unchanged in urine	<6
Volume of distribution (L/kg)	9–13 litres
Half-life – normal/ESRF (hrs)	1.3–1.5/ Unchanged

METABOLISM

Gemfibrozil undergoes oxidation of a ring methyl group to form successively a hydroxymethyl and a carboxyl metabolite (the main metabolite). This metabolite has a low activity compared to the mother compound gemfibrozil and an elimination half-life of approximately 20 hours.

Gemfibrozil is eliminated mainly by metabolism. Approximately 70% of the administered human dose is excreted in the urine, mainly as conjugates of gemfibrozil and its metabolites. Less than 6% of the dose is excreted unchanged in the urine; 6% of the dose is found in faeces.

DOSE IN RENAL IMPAIRMENT GFR (mL/MIN)

20–50	Initially 900 mg daily.
10–20	Initially 900 mg daily. Monitor carefully.
<10	Initially 900 mg daily. Monitor carefully.

DOSE IN PATIENTS UNDERGOING RENAL REPLACEMENT THERAPIES

CAPD	Not dialysed. Dose as in GFR<10 mL/min.
HD	Not dialysed. Dose as in GFR<10 mL/min.
HDF/High flux	Not dialysed. Dose as in GFR<10 mL/min.
CAV/ VVHD	Not dialysed. Dose as in GFR=10–20 mL/min.

IMPORTANT DRUG INTERACTIONS

Potentially hazardous interactions with other drugs

- Antibacterials: increased risk of myopathy with daptomycin – try to avoid concomitant use.
- Anticoagulants: enhances effect of coumarins and phenindione; dose of anticoagulant should be reduced by up to 50% and adjusted by monitoring INR.
- Antidiabetics: may improve glucose tolerance and have an additive effect with insulin or sulphonylureas; rosiglitazone concentration increased – possibly reduce rosiglitazone dose; possibly enhanced effect with nateglinide; increased risk of severe hypoglycaemia with repaglinide – avoid concomitant use.
- Ciclosporin: Parke-Davis have one report on file of an interaction with ciclosporin where serum ciclosporin levels were decreased. No effects on muscle were noted.
- Colchicine: possible increased risk of myopathy.
- Cytotoxics: bexarotene concentration increased – avoid concomitant use.
- Lipid-regulating drugs: increased risk of myopathy in combination with statins and ezetimibe – avoid concomitant use (maximum 20 mg of rosuvastatin).

ADMINISTRATION

RECONSTITUTION
–
ROUTE
- Oral
RATE OF ADMINISTRATION
–
COMMENTS
–

OTHER INFORMATION

- Contraindicated by manufacturer in severe renal impairment.
- Dose in severe renal impairment is from *Drug Prescribing in Renal Failure*, 5th edition, by Aronoff *et al.*
- Adverse effects have not been reported in patients with renal disease, but such patients should start treatment at 900 mg daily, which may be increased after careful assessment of response and renal function.
- Cases of rhabdomyolysis may be increased in those with renal impairment.

- Gemfibrozil alone has caused myalgia and myositis, but the effects appear to occur much more frequently and are more severe when a statin is also used. The combination is therefore not recommended.

Gentamicin

CLINICAL USE

Antibacterial agent

DOSE IN NORMAL RENAL FUNCTION

- Once daily dose: 3–7 mg/kg, dose is then adjusted according to levels
- Endocarditis: 1 mg/kg every 12 hours
- Intrathecal: 1–5 mg daily
- PD peritonitis: see local policy

PHARMACOKINETICS

Molecular weight (daltons)	477.6
% Protein binding	0–30
% Excreted unchanged in urine	90
Volume of distribution (L/kg)	0.3
Half-life – normal/ ESRF (hrs)	2–3/20

METABOLISM

Gentamicin is not metabolised in the body but is excreted unchanged in microbiologically active form predominantly via the kidneys.

DOSE IN RENAL IMPAIRMENT GFR (mL/MIN)

Or use as per local policy
30–70 3–5 mg/kg daily and monitor levels.
10–30 2–3 mg/kg daily and monitor levels.
5–10 2 mg/kg every 48–72 hours according to levels.

DOSE IN PATIENTS UNDERGOING RENAL REPLACEMENT THERAPIES

CAPD	Dialysed. CAPD clearance is about 3 mL/min. Dose as in GFR=5–10 mL/min. Monitor levels.
HD	Dialysed. Dose as in GFR=5–10 mL/min. Give after dialysis.
HDF/High flux	Dialysed. Dose as in GFR=5–10 mL/min. Give after dialysis.
CAV/ VVHD	Dialysed. Dose in GFR=30–70 mL/min according to severity of infection, and measure levels.

IMPORTANT DRUG INTERACTIONS

Potentially hazardous interactions with other drugs

- Antibacterials: increased risk of nephrotoxicity with colistimethate or polymyxins and possibly cephalosporins; increased risk of ototoxicity and nephrotoxicity with capreomycin or vancomycin.
- Ciclosporin: increased risk of nephrotoxicity.
- Cytotoxics: increased risk of nephrotoxicity and possibly of ototoxicity with platinum compounds.
- Diuretics: increased risk of ototoxicity with loop diuretics.
- Muscle relaxants: effects of non-depolarising muscle relaxants and suxamethonium enhanced.
- Parasympathomimetics: antagonism of effect of neostigmine and pyridostigmine.
- Tacrolimus: increased risk of nephrotoxicity.

ADMINISTRATION

RECONSTITUTION
–
ROUTE
- IV, IM, IP, intrathecal
RATE OF ADMINISTRATION
- Bolus IV: over not less than 3 minutes
- Short infusion: 20–30 minutes
- Once daily large infusions over 30–60 minutes
COMMENTS
- Can be added to sodium chloride or glucose 5%.

OTHER INFORMATION

- Concurrent penicillins may result in sub-therapeutic blood levels.
- Monitor blood levels. 1 hour post-dose peak levels must not exceed 10 mg/L. Pre-dose trough levels should be less than 2 mg/L.
- IP therapy commonly used for PD peritonitis. Dose varies according to local protocol and whether CAPD or APD dialysis. Monitoring of blood levels is advisable, as absorption is increased by inflamed peritoneum.
- Potential nephrotoxicity of the drug may worsen residual renal function.
- Long-term concurrent use of gentamicin with teicoplanin causes additive ototoxicity.

Glatiramer acetate

CLINICAL USE

Immunomodulating drug:
- Treatment for patients at a high risk of developing multiple sclerosis and for reduction in relapses in ambulatory patients

DOSE IN NORMAL RENAL FUNCTION

20 mg daily

PHARMACOKINETICS

Molecular weight (daltons)	5000–9000
% Protein binding	Large
% Excreted unchanged in urine	No data
Volume of distribution (L/kg)	No data
Half-life – normal/ ESRF (hrs)	No data

METABOLISM

A substantial fraction of a subcutaneous dose of glatiramer is believed to be hydrolysed locally. Some of the injected dose is also presumed to enter the lymphatic system, either intact or partially hydrolysed.

DOSE IN RENAL IMPAIRMENT GFR (mL/MIN)

20–50	Dose as in normal renal function.
10–20	Dose as in normal renal function. Use with caution.
<10	Dose as in normal renal function. Use with caution.

DOSE IN PATIENTS UNDERGOING RENAL REPLACEMENT THERAPIES

CAPD	Unlikely to be dialysed. Dose as in GFR<10 mL/min.
HD	Unlikely to be dialysed. Dose as in GFR<10 mL/min.
HDF/High flux	Unlikely to be dialysed. Dose as in GFR<10 mL/min.
CAV/ VVHD	Unlikely to be dialysed. Dose as in GFR=10–20 mL/min.

IMPORTANT DRUG INTERACTIONS

Potentially hazardous interactions with other drugs
- None known

ADMINISTRATION

RECONSTITUTION
–
ROUTE
- SC
RATE OF ADMINISTRATION
–

OTHER INFORMATION

- Manufacturer advises use with caution in renal impairment due to lack of studies.

Glibenclamide

CLINICAL USE

Non-insulin dependent diabetes mellitus

DOSE IN NORMAL RENAL FUNCTION

Initially 5 mg daily (elderly patients – avoid) adjusted according to response; maximum 15 mg daily.

PHARMACOKINETICS

Molecular weight (daltons)	494
% Protein binding	97
% Excreted unchanged in urine	<5
Volume of distribution (L/kg)	0.125
Half-life – normal/ ESRF (hrs)	2.1–10/–

METABOLISM

Glibenclamide is metabolised, almost completely, in the liver, the principal metabolite being only very weakly active.

About 50% of a dose is excreted in the urine and 50% via the bile into the faeces.

DOSE IN RENAL IMPAIRMENT GFR (mL/MIN)

20–50	Initial dose of 1.25–2.5 mg once a day. Monitor closely.
10–20	Initial dose of 1.25–2.5 mg once a day. Monitor closely.
<10	Initial dose of 1.25–2.5 mg once a day. Use cautiously, with continuous monitoring.

DOSE IN PATIENTS UNDERGOING RENAL REPLACEMENT THERAPIES

CAPD	Not dialysed. Dose as in GFR<10 mL/min.
HD	Not dialysed. Dose as in GFR<10 mL/min.
HDF/High flux	Unknown dialysability. Dose as in GFR<10 mL/min.
CAV/ VVHD	Unknown dialysability. Dose as in GFR=10–20 mL/min.

IMPORTANT DRUG INTERACTIONS

Potentially hazardous interactions with other drugs

- Analgesics: effects enhanced by NSAIDs.
- Antibacterials: effects enhanced by chloramphenicol, sulphonamides, tetracyclines and trimethoprim; effects possibly enhanced by ciprofloxacin and norfloxacin; effect reduced by rifamycins.
- Anticoagulants: effect possibly enhanced by coumarins; also possibly changes to INR.
- Antifungals: concentration increased by fluconazole and miconazole and possibly voriconazole.
- Bosentan: increased risk of hepatoxicity – avoid concomitant use.
- Ciclosporin: may increase ciclosporin levels.
- Lipid-regulating drugs: absorption reduced by colesevelam; concentration possibly increased by fluvastatin; possibly additive hypoglycaemic effect with fibrates.
- Sulfinpyrazone: enhanced effect of sulphonylureas.

ADMINISTRATION

RECONSTITUTION

–

ROUTE

- Oral

RATE OF ADMINISTRATION

–

COMMENTS

- Take with breakfast.

OTHER INFORMATION

- Metabolites of glibenclamide are only weakly hypoglycaemic; this is not clinically relevant where renal and hepatic functions are normal. If creatinine clearance <10 mL/min, accumulation of metabolite and unchanged drug in plasma may cause prolonged hypoglycaemia.
- Company information states that use is contraindicated in severe renal impairment.
- Dose in renal impairment is from *Drug Dosage in Renal Insufficiency* by Seyffart G.
- Compensatory excretion via bile in faeces occurs in renal impairment.

Gliclazide

CLINICAL USE

Non-insulin dependent diabetes mellitus

DOSE IN NORMAL RENAL FUNCTION

Initially: 40–80 mg daily, with breakfast, adjusted according to response up to 160 mg as a single dose; higher doses should be divided; maximum 320 mg daily.

PHARMACOKINETICS

Molecular weight (daltons)	323.4
% Protein binding	Approx 95
% Excreted unchanged in urine	<5
Volume of distribution (L/kg)	0.24
Half-life – normal/ ESRF (hrs)	10–12 (MR: 12–20)/ Prolonged

METABOLISM

Gliclazide is extensively metabolised in the liver to metabolites that have no significant hypoglycaemic activity. Metabolites and a small amount of unchanged drug are excreted in the urine.

DOSE IN RENAL IMPAIRMENT GFR (mL/MIN)

20–50	Initially 20–40 mg daily. Use with caution and monitor closely. See 'Other information'.
10–20	Initially 20–40 mg daily. Use with caution and monitor closely. See 'Other information'.
<10	Initially 20–40 mg daily. Use with caution and monitor closely. See 'Other information'.

DOSE IN PATIENTS UNDERGOING RENAL REPLACEMENT THERAPIES

CAPD	Unlikely to be dialysed. Dose as in GFR<10 mL/min.
HD	Unlikely to be dialysed. Dose as in GFR<10 mL/min.
HDF/High flux	Unlikely to be dialysed. Dose as in GFR<10 mL/min.
CAV/ VVHD	Unlikely to be dialysed. Dose as in GFR=10–20 mL/min.

IMPORTANT DRUG INTERACTIONS

Potentially hazardous interactions with other drugs

- Analgesics: effects enhanced by NSAIDs.
- Antibacterials: effects enhanced by chloramphenicol, sulphonamides, tetracyclines and trimethoprim; effect reduced by rifamycins.
- Anticoagulants: effect possibly enhanced by coumarins; also possibly changes to INR.
- Antifungals: concentration increased by fluconazole and miconazole and possibly voriconazole – avoid with miconazole.
- Lipid-regulating drugs: possibly additive hypoglycaemic effect with fibrates.
- Sulfinpyrazone: enhanced effect of sulphonylureas.

ADMINISTRATION

RECONSTITUTION

–

ROUTE

- Oral

RATE OF ADMINISTRATION

–

COMMENTS

–

OTHER INFORMATION

- Care should be exercised in patients with hepatic and/or renal impairment, and a small starting dose should be used with careful patient monitoring.
- Company contraindicates prescribing of Diamicron in severe renal impairment, which they define as creatinine clearance below 40 mL/min.
- Doses estimated from evaluation of pharmacokinetic data, use with caution in moderate to severe renal impairment.

Glimepiride

CLINICAL USE

Non-insulin dependent diabetes mellitus

DOSE IN NORMAL RENAL FUNCTION

1–4 mg daily; maximum 6 mg daily taken shortly before or with first main meal.

PHARMACOKINETICS

Molecular weight (daltons)	490.6
% Protein binding	>99
% Excreted unchanged in urine	0 (58–60% as metabolites)
Volume of distribution (L/kg)	0.113
Half-life – normal/ ESRF (hrs)	5–9/Unchanged

METABOLISM

The drug is extensively metabolised in the liver to two main metabolites. The cytochrome P450 isoenzyme CYP2C9 is involved in the formation of a hydroxy derivative, which is further metabolised to a carboxy derivative by cytosolic enzymes. About 60% of a dose is eliminated in the urine and 40% in the faeces.

DOSE IN RENAL IMPAIRMENT GFR (mL/MIN)

20–50	Dose as in normal renal function.
10–20	Initially 1 mg and monitor closely.
<10	Initially 1 mg and monitor closely.

DOSE IN PATIENTS UNDERGOING RENAL REPLACEMENT THERAPIES

CAPD	Unlikely to be dialysed. Dose as in GFR<10 mL/min.
HD	Unlikely to be dialysed. Dose as in GFR<10 mL/min.
HDF/High flux	Unlikely to be dialysed. Dose as in GFR<10 mL/min.
CAV/ VVHD	Unlikely to be dialysed. Dose as in GFR=10–20 mL/min.

IMPORTANT DRUG INTERACTIONS

Potentially hazardous interactions with other drugs
- Analgesics: effects enhanced by NSAIDs.
- Antibacterials: effects enhanced by chloramphenicol, sulphonamides, tetracyclines and trimethoprim; effect reduced by rifamycins.
- Anticoagulants: effect possibly enhanced by coumarins; also possibly changes to INR.
- Antifungals: concentration increased by fluconazole and miconazole and possibly voriconazole.
- Lipid-regulating drugs: possibly additive hypoglycaemic effect with fibrates.
- Sulfinpyrazone: enhanced effect of sulphonylureas.

ADMINISTRATION

RECONSTITUTION
–

ROUTE
- Oral

RATE OF ADMINISTRATION
–

COMMENTS
–

OTHER INFORMATION

- Contraindicated by manufacturer in UK, dosage in severe renal impairment is from US data sheet.

Glipizide

CLINICAL USE

Non-insulin dependent diabetes mellitus

DOSE IN NORMAL RENAL FUNCTION

Initially 2.5–5 mg daily, adjusted according to response; maximum 20 mg daily; up to 15 mg may be given as a single dose before breakfast; higher doses divided.

PHARMACOKINETICS

Molecular weight (daltons)	445.5
% Protein binding	98–99
% Excreted unchanged in urine	<10
Volume of distribution (L/kg)	0.13–0.16
Half-life – normal/ ESRF (hrs)	2–4/–

METABOLISM

The metabolism of glipizide is extensive and occurs mainly in the liver. The primary metabolites are inactive hydroxylation products and polar conjugates and are excreted mainly in the urine. Less than 10% unchanged glipizide is found in urine.

DOSE IN RENAL IMPAIRMENT GFR (mL/MIN)

20–50	Initially 2.5 mg daily. Titrate according to response.
10–20	Initially 2.5 mg daily. Titrate according to response.
<10	Initially 2.5 mg daily. Titrate according to response.

DOSE IN PATIENTS UNDERGOING RENAL REPLACEMENT THERAPIES

CAPD	Unlikely to be dialysed. Dose as in GFR<10 mL/min.
HD	Unlikely to be dialysed. Dose as in GFR<10 mL/min.
HDF/High flux	Unlikely to be dialysed. Dose as in GFR<10 mL/min.
CAV/ VVHD	Unlikely to be dialysed. Dose as in GFR=10–20 mL/min.

IMPORTANT DRUG INTERACTIONS

Potentially hazardous interactions with other drugs

- Analgesics: effects enhanced by NSAIDs.
- Antibacterials: effects enhanced by chloramphenicol, sulphonamides, tetracyclines and trimethoprim; effect reduced by rifamycins.
- Anticoagulants: effect possibly enhanced by coumarins; also possibly changes to INR.
- Antifungals: concentration increased by fluconazole, posaconazole and miconazole and possibly voriconazole – avoid with miconazole.
- Lipid-regulating drugs: possibly additive hypoglycaemic effect with fibrates.
- Ciclosporin: may increase ciclosporin levels.
- Sulfinpyrazone: enhanced effect of sulphonylureas.

ADMINISTRATION

RECONSTITUTION

–

ROUTE

- Oral

RATE OF ADMINISTRATION

–

COMMENTS

–

OTHER INFORMATION

- UK SPC does not recommend the use of glipizide in patients with severe renal insufficiency.
- Doses taken from US data sheet and *Drug Prescribing in Renal Failure*, 5th edition, by Aronoff *et al.*
- Renal or hepatic insufficiency may cause elevated blood levels of glipizide (increased risk of serious hypoglycaemic reactions).

Glyceryl trinitrate

CLINICAL USE

Vasodilator:
- Treatment and prophylaxis of angina, left ventricular failure, hypertension during surgery
- Anal fissures
- Maintenance of venous patency

DOSE IN NORMAL RENAL FUNCTION

- S/L tablets: 0.3–1 mg as required.
- Buccal: 2–10 mg 3 times daily or when required.
- Oral dose depends on preparation used.
- Patches: 5–20 mg every 24 hours.
- Maintenance of venous patency: 5 mg patch
- IV infusion: 10–200 mcg/minute; up to 400 mcg/min may be required during surgery.
- Anal fissures: 0.2–0.8% ointment every 12 hours.

PHARMACOKINETICS

Molecular weight (daltons)	227.1
% Protein binding	30–60
% Excreted unchanged in urine	<1
Volume of distribution (L/kg)	2–3
Half-life – normal/ ESRF (hrs)	1–4 minutes/ Unchanged

METABOLISM

GTN undergoes extensive first-pass metabolism in the liver. It is taken up by smooth muscle cells of blood vessels and the nitrate group is cleaved to inorganic nitrite and then to nitric oxide. This reaction requires the presence of cysteine or another thiol. Glyceryl trinitrate also undergoes hydrolysis in plasma and is rapidly metabolised in the liver by glutathione-organic nitrate reductase to dinitrates and mononitrates.

DOSE IN RENAL IMPAIRMENT GFR (mL/MIN)

20–50	Dose as in normal renal function.
10–20	Dose as in normal renal function.
<10	Dose as in normal renal function.

DOSE IN PATIENTS UNDERGOING RENAL REPLACEMENT THERAPIES

CAPD	Not dialysed. Dose as in normal renal function.
HD	Not dialysed. Dose as in normal renal function.
HDF/High flux	Unknown dialysability. Dose as in normal renal function.
CAV/ VVHD	Not dialysed. Dose as in normal renal function.

IMPORTANT DRUG INTERACTIONS

Potentially hazardous interactions with other drugs
- Anticoagulants: infusion of GTN reduces anticoagulant effect of heparins.
- Antidepressants: tricyclics may reduce effect of sublingual tablets due to dry mouth.
- Antimuscarinics: may reduce effect of sublingual tablets due to dry mouth.
- Sildenafil: hypotensive effect significantly enhanced – avoid concomitant use.
- Tadalafil: hypotensive effect significantly enhanced – avoid concomitant use.
- Vardenafil: hypotensive effect significantly enhanced – avoid concomitant use.

ADMINISTRATION

RECONSTITUTION
–
ROUTE
- IV, buccal, S/L, oral, topical
RATE OF ADMINISTRATION
- 10–400 mcg/minute (depends on response)
COMMENTS
- Compatible with sodium chloride 0.9% and glucose 5%.
- Incompatible with polyvinylchloride bags.

OTHER INFORMATION

- Tolerance may develop; may be minimised by having nitrate-'free' periods.
- IV infusions contain propylene glycol which can cause lactic acidosis – restrict to using for no more than 3 consecutive days.

Goserelin

CLINICAL USE

Synthetic decapeptide analogue of LHRH
- Treatment of advanced prostate cancer, breast cancer, endometriosis and endometrial thinning and uterine fibroids.

DOSE IN NORMAL RENAL FUNCTION

3.6 mg every 28 days or 10.8 mg every 12 weeks.
Duration of treatment varies according to condition being treated.

PHARMACOKINETICS

Molecular weight (daltons)	1269.4 (1329.5 as acetate)
% Protein binding	27
% Excreted unchanged in urine	20[1] (90% as unchanged drug & metabolites)
Volume of distribution (L/kg)	30.5–57.8 litres
Half-life – normal/ ESRF (hrs)	2–4/12[1]

METABOLISM

Metabolised by tissue peptidases and is excreted in urine and bile as unchanged drug and metabolites.

DOSE IN RENAL IMPAIRMENT GFR (mL/MIN)

20–50	Dose as in normal renal function.
10–20	Dose as in normal renal function.
<10	Dose as in normal renal function. Monitor closely.

DOSE IN PATIENTS UNDERGOING RENAL REPLACEMENT THERAPIES

CAPD	Unlikely to be dialysed. Dose as in normal renal function.
HD	Unlikely to be dialysed. Dose as in normal renal function.
HDF/High flux	Unknown dialysability. Dose as in normal renal function.
CAV/ VVHD	Unlikely to be dialysed. Dose as in normal renal function.

IMPORTANT DRUG INTERACTIONS

Potentially hazardous interactions with other drugs
- None known

ADMINISTRATION

RECONSTITUTION
–

ROUTE
- SC

RATE OF ADMINISTRATION
–

COMMENTS
–

OTHER INFORMATION

Reference:
1. *Drug Information Handbook.* 22nd ed. American Pharmacists Association. Lexicomp.

Granisetron

CLINICAL USE

Prevention or treatment of nausea
and vomiting induced by cytotoxic
chemotherapy, radiotherapy, or postoperative
nausea and vomiting (PONV)

DOSE IN NORMAL RENAL FUNCTION

- Cytotoxic chemotherapy or radiotherapy:
  — PO: 1–2 mg within 1 hour before start
    of treatment, then 2 mg daily in 1–2
    divided doses during treatment.
  — IV: 3 mg before start of cytotoxic
    therapy; up to 2 additional 3 mg doses
    can be given within 24 hours no less
    than 10 minutes apart.
  — IV Infusion: 40 mcg/kg (max 3 mg)
    before treatment; repeated once more
    if required.
  — Transdermal: Apply 3.1 mg patch
    24–48 hours before chemotherapy.
- PONV: 1 mg IV before induction of
  anaesthesia; then 1 mg as required
  (maximum 2 mg in one day).

PHARMACOKINETICS

Molecular weight (daltons)	312.4 (348.9 as hydrochloride)
% Protein binding	≈65
% Excreted unchanged in urine	<20
Volume of distribution (L/kg)	3
Half-life – normal/ ESRF (hrs)	4–5/Unchanged

METABOLISM

Granisetron is metabolised primarily in the
liver by oxidation followed by conjugation.
The major compounds are 7-OH-granisetron
and its sulphate and glycuronide conjugates.
Although antiemetic properties have
been observed for 7-OH-granisetron and
indazoline N-desmethyl granisetron, it is
unlikely that these contribute significantly to
the pharmacological activity of granisetron in
man. Clearance is predominantly by hepatic
metabolism. Urinary excretion of unchanged
granisetron averages 12% of dose while that
of metabolites amounts to about 47% of
dose. The remainder is excreted in faeces as
metabolites.

DOSE IN RENAL IMPAIRMENT GFR (mL/MIN)

20–50	Dose as in normal renal function.
10–20	Dose as in normal renal function.
<10	Dose as in normal renal function.

DOSE IN PATIENTS UNDERGOING RENAL REPLACEMENT THERAPIES

CAPD	Unknown dialysability. Dose as in normal renal function.
HD	Unknown dialysability. Dose as in normal renal function. Company recommends timing HD for greater than 2 hours after granisetron dose.
HDF/High flux	Unknown dialysability. Dose as in normal renal function. Company recommends timing HD for greater than 2 hours after granisetron dose.
CAV/ VVHD	Unknown dialysability. Dose as in normal renal function.

IMPORTANT DRUG INTERACTIONS

Potentially hazardous interactions with
other drugs
- None known

ADMINISTRATION

RECONSTITUTION
–
ROUTE
- Oral, IV bolus, IV infusion, transdermal
RATE OF ADMINISTRATION
- IV bolus: diluted in 5 or 15 mL sodium
  chloride 0.9% over not less than
  30 seconds.
- IV infusion: 20–50 mL over 5 minutes.
COMMENTS
- Compatible with sodium chloride 0.9%,
  sodium chloride 0.18% and glucose 4%
  solution, glucose 5%, Hartmann's solution,
  sodium lactate injection, 10% Mannitol.
- Maximum administered dose over
  24 hours should not exceed 9 mg.

OTHER INFORMATION

- No special dosing adjustments necessary
  in patients with renal or hepatic failure.

Griseofulvin

CLINICAL USE

Antifungal agent:
* Dermatophyte infections of the skin, scalp, hair and nails

DOSE IN NORMAL RENAL FUNCTION

500 mg daily, in divided doses or as a single dose, in severe infection dose may be doubled.

PHARMACOKINETICS

Molecular weight (daltons)	352.8
% Protein binding	84
% Excreted unchanged in urine	<1
Volume of distribution (L/kg)	1.2–1.41
Half-life – normal/ ESRF (hrs)	9–24/20

METABOLISM

Griseofulvin is metabolised by the liver mainly to 6-demethylgriseofulvin and its glucuronide conjugate which are excreted in the urine. A large amount of a dose of griseofulvin of reduced particle size appears unchanged in the faeces; less than 1% is excreted unchanged in the urine; some is excreted in the sweat.

DOSE IN RENAL IMPAIRMENT GFR (mL/MIN)

20–50	Dose as in normal renal function.
10–20	Dose as in normal renal function.
<10	Dose as in normal renal function.

DOSE IN PATIENTS UNDERGOING RENAL REPLACEMENT THERAPIES

CAPD	Not dialysed. Dose as in normal renal function.
HD	Not dialysed. Dose as in normal renal function.
HDF/High flux	Not dialysed. Dose as in normal renal function.
CAV/ VVHD	Not dialysed. Dose as in normal renal function.

IMPORTANT DRUG INTERACTIONS

Potentially hazardous interactions with other drugs
* Anticoagulants: metabolism of coumarins accelerated (reduced anticoagulant effect).
* Ciclosporin: griseofulvin possibly reduces ciclosporin concentration. (Two reports of such an interaction in literature.)
* Oestrogens and progestogens: metabolism of oral contraceptives accelerated (reduced contraceptive effect).

ADMINISTRATION

RECONSTITUTION
–
ROUTE
* Oral
RATE OF ADMINISTRATION
–
COMMENTS
–

OTHER INFORMATION

* Use with extreme caution in patients with SLE.
* Griseofulvin is deposited in keratin precursor cells and is concentrated in the stratum corneum of the skin and in the nails and hair, thus preventing fungal invasion of newly formed cells.

Guanethidine monosulphate

CLINICAL USE

Treatment of hypertensive crisis

DOSE IN NORMAL RENAL FUNCTION

10–20 mg, repeated after 3 hours if required

PHARMACOKINETICS

Molecular weight (daltons)	296.4
% Protein binding	<5
% Excreted unchanged in urine	25–60
Volume of distribution (L/kg)	Large
Half-life – normal/ ESRF (hrs)	120–240/Increased

METABOLISM

Guanethidine is partially metabolised in the liver, and is excreted in the urine as metabolites and unchanged guanethidine.

DOSE IN RENAL IMPAIRMENT GFR (mL/MIN)

20–50	Give every 24 hours.
10–20	Give every 24 hours.
<10	Give every 24–36 hours; use with caution.

DOSE IN PATIENTS UNDERGOING RENAL REPLACEMENT THERAPIES

CAPD	Unlikely to be dialysed. Dose as in GFR<10 mL/min.
HD	Unlikely to be dialysed. Dose as in GFR<10 mL/min.
HDF/High flux	Likely dialysability. Dose as in GFR<10 mL/min.
CAV/ VVHD	Unknown dialysability. Dose as in GFR=10–20 mL/min.

IMPORTANT DRUG INTERACTIONS

Potentially hazardous interactions with other drugs
- Anaesthetics: enhanced hypotensive effect.
- Sympathomimetics: hypotensive effect antagonised by ephedrine, isometheptene, metaraminol, methylphenidate, noradrenaline, oxymetazoline, phenylephrine, phenylpropanolamine, pseudoephedrine and xylometazoline.

ADMINISTRATION

RECONSTITUTION

–

ROUTE

- IM

RATE OF ADMINISTRATION

–

COMMENTS

–

OTHER INFORMATION

- Blood pressure should fall within 30 minutes of dose.
- Contraindicated by manufacturer. Doses in renal impairment from *Drug Prescribing in Renal Failure*, 5th edition, by Aronoff *et al.*

Haloperidol

CLINICAL USE

- Sedative in severe anxiety
- Intractable hiccup
- Motor tics
- Nausea and vomiting
- Schizophrenia and other psychoses

DOSE IN NORMAL RENAL FUNCTION

- Anxiety: 0.5 mg twice daily.
- Agitation & restlessness in the elderly: 0.5–1.5 mg once or twice daily.
- Hiccup: 1.5 mg 3 times daily.
- Nausea and vomiting: maximum 10 mg/day in divided doses; SC infusion: 2.5–10 mg daily.
- Schizophrenia: Oral: 1.5–5 mg 2–3 times daily, up to 30 mg daily in resistant cases.
- IM: 2–10 mg initially then every 4–8 hours; maximum 18 mg daily.
- Deep IM: 50–300 mg every 4 weeks; higher doses may sometimes be required.
- Motor tics: 0.5–1.5 mg 3 times daily, increased according to response.

PHARMACOKINETICS

Molecular weight (daltons)	375.9
% Protein binding	92
% Excreted unchanged in urine	1
Volume of distribution (L/kg)	14–21
Half-life – normal/ ESRF (hrs)	12–38/–

METABOLISM

Haloperidol is metabolised in the liver and is excreted in the urine and, via the bile, in the faeces; there is evidence of enterohepatic recycling. Routes of metabolism of haloperidol include oxidative N-dealkylation, particularly via the cytochrome P450 isoenzymes CYP3A4 and CYP2D6, glucuronidation, and reduction of the ketone group to form an alcohol known as reduced haloperidol. Metabolites are ultimately conjugated with glycine and excreted in the urine. There is debate over the pharmacological activity of the metabolites.

DOSE IN RENAL IMPAIRMENT GFR (mL/MIN)

20–50	Dose as in normal renal function.
10–20	Dose as in normal renal function.
<10	Start with lower doses. For single doses use 100% of normal dose. Accumulation with repeated dosage.

DOSE IN PATIENTS UNDERGOING RENAL REPLACEMENT THERAPIES

CAPD	Not dialysed. Dose as in GFR<10 mL/min.
HD	Not dialysed. Dose as in GFR<10 mL/min.
HDF/High flux	Not dialysed. Dose as in GFR<10 mL/min.
CAV/ VVHD	Not dialysed. Dose as in normal renal function.

IMPORTANT DRUG INTERACTIONS

Potentially hazardous interactions with other drugs

- Anaesthetics: enhanced hypotensive effects.
- Analgesics: increased risk of convulsions with tramadol; enhanced hypotensive and sedative effects with opioids; possibly severe drowsiness with indomethacin or acemetacin; increased risk of ventricular arrhythmias with methadone.
- Anti-arrhythmics: increased risk of ventricular arrhythmias with anti-arrhythmics that prolong the QT interval; increased risk of ventricular arrhythmias with amiodarone or disopyramide – avoid concomitant use.
- Antibacterials: increased risk of ventricular arrhythmias with moxifloxacin – avoid concomitant use; concentration reduced by rifampicin.
- Antidepressants: concentration increased by fluoxetine and venlafaxine and possibly fluvoxamine; concentration of tricyclics increased.
- Anti-epileptics: metabolism increased by carbamazepine and phenobarbital; lowered seizure threshold; concentration reduced by phenytoin.
- Antifungals: concentration possibly increased by itraconazole.
- Antimalarials: avoid concomitant use with artemether/lumefantrine and piperaquine with artenimol; possible increased risk of ventricular arrhythmias with mefloquine or quinine – avoid.

- Antipsychotics: avoid concomitant use of depot formulations with clozapine (cannot be withdrawn quickly if neutropenia occurs); increased risk of ventricular arrhythmias with sulpiride and droperidol – avoid with droperidol; concentration possibly increased by chlorpromazine.
- Antivirals: concentration possibly increased with ritonavir; increased risk of ventricular arrhythmias with saquinavir – avoid.
- Anxiolytics and hypnotics: increased sedative effects; concentration increased by alprazolam and buspirone.
- Atomoxetine: increased risk of ventricular arrhythmias.
- Beta-blockers: increased risk of ventricular arrhythmias with sotalol.
- Cytotoxics: increased risk of ventricular arrhythmias with vandetanib – avoid; increased risk of ventricular arrhythmias with arsenic trioxide.
- Lithium: increased risk of extrapyramidal side effects and possibly neurotoxicity.

ADMINISTRATION

RECONSTITUTION

–

ROUTE

- Oral, IM or IV (slow bolus)

RATE OF ADMINISTRATION

–

COMMENTS

–

OTHER INFORMATION

- May cause hypotension and excessive sedation.
- Increased CNS sensitivity in renally impaired patients – start with small doses; metabolites may accumulate.
- Equivalent IV/IM dose = 40% of oral dose.

Heparin

CLINICAL USE

Anticoagulant

DOSE IN NORMAL RENAL FUNCTION

- Treatment of deep vein thrombosis and pulmonary embolism:
  - IV: Loading dose: 5000–10000 units then a continuous intravenous infusion of 18 units/kg/hour.
- Treatment of deep vein thrombosis:
  - SC: 15000 units every 12 hours, dose is adjusted according to laboratory monitoring.
- Prophylaxis: 5000 units every 8–12 hours or according to local protocols

PHARMACOKINETICS

Molecular weight (daltons)	3000–40000
% Protein binding	>90
% Excreted unchanged in urine	0 (up to 50% after large doses)
Volume of distribution (L/kg)	0.06–0.1
Half-life – normal/ ESRF (hrs)	1–6/Slightly prolonged (half-life increases with dose)

METABOLISM

Heparin is taken up by the reticuloendothelial system. It is excreted in the urine, mainly as metabolites, although after large doses up to 50% may be excreted unchanged.

DOSE IN RENAL IMPAIRMENT GFR (mL/MIN)

20–50	Dose as in normal renal function.
10–20	Dose as in normal renal function.
<10	Dose as in normal renal function.

DOSE IN PATIENTS UNDERGOING RENAL REPLACEMENT THERAPIES

CAPD	Not dialysed. Dose as in normal renal function.
HD	Not dialysed. Dose as in normal renal function.
HDF/High flux	Not dialysed. Dose as in normal renal function.
CAV/ VVHD	Not dialysed. Dose as in normal renal function.

IMPORTANT DRUG INTERACTIONS

Potentially hazardous interactions with other drugs

- Analgesics: increased risk of bleeding with NSAIDs – avoid concomitant use with IV diclofenac; increased risk of haemorrhage with ketorolac – avoid concomitant use.
- Nitrates: anticoagulant effect reduced by infusions of glyceryl trinitrate.
- Use with care in patients receiving oral anticoagulants, platelet aggregation inhibitors, aspirin or dextran.

ADMINISTRATION

RECONSTITUTION

–

ROUTE

- IV infusion or bolus, SC

RATE OF ADMINISTRATION

- 18 units/kg/hour, or according to local protocol

COMMENTS

–

OTHER INFORMATION

- Half-life is slightly prolonged in haemodialysis patients after intravenous administration.
- Also used for the maintenance of extracorporeal circuits in cardiopulmonary bypass and haemodialysis.
- 1 mg protamine is required to neutralise 100 IU heparin; give slowly over 10 minutes, and do not exceed a total dose of 50 mg.
- To reduce or prevent fibrin formation in patients on PD, heparin may be added to PD fluid at a concentration of 1000 IU/L.

Hydralazine hydrochloride

CLINICAL USE

Vasodilator antihypertensive agent

DOSE IN NORMAL RENAL FUNCTION

- Oral:
  - Hypertension: 25–50 mg twice daily; maximum daily dose 100 mg in women and slow acetylators, 200 mg in fast acetylators.
  - Heart failure: 25–75 mg 3–4 times daily
- IV: slow IV injection: 5–10 mg over 20 minutes; repeat after 20–30 minutes if necessary.
- Infusion: 200–300 micrograms/minute initially, reducing to 50–150 micrograms/minute.

PHARMACOKINETICS

Molecular weight (daltons)	196.6
% Protein binding	87
% Excreted unchanged in urine	2–14
Volume of distribution (L/kg)	0.5–0.9
Half-life – normal/ ESRF (hrs)	2–4/16

METABOLISM

Hydralazine undergoes considerable first-pass metabolism by acetylation in the gastrointestinal mucosa and liver. The rate of metabolism is genetically determined and depends upon the acetylator status of the individual. Systemic metabolism in the liver is by hydroxylation of the ring system and conjugation with glucuronic acid; most sources suggest that N-acetylation is not of major importance in systemic clearance and that therefore acetylator status does not affect elimination. Hydralazine is excreted mainly in urine as metabolites.

DOSE IN RENAL IMPAIRMENT GFR (mL/MIN)

20–50	Start at low dose and adjust in accordance with response.
10–20	Start at low dose and adjust in accordance with response.
<10	Start at low dose and adjust in accordance with response.

DOSE IN PATIENTS UNDERGOING RENAL REPLACEMENT THERAPIES

CAPD	Not dialysed. Dose as in GFR<10 mL/min.
HD	Not dialysed. Dose as in GFR<10 mL/min.
HDF/High flux	Not dialysed. Dose as in GFR<10 mL/min.
CAV/ VVHD	Not dialysed. Dose as in GFR=10–20 mL/min.

IMPORTANT DRUG INTERACTIONS

Potentially hazardous interactions with other drugs
- Anaesthetics: increased hypotensive effects.

ADMINISTRATION

RECONSTITUTION
- 20 mg with 1 mL water for injection then dilute with 10 mL sodium chloride 0.9% for IV injection or 500 mL sodium chloride 0.9% for IV infusion.

ROUTE
- Oral, IV peripherally

RATE OF ADMINISTRATION
- As above

COMMENTS
- Minimum volume of 60 mg in 60 mL. (UK Critical Care Group, *Minimum Infusion Volumes for Fluid Restricted Critically Ill Patients*, 3rd edition, 2006)

OTHER INFORMATION

- Avoid long-term use in severe renal insufficiency and dialysis patients, due to accumulation of metabolites.

Hydrocortisone acetate

CLINICAL USE

Corticosteroid:
- Local inflammation of joints and soft tissue

DOSE IN NORMAL RENAL FUNCTION

5–50 mg according to joint size.

PHARMACOKINETICS

Molecular weight (daltons)	404.5
% Protein binding	>90
% Excreted unchanged in urine	Minimal
Volume of distribution (L/kg)	0.4–0.7
Half-life – normal/ ESRF (hrs)	Approx 100 minutes/ Unchanged

METABOLISM

Hydrocortisone is metabolised in the liver and most body tissues to hydrogenated and degraded forms such as tetrahydrocortisone and tetrahydrocortisol. These are excreted in the urine, mainly conjugated as glucuronides, with a very small proportion of unchanged hydrocortisone.

DOSE IN RENAL IMPAIRMENT GFR (mL/MIN)

20–50	Dose as in normal renal function.
10–20	Dose as in normal renal function.
<10	Dose as in normal renal function.

DOSE IN PATIENTS UNDERGOING RENAL REPLACEMENT THERAPIES

CAPD	Unlikely to be dialysed. Dose as in normal renal function.
HD	Unlikely to be dialysed. Dose as in normal renal function.
HDF/High flux	Unlikely to be dialysed. Dose as in normal renal function.
CAV/ VVHD	Unlikely to be dialysed. Dose as in normal renal function.

IMPORTANT DRUG INTERACTIONS

Potentially hazardous interactions with other drugs
- Aldesleukin: avoid concomitant use.
- Antibacterials: metabolism accelerated by rifampicin; metabolism possibly inhibited by erythromycin; concentration of isoniazid possibly reduced.
- Anticoagulants: efficacy of coumarins and phenindione may be altered.
- Anti-epileptics: metabolism accelerated by carbamazepine, phenobarbital and phenytoin.
- Antifungals: increased risk of hypokalaemia with amphotericin – avoid concomitant use; metabolism possibly inhibited by itraconazole and ketoconazole.
- Antivirals: concentration possibly increased by ritonavir.
- Ciclosporin: rare reports of convulsions in patients on ciclosporin and high-dose corticosteroids.
- Diuretics: enhanced hypokalaemic effects of acetazolamide, loop diuretics and thiazide diuretics.
- Vaccines: high dose corticosteroids can impair immune response to vaccines – avoid concomitant use with live vaccines.

ADMINISTRATION

RECONSTITUTION
–
ROUTE
- Intra-articular, periarticular
RATE OF ADMINISTRATION
–
COMMENTS
–

OTHER INFORMATION

- Used for its local effects. Systemic absorption occurs slowly.

Hydrocortisone sodium succinate

CLINICAL USE

Corticosteroid:
- Anti-inflammatory agent in respiratory, GI, endocrine disorders, and allergic states
- Shock

DOSE IN NORMAL RENAL FUNCTION

- Oral: 20–30mg in divided doses for replacement
- MR: 20–30mg once daily in the morning
- IV/IM: 100–500mg, 3–4 times in 24 hours, or as required

PHARMACOKINETICS

Molecular weight (daltons)	484.5 (486.4 as sodium phosphate)
% Protein binding	>90
% Excreted unchanged in urine	Minimal
Volume of distribution (L/kg)	0.4–0.7
Half-life – normal/ ESRF (hrs)	Approx 100 minutes/ Unchanged

METABOLISM

Hydrocortisone is metabolised in the liver and most body tissues to hydrogenated and degraded forms such as tetrahydrocortisone and tetrahydrocortisol. These are excreted in the urine, mainly conjugated as glucuronides, with a very small proportion of unchanged hydrocortisone.

DOSE IN RENAL IMPAIRMENT GFR (mL/MIN)

20–50	Dose as in normal renal function.
10–20	Dose as in normal renal function.
<10	Dose as in normal renal function.

DOSE IN PATIENTS UNDERGOING RENAL REPLACEMENT THERAPIES

CAPD	Unlikely to be dialysed. Dose as in normal renal function.
HD	Unlikely to be dialysed. Dose as in normal renal function.
HDF/High flux	Unlikely to be dialysed. Dose as in normal renal function.
CAV/ VVHD	Unlikely to be dialysed. Dose as in normal renal function.

IMPORTANT DRUG INTERACTIONS

Potentially hazardous interactions with other drugs
- Aldesleukin: avoid concomitant use.
- Antibacterials: metabolism accelerated by rifampicin; metabolism possibly inhibited by erythromycin; concentration of isoniazid possibly reduced.
- Anticoagulants: efficacy of coumarins and phenindione may be altered.
- Anti-epileptics: metabolism accelerated by carbamazepine, phenobarbital and phenytoin.
- Antifungals: increased risk of hypokalaemia with amphotericin – avoid concomitant use; metabolism possibly inhibited by itraconazole and ketoconazole.
- Antivirals: concentration possibly increased by ritonavir.
- Ciclosporin: rare reports of convulsions in patients on ciclosporin and high-dose corticosteroids.
- Diuretics: enhanced hypokalaemic effects of acetazolamide, loop diuretics and thiazide diuretics.
- Vaccines: high dose corticosteroids can impair immune response to vaccines – avoid concomitant use with live vaccines.

ADMINISTRATION

RECONSTITUTION
- IV injection, IM injection: add 2mL of sterile water for injection.
- IV infusion: add not more than 2mL water for injection, then add to 100–1000mL (not less than 100mL) glucose 5% or sodium chloride 0.9%.

ROUTE
- IV injection, IV infusion, IM

RATE OF ADMINISTRATION
- IV bolus: 2–3 minutes

COMMENTS
- Minimum volume 100mg in 50mL. (UK Critical Care Group, *Minimum Infusion Volumes for Fluid Restricted Critically Ill Patients*, 3rd edition, 2006)

OTHER INFORMATION

- Non-plasma protein bound hydrocortisone is removed by HD.
- One study has shown that plasma clearance rates of hydrocortisone during haemodialysis were 30–63% higher than after dialysis. No recommendations exist to indicate dosing should be altered to take account of this.

Hydromorphone hydrochloride

CLINICAL USE

Relief of severe cancer pain

DOSE IN NORMAL RENAL FUNCTION

1.3 mg 4 hourly, increasing dose as required.
SR: 4 mg 12 hourly, increasing dose as
required

PHARMACOKINETICS

Molecular weight (daltons)	321.8
% Protein binding	7.1
% Excreted unchanged in urine	6
Volume of distribution (L/kg)	24.4 litres
Half-life – normal/ ESRF (hrs)	2.5/–

METABOLISM

Hydromorphone undergoes extensive
first-pass metabolism. It is extensively
metabolised by glucuronidation in
the liver and excreted in the urine
mainly as conjugated hydromorphone,
dihydroisomorphine, and dihydromorphine.

DOSE IN RENAL IMPAIRMENT GFR (mL/MIN)

20–50	Dose as in normal renal function.
10–20	Reduce dose – start with lowest dose and titrate according to response.
<10	Reduce dose – start with lowest dose and titrate according to response.

DOSE IN PATIENTS UNDERGOING RENAL REPLACEMENT THERAPIES

CAPD	Unknown dialysability. Dose as in GFR<10 mL/min.
HD	Unknown dialysability. Dose as in GFR<10 mL/min.
HDF/High flux	Unknown dialysability. Dose as in GFR<10 mL/min.
CAV/ VVHD	Unknown dialysability. Dose as in GFR=10–20 mL/min.

IMPORTANT DRUG INTERACTIONS

Potentially hazardous interactions with
other drugs
- Alcohol: can cause dose dumping with sustained release preparations.
- Antidepressants: possible CNS excitation or depression with MAOIs – avoid concomitant use and for 2 weeks after stopping MAOI; possible CNS excitation or depression with moclobemide; increased sedative effects with tricyclics.
- Antihistamines: increased sedative effects with sedating antihistamines.
- Antipsychotics: enhanced hypotensive and sedative effects.
- Dopaminergics: avoid with selegiline.
- Sodium oxybate: enhanced effect of sodium oxybate – avoid concomitant use.

ADMINISTRATION

RECONSTITUTION
–
ROUTE
- Oral
RATE OF ADMINISTRATION
–
COMMENTS
–

OTHER INFORMATION

- 1.3 mg of hydromorphone is equivalent to 10 mg oral morphine.
- Metabolites may cause neuroexcitation and cognitive impairment.

Hydroxycarbamide (hydroxyurea)

CLINICAL USE

Antineoplastic agent

DOSE IN NORMAL RENAL FUNCTION

15–35 mg/kg daily
CML: 20–30 mg/kg daily or 80 mg/kg every
3 days
Consult local protocol.

PHARMACOKINETICS

Molecular weight (daltons)	76.05
% Protein binding	75–80
% Excreted unchanged in urine	9–95
Volume of distribution (L/kg)	0.5
Half-life – normal/ESRF (hrs)	2–6/–

METABOLISM

Up to 50% of a dose is metabolised by the
liver; 50% of a dose of hydroxycarbamide
is excreted in urine as metabolites and
unchanged drug. Some is excreted as carbon
dioxide via the lungs or via the urine as
urea. About 80% of a dose is reported to be
excreted in the urine within 12 hours.

DOSE IN RENAL IMPAIRMENT GFR (mL/MIN)

>60	85% of normal dose and titrate to response.[1]
45–60	80% of normal dose and titrate to response.[1]
30–45	75% of normal dose and titrate to response.[1]
10–30	50% of normal dose and titrate to response.
<10	20% of normal dose and titrate to response.

DOSE IN PATIENTS UNDERGOING RENAL REPLACEMENT THERAPIES

CAPD	Likely dialysability. Dose as in GFR<10 mL/min.
HD	Likely dialysability. Dose as in GFR<10 mL/min.
HDF/High flux	Likely dialysability. Dose as in GFR<10 mL/min.
CAV/ VVHD	Likely dialysability. Dose as in GFR=10–30 mL/min.

IMPORTANT DRUG INTERACTIONS

Potentially hazardous interactions with
other drugs
- Antipsychotics: avoid concomitant
  use with clozapine, increased risk of
  agranulocytosis.
- Antivirals: increased toxicity with
  didanosine and stavudine – avoid
  concomitant use.

ADMINISTRATION

RECONSTITUTION
–
ROUTE
- Oral
RATE OF ADMINISTRATION
–
COMMENTS
–

OTHER INFORMATION

- Full blood count, renal and hepatic
  function should be monitored repeatedly
  during treatment.
- Dosage should be based on the patient's
  actual or ideal weight, whichever is less.
- Hydroxyurea has been associated with
  impairment of renal tubular function and
  accompanied by elevation in serum uric
  acid, BUN, and creatinine levels.
- The following formula can be used to
  determine the fraction of normal dose
  used for renally impaired patients:
  Fraction of normal dose = (normal dose) ×
  $\{[f(k_f - 1)] + 1\}$. f = fraction of the original
  dose excreted as active or toxic moiety
  (f = 0.35 for hydroxyurea); k_f = patient's
  creatinine clearance (mL/min) divided by
  120 mL/minute.
- Administer with caution to patients
  with marked renal dysfunction; such
  patients may rapidly develop visual and
  auditory hallucinations and significant
  haematological toxicity.
- Doses in severe renal impairment are from
  Drug Prescribing in Renal Failure, 5th
  edition, by Aronoff *et al.*

Reference:
1. Kintzel PE, Dorr RT. Anticancer drug renal
toxicity and elimination: dosing guidelines
for altered renal function. *Cancer Treat Rev.*
1995; **21**: 33–64.

Hydroxychloroquine sulphate

CLINICAL USE

- Rheumatoid arthritis
- Systemic lupus erythematosus
- Dermatological conditions caused or aggravated by sunlight
- Malaria (unlicensed in UK)

DOSE IN NORMAL RENAL FUNCTION

- 200–400 mg daily in divided doses; maximum of 6.5 mg/kg/day
- Prophylaxis of malaria: 400 mg weekly

PHARMACOKINETICS

Molecular weight (daltons)	434
% Protein binding	30–40
% Excreted unchanged in urine	3
Volume of distribution (L/kg)	Large
Half-life – normal/ESRF (hrs)	5.9–504/–

METABOLISM

Hydroxychloroquine is metabolised to chloroquine, which in turn is extensively metabolised in the liver, mainly to monodesethylchloroquine with smaller amounts of bisdesethylchloroquine (didesethylchloroquinine) and other metabolites being formed. Monodesethylchloroquine has been reported to have some activity against *Plasmodium falciparum*.

Chloroquine and its metabolites are excreted in the urine, with about half of a dose appearing as unchanged drug and about 10% as the monodesethyl metabolite.

DOSE IN RENAL IMPAIRMENT GFR (mL/MIN)

See 'Other information'.
30–50   Maximum 75% of dose.
10–30   25–50% of dose (equivalent of 150 mg daily).
<10   25–50% of dose (equivalent of 50–100 mg daily) – use with caution.

DOSE IN PATIENTS UNDERGOING RENAL REPLACEMENT THERAPIES

CAPD	Not dialysed. Dose as in GFR<10 mL/min.
HD	Not dialysed. Dose as in GFR<10 mL/min.
HDF/High flux	Unknown dialysability. Dose as in GFR<10 mL/min.
CAV/ VVHD	Unknown dialysability. Dose as in GFR=10–30 mL/min.

IMPORTANT DRUG INTERACTIONS

Potentially hazardous interactions with other drugs

- Anti-arrhythmics: increased risk of ventricular arrhythmias with amiodarone – avoid concomitant use.
- Antibacterials: increased risk of ventricular arrhythmias with moxifloxacin – avoid concomitant use.
- Anti-epileptics: antagonism of anticonvulsant effect.
- Antimalarials: increased risk of convulsions with mefloquine; avoid concomitant use with artemether/lumefantrine.
- Antipsychotics: increased risk of ventricular arrhythmias with droperidol – avoid.
- Ciclosporin: increased ciclosporin concentration (increased risk of toxicity).
- Digoxin: possibly increased concentration of digoxin.
- Lanthanum: absorption possibly reduced by lanthanum – give at least 2 hours apart.

ADMINISTRATION

RECONSTITUTION
–
ROUTE
- Oral
RATE OF ADMINISTRATION
–
COMMENTS
–

OTHER INFORMATION

- Take with a meal or a glass of milk.
- Excretory patterns are not well characterised, but hydroxychloroquine and its metabolites are slowly excreted via the kidneys.
- Attempt to avoid prolonged use in renal failure.
- In renal insufficiency, need more than annual eye examinations.
- There is case report of retinal toxicity in a patient who developed CKD 3 while on hydroxychloroquine 400 mg daily.

(Tailor R, Elaraoud I, Good P, *et al.* A case of severe hydroxychloroquine-induced retinal toxicity in a patient with recent onset of renal impairment: a review of the literature on the use of hydroxychloroquine in renal impairment. *Case Reports in Ophthalmological*

Medicine. Volume 2012. http://dx.doi.org/10.1155/2012/182747)

- Doses in renal impairment are from Seyffart, but probably not actually practical to give reduced dose so try giving longer dose intervals.

Hydroxyzine hydrochloride

CLINICAL USE

Antihistamine:
- Pruritus
- Anxiety (short term)

DOSE IN NORMAL RENAL FUNCTION

- Pruritus: 25 mg at night increasing as necessary to 3–4 times a day.
- Anxiety: 50–100 mg 4 times daily.

PHARMACOKINETICS

Molecular weight (daltons)	447.8
% Protein binding	No data
% Excreted unchanged in urine	0
Volume of distribution (L/kg)	19.5
Half-life – normal/ ESRF (hrs)	20/–

METABOLISM

Hydroxyzine is extensively metabolised. The formation of the major metabolite cetirizine, a carboxylic acid metabolite (approximately 45% of the oral dose), is mediated by alcohol dehydrogenase. This metabolite has significant peripheral H1-antagonist properties. The other metabolites identified include a N-dealkylated metabolite, and an O-dealkylated metabolite with a plasma half-life of 59 hours. These pathways are mediated principally by CYP3A4/5. Only 0.8% of the dose is excreted unchanged in urine. The major metabolite cetirizine is excreted mainly unchanged in urine (25% and 16% of the hydroxyzine oral and IM dose, respectively).

DOSE IN RENAL IMPAIRMENT GFR (mL/MIN)

20–50	Dose as in normal renal function.
10–20	Start with 50% of dose and increase if necessary.
<10	Start with 50% of dose and increase if necessary.

DOSE IN PATIENTS UNDERGOING RENAL REPLACEMENT THERAPIES

CAPD	Not dialysed. Dose as in GFR<10 mL/min.
HD	Not dialysed. Dose as in GFR<10 mL/min.
HDF/High flux	Not dialysed. Dose as in GFR<10 mL/min.
CAV/ VVHD	Not dialysed. Dose as in GFR=10–20 mL/min.

IMPORTANT DRUG INTERACTIONS

Potentially hazardous interactions with other drugs
- Analgesics: sedative effects possibly increased with opioid analgesics.

ADMINISTRATION

RECONSTITUTION
–
ROUTE
- Oral
RATE OF ADMINISTRATION
–
COMMENTS
–

OTHER INFORMATION

- Increased possibility of side effects, particularly drowsiness.

Hyoscine butylbromide

CLINICAL USE

- Symptomatic relief of gastrointestinal or genitourinary disorders due to smooth muscle spasm
- Bowel colic
- Excessive respiratory secretions

DOSE IN NORMAL RENAL FUNCTION

- Oral: 20 mg 4 times a day
- Irritable bowel syndrome: 10 mg 3 times a day, increasing to 20 mg 4 times a day if required.
- IV/IM: 20 mg repeated after 30 minutes if required; maximum 100 mg daily.
- Bowel colic: 60–300 mg/24 hours by subcutaneous infusion.
- Excessive respiratory secretions: 20–120 mg/24 hours by subcutaneous infusion.

PHARMACOKINETICS

Molecular weight (daltons)	440.4
% Protein binding	10
% Excreted unchanged in urine	1–2
Volume of distribution (L/kg)	No data
Half-life – normal/ ESRF (hrs)	8/–

METABOLISM

The main metabolic pathway is the hydrolytic cleavage of the ester bond. Orally administered hyoscine butylbromide is excreted in the faeces and in the urine. Studies in man show that 2–5% of radioactive doses is eliminated renally after oral, and 0.7–1.6% after rectal administration. Approximately 90% of recovered radioactivity can be found in the faeces after oral administration. The urinary excretion of hyoscine butylbromide is less than 0.1% of the dose. The metabolites excreted via the renal route bind poorly to muscarinic receptors and are therefore not considered to contribute to the effect of the hyoscine butylbromide.

DOSE IN RENAL IMPAIRMENT GFR (mL/MIN)

20–50	Dose as in normal renal function.
10–20	Dose as in normal renal function.
<10	Dose as in normal renal function.

DOSE IN PATIENTS UNDERGOING RENAL REPLACEMENT THERAPIES

CAPD	Dialysed. Dose as in normal renal function.
HD	Dialysed. Dose as in normal renal function.
HDF/High flux	Dialysed. Dose as in normal renal function.
CAV/VVHD	Dialysed. Dose as in normal renal function.

IMPORTANT DRUG INTERACTIONS

Potentially hazardous interactions with other drugs

- None known

ADMINISTRATION

RECONSTITUTION

–

ROUTE

- Oral, IV, IM, SC

RATE OF ADMINISTRATION

–

COMMENTS

–

OTHER INFORMATION

- Only 2–8% of oral dose is absorbed

Hyoscine hydrobromide

CLINICAL USE

- Motion sickness
- Premedication
- Palliative care
- Hypersalivation with clozapine therapy (unlicensed)

DOSE IN NORMAL RENAL FUNCTION

- Motion sickness:
  — Oral: 150–300 mcg 30 minutes before start of journey then repeat every 6 hours if required; maximum 900 mcg in 24 hours.
  — Topical: 1 patch 5–6 hours before journey replace after 72 hours.
- Hypersalivation: 300 mcg up to 3 times daily.
- Premedication (SC/IM): 200–600 mcg 30–60 minutes before anaesthesia.
- SC Infusions: Excessive secretions & bowel colic (patch can also be used for excessive secretions): 1.2–2 mg over 24 hours.

PHARMACOKINETICS

Molecular weight (daltons)	438.3
% Protein binding	10
% Excreted unchanged in urine	2 (1 – oral, 34 – transdermal)
Volume of distribution (L/kg)	No data
Half-life – normal/ ESRF (hrs)	8/–

METABOLISM

Hyoscine hydrobromide is almost entirely metabolised, probably in the liver; only a small proportion of an oral dose is excreted unchanged in the urine. In one study in man, 3.4% of a single dose, administered by subcutaneous injection was excreted unchanged in urine within 72 hours.

DOSE IN RENAL IMPAIRMENT GFR (mL/MIN)

20–50	Dose as in normal renal function.
10–20	Dose as in normal renal function.
<10	Dose as in normal renal function.

DOSE IN PATIENTS UNDERGOING RENAL REPLACEMENT THERAPIES

CAPD	Dialysed. Dose as in normal renal function.
HD	Dialysed. Dose as in normal renal function.
HDF/High flux	Dialysed. Dose as in normal renal function.
CAV/ VVHD	Dialysed. Dose as in normal renal function.

IMPORTANT DRUG INTERACTIONS

Potentially hazardous interactions with other drugs
- None known

ADMINISTRATION

RECONSTITUTION
–
ROUTE
- Oral, topical, SC, IM
RATE OF ADMINISTRATION
–
COMMENTS
–

OTHER INFORMATION

- Only 2–8% of oral dose is absorbed.
- Manufacturer advises to use with caution in renal impairment.

Ibandronic acid

CLINICAL USE

Bisphosphonate:
- Reduction of bone damage in bone metastases in breast cancer
- Hypercalcaemia of malignancy
- Postmenopausal osteoporosis

DOSE IN NORMAL RENAL FUNCTION

- Oral: 50 mg daily.
- IV: 6 mg every 3–4 weeks.
- Hypercalcaemia of malignancy: 2–4 mg as a single dose, repeated according to serum calcium level.
- Postmenopausal osteoporosis: 150 mg monthly (oral), 3 mg every 3 months (IV bolus).

PHARMACOKINETICS

Molecular weight (daltons)	319.2 (Ibandronate Na 359.2)
% Protein binding	87
% Excreted unchanged in urine	50–60
Volume of distribution (L/kg)	90 litres
Half-life – normal/ ESRF (hrs)	10–72/Insignificantly increased.[1]

METABOLISM

After initial systemic exposure, ibandronic acid rapidly binds to bone or is excreted into urine. There is no evidence that ibandronic acid is metabolised in animals or humans. The absorbed fraction of ibandronic acid is removed from the circulation via bone absorption (estimated to be 40–50% in postmenopausal women) and the remainder is eliminated unchanged by the kidney. The unabsorbed fraction of ibandronic acid is eliminated unchanged in the faeces. Renal clearance accounts for 50–60% of total clearance and is related to creatinine clearance. The difference between the apparent total and renal clearances is considered to reflect the uptake by bone.

DOSE IN RENAL IMPAIRMENT GFR (mL/MIN)

30–50	Oral: 50 mg every 48 hours. IV: 4 mg every 3–4 weeks. See 'Other information'.
10–30	Oral: 50 mg weekly. IV: 4 mg every 3–4 weeks. See 'Other information'.
<10	Oral: 50 mg weekly. IV: 2 mg every 3–4 weeks. See 'Other information'.

DOSE IN PATIENTS UNDERGOING RENAL REPLACEMENT THERAPIES

CAPD	Unknown dialysability. Dose as in GFR<10 mL/min.
HD	Dialysed.[2] Dose as in GFR <10 mL/min.
HDF/High flux	Dialysed.[2] Dose as in GFR <10 mL/min.
CAV/ VVHD	Dialysed. Dose as in GFR=10–30 mL/min.

IMPORTANT DRUG INTERACTIONS

Potentially hazardous interactions with other drugs
- None known

ADMINISTRATION

RECONSTITUTION
–
ROUTE
- Oral, IV infusion, IV bolus
RATE OF ADMINISTRATION
- Infusion: over 15 minutes – 2 hours (depends on indication and renal function)
- IV bolus: over 15–30 seconds
COMMENTS
- Add dose to 100–500 mL glucose 5% or sodium chloride 0.9% (depends on indication and renal function).

OTHER INFORMATION

- Oral bioavailability <1%.
- Swallow tablets whole with a glass of water on an empty stomach, at least 30 minutes before breakfast and any other oral medication.
- The patient should stand or sit upright for at least 60 minutes after taking tablets.
- Don't give infusion over 15 minutes if creatinine clearance <50 mL/min; give in 500 mL over 1 hour.
- Bolus dose is contraindicated if GFR<30 mL/min due to lack of studies.
- One study used a dose of 6 mg over 30 minutes in various degrees of renal impairment with no deterioration in renal function.[1]
- Clearance is reduced in severe renal impairment.

- Due to the high bone-binding effect with ibandronic acid a dose of 2 mg monthly in haemodialysis patients is equivalent to a dose of 4–5 mg in patients with normal renal function.[3]
- May cause osteonecrosis of the jaw similar to other bisphosphonates.

References:
1. Bergner R, Henrich DM, Hoffmann M, *et al*. Renal safety and pharmacokinetics of ibandronate in multiple myeloma patients with or without impaired renal function. *J Clin Pharmacol*. 2007; **47**(8): 942–50.
2. Bergner R, Dill K, Boerner D, *et al*. Elimination of intravenously administered ibandronate in patients on haemodialysis: a monocentre open study. *Nephrol Dial Transplant*. 2002 Jul; **17**(7): 1281–5.
3. Bergner R, Henrich D, Hoffman M, *et al*. High bone-binding capacity of ibandronate in hemodialysis patients. *Int J Clin Pharmacol Res*. 2005; **25**(3): 123–31.

Ibuprofen

CLINICAL USE

NSAID and analgesic

DOSE IN NORMAL RENAL FUNCTION

Initially: 200–400 mg 3–4 times daily, after food. Maximum 2.4 g daily

PHARMACOKINETICS

Molecular weight (daltons)	206.3
% Protein binding	90–99
% Excreted unchanged in urine	1
Volume of distribution (L/kg)	0.14
Half-life – normal/ ESRF (hrs)	2/Unchanged

METABOLISM

Ibuprofen is rapidly excreted in the urine mainly as metabolites and their conjugates. About 1% is excreted in the urine as unchanged ibuprofen and about 14% as conjugated ibuprofen.

DOSE IN RENAL IMPAIRMENT GFR (mL/MIN)

20–50	Dose as in normal renal function, but avoid if possible.
10–20	Dose as in normal renal function, but avoid if possible.
<10	Dose as in normal renal function, but only use if on dialysis.

DOSE IN PATIENTS UNDERGOING RENAL REPLACEMENT THERAPIES

CAPD	Not dialysed. Dose as in normal renal function. See 'Other information'.
HD	Not dialysed. Dose as in normal renal function. See 'Other information'.
HDF/High flux	Not dialysed. Dose as in normal renal function. See 'Other information'.
CAV/VVHD	Not dialysed. Dose as in GFR=10–20 mL/min.

IMPORTANT DRUG INTERACTIONS

Potentially hazardous interactions with other drugs

- ACE inhibitors and angiotensin-II antagonists: antagonism of hypotensive effect; increased risk of nephrotoxicity and hyperkalaemia.
- Analgesics: avoid concomitant use of 2 or more NSAIDs, including aspirin (increased side effects); avoid with ketorolac (increased risk of side effects and haemorrhage); possibly reduced antiplatelet effect with aspirin.
- Antibacterials: possibly increased risk of convulsions with quinolones.
- Anticoagulants: effects of coumarins and phenindione enhanced; possibly increased risk of bleeding with heparins and dabigatran.
- Antidepressants: increased risk of bleeding with SSRIs and venlafaxine.
- Antidiabetic agents: effects of sulphonylureas enhanced.
- Anti-epileptics: possibly increased phenytoin concentration.
- Antivirals: increased risk of haematological toxicity with zidovudine; concentration possibly increased by ritonavir.
- Ciclosporin: may potentiate nephrotoxicity.
- Cytotoxic agents: reduced excretion of methotrexate; increased risk of bleeding with erlotinib.
- Diuretics: increased risk of nephrotoxicity; antagonism of diuretic effect; hyperkalaemia with potassium-sparing diuretics.
- Lithium: excretion decreased.
- Pentoxifylline: increased risk of bleeding.
- Tacrolimus: increased risk of nephrotoxicity.

ADMINISTRATION

RECONSTITUTION

–

ROUTE

- Oral

RATE OF ADMINISTRATION

–

COMMENTS

–

OTHER INFORMATION

- Inhibition of renal prostaglandin synthesis by NSAIDs may interfere with renal function, especially in the presence of existing renal disease – avoid if possible; if not, check serum creatinine 48–72 hours after starting NSAID – if raised, discontinue NSAID therapy.
- Use normal doses in patients with ERF on dialysis if they do not pass any urine.
- Use with caution in renal transplant recipients – can reduce intrarenal autocoid synthesis.

Idarubicin hydrochloride

CLINICAL USE

Antineoplastic agent:
- Acute non-lymphoblastic leukaemia (ANLL)
- 2nd line for acute lymphoblastic leukaemia (ALL), breast cancer
- With other cytotoxic agents in combination chemotherapy regimens

DOSE IN NORMAL RENAL FUNCTION

- IV:
  - ANLL: 12 mg/m^2 daily for 3 days in combination with cytarabine, or 8 mg/m^2 daily for 5 days with or without combination therapy
  - ALL: 12 mg/m^2 daily for 3 days.
- Oral:
  - ANLL: 30 mg/m^2 daily for 3 days as a single agent, or 15–30 mg/m^2 daily for 3 days in combination with other anti-leukaemic agents.
- Breast cancer:
  - 45 mg/m^2 given either as a single dose or divided over 3 consecutive days every 3–4 weeks.
- Maximum cumulative dose is 400 mg/m^2 daily.
- Or see local protocol.

PHARMACOKINETICS

Molecular weight (daltons)	534
% Protein binding	97
% Excreted unchanged in urine	1–2 (4.6% as idarubicinol)
Volume of distribution (L/kg)	64
Half-life – normal/ESRF (hrs)	10–35 (oral), 15 (IV)/–

METABOLISM

- Idarubicin is extensively metabolised, both in the liver and extrahepatically; the principal metabolite, idarubicinol (13-dihydroidarubicin) has equal antineoplastic activity. Peak concentrations of idarubicin and idarubicinol in bone marrow and nucleated blood cells are 400 (idarubicin) and 200 (idarubicinol) times greater than those in plasma; cellular concentrations of drug and metabolite decline with apparent terminal half-lives of 15 and 72 hours respectively, whereas plasma half-lives are reported to be 20 to 22 hours and about 45 hours respectively. Idarubicin is excreted in bile, and to a lesser extent in urine, as unchanged drug and metabolites. 17% (IV)/8% (oral) is recovered in the faeces over 5 days and 16% (IV)/5% (oral) is recovered in the urine over 4 days.

DOSE IN RENAL IMPAIRMENT GFR (mL/MIN)

20–50	Use 75% of dose.
10–20	Use 75% of dose with caution.
<10	Use 50% of dose with caution.

DOSE IN PATIENTS UNDERGOING RENAL REPLACEMENT THERAPIES

CAPD	Not dialysed. Dose as in GFR<10 mL/min.
HD	Not dialysed. Dose as in GFR<10 mL/min.
HDF/High flux	Unknown dialysability. Dose as in GFR<10 mL/min.
CAV/VVHD	Unknown dialysability. Dose as in GFR=10–20 mL/min.

IMPORTANT DRUG INTERACTIONS

Potentially hazardous interactions with other drugs
- Other myelosuppressant medication and radiotherapy: increased risk of myelosuppression.
- Antipsychotics: avoid concomitant use with clozapine, increased risk of agranulocytosis.
- Ciclosporin: concentration increased by ciclosporin.

ADMINISTRATION

RECONSTITUTION
- 5 mL water for injection per 5 mg
ROUTE
- IV, oral, intravesical
RATE OF ADMINISTRATION
- Give via the tubing of a fast running intravenous infusion of sodium chloride 0.9% or glucose 5%, over 5–10 minutes
COMMENTS
- Incompatible with alkaline solutions and heparin.
- Reconstituted solution is physically and chemically stable for 7 days at 2–8°C and 72 hours at room temperature.

- Does not contain any antibacterial preservative so maximum recommended stability is 24 hours.

OTHER INFORMATION

- Contraindicated by manufacturer in severe renal impairment.
- Doses in renal impairment are from *Drug Prescribing in Renal Failure*, 5th edition, by Aronoff *et al.*
- May cause the urine to become red for 1–2 days after administration.

- Oral bioavailability is 18–39%, 29–58% for idarubicinol.
- A phase II study instilled 6.25–12.5 mg of idarubicin diluted in 45 mL of sodium chloride 0.9% (0.125–0.25 mg/mL) into the bladder of patients with resected recurrent bladder cancer although it may not be any more effective than doxorubicin or epirubicin and toxicity may limit its use. (Boccardo F, Cannata D, Cussotto M, *et al.* Intravesical idarubicin: a dose-finding study. *Cancer Chemother Pharmacol.* 1996; **38**(1): 102–5.)

Ifosfamide

CLINICAL USE

Antineoplastic agent:
- Treatment of solid tumours, lymphomas and soft tissue sarcoma

DOSE IN NORMAL RENAL FUNCTION

- Usual total dose for each course is either 8–12 g/m², equally divided as single daily doses over 3–5 days, or 5–6 g/m² (maximum 10 g) given as a 24 hour infusion.
- OR according to local protocol.

PHARMACOKINETICS

Molecular weight (daltons)	261.1
% Protein binding	0
% Excreted unchanged in urine	12–18
Volume of distribution (L/kg)	0.4–0.64
Half-life – normal/ ESRF (hrs)	4–8/–

METABOLISM

The pharmacokinetics of ifosfamide are reported to exhibit considerable inter-individual variation. It is a prodrug that is extensively metabolised, chiefly by cytochrome P450 isoenzymes CYP3A4 and CYP2B6 in the liver, to both active and inactive alkylating metabolites; there is some evidence that metabolism is saturated at very high doses. After repeated doses (fractionated therapy) there is a decrease in the elimination half-life, apparently due to auto-induction of metabolism. It is excreted largely in urine, as unchanged drug (80%) and metabolites.

DOSE IN RENAL IMPAIRMENT GFR (mL/MIN)

>60	80% of normal dose.
30–60	80% of normal dose.
15–30	80% of normal dose.
<15	60% of normal dose.

DOSE IN PATIENTS UNDERGOING RENAL REPLACEMENT THERAPIES

CAPD	Dialysed. Dose as in GFR<15 mL/min. Following dose, do not perform CAPD exchange for 12 hours.
HD	Dialysed. Dose as in GFR<15 mL/min. Dose at minimum of 12 hours before next HD session.
HDF/High flux	Dialysed. Dose as in GFR<15 mL/min. Dose at minimum of 12 hours before next HD session.
CAV/VVHD	Dialysed. Dose as in GFR = 15–30 mL/min.

IMPORTANT DRUG INTERACTIONS

Potentially hazardous interactions with other drugs
- Anticoagulants: possibly enhanced effect of coumarins.
- Antipsychotics: avoid concomitant use with clozapine (increased risk of agranulocytosis).

ADMINISTRATION

RECONSTITUTION
- Reconstitute 1 g vial with 12.5 mL water for injection.
- Reconstitute 2 g vial with 25 mL water for injection. The resultant solution of 8% ifosfamide should NOT be injected directly into the vein.

ROUTE
- IV injection: dilute to less than a 4% solution.
- IV infusion: dilute as detailed below.

RATE OF ADMINISTRATION
- IV infusion:
- Infuse in glucose 5% or sodium chloride 0.9% over 30–120 minutes, or
- Inject directly into a fast running infusion, or
- Made up in 3 L of glucose 5% or sodium chloride 0.9%; each litre should be given over 8 hours.

COMMENTS
–

OTHER INFORMATION

- Nephrotoxicity may occur with oliguria, raised uric acid, increased BUN and serum creatinine, and decreased creatinine clearance.

- Ifosfamide is known to be more nephrotoxic than cyclophosphamide; hence greater caution is advised.
- SPC contraindicates the use of ifosfamide if serum creatinine >120 µmol/L.
- If patient is anuric and on dialysis, neither the ifosfamide nor its metabolites nor Mesna should appear in the urinary tract. The use of Mesna may therefore be unnecessary, although this would be a clinical decision.
- If the patient is passing urine, Mesna should be given to prevent urothelial toxicity.
- Doses from Kintzel PE, Dorr RT. Anticancer drug renal toxicity and elimination: dosing guidelines for altered renal function. *Cancer Treat Rev.* 1995; **21**: 33–64.
  — GFR>60 mL/min 80% of dose
  — GFR=45–60 mL/min 75% of dose
  — GFR=30–45 mL/min 70% of dose
- There are 3 case reports of ifosfamide being used in doses of 1.5–4 g/m^2 in patients on haemodialysis; the main side effect was myelosuppression.
- Latcha S, Maki RG, Schwartz GK, *et al.* Case Report: Ifosfamide may be safely used in patients with end stage renal disease on hemodialysis. *Sarcoma.* 2009; **2009**, Article ID 575629 http://dx.doi.org/10.1155/2009/575629

Reference:
1. Lichtman SM, Wildiers H, Launay-Vacher V, *et al.* International society of geriatric oncology (SIOG) recommendations for the adjustment of dosing in elderly cancer patients with renal insufficiency. *Eur J Cancer.* 2007; **43**: 14–34.

Iloprost

CLINICAL USE

Prostacyclin analogue:
- Treatment of pulmonary arterial hypertension
- Relief of pain, promotion of ulcer-healing and limb salvage in patients with severe peripheral arterial ischaemia (unlicensed product)

DOSE IN NORMAL RENAL FUNCTION

- Pulmonary hypertension:
  - Nebulised: 2.5–5 mcg per inhalation session 6 to 9 times per day
  - IV: Usually 1–8 ng/kg/min, but can use higher doses (up to 25 ng/kg/min) according to response.
- Severe peripheral arterial ischaemia:
  - Dose is adjusted according to individual tolerability within the range of 0.5–2 nanograms/kg/minute over 6 hours daily.

PHARMACOKINETICS

Molecular weight (daltons)	360.5
% Protein binding	≈60
% Excreted unchanged in urine	<5
Volume of distribution (L/kg)	0.6–0.8
Half-life – normal/ESRF (hrs)	0.3–0.5/ Unchanged

METABOLISM

On intravenous infusion iloprost is rapidly cleared from the plasma by oxidation. About 80% of the metabolites are excreted in urine and 20% in the bile.

DOSE IN RENAL IMPAIRMENT GFR (mL/MIN)

20–50	Dose as in normal renal function.
10–20	Dose as in normal renal function.
<10	Dose as in normal renal function.

DOSE IN PATIENTS UNDERGOING RENAL REPLACEMENT THERAPIES

CAPD	Unknown dialysability. Dose as in normal renal function.
HD	Unknown dialysability. Dose as in normal renal function.
HDF/High flux	Unknown dialysability. Dose as in normal renal function.
CAV/ VVHD	Unknown dialysability. Dose as in normal renal function.

IMPORTANT DRUG INTERACTIONS

Potentially hazardous interactions with other drugs
- Anticoagulants: enhanced anticoagulant effect and increased risk of bleeding with heparin, coumarins and phenindione, as iloprost inhibits platelet aggregation.
- Increased risk of bleeding with NSAIDs, aspirin, clopidogrel, eptifibatide and tirofiban.

ADMINISTRATION

RECONSTITUTION
- Dilute 0.1 mg with 500 mL sodium chloride 0.9% or glucose 5%. Final concentration = 0.2 micrograms iloprost/mL.

ROUTE
- Nebulised, IV infusion via peripheral vein or central venous catheter.

RATE OF ADMINISTRATION
- Infuse 0.1 mg over 6 hours daily (see below).

COMMENTS
- Treatment should be started at an infusion rate of 10 mL/hour for 30 minutes, which corresponds to a dose of 0.5 nanograms/ kg/minute for a patient of 65 kg.
- Then increase dose in steps of 10 mL/hour every 30 minutes up to a rate of 40 mL/hour (50 mL/hour if patient's body weight is more than 75 kg).
- If side effects occur (e.g. headache, nausea, or an undesired drop in BP), infusion rate should be reduced until the tolerable dose is found; if side effects are severe, infusion should be interrupted.
- For rest of the treatment period, continue with dose found to be tolerated in the first 2–3 days.

OTHER INFORMATION

- BP and heart rate must be measured at the start of the infusion and after every increase in dose.
- Duration of treatment is up to 4 weeks. Shorter treatment periods (3–5 days) are often sufficient in Raynaud's phenomenon.
- Iloprost infusions can also be used to control blood pressure during a scleroderma hypertensive crisis.
- For fluid-restricted patients, dilute 0.1 mg iloprost with 50 mL sodium chloride 0.9%, and run at a rate of 1–4 mL/hour.
- Toxic by inhalation, contact with skin, and if swallowed.
- Manufacturer advises to use with caution if GFR<30 mL/min due to lack of data.

Imatinib

CLINICAL USE

Tyrosine kinase inhibitor, antineoplastic agent
- Treatment of chronic myeloid leukaemia
- Treatment of metastatic malignant gastro-intestinal stromal tumours
- Treatment of acute lymphoblastic leukaemia

DOSE IN NORMAL RENAL FUNCTION

400–600 mg daily, increasing to a maximum of 400 mg twice daily
Dose depends on indication

PHARMACOKINETICS

Molecular weight (daltons)	589.7 (as mesilate)
% Protein binding	95
% Excreted unchanged in urine	5
Volume of distribution (L/kg)	No data
Half-life – normal/ ESRF (hrs)	18/Unknown

METABOLISM

The main circulating metabolite in humans is the N-demethylated piperazine derivative, which shows similar *in vitro* potency to the parent. Imatinib and the N-demethyl metabolite together accounted for about 65% of the circulating radioactivity (AUC (0–48h)). The remaining circulating radioactivity consisted of a number of minor metabolites. *In vitro* results showed that CYP3A4 was the major human P450 enzyme catalysing the biotransformation of imatinib. Based on the recovery of compound(s) after an oral ^{14}C-labelled dose of imatinib, approximately 81% of the dose was recovered within 7 days in faeces (68% of dose) and urine (13% of dose). Unchanged imatinib accounted for 25% of the dose (5% urine, 20% faeces), the remainder being metabolites.

DOSE IN RENAL IMPAIRMENT GFR (mL/MIN)

20–50	Dose as in normal renal function.
10–20	Dose as in normal renal function. See 'Other information'.
<10	Dose as in normal renal function. See 'Other information'.

DOSE IN PATIENTS UNDERGOING RENAL REPLACEMENT THERAPIES

CAPD	Unlikely to be dialysed. Dose as in GFR<10 mL/min.
HD	Unlikely to be dialysed. Dose as in GFR<10 mL/min.
HDF/High flux	Unlikely to be dialysed. Dose as in GFR<10 mL/min.
CAV/ VVHD	Unknown dialysability. Dose as in GFR=10–20 mL/min.

IMPORTANT DRUG INTERACTIONS

Potentially hazardous interactions with other drugs
- Antibacterials: concentration reduced by rifampicin – avoid concomitant use.
- Anticoagulants: enhanced anticoagulant effect of warfarin, replace with heparin.
- Antidepressants: concentration reduced by St John's wort – avoid.
- Anti-epileptics: concentration reduced by carbamazepine, oxcarbazepine and phenytoin – avoid concomitant use; absorption of phenytoin possibly reduced.
- Antipsychotics: avoid concomitant use with clozapine (increased risk of agranulocytosis).
- Antivirals: avoid with boceprevir.
- Ciclosporin: may increase ciclosporin levels.
- Tacrolimus: may increase tacrolimus levels.

ADMINISTRATION

RECONSTITUTION
–
ROUTE
- Oral
RATE OF ADMINISTRATION
–
COMMENTS
–

OTHER INFORMATION

- Associated with oedema and superficial fluid retention in 50–70% of cases. Probability is increased in patients receiving higher doses, age >65 years, and those with a prior history of cardiac disease. Severe fluid retention (e.g. pleural effusion, pericardial effusion, pulmonary oedema and ascites) has been reported in up to 16% of patients. Can be managed by diuretic therapy, and dose reduction or interruption of imatinib therapy.

- Severe elevation of serum creatinine has been observed in approximately 1% of patients.
- Oral bioavailability is 98%.

Imidapril hydrochloride

CLINICAL USE

Angiotensin-converting enzyme inhibitor:
- Hypertension

DOSE IN NORMAL RENAL FUNCTION

2.5–20 mg once daily

PHARMACOKINETICS

Molecular weight (daltons)	441.9
% Protein binding	85
% Excreted unchanged in urine	9 (as imidaprilat)
Volume of distribution (L/kg)	No data
Half-life – normal/ ESRF (hrs)	2/Increased (>24 hours as imidaprilat)

METABOLISM

Imidapril is a prodrug, and is metabolised in the liver to the diacid imidaprilat, its active metabolite. The bioavailability of imidaprilat is about 42% after oral doses of imidapril. About 40% of an oral dose is excreted in the urine, the rest in the faeces.

DOSE IN RENAL IMPAIRMENT GFR (mL/MIN)

20–50	Initially 2.5 mg daily and adjust according to response.
10–20	Initially 2.5 mg daily and adjust according to response.
<10	Initially 2.5 mg daily and adjust according to response.

DOSE IN PATIENTS UNDERGOING RENAL REPLACEMENT THERAPIES

CAPD	Probably dialysed. Dose as in GFR<10 mL/min.
HD	Dialysed. Dose as in GFR<10 mL/min.
HDF/High flux	Dialysed. Dose as in GFR<10 mL/min.
CAV/ VVHD	Probably dialysed. Dose as in GFR=10–20 mL/min.

IMPORTANT DRUG INTERACTIONS

Potentially hazardous interactions with other drugs
- Anaesthetics: enhanced hypotensive effect.
- Analgesics: antagonism of hypotensive effect and increased risk of renal impairment with NSAIDs; hyperkalaemia with ketorolac and other NSAIDs.
- Ciclosporin: increased risk of hyperkalaemia and nephrotoxicity.
- Diuretics: enhanced hypotensive effect; hyperkalaemia with potassium-sparing diuretics.
- ESAs: increased risk of hyperkalaemia; antagonism of hypotensive effect.
- Gold: flushing and hypotension with sodium aurothiomalate.
- Lithium: reduced excretion, possibility of enhanced lithium toxicity.
- Potassium salts: increased risk of hyperkalaemia.
- Tacrolimus: increased risk of hyperkalaemia and nephrotoxicity.

ADMINISTRATION

RECONSTITUTION
–
ROUTE
- Oral
RATE OF ADMINISTRATION
–
COMMENTS
–

OTHER INFORMATION

- Hyperkalaemia and other side effects are more common in patients with impaired renal function.
- Close monitoring of renal function during therapy is necessary in those with renal insufficiency.
- Renal failure has been reported in association with ACE inhibitors with renal artery stenosis, post renal transplant or congestive heat failure.
- High incidence of anaphylactoid reactions have been reported in patients dialysed with high-flux polyacrylonitrile membranes and treated concomitantly with an ACE inhibitor – combination should therefore be avoided.

Imipramine hydrochloride

CLINICAL USE

Tricyclic antidepressant

DOSE IN NORMAL RENAL FUNCTION

25 mg up to 3 times daily increasing up to 150–200 mg daily; maximum 300 mg in hospital patients.

PHARMACOKINETICS

Molecular weight (daltons)	316.9
% Protein binding	95
% Excreted unchanged in urine	5
Volume of distribution (L/kg)	31
Half-life – normal/ ESRF (hrs)	9–28/–

METABOLISM

Imipramine is extensively demethylated by first-pass metabolism in the liver, to its primary active metabolite, desipramine (desmethylimipramine). Paths of metabolism of both imipramine and desipramine include hydroxylation and *N*-oxidation. About 80% is excreted in the urine and about 20% in the faeces, mainly in the form of inactive metabolites. Urinary excretion of unchanged imipramine and of the active metabolite desipramine is about 5% and 6% respectively. Only small quantities of these are excreted in the faeces.

DOSE IN RENAL IMPAIRMENT GFR (mL/MIN)

20–50	Dose as in normal renal function.
10–20	Dose as in normal renal function.
<10	Dose as in normal renal function.

DOSE IN PATIENTS UNDERGOING RENAL REPLACEMENT THERAPIES

CAPD	Not dialysed. Dose as in normal renal function.
HD	Not dialysed. Dose as in normal renal function.
HDF/High flux	Not dialysed. Dose as in normal renal function.
CAV/ VVHD	Not dialysed. Dose as in normal renal function.

IMPORTANT DRUG INTERACTIONS

Potentially hazardous interactions with other drugs
- Alcohol: increased sedative effect.
- Analgesics: increased risk of CNS toxicity with tramadol; possibly increased risk of side effects with nefopam; possibly increased sedative effects with opioids.
- Anti-arrhythmics: increased risk of ventricular arrhythmias with amiodarone – avoid concomitant use; increased risk of ventricular arrhythmias with disopyramide, flecainide or propafenone; avoid with dronedarone.
- Antibacterials: increased risk of ventricular arrhythmias with moxifloxacin and possibly telithromycin – avoid concomitant use with moxifloxacin.
- Anticoagulants: may alter anticoagulant effect of coumarins.
- Antidepressants: enhanced CNS excitation and hypertension with MAOIs and moclobemide – avoid concomitant use; concentration possibly increased with SSRIs.
- Anti-epileptics: convulsive threshold lowered; concentration reduced by carbamazepine, phenobarbital and possibly phenytoin.
- Antimalarials: avoid concomitant use with artemether/lumefantrine and piperaquine with artenimol.
- Antipsychotics: increased risk of ventricular arrhythmias especially with droperidol and pimozide – avoid; increased antimuscarinic effects with clozapine and phenothiazines; concentration increased by antipsychotics.
- Antivirals: increased risk of ventricular arrhythmias with saquinavir – avoid; concentration possibly increased with ritonavir.
- Atomoxetine: increased risk of ventricular arrhythmias and possibly convulsions.
- Beta-blockers: increased risk of ventricular arrhythmias with sotalol; concentration increased by labetalol and propranolol.
- Clonidine: tricyclics antagonise hypotensive effect; increased risk of hypertension on clonidine withdrawal.
- Dopaminergics: avoid use with entacapone; CNS toxicity reported with selegiline and rasagiline.

- Pentamidine: increased risk of ventricular arrhythmias.
- Sympathomimetics: increased risk of hypertension and arrhythmias with adrenaline and noradrenaline; metabolism possibly inhibited by methylphenidate.

ADMINISTRATION

RECONSTITUTION

–

ROUTE

- Oral

RATE OF ADMINISTRATION

–

COMMENTS

–

OTHER INFORMATION

–

Indapamide

CLINICAL USE

Thiazide-like diuretic:
- Essential hypertension

DOSE IN NORMAL RENAL FUNCTION

2.5 daily in the morning
Modified release: 1.5 mg daily in the morning

PHARMACOKINETICS

Molecular weight (daltons)	365.8
% Protein binding	79
% Excreted unchanged in urine	5–7
Volume of distribution (L/kg)	0.3–1.3
Half-life – normal/ ESRF (hrs)	14–24/Unchanged

METABOLISM

Indapamide is strongly bound to red blood cells, and is taken up by the vascular wall in smooth vascular muscle according to its high lipid solubility. Sixty to seventy per cent of a single oral dose is eliminated by the kidneys and 23% by the gastrointestinal tract. Indapamide is extensively metabolised with 5–7% of unchanged drug found in the urine during the 48 hours following administration. About 16–23% of dose is excreted in the faeces.

DOSE IN RENAL IMPAIRMENT GFR (mL/MIN)

20–50	Dose as in normal renal function.
10–50	Dose as in normal renal function.
<10	Dose as in normal renal function. See 'Other information'.

DOSE IN PATIENTS UNDERGOING RENAL REPLACEMENT THERAPIES

CAPD	Not dialysed. Dose as in GFR<10 mL/min.
HD	Not dialysed. Dose as in GFR<10 mL/min.
HDF/High flux	Not dialysed. Dose as in GFR<10 mL/min.
CAV/ VVHD	Not dialysed. Dose as in normal renal function.

IMPORTANT DRUG INTERACTIONS

Potentially hazardous interactions with other drugs
- Analgesics: increased risk of nephrotoxicity with NSAIDs; antagonism of diuretic effect.
- Anti-arrhythmics: hypokalaemia leads to increased cardiac toxicity; effects of lidocaine and mexiletine antagonised.
- Antibacterials: avoid administration with lymecycline.
- Antidepressants: increased risk of hypokalaemia with reboxetine; enhanced hypotensive effect with MAOIs; increased risk of postural hypotension with tricyclics.
- Anti-epileptics: increased risk of hyponatraemia with carbamazepine.
- Antifungals: increased risk of hypokalaemia with amphotericin.
- Antihypertensives: enhanced hypotensive effect; increased risk of first dose hypotension with post-synaptic alpha-blockers like prazosin; hypokalaemia increases risk of ventricular arrhythmias with sotalol.
- Antipsychotics: hypokalaemia increases risk of ventricular arrhythmias with amisulpride; enhanced hypotensive effect with phenothiazines; hypokalaemia increases risk of ventricular arrhythmias with pimozide – avoid concomitant use.
- Atomoxetine: hypokalaemia increases risk of ventricular arrhythmias.
- Cardiac glycosides: increased toxicity if hypokalaemia occurs.
- Ciclosporin: increased risk of nephrotoxicity and possibly hypomagnesaemia.
- Cytotoxics: increased risk of ventricular arrhythmias due to hypokalaemia with arsenic trioxide; increased risk of nephrotoxicity and ototoxicity with platinum compounds.
- Lithium excretion reduced (increased toxicity).

ADMINISTRATION

RECONSTITUTION
–
ROUTE
- Oral
RATE OF ADMINISTRATION
–
COMMENTS
–

OTHER INFORMATION

- If pre-existing renal insufficiency is aggravated – stop indapamide.
- Doses greater than 2.5 mg daily are not recommended.
- Caution if hypokalaemia develops.
- Ineffective in ERF.
- One-month studies of functionally anephric patients undergoing chronic haemodialysis have not shown evidence of drug accumulation, despite the fact that indapamide is not dialysable.
- Contraindicated by manufacturer in severe renal impairment in UK SPC but not US one.

Indinavir

CLINICAL USE

Protease inhibitor:
● Treatment of HIV infection, in
  combination with a nucleoside reverse
  transcriptase inhibitor

DOSE IN NORMAL RENAL FUNCTION

800 mg every 8 hours

PHARMACOKINETICS

Molecular weight (daltons)	711.9 (as sulphate)
% Protein binding	60
% Excreted unchanged in urine	10.4
Volume of distribution (L/kg)	14
Half-life – normal/ ESRF (hrs)	1.8/Unchanged

METABOLISM

Seven major metabolites have been
identified and the metabolic pathways
were identified as glucuronidation at the
pyridine nitrogen, pyridine-N-oxidation
with and without 3'-hydroxylation on the
indane ring, 3'-hydroxylation of indane,
p-hydroxylation of phenylmethyl moiety, and
N-depyridomethylation with and without
the 3'-hydroxylation. *In vitro* studies with
human liver microsomes indicated that
CYP3A4 is the only P450 isozyme that plays
a major role in the oxidative metabolism
of indinavir. Analysis of plasma and urine
samples from subjects who received indinavir
indicated that indinavir metabolites had little
proteinase inhibitory activity. Less than 20%
of indinavir is excreted renally, about half of
this as unchanged drug. The remainder is
excreted in the faeces.

DOSE IN RENAL IMPAIRMENT GFR (mL/MIN)

20–50	Dose as in normal renal function. Monitor closely.
10–20	Dose as in normal renal function. Monitor closely.
<10	Dose as in normal renal function. Monitor closely.

DOSE IN PATIENTS UNDERGOING RENAL REPLACEMENT THERAPIES

CAPD	Unlikely to be dialysed. Dose as in GFR<10 mL/min.
HD	Not dialysed. Dose as in GFR<10 mL/min.
HDF/High flux	Not dialysed. Dose as in GFR<10 mL/min.
CAV/ VVHD	Unlikely to be dialysed. Dose as in GFR=10–20 mL/min.

IMPORTANT DRUG INTERACTIONS

Potentially hazardous interactions with other
drugs
● Anti-arrhythmics: possibly increased
  amiodarone and flecainide concentration
  – avoid concomitant use.
● Antibacterials: rifampicin increases
  metabolism – avoid concomitant use;
  increased rifabutin concentration – avoid;
  avoid with telithromycin in severe renal
  and hepatic failure.
● Antidepressants: concentration reduced by
  St John's wort (avoid concomitant use).
● Anti-epileptics: concentration possibly
  reduced by carbamazepine, phenytoin
  and phenobarbital, also concentration of
  carbamazepine and phenytoin increased.
● Antifungals: itraconazole and
  ketoconazole inhibits metabolism –
  reduce dose of indinavir to 600 mg every
  8 hours.
● Antimalarials: use artemether/
  lumefantrine with caution; possibly
  increased quinine concentration.
● Antipsychotics: possibly increased risk of
  ventricular arrhythmias with pimozide –
  avoid concomitant use; possibly inhibits
  aripiprazole metabolism – reduce
  aripiprazole dose; possibly increases
  quetiapine concentration – avoid.
● Antivirals: avoid with atazanavir;
  concentration reduced by efavirenz,
  nevirapine and possibly etravirine,
  avoid with etravirine; concentration of
  both drugs increased with darunavir;
  concentration of maraviroc increased,
  consider reducing maraviroc dose;
  concentration increased by ritonavir;
  saquinavir concentration increased.
● Anxiolytics and hypnotics: increased risk
  of prolonged sedation with alprazolam and
  midazolam – avoid concomitant use.
● Ciclosporin: concentration of ciclosporin
  increased.

- Colchicine: possibly increases risk of colchicine toxicity, avoid in hepatic or renal impairment.
- Cytotoxics: possibly increases concentration of axitinib, reduce dose of axitinib; possibly increases concentration of crizotinib and everolimus – avoid; avoid with cabazitaxel and pazopanib; reduce dose of ruxolitinib.
- Ergot alkaloids: risk of ergotism – avoid concomitant use.
- Lipid-regulating drugs: increased risk of myopathy with rosuvastatin and simvastatin – avoid concomitant use; and possibly with atorvastatin.
- 5HT$_1$ agonists: concentration of eletriptan increased – avoid concomitant use.
- Ranolazine: possibly increases ranolazine concentration – avoid.
- Sildenafil: concentration of sildenafil increased – reduce initial sildenafil dose.
- Vardenafil: concentration of vardenafil increased – avoid concomitant use.

ADMINISTRATION

RECONSTITUTION
–
ROUTE
- Oral
RATE OF ADMINISTRATION
–
COMMENTS
- Drink 1.5 litres of water in 24 hours.
- Give 1 hour before, or 2 hours after food, or with a low fat meal with water.

OTHER INFORMATION

- If giving with didanosine, leave 1 hour between each drug.
- Mild renal insufficiency is usually due to crystalluria, but a case of interstitial nephritis has been reported.
- If nephrolithiasis with flank pain occurs (with or without haematuria), temporarily stop therapy (e.g. for 1–3 days).

Indometacin

CLINICAL USE

NSAID:
- Pain and inflammation in rheumatic disease and other musculoskeletal disorders
- Acute gout
- Dysmenorrhoea
- Closure of ductus arteriosus

DOSE IN NORMAL RENAL FUNCTION

- Oral: 50–200 mg daily in divided doses, after food
- PR: 100 mg twice daily if required
- Gout: 150–200 mg daily in divided doses
- Dysmenorrhoea: up to 75 mg daily
- Maximum combined oral and PR: 150–200 mg daily
- MR: 75 mg 1–2 times daily, once daily in dysmenorrhoea

PHARMACOKINETICS

Molecular weight (daltons)	357.8
% Protein binding	90–99
% Excreted unchanged in urine	5–20 (60% as metabolites)
Volume of distribution (L/kg)	0.34–1.57
Half-life – normal/ESRF (hrs)	1–16/Unchanged

METABOLISM

Indometacin is metabolised in the liver primarily by demethylation and deacetylation; it also undergoes glucuronidation and enterohepatic circulation. Indometacin is mainly excreted in the urine, approximately 60%, the pH of the urine can affect this amount. Lesser amounts are excreted in the faeces.

DOSE IN RENAL IMPAIRMENT GFR (mL/MIN)

20–50	Dose as in normal renal function, but avoid if possible.
10–20	Dose as in normal renal function, but avoid if possible.
<10	Dose as in normal renal function, but only use if CKD 5 and on dialysis.

DOSE IN PATIENTS UNDERGOING RENAL REPLACEMENT THERAPIES

CAPD	Not dialysed. Dose as in normal renal function. See 'Other information'.
HD	Not dialysed. Dose as in normal renal function. See 'Other information'.
HDF/High flux	Unlikely to be dialysed. Dose as in normal renal function. See 'Other information'.
CAV/VVHD	Not dialysed. Dose as in GFR=10–20 mL/min.

IMPORTANT DRUG INTERACTIONS

Potentially hazardous interactions with other drugs
- ACE inhibitors and angiotensin-II antagonists: antagonism of hypotensive effect; increased risk of nephrotoxicity and hyperkalaemia.
- Analgesics: avoid concomitant use of 2 or more NSAIDs, including aspirin (increased side effects); avoid with ketorolac (increased risk of side effects and haemorrhage).
- Antibacterials: possibly increased risk of convulsions with quinolones.
- Anticoagulants: effects of coumarins and phenindione enhanced; possibly increased risk of bleeding with heparins and dabigatran.
- Antidepressants: increased risk of bleeding with SSRIs and venlafaxine.
- Antidiabetic agents: effects of sulphonylureas enhanced.
- Anti-epileptic agents: effects of phenytoin enhanced.
- Antipsychotics: possible severe drowsiness with haloperidol.
- Antivirals: increased risk of haematological toxicity with zidovudine; concentration possibly increased by ritonavir.
- Ciclosporin: increased risk of nephrotoxicity.
- Cytotoxic agents: reduced excretion of methotrexate.
- Diuretics: increased risk of nephrotoxicity, hyperkalaemia with potassium-sparing diuretics; antagonism of diuretic effect.
- Lithium: lithium excretion reduced.
- Pentoxifylline: possibly increased risk of bleeding.

- Probenecid: excretion of indometacin reduced.
- Tacrolimus: increased risk of nephrotoxicity.

ADMINISTRATION

RECONSTITUTION

–

ROUTE

- Oral, PR, IV

RATE OF ADMINISTRATION

- 20–30 minutes

COMMENTS

–

OTHER INFORMATION

- Inhibition of renal prostaglandin synthesis by NSAIDs may interfere with renal function, especially in the presence of existing renal disease – avoid if possible; if not, check serum creatinine 48–72 hours after starting NSAID – if raised, discontinue NSAID therapy.
- Use normal doses in patients with ERF on dialysis if they do not pass any urine.
- Use with caution in renal transplant recipients – can reduce intrarenal autocoid synthesis.

Indoramin

CLINICAL USE

Alpha-adrenoceptor blocker:
- Hypertension
- Benign prostatic hyperplasia (BPH)

DOSE IN NORMAL RENAL FUNCTION

- Hypertension: 25 mg twice daily initially, increasing to a maximum of 200 mg daily in 2–3 divided doses.
- Benign prostatic hyperplasia: 20 mg twice daily increasing to a maximum of 100 mg daily in divided doses.

PHARMACOKINETICS

Molecular weight (daltons)	383.9 (as hydrochloride)
% Protein binding	>90
% Excreted unchanged in urine	<2
Volume of distribution (L/kg)	7.4
Half-life – normal/ ESRF (hrs)	5/Increased by 50% (reduced by 40% in HD patients)

METABOLISM

In studies with radiolabelled indoramin at doses of 40–60 mg daily for up to three days, after two or three days 35% of the radioactivity was excreted in the urine and 46% in the faeces. Extensive first pass metabolism was suggested. There is evidence to suggest that some metabolites may have some alpha-adrenoceptor blocking activity.

DOSE IN RENAL IMPAIRMENT GFR (mL/MIN)

20–50	Dose as in normal renal function.
10–20	Dose as in normal renal function.
<10	Dose as in normal renal function. See 'Other information'.

DOSE IN PATIENTS UNDERGOING RENAL REPLACEMENT THERAPIES

CAPD	Not dialysed. Dose as in GFR<10 mL/min.
HD	Not dialysed. Dose as in GFR<10 mL/min.
HDF/High flux	Unknown dialysability. Dose as in GFR<10 mL/min.
CAV/ VVHD	Not dialysed. Dose as in normal renal function.

IMPORTANT DRUG INTERACTIONS

Potentially hazardous interactions with other drugs
- Anaesthetics: enhanced hypotensive effect.
- NSAIDs: antagonism of hypotensive effect.
- Antidepressants: enhanced hypotensive effect, especially with MAOIs and linezolid – avoid concomitant use.
- Beta-blockers: enhanced hypotensive effect; increased risk of first dose hypotensive effect.
- Calcium-channel blockers: enhanced hypotensive effect; increased risk of first dose hypotensive effect.
- Diuretics: enhanced hypotensive effect; increased risk of first dose hypotensive effect.
- Moxisylyte: possibly severe postural hypotension when used in combination.
- Vardenafil, sildenafil and tadalafil: enhanced hypotensive effect – avoid concomitant use.

ADMINISTRATION

RECONSTITUTION
–
ROUTE
- Oral
RATE OF ADMINISTRATION
–
COMMENTS
–

OTHER INFORMATION

- For BPH, 20 mg at night may be adequate in the elderly.
- In the elderly the half-life can be prolonged to 6.6–32.8 hours with a mean of 14.7 hours due to reduced clearance.
- Seyffart recommends a maximum dose of 50 mg daily for patients with severe renal impairment if not on dialysis. Dialysis patients should receive a maximum of 100 mg daily on dialysis days, but 50 mg on non-dialysis days.

Infliximab

CLINICAL USE

Tumour necrosis factor alpha (TNFα)
inhibitor:
- Treatment of Crohn's disease, psoriasis,
  rheumatic diseases & ulcerative colitis

DOSE IN NORMAL RENAL FUNCTION

3–7.5 mg/kg depending on indication

PHARMACOKINETICS

Molecular weight (daltons)	144 190
% Protein binding	No data
% Excreted unchanged in urine	0
Volume of distribution (L/kg)	3–4.1 litres
Half-life – normal/ESRF (hrs)	8–9.5 days/ Unknown

METABOLISM

Most likely removed by opsonisation via the
reticuloendothelial system when bound to
T lymphocytes, or by human antimurine
antibody production.

DOSE IN RENAL IMPAIRMENT GFR (mL/MIN)

20–50	Dose as in normal renal function, use with caution.
10–20	Dose as in normal renal function, use with caution.
<10	Dose as in normal renal function, use with caution.

DOSE IN PATIENTS UNDERGOING RENAL REPLACEMENT THERAPIES

CAPD	Not dialysed. Dose as in GFR<10 mL/min.
HD	Not dialysed. Dose as in GFR<10 mL/min.
HDF/High flux	Not dialysed. Dose as in GFR<10 mL/min.
CAV/ VVHD	Not dialysed. Dose as in GFR=10– 20 mL/min.

IMPORTANT DRUG INTERACTIONS

Potentially hazardous interactions with other
drugs
- Anakinra & abatacept: avoid concomitant
  use.
- Live vaccines: avoid concomitant use.

ADMINISTRATION

RECONSTITUTION
- 10 mL water for injection
ROUTE
- IV
RATE OF ADMINISTRATION
- 2 hours
COMMENTS
- Dilute total volume to 250 mL with sodium
  chloride 0.9%
- Use an infusion set with an in-line, sterile,
  non-pyrogenic, low protein-binding filter
  (pore size 1.2 micrometer or less).

OTHER INFORMATION

- Acute infusion reactions during or within
  1 to 2 hours of infusion are common
  especially with the first or second dose.
  Symptoms include fever, chills, pruritus,
  urticaria, dyspnoea, chest pain, and
  hypertension or hypotension. Mild
  reactions may respond to a reduced rate
  of infusion or a temporary interruption.
  If reactions are more severe, therapy
  should be stopped. Pre-treatment
  with paracetamol, corticosteroids, and
  antihistamines may be considered.
- Infections are common and most often
  affect the upper respiratory tract and the
  urinary tract.
- After repeated doses infliximab has been
  detected in serum for at least 8 weeks.
- A case study has been reported where
  a patient was successfully treated with
  infliximab at a dose of 5 mg/kg for
  psoriatic arthritis.[1]
- Case reports of glomerulonephritis have
  been reported with infliximab.[2]

References:
1. Saougou I, Papagoras C, Markatseli TE,
et al. A case report of a psoriatic arthritis
patient on hemodialysis treated with
tumor necrosis factor blocking agent and a
literature review. Clin Rheumatol. 2010 Dec;
29(12): 1455–9.
2. Stokes MB, Foster K, Markowitz GS, et al.
Development of glomerulonephritis during
anti-TNF-α therapy for rheumatoid arthritis.
Nephrol Dial Transplant. 2005 July; 20(7):
1400–6.

Inositol nicotinate

CLINICAL USE

Peripheral vascular disease
Hyperlipidaemia

DOSE IN NORMAL RENAL FUNCTION

3 g daily in 2–3 divided doses, maximum 4 g
daily

PHARMACOKINETICS

Molecular weight (daltons)	810.7
% Protein binding	High
% Excreted unchanged in urine	No data
Volume of distribution (L/kg)	No data
Half-life – normal/ ESRF (hrs)	24/–

METABOLISM

Inositol nicotinate is believed to be slowly
hydrolysed to nicotinic acid. The main
route of metabolism is then conversion to
N-methylnicotinamide and the 2-pyridone
and 4-pyridone derivatives; nicotinuric acid
is also formed. Small amounts of nicotinic
acid are excreted unchanged in urine.

DOSE IN RENAL IMPAIRMENT GFR (mL/MIN)

30–50	Dose as in normal renal function.
10–30	Dose as in normal renal function.
<10	Dose as in normal renal function.

DOSE IN PATIENTS UNDERGOING RENAL REPLACEMENT THERAPIES

CAPD	Unknown dialysability. Dose as in normal renal function.
HD	Unknown dialysability. Dose as in normal renal function.
HDF/High flux	Unknown dialysability. Dose as in normal renal function.
CAV/ VVHD	Unknown dialysability. Dose as in normal renal function.

IMPORTANT DRUG INTERACTIONS

Potentially hazardous interactions with other
drugs
• None known

ADMINISTRATION

RECONSTITUTION
–

ROUTE
• Oral
RATE OF ADMINISTRATION
–

COMMENTS
–

OTHER INFORMATION
–

Insulin – soluble (Actrapid or Humulin S)

CLINICAL USE

- Hyperglycaemia, control of diabetes mellitus
- Emergency management of hyperkalaemia

DOSE IN NORMAL RENAL FUNCTION

Variable

PHARMACOKINETICS

Molecular weight (daltons)	5808
% Protein binding	5
% Excreted unchanged in urine	0
Volume of distribution (L/kg)	0.15
Half-life – normal/ ESRF (hrs)	2–5/13

METABOLISM

Insulin is rapidly metabolised, mainly in the liver but also in the kidneys and muscle tissue. In the kidneys it is reabsorbed in the proximal tubule and either returned to venous blood or metabolised, with only a small amount excreted unchanged in the urine.

DOSE IN RENAL IMPAIRMENT GFR (mL/MIN)

20–50	Variable
10–20	Variable
<10	Variable

DOSE IN PATIENTS UNDERGOING RENAL REPLACEMENT THERAPIES

CAPD	Not dialysed. Dose according to clinical response.
HD	Not dialysed. Dose according to clinical response.
HDF/High flux	Not dialysed. Dose according to clinical response.
CAV/ VVHD	Not dialysed. Dose according to clinical response.

IMPORTANT DRUG INTERACTIONS

Potentially hazardous interactions with other drugs

- Fibrates: may improve glucose tolerance; additive effect with insulin.

ADMINISTRATION

RECONSTITUTION

–

ROUTE

- IV via CRIP

RATE OF ADMINISTRATION

- Over 30 minutes or as required

COMMENTS

- Add 15–25 IU insulin to 50 mL 50% glucose for treatment of hyperkalaemia.
- For maintenance infusion or sliding scale infusion, add 50 IU insulin to 500 mL 10% glucose and adjust rate according to blood glucose levels.
- Continue infusing insulin/glucose solution at rate of 10 mL/hour according to serum potassium.

OTHER INFORMATION

- Monitor blood glucose.
- Prior to insulin/glucose infusion for hyperkalaemia, give IV 20 mL 10% calcium gluconate to protect myocardium and 50–100 mL 8.4% sodium bicarbonate to correct acidosis.
- Commence calcium resonium 15 g 4 times per day orally.
- Insulin is metabolised renally; therefore, requirements may be reduced in ERF.

Interferon alfa-2a (Roferon A)

CLINICAL USE

1. Hairy cell leukaemia
2. AIDS related Kaposi's sarcoma
3. Chronic myelogenous leukaemia
4. Cutaneous T-cell lymphoma
5. Chronic hepatitis B
6. Chronic hepatitis C
7. Follicular non-Hodgkin's lymphoma
8. Advanced renal cell carcinoma
9. Malignant melanoma

DOSE IN NORMAL RENAL FUNCTION:

1. Hairy cell leukaemia: 1.5–3 million IU daily or 3 times per week
2. AIDS related Kaposi's sarcoma: 3–36 million IU daily or 3 times per week
3. Chronic myelogenous leukaemia: 3–9 million IU daily or 3 times per week
4. Cutaneous T-cell lymphoma: 3–18 million IU daily or 3 times per week
5. Chronic hepatitis B: 2.5–5 million IU/m^2 3 times per week
6. Chronic hepatitis C: 3–6 million IU 3 times per week
7. Follicular non-Hodgkin's lymphoma: 6 million IU/m^2 on days 22–26 of each 28 day cycle
8. Advanced renal cell carcinoma: 9–18 million IU 3 times per week
9. Malignant melanoma 1.5–3 million IU 3 times a week

PHARMACOKINETICS

Molecular weight (daltons)	19 000
% Protein binding	0
% Excreted unchanged in urine	Negligible
Volume of distribution (L/kg)	0.4
Half-life – normal/ ESRF (hrs)	3.7–8.5/–

METABOLISM

Alpha-interferons are totally filtered through the glomeruli and undergo rapid proteolytic degradation during tubular reabsorption, rendering a negligible reappearance of intact alfa interferon in the systemic circulation.

DOSE IN RENAL IMPAIRMENT GFR (mL/MIN)

20–50	Dose as in normal renal function. Monitor renal function closely.
10–20	Dose as in normal renal function. Monitor renal function closely.
<10	Use with great caution. See 'Other information'.

DOSE IN PATIENTS UNDERGOING RENAL REPLACEMENT THERAPIES

CAPD	Not dialysed. Dose as in GFR<10 mL/min.
HD	Not dialysed. Dose as in GFR<10 mL/min.
HDF/High flux	Dialysed. Dose as in GFR<10 mL/ min.
CAV/ VVHD	Not dialysed. Dose as in GFR=10– 20 mL/min.

IMPORTANT DRUG INTERACTIONS

Potentially hazardous interactions with other drugs
- Antivirals: increased risk of peripheral neuropathy with telbivudine.
- Immunosuppressants, e.g. ciclosporin, tacrolimus, sirolimus may have an antagonistic effect.
- Theophylline: metabolism of theophylline reduced, consider reducing dose of theophylline.

ADMINISTRATION

RECONSTITUTION
–
ROUTE
- SC, IM
RATE OF ADMINISTRATION
–
COMMENTS
–

OTHER INFORMATION

- Interferon up-regulates the cell surface presentation of class II histocompatibility antigens, which raises the possibility of drug-induced allograft rejection. There are numerous clinical reports of allograft rejection, acute renal failure and graft loss after interferon therapy. Hence extreme care should be exercised in the use of interferon after renal transplantation.

- In patients undergoing haemodialysis, the interferon molecule may accumulate as it is too large to be dialysed and will not undergo renal degradation. Hence, the dose may need to be adjusted.
- Contraindicated by manufacturer in severe renal impairment.

Interferon alfa-2b

CLINICAL USE

1. Chronic hepatitis B
2. Chronic hepatitis C
3. Hairy cell leukaemia
4. Multiple myeloma
5. Carcinoid tumour
6. Chronic myelogenous leukaemia
7. Follicular lymphoma
8. Malignant melanoma

DOSE IN NORMAL RENAL FUNCTION:

1. Chronic hepatitis B: 5–10 million IU 3 times a week
2. Chronic hepatitis C: 3 million IU 3 times a week
3. Hairy cell leukaemia: 2 million IU/m^2 3 times a week
4. Multiple myeloma: 3 million IU/m^2 3 times a week
5. Carcinoid tumour: 3–9 million IU/m^2 3 times a week
6. Chronic myelogenous leukaemia: 4–5 million IU/m^2 daily
7. Follicular lymphoma: 5 million IU 3 times a week
8. Malignant melanoma 20 million IU/m^2 (IV infusion) daily for 5 days, decreasing to 10 million IU/m^2 (SC) 3 times a week

PHARMACOKINETICS

Molecular weight (daltons)	15 000–21 000
% Protein binding	0
% Excreted unchanged in urine	Negligible
Volume of distribution (L/kg)	0.4
Half-life – normal/ ESRF (hrs)	2.7/–

METABOLISM

Alpha-interferons are totally filtered through the glomeruli and undergo rapid proteolytic degradation during tubular reabsorption, rendering a negligible reappearance of intact alfa interferon in the systemic circulation.

DOSE IN RENAL IMPAIRMENT GFR (mL/MIN)

20–50	Dose as in normal renal function. Monitor renal function closely.
10–20	Dose as in normal renal function. Monitor renal function closely.
<10	Use with great caution. See 'Other information'.

DOSE IN PATIENTS UNDERGOING RENAL REPLACEMENT THERAPIES

CAPD	Not dialysed. Dose as in GFR<10 mL/min.
HD	Not dialysed. Dose as in GFR<10 mL/min.
HDF/High flux	Not dialysed. Dose as in GFR <10 mL/min.
CAV/ VVHD	Not dialysed. Dose as in GFR=10–20 mL/min.

IMPORTANT DRUG INTERACTIONS

Potentially hazardous interactions with other drugs

- Antivirals: increased risk of peripheral neuropathy with telbivudine.
- Immunosuppressants, e.g. ciclosporin, tacrolimus, sirolimus may have an antagonistic effect.
- Administration of interferon in combination with other chemotherapeutic agents, e.g. cytarabine, cyclophosphamide, doxorubicin may lead to increased risk of severe toxicity.
- Theophylline: metabolism of theophylline reduced, consider reducing dose of theophylline.

ADMINISTRATION

RECONSTITUTION
–
ROUTE
- IM, SC, IV
RATE OF ADMINISTRATION
- 20 minutes
COMMENTS
- Add to sodium chloride 0.9%.

OTHER INFORMATION

- Interferon up-regulates the cell surface presentation of class II histocompatibility antigens, which raises the possibility of drug-induced allograft rejection. There are numerous clinical reports of allograft rejection, acute renal failure and graft loss after interferon therapy. Hence extreme care should be exercised in the use of interferon after renal transplantation.
- In patients undergoing haemodialysis, the interferon molecule may accumulate as it is too large to be dialysed and will not undergo renal degradation. Hence, the dose may need to be adjusted.
- Several small controlled trials have examined the efficacy of low-dose interferon therapy (3 MU 3 times a week given after dialysis) for chronic hepatitis C in patients on haemodialysis. Treatment appears to have been remarkably effective, possibly because reduced renal clearance of interferon results in higher and more sustained levels of the drug. (Huraib S, Tanimu D, Romeh SA, *et al.* Inteferon-α in chronic hepatitis C infection in dialysis patients. *Am J Kidney Dis.* 1999; **34**(1): 55–60.)
- Contraindicated by manufacturer in severe renal impairment.

Interferon beta

CLINICAL USE

Treatment of relapsing, remitting multiple sclerosis

DOSE IN NORMAL RENAL FUNCTION

Interferon beta-1 a:
- Avonex: 6 million IU (30 micrograms) once a week
- Rebif: 22–44 micrograms 3 times a week

Interferon beta-1 b:
- Betaferon/Extavia: 8 million IU (250 mcg) every second day

PHARMACOKINETICS

Molecular weight (daltons)	18 500–22 500
% Protein binding	No data
% Excreted unchanged in urine	Negligible. See 'Other information'.
Volume of distribution (L/kg)	3
Half-life – normal/ ESRF (hrs)	5–10/–

METABOLISM

Interferon beta is mainly metabolised and excreted by the liver and the kidneys.

DOSE IN RENAL IMPAIRMENT GFR (mL/MIN)

20–50	Dose as in normal renal function. Monitor renal function.
10–20	Dose as in normal renal function. Monitor renal function.
<10	Use with caution due to risk of accumulation, and monitor renal function.

DOSE IN PATIENTS UNDERGOING RENAL REPLACEMENT THERAPIES

CAPD	Not dialysed. Dose as in GFR<10 mL/min.
HD	Not dialysed. Dose as in GFR<10 mL/min.
HDF/High flux	Not dialysed. Dose as in GFR<10 mL/min.
CAV/ VVHD	Not dialysed. Dose as in GFR=10–20 mL/min.

IMPORTANT DRUG INTERACTIONS

Potentially hazardous interactions with other drugs
- Ciclosporin and tacrolimus: interferon reported to reduce the activity of hepatic cytochrome P450 enzymes.

ADMINISTRATION

RECONSTITUTION
- With diluent provided

ROUTE
- IM (Avonex), SC (Rebif, Betaferon, Extavia)

RATE OF ADMINISTRATION
–

COMMENTS
- Stable for 6 hours at 2–8°C once reconstituted

OTHER INFORMATION

- Pre-treatment with paracetamol is recommended to reduce incidence of flu-like symptoms.
- Vary the site of injection each week.
- Rare cases of lupus erythematosus syndrome have occurred.
- Transient increases in creatinine, potassium, urea, nitrogen and urinary calcium may occur.
- Interferon up-regulates the cell surface presentation of class II histocompatibility antigens, which raises the possibility of drug-induced allograft rejection. There are numerous clinical reports of allograft rejection, acute renal failure and graft loss after interferon therapy. Hence extreme care should be exercised in the use of interferon after renal transplantation.
- In patients undergoing haemodialysis, the interferon molecule may accumulate as it is too large to be dialysed and will not undergo renal degradation. Hence, the dose may need to be adjusted.

Interferon gamma-1b (Immukin)

CLINICAL USE

Adjunct to antibiotics to reduce the frequency of serious infections in patients with chronic granulomatous disease

DOSE IN NORMAL RENAL FUNCTION

50 mcg/m^2 3 times a week
or 1.5 mcg/kg 3 times a week if surface area <0.5 m^2

PHARMACOKINETICS

Molecular weight (daltons)	15000–21000
% Protein binding	No data
% Excreted unchanged in urine	Negligible
Volume of distribution (L/kg)	0.2–0.6
Half-life – normal/ ESRF (hrs)	5.9/–

METABOLISM

The metabolism of cloned interferons falls within the natural handling of proteins. Interferon gamma-1b was not detected in the urine of healthy male subjects following administration via IV, IM or SC routes. *In vitro* hepatic and renal perfusion studies demonstrate that the liver and kidneys are capable of clearing interferon gamma-1b from perfusate.

Interferon is metabolised primarily in the kidney. It is excreted in the urine, but is reabsorbed by the tubules where it undergoes lysosomal degradation.

DOSE IN RENAL IMPAIRMENT GFR (mL/MIN)

20–50	No data on use in renal impairment. Dose as for normal renal function and monitor renal function closely.
10–20	No data on use in renal impairment. Dose as for normal renal function and monitor renal function closely.
<10	Use with caution due to risk of accumulation. Monitor renal function closely.

DOSE IN PATIENTS UNDERGOING RENAL REPLACEMENT THERAPIES

CAPD	Not dialysed. Dose as in GFR<10 mL/min.
HD	Not dialysed. Dose as in GFR<10 mL/min.
HDF/High flux	Not dialysed. Dose as in GFR<10 mL/min.
CAV/ VVHD	Unlikely dialysability. Dose as in GFR=10–20 mL/min.

IMPORTANT DRUG INTERACTIONS

Potentially hazardous interactions with other drugs
• Avoid with vaccines.

ADMINISTRATION

RECONSTITUTION
–
ROUTE
• SC
RATE OF ADMINISTRATION
–
COMMENTS
–

OTHER INFORMATION

• Pre-treatment with paracetamol is recommended to reduce incidence of flu-like symptoms.
• Interferon up-regulates the cell surface presentation of class II histocompatibility antigens, which raises the possibility of drug-induced allograft rejection. There are numerous clinical reports of allograft rejection, acute renal failure and graft loss after interferon therapy. Hence extreme care should be exercised in the use of interferon after renal transplantation.
• In patients undergoing haemodialysis, the interferon molecule may accumulate as it is too large to be dialysed and will not undergo renal degradation. Hence, the dose may need to be adjusted.
• Manufacturer advises to use with caution due to risk of accumulation.

Ipilimumab

CLINICAL USE

Anti-neoplastic agent:
- Treatment of advanced (unresectable or metastatic) melanoma in adults who have received prior therapy

DOSE IN NORMAL RENAL FUNCTION

3 mg/kg every 3 weeks for 4 doses

PHARMACOKINETICS

Molecular weight (daltons)	148 000
% Protein binding	No data
% Excreted unchanged in urine	No data
Volume of distribution (L/kg)	7.22 litres
Half-life – normal/ ESRF (hrs)	15 days/Unchanged

METABOLISM

Most likely removed by opsonisation via the reticuloendothelial system when bound to T lymphocytes, or by human antimurine antibody production.

DOSE IN RENAL IMPAIRMENT GFR (mL/MIN)

20–50	Dose as in normal renal function.
10–20	Dose as in normal renal function. Use with caution.
<10	Dose as in normal renal function. Use with caution.

DOSE IN PATIENTS UNDERGOING RENAL REPLACEMENT THERAPIES

CAPD	Unlikely to be dialysed. Dose as in GFR<10 mL/min.
HD	Unlikely to be dialysed. Dose as in GFR<10 mL/min.
HDF/High flux	Unlikely to be dialysed. Dose as in GFR<10 mL/min.
CAV/ VVHD	Unlikely to be dialysed. Dose as in GFR=10–20 mL/min.

IMPORTANT DRUG INTERACTIONS

Potentially hazardous interactions with other drugs
- None known

ADMINISTRATION

RECONSTITUTION
–
ROUTE
- IV
RATE OF ADMINISTRATION
- Over 90 minutes
COMMENTS
- May be administered undiluted or may be added to sodium chloride 0.9% or glucose 5% to give a concentration of 1–4 mg/mL.
- Give via a low-protein binding in-line filter (pore size of 0.2 μm to 1.2 μm).

OTHER INFORMATION

- No studies have been done in patients with a GFR<22 m/L/min but the pharmacokinetic parameters indicate that it should not accumulate.
- US data sheet does not advise a dose reduction in severe renal impairment.

Ipratropium bromide

CLINICAL USE

Anticholinergic bronchodilator:
- Reversible airways obstruction, particularly in COPD

DOSE IN NORMAL RENAL FUNCTION

- Nebuliser solution: 250–500 micrograms 3–4 times daily
- Inhaler: 20–80 micrograms 3–4 times daily

PHARMACOKINETICS

Molecular weight (daltons)	430.4
% Protein binding	<20
% Excreted unchanged in urine	<1
Volume of distribution (L/kg)	4.6
Half-life – normal/ ESRF (hrs)	1.6/–

METABOLISM

After inhalation, around 10–30% of a dose is deposited in the lungs where it exerts its therapeutic effect. Only a small amount of ipratropium reaches the systemic circulation. The majority of a dose is swallowed but is poorly absorbed from the gastrointestinal tract. Ipratropium and its metabolites are eliminated in the urine and faeces.

DOSE IN RENAL IMPAIRMENT GFR (mL/MIN)

20–50	Dose as in normal renal function.
10–20	Dose as in normal renal function.
<10	Dose as in normal renal function.

DOSE IN PATIENTS UNDERGOING RENAL REPLACEMENT THERAPIES

HD	Not dialysed. Dose as in normal renal function.
HDF/High flux	Not dialysed. Dose as in normal renal function.
CAV/VVHD	Not dialysed. Dose as in normal renal function.

IMPORTANT DRUG INTERACTIONS

Potentially hazardous interactions with other drugs
- None known

ADMINISTRATION

RECONSTITUTION
–
ROUTE
- Inhaled
RATE OF ADMINISTRATION
- Nebuliser: according to nebuliser.
COMMENTS
- The dose of nebuliser solution may need to be diluted in order to obtain a final volume suitable for the nebuliser.
- Sterile sodium chloride 0.9% should be used if dilution is required.

Irbesartan

CLINICAL USE

Angiotensin-II receptor antagonist:
- Hypertension
- Diabetic nephropathy

DOSE IN NORMAL RENAL FUNCTION

75–300 mg daily

PHARMACOKINETICS

Molecular weight (daltons)	428.5
% Protein binding	96
% Excreted unchanged in urine	<2
Volume of distribution (L/kg)	53–93 litres
Half-life – normal/ESRF (hrs)	11–15/ Unchanged

METABOLISM

Following oral or intravenous administration of ^{14}C irbesartan, 80–85% of the circulating plasma radioactivity is attributable to unchanged irbesartan. Irbesartan is metabolised by the liver via glucuronide conjugation and oxidation. The major circulating metabolite is irbesartan glucuronide (approximately 6%). *In vitro* studies indicate that irbesartan is primarily oxidised by the cytochrome P450 enzyme CYP2C9; isoenzyme CYP3A4 has negligible effect. Irbesartan and its metabolites are eliminated by both biliary and renal pathways. After either oral or IV administration of ^{14}C irbesartan, about 20% of the radioactivity is recovered in the urine, and the remainder in the faeces. Less than 2% of the dose is excreted in the urine as unchanged irbesartan.

DOSE IN RENAL IMPAIRMENT GFR (mL/MIN)

20–50	Dose as in normal renal function.
10–20	Dose as in normal renal function.
<10	Dose as in normal renal function.

DOSE IN PATIENTS UNDERGOING RENAL REPLACEMENT THERAPIES

CAPD	Not dialysed. Initial dose 75 mg daily and gradually increase.
HD	Not dialysed. Initial dose 75 mg daily and gradually increase.
HDF/High flux	Unknown dialysability. Initial dose 75 mg daily and gradually increase.
CAV/ VVHD	Unknown dialysability. Initial dose 75 mg daily and gradually increase.

IMPORTANT DRUG INTERACTIONS

Potentially hazardous interactions with other drugs
- Anaesthetics: enhanced hypotensive effect.
- Analgesics: antagonism of hypotensive effect and increased risk of renal impairment with NSAIDs; hyperkalaemia with ketorolac and other NSAIDs.
- Ciclosporin: increased risk of hyperkalaemia and nephrotoxicity.
- Diuretics: enhanced hypotensive effect; hyperkalaemia with potassium-sparing diuretics.
- ESAs: increased risk of hyperkalaemia; antagonism of hypotensive effect.
- Lithium: reduced excretion (possibility of enhanced lithium toxicity).
- Potassium salts: increased risk of hyperkalaemia.
- Tacrolimus: increased risk of hyperkalaemia and nephrotoxicity.

ADMINISTRATION

RECONSTITUTION
–
ROUTE
- Oral
RATE OF ADMINISTRATION
–
COMMENTS
–

OTHER INFORMATION

- Hyperkalaemia and other side effects are more common in patients with impaired renal function.
- Renal failure has been reported in association with angiotensin-II antagonists in patients with renal artery stenosis, post renal transplant, and in those with congestive heart failure.
- Close monitoring of renal function during therapy is necessary in those with renal insufficiency.

Irinotecan hydrochloride

CLINICAL USE

Treatment of metastatic colorectal cancer resistant to fluorouracil, or in conjunction with fluorouracil

DOSE IN NORMAL RENAL FUNCTION

- Without 5-FU: 350 mg/m^2 every 3 weeks
- With 5-FU: 180 mg/m^2 every 2 weeks

PHARMACOKINETICS

Molecular weight (daltons)	677.2
% Protein binding	65
% Excreted unchanged in urine	20
Volume of distribution (L/kg)	110–234 litres/m^2
Half-life – normal/ ESRF (hrs)	14/–

METABOLISM

After intravenous doses it is hydrolysed by carboxylesterase in body tissues to active SN-38 (7-ethyl-10-hydroxycamptothecin). Plasma protein binding for SN-38 is about 95%. SN-38 is mainly eliminated by glucuronidation, predominantly by the enzyme uridine diphosphate glucuronosyltransferase 1A1 (UGT1A1). Irinotecan is also partly metabolised by cytochrome P450 isoenzymes CYP3A4 and perhaps CYP3A5. The majority of an intravenous dose of irinotecan is excreted as unchanged drug, with about 64% in the faeces via the bile. The mean 24 hr urinary excretion of irinotecan and SN-38 (its active metabolite) was 19.9% and 0.25% respectively.

DOSE IN RENAL IMPAIRMENT GFR (mL/MIN)

20–50	Dose as in normal renal function and monitor closely.
10–20	Dose as in normal renal function and monitor closely.
<10	Reduce dose (50–80 mg/m^2) and monitor closely. Increase as tolerated.

DOSE IN PATIENTS UNDERGOING RENAL REPLACEMENT THERAPIES

CAPD	Unlikely to be dialysed. Dose as in GFR<10 mL/min.
HD	Unlikely to be dialysed. Dose as in GFR<10 mL/min.
HDF/High flux	Unlikely to be dialysed. Dose as in GFR<10 mL/min.
CAV/ VVHD	Unlikely to be dialysed. Dose as in GFR=10–20 mL/min.

IMPORTANT DRUG INTERACTIONS

Potentially hazardous interactions with other drugs

- Antidepressants: concentration reduced by St John's wort – avoid.
- Antifungals: concentration reduced by ketoconazole, but active metabolite of irinotecan increased – avoid.
- Antipsychotics: avoid concomitant use with clozapine (increased risk of agranulocytosis).
- Antivirals: metabolism possibly inhibited by atazanavir (increased risk of toxicity).
- Cytotoxics: concentration of active metabolite of irinotecan increased by lapatinib, consider reducing dose of irinotecan; concentration possibly increased by sorafenib.

ADMINISTRATION

RECONSTITUTION
–
ROUTE
- IV infusion
RATE OF ADMINISTRATION
- Over 30–90 minutes
COMMENTS
- Dilute in 250 mL sodium chloride 0.9% or glucose 5%.

OTHER INFORMATION

- Manufacturer advises avoiding use in renal impairment due to lack of data.
- There is a case study from Korea using irinotecan at a dose of 100 mg/m^2 in a haemodialysis patient without any complications. (Dong Min Kim, Hyun Lee Kim, Choon Hae Chung and Chi Young Park. Successful treatment of small-cell lung cancer with irinotecan in a hemodialysis patient with end-stage renal

disease. *Korean J Intern Med.* 2009 March; **24**(1): 73–5.)

- Infrequent reports of renal insufficiency due to inadequate hydration.
- Transient, mild to moderate increase in serum creatinine reported in 7.3% of patients.

Iron dextran 5% solution

CLINICAL USE

- Prophylaxis of iron deficiency anaemia (when oral treatment is ineffective or contraindicated)
- Treatment of iron deficiency during ESA therapy especially if serum ferritin is very low (<50 nanograms/mL)

DOSE IN NORMAL RENAL FUNCTION

- Total iron infusion: Dose of iron dextran (mg) = weight (kg) × [Target Hb (g/L) − Actual Hb (g/L)] × 0.24 + 500 mg iron for iron stores (if body weight >35 kg) 20 mg/kg in a single dose.
- Target haemoglobin level (110 g/L for renal patients as a guide) or 100–200 mg 2 or 3 times a week depending on haemoglobin.
- A test dose is essential. Give 0.5 mL or 25 mg iron over 15 minutes and observe for 60 minutes (15 minutes if using low dose bolus) for anaphylaxis. Have resuscitative equipment and drugs at hand (adrenaline, chlorphenamine and hydrocortisone).

PHARMACOKINETICS

Molecular weight (daltons)	165 000
% Protein binding	0
% Excreted unchanged in urine	<0.2
Volume of distribution (L/kg)	0.031–0.055
Half-life – normal/ ESRF (hrs)	5–20/–

METABOLISM

After intravenous infusion, iron dextran is taken up by the cells of the reticuloendothelial cells, particularly in the liver and spleen. The reticuloendothelial cells gradually separate iron from the iron-dextran complex. Most absorbed iron is bound to transferrin and transported to the bone marrow where it is incorporated into haemoglobin; the remainder is contained within the storage forms, ferritin or haemosiderin, or as myoglobin, with smaller amounts occurring in haem-containing enzymes or in plasma bound to transferrin. Only very small amounts of iron are excreted as the majority released after the destruction of the haemoglobin molecule is reused.

DOSE IN RENAL IMPAIRMENT GFR (mL/MIN)

20–50	Dose as in normal renal function.
10–20	Dose as in normal renal function.
<10	Dose as in normal renal function.

DOSE IN PATIENTS UNDERGOING RENAL REPLACEMENT THERAPIES

CAPD	Not dialysed. Dose as in normal renal function.
HD	Not dialysed. Dose as in normal renal function.
HDF/High flux	Not dialysed. Dose as in normal renal function.
CAV/ VVHD	Not dialysed. Dose as in normal renal function.

IMPORTANT DRUG INTERACTIONS

Potentially hazardous interactions with other drugs
- Dimercaprol: avoid concomitant use.
- Oral iron: reduced absorption of oral iron.

ADMINISTRATION

RECONSTITUTION
–
ROUTE
- IV, IM
RATE OF ADMINISTRATION
- Infusion: 100 mL over 30 minutes
- Bolus: 10 mg/minute
- Total dose infusion: over 4–6 hours; increase rate of infusion to 45–60 drops per minute.
COMMENTS
- Infusion: 100–200 mg in 100 mL sodium chloride or glucose 5%.
- Bolus: add to 10–20 mL sodium chloride or glucose 5%.
- Total dose infusion: add to 500 mL sodium chloride 0.9% or glucose 5%.
- Keep under strict supervision during and for 1 hour after infusion.

OTHER INFORMATION

- Do not give to patients with history of asthma.
- If patients with a history of allergy are prescribed iron dextran, give adequate antihistamine cover prior to administration.
- The dose of iron dextran varies widely from 100 mg per dialysis session for 6–10 sessions, to single doses of 500 mg to 1 g.
- The incidence of anaphylaxis with the Cosmofer brand of iron dextran is significantly lower than with the old Imferon brand, since the iron is complexed to a much shorter dextran chain than was used previously.

Iron isomaltoside 1000

CLINICAL USE

Complex of ferric iron and isomaltosides:
- Treatment of iron deficiency anaemia (when oral treatment is ineffective or contraindicated)

DOSE IN NORMAL RENAL FUNCTION

Dose according to weight

PHARMACOKINETICS

Molecular weight (daltons)	1000
% Protein binding	No data
% Excreted unchanged in urine	0
Volume of distribution (L/kg)	No data
Half-life – normal/ ESRF (hrs)	5/–

METABOLISM

Most absorbed iron is bound to transferrin and transported to the bone marrow where it is incorporated into haemoglobin; the remainder is contained within the storage forms, ferritin or haemosiderin, or as myoglobin, with smaller amounts occurring in haem-containing enzymes or in plasma bound to transferrin. Only very small amounts of iron are excreted as the majority released after the destruction of the haemoglobin molecule is reused.

DOSE IN RENAL IMPAIRMENT GFR (mL/MIN)

20–50	Dose as in normal renal function.
10–20	Dose as in normal renal function.
<10	Dose as in normal renal function.

DOSE IN PATIENTS UNDERGOING RENAL REPLACEMENT THERAPIES

CAPD	Not dialysed. Dose as in normal renal function.
HD	Not dialysed. Dose as in normal renal function.
HDF/High flux	Not dialysed. Dose as in normal renal function.
CAV/ VVHD	Not dialysed. Dose as in normal renal function.

IMPORTANT DRUG INTERACTIONS

Potentially hazardous interactions with other drugs
- Dimercaprol: avoid concomitant use.
- Do not administer with oral iron.

ADMINISTRATION

RECONSTITUTION
–

ROUTE
- IV

RATE OF ADMINISTRATION
- IV bolus (up to 500 mg): 50 mg/min
- IV infusion: up to 1000 mg over 30 minutes
- Doses >20 mg/kg in 2 doses with an interval of at least 1 week

COMMENTS
- Patients should be monitored during and for 30 minutes after administration.

Iron sucrose

CLINICAL USE

- Prophylaxis of iron deficiency anaemia (when oral treatment is ineffective or contraindicated)
- Treatment of iron deficiency during ESA therapy especially if serum ferritin is very low (<50 nanograms/mL)

DOSE IN NORMAL RENAL FUNCTION

According to local protocol. See 'Other information'.

PHARMACOKINETICS

Molecular weight (daltons)	34000–60000
% Protein binding	No data
% Excreted unchanged in urine	<5
Volume of distribution (L/kg)	8 litres
Half-life – normal/ ESRF (hrs)	6/–

METABOLISM

After intravenous infusion, iron sucrose is taken up by the cells of the reticuloendothelial cells, particularly in the liver and spleen. The reticuloendothelial cells gradually separate iron from the iron-sucrose complex. Most absorbed iron is bound to transferrin and transported to the bone marrow where it is incorporated into haemoglobin; the remainder is contained within the storage forms, ferritin or haemosiderin, or as myoglobin, with smaller amounts occurring in haem-containing enzymes or in plasma bound to transferrin. Only very small amounts of iron are excreted as the majority released after the destruction of the haemoglobin molecule is reused.

DOSE IN RENAL IMPAIRMENT GFR (mL/MIN)

20–50	Dose as in normal renal function.
10–20	Dose as in normal renal function.
<10	Dose as in normal renal function.

DOSE IN PATIENTS UNDERGOING RENAL REPLACEMENT THERAPIES

CAPD	Not dialysed. Dose as in normal renal function.
HD	Not dialysed. Dose as in normal renal function.
HDF/High flux	Not dialysed. Dose as in normal renal function.
CAV/ VVHD	Not dialysed. Dose as in normal renal function.

IMPORTANT DRUG INTERACTIONS

Potentially hazardous interactions with other drugs
- Dimercaprol: avoid concomitant use.
- Do not administer with oral iron.

ADMINISTRATION

RECONSTITUTION
–
ROUTE
- IV
RATE OF ADMINISTRATION
- Bolus: 1 mL/minute
- Infusion: in sodium chloride 0.9% at a concentration of 1 mg/mL over 20–30 minutes per 100 mg
COMMENTS
- Doses can be administered via the venous limb of the dialysis machine.
- Patients should be monitored during and for 30 minutes after administration.
- Stable for 24 hours at room temperature.

OTHER INFORMATION

- Some regimes are:
  — 50–300 mg weekly
  — 100 mg once or twice monthly
  — 20–40 mg with each dialysis
- Oral iron can be restarted 5 days after completion of the course of IV iron.

Isoniazid

CLINICAL USE

Antibacterial agent:
- Treatment and prophylaxis of tuberculosis in 'at risk' immunocompromised patients

DOSE IN NORMAL RENAL FUNCTION

- IM/IV: 200–300 mg daily
- Oral: 300 mg daily
- Intermittent regimes: 15 mg/kg 3 times weekly
- Prophylaxis: 100–200 mg daily
- Intrapleural: 50–250 mg
- Intrathecal: 25–50 mg daily

PHARMACOKINETICS

Molecular weight (daltons)	137.1
% Protein binding	0
% Excreted unchanged in urine	4–32
Volume of distribution (L/kg)	0.75
Half-life – normal/ ESRF (hrs)	1.2–3.5/1–17 (depends on acetylator status)

METABOLISM

The primary metabolic route is the acetylation of isoniazid to acetyl-isoniazid by N-acetyltransferase found in the liver and small intestine. Acetyl-isoniazid is then hydrolysed to isonicotinic acid and monoacetylhydrazine; isonicotinic acid is conjugated with glycine to isonicotinyl glycine (isonicotinuric acid) and monoacetylhydrazine is further acetylated to diacetylhydrazine. Some unmetabolised isoniazid is conjugated to hydrazones. The metabolites of isoniazid have no tuberculostatic activity and, apart from possibly monoacetylhydrazine, they are also less toxic. The rate of acetylation of isoniazid and monoacetylhydrazine is genetically determined and there is a bimodal distribution of persons who acetylate them either slowly or rapidly. In patients with normal renal function, over 75% of a dose appears in the urine in 24 hours, mainly as metabolites. Small amounts of drug are also excreted in the faeces.

DOSE IN RENAL IMPAIRMENT GFR (mL/MIN)

20–50	Dose as in normal renal function.
10–20	Dose as in normal renal function.
<10	200–300 mg daily.

DOSE IN PATIENTS UNDERGOING RENAL REPLACEMENT THERAPIES

CAPD	Dialysed. Dose as in GFR<10 mL/min.
HD	Dialysed. Dose as in GFR<10 mL/min.
HDF/High flux	Dialysed. Dose as in GFR<10 mL/min.
CAV/ VVHD	Probably dialysed. Dose as in normal renal function.

IMPORTANT DRUG INTERACTIONS

Potentially hazardous interactions with other drugs
- Anti-epileptics: metabolism of carbamazepine, ethosuximide and phenytoin inhibited (enhanced effect); also with carbamazepine, isoniazid hepatotoxicity possibly increased.

ADMINISTRATION

RECONSTITUTION
- Dilute with water for injection if required.
ROUTE
- Oral, IM, IV, intrapleural, intrathecal
RATE OF ADMINISTRATION
- Not critical. Give by slow IV bolus.
COMMENTS
–

OTHER INFORMATION

- Adjust dose accordingly if hepatic illness, slow/fast acetylator status identified.
- Pyridoxine 10 mg daily has been recommended for prophylaxis of peripheral neuritis.

Isosorbide dinitrate

CLINICAL USE

Vasodilator:
- Prophylaxis and treatment of angina
- Left ventricular failure

DOSE IN NORMAL RENAL FUNCTION

- Oral:
  — Angina: 30–120 mg daily in divided doses;
  — LVF: 40–240 mg daily
- IV: 2–20 mg/hour depending on response

PHARMACOKINETICS

Molecular weight (daltons)	236.1
% Protein binding	<1
% Excreted unchanged in urine	10–20
Volume of distribution (L/kg)	2–4
Half-life – normal/ ESRF (hrs)	0.5–1/–

METABOLISM

Isosorbide dinitrate undergoes extensive first-pass metabolism in the liver. It is taken up by smooth muscle cells of blood vessels and the nitrate group is cleaved to inorganic nitrite and then to nitric oxide. It is also rapidly metabolised in the liver to the major active metabolites isosorbide 2-mononitrate and isosorbide 5-mononitrate. Isosorbide mononitrate is metabolised to inactive metabolites, including isosorbide and isosorbide glucuronide. Only about 2% of isosorbide mononitrate is excreted unchanged in the urine.

DOSE IN RENAL IMPAIRMENT GFR (mL/MIN)

20–50	Dose as in normal renal function.
10–20	Dose as in normal renal function.
<10	Dose as in normal renal function.

DOSE IN PATIENTS UNDERGOING RENAL REPLACEMENT THERAPIES

CAPD	Not dialysed. Dose as in normal renal function.
HD	Dialysed. Dose as in normal renal function.
HDF/High flux	Dialysed. Dose as in normal renal function.
CAV/ VVHD	Dialysed. Dose as in normal renal function.

IMPORTANT DRUG INTERACTIONS

Potentially hazardous interactions with other drugs
- Sildenafil: hypotensive effect significantly enhanced – avoid concomitant use.
- Tadalafil: hypotensive effect significantly enhanced – avoid concomitant use.
- Vardenafil: hypotensive effect significantly enhanced – avoid concomitant use.

ADMINISTRATION

RECONSTITUTION
–
ROUTE
- Oral, IV infusion
RATE OF ADMINISTRATION
- 1 mg/10 mL; 60 mL/hour ≡ 6 mg/hour
- 2 mg/10 mL; 30 mL/hour ≡ 6 mg/hour
COMMENTS
- Dilute using sodium chloride 0.9% or glucose 5% to 1 mg/10 mL or 2 mg/10 mL; final volume 500 mL.
- Use of PVC giving sets and containers should be avoided since significant losses of the active ingredient by absorption can occur.

OTHER INFORMATION

- Both metabolites have longer half-lives than the parent compound.

Isosorbide mononitrate

CLINICAL USE
Vasodilator:
- Treatment and prophylaxis of angina
- Adjunct in congestive heart failure

DOSE IN NORMAL RENAL FUNCTION
20–120 mg/day in divided doses

PHARMACOKINETICS

Molecular weight (daltons)	191.1
% Protein binding	<4
% Excreted unchanged in urine	2
Volume of distribution (L/kg)	0.6
Half-life – normal/ ESRF (hrs)	1.5–5/Unchanged

METABOLISM
Unlike isosorbide dinitrate, isosorbide mononitrate does not undergo first-pass hepatic metabolism. Isosorbide mononitrate is taken up by smooth muscle cells of blood vessels and the nitrate group is cleaved to inorganic nitrite and then to nitric oxide. Isosorbide mononitrate is metabolised to inactive metabolites, including isosorbide and isosorbide glucuronide. Only about 2% of isosorbide mononitrate is excreted unchanged in the urine.

DOSE IN RENAL IMPAIRMENT GFR (mL/MIN)
20–50	Dose as in normal renal function.
10–20	Dose as in normal renal function.
<10	Dose as in normal renal function.

DOSE IN PATIENTS UNDERGOING RENAL REPLACEMENT THERAPIES

CAPD	Not dialysed. Dose as in normal renal function.
HD	Dialysed. Dose as in normal renal function.
HDF/High flux	Dialysed. Dose as in normal renal function.
CAV/ VVHD	Dialysed. Dose as in normal renal function.

IMPORTANT DRUG INTERACTIONS
Potentially hazardous interactions with other drugs
- Sildenafil: hypotensive effect significantly enhanced – avoid concomitant use.
- Tadalafil: hypotensive effect significantly enhanced – avoid concomitant use.
- Vardenafil: hypotensive effect significantly enhanced – avoid concomitant use.

ADMINISTRATION
RECONSTITUTION
–
ROUTE
- Oral
RATE OF ADMINISTRATION
–
COMMENTS
–

OTHER INFORMATION
- Tolerance may develop. This may be minimised by having nitrate-'free' periods.

Isotretinoin

CLINICAL USE

Treatment of nodulo-cystic and conglobate acne, and severe acne which has failed to respond to an adequate course of systemic antibiotics

DOSE IN NORMAL RENAL FUNCTION

- 0.5–1 mg/kg daily in 1–2 divided doses initially
- Maximum cumulative dose: 150 mg/kg per course
- Topically: 1–2 times daily

PHARMACOKINETICS

Molecular weight (daltons)	300.4
% Protein binding	99.9
% Excreted unchanged in urine	As metabolites
Volume of distribution (L/kg)	No data
Half-life – normal/ ESRF (hrs)	10–20/Unchanged

METABOLISM

Isotretinoin undergoes metabolism in the gut wall and first-pass metabolism in the liver. It is metabolised in the liver by CYP2C8, CYP2C9, CYP3A4, and CYP2B6 to its major metabolite 4-oxo-isotretinoin; there is also some isomerisation of isotretinoin to tretinoin. Isotretinoin, tretinoin, and their metabolites undergo enterohepatic recycling. Return to physiological levels of retinoids takes about 2 weeks after stopping therapy. Equal amounts of a dose appear in the faeces, mainly as unchanged drug, and in the urine as metabolites.

DOSE IN RENAL IMPAIRMENT GFR (mL/MIN)

20–50	Dose as in normal renal function.
10–20	Dose as in normal renal function.
<10	Initial dose 10 mg daily and slowly increase as tolerated up to 1 mg/kg daily. See 'Other information'.

DOSE IN PATIENTS UNDERGOING RENAL REPLACEMENT THERAPIES

CAPD	Not dialysed. Dose as in GFR<10 mL/min.
HD	Not dialysed. Dose as in GFR<10 mL/min.
HDF/High flux	Unlikely to be dialysed. Dose as in GFR<10 mL/min.
CAV/ VVHD	Not dialysed. Dose as in normal renal function.

IMPORTANT DRUG INTERACTIONS

Potentially hazardous interactions with other drugs
- Antibacterials: possible increased risk of benign intracranial hypertension with tetracyclines – avoid concomitant use.
- Antifungals: possible increased risk of toxicity with fluconazole, ketoconazole and voriconazole.
- Vitamins: increased risk of hypervitaminosis with vitamin A.

ADMINISTRATION

RECONSTITUTION
–
ROUTE
- Oral, topical (0.05% gel)
RATE OF ADMINISTRATION
–
COMMENTS
–

OTHER INFORMATION

- Since the drug is highly protein bound, it is not expected to be significantly removed by dialysis.
- Monitor for signs of vitamin A toxicity.

Ispaghula husk

CLINICAL USE

Bulk-forming laxative

DOSE IN NORMAL RENAL FUNCTION

- Fibrelief: 1–6 sachets daily in water in 1–3 divided doses
- Fybogel: One sachet (3.5 g) in water twice daily
- Isogel: 2 teaspoonfuls in water 1–2 times daily (constipation), 3 times daily (diarrhoea)
- Regulan: 1 sachet in water 1–3 times daily

PHARMACOKINETICS

Molecular weight (daltons)	–
% Protein binding	0
% Excreted unchanged in urine	0
Volume of distribution (L/kg)	Not absorbed.
Half-life – normal/ ESRF (hrs)	Not absorbed.

METABOLISM

The mode of action of Fybogel is physical and does not depend on absorption into the systemic circulation.

DOSE IN RENAL IMPAIRMENT GFR (mL/MIN)

20–50	Dose as in normal renal function.
10–20	Dose as in normal renal function.
<10	Dose as in normal renal function.

DOSE IN PATIENTS UNDERGOING RENAL REPLACEMENT THERAPIES

CAPD	Not dialysed. Dose as in normal renal function.
HD	Not dialysed. Dose as in normal renal function.
HDF/High flux	Not dialysed. Dose as in normal renal function.
CAV/ VVHD	Not dialysed. Dose as in normal renal function.

IMPORTANT DRUG INTERACTIONS

Potentially hazardous interactions with other drugs
- None known

ADMINISTRATION

RECONSTITUTION
–
ROUTE
- Oral
RATE OF ADMINISTRATION
–
COMMENTS
- Fybogel and regulan should be stirred into 150 mL water and taken as quickly as possible, preferably after meals.
- Additional fluid intake should be maintained.

OTHER INFORMATION

- Fybogel is low in sodium and potassium, containing approximately 0.4 mmol sodium and 0.7 mmol potassium per sachet. It is sugar and gluten free and contains aspartame (contributes to the phenylalanine intake and may affect control of phenylketonuria).
- Orange and lemon/lime flavours of regulan contain: 3.4 g ispaghula husk BP, 0.23 mmol sodium, <1 mmol potassium per sachet and are gluten and sugar free. They also contain aspartame.
- Fibrelief contains aspartame.
- Fluid restrictions in dialysis patients can render these treatments inappropriate.

Isradipine

CLINICAL USE

Calcium-channel blocker:
- Essential hypertension

DOSE IN NORMAL RENAL FUNCTION

Initially 2.5 mg twice daily, increased if necessary to 10 mg twice daily.

PHARMACOKINETICS

Molecular weight (daltons)	371.4
% Protein binding	95
% Excreted unchanged in urine	0
Volume of distribution (L/kg)	3–4
Half-life – normal/ ESRF (hrs)	4–8/10–11

METABOLISM

Isradipine undergoes extensive first pass metabolism resulting in a bioavailability of 15–24%. Isradipine is extensively metabolised in the liver, at least partly by the cytochrome P450 isoenzyme CYP3A4. About 70% of an oral dose is reported to be excreted as metabolites in urine, the remainder in faeces.

DOSE IN RENAL IMPAIRMENT GFR (mL/MIN)

20–50	Dose as in normal renal function.
10–20	Dose as in normal renal function.
<10	Dose as in normal renal function.

DOSE IN PATIENTS UNDERGOING RENAL REPLACEMENT THERAPIES

CAPD	Not dialysed. Dose as in normal renal function.
HD	Not dialysed. Dose as in normal renal function.
HDF/High flux	Not dialysed. Dose as in normal renal function.
CAV/ VVHD	Not dialysed. Dose as in normal renal function.

IMPORTANT DRUG INTERACTIONS

Potentially hazardous interactions with other drugs
- Anaesthetics: enhanced hypotensive effect.
- Antibacterials: metabolism accelerated by rifampicin; metabolism possibly inhibited by clarithromycin, erythromycin & telithromycin.
- Antidepressants: enhanced hypotensive effect with MAOIs.
- Anti-epileptics: effect reduced by carbamazepine, barbiturates, phenytoin and primidone.
- Antifungals: metabolism possibly inhibited by itraconazole and ketoconazole; negative inotropic effect possibly increased with itraconazole.
- Antihypertensives: enhanced hypotensive effect; increased risk of first dose hypotensive effect of post-synaptic alpha-blockers.
- Antivirals: concentration possibly increased by ritonavir.
- Grapefruit juice: concentration increased – avoid concomitant use.
- Theophylline: possibly increased theophylline concentration.

ADMINISTRATION

RECONSTITUTION

–

ROUTE
- Oral

RATE OF ADMINISTRATION

–

COMMENTS

–

OTHER INFORMATION

- In elderly patients, or where hepatic or renal function is impaired, initial dose should be 1.25 mg twice daily. Dose should be increased according to the requirements of the individual patient.

Itraconazole

CLINICAL USE

Antifungal agent

DOSE IN NORMAL RENAL FUNCTION

- Oral: 100–200 mg every 8–24 hours according to indication
- IV: 200 mg every 12–24 hours

PHARMACOKINETICS

Molecular weight (daltons)	705.6
% Protein binding	99.8
% Excreted unchanged in urine	<0.03
Volume of distribution (L/kg)	10
Half-life – normal/ESRF (hrs)	20–40/Unchanged

METABOLISM

Itraconazole is metabolised in the liver mainly by cytochrome P450 isoenzyme CYP3A4. The major metabolite, hydroxyitraconazole, has antifungal activity comparable with that of itraconazole. Itraconazole is excreted mainly as inactive metabolites in urine (35%) and faeces (54%) within one week of an oral solution dose. Renal excretion of itraconazole and the active metabolite hydroxy-itraconazole account for less than 1% of an intravenous dose. Based on an oral radiolabelled dose, faecal excretion of unchanged drug varies between 3% and 18% of the dose. Small amounts are eliminated in the stratum corneum and hair.

DOSE IN RENAL IMPAIRMENT GFR (mL/MIN)

30–50	Oral: Dose as in normal renal function. IV: Use with caution. See 'Other information'.
10–30	Oral: Dose as in normal renal function. IV: Avoid. See 'Other information'.
<10	Oral: Dose as in normal renal function. IV: Avoid. See 'Other information'.

DOSE IN PATIENTS UNDERGOING RENAL REPLACEMENT THERAPIES

CAPD	Not dialysed. Dose as in GFR<10 mL/min.
HD	Not dialysed. Dose as in GFR<10 mL/min.
HDF/High flux	Not dialysed. Dose as in GFR<10 mL/min.
CAV/VVHD	Not dialysed. Dose as in GFR=10–30 mL/min.

IMPORTANT DRUG INTERACTIONS

Potentially hazardous interactions with other drugs

- Aliskiren: concentration of aliskiren increased – avoid.
- Analgesics: possibly inhibits alfentanil metabolism; concentration of fentanyl possibly increased.
- Anti-arrhythmics: avoid concomitant use with disopyramide and dronedarone.
- Antibacterials: metabolism accelerated by rifabutin and rifampicin – avoid; possibly increased rifabutin concentration – reduce rifabutin dose; clarithromycin can increase itraconazole concentration.
- Anticoagulants: avoid with apixaban and rivaroxaban; effect of coumarins enhanced; concentration of dabigatran possibly increased – avoid.
- Antidepressants: avoid concomitant use with reboxetine.
- Antidiabetics: can enhance effects of repaglinide.
- Anti-epileptics: concentration reduced by carbamazepine, phenobarbital and phenytoin – avoid with phenytoin.
- Antihistamines: inhibits mizolastine metabolism – avoid concomitant use.
- Antimalarials: avoid concomitant use with piperaquine with artenimol and artemether/lumefantrine.
- Antipsychotics: possibly increases haloperidol concentration; possibly inhibits metabolism of aripiprazole – reduce aripiprazole dose; increased risk of ventricular arrhythmias with pimozide – avoid concomitant use; possibly increased quetiapine concentration – reduce quetiapine dose.
- Antivirals: concentration reduced by efavirenz and nevirapine; concentration of both drugs possibly increased by fosamprenavir; concentration of indinavir increased – may need to reduce indinavir

dose; with ritonavir concentration of both drugs may be increased; concentration of saquinavir possibly increased; concentration possibly increased by telaprevir; concentration reduced by efavirenz.

- Anxiolytics and hypnotics: concentration of buspirone, midazolam and alprazolam increased – reduce buspirone dose.
- Bosentan: possibly increased bosentan concentration.
- Calcium-channel blockers: negative inotropic effect possibly increased; metabolism of felodipine and possibly dihydropyridines inhibited; avoid concomitant use with lercanidipine.
- Cardiac glycosides: concentration of digoxin increased.
- Ciclosporin: metabolism of ciclosporin inhibited (increased ciclosporin levels).
- Clopidogrel: possibly reduced anti-platelet effect.
- Colchicine: possibly increased risk of colchicine toxicity – avoid in hepatic and renal impairment.
- Cytotoxics: metabolism of busulfan inhibited, increased risk of toxicity; possibly increases axitinib, everolimus, gefitinib and crizotinib concentration – reduce dose of axitinib, avoid with crizotinib & everolimus; possibly increased side effects with cyclophosphamide; avoid with lapatinib, nilotinib, pazopanib and cabazitaxel; reduce dose of ruxolitinib; possibly inhibits metabolism of vinorelbine & vincristine, increased risk of neurotoxicity; increases vinflunine concentration – avoid.
- Diuretics: increased eplerenone levels – avoid concomitant use.
- Ergot alkaloids: increased risk of ergotism – avoid concomitant use.
- $5HT_1$ agonists: increased eletriptan concentration – avoid concomitant use.
- Ivabradine: possibly increased ivabradine levels – reduce initial dose.
- Lipid-lowering drugs: increased risk of myopathy with atorvastatin and simvastatin – avoid concomitant use with simvastatin, and maximum atorvastatin dose 40 mg.[1]

- Ranolazine: possibly increased ranolazine concentration – avoid.
- Sirolimus: concentration increased by itraconazole.
- Tacrolimus: possibly increased tacrolimus levels.
- Ulcer-healing drugs: absorption reduced by histamine H_2 antagonists and proton pump inhibitors.
- Vardenafil: possibly increased vardenafil concentration – avoid concomitant use.

ADMINISTRATION

RECONSTITUTION
–
ROUTE
- Oral, IV infusion
RATE OF ADMINISTRATION
- Over 60 minutes
COMMENTS
- Add 250 mg vial to 50 mL sodium chloride 0.9%, administer 60 mL (increased volume due to large displacement value).

OTHER INFORMATION

- Preparations absorbed at different rates: liquid is absorbed within 2.5 hours, capsules within 2–5 hours.
- Oral bioavailability of itraconazole may be lower in some patients with renal insufficiency, e.g. those receiving CAPD.
- Janssen-Cilag advise no dose alterations for the oral preparation are required in renal impairment as drug is extensively metabolised in the liver, and pharmacokinetics are unchanged in patients with ERF compared to normal.
- Hydroxypropyl-β-cyclodextrin, a required component of Sporanox intravenous formulation, is eliminated through glomerular filtration. Therefore, in patients with creatinine clearance <30 mL/min the use of itraconazole IV is contraindicated in the UK SPC.

Reference:
1. MHRA. *Drug Safety Update*. Statins: interactions and updated advice. August 2012; **6**(1): 2–4.

Ivabradine hydrochloride

CLINICAL USE

Symptomatic treatment of chronic stable angina pectoris in patients with sinus rhythm.
Treatment of mild to severe chronic heart failure

DOSE IN NORMAL RENAL FUNCTION

2.5–7.5 mg twice daily (dose is reduced if heart rate is consistently below 50 beats per minute)

PHARMACOKINETICS

Molecular weight (daltons)	504.5
% Protein binding	70
% Excreted unchanged in urine	4
Volume of distribution (L/kg)	100 litres
Half-life – normal/ESRF (hrs)	2/Unchanged

METABOLISM

Ivabradine is extensively metabolised by the liver and the gut by oxidation through cytochrome P450 3A4 (CYP3A4) only. The major active metabolite is N-desmethyl-ivabradine (S 18982) with an exposure about 40% of that of the parent compound. This active metabolite undergoes further metabolism by CYP3A4. Excretion of metabolites occurs to a similar extent via faeces and urine. About 4% of an oral dose is excreted unchanged in urine.

DOSE IN RENAL IMPAIRMENT GFR (mL/MIN)

20–50	Dose as in normal renal function.
15–20	Dose as in normal renal function.
<15	Dose as in normal renal function. Use with caution.

DOSE IN PATIENTS UNDERGOING RENAL REPLACEMENT THERAPIES

CAPD	Unlikely to be dialysed. Dose as in GFR<15 mL/min.
HD	Unlikely to be dialysed. Dose as in GFR<15 mL/min.
HDF/High flux	Unknown dialysability. Dose as in GFR<15 mL/min.
CAV/VVHD	Unknown dialysability. Dose as in normal renal function.

IMPORTANT DRUG INTERACTIONS

Potentially hazardous interactions with other drugs
- Anti-arrhythmics: increased risk of ventricular arrhythmias with amiodarone and disopyramide.
- Antibacterials: concentration possibly increased by clarithromycin and telithromycin – avoid concomitant use; increased risk of ventricular arrhythmias with erythromycin – avoid concomitant use.
- Antifungals: concentration increased by ketoconazole – avoid concomitant use; concentration increased by fluconazole – reduce initial ivabradine dose; concentration possibly increased by itraconazole – avoid concomitant use.
- Antimalarials: increased risk of ventricular arrhythmias with mefloquine.
- Antipsychotics: increased risk of ventricular arrhythmias with pimozide.
- Antivirals: concentration possibly increased by ritonavir – avoid concomitant use.
- Beta-blockers: increased risk of ventricular arrhythmias with sotalol.
- Calcium-channel blockers: concentration increased by diltiazem and verapamil – avoid concomitant use.
- Grapefruit juice: ivabradine concentration increased.
- Pentamidine: increased risk of ventricular arrhythmias.
- St John's wort: ivabradine concentration reduced – avoid concomitant use.

ADMINISTRATION

RECONSTITUTION
–
ROUTE
- Oral
RATE OF ADMINISTRATION
–
COMMENTS
–

OTHER INFORMATION

- Manufacturer advises to use with caution due to lack of data but in practice has been used in end-stage renal disease at normal doses without any problems.

Ketamine

CLINICAL USE

Anaesthetic agent, analgesic

DOSE IN NORMAL RENAL FUNCTION

- All doses are expressed as the base:
  - 1.15 mg ketamine hydrochloride ≡1 mg of base
- Anaesthesia: IM
  - Short procedures: initially 6.5–13 mg/kg (10 mg/kg usually gives 12–25 minutes of surgical anaesthesia)
  - Painful diagnostic manoeuvres: initially 4 mg/kg
- IV Injection:
  - Initially 1–4.5 mg/kg over at least 60 seconds (2 mg/kg usually gives 5–10 minutes of surgical anaesthesia)
- IV Infusion:
  - Induction total dose of 0.5–2 mg/kg; maintenance 10–45 mcg/kg/min; adjust rate according to response if infusion required.
- Analgesia:
  - IM: 1.5–2 mg/kg
  - IV Infusion: 2–3 mg/kg or infusion rate 5–10 mg/hour of a solution of 5 mg/mL

PHARMACOKINETICS

Molecular weight (daltons)	274.2 (as hydrochloride)
% Protein binding	20–50
% Excreted unchanged in urine	2 (88% as metabolites)
Volume of distribution (L/kg)	4
Half-life – normal/ ESRF (hrs)	2–4/Unchanged

METABOLISM

After intravenous boluses, ketamine shows a bi- or triexponential pattern of elimination. The alpha phase, which lasts about 45 minutes, represents ketamine's anaesthetic action, and is terminated by redistribution from the CNS to peripheral tissues and hepatic biotransformation to an active metabolite norketamine. Other metabolic pathways include hydroxylation of the cyclohexone ring and conjugation with glucuronic acid. Ketamine is excreted mainly in the urine as metabolites.

DOSE IN RENAL IMPAIRMENT GFR (mL/MIN)

20–50	Dose as in normal renal function.
10–20	Dose as in normal renal function.
<10	Dose as in normal renal function.

DOSE IN PATIENTS UNDERGOING RENAL REPLACEMENT THERAPIES

CAPD	Unlikely dialysability. Dose as in normal renal function.
HD	Not dialysed. Dose as in normal renal function.
HDF/High flux	Unknown dialysability. Dose as in normal renal function.
CAV/ VVHD	Not dialysed. Dose as in normal renal function.

IMPORTANT DRUG INTERACTIONS

Potentially hazardous interactions with other drugs

- Adrenergic-neurone blockers: enhanced hypotensive effect.
- Antihypertensives: enhanced hypotensive effect.
- Antidepressants: stop MAOIs 2 weeks before surgery; increased risk of arrhythmias and hypotension with tricyclics.
- Antipsychotics: enhanced hypotensive effect.
- Memantine: increased risk of CNS toxicity, avoid concomitant use.
- Muscle relaxants: enhances effects of atracurium.

ADMINISTRATION

RECONSTITUTION

–

ROUTE
- IV bolus, IV Infusion, IM

RATE OF ADMINISTRATION
- Injection: over at least 60 seconds
- Infusion: Depends on clinical indication.

COMMENTS
- Injection: over at least 60 seconds.
- Infusion: Depends on clinical indication.
- For infusion add to glucose 5% or sodium chloride 0.9%, dilute to 1 mg/mL. In the USA can dilute to 2 mg/mL in fluid restricted patients (Dollery).
- Incompatible with diazepam and barbiturates.
- Use infusion solutions within 24 hours.
- 100 mg/mL strength must be diluted with an equal volume of water for injection,

sodium chloride 0.9% or glucose 5% before use.
- Minimum volume 50 mg/mL (undiluted). (UK Critical Care Group, *Minimum Infusion Volumes for Fluid Restricted Critically Ill Patients*, 3rd edition, 2006)

OTHER INFORMATION

- Contraindicated in patients with severe hypertension; 1–2 mg/kg can increase arterial systolic blood pressure by approximately 20–40 mmHg.
- Avoid in those prone to hallucinations or psychotic disorders.
- 4–10% can be removed by haemodialysis.

Ketoconazole

CLINICAL USE
Antifungal agent

DOSE IN NORMAL RENAL FUNCTION
200–400 mg once daily
See 'Other information'

PHARMACOKINETICS

Molecular weight (daltons)	531.4
% Protein binding	>90
% Excreted unchanged in urine	13
Volume of distribution (L/kg)	0.36
Half-life – normal/ ESRF (hrs)	2/3.3

METABOLISM
Following absorption from the gastro-intestinal tract, ketoconazole is converted into several inactive metabolites. The major identified metabolic pathways are oxidation and degradation of the imidazole and piperazine rings, oxidative O-dealkylation and aromatic hydroxylation. Plasma elimination is biphasic with a half-life of 2 hours during the first 10 hours and 8 hours thereafter. About 13% of the dose is excreted in the urine, of which 2–4% is unchanged drug. The major route of excretion is through the bile into the intestinal tract.

DOSE IN RENAL IMPAIRMENT GFR (mL/MIN)
20–50 Dose as in normal renal function.
10–20 Dose as in normal renal function.
<10   Dose as in normal renal function.

DOSE IN PATIENTS UNDERGOING RENAL REPLACEMENT THERAPIES

CAPD	Not dialysed. Dose as in normal renal function.
HD	Not dialysed. Dose as in normal renal function.
HDF/High flux	Unknown dialysability. Dose as in normal renal function.
CAV/ VVHD	Unknown dialysability. Dose as in normal renal function.

IMPORTANT DRUG INTERACTIONS
Potentially hazardous interactions with other drugs
- Analgesics: inhibits buprenorphine metabolism – reduce buprenorphine dose.
- Anti-arrhythmics: increased risk of ventricular arrhythmias with disopyramide – avoid concomitant use; concentration of dronedarone increased – avoid.
- Antibacterials: metabolism increased by rifampicin; may reduce rifampicin concentration; concentration possibly reduced by isoniazid; avoid concomitant use with telithromycin in severe renal and hepatic impairment.
- Anticoagulants: anticoagulant effect of coumarins enhanced; concentration of apixaban, dabigatran and rivaroxaban increased – avoid.
- Antidepressants: avoid concomitant use with reboxetine; ketoconazole increases concentration of mirtazapine.
- Anti-epileptics: concentration of ketoconazole reduced by phenytoin; concentration of carbamazepine possibly increased.
- Antihistamines: concentration of loratadine possibly increased – avoid; avoid concomitant use with mizolastine; concentration of rupatadine increased.
- Antimalarials: avoid with piperaquine with artenimol and artemether and lumefantrine; concentration of mefloquine increased.
- Antipsychotics: increased risk of ventricular arrhythmias with pimozide – avoid concomitant use; possibly increased concentration of quetiapine – reduce quetiapine dose; inhibits aripiprazole metabolism – reduce aripiprazole dose.
- Antivirals: concentration of both drugs increased with darunavir; inhibits metabolism of indinavir; concentration reduced by nevirapine – avoid concomitant use; ketoconazole and ritonavir can increase concentration of each other; concentration of boceprevir, maraviroc and saquinavir increased; concentration increased by fosamprenavir and possibly concentration of fosamprenavir increased; concentration of both drugs increased with telaprevir.
- Anxiolytics and hypnotics: concentration of alprazolam and midazolam increased (risk of prolonged sedation).

- Calcium-channel blockers: increased concentration of felodipine; avoid with lercanidipine; possibly inhibits metabolism of dihydropyridines.
- Ciclosporin: increased ciclosporin concentration.
- Cilostazol: possibly increased concentration of cilostazol, consider reducing dose.
- Cinacalcet: increased cinacalcet concentration.
- Clopidogrel: possibly reduces anti-platelet effect.
- Colchicine: possibly increases risk of colchicine toxicity, avoid concomitant use in hepatic or renal failure.
- Cytotoxics: concentration of axitinib increased (reduce dose of axitinib); concentration of crizotinib, everolimus, lapatinib and nilotinib increased – avoid; possibly increases concentration of dasatinib; inhibits metabolism of erlotinib and sunitinib; concentration of bortezomib and imatinib increased; avoid with cabazitaxel and pazopanib, reduce dose with ruxolitinib; inhibits active metabolite of temsirolimus – avoid; docetaxel possibly interacts with ketoconazole; possible increased risk of neutropenia with brentuximab; concentration of irinotecan, but active metabolite of irinotecan reduced – avoid; concentration of vinflunine increased – avoid.
- Diuretics: increased eplerenone concentration – avoid concomitant use.
- Domperidone: possibly increased risk of arrhythmias – avoid.
- Ergot alkaloids: increased risk of ergotism with ergotamine and methysergide – avoid concomitant use.
- Fingolimod: concentration of fingolimod increased.
- 5HT$_1$ agonists: increased concentration of eletriptan – avoid concomitant use; increased almotriptan concentration (increased toxicity).
- Ivabradine: concentration of ivabradine increased – avoid concomitant use.
- Lanthanum: reduces absorption of ketoconazole – give at least 2 hours apart.
- Ranolazine: concentration of ranolazine increased – avoid.
- Retinoids: concentration of alitretinoin increased; possibly increased risk of tretinoin toxicity.
- Sirolimus: concentration increased by ketoconazole – avoid concomitant use.
- Statins: possibly increased risk of myopathy with atorvastatin and simvastatin – avoid concomitant use with simvastatin.[1]
- Tacrolimus: increased tacrolimus concentration.
- Theophylline; possibly increased concentration of theophylline.
- Ticagrelor: concentration of ticagrelor increased – avoid.
- Tadalafil & vardenafil: increased concentration of tadalafil and vardenafil, avoid concomitant use.

ADMINISTRATION

RECONSTITUTION
–
ROUTE
- Oral, topical
RATE OF ADMINISTRATION
–
COMMENTS
–

OTHER INFORMATION

- The European Medicines Agency's (EMA) Committee for Medicinal Products for Human Use (CHMP) advise that oral ketoconazole is no longer recommended for fungal infections due to the increased risk of liver damage (26 July 2013).
- Monitor LFTs especially if on long-term treatment.

Reference:
1. MHRA. *Drug Safety Update*. Statins: interactions and updated advice. August 2012; **6**(1): 2–4.

Ketoprofen

CLINICAL USE

NSAID and analgesic

DOSE IN NORMAL RENAL FUNCTION

- Oral: 100–200 mg daily in 2–4 divided doses
- Dysmenorrhoea: 50 mg every 8 hours
- PR: 100 mg at night

PHARMACOKINETICS

Molecular weight (daltons)	254.3
% Protein binding	99
% Excreted unchanged in urine	<1
Volume of distribution (L/kg)	0.1
Half-life – normal/ ESRF (hrs)	1.5–8/5–9

METABOLISM

Two processes are involved in the biotransformation of ketoprofen: one very minor (hydroxylation), and the other largely predominant (conjugation with glucuronic acid). Less than 1% of the dose of ketoprofen administered is recovered in unchanged form in the urine, whereas the glucuronide metabolite accounts for about 65–75%. The drug is excreted as metabolites essentially by the urinary route. The rate of excretion is rapid, since 50% of the dose administered is eliminated in the first 6 hours.

DOSE IN RENAL IMPAIRMENT GFR (mL/MIN)

20–50	Dose as in normal renal function, but avoid if possible.
10–20	Dose as in normal renal function, but avoid if possible.
<10	Dose as in normal renal function, but only use if on dialysis.

DOSE IN PATIENTS UNDERGOING RENAL REPLACEMENT THERAPIES

CAPD	Unlikely to be dialysed. Dose as in normal renal function. See 'Other information'
HD	Unlikely to be dialysed. Dose as in normal renal function. See 'Other information'
HDF/High flux	Unknown dialysability. Dose as in normal renal function. See 'Other information'.
CAV/ VVHD	Unlikely to be dialysed. Dose as in GFR=10–20 mL/min.

IMPORTANT DRUG INTERACTIONS

Potentially hazardous interactions with other drugs

- ACE inhibitors and angiotensin-II antagonists: antagonism of hypotensive effect, increased risk of nephrotoxicity and hyperkalaemia.
- Analgesics: avoid concomitant use of 2 or more NSAIDs, including aspirin (increased side effects); avoid with ketorolac (increased risk of side effects and haemorrhage).
- Antibacterials: possibly increased risk of convulsions with quinolones.
- Anticoagulants: effects of coumarins and phenindione enhanced; possibly increased risk of bleeding with heparins and dabigatran.
- Antidepressants: increased risk of bleeding with SSRIs and venlafaxine.
- Antidiabetic agents: effects of sulphonylureas enhanced.
- Anti-epileptics: possibly increased phenytoin concentration.
- Antivirals: increased risk of haematological toxicity with zidovudine; concentration possibly increased by ritonavir.
- Ciclosporin: may potentiate nephrotoxicity.
- Cytotoxic agents: reduced excretion of methotrexate; increased risk of bleeding with erlotinib.
- Diuretics: increased risk of nephrotoxicity; antagonism of diuretic effect, hyperkalaemia with potassium-sparing diuretics.
- Lithium: excretion decreased.
- Pentoxifylline: increased risk of bleeding.
- Probenecid: excretion reduced by probenecid.
- Tacrolimus: increased risk of nephrotoxicity.

ADMINISTRATION

RECONSTITUTION
–
ROUTE
● Oral, rectal.
RATE OF ADMINISTRATION
–
COMMENTS
–

OTHER INFORMATION

● Combined oral and rectal treatment, maximum total daily dose 200 mg.
● Inhibition of renal prostaglandin synthesis by NSAIDs may interfere with renal function, especially in the presence of existing renal disease – avoid if possible; if not, check serum creatinine 48–72 hours after starting NSAID – if raised, discontinue NSAID therapy.
● Use normal doses in patients with ERF on dialysis if they do not pass any urine.
● Use with caution in renal transplant recipients – can reduce intrarenal autocoid synthesis.
● NSAIDs decrease platelet aggregation.
● Associated with nephrotic syndrome, interstitial nephritis, hyperkalaemia and sodium retention.

Ketorolac trometamol

CLINICAL USE

Short-term management of moderate to severe acute postoperative pain

DOSE IN NORMAL RENAL FUNCTION

- Oral: 10 mg every 4–6 hours (elderly every 6–8 hours); maximum 40 mg daily; maximum duration 7 days.
- IM/IV: initially 10 mg, then 10–30 mg when required every 4–6 hours (every 2 hours in initial postoperative period); maximum 90 mg daily (elderly and patients less than 50 kg: maximum 60 mg daily); maximum duration 2 days.

PHARMACOKINETICS

Molecular weight (daltons)	376.4
% Protein binding	>99
% Excreted unchanged in urine	Approx 60
Volume of distribution (L/kg)	0.15
Half-life – normal/ESRF (hrs)	IM dose: 3.5–9.2/ 5.9–19.2

METABOLISM

The major metabolic pathway is glucuronic acid conjugation; there is some *para*-hydroxylation. About 91.4% of a dose is excreted in urine as unchanged drug and conjugated and hydroxylated metabolites, with a further 6.1% being excreted in the faeces.

DOSE IN RENAL IMPAIRMENT GFR (mL/MIN)

20–50	Maximum 60 mg daily
10–20	Avoid if possible. Use small doses and monitor closely.
<10	Avoid if possible. Use small doses and monitor closely.

DOSE IN PATIENTS UNDERGOING RENAL REPLACEMENT THERAPIES

CAPD	Unlikely to be dialysed. Dose as in GFR<10 mL/min.
HD	Unlikely to be dialysed. Dose as in GFR<10 mL/min.
HDF/High flux	Unknown dialysability. Dose as in GFR<10 mL/min.
CAV/ VVHD	Unknown dialysability. Dose as in GFR=10–20 mL/min.

IMPORTANT DRUG INTERACTIONS

Potentially hazardous interactions with other drugs

- ACE inhibitors and angiotensin-II antagonists: antagonism of hypotensive effect; increased risk of nephrotoxicity and hyperkalaemia.
- Analgesics: avoid concomitant use of 2 or more NSAIDs, including aspirin (increased risk of side effects and haemorrhage).
- Antibacterials: possibly increased risk of convulsions with quinolones.
- Anticoagulants increased risk of bleeding with heparins, dabigatran, phenindione and coumarins – avoid concomitant use; increased risk of haemorrhage with parenteral ketorolac and heparin – avoid concomitant use.
- Antidepressants: increased risk of bleeding with SSRIs and venlafaxine.
- Antidiabetics: effects of sulphonylureas possibly enhanced.
- Anti-epileptics: effect of phenytoin possibly enhanced.
- Antivirals: increased risk of haematological toxicity with zidovudine; concentration possibly increased by ritonavir.
- Ciclosporin: increased risk of nephrotoxicity.
- Cytotoxics: excretion of methotrexate reduced; increased risk of bleeding with erlotinib.
- Diuretics: increased risk of nephrotoxicity; antagonism of diuretic effect; hyperkalaemia with potassium-sparing diuretics.
- Lithium: excretion of lithium reduced – avoid concomitant use.
- Pentoxifylline: risk of ketorolac associated bleeding increased – avoid concomitant use.
- Probenecid: delays excretion of ketorolac – avoid concomitant use.
- Tacrolimus: increased risk of nephrotoxicity.

ADMINISTRATION

RECONSTITUTION

–

ROUTE

- IM, IV, Oral

RATE OF ADMINISTRATION

- IV bolus over no less than 15 seconds.

COMMENTS

- Compatible with sodium chloride 0.9%, glucose 5%, Ringer's, lactated Ringer's or plasmalyte solutions.

OTHER INFORMATION

- Drugs that inhibit prostaglandin biosynthesis (including NSAIDs) have been reported to cause nephrotoxicity, including, but not limited to, glomerular nephritis, interstitial nephritis, renal papillary necrosis, nephrotic syndrome and acute renal failure. In patients with renal, cardiac or hepatic impairment, caution is required since the use of NSAIDs may result in deterioration of renal function.
- Ketorolac and its metabolites are excreted primarily by the kidney.
- Reported renal side effects include increased urinary frequency, oliguria, acute renal failure, hyponatraemia, hyperkalaemia, haemolytic uraemic syndrome, flank pain (with or without haematuria), raised serum urea and creatinine.

Ketotifen

CLINICAL USE

Antihistamine:
- Allergic conditions

DOSE IN NORMAL RENAL FUNCTION

- 1–2 mg twice daily
- Initial dose in readily sedated patients: 0.5–1 mg at night

PHARMACOKINETICS

Molecular weight (daltons)	425.5 (as fumarate)
% Protein binding	75
% Excreted unchanged in urine	1
Volume of distribution (L/kg)	8.8[1]
Half-life – normal/ ESRF (hrs)	21/–

METABOLISM

Undergoes hepatic first-pass metabolism to form inactive metabolites which are mainly excreted in the urine.

DOSE IN RENAL IMPAIRMENT GFR (mL/MIN)

20–50	Dose as in normal renal function.
10–20	Dose as in normal renal function.
<10	Dose as in normal renal function.

DOSE IN PATIENTS UNDERGOING RENAL REPLACEMENT THERAPIES

CAPD	Unknown dialysability. Dose as in normal renal function.
HD	Unknown dialysability. Dose as in normal renal function.
HDF/High flux	Unknown dialysability. Dose as in normal renal function.
CAV/ VVHD	Unknown dialysability. Dose as in normal renal function.

IMPORTANT DRUG INTERACTIONS

Potentially hazardous interactions with other drugs
- Analgesics: sedative effects possibly increased with opioid analgesics.

ADMINISTRATION

RECONSTITUTION
–
ROUTE
- Oral, topical
RATE OF ADMINISTRATION
–
COMMENTS
–

OTHER INFORMATION

- Increased possibility of side effects, particularly drowsiness.
- Bioavailability is 50%.

Reference:
1. www.accessdata.fda.gov/drugsatfda_docs/nda/99/21- 066_ZADITOR%200.025%25_biopharmr.pdf

Klean-Prep

CLINICAL USE

Colonic lavage prior to diagnostic examination or surgical procedures requiring a clean colon

DOSE IN NORMAL RENAL FUNCTION

4 sachets, each reconstituted in 1 litre of water, at a rate of 250 mL every 10–15 minutes.

PHARMACOKINETICS

Molecular weight (daltons)	3350 (Macrogol)
% Protein binding	N/A
% Excreted unchanged in urine	N/A
Volume of distribution (L/kg)	N/A
Half-life – normal/ ESRF (hrs)	N/A

METABOLISM

Macrogol 3350 is unchanged along the gut. It is virtually unabsorbed from the gastro-intestinal tract. Any macrogol 3350 that is absorbed is excreted via the urine.

DOSE IN RENAL IMPAIRMENT GFR (mL/MIN)

20–50	Dose as in normal renal function.
10–20	Dose as in normal renal function.
<10	Dose as in normal renal function.

DOSE IN PATIENTS UNDERGOING RENAL REPLACEMENT THERAPIES

CAPD	Not absorbed. Dose as in normal renal function.
HD	Not absorbed. Dose as in normal renal function.
HDF/High flux	Not absorbed. Dose as in normal renal function.
CAV/ VVHD	Not absorbed. Dose as in normal renal function.

IMPORTANT DRUG INTERACTIONS

Potentially hazardous interactions with other drugs
● None known

ADMINISTRATION

RECONSTITUTION
● Each sachet in 1 litre of water
ROUTE
● Oral
RATE OF ADMINISTRATION
● 250 mL every 15–30 minutes.
● If given via NG tube, rate is 20–30 mL/minute.
COMMENTS
● Klean-Prep is formulated to be hyper-osmotic and draw water into the bowel. None is absorbed systemically.

OTHER INFORMATION

Each sachet of Klean-Prep contains:
— Polyethylene glycol 3350 – 59 g
— Anhydrous sodium sulphate – 5.685 g
— Sodium bicarbonate – 1.685 g
— Sodium chloride – 1.465 g
— Potassium chloride – 0.7425 g
● The electrolyte content of 1 sachet when made up in 1 litre of water is:
— Sodium – 125 mmol
— Sulphate – 40 mmol
— Chloride – 35 mmol
— Bicarbonate – 20 mmol
— Potassium – 10 mmol

Labetalol hydrochloride

CLINICAL USE

Beta-adrenoceptor blocker:
- Hypertensive crisis, hypertension

DOSE IN NORMAL RENAL FUNCTION

- Oral: 50–400 mg twice daily (in 3–4 divided doses if >800 mg daily); maximum 2.4 g daily
- IV infusion: 2 mg/minute until satisfactory response; usual total dose 50–200 mg
- IV bolus: 50 mg over 1 minute, repeated at 5 minute intervals to a total dose of 200 mg
- Pregnancy: 20–160 mg/hour
- Hypertension after an MI: 15–120 mg/hour

PHARMACOKINETICS

Molecular weight (daltons)	364.9
% Protein binding	50
% Excreted unchanged in urine	5
Volume of distribution (L/kg)	5.6
Half-life – normal/ESRF (hrs)	4–8/ Unchanged

METABOLISM

Labetalol is subject to considerable first-pass metabolism. It is metabolised mainly in the liver, the metabolites being excreted in the urine with only small amounts of unchanged labetalol; its major metabolite has not been found to have significant alpha- or beta-blocking effects. Excretion also occurs in the faeces via the bile.

DOSE IN RENAL IMPAIRMENT GFR (mL/MIN)

20–50	Dose as in normal renal function.
10–20	Dose as in normal renal function.
<10	Dose as in normal renal function.

DOSE IN PATIENTS UNDERGOING RENAL REPLACEMENT THERAPIES

CAPD	Not dialysed. Dose as in normal renal function.
HD	Not dialysed. Dose as in normal renal function.
HDF/High flux	Unknown dialysability. Dose as in normal renal function.
CAV/ VVHD	Probably not dialysed. Dose as in normal renal function.

IMPORTANT DRUG INTERACTIONS

Potentially hazardous interactions with other drugs
- Anaesthetics: enhanced hypotensive effect.
- Analgesics: NSAIDs antagonise hypotensive effect.
- Anti-arrhythmics: increased risk of myocardial depression and bradycardia; increased risk of bradycardia, myocardial depression and AV block with amiodarone; increased risk of myocardial depression and bradycardia with flecainide.
- Antidepressants: enhanced hypotensive effect with MAOIs; concentration of imipramine increased.
- Antihypertensives; enhanced hypotensive effect; increased risk of withdrawal hypertension with clonidine; increased risk of first dose hypotensive effect with post-synaptic alpha-blockers such as prazosin.
- Antimalarials: increased risk of bradycardia with mefloquine.
- Antipsychotics enhanced hypotensive effect with phenothiazines.
- Calcium-channel blockers: increased risk of bradycardia and AV block with diltiazem; hypotension and heart failure possible with nifedipine and nisoldipine; asystole, severe hypotension and heart failure with verapamil.
- Cytotoxics: possible increased risk of bradycardia with crizotinib.
- Diuretics: enhanced hypotensive effect.
- Fingolimod: possibly increased risk of bradycardia.
- Moxisylyte: possible severe postural hypotension.
- Sympathomimetics: severe hypertension with adrenaline and noradrenaline and possibly with dobutamine.

ADMINISTRATION

RECONSTITUTION
–

ROUTE
- Oral, IV

RATE OF ADMINISTRATION
- 2 mg/minute initially then titrate according to response or to indication

COMMENTS
- 200 mg labetalol (40 mL) to 200 mL glucose 5%.

● Can be used undiluted. (UK Critical Care
Group, *Minimum Infusion Volumes for
Fluid Restricted Critically Ill Patients*, 3rd
edition, 2006)

OTHER INFORMATION

● No adverse effects on renal function.
● No accumulation in renal impairment.
● Hypoglycaemia can occur in dialysis
patients.
● Tachyphylaxis can occur with prolonged
use.

Lacidipine

CLINICAL USE

Calcium-channel blocker
- Hypertension

DOSE IN NORMAL RENAL FUNCTION

2–6 mg once daily

PHARMACOKINETICS

Molecular weight (daltons)	455.5
% Protein binding	95
% Excreted unchanged in urine	0
Volume of distribution (L/kg)	0.9–2.3
Half-life – normal/ ESRF (hrs)	13–19/–

METABOLISM

Lacidipine undergoes extensive first-pass metabolism in the liver. The drug is eliminated primarily by hepatic metabolism (involving cytochrome P450 CYP3A4).

The principal metabolites possess little, if any, pharmacodynamic activity. Approximately 70% of the administered dose is eliminated as metabolites in the faeces and the remainder as metabolites in the urine.

DOSE IN RENAL IMPAIRMENT GFR (mL/MIN)

20–50	Dose as in normal renal function.
10–20	Dose as in normal renal function.
<10	Dose as in normal renal function.

DOSE IN PATIENTS UNDERGOING RENAL REPLACEMENT THERAPIES

CAPD	Unknown dialysability. Dose as in normal renal function.
HD	Unknown dialysability. Dose as in normal renal function.
HDF/High flux	Unknown dialysability. Dose as in normal renal function.
CAV/ VVHD	Unknown dialysability. Dose as in normal renal function.

IMPORTANT DRUG INTERACTIONS

Potentially hazardous interactions with other drugs
- Anaesthetics: enhanced hypotensive effect.
- Antibacterials: metabolism possibly inhibited by clarithromycin, erythromycin & telithromycin.
- Antidepressants: enhanced hypotensive effect with MAOIs.
- Anti-epileptics: effect possibly reduced by carbamazepine, barbiturates, phenytoin and primidone.
- Antifungals: metabolism possibly inhibited by itraconazole and ketoconazole; negative inotropic effect possibly increased with itraconazole.
- Antihypertensives: enhanced hypotensive effect, increased risk of first dose hypotensive effect of post-synaptic alpha-blockers.
- Antivirals: concentration possibly increased by ritonavir.
- Ciclosporin: 10 kidney transplant patients on ciclosporin, prednisone and azathioprine were given 4 mg lacidipine daily. A very small increase in the trough serum levels (+6%) and AUC (+14%) of the ciclosporin occurred.
- Grapefruit juice: concentration increased – avoid concomitant use.
- Theophylline: possibly increased theophylline concentration.

ADMINISTRATION

RECONSTITUTION

–

ROUTE
- Oral

RATE OF ADMINISTRATION

–

COMMENTS

–

Lacosamide

CLINICAL USE

Anti-epileptic agent

DOSE IN NORMAL RENAL FUNCTION

50–200 mg twice daily

PHARMACOKINETICS

Molecular weight (daltons)	250.3
% Protein binding	<15
% Excreted unchanged in urine	40
Volume of distribution (L/kg)	0.6
Half-life – normal/ ESRF (hrs)	13/–

METABOLISM

The metabolism of lacosamide has not been completely characterised. Lacosamide is a CYP2C19 substrate. Metabolites are inactive.

About 95% of a dose is excreted in the urine, about 40% as unchanged drug and less than 30% as the inactive O-desmethyl metabolite. Less than 0.5% of a dose is excreted in the faeces.

DOSE IN RENAL IMPAIRMENT GFR (mL/MIN)

30–50	Dose as in normal renal function
10–30	Maximum dose 250 mg daily
<10	Titrate slowly, maximum dose 250 mg daily

DOSE IN PATIENTS UNDERGOING RENAL REPLACEMENT THERAPIES

CAPD	Unlikely to be dialysed. Dose as in GFR<10 mL/min.
HD	Dialysed. Dose as in GFR<10 mL/min.
HDF/High flux	Dialysed. Dose as in GFR<10 mL/min.
CAV/VVHD	Dialysed. Dose as in GFR=10–30 mL/min.

IMPORTANT DRUG INTERACTIONS

Potentially hazardous interactions with other drugs

- Antidepressants: anticonvulsant effect antagonised; avoid concomitant use with St John's wort.
- Antimalarials: mefloquine antagonises anticonvulsant effect.
- Antipsychotics: anticonvulsant effect antagonised.
- Orlistat: possibly increased risk of convulsions.

ADMINISTRATION

RECONSTITUTION

–

ROUTE

- Oral, IV infusion

RATE OF ADMINISTRATION

- 15–60 minutes

OTHER INFORMATION

- Metabolite with no known pharmacological activity accumulates in ERF, therefore use with caution.
- Prolongations in PR interval with lacosamide have been observed in clinical studies.
- Infusion contains 2.6 mmol (or 59.8 mg) sodium per vial.
- Tablets have 100% bioavailability.
- The AUC of lacosamide was increased by approximately 30% in mildly and moderately and 60% in severely renal impaired patients and patients with ERF requiring haemodialysis compared to healthy subjects, whereas C_{max} was unaffected.
- Approximately 50% of lacosamide is removed following a 4 hour haemodialysis session.

Lactulose

CLINICAL USE

- Constipation
- Hepatic encephalopathy

DOSE IN NORMAL RENAL FUNCTION

- Constipation: initially 15 mL twice daily; adjust according to requirements.
- Hepatic encephalopathy: 30–50 mL 3 times daily adjusted to produce 2–3 soft stools daily

PHARMACOKINETICS

Molecular weight (daltons)	342.3
% Protein binding	No data
% Excreted unchanged in urine	<3
Volume of distribution (L/kg)	N/A – not absorbed.
Half-life – normal/ ESRF (hrs)	No data

METABOLISM

Lactulose passes essentially unchanged into the large intestine where it is metabolised by saccharolytic bacteria with the formation of simple organic acids, mainly lactic acid and small amounts of acetic and formic acids. A small amount of absorbed lactulose is subsequently excreted unchanged in the urine.

DOSE IN RENAL IMPAIRMENT GFR (mL/MIN)

20–50	Dose as in normal renal function.
10–20	Dose as in normal renal function.
<10	Dose as in normal renal function.

DOSE IN PATIENTS UNDERGOING RENAL REPLACEMENT THERAPIES

CAPD	Not dialysed. Dose as in normal renal function.
HD	Not dialysed. Dose as in normal renal function.
HDF/High flux	Not dialysed. Dose as in normal renal function.
CAV/ VVHD	Not dialysed. Dose as in normal renal function.

IMPORTANT DRUG INTERACTIONS

Potentially hazardous interactions with other drugs
- None known

ADMINISTRATION

RECONSTITUTION
–
ROUTE
- Oral
RATE OF ADMINISTRATION
–
COMMENTS
–

OTHER INFORMATION

- May take up to 72 hours to work.
- Not significantly absorbed from GIT.
- Safe for diabetics (lactulose is converted to lactic, formic and acetic acid in the bowel).
- Osmotic and bulking effect.

Lamivudine

CAPD	Not dialysed. Dose as in GFR<5 mL/min.
HD	Dialysed. Dose as in GFR<5 mL/min.
HDF/High flux	Dialysed. Dose as in GFR<5 mL/min.
CAV/VVHD	Unknown dialysability. Dose as in GFR=5–15 mL/min.

CLINICAL USE

Nucleoside reverse transcriptase inhibitor
- Treatment of HIV in combination with other antiretroviral drugs
- Treatment of chronic hepatitis B in adults

DOSE IN NORMAL RENAL FUNCTION

- HIV: 150 mg twice daily or 300 mg daily.
- Hepatitis B: 100 mg daily.

PHARMACOKINETICS

Molecular weight (daltons)	229.3
% Protein binding	<36
% Excreted unchanged in urine	70
Volume of distribution (L/kg)	1.3
Half-life – normal/ESRF (hrs)	5–7/20

METABOLISM

Lamivudine is metabolised intracellularly to the active antiviral triphosphate. Hepatic metabolism is low (5–10%) and the majority of lamivudine is excreted unchanged in the urine via glomerular filtration and active secretion (organic cationic transport system).

DOSE IN RENAL IMPAIRMENT GFR (mL/MIN)

See 'Other information'.

30–50	HIV: 150 mg daily. Hepatitis B: 100 mg stat then 50 mg daily.
15–30	HIV: 150 mg stat then 100 mg daily. Hepatitis B: 100 mg stat then 25 mg daily.
5–15	HIV: 150 mg stat then 50 mg daily. Hepatitis B: 35 mg stat then 15 mg daily.
<5	HIV: 50 mg stat then 25–50 mg daily.[1,2] Hepatitis B: 35 mg stat then 10 mg daily.

IMPORTANT DRUG INTERACTIONS

Potentially hazardous interactions with other drugs
- Trimethoprim: inhibits excretion of lamivudine – avoid concomitant use of high dose co-trimoxazole.
- Antivirals: avoid concomitant use with foscarnet, emtricitabine and IV ganciclovir.

ADMINISTRATION

RECONSTITUTION

–

ROUTE
- Oral

RATE OF ADMINISTRATION

–

COMMENTS
- Administer with or without food.

OTHER INFORMATION

- 15 mL of oral suspension contains 3 g of sucrose.
- Dosage from Bennett (5th edition):
GFR>50 mL/min: 100% of dose
GFR=10–50 mL/min: 150 mg loading dose then 50–150 mg daily
GFR<10 mL/min: 50 mg loading dose then 25–50 mg daily

References:
1. Izzedine H, Launay-Vacher V, Baumelou A, *et al.* An appraisal of antiretroviral drugs in haemodialysis. *Kidney International.* 2001; **66**: 821–30.
2. Hilts AE, Fish DN. Dosage adjustments of antiretroviral agents in patients with organ dysfunction. *Am J Health-Syst Pharm.* 1998; **55**: 2528–33.

Lamotrigine

CLINICAL USE

- Monotherapy and adjunctive treatment of partial seizures, and primary and secondary generalised tonic-clonic seizures
- Prevention of depressive episodes in bipolar disease
- Trigeminal neuralgia (unlicensed)

DOSE IN NORMAL RENAL FUNCTION

25–200 mg daily in 1–2 divided doses, according to clinical indication. Maximum 500 mg daily; 700 mg with enzyme-inducing drugs

PHARMACOKINETICS

Molecular weight (daltons)	256.1
% Protein binding	55
% Excreted unchanged in urine	<10
Volume of distribution (L/kg)	0.92–1.22
Half-life – normal/ ESRF (hrs)	24–35/Unchanged

METABOLISM

Lamotrigine is extensively metabolised in the liver by UDP-glucuronyl transferases and excreted almost entirely in urine, principally as an inactive glucuronide conjugate. It slightly induces its own metabolism. Only about 2% of lamotrigine-related material is excreted in faeces.

DOSE IN RENAL IMPAIRMENT GFR (mL/MIN)

20–50	Caution. Start with 75% of dose and monitor closely.
10–20	Caution. Start with 75% of dose and monitor closely.
<10	Caution. Start with low doses and monitor closely.

DOSE IN PATIENTS UNDERGOING RENAL REPLACEMENT THERAPIES

CAPD	Unlikely dialysability. Dose as in GFR<10 mL/min.
HD	Not dialysed. Dose as in GFR<10 mL/min.
HDF/High flux	Unknown dialysability. Dose as in GFR<10 mL/min.
CAV/ VVHD	Unknown dialysability. Dose as in GFR=10–20 mL/min.

IMPORTANT DRUG INTERACTIONS

Potentially hazardous interactions with other drugs

- Antibacterials: concentration reduced by rifampicin.
- Antidepressants: antagonism of anticonvulsant effect; avoid with St John's wort.
- Antiepileptics: concentration reduced by carbamazepine, phenobarbital and phenytoin, also possibility of increased concentration of active carbamazepine metabolite; concentration increased by valproate – reduce lamotrigine dose.
- Antimalarials: mefloquine antagonises anticonvulsant effect.
- Antipsychotics: anticonvulsant effect antagonised.
- Oestrogens: concentration of lamotrigine reduced and the dose may need to be increased by as much as 2-fold.
- Orlistat: possibly increased risk of convulsions.

ADMINISTRATION

RECONSTITUTION

–

ROUTE

- Oral

RATE OF ADMINISTRATION

–

COMMENTS

–

OTHER INFORMATION

- Pharmacokinetic studies using single doses in subjects with renal failure indicate that lamotrigine pharmacokinetics are little affected, but plasma concentrations of the major glucuronide metabolite increase almost 8-fold due to reduced renal clearance.
- The 2-N-glucuronide is inactive and accounts for 75–90% of the metabolised drug present in the urine. Although the metabolite is inactive the consequences of accumulation are unknown; hence the company advises caution with the use of lamotrigine in renal impairment.

- Doses in renal impairment are from *Drug Prescribing in Renal Failure*, 5th edition, by Aronoff *et al.*
- The half-life of lamotrigine is affected by other drugs; reduced to 14 hours when given with enzyme-inducing drugs, e.g. carbamazepine and phenytoin, and is increased to approximately 70 hours when co-administered with sodium valproate alone.

Lanreotide

CLINICAL USE

Treatment of neuroendocrine & thyroid tumours and acromegaly

DOSE IN NORMAL RENAL FUNCTION

- LA: Neuroendocrine tumours and acromegaly: 30 mg every 14 days, increased to every 7–10 days according to response.
- Thyroid tumours: 30 mg every 14 days, increased to every 10 days according to response.
- Autogel: Acromegaly: 60 mg every 28 days, adjusted according to response.
- Neuroendocrine tumours: 60–120 mg every 28 days, adjusted according to response.

PHARMACOKINETICS

Molecular weight (daltons)	1096.3
% Protein binding	Unknown
% Excreted unchanged in urine	<5
Volume of distribution (L/kg)	16.1 litres
Half-life – normal/ ESRF (hrs)	2.5 (Depot 5–30 days)/5 (Depot 10–60)

METABOLISM

No data.

DOSE IN RENAL IMPAIRMENT GFR (mL/MIN)

20–50	Dose as in normal renal function.
10–20	Dose as in normal renal function.
<10	Dose as in normal renal function.

DOSE IN PATIENTS UNDERGOING RENAL REPLACEMENT THERAPIES

CAPD	Unknown dialysability. Dose as in normal renal function.
HD	Dialysed. Dose as in normal renal function.
HDF/High flux	Dialysed. Dose as in normal renal function.
CAV/ VVHD	Dialysed. Dose as in normal renal function.

IMPORTANT DRUG INTERACTIONS

Potentially hazardous interactions with other drugs
- Ciclosporin: ciclosporin concentration reduced.

ADMINISTRATION

RECONSTITUTION
–
ROUTE
- LA: IM; Autogel: SC
RATE OF ADMINISTRATION
–

OTHER INFORMATION

- Due to a wide therapeutic window, lanreotide may be given at the normal starting dose and then adjusted according to response despite reduced clearance in renal impairment.
- Bioavailability is 55–80% depending on product.

Lansoprazole

CLINICAL USE

Gastric acid suppression

DOSE IN NORMAL RENAL FUNCTION

- 5–30 mg daily in the morning; duration dependent on indication.
- Zollinger-Ellison syndrome: initially 60 mg daily; adjust according to response (if >120 mg, give in 2 divided doses).

PHARMACOKINETICS

Molecular weight (daltons)	369.4
% Protein binding	97
% Excreted unchanged in urine	0 (15–30 as metabolites)
Volume of distribution (L/kg)	25–33 litres
Half-life – normal/ ESRF (hrs)	1–2/Unchanged

METABOLISM

Lansoprazole is extensively metabolised in the liver, primarily by cytochrome P450 isoenzyme CYP2C19 to form 5-hydroxyl-lansoprazole and by CYP3A4 to form lansoprazole sulfone. The metabolites are excreted by both the renal and biliary route. A study with ^{14}C-labelled lansoprazole indicated that approximately one-third of the administered radiation was excreted in the urine and two-thirds was recovered in the faeces.

DOSE IN RENAL IMPAIRMENT GFR (mL/MIN)

20–50	Dose as in normal renal function.
10–20	Dose as in normal renal function.
<10	Dose as in normal renal function.

DOSE IN PATIENTS UNDERGOING RENAL REPLACEMENT THERAPIES

CAPD	Unlikely to be dialysed. Dose as in normal renal function.
HD	Not dialysed. Dose as in normal renal function.
HDF/High flux	Unknown dialysability. Dose as in normal renal function.
CAV/ VVHD	Unknown dialysability, probably not removed. Dose as in normal renal function.

IMPORTANT DRUG INTERACTIONS

Potentially hazardous interactions with other drugs
- Antifungals: absorption of itraconazole and ketoconazole reduced; avoid with posaconazole.
- Antivirals: concentration of atazanavir and rilpivirine reduced – avoid concomitant use; concentration of raltegravir and saquinavir possibly increased – avoid.
- Ciclosporin: theoretical, interaction unlikely – little information available.
- Clopidogrel: possibly reduced anti-platelet effect.
- Cytotoxics: possibly reduced excretion of methotrexate; avoid with erlotinib and vandetanib; possibly reduced lapatinib absorption; possibly reduced absorption of pazopanib.
- Tacrolimus: may increase tacrolimus concentration.
- Ulipristal: reduced contraceptive effect, avoid with high dose ulipristal.

ADMINISTRATION

RECONSTITUTION
–
ROUTE
- Oral
RATE OF ADMINISTRATION
–
COMMENTS
–

Lanthanum carbonate

CLINICAL USE

Phosphate binder in patients with CKD 5

DOSE IN NORMAL RENAL FUNCTION

Usually 500 mg – 1 g 3 times a day with meals.
Maximum 3750 mg daily

PHARMACOKINETICS

Molecular weight (daltons)	457.8
% Protein binding	>99.7
% Excreted unchanged in urine	Negligible
Volume of distribution (L/kg)	Not absorbed
Half-life – normal/ ESRF (hrs)	36/–

METABOLISM

Lanthanum carbonate is poorly absorbed from the gastrointestinal tract, with an absolute oral bioavailability of less than 1%. The small fraction that is absorbed is more than 99% bound to plasma proteins and is widely distributed in the tissues, particularly the bones, the liver, and the gastrointestinal tract. Lanthanum is not metabolised.
It is excreted mainly in the faeces with only around 0.000031% of an oral dose excreted via the urine in healthy subjects (renal clearance approximately 1 mL/min, representing <2% of total plasma clearance).

DOSE IN RENAL IMPAIRMENT GFR (mL/MIN)

20–50	Dose as in normal renal function.
10–20	Dose as in normal renal function.
<10	Dose as in normal renal function.

DOSE IN PATIENTS UNDERGOING RENAL REPLACEMENT THERAPIES

CAPD	Not dialysed. Dose as in normal renal function.
HD	Not dialysed. Dose as in normal renal function.
HDF/High flux	Not dialysed. Dose as in normal renal function.
CAV/ VVHD	Not dialysed. Dose as in normal renal function.

IMPORTANT DRUG INTERACTIONS

Potentially hazardous interactions with other drugs
- Antibacterials: possibly reduces absorption of quinolones – give at least 2 hours before or 4 hours after lanthanum.
- Antifungals: absorption of ketoconazole reduced – give at least 2 hours apart.
- Antimalarials: absorption of chloroquine and hydroxychloroquine possibly reduced – give at least 2 hours apart.
- Thyroid hormones: reduces absorption of levothyroxine – give at least 2 hours apart.

ADMINISTRATION

RECONSTITUTION
–
ROUTE
- Oral
RATE OF ADMINISTRATION
–
COMMENTS
- Must be chewed WITH food; do not take before meals.

OTHER INFORMATION

- Following ingestion, lanthanum carbonate is converted in the GI tract to the insoluble lanthanum phosphate, which is not readily absorbed into the blood.
- Tablets can be crushed and put down a NG tube. (Kitajima Y, Takahashi T, Sato Y, Nakaya Y. Efficacy of crushed lanthanum carbonate for hyperphosphataemia in hemodialysis patients undergoing tube feeding. *Nephrol Dial Transplant.* 2011; 4: 253–5.)
- Sachets should be mixed with soft food and consumed within 15 minutes.
- Bioavailability of drugs administered concomitantly may be reduced due to binding by lanthanum carbonate.
- Very little is absorbed.
- If not taken with meals, may result in vomiting.

Lapatinib

CLINICAL USE

Tyrosine kinase inhibitor
● Treatment of advanced or metastatic breast cancer in combination with capecitabine

DOSE IN NORMAL RENAL FUNCTION

1.25 g daily
In combination with an aromatase inhibitor: 1.5 g once daily

PHARMACOKINETICS

Molecular weight (daltons)	943.5 (as tosilate)
% Protein binding	>99
% Excreted unchanged in urine	<2
Volume of distribution (L/kg)	No data
Half-life – normal/ ESRF (hrs)	24/–

METABOLISM

Extensive hepatic metabolism, mainly by cytochrome P450 isoenzymes CYP3A4 and CYP3A5; CYP2C19 and CYP2C8 account for some minor metabolism.

About 27% and 14% of an oral dose is recovered in the faeces, as parent lapatinib and metabolites, respectively; renal excretion is negligible.

DOSE IN RENAL IMPAIRMENT GFR (mL/MIN)

20–50	Dose as in normal renal function.
10–20	Dose as in normal renal function.
<10	Dose as in normal renal function. Use with caution.

DOSE IN PATIENTS UNDERGOING RENAL REPLACEMENT THERAPIES

CAPD	Unlikely dialysability. Dose as in GFR<10 mL/min.
HD	Unlikely dialysability. Dose as in GFR<10 mL/min.
HDF/High flux	Unlikely dialysability. Dose as in GFR<10 mL/min.
CAV/ VVHD	Unlikely dialysability. Dose as in normal renal function.

IMPORTANT DRUG INTERACTIONS

Potentially hazardous interactions with other drugs
● Antibacterials: avoid concomitant use with rifabutin, rifampicin and telithromycin.
● Antidepressants: avoid concomitant use with St John's wort.
● Antidiabetics: avoid concomitant use with repaglinide.
● Antiepileptics: concentration reduced by carbamazepine, avoid concomitant use; possibly reduced phenytoin concentration, avoid concomitant use.
● Antifungals: concentration increased by ketoconazole, avoid concomitant use; avoid concomitant use with itraconazole, posaconazole and voriconazole.
● Antipsychotics: avoid concomitant use with clozapine (increased risk of agranulocytosis); avoid concomitant use with pimozide.
● Antivirals: avoid concomitant use with boceprevir, ritonavir and saquinavir.
● Cytotoxics: concentration of pazopanib increased; possible increased risk of neutropenia with docetaxel and paclitaxel; concentration of active metabolite of irinotecan increased, consider reducing irinotecan dose.
● Grapefruit juice: avoid concomitant use.

ADMINISTRATION

RECONSTITUTION
–
ROUTE
● Oral
RATE OF ADMINISTRATION
–
COMMENTS
● Take either at least one hour before, or at least one hour after food; food increases absorption.

OTHER INFORMATION

● No experience in severe renal impairment hence use with caution.

Leflunomide

CLINICAL USE

Disease modifying agent
- Active rheumatoid arthritis
- Psoriatic arthritis

DOSE IN NORMAL RENAL FUNCTION

- Rheumatoid arthritis: 100 mg daily for 3 days then 10–20 mg daily
- Psoriatic arthritis: 100 mg daily for 3 days then 20 mg daily

PHARMACOKINETICS

Molecular weight (daltons)	270.2
% Protein binding	>99
% Excreted unchanged in urine	0
Volume of distribution (L/kg)	11 litres
Half-life – normal/ ESRF (hrs)	2 weeks (metabolite)/ Unchanged

METABOLISM

After oral doses leflunomide undergoes rapid first-pass metabolism in the liver and gut wall to teriflunomide (A-771726), which is responsible for the majority of the *in vivo* activity. Teriflunomide is mostly eliminated as unchanged drug in the bile and as metabolites in the urine. It is thought to undergo enterohepatic recycling and has an elimination half-life of about 18 to 19 days after repeated oral doses.

DOSE IN RENAL IMPAIRMENT GFR (mL/MIN)

20–50	Dose as in normal renal function.
10–20	Use with caution. See 'Other information'.
<10	Use with caution. See 'Other information'.

DOSE IN PATIENTS UNDERGOING RENAL REPLACEMENT THERAPIES

CAPD	Not dialysed. Use with caution.
HD	Not dialysed. Use with caution.
HDF/High flux	Not dialysed. Use with caution.
CAV/ VVHD	Not dialysed. Use with caution.

IMPORTANT DRUG INTERACTIONS

Potentially hazardous interactions with other drugs
- Hepatotoxic or haemotoxic drugs: increased risk of toxicity.
- Cytotoxics: risk of toxicity with methotrexate.
- Lipid-lowering agents: effect significantly reduced by cholestyramine – avoid.
- Live vaccines: avoid concomitant use.

ADMINISTRATION

RECONSTITUTION
–
ROUTE
- Oral
RATE OF ADMINISTRATION
–
COMMENTS
- Administer with food.

OTHER INFORMATION

- Contraindicated in moderate to severe renal impairment by UK manufacturer due to insufficient evidence.
- US licence says it can be used in renal impairment with caution.
- Protein binding is variable in CKD.
- In haemodialysis and PD the free fraction of the active metabolite in plasma is doubled.
- A case study from Beaman used leflunomide in a haemodialysis patient at a dose of 100 mg loading dose followed by 10 mg daily which was later increased to 20 mg daily but then reduced to 15 mg daily due to altered hepatic function. He concluded that it could be safely used in haemodialysis patients. (Beaman JM, Hackett LP, Luxton G, *et al.* Effect of hemodialysis on leflunomide plasma concentrations. *Ann Pharmacother.* 2002 Jan; **36**(1): 75–7.)

Lenalidomide

CLINICAL USE

Treatment of multiple myeloma in combination with dexamethasone and myelodysplastic syndrome

DOSE IN NORMAL RENAL FUNCTION

- Myeloma: 25 mg daily on days 1–21 of a 28 day cycle; reduce dose if patient has neutropenia or thrombocytopenia; see data sheet.
- Myelodysplastic syndrome: 10 mg once daily initially, dose is then adjusted according to neutropenia and thrombocytopenia.

PHARMACOKINETICS

Molecular weight (daltons)	259.3
% Protein binding	22.7–29.2
% Excreted unchanged in urine	65–85
Volume of distribution (L/kg)	86 litres
Half-life – normal/ ESRF (hrs)	3.5/>9

METABOLISM

Lenalidomide is poorly metabolised as 82% of the dose is excreted unchanged in urine. Hydroxy-lenalidomide and N-acetyl-lenalidomide represent 4.59% and 1.83% of the excreted dose, respectively. The renal clearance of lenalidomide exceeds the glomerular filtration rate and therefore is at least actively secreted to some extent. Approximately 4% of lenalidomide is eliminated in faeces.

DOSE IN RENAL IMPAIRMENT GFR (mL/MIN)

30–50	Myeloma: 10 mg daily, increasing to 15 mg after 2 cycles if patient is not responding. Myelodysplastic syndrome: Initially 5 mg once daily.
<30	Myeloma: 15 mg every 48 hours, can be increased to 10 mg daily if patient is not responding. Myelodysplastic syndrome: Initially 2.5 mg once daily.

DOSE IN PATIENTS UNDERGOING RENAL REPLACEMENT THERAPIES

CAPD	Probably dialysed. Myeloma: 15 mg 2–3 times a week or 5 mg daily; Myelodysplastic syndrome: Dose as in GFR<30 mL/min.
HD	Probably dialysed. Myeloma: 15 mg 2–3 times a week post dialysis or 5 mg daily; Myelodysplastic syndrome: Dose as in GFR<30 mL/min.
HDF/High flux	Probably dialysed. Myeloma: 15 mg 2–3 times a week post dialysis or 5 mg daily; Myelodysplastic syndrome: Dose as in GFR<30 mL/min.
CAV/ VVHD	Probably dialysed. Dose as in GFR=30–50 mL/min.

IMPORTANT DRUG INTERACTIONS

Potentially hazardous interactions with other drugs
- Cardiac glycosides: possibly increases concentration of digoxin.

ADMINISTRATION

RECONSTITUTION
–

ROUTE
- Oral

RATE OF ADMINISTRATION
–

COMMENTS
–

OTHER INFORMATION

- May cause acute renal failure – monitor renal function during treatment.
- Patients with renal impairment are more likely to develop side effects.

Lenograstim

CLINICAL USE

Recombinant human granulocyte-colony
stimulating factor (rHuG-CSF):
- Reduction of duration of neutropenia

DOSE IN NORMAL RENAL FUNCTION

- Cytotoxic neutropenia: 150 mcg/m^2
  (19.2 MIU/m^2) daily SC
- Mobilisation of peripheral blood
  progenitor cells: 10 mcg/kg (1.28 MIU/
  kg) daily
- Bone marrow transplant: 150 mcg/m^2
  (19.2 MIU/m^2) daily as an IV infusion or
  SC injection

PHARMACOKINETICS

Molecular weight (daltons)	20 000
% Protein binding	No data
% Excreted unchanged in urine	<1
Volume of distribution (L/kg)	1
Half-life – normal/ ESRF (hrs)	3–4

METABOLISM

Lenograstim is primarily eliminated by
the kidney and neutrophils/neutrophil
precursors; the latter presumably involves
binding of the growth factor to the G-CSF
receptor on the cell surface, internalisation
of the growth factor-receptor complexes via
endocytosis, and subsequent degradation
inside the cells. During chemotherapy-
induced neutropenia, the clearance of
lenograstim is significantly reduced and the
concentration of lenograstim is sustained
until onset of neutrophil recovery.

DOSE IN RENAL IMPAIRMENT GFR (mL/MIN)

20–50	Dose as in normal renal function.
10–20	Dose as in normal renal function.
<10	Dose as in normal renal function.

DOSE IN PATIENTS UNDERGOING RENAL REPLACEMENT THERAPIES

CAPD	Not dialysed. Dose as in normal renal function.
HD	Not dialysed. Dose as in normal renal function.
HDF/High flux	Unlikely to be dialysed. Dose as in normal renal function.
CAV/ VVHD	Not dialysed. Dose as in normal renal function.

IMPORTANT DRUG INTERACTIONS

Potentially hazardous interactions with other
drugs
- None known

ADMINISTRATION

RECONSTITUTION
- Water for injection (1 mL)
ROUTE
- SC, IV
RATE OF ADMINISTRATION
- 30 minutes
COMMENTS
- Dilute lenograstim-13.4 in up to 50 mL
  sodium chloride 0.9%.
- Dilute lenograstim-33.6 in up to 100 mL
  sodium chloride 0.9%.

Lercanidipine hydrochloride

CLINICAL USE

Calcium-channel antagonist
- Mild to moderate hypertension

DOSE IN NORMAL RENAL FUNCTION

10–20 mg daily

PHARMACOKINETICS

Molecular weight (daltons)	648.2
% Protein binding	>98
% Excreted unchanged in urine	50 (as metabolites)
Volume of distribution (L/kg)	No data
Half-life – normal/ ESRF (hrs)	8–10/Increased

METABOLISM

Lercanidipine undergoes extensive first pass metabolism. Lercanidipine is extensively metabolised by CYP3A4; no parent drug is found in the urine or the faeces. It is predominantly converted to inactive metabolites and about 50% of the dose is excreted in the urine, and 50% via the faeces.

DOSE IN RENAL IMPAIRMENT GFR (mL/MIN)

20–50	Use small doses and titrate to response.
10–20	Use small doses and titrate to response.
<10	Use small doses and titrate to response.

DOSE IN PATIENTS UNDERGOING RENAL REPLACEMENT THERAPIES

CAPD	Unlikely to be dialysed. Dose as in GFR<10 mL/min.
HD	Unknown dialysability. Dose as in GFR<10 mL/min.
HDF/High flux	Unknown dialysability. Dose as in GFR<10 mL/min.
CAV/ VVHD	Unlikely to be dialysed. Dose as in GFR=10–20 mL/min.

IMPORTANT DRUG INTERACTIONS

Potentially hazardous interactions with other drugs
- Anaesthetics: enhanced hypotensive effect.
- Antibacterials: metabolism possibly inhibited by clarithromycin, erythromycin & telithromycin avoid concomitant use with erythromycin.
- Antidepressants: enhanced hypotensive effect with MAOIs.
- Anti-epileptics: effect reduced by carbamazepine, barbiturates, phenytoin and primidone.
- Antifungals: metabolism possibly inhibited by itraconazole and ketoconazole – avoid concomitant use; negative inotropic effect possibly increased with itraconazole.
- Antihypertensives: enhanced hypotensive effect, increased risk of first dose hypotensive effect of post-synaptic alpha-blockers.
- Antivirals: concentration increased by ritonavir – avoid concomitant use.
- Cardiac glycosides: digoxin concentration increased.
- Ciclosporin: concentration of both drugs may be increased – avoid concomitant use.
- Grapefruit juice: concentration increased – avoid concomitant use.
- Theophylline: possibly increased theophylline concentration.

ADMINISTRATION

RECONSTITUTION
–
ROUTE
- Oral
RATE OF ADMINISTRATION
–
COMMENTS
- Take before food.

OTHER INFORMATION

Causes less peripheral oedema than other calcium-channel blockers.

Letrozole

CLINICAL USE

Treatment of breast cancer

DOSE IN NORMAL RENAL FUNCTION

2.5 mg daily

PHARMACOKINETICS

Molecular weight (daltons)	285.3
% Protein binding	60
% Excreted unchanged in urine	6
Volume of distribution (L/kg)	1.87
Half-life – normal/ ESRF (hrs)	48/Unchanged

METABOLISM

Metabolic clearance via the cytochrome P450 isoenzymes 3A4 and 2A6 to a pharmacologically inactive carbinol metabolite is the major elimination pathway of letrozole. Formation of minor unidentified metabolites and direct renal and faecal excretion play only a minor role in the overall elimination of letrozole. Within 2 weeks after administration of 2.5 mg ^{14}C-labelled letrozole to healthy postmenopausal volunteers, 88.2±7.6% of the radioactivity was recovered in urine and 3.8±0.9% in faeces. At least 75% of the radioactivity recovered in urine up to 216 hours (84.7±7.8% of the dose) was attributed to the glucuronide of the carbinol metabolite, about 9% to two unidentified metabolites, and 6% to unchanged letrozole.

DOSE IN RENAL IMPAIRMENT GFR (mL/MIN)

20–50	Dose as in normal renal function.
10–20	Dose as in normal renal function.
<10	Dose as in normal renal function. See 'Other information'.

DOSE IN PATIENTS UNDERGOING RENAL REPLACEMENT THERAPIES

CAPD	Probably dialysed. Dose as in GFR<10 mL/min.
HD	Dialysed. Dose as in GFR<10 mL/min.
HDF/High flux	Dialysed. Dose as in GFR<10 mL/min.
CAV/ VVHD	Probably dialysed. Dose as in normal renal function.

IMPORTANT DRUG INTERACTIONS

Potentially hazardous interactions with other drugs
- None known

ADMINISTRATION

RECONSTITUTION

–

ROUTE
- Oral

RATE OF ADMINISTRATION

–

COMMENTS

–

OTHER INFORMATION

- Manufacturer advises to use with caution if GFR<10 mL/min due to lack of data. In studies down to a GFR of 9 mL/min there were no differences in the pharmacokinetics of letrozole.
- From personal experience, letrozole can be used in patients with end-stage renal impairment and those on renal replacement therapies in normal doses.

Leuprorelin acetate

CLINICAL USE

Treatment of advanced prostate cancer and endometriosis

DOSE IN NORMAL RENAL FUNCTION

- 11.25 mg every 3 months (SC depot injection, prostate cancer only).
- Or 3.75 mg every 4 weeks.
- Endometriosis: 3.75 mg every month or 11.25 mg every 3 months for maximum 6 months (not to be repeated).

PHARMACOKINETICS

Molecular weight (daltons)	1269.5
% Protein binding	43–49
% Excreted unchanged in urine	<5 (+ metabolites)
Volume of distribution (L/kg)	27 litres
Half-life – normal/ ESRF (hrs)	3/Increased

METABOLISM

Leuprorelin binds to the LHRH receptors and is rapidly degraded by peptidases, then excreted in the urine.

DOSE IN RENAL IMPAIRMENT GFR (mL/MIN)

20–50	Dose as in normal renal function.
10–20	Dose as in normal renal function.
<10	Dose as in normal renal function.

DOSE IN PATIENTS UNDERGOING RENAL REPLACEMENT THERAPIES

CAPD	Unlikely to be dialysed. Dose as in normal renal function.
HD	Unlikely to be dialysed. Dose as in normal renal function.
HDF/High flux	Unknown dialysability. Dose as in normal renal function.
CAV/ VVHD	Unlikely to be dialysed. Dose as in normal renal function.

IMPORTANT DRUG INTERACTIONS

Potentially hazardous interactions with other drugs
- None known

ADMINISTRATION

RECONSTITUTION
- With diluent provided
ROUTE
- IM, SC depot
RATE OF ADMINISTRATION
–
COMMENTS
–

OTHER INFORMATION

- Women on dialysis may be at greater risk of ovarian hyperstimulation, possibly because dialysis affects circulating leuprorelin concentration so endogenous gonadotrophins were still excreted. Alternatively, haemodialysis patients may have increased responsiveness to endogenous gonadotrophins.

Levamisole (unlicensed product)

CLINICAL USE

Treatment of roundworm (*Ascaris lumbricoides*)

DOSE IN NORMAL RENAL FUNCTION

2.5 mg/kg as a single dose

PHARMACOKINETICS

Molecular weight (daltons)	204.3
% Protein binding	19–26
% Excreted unchanged in urine	5
Volume of distribution (L/kg)	100–120 litres
Half-life – normal/ ESRF (hrs)	3–4 (16 for metabolites)/–

METABOLISM

Levamisole is extensively metabolised in the liver. It is excreted mainly in the urine as metabolites and a small proportion in the faeces. About 70% of a dose is excreted in the urine over 3 days, with about 5% as unchanged levamisole.

DOSE IN RENAL IMPAIRMENT GFR (mL/MIN)

20–50	Dose as in normal renal function.
10–20	Dose as in normal renal function.
<10	Dose as in normal renal function.

DOSE IN PATIENTS UNDERGOING RENAL REPLACEMENT THERAPIES

CAPD	Unknown dialysability. Dose as in normal renal function.
HD	Unknown dialysability. Dose as in normal renal function.
HDF/High flux	Unknown dialysability. Dose as in normal renal function.
CAV/ VVHD	Unknown dialysability. Dose as in normal renal function.

IMPORTANT DRUG INTERACTIONS

Potentially hazardous interactions with other drugs
- Alcohol: may produce a disulfiram-like reaction
- Phenytoin: increased levels of phenytoin have been reported
- Warfarin: enhanced INR

ADMINISTRATION

RECONSTITUTION

–

ROUTE
- Oral

RATE OF ADMINISTRATION

–

COMMENTS

–

OTHER INFORMATION

- Available on a named patient basis from IDIS.
- Avoid in patients with pre-existing blood disorders.
- Has been successfully used to treat relapsing nephrotic syndrome in children at a dose of 2.5 mg/kg/alternate day. (Al-Saran K, Mirza K, Al-Ghanam G, *et al.* Experience with levamisole in frequently relapsing, steroid-dependent nephritic syndrome. *Pediatr Nephrol.* 2006 Feb; **21**(2): 201–5).
- Has also been used in haemodialysis patients to enhance response to hepatitis B vaccine at a dose of 80 mg after each dialysis session for 4 months. (Kayatas M. Levamisole treatment enhances protective antibody response to hepatitis B vaccine in hemodialysis patients. *Artif Organs.* 2002 Jun; **26**(6): 492–6.)

Levetiracetam

CLINICAL USE

Anti-epileptic agent

DOSE IN NORMAL RENAL FUNCTION

250 mg – 1.5 g twice daily

PHARMACOKINETICS

Molecular weight (daltons)	170.2
% Protein binding	<10
% Excreted unchanged in urine	66 (95% drug + metabolite)
Volume of distribution (L/kg)	0.5–0.7
Half-life – normal/ ESRF (hrs)	6–8/25

METABOLISM

Levetiracetam is not extensively metabolised in humans. The major metabolic pathway (24% of the dose) is an enzymatic hydrolysis of the acetamide group, to form the primary metabolite, ucb L057, which is pharmacologically inactive.

Two minor metabolites have also been identified. One was obtained by hydroxylation of the pyrrolidone ring (1.6% of the dose) and the other one by opening of the pyrrolidone ring (0.9% of the dose).

The major route of excretion was via urine, accounting for a mean 95% of the dose (approximately 93% of the dose was excreted within 48 hours). The cumulative urinary excretion of levetiracetam and its primary metabolite accounted for 66% and 24% of the dose, respectively, during the first 48 hours. Excretion via faeces accounted for only 0.3% of the dose.

Levetiracetam is excreted by glomerular filtration with subsequent tubular reabsorption and that the primary metabolite is also excreted by active tubular secretion in addition to glomerular filtration.

DOSE IN RENAL IMPAIRMENT GFR (mL/MIN)

50–79	500–1000 mg twice daily
30–49	250–750 mg twice daily
<30	250–500 mg twice daily

DOSE IN PATIENTS UNDERGOING RENAL REPLACEMENT THERAPIES

CAPD	Likely dialysability. 750 mg loading dose then 500–1000 mg daily.
HD	Dialysed. 750 mg loading dose then 500–1000 mg once daily.
HDF/High flux	Dialysed. 750 mg loading dose then 500–1000 mg once daily.
CAV/ VVHD	Likely dialysability. Dose as in GFR=30–49 mL/min.

IMPORTANT DRUG INTERACTIONS

Potentially hazardous interactions with other drugs

- Antidepressants: antagonism of anticonvulsant effect (convulsive threshold lowered); avoid with St John's wort.
- Antimalarials: mefloquine antagonises anticonvulsant effect.
- Antipsychotics: convulsant effect antagonised.
- Orlistat: possibly increased risk of convulsions.

ADMINISTRATION

RECONSTITUTION

–

ROUTE

- Oral, IV

RATE OF ADMINISTRATION

- 15 minutes

COMMENTS

- Dilute in 100 mL sodium chloride or glucose 5%.

OTHER INFORMATION

- 51% of the dose is removed with 4 hours of haemodialysis.
- The inactive metabolite (ucb L057) accumulates in renal failure.

Levocetirizine hydrochloride

CLINICAL USE

Antihistamine
- Symptomatic relief of allergy such as hay fever, urticaria

DOSE IN NORMAL RENAL FUNCTION

5 mg daily

PHARMACOKINETICS

Molecular weight (daltons)	461.8
% Protein binding	90
% Excreted unchanged in urine	85.4 (includes metabolites)
Volume of distribution (L/kg)	0.4
Half-life – normal/ ESRF (hrs)	6–9.8/Increased

METABOLISM

The extent of metabolism of levocetirizine in humans is less than 14% of the dose. Metabolic pathways include aromatic oxidation, N- and O-dealkylation and taurine conjugation. Dealkylation pathways are primarily mediated by CYP 3A4 while aromatic oxidation involved multiple and/or unidentified CYP isoforms. The major route of excretion of levocetirizine and metabolites is via urine, accounting for a mean of 85.4% of the dose. Excretion via faeces accounts for only 12.9% of the dose. Levocetirizine is excreted both by glomerular filtration and active tubular secretion.

DOSE IN RENAL IMPAIRMENT GFR (mL/MIN)

30–50	5 mg every 48 hours. See 'Other information'.
10–30	5 mg every 72 hours. See 'Other information'.
<10	5 mg every 72 hours. See 'Other information'.

DOSE IN PATIENTS UNDERGOING RENAL REPLACEMENT THERAPIES

CAPD	Unlikely dialysability. Dose as in GFR<10 mL/min.
HD	Not dialysed. Dose as in GFR<10 mL/min.
HDF/High flux	Unknown dialysability. Dose as in GFR<10 mL/min.
CAV/ VVHD	Unlikely dialysability. Dose as in GFR=10–30 mL/min.

IMPORTANT DRUG INTERACTIONS

Potentially hazardous interactions with other drugs
- Antivirals: concentration possibly increased by ritonavir

ADMINISTRATION

RECONSTITUTION
–
ROUTE
- Oral
RATE OF ADMINISTRATION
–
COMMENTS
–

OTHER INFORMATION

- Manufacturer recommends to avoid in GFR<10 mL/min, but anecdotally it has been used at normal dose in haemodialysis patients.
- Less than 10% is removed during a 4 hour haemodialysis session.

Levofloxacin

CLINICAL USE

Antibacterial agent

DOSE IN NORMAL RENAL FUNCTION

250–500 mg once or twice a day (varies depending on indication).

PHARMACOKINETICS

Molecular weight (daltons)	361.4
% Protein binding	30–40
% Excreted unchanged in urine	>85
Volume of distribution (L/kg)	1.1–1.5
Half-life – normal/ ESRF (hrs)	6–8/35

METABOLISM

Levofloxacin is metabolised to a very small extent, the metabolites being desmethyl-levofloxacin and levofloxacin N-oxide. These metabolites account for <5% of the dose and are excreted in urine. Excretion is primarily by the renal route (>85% of the administered dose).

DOSE IN RENAL IMPAIRMENT GFR (mL/MIN)

20–50	Initial dose 250–500 mg then 125 mg 12–24 hourly. See 'Other information'.
10–20	Initial dose 250–500 mg then 125 mg 12–48 hourly. See 'Other information'.
<10	Initial dose 250–500 mg then 125 mg 12–48 hourly. See 'Other information'.

DOSE IN PATIENTS UNDERGOING RENAL REPLACEMENT THERAPIES

CAPD	Not dialysed. Dose as in GFR<10 mL/min.
HD	Not dialysed. Dose as in GFR<10 mL/min.
HDF/High flux	Not dialysed. Dose as in GFR<10 mL/min.
CAV/ VVHD	Not dialysed. Loading dose: 500 mg then 250 mg every 24 hours.[1]

IMPORTANT DRUG INTERACTIONS

Potentially hazardous interactions with other drugs

- Analgesics: possibly increased risk of convulsions with NSAIDs.
- Anti-arrhythmics: increased risk of ventricular arrhythmias with amiodarone – avoid.
- Anticoagulants: anticoagulant effect of coumarins and phenindione enhanced.
- Antimalarials: manufacturer advises avoid concomitant use with artemether and lumefantrine.
- Ciclosporin: half-life of ciclosporin increased by 33%; increased risk of nephrotoxicity.
- Cytotoxics: increased risk of ventricular arrhythmias with arsenic trioxide.
- Tacrolimus: may increase tacrolimus concentration.
- Theophylline: possibly increased risk of convulsions.

ADMINISTRATION

RECONSTITUTION
–
ROUTE
- Oral, IV
RATE OF ADMINISTRATION
- 30 minutes per 250 mg
COMMENTS
–

OTHER INFORMATION

- Dose and frequency depend on indication.
- *Drug Prescribing in Renal Failure*, 5th edition, by Aronoff *et al.* suggests:
  — GFR=10–50 mL/min: 500–750 mg stat followed by 250–750 mg every 24–48 hours
  — GFR<10 mL/min: 500 mg stat followed by 250–500 mg every 48 hours.

Reference:
1. Trotman RL, Williamson JC, Shoemaker DM, *et al.* Antibiotic dosing in critically ill adult patients receiving continuous renal replacement therapy. *Clin Infect Dis.* 2005 Oct 15; **41**: 1159–66.

Levomepromazine (methotrimeprazine)

CLINICAL USE

- Treatment of schizophrenia
- Adjunctive treatment in palliative care
- Nausea and vomiting

DOSE IN NORMAL RENAL FUNCTION

- Schizophrenia: Oral, initially 25–50 mg daily, increasing to 100–200 mg in 3 divided doses; maximum dose 1 g daily.
- Palliative care:
  - Oral/SC: 12.5–50 mg every 4–8 hours
  - IM/IV: 12.5–50 mg every 6–8 hours
  - SC Infusion: 5–200 mg daily

PHARMACOKINETICS

Molecular weight (daltons)	328.5
% Protein binding	No data
% Excreted unchanged in urine	1
Volume of distribution (L/kg)	23–42
Half-life – normal/ ESRF (hrs)	30/–

METABOLISM

Levomepromazine is metabolised in the liver and degraded to a sulfoxide, a glucuronide and a demethyl-moiety. It is eliminated via urine and faeces.

DOSE IN RENAL IMPAIRMENT GFR (mL/MIN)

20–50	Dose as in normal renal function.
10–20	Dose as in normal renal function.
<10	Start with small dose and increase as necessary.

DOSE IN PATIENTS UNDERGOING RENAL REPLACEMENT THERAPIES

CAPD	Unknown dialysability. Dose as in GFR<10 mL/min.
HD	Unknown dialysability. Dose as in GFR<10 mL/min.
HDF/High flux	Unknown dialysability. Dose as in GFR<10 mL/min.
CAV/ VVHD	Unknown dialysability. Dose as in normal renal function.

IMPORTANT DRUG INTERACTIONS

Potentially hazardous interactions with other drugs

- Anaesthetics: enhanced hypotensive effect.
- Analgesics: increased risk of convulsions with tramadol; increased hypotension and sedation with opioid analgesics.
- Anti-arrhythmics: increased risk of ventricular arrhythmias due to prolongation of QT interval; increased risk of ventricular arrhythmias with amiodarone, disopyramide and dronedarone – avoid concomitant use.
- Antibacterials: increased risk of ventricular arrhythmias with moxifloxacin – avoid concomitant administration.
- Antidepressants: possibly increased concentration of tricyclics, increased antimuscarinic effects and ventricular arrhythmias; avoid concomitant administration with MAOIs (2 fatalities have been reported).
- Anticonvulsant: lowers anticonvulsant threshold.
- Antimalarials: avoid concomitant use with artemether/lumefantrine.
- Antipsychotics: increased risk of ventricular arrhythmias with pimozide – avoid concomitant use.
- Antivirals: concentration possibly increased by ritonavir.
- Antihypertensives: enhanced hypotensive effect; increased risk of ventricular arrhythmias with sotalol.
- Antimalarials: avoid concomitant use with artemether/lumefantrine and piperaquine with artenimol.
- Antipsychotics: increased risk of ventricular arrhythmias with droperidol – avoid concomitant use.
- Anxiolytics and hypnotics: increased sedation.
- Cytotoxics: increased risk of ventricular arrhythmias with arsenic trioxide.
- Diuretics: enhanced hypotensive effect.
- Lithium: increased risk of extrapyramidal effects and neurotoxicity.
- Pentamidine: increased risk of ventricular arrhythmias – avoid concomitant use.

ADMINISTRATION

RECONSTITUTION

–

ROUTE

- Oral, IV, IM, SC

RATE OF ADMINISTRATION

–

COMMENTS

- For a subcutaneous infusion dilute in sodium chloride 0.9% and give via a syringe driver.
- Compatible with diamorphine.
- For IV injection, dilute with an equal volume of sodium chloride 0.9%.

OTHER INFORMATION

- In renal disease there is an increased risk of cerebral sensitivity.

Levothyroxine sodium (thyroxine)

CLINICAL USE

Hypothyroidism

DOSE IN NORMAL RENAL FUNCTION

25–300 micrograms daily depending on thyroid hormone levels

PHARMACOKINETICS

Molecular weight (daltons)	798.9
% Protein binding	99.97
% Excreted unchanged in urine	30–55
Volume of distribution (L/kg)	8.7–9.7
Half-life – normal/ ESRF (hrs)	6–7 days/Unchanged

METABOLISM

Levothyroxine is mainly metabolised in the liver and kidney to triiodothyronine (liothyronine) and, about 40%, to inactive reverse triiodothyronine (reverse T_3), both of which undergo further deiodination to inactive metabolites. Further metabolites result from conjugation and decarboxylation; tetra-iodothyroacetic acid (tetrac) is one such metabolite. Further hydrolysis of the conjugates releases free hormone, which can be reabsorbed in the intestine to undergo enterohepatic recycling. Some conjugates reach the colon unchanged, then undergo hydrolysis, and are eliminated in the faeces as free hormone. Levothyroxine is mainly eliminated by the kidneys as free drug, deiodinated metabolites, or conjugates.

DOSE IN RENAL IMPAIRMENT GFR (mL/MIN)

20–50	Dose as in normal renal function.
10–20	Dose as in normal renal function.
<10	Dose as in normal renal function.

DOSE IN PATIENTS UNDERGOING RENAL REPLACEMENT THERAPIES

CAPD	Not dialysed. Dose as in normal renal function.
HD	Not dialysed. Dose as in normal renal function.
HDF/High flux	Not dialysed. Dose as in normal renal function.
CAV/ VVHD	Not dialysed. Dose as in normal renal function.

IMPORTANT DRUG INTERACTIONS

Potentially hazardous interactions with other drugs

- Anticoagulants: effect of coumarins and phenindione enhanced.
- Lanthanum: absorption reduced by lanthanum, give at least 2 hours apart.
- Sevelamer: absorption reduced by sevelamer.

ADMINISTRATION

RECONSTITUTION

–

ROUTE

- Oral

RATE OF ADMINISTRATION

–

COMMENTS

–

OTHER INFORMATION

- Uraemic toxins may result in inhibition of the enzyme associated with conversion of L-thyroxine to liothyronine.

Lidocaine hydrochloride (Lignocaine)

CLINICAL USE

- Local anaesthetic
- Ventricular arrhythmias

DOSE IN NORMAL RENAL FUNCTION

- Local anaesthetic: usually 1% or 2% solutions used, according to patient's weight and procedure.
- Ventricular arrhythmias: 100 mg as a bolus in patients without gross circulatory impairment (50 mg in lighter patients or in severely impaired circulation), followed by an infusion of 4 mg/min for 30 minutes, 2 mg/min for 2 hours, then 1 mg/min or according to local policy.

PHARMACOKINETICS

Molecular weight (daltons)	288.8
% Protein binding	66
% Excreted unchanged in urine	<10
Volume of distribution (L/kg)	1.3
Half-life – normal/ ESRF (hrs)	1–2/1.3–3

METABOLISM

Lidocaine is largely metabolised in the liver. First-pass metabolism is extensive and bioavailability is about 35% after oral doses. Metabolism in the liver is rapid and about 90% of a given dose is dealkylated to form monoethylglycinexylidide and glycinexylidide. Both of these metabolites may contribute to the therapeutic and toxic effects of lidocaine and since their half-lives are longer than that of lidocaine, accumulation, particularly of glycinexylidide, may occur during prolonged infusions. Further metabolism occurs and metabolites are excreted in the urine with less than 10% of unchanged lidocaine.

DOSE IN RENAL IMPAIRMENT GFR (mL/MIN)

20–50	Dose as in normal renal function.
10–20	Dose as in normal renal function.
<10	Dose as in normal renal function.

DOSE IN PATIENTS UNDERGOING RENAL REPLACEMENT THERAPIES

CAPD	Unlikely to be dialysed. Dose as in normal renal function.
HD	Not dialysed. Dose as in normal renal function.
HDF/High flux	Unknown dialysability. Dose as in normal renal function.
CAV/ VVHD	Not dialysed. Dose as in normal renal function.

IMPORTANT DRUG INTERACTIONS

Potentially hazardous interactions with other drugs

- Anti-arrhythmics: increased risk of myocardial depression.
- Antipsychotics: increased risk of ventricular arrhythmias with antipsychotics that prolong the QT interval.
- Antivirals: concentration possibly increased by atazanavir, darunavir, fosamprenavir and lopinavir – avoid concomitant use with amprenavir and darunavir; increased risk of ventricular arrhythmias with saquinavir – avoid; use IV lidocaine with caution with telaprevir.
- Beta-blockers: increased risk of myocardial depression; increased risk of lidocaine toxicity with propranolol.
- Diuretics: effects antagonised by hypokalaemia.
- Ulcer-healing drugs: concentration increased by cimetidine, increased toxicity.

ADMINISTRATION

RECONSTITUTION

–

ROUTE

- IV, SC, topical

RATE OF ADMINISTRATION

- According to dose

COMMENTS

- Usually 1–2 mg/mL in glucose 5%
- Minimum volume 8–20 mg/mL but watch for extravasation. (UK Critical Care Group, *Minimum Infusion Volumes for Fluid Restricted Critically Ill Patients*, 3rd edition, 2006.

OTHER INFORMATION

- IV injection only lasts for 15–20 minutes.
- Pharmacokinetic data: Lee CS, Marbury TC. Drug therapy in patients undergoing haemodialysis: clinical pharmacokinetic considerations. *Clin Pharmacokinet*. 1984; **9**: 42–66.

Linagliptin

CLINICAL USE

Type-2 diabetes mellitus

DOSE IN NORMAL RENAL FUNCTION

5 mg once daily

PHARMACOKINETICS

Molecular weight (daltons)	472.6
% Protein binding	75–99 (concentration dependent)
% Excreted unchanged in urine	5
Volume of distribution (L/kg)	1110 litres
Half-life – normal/ ESRF (hrs)	12/–

METABOLISM

Minimal metabolism to inactive metabolites. Approximately 80% is eliminated in the faeces and 5% in the urine.

DOSE IN RENAL IMPAIRMENT GFR (mL/MIN)

20–50	Dose as in normal renal function.
10–20	Dose as in normal renal function.
<10	Dose as in normal renal function.

DOSE IN PATIENTS UNDERGOING RENAL REPLACEMENT THERAPIES

CAPD	Not dialysed. Dose as in normal renal function.
HD	Not dialysed. Dose as in normal renal function.
HDF/High flux	Not dialysed. Dose as in normal renal function.
CAV/ VVHD	Not dialysed. Dose as in normal renal function.

IMPORTANT DRUG INTERACTIONS

Potentially hazardous interactions with other drugs
- Antibacterials: effects possibly reduced by rifampicin.

ADMINISTRATION

RECONSTITUTION

–

ROUTE
- Oral

RATE OF ADMINISTRATION

–

OTHER INFORMATION

- Bioavailability is 30%.
- In moderate renal failure, a moderate increase in exposure of about 1.7 fold was observed compared with control. Exposure in T2DM patients with severe renal failure was increased by about 1.4 fold compared to T2DM patients with normal renal function. Steady-state predictions for AUC of linagliptin in patients with ESRD indicated comparable exposure to that of patients with moderate or severe renal impairment.

Linezolid

CLINICAL USE

Antibacterial agent

DOSE IN NORMAL RENAL FUNCTION

600 mg twice daily

PHARMACOKINETICS

Molecular weight (daltons)	337.3
% Protein binding	31
% Excreted unchanged in urine	30
Volume of distribution (L/kg)	0.6
Half-life – normal/ ESRF (hrs)	5–7/Unchanged

METABOLISM

Linezolid is primarily metabolised by oxidation of the morpholine ring resulting mainly in the formation of two inactive open-ring carboxylic acid derivatives: the aminoethoxyacetic acid metabolite (PNU-142300) and the hydroxyethyl glycine metabolite (PNU-142586). The hydroxyethyl glycine metabolite (PNU-142586) is the predominant human metabolite and is believed to be formed by a non-enzymatic process. The aminoethoxyacetic acid metabolite (PNU-142300) is less abundant. Other minor, inactive metabolites have been characterised.

In patients with normal renal function or mild to moderate renal insufficiency, linezolid is primarily excreted under steady-state conditions in the urine as PNU-142586 (40%), parent drug (30%) and PNU-142300 (10%). Virtually no parent drug is found in the faeces while approximately 6% and 3% of each dose appears as PNU-142586 and PNU-142300, respectively. Non-renal clearance accounts for approximately 65% of the total clearance of linezolid.

DOSE IN RENAL IMPAIRMENT GFR (mL/MIN)

20–50	Dose as in normal renal function.
10–20	Dose as in normal renal function.
<10	Dose as in normal renal function, but monitor closely. See 'Other information'.

DOSE IN PATIENTS UNDERGOING RENAL REPLACEMENT THERAPIES

CAPD	Likely to be dialysed. Dose as in GFR<10 mL/min.
HD	Dialysed. Dose as in GFR<10 mL/min.
HDF/High flux	Dialysed. Dose as in GFR<10 mL/min.
CAV/ VVHD	Dialysed. Dose as in normal renal function.
CVVHDF	Dialysed. Dose as in normal renal function.[1]

IMPORTANT DRUG INTERACTIONS

Potentially hazardous interactions with other drugs

- Antidepressants: increased risk of serotonergic syndrome with SSRIs and tricyclics; avoid concomitant use with MAOIs and moclobemide.
- Selegiline: avoid concomitant use.
- Sympathomimetics: enhanced hypertensive effect with adrenaline, noradrenaline, dopamine, dobutamine, phenylpropanolamine and pseudoephedrine – use with caution.

ADMINISTRATION

RECONSTITUTION

–

ROUTE

- Oral, IV

RATE OF ADMINISTRATION

- Over 30–120 minutes

COMMENTS

–

OTHER INFORMATION

- 30% of dose is removed by a 3 hour haemodialysis session.
- After single doses of 600 mg, there was a 7–8-fold increase in exposure to the two primary metabolites of linezolid in the plasma of patients with severe renal insufficiency (i.e. creatinine clearance <30 mL/min). However, there was no increase in AUC of parent drug. Although there is some removal of the major metabolites of linezolid by haemodialysis, metabolite plasma levels after single 600 mg doses were still considerably higher following dialysis than those observed in patients with normal renal function or mild to moderate renal insufficiency.

- In 24 patients with severe renal insufficiency, 21 of whom were on regular haemodialysis, peak plasma concentrations of the two major metabolites after several days dosing were about 10 fold those seen in patients with normal renal function. Peak plasma levels of linezolid were not affected.
- In patients with GFR<10 mL/min, if platelet count drops on a dose of 600 mg twice daily, consider reducing dose to 600 mg once daily.
- Two metabolites accumulate in renal failure which have MAOI activity but no antibacterial activity – monitor patients closely.
- There is 5 mmol sodium per 300 mL infusion.
- Linezolid is a weak, reversible non-selective inhibitor of MAO therefore can be used with drugs not normally given with MAOIs (e.g. SSRIs) but monitor closely.

- In patients who have been on linezolid for longer than 28 days, there have been reports of peripheral neuropathy and/or optic neuropathy occasionally leading to loss of vision, anaemia requiring transfusions, and lactic acidosis – visual function should be monitored in these patients.
- After oral or IV administration, adequate drug concentrations can be found in PF fluid to treat VRE peritonitis. (Salzer W. Antimicrobial-resistant gram-positive bacteria in PD peritonitis. *Perit Dial Int.* 2005; **25**: 313–19.)

Reference:

1. Kraft MD, Pasko DA, DePestel DD, *et al.* Linezolid clearance during continuous venovenous hemodiafiltration: a case report. *Pharmacotherapy.* 2003; **23**(8): 1071–5.

Liothyronine sodium (triiodothyronine)

CLINICAL USE

Hypothyroidism

DOSE IN NORMAL RENAL FUNCTION

- Oral: 10–20 micrograms daily, increased to 60 micrograms in 2–3 divided doses.
- IV: 5–20 micrograms every 4–12 hours, or 50 micrograms initially then 25 micrograms every 8 hours, reducing to 25 micrograms twice a day.

PHARMACOKINETICS

Molecular weight (daltons)	673
% Protein binding	<99
% Excreted unchanged in urine	2.5
Volume of distribution (L/kg)	0.1–0.2
Half-life – normal/ ESRF (hrs)	24–48/–

METABOLISM

Liothyronine is metabolised by deiodination to inactive diiodothyronine and mono-iodothyronine. Iodine released by deiodination is largely reused within the thyroid cells. Further metabolites result from conjugation and decarboxylation; tiratricol (triac) is one such metabolite.

DOSE IN RENAL IMPAIRMENT GFR (mL/MIN)

20–50	Dose as in normal renal function.
20–10	Dose as in normal renal function.
<10	Dose as in normal renal function.

DOSE IN PATIENTS UNDERGOING RENAL REPLACEMENT THERAPIES

CAPD	Not dialysed. Dose as in normal renal function.
HD	Not dialysed. Dose as in normal renal function.
HDF/High flux	Not dialysed. Dose as in normal renal function.
CAV/ VVHD	Not dialysed. Dose as in normal renal function.

IMPORTANT DRUG INTERACTIONS

Potentially hazardous interactions with other drugs

- Anticoagulants: effect of coumarins and phenindione enhanced.

ADMINISTRATION

RECONSTITUTION
- Dissolve with 1–2 mL water for injection.

ROUTE
- IV, oral

RATE OF ADMINISTRATION
- Slow bolus

COMMENTS
- Alkaline solution – may cause irritation if given IM.

OTHER INFORMATION

- 20 mcg of liothyronine is equivalent to 100 mcg of levothyroxine.
- Protein-losing states, such as nephrotic syndrome, will result in a decrease in total T3 and T4.
- Thyroxine (T4) is the drug of choice in hypothyroidism, but T3 can be useful due to its rapid onset of action.
- Elderly patients should receive smaller initial doses.

Liraglutide

CLINICAL USE

Glucogen-like peptide-1 analogue
● Treatment of type 2 diabetes mellitus in combination with other antidiabetic therapy

DOSE IN NORMAL RENAL FUNCTION

0.6–1.8 mg daily

PHARMACOKINETICS

Molecular weight (daltons)	3751.3
% Protein binding	>98
% Excreted unchanged in urine	Minimal (6% as metabolites)
Volume of distribution (L/kg)	0.07
Half-life – normal/ ESRF (hrs)	13/–

METABOLISM

Liraglutide is metabolised in a similar manner to large proteins without a specific organ having been identified as major route of elimination. Only 2 minor metabolites have been identified. No specific organ has been identified as a major route of elimination.

DOSE IN RENAL IMPAIRMENT GFR (mL/MIN)

20–60	Dose as in normal renal function. See 'Other information'.[1,2]
10–20	Dose as in normal renal function. See 'Other information'.[1,2]
<10	Dose as in normal renal function. See 'Other information'.[1,2]

DOSE IN PATIENTS UNDERGOING RENAL REPLACEMENT THERAPIES

CAPD	Not dialysed. Dose as in normal renal function.
HD	Not dialysed. Dose as in normal renal function.
HDF/High flux	Unlikely to be dialysed. Dose as in normal renal function.
CAV/ VVHD	Unlikely to be dialysed. Dose as in normal renal function.

IMPORTANT DRUG INTERACTIONS

Potentially hazardous interactions with other drugs
● None known

ADMINISTRATION

RECONSTITUTION
–

ROUTE
● SC

RATE OF ADMINISTRATION
–

COMMENTS
● Can be given at any time of day independent of meals
● Dose of concomitant sulphonylurea may need reduced.

OTHER INFORMATION

● Not recommended in GFR<60 mL/ min by UK manufacturer due to lack of experience.
● Maximum concentration is reached 8 12 hours post dose.
● Bioavailability is 55%.
● Liraglutide exposure was lowered by 33%, 14%, 27% and 28%, respectively, in subjects with mild (creatinine clearance, GFR 50–80 mL/min), moderate (GFR 30–50 mL/min), and severe (GFR <30 mL/ min) renal impairment and in people on dialysis.
● Can cause acute kidney injury requiring haemodialysis, therefore use with caution.

References:
1. Liraglutide. Trial ID: NN2211–1329. Clinical Trial Report. Report Synopsis. Novo Nordisk 28/1/2008.
2. Thong KY, Walton C, Ryder REJ. Liraglutide is safe and effective in mild or moderate renal impairment: the Association of British Clinical Diabetologists (ABCD) Nationwide Liraglutide Audit. Presented at the American Diabetes Association, 8–12 June 2012, Philadelphia, PA, USA.

Lisinopril

CLINICAL USE

Angiotensin-converting enzyme inhibitor:
- Hypertension, heart failure, following myocardial infarction in haemodynamically stable patients
- Diabetic nephropathy

DOSE IN NORMAL RENAL FUNCTION

2.5–80 mg daily
After a myocardial infarction: 2.5–10 mg daily

PHARMACOKINETICS

Molecular weight (daltons)	441.5
% Protein binding	0
% Excreted unchanged in urine	80–90
Volume of distribution (L/kg)	0.44–0.51
Half-life – normal/ ESRF (hrs)	12/40–50

METABOLISM

Lisinopril does not undergo significant metabolism and is excreted unchanged predominantly in the urine.

DOSE IN RENAL IMPAIRMENT GFR (mL/MIN)

20–50	Initial dose 2.5 mg daily and titrate according to response.
10–20	Initial dose 2.5 mg daily and titrate according to response.
<10	Initial dose 2.5 mg daily and titrate according to response.

DOSE IN PATIENTS UNDERGOING RENAL REPLACEMENT THERAPIES

CAPD	Unknown dialysability. Dose as in GFR<10 mL/min.
HD	Dialysed. Dose as in GFR<10 mL/min.
HDF/High flux	Dialysed. Dose as in GFR<10 mL/min.
CAV/ VVHD	Unknown dialysability. Dose as in GFR=10–20 mL/min.

IMPORTANT DRUG INTERACTIONS

Potentially hazardous interactions with other drugs
- Anaesthetics: enhanced hypotensive effect.
- Analgesics: antagonism of hypotensive effect and increased risk of renal impairment with NSAIDs; hyperkalaemia with ketorolac and other NSAIDs.
- Ciclosporin: increased risk of hyperkalaemia and nephrotoxicity.
- Diuretics: enhanced hypotensive effect; hyperkalaemia with potassium-sparing diuretics.
- ESAs: increased risk of hyperkalaemia; antagonism of hypotensive effect.
- Gold: flushing and hypotension with sodium aurothiomalate.
- Lithium: reduced excretion (possibility of enhanced lithium toxicity).
- Potassium salts: increased risk of hyperkalaemia.
- Tacrolimus: increased risk of hyperkalaemia and nephrotoxicity.

ADMINISTRATION

RECONSTITUTION
–
ROUTE
- Oral
RATE OF ADMINISTRATION
--
COMMENTS
–

OTHER INFORMATION

- Close monitoring of renal function during therapy is necessary in those with renal insufficiency.
- Renal failure has been reported in association with ACE inhibitors and has been mainly in patients with severe congestive heart failure, renal artery stenosis, and post renal transplant.
- High incidence of anaphylactoid reactions has been reported in patients dialysed with high-flux polyacrylonitrile membranes and treated concomitantly with an ACE inhibitor – this combination should therefore be avoided.
- Hyperkalaemia and other side effects are more common in patients with impaired renal function.

Lithium carbonate

CLINICAL USE

- Treatment and prophylaxis of mania, manic depressive illness, and recurrent depression
- Aggressive or self-mutilating behaviour

DOSE IN NORMAL RENAL FUNCTION

See individual preparations. Adjust according to lithium plasma concentration.

PHARMACOKINETICS

Molecular weight (daltons)	73.9
% Protein binding	0
% Excreted unchanged in urine	95
Volume of distribution (L/kg)	0.5–0.9
Half-life – normal/ ESRF (hrs)	12–24/40–50

METABOLISM

Lithium is excreted mainly unchanged in the urine; only a small amount can be detected in the faeces, saliva, and sweat.

DOSE IN RENAL IMPAIRMENT GFR (mL/MIN)

Contraindicated in renal impairment.

20–50	Avoid if possible, or reduce dose to 50–75% and monitor plasma concentration carefully.
10–20	Avoid if possible, or reduce dose to 50–75% and monitor plasma concentration carefully.
<10	Avoid if possible, or reduce dose to 25–50% and monitor plasma concentration carefully.

DOSE IN PATIENTS UNDERGOING RENAL REPLACEMENT THERAPIES

CAPD	Dialysed in lithium intoxication. Dose as in GFR<10 mL/min.
HD	Dialysed in lithium intoxication. Dose as in GFR<10 mL/min.
HDF/High flux	Dialysed in lithium intoxication. Dose as in GFR<10 mL/min.
CAV/ VVHD	Dialysed. Dose as in GFR=10–20 mL/min.

IMPORTANT DRUG INTERACTIONS

Potentially hazardous interactions with other drugs

- ACE inhibitors and angiotensin-II antagonists: lithium excretion reduced – avoid.
- Analgesics: NSAIDs and ketorolac reduce excretion of lithium.
- Anti-arrhythmics: increased risk of ventricular arrhythmias with amiodarone – avoid concomitant use.
- Antidepressants: increased risk of CNS effects with SSRIs; risk of toxicity with tricyclics; possible increased serotonergic effects with venlafaxine.
- Antipsychotics: increased risk of extrapyramidal side effects and possibly neurotoxicity with clozapine, flupentixol, haloperidol, phenothiazines or zuclopenthixol; increased risk of extrapyramidal side effects with sulpiride; possible risk of toxicity with olanzapine.
- Cytotoxics: increased risk of ventricular arrhythmias with arsenic trioxide.
- Diuretics: lithium excretion reduced by loop diuretics, potassium-sparing diuretics, aldosterone antagonists and thiazides; lithium excretion increased by acetazolamide.
- Methyldopa: neurotoxicity may occur without increased lithium levels.

ADMINISTRATION

RECONSTITUTION
–

ROUTE
- Oral

RATE OF ADMINISTRATION
–

COMMENTS
- Different preparations vary widely in bioavailability; a change in the preparation used requires the same precautions as initiation of treatment.

OTHER INFORMATION

- Contraindicated by manufacturer in severe renal impairment and use with caution in mild to moderate renal impairment.
- Doses are adjusted to achieve lithium plasma concentrations of 0.4–1 mmol/L (lower end of range for maintenance therapy in elderly patients) in samples

- taken 12 hours after the preceding dose. It takes 4–7 days to reach steady state.
- Doses in renal impairment are from *Drug Prescribing in Renal Failure*, 5th edition, by Aronoff *et al.*
- Long-term treatment may result in permanent changes in kidney histology and impairment of renal function. High serum concentration of lithium, including episodes of acute lithium toxicity, may aggravate these changes. The minimum clinically effective dose of lithium should always be used.
- Lithium generally should not be used in patients with severe renal disease because of increased risk of toxicity.

- Dialysability: serum lithium concentrations rebound within 5–8 hours post haemodialysis because of redistribution of the drug, often necessitating repeated courses of haemodialysis. Peritoneal dialysis is less effective at removing lithium and is only used if haemodialysis is not possible.
- Up to one-third of patients on lithium may develop polyuria, usually due to lithium blocking the effect of ADH. This reaction is reversible on withdrawal of lithium therapy.

Lofepramine

CLINICAL USE

Tricyclic antidepressant

DOSE IN NORMAL RENAL FUNCTION

140–210 mg daily in 2–3 divided doses

PHARMACOKINETICS

Molecular weight (daltons)	455.4 (as hydrochloride)
% Protein binding	99
% Excreted unchanged in urine	Mainly as metabolites
Volume of distribution (L/kg)	Large
Half-life – normal/ ESRF (hrs)	1.7–5/–

METABOLISM

Lofepramine is metabolised in the liver by cleavage of the p-chlorophenacyl group from the lofepramine molecule leaving desmethylimipramine (DMI). The latter is pharmacologically active. The p-chlorobenzoyl portion is mainly metabolised to p-chlorobenzoic acid which is then conjugated with glycine. The conjugate is excreted mostly in the urine. DMI has been found excreted in the faeces.

DOSE IN RENAL IMPAIRMENT GFR (mL/MIN)

20–50	Dose as in normal renal function.
10–20	Dose as in normal renal function.
<10	Start with a small dose and titrate slowly.

DOSE IN PATIENTS UNDERGOING RENAL REPLACEMENT THERAPIES

CAPD	Unknown dialysability. Dose as in GFR<10 mL/min.
HD	Unknown dialysability. Dose as in GFR<10 mL/min.
HDF/High flux	Unknown dialysability. Dose as in GFR<10 mL/min.
CAV/ VVHD	Unknown dialysability. Dose as in normal renal function.

IMPORTANT DRUG INTERACTIONS

Potentially hazardous interactions with other drugs

- Alcohol: increased sedative effect.
- Analgesics: increased risk of CNS toxicity with tramadol; possibly increased risk of side effects with nefopam; possibly increased sedative effects with opioids.
- Anti-arrhythmics: increased risk of ventricular arrhythmias with amiodarone – avoid concomitant use; increased risk of ventricular arrhythmias with disopyramide, flecainide or propafenone; avoid with dronedarone.
- Antibacterials: increased risk of ventricular arrhythmias with moxifloxacin and possibly telithromycin – avoid concomitant use with moxifloxacin.
- Anticoagulants: may enhance or reduce anticoagulant effect of coumarins.
- Antidepressants: enhanced CNS excitation and hypertension with MAOIs and moclobemide; concentration possibly increased with SSRIs.
- Anti-epileptics: convulsive threshold lowered; concentration reduced by carbamazepine, phenobarbital and possibly phenytoin.
- Antimalarials: avoid concomitant use with artemether/lumefantrine and piperaquine with artenimol.
- Antipsychotics: increased risk of ventricular arrhythmias especially with droperidol and pimozide – avoid; increased antimuscarinic effects with clozapine and phenothiazines; concentration increased by antipsychotics.
- Antivirals: increased risk of ventricular arrhythmias with saquinavir – avoid; concentration possibly increased with ritonavir.
- Atomoxetine: increased risk of ventricular arrhythmias; possibly increased risk of convulsions.
- Beta-blockers: increased risk of ventricular arrhythmias with sotalol.
- Clonidine: tricyclics antagonise hypotensive effect; increased risk of hypertension on clonidine withdrawal.
- Dopaminergics: avoid use with entacapone; CNS toxicity reported with selegiline and rasagiline.
- Pentamidine: increased risk of ventricular arrhythmias.
- Sympathomimetics: increased risk of hypertension and arrhythmias with adrenaline and noradrenaline; metabolism possibly inhibited by methylphenidate.

ADMINISTRATION

RECONSTITUTION

–

ROUTE

● Oral

RATE OF ADMINISTRATION

–

COMMENTS

–

OTHER INFORMATION

● Contraindicated by manufacturer in severe renal impairment due to lack of data.

Lomitapide

CLINICAL USE

Adjunctive treatment of homozygous familial hypercholesterolemia

DOSE IN NORMAL RENAL FUNCTION

5–60 mg once daily

PHARMACOKINETICS

Molecular weight (daltons)	693.7 (789.8 as mesilate)
% Protein binding	99.8
% Excreted unchanged in urine	52.9–59.5
Volume of distribution (L/kg)	985–1292 litres
Half-life – normal/ ESRF (hrs)	39.7/79.4

METABOLISM

Lomitapide is metabolised extensively by the liver via oxidation, oxidative N-dealkylation, glucuronide conjugation, and piperidine ring opening. Cytochrome P450 (CYP) 3A4 metabolises lomitapide to its major metabolites, M1 and M3, as detected in plasma. The oxidative N-dealkylation pathway breaks the lomitapide molecule into M1 and M3. M1 is the moiety that retains the piperidine ring, whereas M3 retains the rest of the lomitapide molecule *in vitro*. CYPs 1A2, 2B6, 2C8, and 2C19 may metabolise lomitapide to a small extent to M1. M1 and M3 do not inhibit activity of microsomal triglyceride transfer protein *in vitro*.

Just over half of a dose is excreted in the urine and about a third in the faeces.

DOSE IN RENAL IMPAIRMENT GFR (mL/MIN)

20–50	Dose as in normal renal function. Use with caution.
10–20	Dose as in normal renal function. Use with caution.
<10	Maximum dose 40 mg daily.

DOSE IN PATIENTS UNDERGOING RENAL REPLACEMENT THERAPIES

CAPD	Unlikely to be dialysed. Dose as in GFR<10 mL/min.
HD	Unlikely to be dialysed. Dose as in GFR<10 mL/min.
HDF/High flux	Unlikely to be dialysed. Dose as in GFR<10 mL/min.
CAV/ VVHD	Unlikely to be dialysed. Dose as in GFR=10–20 mL/min.

IMPORTANT DRUG INTERACTIONS

Potentially hazardous interactions with other drugs
- Anticoagulants: increases warfarin concentration.
- Lipid lowering agents: reduce simvastatin dose by 50% if used together.

ADMINISTRATION

RECONSTITUTION
–

ROUTE
- Oral

RATE OF ADMINISTRATION
–

COMMENTS
- Administer at least 2 hours after evening meal as food can increase GI side effects.

OTHER INFORMATION

- Use with caution in renal impairment due to lack of studies.
- Can cause deranged LFTs.
- Exposure is increased by 50% in renal impairment.
- Oral bioavailability is approximately 7%.

Lomustine

CLINICAL USE

Treatment of Hodgkin's disease and certain solid tumours

DOSE IN NORMAL RENAL FUNCTION

120–130 mg/m^2 every 6–8 weeks if used alone; lower dose is used in combination treatment and compromised bone marrow function.

PHARMACOKINETICS

Molecular weight (daltons)	233.7
% Protein binding	60
% Excreted unchanged in urine	50 (as metabolites)
Volume of distribution (L/kg)	No data
Half-life – normal/ ESRF (hrs)	16–48 (metabolites)/–

METABOLISM

After oral application of radioactive marked lomustine approximately 15–30% of the measured radioactivity in the plasma can be detected in the cerebrospinal fluid. Lomustine is rapidly metabolised through hepatic microsomal enzymes and the metabolites are excreted mainly via the kidneys. About half a dose is excreted as metabolites in the urine within 24 hours and about 75% is excreted within 4 days. In addition, 10% is excreted as CO_2 and <5% excreted in the faeces. Lomustine cannot be detected in its active form in the urine at any time.

DOSE IN RENAL IMPAIRMENT GFR (mL/MIN)

45–60	75% of dose
30–45	50–70% of dose
<30	Not recommended. See 'Other information'.

DOSE IN PATIENTS UNDERGOING RENAL REPLACEMENT THERAPIES

CAPD	Unlikely to be dialysed. Avoid.
HD	Not dialysed. Avoid. See 'Other information'.
HDF/High flux	Unknown dialysability. Avoid. See 'Other information'.
CAV/ VVHD	Unlikely to be dialysed. Avoid. See 'Other information'.

IMPORTANT DRUG INTERACTIONS

Potentially hazardous interactions with other drugs

- Antipsychotics: avoid concomitant use with clozapine (increased risk of agranulocytosis).

ADMINISTRATION

RECONSTITUTION

–

ROUTE

- Oral

RATE OF ADMINISTRATION

–

COMMENTS

–

OTHER INFORMATION

- Bone marrow toxicity is delayed.
- Contraindicated by manufacturer in severe renal impairment in the UK but not in the US.
- Dosage from BC Cancer Agency: Accessed 17/9/13 GFR=10–50 mL/min, give 75% of previous dose. GFR<10 mL/min, give 50% of previous dose.
- Doses in renal failure from Kintzel PE, Dorr RT. Anticancer drug renal toxicity and elimination: dosing guidelines for altered renal function. *Cancer Treat Rev.* 1995; **21**: 33–64.

Loperamide hydrochloride

CLINICAL USE

Antidiarrhoeal agent

DOSE IN NORMAL RENAL FUNCTION

4 mg stat, then 2 mg after each loose stool; maximum 16 mg daily

PHARMACOKINETICS

Molecular weight (daltons)	513.5
% Protein binding	80
% Excreted unchanged in urine	<10
Volume of distribution (L/kg)	No data
Half-life – normal/ ESRF (hrs)	9–14/–

METABOLISM

Loperamide undergoes extensive first pass metabolism in the liver, where it is predominantly metabolised to inactive metabolites, conjugated and excreted via the bile. Oxidative N-demethylation is the main metabolic pathway for loperamide, and is mediated mainly through CYP3A4 and CYP2C8. Excretion of the unchanged loperamide and the metabolites mainly occurs through the faeces.

DOSE IN RENAL IMPAIRMENT GFR (mL/MIN)

20–50	Dose as in normal renal function.
10–20	Dose as in normal renal function.
<10	Dose as in normal renal function. See 'Other information'.

DOSE IN PATIENTS UNDERGOING RENAL REPLACEMENT THERAPIES

CAPD	Unlikely to be dialysed. Dose as in GFR<10 mL/min.
HD	Unlikely to be dialysed. Dose as in GFR<10 mL/min.
HDF/High flux	Unknown dialysability. Dose as in GFR<10 mL/min.
CAV/ VVHD	Unlikely to be dialysed. Dose as in normal renal function.

IMPORTANT DRUG INTERACTIONS

Potentially hazardous interactions with other drugs
- None known

ADMINISTRATION

RECONSTITUTION

–

ROUTE
- Oral

RATE OF ADMINISTRATION

–

COMMENTS

–

OTHER INFORMATION

- In normal doses loperamide may cause excessive drowsiness in CKD 5.

Lopinavir

CLINICAL USE

Protease inhibitor:
- Treatment of HIV infected patients, in combination with other antiretroviral agents

DOSE IN NORMAL RENAL FUNCTION

2 tablets twice daily or 4 tablets once daily (in combination with ritonavir, Kaletra®), or 5 mL twice daily.

PHARMACOKINETICS

Molecular weight (daltons)	628.8
% Protein binding	98–99
% Excreted unchanged in urine	2.2
Volume of distribution (L/kg)	0.5
Half-life – normal/ESRF (hrs)	5–6/12–17

METABOLISM

Lopinavir is extensively metabolised, mainly by oxidation by cytochrome P450 isoenzyme CYP3A4; 13 metabolites have been identified with some, such as 4-oxylopinavir and 4-hydroxylopinavir, having antiviral activity. Lopinavir is mainly excreted in faeces and to a smaller extent in the urine; unchanged lopinavir accounts for about 2.2% of a dose excreted in the urine and 19.8% in the faeces. After multiple dosing, less than 3% of the absorbed lopinavir dose is excreted unchanged in the urine.

DOSE IN RENAL IMPAIRMENT GFR (mL/MIN)

20–50	Dose as in normal renal function.
10–20	Dose as in normal renal function.
<10	Dose as in normal renal function.

DOSE IN PATIENTS UNDERGOING RENAL REPLACEMENT THERAPIES

CAPD	Unlikely to be dialysed. Dose as in normal renal function.
HD	Unlikely to be dialysed. Dose as in normal renal function.
HDF/High flux	Unlikely to be dialysed. Dose as in normal renal function.
CAV/VVHD	Unknown dialysability. Dose as in normal renal function.

IMPORTANT DRUG INTERACTIONS

Potentially hazardous interactions with other drugs

In combination with ritonavir – see ritonavir interactions.
- Anti-arrhythmics: increased risk of ventricular arrhythmias with flecainide – avoid; possibly increased lidocaine concentration.
- Antibacterials: concentration reduced by rifampicin – avoid concomitant use; avoid concomitant use with telithromycin in severe renal and hepatic impairment.
- Antidepressants: concentration reduced by St John's wort – avoid concomitant use.
- Anti-epileptics: concentration possibly reduced by carbamazepine, phenytoin and phenobarbital.
- Antimalarials: use artemether/lumefantrine with caution.
- Antipsychotics: possibly inhibits metabolism of aripiprazole – reduce dose of aripiprazole; possibly increases quetiapine concentration – avoid.
- Antivirals: avoid with boceprevir and telaprevir; fosamprenavir concentration reduced – avoid; concentration reduced by efavirenz and tipranavir; concentration possibly reduced by nevirapine, consider increasing lopinavir dose; increased risk of ventricular arrhythmias with saquinavir – avoid; concentration of tenofovir increased; concentration increased by darunavir and darunavir concentration reduced – avoid; concentration of maraviroc increased, consider reducing maraviroc dose.
- Ciclosporin: may increase concentration of ciclosporin.
- Cytotoxics: reduce dose of ruxolitinib.
- Ranolazine: possibly increases ranolazine concentration – avoid.
- Sirolimus: may increase concentration of sirolimus.
- Statins: increased risk of myopathy with atorvastatin; possibly increased risk of myopathy with rosuvastatin and simvastatin – avoid concomitant use.
- Tacrolimus: may increase concentration of tacrolimus.

ADMINISTRATION

RECONSTITUTION

–

ROUTE

● Oral

RATE OF ADMINISTRATION

–

COMMENTS

● Take with food.

OTHER INFORMATION

–

Loratadine

CLINICAL USE

Antihistamine:
- Symptomatic relief of allergy such as hay fever, urticaria

DOSE IN NORMAL RENAL FUNCTION

10 mg daily

PHARMACOKINETICS

Molecular weight (daltons)	382.9
% Protein binding	97–99
% Excreted unchanged in urine	40
Volume of distribution (L/kg)	No data
Half-life – normal/ ESRF (hrs)	12–15/Unchanged

METABOLISM

Loratadine undergoes an extensive first pass metabolism, mainly by CYP3A4 and CYP2D6. The major metabolite, desloratadine, is pharmacologically active and responsible for a large part of the clinical effect.

Approximately 40% of the dose is excreted in the urine and 42% in the faeces over a 10 day period and mainly in the form of conjugated metabolites.

Approximately 27% of the dose is eliminated in the urine during the first 24 hours. Less than 1% of the active substance is excreted unchanged in the active form, as loratadine or desloratadine.

DOSE IN RENAL IMPAIRMENT GFR (mL/MIN)

20–50	Dose as in normal renal function.
10–20	Dose as in normal renal function.
<10	Dose as in normal renal function.

DOSE IN PATIENTS UNDERGOING RENAL REPLACEMENT THERAPIES

CAPD	Not dialysed. Dose as in normal renal function.
HD	Not dialysed. Dose as in normal renal function.
HDF/High flux	Unknown dialysability. Dose as in normal renal function.
CAV/ VVHD	Unlikely to be dialysed. Dose as in normal renal function.

IMPORTANT DRUG INTERACTIONS

Potentially hazardous interactions with other drugs
- Antibacterials: concentration possibly increased by erythromycin.
- Antifungals: concentration of loratadine possibly increased by ketoconazole – avoid concomitant use.
- Antivirals: concentration possibly increased by ritonavir.

ADMINISTRATION

RECONSTITUTION
–
ROUTE
- Oral
RATE OF ADMINISTRATION
–
COMMENTS
–

OTHER INFORMATION

- Patients with renal impairment are at increased risk of sedation.

Lorazepam

CLINICAL USE

Benzodiazepine:
- Short-term use in anxiety or insomnia
- Status epilepticus
- Perioperative

DOSE IN NORMAL RENAL FUNCTION

- Anxiety: 1–4 mg daily in divided doses.
- Insomnia associated with anxiety: 1–2 mg at bedtime.
- Acute panic attacks: (IV/IM): 25–30 mcg/kg; repeat 6 hourly if required; usual range 1.5–2.5 mg.
- Status epilepticus: 4 mg IV repeated once after 10 minutes.

PHARMACOKINETICS

Molecular weight (daltons)	321.2
% Protein binding	85
% Excreted unchanged in urine	<1
Volume of distribution (L/kg)	0.9–1.3
Half-life – normal/ ESRF (hrs)	10–20/32–70

METABOLISM

Lorazepam is metabolised in the liver to the inactive glucuronide, and excreted in the urine.

DOSE IN RENAL IMPAIRMENT GFR (mL/MIN)

20–50	Dose as in normal renal function.
10–20	Dose as in normal renal function.
<10	Dose as in normal renal function. Start with small doses.

DOSE IN PATIENTS UNDERGOING RENAL REPLACEMENT THERAPIES

CAPD	Unlikely dialysability. Dose as in GFR<10 mL/min.
HD	Not dialysed. Dose as in GFR<10 mL/min.
HDF/High flux	Unknown dialysability. Dose as in GFR<10 mL/min.
CAV/ VVHD	Not dialysed. Dose as in normal renal function.

IMPORTANT DRUG INTERACTIONS

Potentially hazardous interactions with other drugs
- Antibacterials: metabolism possibly increased by rifampicin.
- Antipsychotics: increased sedative effects; increased risk of hypotension, bradycardia and respiratory depression when parenteral benzodiazepines are given with IM olanzapine; risk of serious adverse effects in combination with clozapine.
- Antivirals: concentration possibly increased by ritonavir.
- Disulfiram: metabolism inhibited, increased sedative effects.
- Sodium oxybate: enhanced effects of sodium oxybate – avoid.
- Ulcer-healing drugs: metabolism inhibited by cimetidine.

ADMINISTRATION

ROUTE
- Oral, IV, IM, sublingual

RATE OF ADMINISTRATION
- Slow IV bolus

COMMENTS
- Onset of effect after IM injection is similar to oral administration.
- IV route preferred over IM route.
- Dilute 1:1 with sodium chloride 0.9% or water for injection.
- Can be used undiluted. (UK Critical Care Group, *Minimum Infusion Volumes for Fluid Restricted Critically Ill Patients*, 3rd edition, 2006)

OTHER INFORMATION

- Patients with impaired renal or hepatic function should be monitored frequently and have their dosage adjusted carefully according to response. Lower doses may be sufficient in these patients.
- Lorazepam as intact drug is not removed by dialysis. The glucuronide metabolite is highly dialysable, but is pharmacologically inactive.
- Increased CNS sensitivity in patients with renal impairment.

Lormetazepam

CLINICAL USE

Benzodiazepine:
- Insomnia (short term use)

DOSE IN NORMAL RENAL FUNCTION

0.5–1.5 mg at night

PHARMACOKINETICS

Molecular weight (daltons)	335.2
% Protein binding	85
% Excreted unchanged in urine	<6 (86 as metabolites)
Volume of distribution (L/kg)	4.6
Half-life – normal/ ESRF (hrs)	11–16/Unchanged

METABOLISM

Lormetazepam is metabolised in the liver to the inactive glucuronide, and excreted in the urine.

DOSE IN RENAL IMPAIRMENT GFR (mL/MIN)

20–50	Dose as in normal renal function.
10–20	Dose as in normal renal function. Start with small doses.
<10	Dose as in normal renal function. Start with small doses.

DOSE IN PATIENTS UNDERGOING RENAL REPLACEMENT THERAPIES

CAPD	Not dialysed. Dose as in GFR<10 mL/min.
HD	Not dialysed. Dose as in GFR<10 mL/min.
HDF/High flux	Unknown dialysability. Dose as in GFR<10 mL/min.
CAV/ VVHD	Unknown dialysability. Dose as in GFR=10–20 mL/min.

IMPORTANT DRUG INTERACTIONS

Potentially hazardous interactions with other drugs
- Antibacterials: metabolism possibly increased by rifampicin.
- Antipsychotics: increased sedative effects; risk of serious adverse effects in combination with clozapine.
- Antivirals: concentration possibly increased by ritonavir.
- Disulfiram: metabolism inhibited, increased sedative effects.
- Sodium oxybate: enhanced effect – avoid concomitant use.

ADMINISTRATION

RECONSTITUTION
–
ROUTE
- Oral
RATE OF ADMINISTRATION
–
COMMENTS
–

OTHER INFORMATION

- Increased CNS sensitivity in renal impairment.
- Long-term use may lead to dependence and withdrawal symptoms in certain patients.
- The half-life of the glucuronide metabolite is increased in renal impairment.

Losartan potassium

CLINICAL USE

Angiotensin-II receptor antagonist:
- Hypertension
- Type 2 diabetic nephropathy
- Heart failure

DOSE IN NORMAL RENAL FUNCTION

25–100 mg daily
Heart failure: 12.5–150 mg once daily

PHARMACOKINETICS

Molecular weight (daltons)	461
% Protein binding	>98
% Excreted unchanged in urine	4
Volume of distribution (L/kg)	0.4
Half-life – normal/ ESRF (hrs)	1.5–2.5 (active metabolite 3–9)/4–6

METABOLISM

Losartan undergoes substantial first-pass metabolism resulting in a systemic bioavailability of about 33%. It is metabolised to an active carboxylic acid metabolite E-3174 (EXP-3174), which has greater pharmacological activity than losartan; some inactive metabolites are also formed. Metabolism is mainly by cytochrome P450 isoenzymes CYP2C9 and CYP3A4. Losartan is excreted in the urine, and in the faeces via bile, as unchanged drug and metabolites. About 4% of an oral dose is excreted unchanged in urine and about 6% is excreted in urine as the active metabolite.

DOSE IN RENAL IMPAIRMENT GFR (mL/MIN)

20–50	Dose as in normal renal function.
10–20	Initial dose 25 mg and titrate according to response.
<10	Initial dose 25 mg and titrate according to response.

DOSE IN PATIENTS UNDERGOING RENAL REPLACEMENT THERAPIES

CAPD	Not dialysed. Dose as in GFR<10 mL/min.
HD	Not dialysed. Dose as in GFR<10 mL/min.
HDF/High flux	Not dialysed. Dose as in GFR<10 mL/min.
CAV/ VVHD	Not dialysed. Dose as in GFR=10–20 mL/min.

IMPORTANT DRUG INTERACTIONS

Potentially hazardous interactions with other drugs
- Anaesthetics: enhanced hypotensive effect.
- Analgesics: antagonism of hypotensive effect and increased risk of renal impairment with NSAIDs; hyperkalaemia with ketorolac and other NSAIDs.
- Ciclosporin: increased risk of hyperkalaemia and nephrotoxicity.
- Diuretics: enhanced hypotensive effect; hyperkalaemia with potassium-sparing diuretics.
- ESAs: increased risk of hyperkalaemia; antagonism of hypotensive effect.
- Lithium: reduced excretion (possibility of enhanced lithium toxicity).
- Potassium salts: increased risk of hyperkalaemia.
- Tacrolimus: increased risk of hyperkalaemia and nephrotoxicity.

ADMINISTRATION

RECONSTITUTION
–
ROUTE
- Oral
RATE OF ADMINISTRATION
–
COMMENTS
–

OTHER INFORMATION

- Adverse reactions, especially hyperkalaemia, are more common in patients with renal impairment.
- Renal failure has been reported in association with angiotensin-II antagonists in patients with renal artery stenosis, post renal transplant, and in those with congestive heart failure.
- Close monitoring of renal function during therapy is necessary in those with renal insufficiency.

Lymecycline

CLINICAL USE

Antibacterial agent:
- Also used for treatment of acne

DOSE IN NORMAL RENAL FUNCTION

- 408 mg (1 capsule) twice daily, increasing to 3–4 capsules daily in severe infections.
- Acne: 408 mg daily for at least 8 weeks.

PHARMACOKINETICS

Molecular weight (daltons)	602.6
% Protein binding	Approx 25–60
% Excreted unchanged in urine	25
Volume of distribution (L/kg)	Approx 1.3–1.7
Half-life – normal/ ESRF (hrs)	10/Increased

METABOLISM

The tetracyclines are excreted in the urine and in the faeces. Renal clearance is by glomerular filtration. Up to 60% of an intravenous dose, and up to 55% of an oral dose, is eliminated unchanged in the urine. Usually between 40% and 70% of a dose is excreted in the urine; urinary excretion is increased if urine is alkalinised.

DOSE IN RENAL IMPAIRMENT GFR (mL/MIN)

20–50	Dose as in normal renal function.
10–20	Dose as in normal renal function.
<10	Avoid. See 'Other information'.

DOSE IN PATIENTS UNDERGOING RENAL REPLACEMENT THERAPIES

CAPD	Not dialysed. Dose as in GFR<10 mL/min.
HD	Not dialysed. Dose as in GFR<10 mL/min.
HDF/High flux	Unknown dialysability. Dose as in GFR<10 mL/min.
CAV/ VVHD	Unlikely to be dialysed. Dose as in normal renal function.

IMPORTANT DRUG INTERACTIONS

Potentially hazardous interactions with other drugs
- Anticoagulants: possibly enhanced anticoagulant effect of coumarins and phenindione.
- Oestrogens: possibly reduce contraceptive effects of oestrogens (risk probably small).
- Retinoids: possible increased risk of benign intracranial hypertension – avoid concomitant use.

ADMINISTRATION

RECONSTITUTION
–
ROUTE
- Oral
RATE OF ADMINISTRATION
–
COMMENTS
- Do not take iron preparations, indigestion remedies or phosphate binders at the same time of day as lymecycline.

OTHER INFORMATION

- Lymecycline is a tetracycline derivative.
- 408 mg lymecycline ≡ 300 mg tetracycline.
- Contraindicated by manufacturer in severe renal impairment as lymecycline is mainly excreted by the kidneys.
- Irish medicines board advises to use a lower dose in moderate renal impairment and to avoid in severe renal impairment.

Maraviroc

CLINICAL USE

CCR5 antagonist:
- Treatment of HIV infection in combination with other antiretrovirals

DOSE IN NORMAL RENAL FUNCTION

150–300 mg twice daily

PHARMACOKINETICS

Molecular weight (daltons)	513.7
% Protein binding	76
% Excreted unchanged in urine	8 (20% as unchanged drug and metabolites)
Volume of distribution (L/kg)	194 litres
Half-life – normal/ ESRF (hrs)	13.2/–

METABOLISM

Metabolised in the liver by cytochrome P450 3A4 to metabolites which are inactive against HIV.

It is excreted in both urine (20%) and faeces (76%) as unchanged drug and metabolites.

DOSE IN RENAL IMPAIRMENT GFR (mL/MIN)

20–80	If administered without potent CYP3A4 inhibitors dose as in normal renal function. If administered with potent CYP3A4 inhibitors: 150 mg daily.
10–20	If administered without potent CYP3A4 inhibitors dose as in normal renal function. If administered with potent CYP3A4 inhibitors: 150 mg daily.
<10	If administered without potent CYP3A4 inhibitors dose as in normal renal function. If administered with potent CYP3A4 inhibitors: 150 mg daily.

DOSE IN PATIENTS UNDERGOING RENAL REPLACEMENT THERAPIES

CAPD	Unknown dialysability. Dose as in GFR<10 mL/min.
HD	Some dialysability. Dose as in GFR<10 mL/min.
HDF/High flux	Probably dialysed Dose as in GFR<10 mL/min.
CAV/ VVHD	Some dialysability. Dose as in GFR=10–20 mL/min.

IMPORTANT DRUG INTERACTIONS

Potentially hazardous interactions with other drugs
- Antibacterials: concentration possibly increased by clarithromycin and telithromycin, consider reducing dose of maraviroc; concentration reduced by rifampicin, consider increasing dose of maraviroc.
- Antidepressants: concentration possibly reduced by St John's wort – avoid
- Antifungals: concentration increased by atazanavir, darunavir, indinavir, lopinavir and saquinavir, consider reducing dose of maraviroc; concentration possibly reduced by efavirenz, consider increasing dose of maraviroc; concentration possibly reduced by etravirine; concentration increased by ritonavir.

ADMINISTRATION

RECONSTITUTION
–
ROUTE
- Oral
RATE OF ADMINISTRATION
–

OTHER INFORMATION

- Increased risk of postural hypotension in renal impairment especially if co-administered with potent CYP3A4 inhibitors.
- Bioavailability is 23–33%.

Mebendazole

Treatment of threadworm, roundworm, whipworm, hookworm infections and echinococcosis

DOSE IN NORMAL RENAL FUNCTION

- Threadworm: 100 mg as a single dose; if re-infection occurs repeat after 2 weeks.
- Whipworm, roundworm, hookworm: 100 mg twice daily for 3 days.
- Echinococcosis: 40–50 mg/kg daily for at least 3–6 months.

PHARMACOKINETICS

Molecular weight (daltons)	295.3
% Protein binding	95
% Excreted unchanged in urine	2
Volume of distribution (L/kg)	1–1.2
Half-life – normal/ ESRF (hrs)	0.93/–

METABOLISM

Mebendazole undergoes extensive first-pass metabolism in the liver. Mebendazole, the conjugated forms of mebendazole, and its metabolites are excreted in the urine and bile.

DOSE IN RENAL IMPAIRMENT GFR (mL/MIN)

20–50	Dose as in normal renal function.
10–20	Dose as in normal renal function.
<10	Dose as in normal renal function.

DOSE IN PATIENTS UNDERGOING RENAL REPLACEMENT THERAPIES

CAPD	Unlikely to be dialysed. Dose as in normal renal function.
HD	Unlikely to be dialysed. Dose as in normal renal function.
HDF/High flux	Unknown dialysability. Dose as in normal renal function.
CAV/ VVHD	Unlikely to be dialysed. Dose as in normal renal function.

IMPORTANT DRUG INTERACTIONS

Potentially hazardous interactions with other drugs

- Cimetidine: possibly inhibits metabolism of mebendazole.
- Phenytoin, carbamazepine and phenobarbital: lower mebendazole concentrations, only relevant when being used in high doses for echinococcosis.

ADMINISTRATION

RECONSTITUTION

–

ROUTE

- Oral

RATE OF ADMINISTRATION

–

COMMENTS

–

OTHER INFORMATION

- Contraindicated in pregnancy.
- Poorly absorbed from the gastrointestinal tract (5–10%).

Medroxyprogesterone acetate

CLINICAL USE

Progestogen
- Cachexia (unlicensed), contraception, epilepsy, male hypersexuality, malignant neoplasms, respiratory disorders, sickle-cell disease, dysfunctional uterine bleeding, endometriosis

DOSE IN NORMAL RENAL FUNCTION

- Cachexia (unlicensed): 500 mg twice daily[1]
- Contraception: 150 mg (deep IM) within first 5 days of cycle or within first 5 days after parturition, repeated every 12 weeks
- Breast cancer: Oral: 400–1500 mg daily
- Other hormone sensitive malignancies: Oral: 100–600 mg daily
- Endometrial & renal cell cancer: 200–600 mg daily
- Dysfunctional uterine bleeding: 2.5–10 mg daily for 5–10 days beginning on day 16–21 of cycle, repeated for 2–3 cycles
- Endometriosis: 10 mg 3 times a day for 90 consecutive days, beginning on day 1 of cycle
- Progestogenic opposition of oestrogen HRT: 10 mg daily for the last 14 days of each 28 day oestrogen HRT cycle
- See product literature for more specific information.

PHARMACOKINETICS

Molecular weight (daltons)	386.5
% Protein binding	94
% Excreted unchanged in urine	<5
Volume of distribution (L/kg)	>20 litres
Half-life – normal/ESRF (hrs)	24–48 (up to 50 days after IM administration)/–

METABOLISM

Medroxyprogesterone is mainly metabolised in the liver and excreted mainly as glucuronide conjugates in the urine and faeces.

DOSE IN RENAL IMPAIRMENT GFR (mL/MIN)

20–50	Dose as in normal renal function.
10–20	Dose as in normal renal function.
<10	Dose as in normal renal function. Monitor carefully.

DOSE IN PATIENTS UNDERGOING RENAL REPLACEMENT THERAPIES

CAPD	Unlikely to be dialysed. Dose as in GFR<10 mL/min.
HD	Unlikely to be dialysed. Dose as in GFR<10 mL/min.
HDF/High flux	Unlikely to be dialysed. Dose as in GFR<10 mL/min.
CAV/VVHD	Unlikely to be dialysed. Dose as in normal renal function.

IMPORTANT DRUG INTERACTIONS

Potentially hazardous interactions with other drugs
- Antibacterials: metabolism of progestogens accelerated by rifamycins (reduced contraceptive effect).
- Anticoagulants: progestogens antagonise anticoagulant effect of phenindione and may enhance or reduce effect of coumarins.
- Antidepressants: contraceptive effect reduced by St John's wort – avoid concomitant use.
- Anti-epileptics: metabolism accelerated by carbamazepine, eslicarbazepine, oxcarbazepine, phenytoin, phenobarbital, rufinamide and topiramate (reduced contraceptive effect); concentration reduced by high dose perampanel.
- Antivirals: contraceptive effect possibly reduced by efavirenz; metabolism accelerated by nevirapine (reduced contraceptive effect).
- Aprepitant: possible contraceptive failure.
- Bosentan: possible contraceptive failure.
- Ciclosporin: progestogens inhibit metabolism of ciclosporin (increased plasma concentration).
- Cytotoxics: possibly reduced contraceptive effect with crizotinib and vemurafenib.
- Dopaminergics: concentration of selegiline increased – avoid concomitant use.
- Tacrolimus: contraceptive effect of progestogens possibly reduced by tacrolimus.
- Ulipristal: contraceptive effect possibly reduced.

ADMINISTRATION

RECONSTITUTION
–
ROUTE
- Oral, IM
RATE OF ADMINISTRATION
–

COMMENTS
–

OTHER INFORMATION

- Do not use in patients with porphyria.

Reference:
1. Simons JP, Aaronson NK, Vansteenkiste JP, *et al.* Effects of medroxyprogesterone acetate on appetite, weight and quality of life in advanced-stage non-hormone-sensitive cancer: a placebo controlled multicenter study. *J Clin Oncol.* 1996; **14**: 1077–84.

Mefenamic acid

CLINICAL USE

NSAID:
- Mild to moderate rheumatic pain
- Dysmenorrhoea and menorrhagia

DOSE IN NORMAL RENAL FUNCTION

500 mg 3 times a day

PHARMACOKINETICS

Molecular weight (daltons)	241.3
% Protein binding	99
% Excreted unchanged in urine	6
Volume of distribution (L/kg)	1.06
Half-life – normal/ ESRF (hrs)	2–4/Unchanged

METABOLISM

Metabolised in the liver by the cytochrome P450 isoenzyme CYP2C9 to 3-hydroxymethyl mefenamic acid, which may then be oxidised to 3-carboxymefenamic acid. Over 50% of a dose may be recovered in the urine, as unchanged drug or, mainly, as conjugates of mefenamic acid and its metabolites.

DOSE IN RENAL IMPAIRMENT GFR (mL/MIN)

20–50	Dose as in normal renal function, but avoid if possible.
10–20	Dose as in normal renal function, but avoid if possible.
<10	Dose as in normal renal function, but only use if on dialysis.

DOSE IN PATIENTS UNDERGOING RENAL REPLACEMENT THERAPIES

CAPD	Unlikely to be dialysed. Dose as in normal renal function. See 'Other information'.
HD	Not dialysed. Dose as in normal renal function. See 'Other information'.
HDF/High flux	Unknown dialysability. Dose as in normal renal function. See 'Other information'.
CAV/ VVHD	Unlikely to be dialysed. Dose as in GFR=10–20 mL/min.

IMPORTANT DRUG INTERACTIONS

Potentially hazardous interactions with other drugs
- ACE inhibitors and angiotensin-II antagonists: antagonism of hypotensive effect; increased risk of nephrotoxicity and hyperkalaemia.
- Analgesics: avoid concomitant use of 2 or more NSAIDs, including aspirin (increased side effects); avoid with ketorolac (increased risk of side effects and haemorrhage).
- Antibacterials: possibly increased risk of convulsions with quinolones.
- Anticoagulants: effects of coumarins and phenindione enhanced; possibly increased risk of bleeding with heparins and dabigatran.
- Antidepressants: increased risk of bleeding with SSRIs and venlafaxine.
- Antidiabetic agents: effects of sulphonylureas enhanced.
- Anti-epileptics: possibly increased phenytoin concentration.
- Antivirals: increased risk of haematological toxicity with zidovudine; concentration possibly increased by ritonavir.
- Ciclosporin: may potentiate nephrotoxicity.
- Cytotoxic agents: reduced excretion of methotrexate; increased risk of bleeding with erlotinib.
- Diuretics: increased risk of nephrotoxicity; antagonism of diuretic effect; hyperkalaemia with potassium-sparing diuretics.
- Lithium: excretion decreased.
- Pentoxifylline: increased risk of bleeding.
- Tacrolimus: increased risk of nephrotoxicity.

ADMINISTRATION

RECONSTITUTION
–

ROUTE
- Oral

RATE OF ADMINISTRATION
–

COMMENTS
–

OTHER INFORMATION

- As with other prostaglandin inhibitors, allergic glomerulonephritis has occurred occasionally. There have also been reports of acute interstitial nephritis with haematuria and proteinuria and occasionally nephrotic syndrome.
- Inhibition of renal prostaglandin synthesis by NSAIDs may interfere with renal function, especially in the presence of existing renal disease – avoid use if possible; if not, check serum creatinine 48–72 hours after starting NSAID – if raised, discontinue NSAID therapy.
- Use with caution in renal transplant recipients (can reduce intrarenal autocoid synthesis).
- Use normal doses in patients with CKD 5 on dialysis if they do not pass any urine.

Mefloquine

CLINICAL USE

Malaria prophylaxis and treatment

DOSE IN NORMAL RENAL FUNCTION

- Prophylaxis: 250 mg weekly
- Treatment:
  — Non-immune patients: 20–25 mg/kg in 2–3 divided doses; maximum 1.5 g
  — Partially immune patients: 15 mg/kg in 2–3 divided doses

PHARMACOKINETICS

Molecular weight (daltons)	414.8 (as hydrochloride)
% Protein binding	98
% Excreted unchanged in urine	9 (+4% metabolites)
Volume of distribution (L/kg)	20
Half-life – normal/ ESRF (hrs)	21 days/–

METABOLISM

Mefloquine is extensively metabolised in the liver by the cytochrome P450 isoenzyme CYP3A4. There is evidence that mefloquine is excreted mainly in the bile and faeces. In volunteers, urinary excretion of unchanged mefloquine and its main metabolite accounted for about 9% and 4% of the dose, respectively.

DOSE IN RENAL IMPAIRMENT GFR (mL/MIN)

20–50	Dose as in normal renal function.
10–20	Dose as in normal renal function.
<10	Use with caution. Prophylaxis: Dose as in normal renal function.

DOSE IN PATIENTS UNDERGOING RENAL REPLACEMENT THERAPIES

CAPD	Not dialysed. Dose as in GFR<10 mL/min.
HD	Not dialysed. Dose as in GFR<10 mL/min.
HDF/High flux	Not dialysed. Dose as in GFR<10 mL/min.
CAV/ VVHD	Not dialysed. Dose as in normal renal function.

IMPORTANT DRUG INTERACTIONS

Potentially hazardous interactions with other drugs

- Anti-arrhythmics: increased risk of ventricular arrhythmias with amiodarone – avoid concomitant use.
- Antibacterials: increased risk of ventricular arrhythmias with moxifloxacin – avoid concomitant use; concentration reduced by rifampicin – avoid.
- Anti-epileptics: antagonism of anticonvulsant effect.
- Antimalarials: increased risk of convulsions with chloroquine, hydroxychloroquine and quinine; avoid concomitant use with artemether and lumefantrine.
- Antipsychotics: increased risk of ventricular arrhythmias with haloperidol and pimozide – avoid concomitant use.
- Atomoxetine: increased risk of ventricular arrhythmias.
- Ivabradine: increased risk of ventricular arrhythmias.

ADMINISTRATION

RECONSTITUTION

–

ROUTE

- Oral

RATE OF ADMINISTRATION

–

COMMENTS

–

OTHER INFORMATION

- Start prophylaxis 1–3 weeks before arriving in malarial area and continue for 4 weeks after leaving the malarial area.
- Increased risk of convulsions in patients with epilepsy.
- Contraindicated by manufacturer due to lack of experience in severe renal impairment.
- Doses in renal impairment are from *Drug Prescribing in Renal Failure*, 5th edition, by Aronoff *et al.*

Megestrol acetate

CLINICAL USE

Progestogen:
- Treatment of breast cancer, cachexia (unlicensed)

DOSE IN NORMAL RENAL FUNCTION

160 mg daily.

PHARMACOKINETICS

Molecular weight (daltons)	384.5
% Protein binding	Highly
% Excreted unchanged in urine	56.5–78.4 (5–8% as metabolites)
Volume of distribution (L/kg)	No data
Half-life – normal/ ESRF (hrs)	34/–

METABOLISM

It undergoes hepatic metabolism, with 57–78% of a dose being excreted in the urine and 8–30% in the faeces.

DOSE IN RENAL IMPAIRMENT GFR (mL/MIN)

20–50	Dose as in normal renal function.
10–20	Dose as in normal renal function.
<10	Dose as in normal renal function. Monitor carefully.

DOSE IN PATIENTS UNDERGOING RENAL REPLACEMENT THERAPIES

CAPD	Unlikely to be dialysed. Dose as in GFR<10 mL/min.
HD	Unlikely to be dialysed. Dose as in GFR<10 mL/min.
HDF/High flux	Unlikely to be dialysed. Dose as in GFR<10 mL/min.
CAV/ VVHD	Unlikely to be dialysed. Dose as in normal renal function.

IMPORTANT DRUG INTERACTIONS

Potentially hazardous interactions with other drugs
- Antibacterials: metabolism of progestogens accelerated by rifamycins.
- Anticoagulants: progestogens antagonise anticoagulant effect of phenindione; may enhance or reduce anticoagulant effect of coumarins.
- Anti-epileptics: metabolism accelerated by carbamazepine, eslicarbazepine, oxcarbazepine, phenobarbital, phenytoin, rufinamide and topiramate; concentration reduced by high dose perampanel.
- Ciclosporin: progestogens inhibit metabolism of ciclosporin (increased plasma concentration).
- Dopaminergics: concentration of selegiline increased – avoid concomitant use.

ADMINISTRATION

RECONSTITUTION
–
ROUTE
- Oral
RATE OF ADMINISTRATION
–
COMMENTS
–

OTHER INFORMATION

- Increased risk of toxic reactions in renal impairment.

Melatonin

CLINICAL USE

Melatonin receptor agonist:
- Short-term use for insomnia

DOSE IN NORMAL RENAL FUNCTION

2 mg once daily 1–2 hours before bedtime

PHARMACOKINETICS

Molecular weight (daltons)	232.3
% Protein binding	60
% Excreted unchanged in urine	2
Volume of distribution (L/kg)	65–88 litres (as metabolites)
Half-life – normal/ ESRF (hrs)	3.5–4/Unchanged

METABOLISM

Metabolised in the liver to form inactive metabolites.

DOSE IN RENAL IMPAIRMENT GFR (mL/MIN)

20–50	Dose as in normal renal function.
10–20	Dose as in normal renal function.
<10	Dose as in normal renal function. Use with caution.

DOSE IN PATIENTS UNDERGOING RENAL REPLACEMENT THERAPIES

CAPD	Dialysed. Dose as in GFR<10 mL/min.
HD	Dialysed. Dose as in GFR<10 mL/min.
HDF/High flux	Dialysed. Dose as in GFR<10 mL/min.
CAV/VVHD	Dialysed. Dose as in normal renal function.

IMPORTANT DRUG INTERACTIONS

Potentially hazardous interactions with other drugs
- Antidepressants: increased sedative effects with mirtazapine or tricyclics.
- Antipsychotics: enhanced sedative effects.
- Antivirals: concentration possibly increased by ritonavir.

ADMINISTRATION

RECONSTITUTION
–
ROUTE
- Oral
RATE OF ADMINISTRATION
–
COMMENTS
–

OTHER INFORMATION

- Manufacturer advises to use with caution in severe renal impairment due to lack of studies.
- Oral bioavailability is 15%.

Meloxicam

CLINICAL USE

Cox II inhibitor and analgesic

DOSE IN NORMAL RENAL FUNCTION

7. 5–15 mg daily

PHARMACOKINETICS

Molecular weight (daltons)	351.4
% Protein binding	99
% Excreted unchanged in urine	3
Volume of distribution (L/kg)	11 litres
Half-life – normal/ ESRF (hrs)	20/–

METABOLISM

Extensively metabolised by cytochrome P450 isoenzyme CYP2C9 and to a lesser degree by CYP3A4, mainly by oxidation to its major metabolite, 5'-carboxymeloxicam. Meloxicam, in the form of metabolites, is excreted in similar amounts in the urine and in the faeces.

DOSE IN RENAL IMPAIRMENT GFR (mL/MIN)

20–50	Dose as in normal renal function.
10–20	Dose as in normal renal function, but avoid if possible.
<10	Dose as in normal renal function, but avoid if possible. Only use if on dialysis.

DOSE IN PATIENTS UNDERGOING RENAL REPLACEMENT THERAPIES

CAPD	Not dialysed. Dose as in normal renal function. See 'Other information'.
HD	Not dialysed. Dose as in normal renal function. See 'Other information'.
HDF/High flux	Unlikely to be dialysed. Dose as in normal renal function. See 'Other information'.
CAV/ VVHD	Not dialysed. Dose as in GFR=10–20mL/min.

IMPORTANT DRUG INTERACTIONS

Potentially hazardous interactions with other drugs

- ACE inhibitors and angiotensin-II antagonists: antagonism of hypotensive effect; increased risk of nephrotoxicity and hyperkalaemia.
- Analgesics: avoid concomitant use of 2 or more NSAIDs, including aspirin (increased side effects); avoid with ketorolac (increased risk of side effects and haemorrhage).
- Antibacterials: possibly increased risk of convulsions with quinolones.
- Anticoagulants: effects of coumarins and phenindione enhanced; possibly increased risk of bleeding with heparins and dabigatran.
- Antidepressants: increased risk of bleeding with SSRIs and venlafaxine.
- Antidiabetic agents: effects of sulphonylureas enhanced.
- Anti-epileptics: possibly increased phenytoin concentration.
- Antivirals: increased risk of haematological toxicity with zidovudine; concentration possibly increased by ritonavir.
- Ciclosporin: may potentiate nephrotoxicity.
- Cytotoxic agents: reduced excretion of methotrexate; increased risk of bleeding with erlotinib.
- Diuretics: increased risk of nephrotoxicity; antagonism of diuretic effect; hyperkalaemia with potassium-sparing diuretics.
- Lithium: decreased excretion leading to increased lithium levels.
- Pentoxifylline: possibly increased risk of bleeding.
- Tacrolimus: possibly increased risk of nephrotoxicity.

ADMINISTRATION

RECONSTITUTION

–

ROUTE

- Oral

RATE OF ADMINISTRATION

–

COMMENTS

–

OTHER INFORMATION

- Clinical trials have shown renal effects similar to those observed with comparative NSAIDs. Monitor patient for deterioration in renal function and fluid retention.
- Inhibition of renal prostaglandin synthesis by NSAIDs may interfere with renal function, especially in the presence of existing renal disease – avoid if possible; if not, check serum creatinine 48–72 hours after starting NSAID – if raised, discontinue NSAID therapy.
- Use with caution in renal transplant recipients (can reduce intrarenal autocoid synthesis).
- Meloxicam should be used with caution in uraemic patients predisposed to gastrointestinal bleeding or uraemic coagulopathies.
- Use normal doses in patients with CKD 5 on dialysis if they do not pass any urine.

Melphalan

CLINICAL USE

Alkylating agent:
- Myelomas
- Solid tumours
- Lymphomas
- Polycythaemia vera

DOSE IN NORMAL RENAL FUNCTION

- Orally: 150–200 micrograms/kg daily
  - Polycythaemia vera: 6–10 mg daily, reduced after 5–7 days to 2–4 mg daily, then further reduced to 2–6 mg per week
- IV administration: 16–200 mg/m^2 according to indication and local protocol

PHARMACOKINETICS

Molecular weight (daltons)	305.2
% Protein binding	60–90
% Excreted unchanged in urine	11
Volume of distribution (L/kg)	0.5
Half-life – normal/ ESRF (hrs)	0.5–2.5/4–6

METABOLISM

Spontaneous hydrolysis degradation rather than enzymatic metabolism. Percentage of dose excreted in the urine as active or toxic moiety ranges from 11% to 93%; 20–50% excreted in the faeces within 6 days.

DOSE IN RENAL IMPAIRMENT GFR (mL/MIN)

20–50	75% of dose. See 'Other information'.
10–20	75% of dose. See 'Other information'.
<10	50% of dose. See 'Other information'.

DOSE IN PATIENTS UNDERGOING RENAL REPLACEMENT THERAPIES

CAPD	Not dialysed. Dose as in GFR<10 mL/min.
HD	Not dialysed. Dose as in GFR<10 mL/min.
HDF/High flux	Unknown dialysability. Dose as in GFR<10 mL/min.
CAV/ VVHD	Unknown dialysability. Dose as in GFR=10–20 mL/min.

IMPORTANT DRUG INTERACTIONS

Potentially hazardous interactions with other drugs
- Antipsychotics: avoid concomitant use with clozapine (increased risk of agranulocytosis).
- Ciclosporin: increased risk of nephrotoxicity.

ADMINISTRATION

RECONSTITUTION
- 10 mL of provided diluent

ROUTE
- IV, oral

RATE OF ADMINISTRATION
- Inject slowly into a fast running infusion solution or via an infusion bag.

COMMENTS
- Further dilution with sodium chloride 0.9%.

OTHER INFORMATION

- Melphalan clearance, though variable, is decreased in renal impairment.
- Incomplete and variable oral absorption – 25–89% post oral dose; AUC decreased by 39% when taken with food.
- Doses from BC Cancer Agency (accessed 18 September 2013).
- Manufacturer states that currently available pharmacokinetic data do not justify an absolute recommendation on dosage reduction when administering melphalan tablets to patients with moderate to severe renal impairment, but it may be prudent to use a reduced dosage initially until tolerance is established.
- When melphalan injection is used at conventional IV dosage (8–40 mg/m^2 BSA) in patients with moderate to severe renal impairment, it is recommended that the initial dose should be reduced by 50% and subsequent dosage be determined by the degree of haematological suppression.
- For high IV doses of melphalan (100–240 mg/m^2 BSA), the need for dose reduction depends upon the degree of renal impairment, whether autologous bone marrow stem cells are re-infused, and therapeutic need. High dose melphalan is not recommended in patients with more severe renal impairment (EDTA clearance less than 30 mL/minute).
- It should be borne in mind that dose reduction of melphalan in renal impairment is somewhat arbitrary. At

moderate doses, where melphalan is used as part of a combined regimen, dosage reductions of up to 50% may be appropriate. However, at high doses, e.g. conditioning for bone marrow transplant, there is a risk of underdosing the patient and not achieving the desired therapeutic effect, so the dose should be reduced with caution in these instances.

- Adequate hydration and forced diuresis may be necessary in patients with poor renal function.
- In myeloma patients with renal damage, temporary but significant increases in blood urea levels have been observed during melphalan therapy.

Memantine

CLINICAL USE

NMDA-receptor antagonist:
- Treatment of moderate to severe dementia in Alzheimer's disease

DOSE IN NORMAL RENAL FUNCTION

5–20 mg daily

PHARMACOKINETICS

Molecular weight (daltons)	215.8
% Protein binding	45
% Excreted unchanged in urine	48 (74% plus metabolites)
Volume of distribution (L/kg)	10
Half-life – normal/ ESRF (hrs)	60–100/117–156[1]

METABOLISM

Memantine undergoes partial hepatic metabolism to form mainly three polar metabolites which possess minimal NMDA receptor antagonistic activity: the N-glucuronide conjugate, 6-hydroxy memantine, and 1-nitroso-deaminated memantine. Renal clearance involves active tubular secretion moderated by pH dependent tubular reabsorption.

DOSE IN RENAL IMPAIRMENT GFR (mL/MIN)

30–50	10 mg daily, if tolerated can be increased gradually to 20 mg.
5–29	10 mg daily.
<5	10 mg daily.

DOSE IN PATIENTS UNDERGOING RENAL REPLACEMENT THERAPIES

CAPD	Dialysed. Dose as in GFR<5 mL/min.
HD	Dialysed. Dose as in GFR<5 mL/min.
HDF/High flux	Dialysed. Dose as in GFR<5 mL/min.
CAV/ VVHD	Dialysed. Dose as in GFR=5–29 mL/min.

IMPORTANT DRUG INTERACTIONS

Potentially hazardous interactions with other drugs
- Anaesthetics: increased risk of CNS toxicity with ketamine – avoid concomitant use.
- Analgesics: increased risk of CNS toxicity with dextromethorphan – avoid concomitant use.
- Dopaminergics: possibly enhances effects of dopaminergics & selegiline; increased risk of CNS toxicity with amantadine – avoid concomitant use.

ADMINISTRATION

RECONSTITUTION
–
ROUTE
- Oral
RATE OF ADMINISTRATION
–

OTHER INFORMATION

- Bioavailability is 100%.
- Mean AUC0-∞ increased by 4%, 60%, and 115% in subjects with mild, moderate, and severe renal impairment, respectively, compared to healthy subjects. The terminal elimination half-life increased by 18%, 41%, and 95% in subjects with mild, moderate, and severe renal impairment, respectively, compared to healthy subjects.

Reference:
1. *Drug Information Handbook*. 22nd ed. American Pharmacists Association. Lexicomp.

Mepacrine hydrochloride (unlicensed product)

CLINICAL USE

- Giardiasis
- Discoid lupus erythematosus

DOSE IN NORMAL RENAL FUNCTION

100 mg every 8 hours for 5–7 days

PHARMACOKINETICS

Molecular weight (daltons)	508.9
% Protein binding	80–90
% Excreted unchanged in urine	<11
Volume of distribution (L/kg)	Large
Half-life – normal/ ESRF (hrs)	5–14 days/–

METABOLISM

Mepacrine is excreted slowly mainly in the urine, with an elimination half-life of 5 days, and is still detectable in the urine after 2 months.

DOSE IN RENAL IMPAIRMENT GFR (mL/MIN)

20–50	Dose as in normal renal function.
10–20	Dose as in normal renal function.
<10	Dose as in normal renal function.

DOSE IN PATIENTS UNDERGOING RENAL REPLACEMENT THERAPIES

CAPD	Unlikely to be dialysed. Dose as in normal renal function.
HD	Unlikely to be dialysed. Dose as in normal renal function.
HDF/High flux	Unlikely to be dialysed. Dose as in normal renal function.
CAV/ VVHD	Unlikely to be dialysed. Dose as in normal renal function.

IMPORTANT DRUG INTERACTIONS

Potentially hazardous interactions with other drugs

- Alcohol: can cause a mild disulfiram reaction.
- Antimalarials: increased concentration of primaquine (increased risk of toxicity).

ADMINISTRATION

RECONSTITUTION

–

ROUTE

- Oral

RATE OF ADMINISTRATION

–

COMMENTS

–

OTHER INFORMATION

- Still detectable in the urine after 2 months.

Meptazinol

CLINICAL USE

Opioid analgesic used for moderate to severe pain

DOSE IN NORMAL RENAL FUNCTION

- Oral: 200 mg every 3–6 hours
- IM: 75–100 mg every 2–4 hours; obstetric analgesia: 100–150 mg depending on patient's weight (2 mg/kg)
- Slow IV: 50–100 mg every 2–4 hours

PHARMACOKINETICS

Molecular weight (daltons)	269.8 (as hydrochloride)
% Protein binding	27
% Excreted unchanged in urine	<5
Volume of distribution (L/kg)	3.1
Half-life – normal/ ESRF (hrs)	1.4–4/–

METABOLISM

Meptazinol is extensively metabolised in the liver and is excreted mainly in the urine as the glucuronide conjugate. Less than 10% of a dose has been recovered from the faeces.

DOSE IN RENAL IMPAIRMENT GFR (mL/MIN)

20–50	Dose as in normal renal function.
10–20	Dose as in normal renal function.
<10	Dose as in normal renal function. Start with low doses.

DOSE IN PATIENTS UNDERGOING RENAL REPLACEMENT THERAPIES

CAPD	Unknown dialysability. Dose as in GFR<10 mL/min.
HD	Likely dialysability. Dose as in GFR<10 mL/min.
HDF/High flux	Likely dialysability. Dose as in GFR<10 mL/min.
CAV/ VVHD	Unknown dialysability. Dose as in normal renal function.

IMPORTANT DRUG INTERACTIONS

Potentially hazardous interactions with other drugs

- Antidepressants: possible CNS excitation or depression with MAOIs – avoid concomitant use; possible CNS excitation or depression with moclobemide; possibly increased sedative effects with tricyclics.
- Antihistamines: increased sedative effects with sedating antihistamines.
- Antipsychotics: enhanced hypotensive and sedative effects.
- Dopaminergics: avoid with selegiline.
- Sodium oxybate: enhanced effect of sodium oxybate – avoid concomitant use.

ADMINISTRATION

RECONSTITUTION
–
ROUTE
- Oral, IV, IM
RATE OF ADMINISTRATION
–
COMMENTS
–

OTHER INFORMATION

- Oral and IM peak analgesic effect occurs within 30–60 minutes and last for 3–4 hours.
- IV works immediately and lasts for at least 1 hour.

Mercaptopurine

CLINICAL USE

Antineoplastic agent:
● Acute leukaemias
● Inflammatory bowel disease (unlicensed)

DOSE IN NORMAL RENAL FUNCTION

● Initially 2.5 mg/kg/day, but the dose and duration of administration depend on the nature and dosage of other cytotoxic agents given in conjunction.
● Crohn's disease or ulcerative colitis: 1–1.5 mg/kg daily, some patients may respond to a lower dose.

PHARMACOKINETICS

Molecular weight (daltons)	170.2
% Protein binding	20
% Excreted unchanged in urine	7
Volume of distribution (L/kg)	0.1–1.7
Half-life – normal/ ESRF (hrs)	1–1.5/–

METABOLISM

Extensively metabolised by first pass metabolism in the liver via intracellular activation to an active metabolite.

At conventional doses clearance is primarily hepatic. Renal clearance may become important at high doses.

The active metabolites have a longer half-life than the parent drug. The main method of elimination for 6-mercaptopurine is by metabolic alteration. The kidneys eliminate approximately 7% of 6-mercaptopurine unaltered within 12 hours of the drug being administered. Xanthine oxidase is the main catabolic enzyme of 6-mercaptopurine and it converts the drug into the inactive metabolite, 6-thiouric acid. This is excreted in the urine.

DOSE IN RENAL IMPAIRMENT GFR (mL/MIN)

20–50	Caution – reduce dose. See 'Other information'.
10–20	Caution – reduce dose. See 'Other information'.
<10	Caution – reduce dose. See 'Other information'.

DOSE IN PATIENTS UNDERGOING RENAL REPLACEMENT THERAPIES

CAPD	Unknown dialysability. Dose as in GFR<10 mL/min.
HD	Dialysed. Dose as in GFR<10 mL/min.
HDF/High flux	Dialysed. Dose as in GFR<10 mL/min.
CAV/ VVHD	Dialysed. Dose as in GFR=10– 20 mL/min.

IMPORTANT DRUG INTERACTIONS

Potentially hazardous interactions with other drugs
● Allopurinol: decreased rate of metabolism of mercaptopurine – reduce dose of mercaptopurine to a quarter of normal dose.
● Antibacterials: increased risk of haematological toxicity with co-trimoxazole and trimethoprim.
● Anticoagulants: possibly reduced anticoagulant effect of coumarins.
● Antipsychotics: avoid concomitant use with clozapine (increased risk of agranulocytosis).
● Febuxostat: avoid concomitant use.

ADMINISTRATION

RECONSTITUTION
–
ROUTE
● Oral
RATE OF ADMINISTRATION
–
COMMENTS
–

OTHER INFORMATION

● Absorption of an oral dose is incomplete, averaging ~50%. This is largely due to first pass metabolism (less when given with food). There is enormous inter-individual variability in absorption, which can result in a 5-fold variation in AUC.
● Manufacturer recommends reducing the dose in patients with impaired hepatic or renal function, although no specific dosing guidelines are available due to lack of data.
● The following dosing intervals have been suggested in renal impairment: 24–36 hrs for CRCL of 50–80 mL/min, and 48 hrs for CRCL of 10–50 mL/min. (Summerhayes M, Daniels S (ed). *Practical Chemotherapy*

– a multidisciplinary guide. 1st ed. Oxford: Radcliffe Medical Press Ltd. 2003. p. 384)

- A recent study on anti-cancer drug renal toxicity and elimination concluded that the dose of 6 mercaptopurine does not require modification in patients with decreased renal function (except in conjunction with allopurinol). This study also gives percentage excreted unchanged in urine as 21%. (Kintzel PE, Dorr RT. Anticancer drug renal toxicity and elimination: dosing guidelines for altered renal function. *Cancer Treat Rev.* 1995; **21**: 33–64).

Meropenem

CLINICAL USE

Antibacterial agent

DOSE IN NORMAL RENAL FUNCTION

500 mg – 1 g every 8 hours
Higher doses used in cystic fibrosis and
meningitis (up to 2 g every 8 hours)

PHARMACOKINETICS

Molecular weight (daltons)	437.5
% Protein binding	2
% Excreted unchanged in urine	70
Volume of distribution (L/kg)	0.35[1]
Half-life – normal/ ESRF (hrs)	1/6–13.7[2]

METABOLISM

Meropenem is more stable to renal
dehydropeptidase I than imipenem but
undergoes some renal metabolism, and
is mainly excreted in the urine by tubular
secretion and glomerular filtration. About
70% of a dose is recovered unchanged in the
urine over a 12-hour period. Meropenem
is reported to have one metabolite (ICI-
213689), which is inactive and is excreted in
the urine.

DOSE IN RENAL IMPAIRMENT GFR (mL/MIN)

26–50	500 mg – 2 g every 12 hours.
10–20	500 mg – 1 g every 12 hours or 500 mg every 8 hours.
<10	500 mg – 1 g every 24 hours.

DOSE IN PATIENTS UNDERGOING RENAL REPLACEMENT THERAPIES

CAPD	Dialysed. Dose as in GFR<10 mL/min.
HD	Dialysed. Dose as in GFR<10 mL/min or 1–2 g post dialysis.[2]
HDF/High flux	Dialysed. Dose as in GFR<10 mL/min.
CAV/VVH/ HD[1,2]	Dialysed. 0.5–1 g every 8 hours[2,3] or 1 g every 12 hours.[1]
CVVHDF	1 g every 12 hours.[3]

IMPORTANT DRUG INTERACTIONS

Potentially hazardous interactions with other
drugs
- Anti-epileptics: concentration of valproate reduced – avoid.
- Probenecid: avoid concomitant use.

ADMINISTRATION

RECONSTITUTION
- Add 5 mL water for injection to each 250 mg of meropenem.
ROUTE
- Bolus: 5 minutes
- IV Infusion: 15–30 minutes
COMMENTS
- Further dilute in 50–200 mL sodium chloride 0.9%, glucose 5% or glucose 10% if for infusion.
- Stable for 24 hours once reconstituted.
- Minimum volume 1 g in 10 mL. (UK Critical Care Group, *Minimum Infusion Volumes for Fluid Restricted Critically Ill Patients*, 3rd edition, 2006)

OTHER INFORMATION

- Each 1 g vial contains 3.9 mmol of sodium.
- Has less potential to induce seizures than imipenem.
- Has been used intraperitoneally for peritoneal dialysis Pseudomonas peritonitis at a concentration of 100 mg/L.
- 50% is removed by CVVHF, 13–53% by CVVHDF, 50% by intermittent HD.[2]
- Differences in renal replacement doses are due to the different flow rates used in the studies.

References:
1. Giles LJ, Jennings AC, Thomson AH, *et al.*
Pharmacokinetics of meropenem in intensive
care unit patients receiving continuous venovenous hemofiltration or hemodiafiltration.
Crit Care Med. 2000; **28**(3): 632–7.
2. Thalhammer F, Hörl WH.
Pharmacokinetics of meropenem in patients
with renal failure and patients receiving renal
replacement therapy. *Clin Pharmacokinet.*
2000; **39**(4): 271–9.
3. Valtonen M, Backman JT, Neuvonen
PJ. Elimination of meropenem during
continuous veno-venous haemofiltration and
haemodiafiltration in patients with acute
renal failure. *J Antimicrob Chemother.* 2000;
45(5): 701–4.

Mesalazine

CLINICAL USE

Induction and maintenance of remission in ulcerative colitis

DOSE IN NORMAL RENAL FUNCTION

Dose depends on preparation

PHARMACOKINETICS

Molecular weight (daltons)	153.1
% Protein binding	40–50
% Excreted unchanged in urine	No data
Volume of distribution (L/kg)	no data
Half-life – normal/ ESRF (hrs)	0.6/–

METABOLISM

The absorbed part of mesalazine is almost completely acetylated in the gut wall and in the liver to acetyl-5-aminosalicylic acid. The acetylated metabolite is excreted mainly in urine by tubular secretion, with traces of the parent compound.

DOSE IN RENAL IMPAIRMENT GFR (mL/MIN)

20–50	Caution – use only if necessary. Start with low dose and increase according to response.
10–20	Caution – use only if necessary. Start with low dose and monitor closely.
<10	Caution – use only if necessary. Start with low dose and monitor closely.

DOSE IN PATIENTS UNDERGOING RENAL REPLACEMENT THERAPIES

CAPD	Unlikely to be dialysed. Dose as in GFR<10 mL/min.
HD	Unlikely to be dialysed. Dose as in GFR<10 mL/min.
HDF/High flux	Unknown dialysability. Dose as in GFR<10 mL/min.
CAV/ VVHD	Unknown dialysability. Dose as in GFR=10–20 mL/min.

IMPORTANT DRUG INTERACTIONS

Potentially hazardous interactions with other drugs
* None known

ADMINISTRATION

RECONSTITUTION
–
ROUTE
* Oral, PR
RATE OF ADMINISTRATION
–
COMMENTS
–

OTHER INFORMATION

* Contraindicated by manufacturer if GFR<20 mL/min.
* Nephrotoxicity has been reported.
* Mesalazine is best avoided in patients with established renal impairment, but if necessary should be used with caution, and the patient carefully monitored.

Mesna

CLINICAL USE

Prophylaxis of urothelial toxicity in patients treated with ifosfamide or cyclophosphamide

DOSE IN NORMAL RENAL FUNCTION

Dose and timing depends on cytotoxic agent and on route of administration of mesna.

PHARMACOKINETICS

Molecular weight (daltons)	164.2
% Protein binding	70
% Excreted unchanged in urine	32
Volume of distribution (L/kg)	0.65
Half-life – normal/ ESRF (hrs)	0.3/–

METABOLISM

Rapidly metabolised in the liver to the disulfide, dimesna, and is excreted in the urine as both metabolite and unchanged drug; dimesna is reduced back to mesna, which is the active form, in the kidney.

DOSE IN RENAL IMPAIRMENT GFR (mL/MIN)

20–50	Dose as in normal renal function. See 'Other information'.
10–20	Dose as in normal renal function. See 'Other information'.
<10	Dose as in normal renal function. See 'Other information'.

DOSE IN PATIENTS UNDERGOING RENAL REPLACEMENT THERAPIES

CAPD	Unknown dialysability. Dose as in GFR<10 mL/min.
HD	Probably dialysed. Dose as in GFR<10 mL/min.
HDF/High flux	Probably dialysed. Dose as in GFR<10 mL/min.
CAV/ VVHD	Probably dialysed. Dose as in GFR=10–20 mL/min.

IMPORTANT DRUG INTERACTIONS

Potentially hazardous interactions with other drugs
- None known

ADMINISTRATION

RECONSTITUTION
–
ROUTE
- Oral, IV bolus, IV infusion
RATE OF ADMINISTRATION
- IV bolus: over 15–30 minutes
- IV infusion: over 12–24 hours
COMMENTS
- Compatible with sodium chloride 0.9% and glucose 5%.
- Mesna injection can be administered orally in orange juice or cola to improve palatability.

OTHER INFORMATION

- Doses in renal impairment are from *Drug Prescribing in Renal Failure*, 5th edition, by Aronoff *et al.*
- Urinary output should be maintained at 100 mL/hr (as required for oxazaphosphorine treatment).
- The dose of mesna is dependent on the dose of oxazaphosphorine, e.g. reduce dose of cyclophosphamide to 50% of normal if GFR <10 mL/min; hence, dose of mesna will consequently be reduced.
- From what is known about the pharmacokinetics and mechanism of action of mesna, its availability in the urinary tract depends on renal function.
- In the case of completely anuric patients (extremely rare) neither cyclophosphamide nor its metabolites should appear in the urinary tract: the use of mesna concomitantly may therefore be unnecessary in anuric patients. If there is any risk of cyclophosphamide or its metabolites entering the urinary tract, mesna should probably be given to prevent urothelial toxicity.
- Limited kinetic information would suggest mesna would be eliminated by haemodialysis.

Metformin hydrochloride

CLINICAL USE

- Non-insulin dependent diabetes mellitus
- Polycystic ovary syndrome

DOSE IN NORMAL RENAL FUNCTION

- 500 mg 3 times a day; maximum 2 g daily in divided doses
- Polycystic ovary syndrome: 1.5–1.7 g daily in 2–3 divided doses
- MR: 500 mg – 2 g daily in 1–2 divided doses

PHARMACOKINETICS

Molecular weight (daltons)	165.6
% Protein binding	Negligible
% Excreted unchanged in urine	100
Volume of distribution (L/kg)	1–4
Half-life – normal/ ESRF (hrs)	2–6/prolonged

METABOLISM

Metformin is not metabolised to any great extent, and is entirely excreted unchanged in the urine.

DOSE IN RENAL IMPAIRMENT GFR (mL/MIN)

40–50	25–50% of dose
10–40	25% of dose. See 'Other information'.
<10	Avoid. See 'Other information'.

DOSE IN PATIENTS UNDERGOING RENAL REPLACEMENT THERAPIES

CAPD	Unknown dialysability. Avoid.
HD	Dialysed. Avoid.
HDF/High flux	Dialysed. Avoid.
CAV/ VVHD	Probably dialysed. Avoid.

IMPORTANT DRUG INTERACTIONS

Potentially hazardous interactions with other drugs
- Alcohol: increased risk of lactic acidosis.
- Cimetidine: Inhibits renal excretion of metformin.

ADMINISTRATION

RECONSTITUTION

–

ROUTE
- Oral

RATE OF ADMINISTRATION

–

COMMENTS

–

OTHER INFORMATION

- Doses in renal impairment are from *Drug Prescribing in Renal Failure*, 5th edition, by Aronoff *et al.*
- Lactic acidosis is a rare but serious metabolic complication that can occur due to metformin accumulation. Reported cases have occurred primarily in diabetic patients with significant renal impairment.
- Contraindicated by manufacturer if GFR<60 mL/min.
- A recent paper debates how safe metformin is in renal disease and suggests it can be used in patients with GFR>30 mL/min with careful monitoring and query the data which says it commonly causes lactic acidosis. (Herrington WG, Levy JB. Metformin: effective and safe in renal disease? *Urol Nephrol.* 2008; **40**: 411–17)
- As metformin is renally excreted eGFR values should be determined before initiating treatment and regularly thereafter:
  — at least annually in patients with normal renal function
  — at least 2–4 times a year in patients with an eGFR at the lower limit of normal and in elderly subjects.
- Special caution should be exercised in the elderly in situations where renal function may become impaired, e.g. initiating therapy with antihypertensives, diuretics or NSAIDs.

Methadone hydrochloride

CLINICAL USE

- Treatment of opioid drug addiction
- Analgesic for moderate to severe pain

DOSE IN NORMAL RENAL FUNCTION

- Opioid addiction: 10–40mg per day, increasing by 10mg per day until there are no signs of withdrawal or intoxication; reduce gradually.
- Analgesia: 5–10mg every 6–8 hours.

PHARMACOKINETICS

Molecular weight (daltons)	346.9
% Protein binding	60–90
% Excreted unchanged in urine	15–60
Volume of distribution (L/kg)	3–6
Half-life – normal/ ESRF (hrs)	13–47/–

METABOLISM

Metabolised in the liver to the major metabolite 2-ethylidine-1,5-dimethyl-3,3-diphenylpyrrolidine and the minor metabolite 2-ethyl-3,3-diphenyl-5-methylpyrrolidine, both of them inactive. Two other metabolites have also been identified.

These metabolites are excreted in the faeces and urine with unchanged methadone

DOSE IN RENAL IMPAIRMENT GFR (mL/MIN)

20–50	Dose as in normal renal function.
10–20	Dose as in normal renal function.
<10	50–75% of normal dose, and titrate according to response.

DOSE IN PATIENTS UNDERGOING RENAL REPLACEMENT THERAPIES

CAPD	Not dialysed. Dose as in GFR<10mL/min.
HD	Not dialysed. Dose as in GFR<10mL/min.
HDF/High flux	Dialysed. Dose as in GFR<10mL/min.
CAV/ VVHD	Unknown dialysability. Dose as in normal renal function.

IMPORTANT DRUG INTERACTIONS

Potentially hazardous interactions with other drugs

- Antibacterials: metabolism increased by rifampicin; increased risk of ventricular arrhythmias with telithromycin.
- Antidepressants: concentration possibly increased by fluoxetine, fluvoxamine, paroxetine and sertraline; possible CNS excitation or depression with MAOIs and moclobemide – avoid concomitant use; possibly increased sedative effects with tricyclics; concentration possibly reduced by St John's wort.
- Anti-epileptics: concentration reduced by carbamazepine, phenobarbital and phenytoin.
- Antifungals: concentration increased by fluconazole and voriconazole – may need to reduce methadone dose with voriconazole.
- Antihistamines: increased sedative effects with sedating antihistamines.
- Antimalarials: increased risk of ventricular arrhythmias with piperaquine with artenimol – avoid.
- Antipsychotics: enhanced hypotensive and sedative effects; increased risk of ventricular arrhythmias with antipsychotics that prolong the QT interval – avoid with amisulpride.
- Antivirals: methadone possibly increases concentration of zidovudine; concentration reduced by efavirenz, fosamprenavir and ritonavir; concentration possibly reduced by abacavir, nevirapine and rilpivirine; concentration possibly affected by boceprevir; concentration of didanosine possibly reduced; increased risk of ventricular arrhythmias with saquinavir and telaprevir – avoid with saquinavir and use with caution with telaprevir.
- Atomoxetine: increased risk of ventricular arrhythmias.
- Cytotoxics: possible increased risk of ventricular arrhythmias with vandetanib.
- Dopaminergics: avoid with selegiline.
- Sodium oxybate: enhanced effect of sodium oxybate – avoid concomitant use.

ADMINISTRATION

RECONSTITUTION

–

ROUTE

- IM, SC, oral

RATE OF ADMINISTRATION

–

COMMENTS

- Methadone is probably not suitable to be used as an analgesic for patients with severe renal impairment.

OTHER INFORMATION

- Dose in severe renal impairment is from *Drug Prescribing in Renal Failure*, 5th edition, by Aronoff *et al.*
- Overdosage with methadone can be reversed using naloxone.
- Risk of QT interval prolongation especially with high doses and concomitant risk factors.

Methenamine hippurate

CLINICAL USE

Antibacterial agent

DOSE IN NORMAL RENAL FUNCTION

1 g every 8–12 hours

PHARMACOKINETICS

Molecular weight (daltons)	319.4
% Protein binding	No data
% Excreted unchanged in urine	80–90
Volume of distribution (L/kg)	No data
Half-life – normal/ ESRF (hrs)	4/–

METABOLISM

Under acid conditions methenamine is slowly hydrolysed to formaldehyde and ammonia. Almost no hydrolysis of methenamine takes place at physiological pH, and it is therefore virtually inactive in the body. Methenamine is rapidly and almost completely eliminated in the urine, and provided this is acidic (preferably below pH 5.5) bactericidal concentrations of formaldehyde occur. Because of the time taken for hydrolysis, however, these do not occur until the urine reaches the bladder.

DOSE IN RENAL IMPAIRMENT GFR (mL/MIN)

20–50	Dose as in normal renal function.
10–20	Dose as in normal renal function.
<10	Avoid. See 'Other information'.

DOSE IN PATIENTS UNDERGOING RENAL REPLACEMENT THERAPIES

CAPD	Unknown dialysability. Avoid. See 'Other information'.
HD	Unknown dialysability. Avoid. See 'Other information'.
HDF/High flux	Unknown dialysability. Avoid. See 'Other information'.
CAV/ VVHD	Unknown dialysability. Dose as in normal renal function.

IMPORTANT DRUG INTERACTIONS

Potentially hazardous interactions with other drugs

- Antibacterials: increased risk of crystalluria with sulphonamides.
- Diuretics: effects antagonised by acetazolamide.

ADMINISTRATION

RECONSTITUTION

–

ROUTE

- Oral

RATE OF ADMINISTRATION

–

COMMENTS

–

OTHER INFORMATION

- Avoid hippurate salt in renal impairment due to the risk of hippurate crystalluria.
- Methenamine is not recommended in severe renal impairment as urinary concentrations are too low for it to be effective.
- Contraindicated in metabolic acidosis, severe dehydration, renal parenchymal infections and hepatic failure.

Methotrexate

CLINICAL USE

Antineoplastic agent:
- Severe rheumatoid arthritis
- Severe uncontrolled psoriasis
- Crohn's disease (unlicensed)
- Neoplastic disease

DOSE IN NORMAL RENAL FUNCTION

- Rheumatoid arthritis:
  - Oral: 7.5–20 mg once weekly
  - IM, IV, SC: 7.5–25 mg once weekly.
- Psoriasis: (Oral, IM, IV, SC) 10–30 mg once weekly, adjusted to response.
- Crohn's disease (unlicensed): Oral: 10–25 mg once weekly; IM: Induction: 25 mg once weekly; Maintenance: 15 mg once weekly
- Neoplastic disease: Dose by weight or surface area according to specific indication.

PHARMACOKINETICS

Molecular weight (daltons)	454.4
% Protein binding	45–60
% Excreted unchanged in urine	80–90
Volume of distribution (L/kg)	0.4–0.8
Half-life – normal/ ESRF (hrs)	2–17/Increased

METABOLISM

Metabolism is via liver and intracellular metabolism to polyglutamated products. Methotrexate does not appear to undergo significant metabolism at low doses; after high-dose therapy the 7-hydroxy metabolite has been detected. Methotrexate may be partly metabolised by the intestinal flora after oral doses. It is excreted mainly in the urine (90%), by glomerular filtration and active tubular secretion. Small amounts are excreted in bile and found in faeces; there is some evidence for enterohepatic recirculation.

DOSE IN RENAL IMPAIRMENT GFR (mL/MIN)

20–50	50% of normal dose. See 'Other information'.
10–20	50% of normal dose. See 'Other information'.
<10	Contraindicated. See 'Other information'.

DOSE IN PATIENTS UNDERGOING RENAL REPLACEMENT THERAPIES

CAPD	Not dialysed. Contraindicated.
HD	Dialysed. Haemodialysis clearance is 38–40 mL/minute. 50% of normal dose at least 12 hours before next dialysis. Use with caution.
HDF/High flux	Dialysed. 50% of normal dose at least 12 hours before next dialysis. Use with caution.
CAV/ VVHD	Unknown dialysability. Dose as in GFR=10–20 mL/min.

IMPORTANT DRUG INTERACTIONS

Potentially hazardous interactions with other drugs
- Anaesthetics: antifolate effect increased by nitrous oxide – avoid concomitant use.
- Analgesics: increased risk of toxicity with NSAIDs – avoid.
- Antibacterials: absorption possibly reduced by neomycin; antifolate effect increased with co-trimoxazole and trimethoprim; penicillins and possibly ciprofloxacin reduce excretion of methotrexate (increased risk of toxicity); increased haematological toxicity with doxycycline, sulfonamides and tetracycline.
- Antimalarials: antifolate effect enhanced by pyrimethamine.
- Antipsychotics: avoid concomitant use with clozapine (increased risk of agranulocytosis).
- Ciclosporin: methotrexate may inhibit the clearance of ciclosporin or its metabolites; ciclosporin may inhibit methotrexate elimination.
- Corticosteroids: increased risk of haematological toxicity.
- Cytotoxics: increased pulmonary toxicity with cisplatin.
- Leflunomide: risk of toxicity.
- Probenecid: excretion of methotrexate reduced.

- Retinoids: concentration increased by acitretin, also increased hepatotoxicity – avoid concomitant use.

ADMINISTRATION

RECONSTITUTION
- Compatible with glucose 5%, sodium chloride 0.9%, compound sodium lactate, or Ringer's solution.

ROUTE
- Oral, IM, SC, IV (bolus injection or infusion), intrathecal, intra-arterial, intraventricular

RATE OF ADMINISTRATION
- Slow IV injection

COMMENTS
- High-dose methotrexate may cause precipitation of methotrexate or its metabolites in renal tubules. A high fluid throughput and alkalinisation of urine, using sodium bicarbonate if necessary, is recommended.

OTHER INFORMATION

- Renal function should be closely monitored throughout treatment. If there is any deterioration in renal function methotrexate must be discontinued and discussed with the consultant who started treatment.
- Doses in renal impairment are from *Drug Prescribing in Renal Failure*, 5th edition, by Aronoff et al.
- The dose is well absorbed at doses <30 mg/m^2 – bioavailability is decreased by food and milk.

- Calcium folinate (calcium leucovorin) is a potent agent for neutralising the immediate toxic effects of methotrexate on the haematopoietic system.
- Calcium folinate rescue may begin 24/32/36 hours post start of methotrexate therapy, according to local protocol. Doses of up to 120 mg may be given over 12–24 hours by IM or IV injection or infusion, followed by 12–15 mg IM, or 15 mg orally every 6 hours for the next 48 hours.
- An approximate correction for renal function may be made by reducing the dose in proportion to the reduction in creatinine clearance based on a normal creatinine clearance of 60 mL/minute/m^2.
- Alternative dosing regimen:

CRCL (mL/min)	Dose
>80	100%
60	65%
45	50%
<30	Avoid

Doses in renal failure from Kintzel PE, Dorr RT. Anticancer drug renal toxicity and elimination: dosing guidelines for altered renal function. *Cancer Treat Rev.* 1995; **21**: 33–64.

BC Cancer agency suggest (accessed 19 September 2013):
GFR=61–80: 75% of dose,
GFR=51–60: 70% of dose,
GFR=10–50: 30–50% of dose,
GFR<10: Avoid.

Methyldopa

CLINICAL USE

Hypertension

DOSE IN NORMAL RENAL FUNCTION

250 mg 2–3 times a day, increasing to a
maximum dose of 3 g daily
- Elderly: 125 mg twice daily to a maximum
  of 2 g daily

PHARMACOKINETICS

Molecular weight (daltons)	238.2
% Protein binding	<15
% Excreted unchanged in urine	25–40
Volume of distribution (L/kg)	0.5
Half-life – normal/ ESRF (hrs)	1.6–2/6–16

METABOLISM

Methyldopa is extensively metabolised in
the liver to form active metabolites with a
long half-life. It is excreted in urine mainly as
unchanged drug and the O-sulfate conjugate.

DOSE IN RENAL IMPAIRMENT GFR (mL/MIN)

20–50	Dose as in normal renal function and adjust according to response.
10–20	Dose as in normal renal function and adjust according to response.
<10	Dose as in normal renal function and adjust according to response.

DOSE IN PATIENTS UNDERGOING RENAL REPLACEMENT THERAPIES

CAPD	Dialysed. Dose as in GFR<10 mL/min.
HD	Dialysed. Dose as in GFR<10 mL/min.
HDF/High flux	Dialysed. Dose as in GFR<10 mL/min.
CAV/VVHD	Probably dialysed. Dose as in GFR=10–20 mL/min.

IMPORTANT DRUG INTERACTIONS

Potentially hazardous interactions with other
drugs
- Anaesthetics: enhanced hypotensive effect.
- Antidepressants: avoid concomitant use
  with MAOIs.
- Lithium: neurotoxicity (without increased
  plasma-lithium concentrations).
- Salbutamol: acute hypotension reported
  with salbutamol infusions.

ADMINISTRATION

RECONSTITUTION

–

ROUTE
- Oral

RATE OF ADMINISTRATION

–

COMMENTS

–

OTHER INFORMATION

- Interferes with serum creatinine
  measurement.
- Orthostatic hypotension more common in
  renally impaired patients.

Methylprednisolone

CLINICAL USE

Corticosteroid:
- Suppression of inflammatory and allergic disorder
- Immunosuppressant
- Rheumatic disease
- Cerebral oedema

DOSE IN NORMAL RENAL FUNCTION

- Oral: 2–40 mg daily
- IM/IV: 10–500 mg
- Graft rejection: up to 1 g daily for up to 3 days. See 'Other information'.
- IM depot: 40–120 mg into gluteal muscle, repeated after 2–3 weeks if required

PHARMACOKINETICS

Molecular weight (daltons)	375
% Protein binding	40–60
% Excreted unchanged in urine	<10
Volume of distribution (L/kg)	1.2–1.5
Half-life – normal/ESRF (hrs)	2.4–3.5/ Unchanged

METABOLISM

Metabolism in the liver occurs primarily via the CYP3A4 enzyme to inactive metabolites, which are excreted in the urine.

DOSE IN RENAL IMPAIRMENT GFR (mL/MIN)

20–50	Dose as in normal renal function.
10–20	Dose as in normal renal function.
<10	Dose as in normal renal function.

DOSE IN PATIENTS UNDERGOING RENAL REPLACEMENT THERAPIES

CAPD	Dialysed. Dose as in normal renal function.
HD	Dialysed. Dose as in normal renal function.
HDF/High flux	Dialysed. Dose as in normal renal function.
CAV/ VVHD	Dialysed. Dose as in normal renal function.

IMPORTANT DRUG INTERACTIONS

Potentially hazardous interactions with other drugs
- Aldesleukin: avoid concomitant use.
- Antibacterials: metabolism accelerated by rifampicin; metabolism inhibited by erythromycin and possibly clarithromycin; concentration of isoniazid possibly reduced.
- Anticoagulants: efficacy of coumarins and phenindione may be altered.
- Anti-epileptics: metabolism accelerated by carbamazepine, phenobarbital and phenytoin.
- Antifungals: increased risk of hypokalaemia with amphotericin – avoid concomitant use; metabolism inhibited by ketoconazole and possibly itraconazole.
- Antivirals: concentration possibly increased by ritonavir.
- Ciclosporin: rare reports of convulsions in patients on ciclosporin and high-dose corticosteroids; levels of ciclosporin increased with high dose methylprednisolone.
- Diuretics: enhanced hypokalaemic effects of acetazolamide, loop diuretics and thiazide diuretics.
- Vaccines: high dose corticosteroids can impair immune response to vaccines; avoid concomitant use with live vaccines.

ADMINISTRATION

RECONSTITUTION
- Use solvent supplied (Solu-medrone) or see manufacturer's recommendations.

ROUTE
- Oral, IM, IV peripherally or centrally

RATE OF ADMINISTRATION
- 30 minutes

COMMENTS
- NB: Rapid bolus injection may be associated with arrhythmias or cardiovascular collapse.

OTHER INFORMATION

- A single dose of 500 mg –1 g is often given at transplantation.
- Three 500 mg – 1 g doses at 24 hour intervals are often used as first line for reversal of acute rejection episodes. (Some units use 300–500 mg daily for 3 days.)
- Anecdotally, possesses less mineralocorticoid activity than equipotent doses of prednisolone.

Metoclopramide hydrochloride

CLINICAL USE

Nausea and vomiting

DOSE IN NORMAL RENAL FUNCTION

10 mg 3 times a day.
- Use in patients under 20 years should be restricted.

PHARMACOKINETICS

Molecular weight (daltons)	354.3
% Protein binding	13–22
% Excreted unchanged in urine	20–30
Volume of distribution (L/kg)	3.5
Half-life – normal/ ESRF (hrs)	4–6/15

METABOLISM

Metoclopramide undergoes first-pass hepatic metabolism. It is excreted in the urine, about 85% of a dose being eliminated in 72 hours, 20% as unchanged metoclopramide and the remainder as sulfate or glucuronide conjugates, or as metabolites. About 5% of a dose is excreted in faeces via the bile.

DOSE IN RENAL IMPAIRMENT GFR (mL/MIN)

20–50	Dose as in normal renal function.
10–20	Dose as in normal renal function.
<10	Dose as in normal renal function.

DOSE IN PATIENTS UNDERGOING RENAL REPLACEMENT THERAPIES

CAPD	Not dialysed. Dose as in normal renal function.
HD	Dialysed. Dose as in normal renal function.
HDF/High flux	Dialysed. Dose as in normal renal function.
CAV/ VVHD	Dialysed. Dose as in normal renal function.

IMPORTANT DRUG INTERACTIONS

Potentially hazardous interactions with other drugs
- Ciclosporin: increased ciclosporin blood levels.

ADMINISTRATION

RECONSTITUTION
–

ROUTE
- Oral, IV, IM

RATE OF ADMINISTRATION
- 1–2 minutes

COMMENTS
–

OTHER INFORMATION

- Increased risk of extrapyramidal reactions in severe renal impairment.
- Can be used for hiccups at a dose of 10 mg 3 times a day.

Metolazone (unlicensed)

CLINICAL USE

Thiazide diuretic, acts synergistically with loop diuretics:
- Oedema
- Hypertension

DOSE IN NORMAL RENAL FUNCTION

- Oedema: 5–10 mg, increased to 20 mg daily; maximum 80 mg daily
- Hypertension: 5 mg initially; maintenance: 5 mg on alternate days

PHARMACOKINETICS

Molecular weight (daltons)	365.8
% Protein binding	95
% Excreted unchanged in urine	80–95
Volume of distribution (L/kg)	1.6
Half-life – normal/ ESRF (hrs)	8–10/–

METABOLISM

Minimal metabolism in the kidney. About 70–80% of the amount of metolazone absorbed is excreted in the urine, of which 80–95% is excreted unchanged. The remainder is excreted in the bile and some enterohepatic circulation has been reported.

DOSE IN RENAL IMPAIRMENT GFR (mL/MIN)

20–50	Dose as in normal renal function.
10–20	Dose as in normal renal function.
<10	Dose as in normal renal function.

DOSE IN PATIENTS UNDERGOING RENAL REPLACEMENT THERAPIES

CAPD	Unlikely to be dialysed. Dose as in normal renal function.
HD	Not dialysed. Dose as in normal renal function.
HDF/High flux	Unknown dialysability. Dose as in normal renal function.
CAV/ VVHD	Not dialysed. Dose as in normal renal function.

IMPORTANT DRUG INTERACTIONS

Potentially hazardous interactions with other drugs

- Analgesics: increased risk of nephrotoxicity with NSAIDs; antagonism of diuretic effect.
- Anti-arrhythmics: hypokalaemia leads to increased cardiac toxicity; effects of lidocaine and mexiletine antagonised.
- Antibacterials: avoid administration with lymecycline.
- Antidepressants: increased risk of hypokalaemia with reboxetine; enhanced hypotensive effect with MAOIs; increased risk of postural hypotension with tricyclics.
- Anti-epileptics: increased risk of hyponatraemia with carbamazepine.
- Antifungals: increased risk of hypokalaemia with amphotericin.
- Antihypertensives: enhanced hypotensive effect; increased risk of first dose hypotension with post-synaptic alpha-blockers like prazosin; hypokalaemia increases risk of ventricular arrhythmias with sotalol.
- Antipsychotics: hypokalaemia increases risk of ventricular arrhythmias with amisulpride; enhanced hypotensive effect with phenothiazines; hypokalaemia increases risk of ventricular arrhythmias with pimozide – avoid concomitant use.
- Atomoxetine: hypokalaemia increases risk of ventricular arrhythmias.
- Cardiac glycosides: increased toxicity if hypokalaemia occurs.
- Ciclosporin: increased risk of nephrotoxicity and possibly hypomagnesaemia.
- Cytotoxics: increased risk of ventricular arrhythmias due to hypokalaemia with arsenic trioxide; increased risk of nephrotoxicity and ototoxicity with platinum compounds.
- Lithium excretion reduced, increased toxicity.

ADMINISTRATION

RECONSTITUTION
–

ROUTE
- Oral

RATE OF ADMINISTRATION
–

COMMENTS
–

OTHER INFORMATION

- May result in profound diuresis. Monitor patient's fluid balance carefully.
- Monitor for hypokalaemia.
- In patients with creatinine clearance less than 50 mL/minute there is no clinical evidence of accumulation.

Metoprolol tartrate

CLINICAL USE

Beta-adrenoceptor blocker:
- Hypertension
- Angina
- Cardiac arrhythmias
- Migraine prophylaxis
- Hyperthyroidism

DOSE IN NORMAL RENAL FUNCTION

Oral:
- Hypertension: 100–400 mg daily in divided doses
- Angina: 50–100 mg 2–3 times daily
- Arrhythmias: 100–300 mg in 2–3 divided doses
- Migraine: 100–200 mg daily in divided doses
- Hyperthyroidism: 50 mg 4 times daily

IV: 5 mg repeated after 5 minutes to a total dose of 10–15 mg
In surgery: 2–4 mg by slow IV injection then 2 mg as required to a maximum of 10 mg

PHARMACOKINETICS

Molecular weight (daltons)	684.8
% Protein binding	10–12
% Excreted unchanged in urine	5–10
Volume of distribution (L/kg)	5.6
Half-life – normal/ ESRF (hrs)	1–9 (av: 3.5)/ Unchanged

METABOLISM

Extensively metabolised in the liver, mainly by the cytochrome P450 isoenzyme CYP2D6, and undergoes oxidative deamination, O-dealkylation followed by oxidation, and aliphatic hydroxylation.

The metabolites are excreted in the urine with only small amounts of unchanged metoprolol.

DOSE IN RENAL IMPAIRMENT GFR (mL/MIN)

20–50	Dose as in normal renal function.
10–20	Start with small doses and titrate in accordance with response.
<10	Start with small doses and titrate in accordance with response.

DOSE IN PATIENTS UNDERGOING RENAL REPLACEMENT THERAPIES

CAPD	Not dialysed. Dose as in GFR<10 mL/min.
HD	Not dialysed. Dose as in GFR<10 mL/min.
HDF/High flux	Dialysed. Dose as in GFR<10 mL/min.
CAV/ VVHD	Probably dialysed. Dose as in GFR=10–20 mL/min.

IMPORTANT DRUG INTERACTIONS

Potentially hazardous interactions with other drugs
- Anaesthetics: enhanced hypotensive effect.
- Analgesics: NSAIDs antagonise hypotensive effect.
- Anti-arrhythmics: increased risk of myocardial depression and bradycardia; increased risk of bradycardia, myocardial depression and AV block with amiodarone; increased risk of myocardial depression and bradycardia with flecainide; concentration increased by propafenone and dronedarone.
- Antibacterials: concentration reduced by rifampicin.
- Antidepressants: enhanced hypotensive effect with MAOIs; concentration increased by citalopram and escitalopram and possibly by paroxetine.
- Antihypertensives; enhanced hypotensive effect; increased risk of withdrawal hypertension with clonidine; increased risk of first dose hypotensive effect with post-synaptic alpha-blockers such as prazosin.
- Antimalarials: increased risk of bradycardia with mefloquine; avoid with artemether/lumefantrine.
- Antipsychotics enhanced hypotensive effect with phenothiazines.
- Antivirals: avoid concomitant use with tipranavir in heart failure.
- Calcium-channel blockers: increased risk of bradycardia and AV block with diltiazem; hypotension and heart failure possible with nifedipine and nisoldipine; asystole, severe hypotension and heart failure with verapamil.
- Cytotoxics: possible increased risk of bradycardia with crizotinib.

- Diuretics: enhanced hypotensive effect.
- Fingolimod: possibly increased risk of bradycardia.
- Moxisylyte: possible severe postural hypotension.
- Sympathomimetics: severe hypertension with adrenaline and noradrenaline and possibly with dobutamine.

ADMINISTRATION

RECONSTITUTION

–

ROUTE

- Oral, IV

RATE OF ADMINISTRATION

- For bolus injection, 1–2 mg/minute or by continuous infusion via CRIP

COMMENTS

- A total dose of 10–15 mg IV is usually sufficient.

OTHER INFORMATION

- Can cause hypoglycaemia in dialysis patients.
- Accumulation of the metabolites will occur in renal failure, but does not seem to cause any side effects.

Metronidazole

CLINICAL USE

Antibiotic:
- Anaerobic and protozoal infections

DOSE IN NORMAL RENAL FUNCTION

- Oral: 200–500 mg every 8–12 hours
- IV: 500 mg every 8 hours
- PR: 1 g every 8–12 hours

PHARMACOKINETICS

Molecular weight (daltons)	171.2
% Protein binding	10–20
% Excreted unchanged in urine	20
Volume of distribution (L/kg)	0.7–1.5
Half-life – normal/ ESRF (hrs)	5.6–11.4/7–21

METABOLISM

Metabolised in the liver by side-chain oxidation and glucuronide formation. The main hydroxy metabolite has antibacterial activity and is detected in plasma and urine, the acid metabolite has virtually no antibacterial activity and is often not detected in plasma, but is excreted in urine. Small amounts of reduced metabolites, acetamide and N-(2-hydroxyethyl)oxamic acid (HOA), have also been detected in urine and are probably formed by the intestinal flora.

Active metabolites have long half-life in renal impairment.

DOSE IN RENAL IMPAIRMENT GFR (mL/MIN)

20–50	Dose as in normal renal function.
10–20	Dose as in normal renal function.
<10	Dose as in normal renal function.

DOSE IN PATIENTS UNDERGOING RENAL REPLACEMENT THERAPIES

CAPD	Not dialysed. Dose as in normal renal function.
HD	Dialysed. Dose as in normal renal function.
HDF/High flux	Dialysed. Dose as in normal renal function.
CAV/VVHD	Unknown dialysability. Dose as in normal renal function.

IMPORTANT DRUG INTERACTIONS

Potentially hazardous interactions with other drugs
- Alcohol: disulfiram-like reaction.
- Anticoagulants: effects of coumarins enhanced.
- Anti-epileptics: metabolism of phenytoin inhibited; concentration reduced by phenobarbital.
- Ciclosporin: raised blood level of ciclosporin.
- Cytotoxics: busulfan concentration increased; metabolism of fluorouracil inhibited.

ADMINISTRATION

RECONSTITUTION
–
ROUTE
- IV, Oral, PR
RATE OF ADMINISTRATION
- IV: 5 mL/minute, i.e. 500 mg over 20 minutes
COMMENTS
–

OTHER INFORMATION

- Increased incidence of GIT reactions and vestibular toxicity in renal failure.
- Drug induced lupus is a rare adverse drug reaction.
- Rectally: dose frequency reduced to 12 hours after 3 days.
- 500 mg/100 mL infusion provides 14 mmol sodium.

Mexiletine hydrochloride (unlicensed)

CLINICAL USE

Life-threatening ventricular arrhythmias, especially after a myocardial infarction

DOSE IN NORMAL RENAL FUNCTION

- Oral: 400 mg loading dose, followed by 200–300 mg 3 times daily commencing 2 hours after the loading dose. Maximum 1.2 g daily
- IV injection: 100–250 mg at a rate of 25 mg/minute with ECG monitoring, followed by an infusion of 250 mg as a 0.1% solution over 1 hour, 125 mg/hour for 2 hours then 500 micrograms/minute thereafter.

PHARMACOKINETICS

Molecular weight (daltons)	215.7
% Protein binding	50–70
% Excreted unchanged in urine	10
Volume of distribution (L/kg)	5–7
Half-life – normal/ ESRF (hrs)	5–17/16

METABOLISM

Mexiletine is metabolised in the liver to several metabolites; metabolism may involve cytochrome P450 isoenzymes CYP1A2, CYP2D6, and CYP3A4, and genetic polymorphism in relation to CYP2D6 has been identified. Mexiletine is excreted in the urine, mainly in the form of its metabolites with about 10% excreted unchanged; clearance is increased in acid urine.

DOSE IN RENAL IMPAIRMENT GFR (mL/MIN)

20–50	Dose as in normal renal function.
10–20	Dose as in normal renal function.
<10	50–100% of normal dose and titrate according to response.

DOSE IN PATIENTS UNDERGOING RENAL REPLACEMENT THERAPIES

CAPD	Not dialysed. Dose as in GFR<10 mL/min.
HD	Not dialysed. Dose as in GFR<10 mL/min.
HDF/High flux	Dialysed. Dose as in GFR<10 mL/min.
CAV/ VVHD	Not dialysed. Dose as in normal renal function.

IMPORTANT DRUG INTERACTIONS

Potentially hazardous interactions with other drugs
- Analgesics: opioids delay absorption.
- Anti-arrhythmics: increased myocardial depression with any combination of anti-arrhythmics.
- Antidepressants: metabolism inhibited by fluvoxamine (increased toxicity).
- Antihistamines: increased risk of ventricular arrhythmias with mizolastine – avoid concomitant use.
- Antipsychotics: increased risk of ventricular arrhythmias with antipsychotics that prolong the QT interval.
- Antivirals: possibly increased risk of arrhythmias with ritonavir and tipranavir.
- Beta-blockers: increased myocardial depression.
- Diuretics: action of mexiletine antagonised by hypokalaemia.

ADMINISTRATION

RECONSTITUTION

–

ROUTE
- IV infusion, Oral.

RATE OF ADMINISTRATION
- Variable

COMMENTS
- Add 250–500 mg mexiletine to 500 mL of infusion solution, e.g. sodium chloride 0.9%, glucose 5%, sodium bicarbonate 8.4%, sodium lactate, sodium chloride 0.9% with potassium chloride 0.3% or 0.6%.

OTHER INFORMATION

- *Drug Prescribing in Renal Failure*, 5th edition, by Aronoff *et al.* suggest using 100% of dose in renal impairment.
- Mexiletine has a narrow therapeutic index. Its therapeutic effect has been correlated with plasma concentrations of 0. 5–2 micrograms per mL.
- Rate of elimination increased with acidic urine.
- Injection can be given orally; however, due to local anaesthetic effect, care needed with hot foods.
- Available from 'special order' manufacturers.

Micafungin

CLINICAL USE

Antimycotic:
- Treatment of invasive candidiasis.
- Treatment of oesophageal candidiasis
- Prophylaxis of *Candida* infection in patients undergoing allogeneic haematopoietic stem cell transplantation or patients who are expected to have neutropenia

DOSE IN NORMAL RENAL FUNCTION

Weight >40 kg: 50–200 mg once daily
Weight <40 kg: 1–4 mg/kg
(Dose depends on indication)

PHARMACOKINETICS

Molecular weight (daltons)	1292.3 (as sodium salt)
% Protein binding	>99
% Excreted unchanged in urine	11.6
Volume of distribution (L/kg)	0.28–0.5
Half-life – normal/ESRF (hrs)	10–17/Unchanged

METABOLISM

Metabolised in the liver by arylsulfatase to its catechol form and further metabolised to the methoxy form by catechol-O-methyltransferase. Some hydroxylation to micafungin via cytochrome P450 isoenzymes also occurs. Exposure to these metabolites is low and metabolites do not contribute to the overall efficacy of micafungin.

After 28 days about 71% of a dose is recovered in the faeces and 12% in the urine.

DOSE IN RENAL IMPAIRMENT GFR (mL/MIN)

20–50	Dose as in normal renal function.
10–20	Dose as in normal renal function.
<10	Dose as in normal renal function.

DOSE IN PATIENTS UNDERGOING RENAL REPLACEMENT THERAPIES

CAPD	Not dialysed. Dose as in normal renal function.
HD	Not dialysed. Dose as in normal renal function.
HDF/High flux	Not dialysed. Dose as in normal renal function.
CAV/VVHD	Not dialysed. Dose as in normal renal function.

IMPORTANT DRUG INTERACTIONS

Potentially hazardous interactions with other drugs
- Ciclosporin: possibly increases ciclosporin concentration.
- Sirolimus: increases sirolimus concentration.

ADMINISTRATION

RECONSTITUTION
- 5 mL sodium chloride 0.9% or glucose 5%

ROUTE
- IV

RATE OF ADMINISTRATION
- Over 60 minutes

COMMENTS
- Add dose to 100 mL sodium chloride 0.9% or glucose 5%

OTHER INFORMATION

- Isolated cases of renal dysfunction or acute kidney injury have occurred in patients taking micafungin.

Miconazole

CLINICAL USE

Antifungal agent

DOSE IN NORMAL RENAL FUNCTION

- Oral gel: 5–10 mL in mouth, after food, 4 times daily
- Buccal: 50 mg daily

PHARMACOKINETICS

Molecular weight (daltons)	416.1
% Protein binding	90
% Excreted unchanged in urine	1
Volume of distribution (L/kg)	20
Half-life – normal/ ESRF (hrs)	24/Unchanged

METABOLISM

Miconazole is metabolised in the liver to inactive metabolites; 10–20% of an oral dose is excreted in the urine as metabolites. About 50% of an oral dose may be excreted mainly unchanged in the faeces.

DOSE IN RENAL IMPAIRMENT GFR (mL/MIN)

20–50	Dose as in normal renal function.
10–20	Dose as in normal renal function.
<10	Dose as in normal renal function.

DOSE IN PATIENTS UNDERGOING RENAL REPLACEMENT THERAPIES

CAPD	Not dialysed. Dose as in normal renal function.
HD	Not dialysed. Dose as in normal renal function.
HDF/High flux	Unknown dialysability. Dose as in normal renal function.
CAV/ VVHD	Unlikely to be significantly dialysed. Dose as in normal renal function.

IMPORTANT DRUG INTERACTIONS

Potentially hazardous interactions with other drugs

- Anticoagulants: effect of coumarins enhanced.
- Antidepressants: avoid concomitant use with reboxetine.
- Antidiabetics: enhances hypoglycaemic effect of gliclazide and glipizide; concentration of sulphonylureas increased.
- Antiepileptics: effect of phenytoin enhanced; possibly increased carbamazepine concentration.
- Antihistamines: avoid concomitant use with mizolastine, risk of ventricular arrhythmias.
- Antimalarials: avoid concomitant use with piperaquine with artenimol and artemether with lumefantrine.
- Antipsychotics: increased risk of ventricular arrhythmias with pimozide – avoid concomitant use; possibly increased concentration of quetiapine – reduce quetiapine dose.
- Antivirals: concentration of saquinavir possibly increased.
- Ciclosporin: possibly increased ciclosporin concentration.
- Ergot alkaloids: increased risk of ergotism with ergotamine and methysergide – avoid concomitant use.
- Sirolimus: concentration increased by miconazole.
- Statins: possibly increased risk of myopathy with atorvastatin and simvastatin – avoid concomitant use with simvastatin.
- Tacrolimus: possibly increased tacrolimus concentration.

ADMINISTRATION

RECONSTITUTION

–

ROUTE

- Oral gel, buccal, topical

RATE OF ADMINISTRATION

–

COMMENTS

–

OTHER INFORMATION

- There is little absorption through skin or mucous membranes when miconazole nitrate is applied topically.
- 50% removed during haemodialysis.

Midazolam

CLINICAL USE

Benzodiazepine:
- Sedation with amnesia in conjunction with local anaesthesia, premedication, induction
- Status epilepticus (unlicensed)

DOSE IN NORMAL RENAL FUNCTION

See SPC for dosing guidelines.
Status epilepticus: Buccal: 10 mg repeated once after 10 minutes if required

PHARMACOKINETICS

Molecular weight (daltons)	325.8 (362.2 as hydrochloride)
% Protein binding	96–98
% Excreted unchanged in urine	<1
Volume of distribution (L/kg)	0.7–1.2
Half-life – normal/ ESRF (hrs)	2–7/Unchanged

METABOLISM

Metabolised in the liver via the cytochrome P450 isoenzyme CYP3A4. The major metabolite, alpha-hydroxymidazolam has some activity; its half-life is less than 1 hour. Midazolam metabolites are excreted in the urine, mainly as glucuronide conjugates.

DOSE IN RENAL IMPAIRMENT GFR (mL/MIN)

20–50	Dose as in normal renal function.
10–20	Dose as in normal renal function.
<10	Use sparingly and titrate according to response. Only bolus doses, not continuous infusion.

DOSE IN PATIENTS UNDERGOING RENAL REPLACEMENT THERAPIES

CAPD	Unlikely to be dialysed. Dose as in GFR<10 mL/min.
HD	Not dialysed. Dose as in GFR<10 mL/min.
HDF/High flux	Unknown dialysability. Dose as in GFR<10 mL/min.
CAV/ VVHD	Unknown dialysability. Dose as in normal renal function.

IMPORTANT DRUG INTERACTIONS

Potentially hazardous interactions with other drugs
- Antibacterials: concentration increased by erythromycin, clarithromycin and telithromycin (profound sedation); metabolism possibly accelerated by rifampicin.
- Antidepressants: concentration of oral midazolam possibly reduced by St John's wort.
- Antifungals: concentration increased by itraconazole, fluconazole, ketoconazole, posaconazole and voriconazole (prolonged sedative effect).
- Antipsychotics: increased sedative effects; increased risk of hypotension, bradycardia and respiratory depression when parenteral benzodiazepines are given with IM olanzapine.
- Antivirals: concentration increased by atazanavir, boceprevir, efavirenz, indinavir, fosamprenavir, ritonavir, saquinavir and telaprevir increase risk of prolonged sedation avoid with oral midazolam.
- Ciclosporin: *in vitro* studies suggested that ciclosporin could inhibit the metabolism of midazolam. However, blood ciclosporin concentrations in patients given ciclosporin to prevent graft rejection were considered too low to result in an interaction.
- Cytotoxics: concentration increased by crizotinib and nilotinib.
- Sodium oxybate: enhanced effects of sodium oxybate – avoid.

ADMINISTRATION

RECONSTITUTION
–
ROUTE
- IV, IM, Buccal
RATE OF ADMINISTRATION
- 1–10 mL/hour according to response
COMMENTS
- Can be used undiluted.
- Compatible with glucose 5%, sodium chloride 0.9%.

OTHER INFORMATION

- Protein binding of midazolam is decreased in ERF; hence more unbound drug is available to produce CNS effects, so a decrease in dose is recommended.
- CSM has received reports of respiratory depression, sometimes associated with

severe hypotension, following intravenous administration.

- Caution when used for sedation in severe renal impairment especially when used with opiates and/or neuromuscular blocking agents – monitor sedation and titrate to response.

- Increased CNS sensitivity in patients with renal impairment.
- One study reports midazolam as having a sieving coefficient = 0.06 and unlikely to be removed by haemofiltration.
- Midazolam injection can be administered by the buccal route (unlicensed).

Midodrine hydrochloride (unlicensed)

CLINICAL USE

Treatment of orthostatic hypotension, including dialysis-related hypotension

DOSE IN NORMAL RENAL FUNCTION

2.5 mg twice daily up to 10 mg 3 times a day

PHARMACOKINETICS

Molecular weight (daltons)	290.7
% Protein binding	Negligible
% Excreted unchanged in urine	2
Volume of distribution (L/kg)	No data
Half-life – normal/ ESRF (hrs)	25 minutes (3 hours for active metabolite)/ increased (9 for active metabolite)

METABOLISM

Undergoes enzymatic hydrolysis in the systemic circulation to an active metabolite (desglymidodrine).

DOSE IN RENAL IMPAIRMENT GFR (mL/MIN)

20–50	Dose as in normal renal function.
10–20	Dose as in normal renal function. Start with a lower dose and titrate according to response.
<10	Dose as in normal renal function. Start with a lower dose and titrate according to response.

DOSE IN PATIENTS UNDERGOING RENAL REPLACEMENT THERAPIES

CAPD	Dialysed. Dose as in GFR<10 mL/ min.
HD	Dialysed. Initial dose, 2.5 mg if <70 kg, 5 mg if >70 kg. See 'Other information'.
HDF/High flux	Dialysed. Initial dose, 2.5 mg if <70 kg, 5 mg if >70 kg. See 'Other information'.
CAV/ VVHD	Dialysed. Dose as in GFR=10– 20 mL/min.

IMPORTANT DRUG INTERACTIONS

Potentially hazardous interactions with other drugs
- Adrenergic neurone blockers: midodrine antagonises hypotensive effect.
- Risk of arrhythmias if given with volatile anaesthetics.
- Risk of arrhythmias and hypertension if given with tricyclic antidepressants and MAOIs and moclobemide.
- Antihypertensives: antagonise hypertensive effect of midodrine.
- Risk of severe hypertension if given with beta-blockers.
- Dopaminergics: avoid with rasagiline and selegiline.
- Other drugs which increase blood pressure: enhanced hypertensive effect.

ADMINISTRATION

RECONSTITUTION
–

ROUTE
- Oral

RATE OF ADMINISTRATION
–

COMMENTS
- Take last dose at least 4 hours before bed.

OTHER INFORMATION

- After dialysis only 15% of drug remaining, so effectively removed by dialysis.
- Hypertension post dialysis is not a problem because drug is dialysed out.
- Peak levels occur 30 minutes after administration (60 minutes for active metabolite) so give 30 minutes before dialysis – avoid in patients with active coronary ischaemia.
- 93% bioavailability.
- For haemodialysis patients, start at a low dose and increase to a maximum of 30 mg; a second dose can be given midway through dialysis (maximum dose 10 mg).
- Contraindicated in severe organic heart disease, urinary retention, phaeochromocytoma and thyrotoxicosis.

Mifamurtide

CLINICAL USE

Antineoplastic agent:
- Treatment of metastatic osteosarcoma

DOSE IN NORMAL RENAL FUNCTION

$2 \, mg/m^2$ initially twice weekly, reduced to once weekly after 12 weeks

PHARMACOKINETICS

Molecular weight (daltons)	1237.5
% Protein binding	No data
% Excreted unchanged in urine	No data
Volume of distribution (L/kg)	25.9 litres[1]
Half-life – normal/ ESRF (hrs)	1.65–2.45/Unchanged

METABOLISM

The cells of the reticuloendothelial system clear mifamurtide liposomes by phagocytosis.

DOSE IN RENAL IMPAIRMENT GFR (mL/MIN)

30–50	Dose as in normal renal function.
10–30	Dose as in normal renal function. Use with caution.
<10	Dose as in normal renal function. Use with caution.

DOSE IN PATIENTS UNDERGOING RENAL REPLACEMENT THERAPIES

CAPD	Unlikely to be dialysed. Dose as in GFR<10 mL/min.
HD	Unlikely to be dialysed. Dose as in GFR<10 mL/min.
HDF/High flux	Unlikely to be dialysed. Dose as in GFR<10 mL/min.
CAV/ VVHD	Unlikely to be dialysed. Dose as in GFR=10–30 mL/min.

IMPORTANT DRUG INTERACTIONS

Potentially hazardous interactions with other drugs
- Analgesics: avoid with high dose NSAIDs.
- Ciclosporin: avoid concomitant use.
- Corticosteroids: avoid concomitant use.
- Tacrolimus: avoid concomitant use.

ADMINISTRATION

RECONSTITUTION
- 50 mL sodium chloride 0.9%
ROUTE
- IV infusion
RATE OF ADMINISTRATION
- 1 hour
COMMENTS
- Use filter provided.
- Appropriate dose is further diluted in 50 mL sodium chloride 0.9%.

OTHER INFORMATION

- Manufacturer advises to use with caution in severe renal impairment due to lack of studies.
- There was no difference in pharmacokinetics in GFR down to 30 mL/ min compared to healthy volunteers.

Reference:
1. Venkatakrishnan K, Liu Y, Noe D, *et al.* Total and non-liposome associated muramyl tripeptide-phosphatidyl ethanolamine pharmacokinetics following intravenous infusion of liposomal mifamurtide to healthy adults. Poster presented at the 24th EORTC-NCI-AACR Symposium on Molecular Targets and Cancer Therapeutics, Dublin, Ireland, November 6–9, 2012.

Minocycline

CLINICAL USE

Antibacterial agent

DOSE IN NORMAL RENAL FUNCTION

100 mg twice daily
- Acne: 100 mg daily in 1 or 2 divided doses

PHARMACOKINETICS

Molecular weight (daltons)	457.5
% Protein binding	75
% Excreted unchanged in urine	5–10
Volume of distribution (L/kg)	1–1.5
Half-life – normal/ ESRF (hrs)	11–26/12–18

METABOLISM

Undergoes some metabolism in the liver, mainly to 9-hydroxyminocycline.

DOSE IN RENAL IMPAIRMENT GFR (mL/MIN)

20–50	Dose as in normal renal function.
10–20	Dose as in normal renal function.
<10	Dose as in normal renal function.

DOSE IN PATIENTS UNDERGOING RENAL REPLACEMENT THERAPIES

CAPD	Not dialysed. Dose as in normal renal function.
HD	Not dialysed. Dose as in normal renal function.
HDF/High flux	Unknown dialysability. Dose as in normal renal function.
CAV/ VVHD	Unlikely to be dialysed. Dose as in normal renal function.

IMPORTANT DRUG INTERACTIONS

Potentially hazardous interactions with other drugs
- Anticoagulants: possibly enhanced anticoagulant effect of coumarins and phenindione.
- Oestrogens: possibly reduced contraceptive effect of oestrogens (risk probably small).
- Retinoids: possibly increased risk of benign intracranial hypertension – avoid concomitant use.

ADMINISTRATION

RECONSTITUTION
–
ROUTE
- Oral
RATE OF ADMINISTRATION
–

COMMENTS
- Do not take iron preparations, indigestion remedies or phosphate binders at the same time of day as minocycline.

Minoxidil

CLINICAL USE

- Severe hypertension (in addition to a diuretic and a beta-blocker)
- Male pattern baldness

DOSE IN NORMAL RENAL FUNCTION

- Initially 5 mg (elderly 2.5 mg) daily in 1–2 doses increased by 5–10 mg every 3 or more days; maximum 100 mg daily.
- Male pattern baldness: 1 mL twice daily.

PHARMACOKINETICS

Molecular weight (daltons)	209.2
% Protein binding	0
% Excreted unchanged in urine	15–20
Volume of distribution (L/kg)	2–3
Half-life – normal/ ESRF (hrs)	4.2/8.9

METABOLISM

Extensively metabolised by the liver. It requires sulphation to become active, but the major metabolite is a glucuronide conjugate.

Excreted mainly in the urine in the form of metabolites. Minoxidil and its metabolites are dialysable, although the pharmacological effect is not reversed.

DOSE IN RENAL IMPAIRMENT GFR (mL/MIN)

20–50	Start with small doses and titrate according to response. See 'Other information'.
10–20	Start with small doses and titrate according to response. See 'Other information'.
<10	Start with small doses and titrate according to response. See 'Other information'.

DOSE IN PATIENTS UNDERGOING RENAL REPLACEMENT THERAPIES

CAPD	Dialysed. Dose as in GFR<10 mL/min.
HD	Dialysed. Dose as in GFR<10 mL/min.
HDF/High flux	Dialysed. Dose as in GFR<10 mL/min.
CAV/ VVHD	Dialysed. Dose as in GFR=10–20 mL/min.

IMPORTANT DRUG INTERACTIONS

Potentially hazardous interactions with other drugs
- Anaesthetics: enhanced hypotensive effect.

ADMINISTRATION

RECONSTITUTION
–
ROUTE
- Oral
RATE OF ADMINISTRATION
–
COMMENTS
–

OTHER INFORMATION

- A study of the pharmacokinetics of minoxidil in patients with varying degrees of renal impairment found that the non-renal clearance was also impaired as renal function worsened. Substantial accumulation of minoxidil might occur in these patients during multiple-dose therapy. Recommended that minoxidil therapy be initiated with smaller doses or a longer dose interval in patients with significant renal impairment.
- Minoxidil is a peripheral vasodilator and should be given in conjunction with a diuretic to control salt and water retention, and a beta-blocker to control reflex tachycardia. Patients on dialysis do not need to be given minoxidil in conjunction with a diuretic.
- Following topical application, between 0.3% and 4.5% of the total applied dose of minoxidil is absorbed from intact scalp.

Mirabegron

CLINICAL USE

Potent and selective beta 3-adrenoceptor agonist:
- Urinary frequency, urgency and incontinence

DOSE IN NORMAL RENAL FUNCTION

50 mg daily

PHARMACOKINETICS

Molecular weight (daltons)	396.5
% Protein binding	71
% Excreted unchanged in urine	25
Volume of distribution (L/kg)	1670 litres
Half-life – normal/ ESRF (hrs)	50/Increased

METABOLISM

Metabolised via multiple pathways involving dealkylation, oxidation, (direct) glucuronidation, and amide hydrolysis.

Renal elimination of mirabegron is primarily through active tubular secretion along with glomerular filtration.

DOSE IN RENAL IMPAIRMENT GFR (mL/MIN)

60–30	Dose as in normal renal function. 25 mg with CYP 3A inhibitors.
15–29	25 mg daily. Avoid with CYP 3A inhibitors.
<15	25 mg daily. Avoid with CYP 3A inhibitors. See 'Other information'.

DOSE IN PATIENTS UNDERGOING RENAL REPLACEMENT THERAPIES

CAPD	Unlikely to be dialysed. Dose as in GFR<15 mL/min.
HD	Unlikely to be dialysed. Dose as in GFR<15 mL/min.
HDF/High flux	Unlikely to be dialysed. Dose as in GFR<15 mL/min.
CAV/ VVHD	Unlikely to be dialysed. Dose as in GFR=15–29 mL/min.

ADMINISTRATION

RECONSTITUTION
–
ROUTE
- Oral
RATE OF ADMINISTRATION
–

OTHER INFORMATION

- Not recommended by manufacturer in severe renal impairment due to lack of information.
- Oral bioavailability is 29–35% depending on dose.
- In patients with severe renal impairment (eGFR 15 to 29 mL/min/1.73 m^2), mean C_{max} and AUC values were 92% and 118% higher compared to healthy subjects with normal renal function.

Mircera

CLINICAL USE

Management of anaemia associated with renal impairment in pre-dialysis and dialysis patients

DOSE IN NORMAL RENAL FUNCTION

- ESA-naive patients: 0.6 mcg/kg every 2 weeks or 1.2 mcg/kg every 4 weeks, changing by 25% according to response; once stable change to monthly dosing.
- Target haemoglobin usually 10–12 g/dL.
- If previously on an ESA: 120–360 mcg monthly depending on previous ESA dose, and adjust according to response.

PHARMACOKINETICS

Molecular weight (daltons)	60 000
% Protein binding	No data
% Excreted unchanged in urine	Unlikely
Volume of distribution (L/kg)	3–5.4 litres
Half-life – normal/ ESRF (hrs)	IV: 134/Unchanged SC: 139 (142 if not on dialysis)/Unchanged

METABOLISM

The metabolic fate of both endogenous and recombinant erythropoietin is poorly understood. Current evidence from studies in animals suggests that hepatic metabolism contributes only minimally to elimination of the *intact* hormone, but desialylated epoetin (i.e. terminal sialic acid groups removed) appears to undergo substantial hepatic clearance via metabolic pathways and/or binding. Desialylation and/or removal of the oligosaccharide side chains of erythropoietin appear to occur principally in the liver; bone marrow also may have a role in catabolism of the hormone. Elimination of desialylated drug by the kidneys, bone marrow, and spleen also may occur; results of animal studies suggest that proximal renal tubular secretion may be involved in renal elimination.

DOSE IN RENAL IMPAIRMENT GFR (mL/MIN)

20–50	Dose as in normal renal function.
10–20	Dose as in normal renal function.
<10	Dose as in normal renal function.

DOSE IN PATIENTS UNDERGOING RENAL REPLACEMENT THERAPIES

CAPD	Not dialysed. Dose as in normal renal function.
HD	Not dialysed. Dose as in normal renal function.
HDF/High flux	Not dialysed. Dose as in normal renal function.
CAV/ VVHD	Not dialysed. Dose as in normal renal function.

IMPORTANT DRUG INTERACTIONS

Potentially hazardous interactions with other drugs
- Risk of hyperkalaemia with ACE inhibitors and angiotensin-II antagonists.

ADMINISTRATION

RECONSTITUTION
–
ROUTE
- SC, IV
RATE OF ADMINISTRATION
–
COMMENTS

OTHER INFORMATION

- Pre-treatment checks and appropriate correction/treatment needed for iron, folate and B12 deficiencies, infection, inflammation or aluminium toxicity to produce optimum response to therapy.
- Concomitant iron therapy (200–300 mg elemental oral iron) needed daily. IV iron may be needed for patients with very low serum ferritin (<100 nanograms/mL).
- May increase heparin requirement during HD.
- Reported association of pure red cell aplasia (PRCA) with epoetin therapy – very rare; due to failed production of red blood cell precursors in the bone marrow, resulting in profound anaemia. Possibly due to an immune response to the protein backbone of R-HuEPO. Resulting antibodies render the patient unresponsive to the therapeutic effects of all epoetins and darbepoetin.

Mirtazapine

CLINICAL USE

Antidepressant

DOSE IN NORMAL RENAL FUNCTION

15–45 mg daily in 1 or 2 divided doses

PHARMACOKINETICS

Molecular weight (daltons)	265.4
% Protein binding	85
% Excreted unchanged in urine	75
Volume of distribution (L/kg)	107 litres
Half-life – normal/ ESRF (hrs)	20–40/Increased

METABOLISM

Extensively metabolised in the liver via CYP2D6, CYP1A2, and CYP3A4. The major biotransformation pathways are demethylation and oxidation followed by glucuronide conjugation. The N-desmethyl metabolite is pharmacologically active. Elimination is via urine (75%) and faeces (15%).

DOSE IN RENAL IMPAIRMENT GFR (mL/MIN)

20–40	Dose as in normal renal function.
10–20	Start at low dose and monitor closely.
<10	Start at low dose and monitor closely.

DOSE IN PATIENTS UNDERGOING RENAL REPLACEMENT THERAPIES

CAPD	Unlikely to be dialysed. Dose as in GFR<10 mL/min.
HD	Unlikely to be dialysed. Dose as in GFR<10 mL/min.
HDF/High flux	Unknown dialysability. Dose as in GFR<10 mL/min.
CAV/ VVHD	Unlikely to be dialysed. Dose as in GFR=10–20 mL/min.

IMPORTANT DRUG INTERACTIONS

Potentially hazardous interactions with other drugs

- Alcohol: increased sedative effect.
- Antidepressants: possibly increased risk of serotonergic effects with fluoxetine, fluvoxamine or venlafaxine; CNS excitation and hypertension with MAOI and moclobemide – avoid concomitant use.
- Antimalarials: avoid concomitant use with artemether and lumefantrine and piperaquine with artenimol.
- Methylthioninium: risk of CNS toxicity – avoid if possible.

ADMINISTRATION

RECONSTITUTION

–

ROUTE

- Oral

RATE OF ADMINISTRATION

–

COMMENTS

–

Misoprostol

CLINICAL USE

- Benign gastric and duodenal ulceration and NSAID-associated ulceration
- Prophylaxis of NSAID-induced ulceration

DOSE IN NORMAL RENAL FUNCTION

- Treatment: 800 mcg daily in 2 or 4 divided doses
- Prophylaxis: 200 mcg 2–4 times daily

PHARMACOKINETICS

Molecular weight (daltons)	382.5
% Protein binding	<90 (as Misoprostol acid)
% Excreted unchanged in urine	<1
Volume of distribution (L/kg)	858 litres
Half-life – normal/ ESRF (hrs)	20–40 minutes/ 40–80 minutes (as Misoprostol acid)

METABOLISM

Rapidly metabolised to its active form (misoprostol acid) after oral doses. Misoprostol acid is further metabolised by oxidation in several body organs and is excreted mainly in the urine.

DOSE IN RENAL IMPAIRMENT GFR (mL/MIN)

10–50	Dose as in normal renal function.
10–20	Dose as in normal renal function.
<10	Dose as in normal renal function.

DOSE IN PATIENTS UNDERGOING RENAL REPLACEMENT THERAPIES

CAPD	Unlikely to be dialysed. Dose as in normal renal function.
HD	Unlikely to be dialysed. Dose as in normal renal function.
HDF/High flux	Unknown dialysability. Dose as in normal renal function.
CAV/ VVHD	Unlikely to be dialysed. Dose as in normal renal function.

IMPORTANT DRUG INTERACTIONS

Potentially hazardous interactions with other drugs
- None known

ADMINISTRATION

RECONSTITUTION
–
ROUTE
- Oral
RATE OF ADMINISTRATION
–
COMMENTS
–

OTHER INFORMATION

- Plasma concentrations of misoprostol are generally undetectable due to its rapid metabolic conversion to misoprostol acid.
- Dosage adjustment is not usually necessary in patients with varying degrees of renal impairment, even though there is an approximate doubling of half-life, maximum plasma concentration and area under the curve. If renal patients are unable to tolerate it, the dose can be reduced.

Mitomycin

CLINICAL USE

Cytotoxic antibiotic used in a range of neoplastic conditions

DOSE IN NORMAL RENAL FUNCTION

- IV: Some regimens use an initial dose of 10–20 mg/m^2, others use 4–10 mg or 0.06–0.15 mg/kg given every 1–6 weeks, depending on concurrent therapy and bone marrow recovery
- For instillation into bladder: 20–40 mg

PHARMACOKINETICS

Molecular weight (daltons)	334.3
% Protein binding	No data
% Excreted unchanged in urine	10
Volume of distribution (L/kg)	0.5
Half-life – normal/ ESRF (hrs)	50 minutes/–

METABOLISM

Mitomycin is a prodrug, and is activated *in vivo* by metabolism mainly in the liver to a bifunctional and trifunctional alkylating agent. Binding to DNA leads to cross-linking and inhibition of DNA synthesis and function. Rate of clearance is inversely proportional to the maximum serum concentration, due to saturation of the degradative pathways. Approximately 10% is excreted unchanged in the urine. Since metabolic pathways are saturated at low doses, the percentage dose excreted in the urine increases with increasing dose.

DOSE IN RENAL IMPAIRMENT GFR (mL/MIN)

20–50	Dose as in normal renal function.
10–20	Dose as in normal renal function.
<10	75% of normal dose.

DOSE IN PATIENTS UNDERGOING RENAL REPLACEMENT THERAPIES

CAPD	Unknown dialysability. Dose as in GFR<10 mL/min.
HD	Unknown dialysability. Dose as in GFR<10 mL/min.
HDF/High flux	Unknown dialysability. Dose as in GFR<10 mL/min.
CAV/ VVHD	Unknown dialysability. Dose as in normal renal function.

IMPORTANT DRUG INTERACTIONS

Potentially hazardous interactions with other drugs
- Antipsychotics: avoid concomitant use with clozapine (increased risk of agranulocytosis).

ADMINISTRATION

RECONSTITUTION
- With water for injection or sodium chloride 0.9%; 5 mL for the 2 mg vial, at least 10 mL for the 10 mg vial and at least 20 mL for the 20 mg vial.

ROUTE
- IV injection, intra-arterial, bladder instillation

RATE OF ADMINISTRATION
- Bolus injection over 3–5 minutes (1 mL/min)
- Infusion over 15–30 minutes

COMMENTS
–

OTHER INFORMATION

- Dose in severe renal impairment is from *Drug Prescribing in Renal Failure*, 5th edition, by Aronoff *et al.*
- A syndrome of thrombotic microangiopathy resembling haemolytic-uraemic syndrome has been seen in patients receiving mitomycin, either alone or, more frequently, combined with other agents. Symptoms of haemolysis and renal failure may be accompanied by ATN and cardiovascular problems, pulmonary oedema and neurological symptoms.
- Principal toxicity of mitomycin-C is bone marrow suppression. The nadir is usually around 4 weeks after treatment and toxicity is cumulative, with increasing risk after each course of treatment.

Mitotane

CLINICAL USE

Antineoplastic agent
● Treatment of advanced or inoperable adrenocortical carcinoma

DOSE IN NORMAL RENAL FUNCTION

2–3 g daily (up to 6 g daily in severe illness) in 2–3 divided doses adjusted according to plasma mitotane concentration
Consult relevant local protocol.

PHARMACOKINETICS

Molecular weight (daltons)	320
% Protein binding	6
% Excreted unchanged in urine	0 (10–25% as metabolites)
Volume of distribution (L/kg)	Large
Half-life – normal/ ESRF (hrs)	18–159 days/–

METABOLISM

Metabolised in the liver and other tissues and excreted as metabolites in urine and bile. From 10% to 25% of a dose has been recovered in the urine as a water-soluble metabolite and 1–17% in the faeces as metabolites.

DOSE IN RENAL IMPAIRMENT GFR (mL/MIN)

20–50	Use with caution and monitor levels.
10–20	Use with caution and monitor levels.
<10	Avoid. See 'Other information'.

DOSE IN PATIENTS UNDERGOING RENAL REPLACEMENT THERAPIES

CAPD	Not dialysed. Dose as in GFR<10 mL/min.
HD	Not dialysed. Dose as in GFR<10 mL/min.
HDF/High flux	Not dialysed. Dose as in GFR<10 mL/min.
CAV/ VVHD	Not dialysed. Dose as in GFR=10–20 mL/min.

IMPORTANT DRUG INTERACTIONS

Potentially hazardous interactions with other drugs
● Anticoagulants: possibly reduced anticoagulant effect of coumarins.
● Antipsychotics: avoid concomitant use with clozapine (increased risk of agranulocytosis).
● Diuretics: avoid with spironolactone.

ADMINISTRATION

RECONSTITUTION
–
ROUTE
● Oral
RATE OF ADMINISTRATION
–
COMMENTS
–

OTHER INFORMATION

● Aim for plasma mitotane levels of 14–20 mg/l.
● There is no experience of mitotane in patients with renal failure so manufacturer is unable to advise on dosing.
● No reduction for renal failure in American data sheet.

Mitoxantrone

CLINICAL USE

Antineoplastic agent:
- Metastatic breast cancer
- Non-Hodgkin's lymphoma
- Adult acute non-lymphocytic leukaemia

DOSE IN NORMAL RENAL FUNCTION

- Metastatic breast cancer, non-Hodgkin's lymphoma and hepatoma: 14 mg/m^2 every 21 days (12 mg/m^2 or less if inadequate bone marrow reserves)
- Adult acute non-lymphocytic leukaemia: 12 mg/m^2 for 5 consecutive days
- For untreated patients in combination with cytarabine: 10–12 mg/m^2 daily for 3 days
- Or according to local protocol

PHARMACOKINETICS

Molecular weight (daltons)	517.4 (as hydrochloride)
% Protein binding	78
% Excreted unchanged in urine	7
Volume of distribution (L/kg)	1000 L/m^2
Half-life – normal/ ESRF (hrs)	5–18 days/–

METABOLISM

Extensive metabolism in the liver. Excretion is predominantly via the bile and faeces. 5–10% of a dose is excreted in the urine and 13–25% in the faeces, within 5 days.

DOSE IN RENAL IMPAIRMENT GFR (mL/MIN)

20–50	Dose as in normal renal function.
10–20	Dose as in normal renal function.
<10	Dose as in normal renal function.

DOSE IN PATIENTS UNDERGOING RENAL REPLACEMENT THERAPIES

CAPD	Not dialysed. Dose as in normal renal function.
HD	Not dialysed. Dose as in normal renal function.
HDF/High flux	Not dialysed. Dose as in normal renal function.
CAV/ VVHD	Not dialysed. Dose as in normal renal function.

IMPORTANT DRUG INTERACTIONS

Potentially hazardous interactions with other drugs
- Other antineoplastic agents: enhanced myelosuppression – when used in combination reduce mitoxantrone dose by 2–4 mg/m^2.
- Antipsychotics: avoid concomitant use with clozapine, increased risk of agranulocytosis.
- Cardiotoxic drugs: increased risk of cardiac toxicity.
- Ciclosporin: excretion of mitoxantrone reduced.

ADMINISTRATION

RECONSTITUTION
–
ROUTE
- IV infusion
RATE OF ADMINISTRATION
- At least 3 minutes
COMMENTS
- Dilute to at least 50 mL in sodium chloride 0.9%, glucose 5% or sodium chloride 0.18% and glucose 4%.

OTHER INFORMATION

- Has been administered intraperitoneally at a dose of 28–38 mg/m^2 every 3–4 weeks although some people advise a maximum dose of only 30 mg/m^2 per month with a dwell time of 1–4 hours. (Alberts DS, Surwit EA, Peng YM, *et al.* Phase I clinical and pharmacokinetic study of mitoxantrone given to patients by intraperitoneal administration. *Cancer Res.* 1988; **48**(20): 5874–7).

Mivacurium

CLINICAL USE

Non-depolarising muscle relaxant of short duration

DOSE IN NORMAL RENAL FUNCTION

- IV injection: 70–250 micrograms/kg; maintenance 100 micrograms/kg every 15 minutes
- IV infusion: maintenance of block 8–10 micrograms/kg/minute, adjusted to maintenance dose of 6–7 micrograms/kg/minute according to response

PHARMACOKINETICS

Molecular weight (daltons)	1029; (1100.2 as chloride)
% Protein binding	No data
% Excreted unchanged in urine	<10
Volume of distribution (L/kg)	0.1–0.3
Half-life – normal/ ESRF (hrs)	2–10 minutes/–

METABOLISM

Mivacurium is a mixture of three stereoisomers, two of which (cis-trans and trans-trans) are considered to account for most of the neuromuscular blocking effect. All three isomers are inactivated by plasma cholinesterase. Renal and hepatic mechanisms are involved in their elimination with excretion in urine and bile.

DOSE IN RENAL IMPAIRMENT GFR (mL/MIN)

20–50	Initially 50% and adjust to response. Slower infusion rate may be required.
10–20	Initially 50% and adjust to response. Slower infusion rate may be required.
<10	Initially 50% and adjust to response. See 'Other information'.

DOSE IN PATIENTS UNDERGOING RENAL REPLACEMENT THERAPIES

CAPD	Unknown dialysability. Adjust infusion to response.
HD	Unknown dialysability. Adjust infusion to response.
HDF/High flux	Unknown dialysability. Adjust infusion to response.
CAV/ VVHD	Unknown dialysability. Adjust infusion to response.

IMPORTANT DRUG INTERACTIONS

Potentially hazardous interactions with other drugs

- Anaesthetics: enhanced muscle relaxant effect.
- Anti-arrhythmics: procainamide enhances muscle relaxant effect.
- Antibacterials: effect enhanced by aminoglycosides, clindamycin, polymyxins and piperacillin.
- Anti-epileptics: muscle relaxant effects antagonised by carbamazepine; effects reduced by long-term use of phenytoin but might be increased by acute use.
- Botulinum toxin: neuromuscular blockade enhanced, (risk of toxicity).

ADMINISTRATION

RECONSTITUTION
–
ROUTE
- IV bolus, IV infusion
RATE OF ADMINISTRATION
- IV bolus: Doses of up to 0.15 mg/kg may be administered over 5–15 seconds. Higher doses should be administered over 30 seconds.
COMMENTS
- Compatible with sodium chloride 0.9%; glucose 5%; dilute to 500 micrograms/mL.
- Compatible with fentanyl, alfentanil, droperidol and midazolam.

OTHER INFORMATION

- Doses in renal impairment are from *Drug Prescribing in Renal Failure*, 5th edition, by Aronoff *et al.*
- Spontaneous recovery is complete in approximately 15 minutes and is independent of dose administered.
- In patients with CKD 5 the clinically effective duration of block produced by 0.15 mg/kg is approximately 1.5 times longer than in patients with normal renal

function; hence, dosage should be adjusted according to individual clinical response.

- Results from a study comparing 20 anephric patients with 20 healthy patients highlight the need for reduced dosages of Mivacron in patients with renal failure: patients with renal failure had a slightly shorter time to maximum depression of T1/T0, a slower recovery of T1/T0 to 5% (15.3 vs 9.8 min), required a slower infusion rate (6.3 vs 10.4 micrograms/kg/min) and experienced slower spontaneous recovery (12.2 vs 7.7 min). The drug company has no specific guidelines as to the extent of dose reduction required.

Mizolastine

CLINICAL USE

Antihistamine:
Symptomatic relief of allergy, e.g. hay fever, urticaria

DOSE IN NORMAL RENAL FUNCTION

10 mg daily

PHARMACOKINETICS

Molecular weight (daltons)	432.5
% Protein binding	98.4
% Excreted unchanged in urine	<0.5
Volume of distribution (L/kg)	1.4
Half-life – normal/ ESRF (hrs)	13/–

METABOLISM

Mainly metabolised by glucuronidation although other metabolic pathways are involved, including metabolism by the cytochrome P450 isoenzyme CYP3A4, with the formation of inactive hydroxylated metabolites.

DOSE IN RENAL IMPAIRMENT GFR (mL/MIN)

20–50	Dose as in normal renal function.
10–20	Dose as in normal renal function.
<10	Dose as in normal renal function.

DOSE IN PATIENTS UNDERGOING RENAL REPLACEMENT THERAPIES

CAPD	Not dialysed. Dose as in normal renal function.
HD	Not dialysed. Dose as in normal renal function.
HDF/High flux	Not dialysed. Dose as in normal renal function.
CAV/ VVHD	Not dialysed. Dose as in normal renal function.

IMPORTANT DRUG INTERACTIONS

Potentially hazardous interactions with other drugs

- Anti-arrhythmics: increased risk of ventricular arrhythmias – avoid concomitant use with amiodarone, disopyramide, flecainide, mexiletine, procainamide and propafenone.
- Antibacterials: metabolism possibly inhibited by macrolides – avoid concomitant use; increased risk of ventricular arrhythmias with moxifloxacin – avoid concomitant use.
- Antifungals: metabolism inhibited by itraconazole and ketoconazole and possibly imidazoles – avoid concomitant use.
- Antimalarials: avoid with piperaquine with artenimol.
- Antivirals: concentration possibly increased by ritonavir; increased risk of ventricular arrhythmias with saquinavir – avoid.
- Beta-blockers: increased risk of ventricular arrhythmias with sotalol – avoid concomitant use.
- Ciclosporin: use with caution due to inhibition of ciclosporin metabolism.
- Cytotoxics: possible increased risk of ventricular arrhythmias with vandetanib.
- Avoid concomitant treatment with any drug that could prolong QT interval.
- Caution with drugs that inhibit cytochrome P450 enzymes (may elevate mizolastine levels).

ADMINISTRATION

RECONSTITUTION
–
ROUTE
- Oral
RATE OF ADMINISTRATION
–
COMMENTS
–

OTHER INFORMATION

- Contraindicated in patients with electrolyte imbalances, particularly hypokalaemia.

Moclobemide

CLINICAL USE

Reversible MAOI:
- Depression
- Social phobia

DOSE IN NORMAL RENAL FUNCTION

- Depression: 150–600 mg daily in divided doses
- Social phobia: 300 mg twice daily

PHARMACOKINETICS

Molecular weight (daltons)	268.7
% Protein binding	50
% Excreted unchanged in urine	<1
Volume of distribution (L/kg)	1
Half-life – normal/ ESRF (hrs)	2–4/Unchanged

METABOLISM

Moclobemide is extensively metabolised in the liver, partly by the cytochrome P450 isoenzymes CYP2C19 and CYP2D6. Metabolites of moclobemide and a small amount of unchanged drug are excreted in the urine.

DOSE IN RENAL IMPAIRMENT GFR (mL/MIN)

20–50	Dose as in normal renal function.
10–20	Dose as in normal renal function.
<10	Dose as in normal renal function.

DOSE IN PATIENTS UNDERGOING RENAL REPLACEMENT THERAPIES

CAPD	Likely dialysability. Dose as in normal renal function.
HD	Likely dialysability. Dose as in normal renal function.
HDF/High flux	Likely dialysability. Dose as in normal renal function.
CAV/ VVHD	Likely dialysability. Dose as in normal renal function.

IMPORTANT DRUG INTERACTIONS

Potentially hazardous interactions with other drugs
- Analgesics: possible CNS excitation or depression with dextromethorphan or pethidine – avoid concomitant use; possible CNS excitation or depression with opioid analgesics.
- Antidepressants: avoid concomitant use; possible increased serotonergic effects with duloxetine.
- Antimalarials: avoid concomitant use with artemether/lumefantrine and piperaquine with artenimol.
- Bupropion: avoid concomitant use.
- Clopidogrel: anti-platelet effect possibly reduced.
- Dopaminergics: use with caution with entacapone; increased side effects with levodopa; avoid concomitant use with selegiline.
- 5HT$_1$ agonists: increased CNS toxicity with rizatriptan and sumatriptan – avoid concomitant use; increased CNS toxicity with zolmitriptan – reduce zolmitriptan dose.
- Sympathomimetics: risk of hypertensive crisis.

ADMINISTRATION

RECONSTITUTION

–

ROUTE
- Oral

RATE OF ADMINISTRATION

–

COMMENTS
- Take after food.

OTHER INFORMATION

- Hyponatraemia has been reported (especially in elderly patients) due to inappropriate secretion of antidiuretic hormone.

Modafinil

CLINICAL USE

Excessive daytime drowsiness associated with narcolepsy and obstructive sleep apnoea

DOSE IN NORMAL RENAL FUNCTION

200–400 mg daily in 1 or 2 divided doses

PHARMACOKINETICS

Molecular weight (daltons)	273.4
% Protein binding	60
% Excreted unchanged in urine	<10
Volume of distribution (L/kg)	0.9
Half-life – normal/ ESRF (hrs)	15/–

METABOLISM

Metabolised in the liver, partly by the cytochrome P450 isoenzymes CYP3A4 and CYP3A5; two major metabolites have been identified: acid modafinil and modafinil sulfone, both of which are inactive. Excretion is mainly through the kidneys with less than 10% of the dose being eliminated unchanged.

DOSE IN RENAL IMPAIRMENT GFR (mL/MIN)

20–50	Dose as in normal renal function.
10–20	Dose as in normal renal function.
<10	Start at 50% normal dose and increase according to response.

DOSE IN PATIENTS UNDERGOING RENAL REPLACEMENT THERAPIES

CAPD	Unknown dialysability. Dose as in GFR<10 mL/min.
HD	Unknown dialysability. Dose as in GFR<10 mL/min.
HDF/High flux	Unknown dialysability. Dose as in GFR<10 mL/min.
CAV/ VVHD	Unknown dialysability. Dose as in normal renal function.

IMPORTANT DRUG INTERACTIONS

Potentially hazardous interactions with other drugs

- Ciclosporin: reduced ciclosporin concentration.
- Oestrogens: metabolism accelerated (reduced contraceptive effect).

ADMINISTRATION

RECONSTITUTION

–

ROUTE

- Oral

RATE OF ADMINISTRATION

–

COMMENTS

–

OTHER INFORMATION

- Recommended that modafinil not be used in patients with left ventricular hypertrophy or ischaemic ECG changes.
- Modafinil is not recommended in severe renal impairment by the manufacturer due to lack of data. In single dose studies with 200 mg modafinil, at a GFR<20 mL/min there was no difference in the pharmacokinetics although there was a 9-fold increase in exposure to the inactive metabolite.

Moexipril hydrochloride

CLINICAL USE

Angiotensin-converting enzyme inhibitor:
- Hypertension

DOSE IN NORMAL RENAL FUNCTION

3.75–30 mg daily

PHARMACOKINETICS

Molecular weight (daltons)	535
% Protein binding	50
% Excreted unchanged in urine	1
Volume of distribution (L/kg)	183 litres
Half-life – normal/ ESRF (hrs)	12 (of active metabolite)/Increased

METABOLISM

Moexipril is a prodrug that is converted to an active metabolite, moexiprilat, in the gastrointestinal mucosa and liver. Moexipril is excreted mainly in the urine as moexiprilat, unchanged drug, and other metabolites; some moexiprilat may also be excreted in the faeces.

DOSE IN RENAL IMPAIRMENT GFR (mL/MIN)

20–40	Start with low dose and adjust according to response.
10–20	Start with low dose and adjust according to response.
<10	Start with low dose and adjust according to response.

DOSE IN PATIENTS UNDERGOING RENAL REPLACEMENT THERAPIES

CAPD	Unknown dialysability. Dose as in GFR<10 mL/min.
HD	Unknown dialysability. Dose as in GFR<10 mL/min.
HDF/High flux	Unknown dialysability. Dose as in GFR<10 mL/min.
CAV/ VVHD	Unknown dialysability. Dose as in GFR=10–20 mL/min.

IMPORTANT DRUG INTERACTIONS

Potentially hazardous interactions with other drugs
- Anaesthetics: enhanced hypotensive effect.
- Analgesics: antagonism of hypotensive effect and increased risk of renal impairment with NSAIDs; hyperkalaemia with ketorolac and other NSAIDs.
- Ciclosporin: increased risk of hyperkalaemia and nephrotoxicity.
- Diuretics: enhanced hypotensive effect; hyperkalaemia with potassium-sparing diuretics.
- ESAs: increased risk of hyperkalaemia; antagonism of hypotensive effect.
- Gold: flushing and hypotension with sodium aurothiomalate.
- Lithium: reduced excretion (possibility of enhanced lithium toxicity).
- Potassium salts: increased risk of hyperkalaemia.
- Tacrolimus: increased risk of hyperkalaemia and nephrotoxicity.

ADMINISTRATION

RECONSTITUTION
–

ROUTE
- Oral

RATE OF ADMINISTRATION
–

COMMENTS
–

OTHER INFORMATION

- Close monitoring of renal function during therapy is necessary in those with renal insufficiency.
- Renal failure has been reported in association with ACE inhibitors, mainly in patients with severe congestive heart failure, renal artery stenosis, or post renal transplant.
- High incidence of anaphylactoid reactions has been reported in patients dialysed with high-flux polyacrylonitrile membranes and treated concomitantly with an ACE inhibitor. This combination should therefore be avoided.
- Hyperkalaemia and other side effects are more common in patients with impaired renal function.

Montelukast

CLINICAL USE

Leukotriene receptor antagonist:
- Prophylaxis of asthma
- Seasonal allergic rhinitis

DOSE IN NORMAL RENAL FUNCTION

10 mg at night.

PHARMACOKINETICS

Molecular weight (daltons)	608.2 (as sodium salt)
% Protein binding	>99
% Excreted unchanged in urine	<0.2
Volume of distribution (L/kg)	8–11 litres
Half-life – normal/ ESRF (hrs)	2.7–5.5/–

METABOLISM

Extensively metabolised in the liver by cytochrome P450 isoenzymes CYP3A4, CYP2A6, and CYP2C9.

Excreted principally in the faeces via the bile.

Metabolites have minimal therapeutic activity.

DOSE IN RENAL IMPAIRMENT GFR (mL/MIN)

20–50	Dose as in normal renal function.
10–20	Dose as in normal renal function.
<10	Dose as in normal renal function.

DOSE IN PATIENTS UNDERGOING RENAL REPLACEMENT THERAPIES

CAPD	Not dialysed. Dose as in normal renal function.
HD	Not dialysed. Dose as in normal renal function.
HDF/High flux	Not dialysed. Dose as in normal renal function.
CAV/ VVHD	Not dialysed. Dose as in normal renal function.

IMPORTANT DRUG INTERACTIONS

Potentially hazardous interactions with other drugs
- None known

ADMINISTRATION

RECONSTITUTION
–

ROUTE
- Oral

RATE OF ADMINISTRATION
–

COMMENTS
–

Morphine

CLINICAL USE

Opiate analgesic

DOSE IN NORMAL RENAL FUNCTION

- 5–20 mg every 4 hours (higher in very severe pain or terminal illness)
- PR: 15–30 mg every 4 hours
- SR/XL: according to preparation every 12 or 24 hours

PHARMACOKINETICS

Molecular weight (daltons)	285.3 (758.8 as sulphate); (774.8 as tartrate)
% Protein binding	20–35
% Excreted unchanged in urine	10
Volume of distribution (L/kg)	3–5
Half-life – normal/ ESRF (hrs)	2–3/Unchanged

METABOLISM

Extensive first-pass metabolism in the liver and gut. The majority of a dose of morphine is conjugated with glucuronic acid in the liver and gut to produce morphine-3-glucuronide and morphine-6-glucuronide (active). Other active metabolites include normorphine, codeine, and morphine ethereal sulphate. After an oral dose, about 60% is excreted in the urine in 24 hours, with about 3% excreted as free morphine in 48 hours. After a parenteral dose, about 90% is excreted in 24 hours, with about 10% as free morphine, 65 to 70% as conjugated morphine, 1% as normorphine and 3% as normorphine glucuronide. Up to 10% of a dose may be excreted in the bile.

DOSE IN RENAL IMPAIRMENT GFR (mL/MIN)

20–50	75% of normal dose
10–20	Use small doses (50% of dose), e.g. 2.5–5 mg and extended dosing intervals. Titrate according to response.
<10	Use small doses (50% of dose), e.g. 1.25–2.5 mg and extended dosing intervals. Titrate according to response.

DOSE IN PATIENTS UNDERGOING RENAL REPLACEMENT THERAPIES

CAPD	Not dialysed. Dose as in GFR<10 mL/min.
HD	Dialysed – active metabolite removed significantly. Dose as in GFR<10 mL/min.
HDF/High flux	Dialysed – active metabolite removed significantly. Dose as in GFR<10 mL/min.
CAV/ VVHD	Dialysed. Dose as in GFR=10–20 mL/min.

IMPORTANT DRUG INTERACTIONS

Potentially hazardous interactions with other drugs

- Antibacterials: metabolism increased by rifampicin.
- Antidepressants: possible CNS excitation or depression with MAOIs – avoid concomitant use, and for 2 weeks after stopping MAOI; possible CNS excitation or depression with moclobemide; increased sedative effects with tricyclics.
- Anti-epileptics: increases bioavailability of gabapentin.
- Antihistamines: increased sedative effects with sedating antihistamines.
- Antipsychotics: enhanced hypotensive and sedative effects.
- Antivirals: concentration possibly reduced by ritonavir.
- Dopaminergics: avoid with selegiline.
- Sodium oxybate: enhanced effect of sodium oxybate – avoid concomitant use.

ADMINISTRATION

RECONSTITUTION

–

ROUTE

- Oral, SC, IM, IV, PR

RATE OF ADMINISTRATION

- 2 mg/minute (Titrate according to response.)

COMMENTS

–

OTHER INFORMATION

- Doses in renal impairment are from *Drug Prescribing in Renal Failure*, 5th edition, by Aronoff *et al.*
- Extreme caution with all opiates in patients with impaired renal function.
- Potential accumulation of morphine-6-glucuronide (a renally excreted active

metabolite, more potent than morphine) and morphine-3-glucuronide. Half-life of morphine-6-glucuronide is increased from 3–5 hours in normal renal function to about 50 hours in ERF.

- ENSURE NALOXONE READILY AVAILABLE.

- Some units avoid slow release oral preparations as any side effects may be prolonged.

Movicol (active ingredient is the osmotic laxative polyethylene glycol)

CLINICAL USE

Laxative

DOSE IN NORMAL RENAL FUNCTION

- 1–3 sachets daily in divided doses in 125 mL of water
- Maintenance: 1–2 sachets daily
- Faecal impaction: 4 sachets on 1st day increasing up to 8 sachets daily

PHARMACOKINETICS

Molecular weight (daltons)	3350
% Protein binding	Not absorbed.
% Excreted unchanged in urine	Not absorbed.
Volume of distribution (L/kg)	Not absorbed.
Half-life – normal/ ESRF (hrs)	Not absorbed.

METABOLISM

Not absorbed systemically.

DOSE IN RENAL IMPAIRMENT GFR (mL/MIN)

20–50	Dose as in normal renal function.
10–20	Dose as in normal renal function.
<10	Dose as in normal renal function.

DOSE IN PATIENTS UNDERGOING RENAL REPLACEMENT THERAPIES

CAPD	Not dialysed. Dose as in normal renal function.
HD	Not dialysed. Dose as in normal renal function.
HDF/High flux	Not dialysed. Dose as in normal renal function.
CAV/ VVHD	Not dialysed. Dose as in normal renal function.

IMPORTANT DRUG INTERACTIONS

Potentially hazardous interactions with other drugs
- None known

ADMINISTRATION

RECONSTITUTION
–
ROUTE
- Oral
RATE OF ADMINISTRATION
–
COMMENTS
–

OTHER INFORMATION

- Movicol contains polyethylene glycol, sodium chloride, sodium bicarbonate and potassium chloride.
- Electrolyte content of a sachet when made up with 125 mL water is:
  - Sodium 65 mmol/L
  - Chloride 53 mmol/L
  - Potassium 5.4 mmol/L
  - Bicarbonate 17 mmol/L
- Sachets are formulated to ensure that there is virtually no net gain or loss of sodium, potassium or water.

Moxifloxacin

CLINICAL USE

Antibacterial agent

DOSE IN NORMAL RENAL FUNCTION

400 mg once daily

PHARMACOKINETICS

Molecular weight (daltons)	437.9 (as hydrochloride)
% Protein binding	30–50
% Excreted unchanged in urine	19
Volume of distribution (L/kg)	2
Half-life – normal/ ESRF (hrs)	12/Unchanged

METABOLISM

Metabolised mainly via sulphate and glucuronide conjugation, and is excreted in the urine and the faeces as unchanged drug and as metabolites, the sulphate conjugate mainly in the faeces and the glucuronide exclusively in the urine.

DOSE IN RENAL IMPAIRMENT GFR (mL/MIN)

30–50	Dose as in normal renal function.
10–30	Dose as in normal renal function.
<10	Dose as in normal renal function.

DOSE IN PATIENTS UNDERGOING RENAL REPLACEMENT THERAPIES

CAPD	Unknown dialysability. Dose as in normal renal function.
HD	Unknown dialysability. Dose as in normal renal function.
HDF/High flux	Unknown dialysability. Dose as in normal renal function.
CAV/ VVHD	Unknown dialysability. Dose as in normal renal function.

IMPORTANT DRUG INTERACTIONS

Potentially hazardous interactions with other drugs
- Analgesics: increased risk of convulsions with NSAIDs.
- Anti-arrhythmics: increased risk of ventricular arrhythmias with amiodarone, disopyramide and procainamide – avoid concomitant use.
- Antibacterials: increased risk of ventricular arrhythmias with parenteral erythromycin – avoid concomitant use; increased risk of ventricular arrhythmias with telithromycin.
- Anticoagulants: anticoagulant effect enhanced.
- Antidepressants: increased risk of ventricular arrhythmias with tricyclics – avoid concomitant use.
- Antihistamines: increased risk of ventricular arrhythmias with mizolastine – avoid concomitant use.
- Antimalarials: increased risk of ventricular arrhythmias with chloroquine, hydroxychloroquine, mefloquine or quinine – avoid concomitant use; avoid concomitant use with artemether with lumefantrine and piperaquine with artenimol.
- Antipsychotics: increased risk of ventricular arrhythmias with benperidol, droperidol, haloperidol, phenothiazines, pimozide or zuclopenthixol – avoid concomitant use.
- Antivirals: increased risk of ventricular arrhythmias with saquinavir – avoid.
- Atomoxetine: increased risk of ventricular arrhythmias – avoid.
- Beta-blockers: increased risk of ventricular arrhythmias with sotalol – avoid concomitant use.
- Ciclosporin: some reports of increased nephrotoxicity.
- Cytotoxics: increased risk of ventricular arrhythmias with arsenic trioxide and vandetanib, avoid with vandetanib.
- Pentamidine: increased risk of ventricular arrhythmias – avoid concomitant use.
- Theophylline: possibly increased risk of convulsions.

ADMINISTRATION

RECONSTITUTION

–

ROUTE
- Oral

RATE OF ADMINISTRATION

–

COMMENTS
- Do not take milk, iron preparations, indigestion remedies or phosphate binders at the same time as moxifloxacin.

OTHER INFORMATION

Oral bioavailability is 90%.

Moxisylyte (thymoxamine)

CLINICAL USE

Primary Raynaud's syndrome

DOSE IN NORMAL RENAL FUNCTION

40–80 mg 4 times daily

PHARMACOKINETICS

Molecular weight (daltons)	315.8
% Protein binding	No data
% Excreted unchanged in urine	<1
Volume of distribution (L/kg)	Low[1]
Half-life – normal/ ESRF (hrs)	1–2/–

METABOLISM

Rapidly converted to desacetylmoxisylyte (metabolite I) and desmethyldesacetylmoxisylyte (metabolite II) which are pharmacologically active. These are then further metabolised to the sulphate and glucuronide conjugates of metabolites I and II. Excretion is almost exclusively via the kidneys.

DOSE IN RENAL IMPAIRMENT GFR (mL/MIN)

25–50	Dose as in normal renal function.
10–25	Dose as in normal renal function.
<10	Dose as in normal renal function.

DOSE IN PATIENTS UNDERGOING RENAL REPLACEMENT THERAPIES

CAPD	Unlikely to be dialysed. Dose as in normal renal function.
HD	Unlikely to be dialysed. Dose as in normal renal function.
HDF/High flux	Unlikely to be dialysed. Dose as in normal renal function.
CAV/ VVHD	Unlikely to be dialysed. Dose as in normal renal function.

IMPORTANT DRUG INTERACTIONS

Potentially hazardous interactions with other drugs
- Alpha-blockers: possibly severe postural hypotension when given in combination.
- Beta-blockers: possibly severe postural hypotension when given in combination.

ADMINISTRATION

RECONSTITUTION
–
ROUTE
- Oral
RATE OF ADMINISTRATION
–
COMMENTS
–

OTHER INFORMATION

- Theoretically may decrease insulin requirements in diabetics.

Reference:
1. Marquer C, Bressole F. Moxisylyte: a review of its pharmacodynamic and pharmacokinetic properties, and its therapeutic use in impotence. *Fundam Clin Pharmacol.* 1998; **12**: 377–87.

Moxonidine

CLINICAL USE

Antihypertensive agent (centrally acting agonist at I_1 receptor, imidazoline and alpha-2 adrenoceptors)

DOSE IN NORMAL RENAL FUNCTION

200–600 mcg daily
(Doses >400 mcg should be in 2 divided doses)

PHARMACOKINETICS

Molecular weight (daltons)	241.7
% Protein binding	7
% Excreted unchanged in urine	50–75
Volume of distribution (L/kg)	1.8
Half-life – normal/ ESRF (hrs)	2–3/6.9 +/−3.7

METABOLISM

10–20% metabolised, predominantly to 4,5-dehydromoxonidine and to an aminomethanamidine derivative both of which are much less active than moxonidine. Moxonidine and its metabolites are almost entirely eliminated via the kidney. More than 90% of the dose is eliminated in the first 24 hours via the kidney, while approximately 1% is eliminated in the faeces.

DOSE IN RENAL IMPAIRMENT GFR (mL/MIN)

30–60	Dose as in normal renal function.
10–30	Dose as in normal renal function.
<10	Dose as in normal renal function.

DOSE IN PATIENTS UNDERGOING RENAL REPLACEMENT THERAPIES

CAPD	Probably dialysed. Dose as in normal renal function.
HD	Probably dialysed. Dose as in normal renal function.
HDF/High flux	Probably dialysed. Dose as in normal renal function.
CAV/ VVHD	Probably dialysed. Dose as in normal renal function.

IMPORTANT DRUG INTERACTIONS

Potentially hazardous interactions with other drugs
● None known

ADMINISTRATION

RECONSTITUTION
–
ROUTE
● Oral
RATE OF ADMINISTRATION
–
COMMENTS
–

OTHER INFORMATION

● In moderately impaired renal function (GFR=30–60 mL/min) AUC is increased by 85% and clearance decreased by 52%; therefore, monitor patient closely.
● Anecdotal evidence suggests that moxonidine can be used safely at standard doses in patients with all degrees of renal impairment.
● One paper suggests that moxonidine can be used in patients with severe renal failure, at a dose of 300 mcg daily. (Kirch W, Hutt HJ, Planitz V. The influence of renal function on clinical pharmacokinetics of moxonidine. *Clin Pharmacokinet.* 1988; **15**: 245–53.)

Muromonab CD3 (OKT3) (unlicensed)

CLINICAL USE

- Steroid resistant acute transplant rejection
- Prophylaxis of rejection in sensitised patients

DOSE IN NORMAL RENAL FUNCTION

5 mg daily for 10–14 days (10 days most common)

PHARMACOKINETICS

Molecular weight (daltons)	50 000 (Heavy chain) + 25 000 (Light chain)
% Protein binding	No data
% Excreted unchanged in urine	No data
Volume of distribution (L/kg)	0.093
Half-life – normal/ ESRF (hrs)	18–36/–

METABOLISM

Most likely removed by opsonisation via the reticuloendothelial system when bound to T lymphocytes, or by human antimurine antibody production.

DOSE IN RENAL IMPAIRMENT GFR (mL/MIN)

20–50	Dose as in normal renal function.
10–20	Dose as in normal renal function.
<10	Dose as in normal renal function.

DOSE IN PATIENTS UNDERGOING RENAL REPLACEMENT THERAPIES

CAPD	Unlikely to be dialysed. Dose as in normal renal function.
HD	Not dialysed. Dose as in normal renal function.
HDF/High flux	Unknown dialysability. Dose as in normal renal function.
CAV/ VVHD	Unknown dialysability. Dose as in normal renal function.

IMPORTANT DRUG INTERACTIONS

Potentially hazardous interactions with other drugs

- Ciclosporin: increases ciclosporin plasma levels.
- Indomethacin: may increase risk of encephalopathy.
- Volatile anaesthetics/drugs that decrease cardiac contractility: increase risk of developing cardiovascular problems.

ADMINISTRATION

RECONSTITUTION
–
ROUTE
- IV
RATE OF ADMINISTRATION
- FAST over less than 1 minute
COMMENTS
- NB Doctor administration recommended

OTHER INFORMATION

*** ENSURE PATIENT IS NOT FLUID OVERLOADED PRIOR TO ADMINISTRATION ***

- Possible future scope for dose titration according to CD3 or absolute T-cell count.
- Reduce or stop other immunosuppressant therapy during treatment, and resume 3 days prior to cessation of OKT3.
- IV methylprednisolone sodium succinate (8 mg/kg given 1–4 hours prior to the first dose of OKT3) is strongly recommended to decrease the incidence and severity of reactions to the first dose. Paracetamol and antihistamines given concomitantly with OKT3 may also help to reduce some early reactions.
- Side effects pronounced: WARN PATIENT.

Mycophenolate

CLINICAL USE

- Mycophenolate sodium: for renal transplantation
- Mycophenolate mofetil: prophylaxis against acute transplant rejection; autoimmune renal diseases.

DOSE IN NORMAL RENAL FUNCTION

- Mycophenolate sodium: 720 mg twice daily
- Mycophenolate mofetil: 1–1.5 g twice a day

PHARMACOKINETICS

Molecular weight (daltons)	320.3 (Mycophenolic acid) 433.5 (as mofetil) 342.3 (as sodium)
% Protein binding	97
% Excreted unchanged in urine	<1
Volume of distribution (L/kg)	3.6–4
Half-life – normal/ ESRF (hrs)	12–17.9/–

METABOLISM

Mycophenolate undergoes presystemic metabolism in the liver to active mycophenolic acid (MPA). MPA undergoes enterohepatic recirculation and secondary increases in plasma MPA concentrations are seen; these have been reported at between 6 to 12 hours after a dose of mycophenolate mofetil, and at between 6 to 8 hours after a dose of mycophenolate sodium. MPA is metabolised by glucuronidation to the inactive mycophenolic acid glucuronide. The majority of a dose of mycophenolate is excreted in the urine as this glucuronide, with negligible amounts of MPA; about 6% of a dose is recovered in faeces.

DOSE IN RENAL IMPAIRMENT GFR (mL/MIN)

25–50	Dose as in normal renal function.
10–25	Mycophenolate mofetil: 1 g twice a day, starting immediately post transplant. Mycophenolate sodium: Maximum 1440 mg daily, starting immediately post transplant.
<10	Mycophenolate mofetil: 1 g twice a day, starting immediately post transplant. Mycophenolate sodium: Maximum 1440 mg daily, starting immediately post transplant.

DOSE IN PATIENTS UNDERGOING RENAL REPLACEMENT THERAPIES

CAPD	Not dialysed. Dose as in GFR<10 mL/min.
HD	Not dialysed. Dose as in GFR<10 mL/min.
HDF/High flux	Unknown dialysability. Dose as in GFR<10 mL/min.
CAV/ VVHD	Not dialysed. Dose as in normal renal function.

IMPORTANT DRUG INTERACTIONS

Potentially hazardous interactions with other drugs

- Antipsychotics: avoid concomitant use with clozapine (increased risk of agranulocytosis).
- Antivirals: higher concentrations of both mycophenolate and aciclovir or ganciclovir when the two are prescribed concomitantly.
- Antacids: absorption of mycophenolate decreased in presence of magnesium and aluminium salts.
- Antibacterials: bioavailability of mycophenolate possibly reduced by metronidazole and norfloxacin; concentration of active metabolite reduced by rifampicin.
- Cholestyramine: 40% reduction in oral bioavailability of mycophenolate.
- Ciclosporin: some studies show that ciclosporin decreases plasma MPA AUC levels; other studies show increases – no dose change required.
- Iron preparations: may significantly reduce absorption of mycophenolate.
- Sevelamer: reduced levels of mycophenolate.
- Tacrolimus: increases MPA concentrations – no dose change required but monitor closely.
- See 'Other information'.

ADMINISTRATION

RECONSTITUTION
- Add 14 mL of glucose 5% per 500 mg vial
ROUTE
- Oral, IV
RATE OF ADMINISTRATION
- Over 2 hours

COMMENTS

- Dilute reconstituted solution further with glucose 5% to achieve a concentration of 6 mg/mL.

OTHER INFORMATION

- If neutrophil count drops below $1.3 \times 10^3/\mu L$, consider suspending MMF therapy.
- No dosage reduction is required in the event of a transplant rejection episode.
- Mycophenolate sodium 720 mg is approximately equivalent to 1 g mycophenolate mofetil.
- In patients receiving mycophenolate mofetil, reduction in pre-dose concentration of the active metabolite mycophenolic acid (MPA) of approximately 50% has been reported after starting oral co-amoxiclav. The change in pre-dose level may not accurately represent changes in overall MPA exposure. Therefore, a change in the dose of mycophenolate mofetil should not normally be necessary in the absence of clinical evidence of graft dysfunction. However, close clinical monitoring should be performed during the combination and shortly after antibiotic treatment.

Nabumetone

CLINICAL USE

NSAID and analgesic

DOSE IN NORMAL RENAL FUNCTION

1 g at night; in severe conditions 0.5–1 g in the morning as well; elderly 0.5–1 g daily

PHARMACOKINETICS

Molecular weight (daltons)	228.3
% Protein binding	>99
% Excreted unchanged in urine	<1
Volume of distribution (L/kg)	0.11
Half-life – normal/ESRF (hrs)	24/39[1]

METABOLISM

Nabumetone is rapidly metabolised in the liver to the main active metabolite 6-methoxy-2-naphthylacetic acid (6-MNA). The metabolite is a potent inhibitor of prostaglandin synthesis. Excretion of the metabolite is predominantly in the urine.

DOSE IN RENAL IMPAIRMENT GFR (mL/MIN)

20–50	Dose as in normal renal function, but avoid if possible
10–20	0.5–1 g daily, but avoid if possible
<10	0.5–1 g daily, but only use if on dialysis. See 'Other information'.

DOSE IN PATIENTS UNDERGOING RENAL REPLACEMENT THERAPIES

CAPD	Not dialysed. Dose as in GFR<10 mL/min.
HD	Not dialysed. Dose as in GFR<10 mL/min.
HDF/High flux	Not dialysed. Dose as in GFR<10 mL/min.
CAV/ VVHD	Not dialysed. Dose as in GFR=10–20 mL/min.

IMPORTANT DRUG INTERACTIONS

Potentially hazardous interactions with other drugs

- ACE inhibitors and angiotensin-II antagonists: antagonism of hypotensive effect; increased risk of nephrotoxicity and hyperkalaemia.
- Analgesics: avoid concomitant use of 2 or more NSAIDs, including aspirin (increased side effects); avoid with ketorolac (increased risk of side effects and haemorrhage).
- Antibacterials: possibly increased risk of convulsions with quinolones.
- Anticoagulants: effects of coumarins and phenindione enhanced; possibly increased risk of bleeding with heparins and dabigatran.
- Antidepressants: increased risk of bleeding with SSRIs and venlafaxine.
- Antidiabetic agents: effects of sulphonylureas enhanced.
- Anti-epileptics: possibly increased phenytoin concentration.
- Antivirals: increased risk of haematological toxicity with zidovudine; concentration possibly increased by ritonavir.
- Ciclosporin: may potentiate nephrotoxicity.
- Cytotoxic agents: reduced excretion of methotrexate; increased risk of bleeding with erlotinib.
- Diuretics: increased risk of nephrotoxicity; antagonism of diuretic effect; hyperkalaemia with potassium-sparing diuretics.
- Lithium: excretion decreased.
- Pentoxifylline: increased risk of bleeding.
- Tacrolimus: increased risk of nephrotoxicity.

ADMINISTRATION

RECONSTITUTION

–

ROUTE

- Oral

RATE OF ADMINISTRATION

–

COMMENTS

–

OTHER INFORMATION

- The SPC recommends a dose reduction if creatinine clearance <30 mL/minute; however, an article by Brier et al. concluded that dosage adjustments may not be necessary with decreased renal function. The authors found an increase in the elimination half-life of 6-MNA, but stated that the increased half-life in patients with renal failure is offset by changes in the apparent volume of distribution that prevent the accumulation of 6-MNA. (Brier ME, Sloan RS, Aronoff

GR. Population pharmacokinetics of the active metabolite of nabumetone in renal dysfunction. *Clin Pharmacol Ther.* 1995 Jun; **57**(6): 622–7.)

- *Drug Prescribing in Renal Failure*, 5th edition, by Aronoff *et al.* recommends 50–100% of dose.

- Inhibition of renal prostaglandin synthesis by NSAIDs may interfere with renal function, especially in the presence of existing renal disease – avoid if possible; if not, check serum creatinine 48–72 hours after starting NSAID – if increased, discontinue NSAID therapy.

- Use normal doses in patients with CKD 5 on dialysis if they do not pass any urine.

- Use with caution in renal transplant recipients – can reduce intrarenal autocoid synthesis.

Reference:

1. Fillastre JP, Singlas E. Pharmacokinetics of newer drugs in patients with renal impairment (part I). *Clin Pharmacokinet.* 1991; **20**(4): 293–310.

Nadolol

CLINICAL USE

Beta-adrenoceptor blocker:
- Hypertension
- Angina
- Arrhythmias
- Migraine
- Thyrotoxicosis

DOSE IN NORMAL RENAL FUNCTION

- Hypertension: 80–240 mg per day
- Angina, arrhythmias, migraine: 40–160 mg daily
- Thyrotoxicosis: 80–160 mg daily

PHARMACOKINETICS

Molecular weight (daltons)	309.4
% Protein binding	30
% Excreted unchanged in urine	73
Volume of distribution (L/kg)	1.9
Half-life – normal/ ESRF (hrs)	12–24/45

METABOLISM

Unlike most other beta-blockers, nadolol is not metabolised and is excreted unchanged mainly by the kidneys.

DOSE IN RENAL IMPAIRMENT GFR (mL/MIN)

20–50	Start with low dose and increase according to response.
10–20	Start with low dose and increase according to response.
<10	Start with low dose and increase according to response.

DOSE IN PATIENTS UNDERGOING RENAL REPLACEMENT THERAPIES

CAPD	Dialysed. Dose as in GFR<10 mL/ min.
HD	Dialysed. Dose as in GFR<10 mL/ min.
HDF/High flux	Dialysed. Dose as in GFR<10 mL/ min.
CAV/ VVHD	Dialysed. Dose as in GFR=10– 20 mL/min.

IMPORTANT DRUG INTERACTIONS

Potentially hazardous interactions with other drugs
- Anaesthetics: enhanced hypotensive effect.
- Analgesics: NSAIDs antagonise hypotensive effect.
- Anti-arrhythmics: increased risk of myocardial depression and bradycardia; increased risk of bradycardia, myocardial depression and AV block with amiodarone; increased risk of myocardial depression and bradycardia with flecainide.
- Antidepressants: enhanced hypotensive effect with MAOIs.
- Antihypertensives: enhanced hypotensive effect; increased risk of withdrawal hypertension with clonidine; increased risk of first dose hypotensive effect with post-synaptic alpha-blockers such as prazosin.
- Antimalarials: increased risk of bradycardia with mefloquine.
- Antipsychotics enhanced hypotensive effect with phenothiazines.
- Calcium-channel blockers: increased risk of bradycardia and AV block with diltiazem; hypotension and heart failure possible with nifedipine and nisoldipine; asystole, severe hypotension and heart failure with verapamil.
- Cytotoxics: possible increased risk of bradycardia with crizotinib.
- Diuretics: enhanced hypotensive effect.
- Fingolimod: possibly increased risk of bradycardia.
- Moxisylyte: possible severe postural hypotension.
- Sympathomimetics: severe hypertension with adrenaline and noradrenaline and possibly with dobutamine.

ADMINISTRATION

RECONSTITUTION
–
ROUTE
- Oral
RATE OF ADMINISTRATION
–
COMMENTS
–

OTHER INFORMATION

- SPC guidelines for increasing dosing interval for patients with renal impairment may be impractical with respect to patient compliance.
- UK SPC provides no guidance in renal impairment.
- US SPC advises:
  - GFR=31–50: every 24–36 hours
  - GFR=10–30: every 24–48 hours
  - GFR<10: 40–60 hours.

Naftidrofuryl oxalate

CLINICAL USE

Vasodilator:
- Peripheral and cerebral vascular disease

DOSE IN NORMAL RENAL FUNCTION

- Peripheral vascular disease: 100–200 mg 3 times daily
- Cerebral vascular disease: 100 mg 3 times daily

PHARMACOKINETICS

Molecular weight (daltons)	473.6
% Protein binding	60–65
% Excreted unchanged in urine	<1 (mainly as metabolites)
Volume of distribution (L/kg)	61.5 litres
Half-life – normal/ ESRF (hrs)	1–2/3.5

METABOLISM

Metabolised by plasma pseudo-cholinesterases to three active metabolites.[1]

DOSE IN RENAL IMPAIRMENT GFR (mL/MIN)

20–50	Dose as in normal renal function.
10–20	Dose as in normal renal function. Start with low doses.
<10	Dose as in normal renal function. Start with low doses.

DOSE IN PATIENTS UNDERGOING RENAL REPLACEMENT THERAPIES

CAPD	Unlikely to be dialysed. Dose as in GFR<10 mL/min.
HD	Dialysed. Dose as in GFR<10 mL/min.
HDF/High flux	Dialysed. Dose as in GFR<10 mL/min.
CAV/ VVHD	Unlikely to be dialysed. Dose as in GFR=10–20 mL/min.

IMPORTANT DRUG INTERACTIONS

Potentially hazardous interactions with other drugs
- None known

ADMINISTRATION

RECONSTITUTION
–
ROUTE
- Oral
RATE OF ADMINISTRATION
–
COMMENTS
–

OTHER INFORMATION

- IV preparation was withdrawn due to increased risk of cardiac and neurological toxicity. It has also been associated with acute renal failure secondary to oxalate crystallisation in the renal tubules.

Reference:
1. Barradell LB, Brogden RN. Oral naftidrofuryl. *Drugs & Aging.* 1996; **8**(4): 299–322.

Nalidixic acid

CLINICAL USE

Antibacterial agent

DOSE IN NORMAL RENAL FUNCTION

600–900 mg every 6 hours

PHARMACOKINETICS

Molecular weight (daltons)	232.2
% Protein binding	93–97
% Excreted unchanged in urine	11–33 (80–90% as inactive metabolites)
Volume of distribution (L/kg)	0.47–0.55
Half-life – normal/ ESRF (hrs)	6–8/21

METABOLISM

Nalidixic acid is partially metabolised in the liver to hydroxynalidixic acid, which has antibacterial activity similar to that of nalidixic acid and accounts for about 30% of active drug in the blood. Both nalidixic acid and hydroxynalidixic acid are rapidly metabolised to inactive glucuronide and dicarboxylic acid derivatives; the major inactive metabolite 7-carboxynalidixic acid is usually only detected in urine.

DOSE IN RENAL IMPAIRMENT GFR (mL/MIN)

20–50	Dose as in normal renal function.
10–20	Dose as in normal renal function.
<10	Avoid. See 'Other information'.

DOSE IN PATIENTS UNDERGOING RENAL REPLACEMENT THERAPIES

CAPD	Unlikely to be dialysed. Dose as in GFR<10 mL/min.
HD	Unlikely to be dialysed. Dose as in GFR<10 mL/min.
HDF/High flux	Unlikely to be dialysed. Dose as in GFR<10 mL/min.
CAV/ VVHD	Unknown dialysability. Dose as in normal renal function.

IMPORTANT DRUG INTERACTIONS

Potentially hazardous interactions with other drugs
- Analgesics: increased risk of convulsions with NSAIDs.
- Antibacterials: possibly antagonised by nitrofurantoin.
- Anticoagulants: anticoagulant effect of coumarins enhanced.
- Ciclosporin: Increased risk of nephrotoxicity.
- Cytotoxics: increases risk of melphalan toxicity.
- Antimalarials: manufacturer of artemether with lumefantrine advises avoid concomitant use.
- Theophylline: possibly increased risk of convulsions.

ADMINISTRATION

RECONSTITUTION
–
ROUTE
- Oral
RATE OF ADMINISTRATION
–
COMMENTS
–

OTHER INFORMATION

- Avoid in severe renal impairment because the concentration in the urine is inadequate, and risk of monoglucuronide metabolite toxicity.

Nalmefene hydrochloride dihydrate

CLINICAL USE

Opioid system modulator
- Reduction of alcohol consumption.

DOSE IN NORMAL RENAL FUNCTION

ONE tablet daily if at risk of drinking

PHARMACOKINETICS

Molecular weight (daltons)	375.9
% Protein binding	30
% Excreted unchanged in urine	<3
Volume of distribution (L/kg)	3200 litres
Half-life – normal/ ESRF (hrs)	10/26

METABOLISM

It is metabolised in the liver, mainly to the inactive glucuronide, and is excreted in the urine (54%). Some of the dose is excreted in the faeces and it may undergo enterohepatic recycling.

DOSE IN RENAL IMPAIRMENT GFR (mL/MIN)

30–50	Dose as in normal renal function.
<30	Avoid.

DOSE IN PATIENTS UNDERGOING RENAL REPLACEMENT THERAPIES

CAPD	Likely to be dialysed. Avoid.
HD	Likely to be dialysed. Avoid.
HDF/High flux	Likely to be dialysed. Avoid.
CAV/ VVHD	Likely to be dialysed. Avoid.

IMPORTANT DRUG INTERACTIONS

Potentially hazardous interactions with other drugs
- None known

ADMINISTRATION

RECONSTITUTION
–
ROUTE
- Oral
RATE OF ADMINISTRATION
–

OTHER INFORMATION

- Contraindicated by manufacturer if GFR<30mL/min as no studies have been done.
- Oral bioavailability is 41%.

Naloxone hydrochloride

CLINICAL USE

Reversal of opioid-induced respiratory depression

DOSE IN NORMAL RENAL FUNCTION

See 'Other information'.

PHARMACOKINETICS

Molecular weight (daltons)	363.8
% Protein binding	54
% Excreted unchanged in urine	0
Volume of distribution (L/kg)	3
Half-life – normal/ ESRF (hrs)	1–1.5/Unchanged

METABOLISM

Naloxone hydrochloride is rapidly metabolised in the liver, mainly by conjugation with glucuronic acid to naloxone-3-glucuronide, which is excreted in the urine.

DOSE IN RENAL IMPAIRMENT GFR (mL/MIN)

20–50	Dose as in normal renal function.
10–20	Dose as in normal renal function.
<10	Dose as in normal renal function.

DOSE IN PATIENTS UNDERGOING RENAL REPLACEMENT THERAPIES

CAPD	Unknown dialysability. Dose as in normal renal function.
HD	Unknown dialysability. Dose as in normal renal function.
HDF/High flux	Unknown dialysability. Dose as in normal renal function.
CAV/ VVHD	Unknown dialysability. Dose as in normal renal function.

IMPORTANT DRUG INTERACTIONS

Potentially hazardous interactions with other drugs
- None known

ADMINISTRATION

RECONSTITUTION
–
ROUTE
- IV, IM, SC. IV more rapid response
RATE OF ADMINISTRATION
- Rapid if bolus injection
COMMENTS
–

OTHER INFORMATION

- IV Postoperative use: Give 1.5–3 micrograms/kg; if response inadequate, increments of 100 micrograms every 2 minutes. Further dose by IM injection if needed.
- OR Dilute 400 micrograms in 100 mL sodium chloride 0.9% or glucose 5% (4 micrograms/mL) and give by continuous infusion. Titrate dose according to response.
- Opioid overdosage: initial dose of 400–2000 micrograms IV; may be repeated at 2–3 minute intervals if the desired degree of counteraction and improvement in respiratory function is not obtained. (If no response after 10 mg then question the diagnosis of opioid induced toxicity.) OR give as an infusion: 4 mg in 20 mL (200 mcg/mL solution) (unlicensed).

Naltrexone hydrochloride

CLINICAL USE

Opioid antagonist:
- Adjunctive prophylactic treatment in patients previously opioid dependant.
- Treatment of alcohol dependence.

DOSE IN NORMAL RENAL FUNCTION

- Opioid dependence: Initially 25 mg daily then 50 mg once daily
- Alcohol dependence: 50 mg once daily
- There is an option for a 3 times a week regimen if compliance may be an issue.

PHARMACOKINETICS

Molecular weight (daltons)	377.9
% Protein binding	21
% Excreted unchanged in urine	<2
Volume of distribution (L/kg)	1350 litres (IV)
Half-life – normal/ ESRF (hrs)	4 (13 for active metabolite)

METABOLISM

Naltrexone is well absorbed from the gastrointestinal tract but is subject to considerable first-pass metabolism and may undergo enterohepatic recycling. It is extensively metabolised in the liver and the major metabolite, 6-β-naltrexol, may also possess weak opioid antagonist activity. It is excreted mainly in the urine, <5% is excreted in the faeces.

The renal clearance for naltrexone ranges from 30 to 127 mL/min and suggests that renal elimination is primarily by glomerular filtration.

DOSE IN RENAL IMPAIRMENT GFR (mL/MIN)

20–50	Dose as in normal renal function.
10–20	Use with caution.
<10	Use with caution.

DOSE IN PATIENTS UNDERGOING RENAL REPLACEMENT THERAPIES

CAPD	Likely dialysability. Dose as in GFR<10 mL/min.
HD	Likely dialysability. Dose as in GFR<10 mL/min.
HDF/High flux	Likely dialysability. Dose as in GFR<10 mL/min.
CAV/ VVHD	Likely dialysability. Dose as in GFR=10–20 mL/min.

IMPORTANT DRUG INTERACTIONS

Potentially hazardous interactions with other drugs
- Opioids: avoid concomitant use.

ADMINISTRATION

RECONSTITUTION
–

ROUTE
- Oral

RATE OF ADMINISTRATION
–

OTHER INFORMATION

- Contraindicated in UK SPC in severe renal impairment due to lack of studies. Use with caution advised in New Zealand and US data sheets as naltrexone and its metabolites are renally excreted.
- A naloxone test must first be done to ensure patients do not have any opioids in their system.
- Oral bioavailability varies from 5% to 40%.

Naproxen

CLINICAL USE

NSAID and analgesic

DOSE IN NORMAL RENAL FUNCTION

- Rheumatic disease: 0.5–1 g in 1–2 divided doses
- Musculoskeletal disorders and dysmenorrhoea: 500 mg initially then 250 mg every 6–8 hours; maximum 1.25 g daily
- Gout: 750 mg initially then 250 mg every 8 hours

PHARMACOKINETICS

Molecular weight (daltons)	230.3
% Protein binding	99
% Excreted unchanged in urine	<1
Volume of distribution (L/kg)	0.16
Half-life – normal/ESRF (hrs)	12–15/ Unchanged

METABOLISM

Naproxen is extensively metabolised in the liver to 6–0-desmethyl naproxen. Both naproxen and 6–0-desmethyl naproxen are further metabolised to their respective acylglucuronide conjugated metabolites. About 95% of a dose is excreted in urine as naproxen and 6-O-desmethylnaproxen and their conjugates. Less than 5% of a dose appears in the faeces.

DOSE IN RENAL IMPAIRMENT GFR (mL/MIN)

20–50	Dose as in normal renal function, but avoid if possible.
10–20	Dose as in normal renal function, but avoid if possible.
<10	Dose as in normal renal function, but only use if on dialysis. See 'Other information'.

DOSE IN PATIENTS UNDERGOING RENAL REPLACEMENT THERAPIES

CAPD	Slightly dialysed. Dose as in GFR<10 mL/min.
HD	Not dialysed. Dose as in GFR<10 mL/min.
HDF/High flux	Unknown dialysability. Dose as in GFR<10 mL/min.
CAV/ VVHD	Slightly dialysed. Dose as in GFR=10–20 mL/min.

IMPORTANT DRUG INTERACTIONS

Potentially hazardous interactions with other drugs

- ACE inhibitors and angiotensin-II antagonists: antagonism of hypotensive effect; increased risk of nephrotoxicity and hyperkalaemia.
- Analgesics: avoid concomitant use of two or more NSAIDs, including aspirin (increased side effects); avoid with ketorolac (increased risk of side effects and haemorrhage).
- Antibacterials: possibly increased risk of convulsions with quinolones.
- Anticoagulants: effects of coumarins and phenindione enhanced; possibly increased risk of bleeding with heparins and dabigatran.
- Antidepressants: increased risk of bleeding with SSRIs and venlafaxine.
- Antidiabetic agents: effects of sulphonylureas enhanced.
- Anti-epileptics: possibly increased phenytoin concentration.
- Antivirals: increased risk of haematological toxicity with zidovudine; concentration possibly increased by ritonavir.
- Ciclosporin: may potentiate nephrotoxicity.
- Cytotoxic agents: reduced excretion of methotrexate; increased risk of bleeding with erlotinib.
- Diuretics: increased risk of nephrotoxicity; antagonism of diuretic effect; hyperkalaemia with potassium-sparing diuretics.
- Lithium: excretion decreased.
- Pentoxifylline: increased risk of bleeding.
- Probenecid: excretion reduced by probenecid.
- Tacrolimus: increased risk of nephrotoxicity.

ADMINISTRATION

RECONSTITUTION

–

ROUTE

- Oral

RATE OF ADMINISTRATION

–

COMMENTS

–

OTHER INFORMATION

- Associated with an intermediate risk of side effects.

- Inhibition of renal prostaglandin synthesis by NSAIDs may interfere with renal function, especially in the presence of existing renal disease – avoid if possible; if not, check serum creatinine 48–72 hours after starting NSAID – if raised, discontinue NSAID therapy. Use normal doses in patients with CKD 5 on dialysis and who do not pass any urine.
- Use with caution in renal transplant recipients (can reduce intrarenal autocoid synthesis).

Naratriptan

CLINICAL USE

$5HT_1$ receptor agonist:
- Acute treatment of migraine

DOSE IN NORMAL RENAL FUNCTION

2.5 mg. Dose may be repeated after 4 hours; maximum 5 mg/24 hours

PHARMACOKINETICS

Molecular weight (daltons)	371.9 (as hydrochloride)
% Protein binding	29
% Excreted unchanged in urine	50
Volume of distribution (L/kg)	170 litres
Half-life – normal/ ESRF (hrs)	6/11

METABOLISM

Naratriptan undergoes some hepatic metabolism via a wide range of cytochrome P450 isoenzymes to form inactive metabolites. Naratriptan is excreted by glomerular filtration and active secretion into the renal tubules.

It is mainly excreted in the urine with 50% of a dose being recovered as unchanged drug and 30% as inactive metabolites.

DOSE IN RENAL IMPAIRMENT GFR (mL/MIN)

20–50	Maximum 2.5 mg daily.
15–20	Maximum 2.5 mg daily.
<15	Use with caution – maximum 2.5 mg daily.

DOSE IN PATIENTS UNDERGOING RENAL REPLACEMENT THERAPIES

CAPD	Likely dialysability. Dose as for GFR<15 mL/min.
HD	Likely dialysability. Dose as for GFR<15 mL/min.
HDF/High flux	Likely dialysability. Dose as for GFR<15 mL/min.
CAV/ VVHD	Unknown dialysability. Dose as for GFR=15–20 mL/min.

IMPORTANT DRUG INTERACTIONS

Potentially hazardous interactions with other drugs
- Antidepressants: increased CNS toxicity with citalopram – avoid; possibly increased serotonergic effects with duloxetine, SSRIs and venlafaxine; increased serotonergic effects with St John's wort – avoid concomitant use.
- Ergot alkaloids: increased risk of vasospasm – avoid concomitant use.

ADMINISTRATION

RECONSTITUTION
–
ROUTE
- Oral
RATE OF ADMINISTRATION
–
COMMENTS
–

OTHER INFORMATION

- Do not take second dose at 4 hours during an attack if the first dose was ineffectual.
- Contraindicated by manufacturer if GFR<15 mL/min due to reduced clearance therefore use with caution.
- Studies in patients with impaired renal function (GFR=18–115 mL/min) showed an 80% increase in half-life and a 50% decrease in clearance compared with matched individuals with normal renal function.

Natalizumab

CLINICAL USE

Monoclonal antibody:
- Treatment of relapsing-remitting multiple sclerosis

DOSE IN NORMAL RENAL FUNCTION

300 mg every 4 weeks

PHARMACOKINETICS

Molecular weight (daltons)	149 000
% Protein binding	No data
% Excreted unchanged in urine	No data
Volume of distribution (L/kg)	3.8–7.6 litres
Half-life – normal/ ESRF (hrs)	7–15 days

METABOLISM

Most likely removed by opsonisation via the reticuloendothelial system when bound to leukocytes.

DOSE IN RENAL IMPAIRMENT GFR (mL/MIN)

20–50	Dose as in normal renal function.
10–20	Dose as in normal renal function.
<10	Dose as in normal renal function.

DOSE IN PATIENTS UNDERGOING RENAL REPLACEMENT THERAPIES

CAPD	Not dialysed. Dose as in normal renal function.
HD	Not dialysed. Dose as in normal renal function.
HDF/High flux	Not dialysed. Dose as in normal renal function.
CAV/ VVHD	Not dialysed. Dose as in normal renal function.

IMPORTANT DRUG INTERACTIONS

Potentially hazardous interactions with other drugs
- Avoid concomitant administration with beta-interferons or glatiramer acetate.

ADMINISTRATION

RECONSTITUTION
–
ROUTE
- IV infusion
RATE OF ADMINISTRATION
- 60 minutes (2 mL/min)
COMMENTS
- Dilute in 100 mL sodium chloride 0.9%.
- Use within 8 hours of preparation.

OTHER INFORMATION

- No studies have been conducted in renal impairment but the mechanism for elimination and pharmacokinetics suggest that dose adjustment would not be necessary in patients with renal impairment.
- The effect of plasma exchange on natalizumab clearance and pharmacodynamics was evaluated in a study of 12 MS patients. Estimates of the total natalizumab removal after 3 plasma exchanges (over a 5–8 day interval) was approximately 70–80%. The impact of plasma exchange on the restitution of lymphocyte migration and ultimately its clinical usefulness is unknown.

Nateglinide

CLINICAL USE

Treatment of type 2 diabetes in combination with metformin

DOSE IN NORMAL RENAL FUNCTION

60–180 mg 3 times daily

PHARMACOKINETICS

Molecular weight (daltons)	317.4
% Protein binding	97–99
% Excreted unchanged in urine	6–16
Volume of distribution (L/kg)	0.17–0.2
Half-life – normal/ ESRF (hrs)	1.5/Unchanged

METABOLISM

Nateglinide is mainly metabolised in the liver by cytochrome P450 isoenzyme CYP2C9, and to a lesser extent by CYP3A4. The major metabolites are less potent than nateglinide. The parent drug and metabolites are mainly excreted in the urine but about 10% is eliminated in the faeces.

DOSE IN RENAL IMPAIRMENT GFR (mL/MIN)

30–50	Dose as in normal renal function.
15–30	Dose as in normal renal function.
<15	Start at a low dose and increase according to response.

DOSE IN PATIENTS UNDERGOING RENAL REPLACEMENT THERAPIES

CAPD	Not dialysed. Dose as in GFR<15 mL/min.
HD	Not dialysed. Dose as in GFR<15 mL/min.
HDF/High flux	Not dialysed. Dose as in GFR<15 mL/min.
CAV/ VVHD	Not dialysed. Dose as in normal renal function.

IMPORTANT DRUG INTERACTIONS

Potentially hazardous interactions with other drugs
- Antibacterials: concentration reduced by rifampicin.
- Antifungals: hypoglycaemic effect possibly enhanced by fluconazole.
- Lipid-lowering agents: hypoglycaemic effect possibly enhanced by gemfibrozil.

ADMINISTRATION

RECONSTITUTION
–
ROUTE
- Oral
RATE OF ADMINISTRATION
–

COMMENTS
–

OTHER INFORMATION

- Although there is a 49% decrease in C_{max} of nateglinide in dialysis patients, the systemic availability and half-life in diabetic subjects with moderate to severe renal insufficiency (creatinine clearance=15–50 mL/min) was comparable between renal subjects requiring haemodialysis and healthy subjects. Although safety was not compromised in this population, dose adjustment may be required in view of low C_{max}.
- Metabolite removed by dialysis.

Nebivolol

CLINICAL USE

Beta-adrenoceptor blocker:
- Essential hypertension
- Adjunct in heart failure

DOSE IN NORMAL RENAL FUNCTION

- Hypertension: 2.5–5 mg once daily.
- Adjunct in heart failure: 1.25–10 mg once daily.

PHARMACOKINETICS

Molecular weight (daltons)	405.4 (441.9 as hydrochloride)
% Protein binding	98
% Excreted unchanged in urine	<0.5
Volume of distribution (L/kg)	11.2
Half-life – normal/ ESRF (hrs)	10 (32–34 in poor hydroxylators)/–

METABOLISM

Nebivolol is extensively metabolised in the liver by acyclic and aromatic hydroxylation, N-dealkylation, and glucuronidation. Hydroxylation is by cytochrome P450 isoenzyme CYP2D6, partly to active hydroxy-metabolites.

It is excreted in the urine and faeces, almost entirely as metabolites.

DOSE IN RENAL IMPAIRMENT GFR (mL/MIN)

20–50	Initial dose 2.5 mg and adjust according to response.
10–20	Initial dose 2.5 mg and adjust according to response.
<10	Initial dose 2.5 mg and adjust according to response.

DOSE IN PATIENTS UNDERGOING RENAL REPLACEMENT THERAPIES

CAPD	Not dialysed. Dose as in GFR<10 mL/min.
HD	Not dialysed. Dose as in GFR<10 mL/min.
HDF/High flux	Unknown dialysability. Dose as in GFR<10 mL/min.
CAV/ VVHD	Not dialysed. Dose as in GFR=10–20 mL/min.

IMPORTANT DRUG INTERACTIONS

Potentially hazardous interactions with other drugs
- Anaesthetics: enhanced hypotensive effect.
- Analgesics: NSAIDs antagonise hypotensive effect.
- Anti-arrhythmics: increased risk of myocardial depression and bradycardia; increased risk of bradycardia, myocardial depression and AV block with amiodarone; increased risk of myocardial depression and bradycardia with flecainide.
- Antidepressants: enhanced hypotensive effect with MAOIs.
- Antihypertensives: enhanced hypotensive effect; increased risk of withdrawal hypertension with clonidine; increased risk of first dose hypotensive effect with post-synaptic alpha-blockers such as prazosin.
- Antimalarials: increased risk of bradycardia with mefloquine.
- Antipsychotics: enhanced hypotensive effect with phenothiazines.
- Calcium-channel blockers: increased risk of bradycardia and AV block with diltiazem; hypotension and heart failure possible with nifedipine and nisoldipine; asystole, severe hypotension and heart failure with verapamil.
- Cytotoxics: possible increased risk of bradycardia with crizotinib.
- Diuretics: enhanced hypotensive effect.
- Fingolimod: possibly increased risk of bradycardia.
- Moxisylyte: possible severe postural hypotension.
- Sympathomimetics: severe hypertension with adrenaline and noradrenaline and possibly with dobutamine.

ADMINISTRATION

RECONSTITUTION
–

ROUTE
- Oral

RATE OF ADMINISTRATION
–

COMMENTS
–

OTHER INFORMATION

- 38% of the dose is excreted in the urine as active metabolites.
- In a trial of 10 patients with renal artery stenosis given nebivolol 5 mg daily, plasma renin activity significantly decreased, although serum aldosterone levels did not change to any great extent. In addition, there was no change in effective renal plasma flow, GFR, renal blood flow, or renal vascular resistance. Renal function remained well-preserved.

Nefopam hydrochloride

CLINICAL USE

Analgesic for moderate pain

DOSE IN NORMAL RENAL FUNCTION

Oral: 30–90 mg 3 times a day

PHARMACOKINETICS

Molecular weight (daltons)	289.8
% Protein binding	73
% Excreted unchanged in urine	<5
Volume of distribution (L/kg)	No data
Half-life – normal/ ESRF (hrs)	4/–

METABOLISM

Extensively metabolised in the liver to produce active metabolites. It is mainly excreted in the urine, with less than 5% of a dose excreted unchanged. About 8% of a dose is excreted via the faeces.

DOSE IN RENAL IMPAIRMENT GFR (mL/MIN)

20–50	Dose as in normal renal function.
10–20	Dose as in normal renal function.
<10	Dose as in normal renal function. See 'Other information'.

DOSE IN PATIENTS UNDERGOING RENAL REPLACEMENT THERAPIES

CAPD	Unknown dialysability. Dose as in GFR<10 mL/min.
HD	Unlikely to be dialysed. Dose as in GFR<10 mL/min.
HDF/High flux	Unknown dialysability. Dose as in GFR<10 mL/min.
CAV/ VVHD	Unknown dialysability. Dose as in normal renal function.

IMPORTANT DRUG INTERACTIONS

Potentially hazardous interactions with other drugs
- Antidepressants: avoid MAOIs; tricyclics possibly increased risk of side effects.

ADMINISTRATION

RECONSTITUTION
–
ROUTE
- Oral
RATE OF ADMINISTRATION
–
COMMENTS
–

OTHER INFORMATION

- Avoid repeated or chronic administration in end stage renal disease and dialysis patients.
- In the elderly a dose of 30 mg 8 hourly is recommended due to reduced metabolism and increased susceptibility to side effects. Renal patients may also have reduced metabolism and excretion so may also have the same problems – always start with the lower dose.
- Avoid in convulsive disorders.

Nelarabine

CLINICAL USE

Antineoplastic agent:
- T-cell acute lymphoblastic leukaemia (T-ALL)
- T-cell lymphoblastic lymphoma (T-LBL)

DOSE IN NORMAL RENAL FUNCTION

IV: 1.5 g/m^2 on days 1, 3 & 5; repeated every 21 days
Consult relevant local protocol.

PHARMACOKINETICS

Molecular weight (daltons)	297.3
% Protein binding	<25
% Excreted unchanged in urine	5.3 (23.2 as metabolite)
Volume of distribution (L/kg)	115 L/m^2
Half-life – normal/ ESRF (hrs)	30 minutes/–

METABOLISM

Nelarabine is a prodrug of the deoxyguanosine analogue ara-G.

Extensive metabolism by O-demethylation by adenosine deaminase to form ara-G, which undergoes hydrolysis to form guanine. In addition, some nelarabine is hydrolysed to form methylguanine, which is O-demethylated to form guanine. Guanine is N-deaminated to form xanthine, which is further oxidised to yield uric acid.

Nelarabine and ara-G are partially eliminated by the kidneys.

DOSE IN RENAL IMPAIRMENT GFR (mL/MIN)

30–50	Dose as in normal renal function. Monitor closely.
10–30	Dose as in normal renal function. Monitor closely.
<10	Dose as in normal renal function. Monitor closely. Use with caution.

DOSE IN PATIENTS UNDERGOING RENAL REPLACEMENT THERAPIES

CAPD	Unlikely to be dialysed. Dose as in GFR<10 mL/min.
HD	Unlikely to be dialysed. Dose as in GFR<10 mL/min.
HDF/High flux	Unknown dialysability. Dose as in GFR<10 mL/min.
CAV/ VVHD	Unlikely to be dialysed. Dose as in GFR=10–30 mL/min.

IMPORTANT DRUG INTERACTIONS

Potentially hazardous interactions with other drugs
- None known

ADMINISTRATION

RECONSTITUTION
–
ROUTE
- IV infusion
RATE OF ADMINISTRATION
- 2 hours
COMMENTS
- Nelarabine must NOT be diluted prior to administration. The appropriate dose must be transferred into polyvinylchloride or ethyl vinyl acetate infusion bags or glass containers.

OTHER INFORMATION

- No studies have been done in renal impairment (GFR<50 mL/min). Patients with renal impairment are more at risk of toxicities. So monitor closely.
- Contains 1.725 mg/mL (75 micromoles) of sodium.
- Severe neurotoxicity is a dose-limiting side effect.
- The mean apparent clearance of ara-G was about 15% and 40% lower in patients with mild and moderate renal impairment, respectively, than in patients with normal renal function.

Neomycin sulphate

CLINICAL USE

Antibacterial agent:
- Bowel sterilisation before surgery
- Hepatic coma

DOSE IN NORMAL RENAL FUNCTION

- Bowel sterilisation: 1 g every hour for 4 hours, then 1 g every 4 hours for 2–3 days
- Hepatic coma: up to 4 g daily in divided doses usually for 5–7 days

PHARMACOKINETICS

Molecular weight (daltons)	711.7
% Protein binding	0–30
% Excreted unchanged in urine	30–50
Volume of distribution (L/kg)	0.25
Half-life – normal/ ESRF (hrs)	2–3/12–24

METABOLISM

Only 3% of dose is absorbed. Approximately 97% of an oral dose is excreted unchanged in the faeces.

DOSE IN RENAL IMPAIRMENT GFR (mL/MIN)

20–50	Dose as in normal renal function. Use with caution and monitor renal function.
10–20	Dose as in normal renal function. Use with caution and monitor renal function.
<10	Dose as in normal renal function. Use with caution and monitor renal function.

DOSE IN PATIENTS UNDERGOING RENAL REPLACEMENT THERAPIES

CAPD	Dialysed. Dose as in GFR<10 mL/min.
HD	Dialysed. Dose as in GFR<10 mL/min.
HDF/High flux	Dialysed. Dose as in GFR<10 mL/min.
CAV/ VVHD	Dialysed. Dose as in GFR=10–20 mL/min.

IMPORTANT DRUG INTERACTIONS

Potentially hazardous interactions with other drugs
- Antibacterials: absorption of phenoxymethylpenicillin reduced; increased risk of nephrotoxicity with colistimethate or polymyxins and possibly cephalosporins; increased risk of ototoxicity and nephrotoxicity with capreomycin or vancomycin.
- Anticoagulants: altered INR with coumarins or phenindione.
- Ciclosporin: increased risk of nephrotoxicity.
- Cytotoxics: possibly reduced methotrexate absorption; bioavailability of sorafenib reduced; increased risk of nephrotoxicity and possibly of ototoxicity with platinum compounds.
- Diuretics: increased risk of ototoxicity with loop diuretics.
- Muscle relaxants: enhanced effects of suxamethonium and non-depolarising muscle relaxants.
- Parasympathomimetics: antagonism of effect of neostigmine and pyridostigmine.
- Tacrolimus: increased risk of nephrotoxicity.

ADMINISTRATION

RECONSTITUTION
–
ROUTE
- Oral, topical
RATE OF ADMINISTRATION
–
COMMENTS
–

OTHER INFORMATION

- Impaired GI motility may increase absorption of the drug; therefore, possible that prolonged therapy could result in ototoxicity and nephrotoxicity, particularly in patients with a degree of renal failure.
- If renal impairment occurs the dose should be reduced or treatment discontinued.
- High doses associated with nephrotoxicity and ototoxicity.
- In mild renal failure, i.e. a GFR>50 mL/min, the frequency should be reduced to every 6 hours.

Neostigmine

CLINICAL USE

- Myasthenia gravis
- Antagonist to non-depolarising neuromuscular blockade

DOSE IN NORMAL RENAL FUNCTION

- Myasthenia gravis: Oral: neostigmine bromide 15–30 mg at suitable intervals throughout day – total daily dose 75–300 mg
- Neostigmine metilsulfate, IM, SC, 1–2.5 mg – usual total daily dose 5–20 mg
- Antagonist to non-depolarising neuromuscular blockade: 50–70 mcg/kg over 1 minute; maximum dose 5 mg

PHARMACOKINETICS

Molecular weight (daltons)	223.3 (303.2 as bromide); (334.4 as metilsulphate)
% Protein binding	15–25
% Excreted unchanged in urine	50
Volume of distribution (L/kg)	0.5–1
Half-life – normal/ ESRF (hrs)	0.8–1.5/3

METABOLISM

Poorly absorbed orally. Neostigmine undergoes hydrolysis by cholinesterases and is also metabolised in the liver. Neostigmine is rapidly eliminated and is excreted in the urine both as unchanged drug and metabolites.

DOSE IN RENAL IMPAIRMENT GFR (mL/MIN)

20–50	50–100% of normal dose
10–20	50–100% of normal dose
<10	25–100% of normal dose

DOSE IN PATIENTS UNDERGOING RENAL REPLACEMENT THERAPIES

CAPD	Unknown dialysability. Dose as in GFR<10 mL/min.
HD	Unknown dialysability. Dose as in GFR<10 mL/min.
HDF/High flux	Unknown dialysability. Dose as in GFR<10 mL/min.
CAV/ VVHD	Unknown dialysability. Dose as in GFR=10–20 mL/min.

IMPORTANT DRUG INTERACTIONS

Potentially hazardous interactions with other drugs
- Aminoglycosides, clindamycin and polymyxins antagonise effects of neostigmine.

ADMINISTRATION

RECONSTITUTION
–
ROUTE
- Neostigmine bromide: Oral
- Neostigmine metilsulfate: SC, IM, IV
RATE OF ADMINISTRATION
- IV: Very slowly
COMMENTS
–

OTHER INFORMATION

- Neostigmine 0.5 mg IV = 1–1.5 mg IM/SC =15 mg orally.
- When used for reversal of non-depolarising neuromuscular blockade, atropine (0.6–1.2 mg IV) or glycopyrronium should be given before or with neostigmine in order to prevent bradycardia, excessive salivation and other muscarinic actions of neostigmine.
- The physicochemical nature of neostigmine may tend to encourage its removal by various renal replacement therapies.
- No dose reduction is advised in SPC but a dose reduction is suggested in *Drug Prescribing in Renal Failure*, 5th edition, by Aronoff *et al.*

Nevirapine

CLINICAL USE

Non-nucleoside reverse transcriptase inhibitor:
- Treatment of progressive or advanced HIV infection in combination with at least two other antivirals

DOSE IN NORMAL RENAL FUNCTION

- 200 mg daily, increasing to twice daily after 14 days if tolerated
- MR: 400 mg once daily

PHARMACOKINETICS

Molecular weight (daltons)	266.3
% Protein binding	60
% Excreted unchanged in urine	<3
Volume of distribution (L/kg)	1.12–1.3
Half-life – normal/ ESRF (hrs)	45 (single dose) 25–30 (multiple dosing)/ Unchanged

METABOLISM

Nevirapine is extensively metabolised by hepatic microsomal enzymes, mainly by the cytochrome P450 isoenzymes CYP3A4 and CYP2B6, to several inactive hydroxylated metabolites. Auto-induction of these enzymes results in a 1.5- to 2-fold increase in apparent oral clearance after 2 to 4 weeks at usual dosage, and a decrease in terminal half-life from 45 hours to 25 to 30 hours over the same period. Nevirapine is mainly excreted in the urine as glucuronide conjugates of the hydroxylated metabolites.

DOSE IN RENAL IMPAIRMENT GFR (mL/MIN)

20–50	Dose as in normal renal function.
10–20	Dose as in normal renal function.
<10	Dose as in normal renal function. See 'Other information'.

DOSE IN PATIENTS UNDERGOING RENAL REPLACEMENT THERAPIES

CAPD	Dialysed. Dose as in GFR<10 mL/min.
HD	Dialysed. Dose as in GFR<10 mL/min.
HDF/High flux	Dialysed. Dose as in GFR<10 mL/min.
CAV/VVHD	Unknown dialysability. Dose as in normal renal function.

IMPORTANT DRUG INTERACTIONS

Potentially hazardous interactions with other drugs
- Antibacterials: reduces concentration of clarithromycin, but concentration of active metabolite increased, also concentration of nevirapine increased; concentration decreased by rifampicin – avoid concomitant use; possibly increased rifabutin concentration.
- Anticoagulants: may increase or reduce effect of warfarin.
- Antidepressants: concentration reduced by St John's wort – avoid concomitant use.
- Antifungals: concentration of ketoconazole reduced – avoid concomitant use; concentration increased by fluconazole; possibly reduced caspofungin and itraconazole concentration – may need to increase caspofungin and itraconazole dose.
- Antipsychotics: possibly reduced aripiprazole concentration – increase aripiprazole dose.
- Antivirals: concentration of indinavir and efavirenz reduced and possibly etravirine, fosamprenavir, lopinavir and atazanavir – avoid concomitant use with atazanavir and etravirine, consider increasing lopinavir dose.
- Oestrogens and progestogens: accelerated metabolism (reduced contraceptive effect).

ADMINISTRATION

RECONSTITUTION
–
ROUTE
- Oral
RATE OF ADMINISTRATION
–
COMMENTS
–

OTHER INFORMATION

- Little data available on the use of nevirapine in renal failure, but need for dose adjustment is unlikely due to the pharmacokinetics of nevirapine. Use with caution.

- There was a preliminary study of haemodialysis patients which showed that a normal dose was not associated with increased side effects. (Izzedine H, Launay-Vacher V, Aymard G, *et al.* Pharmacokinetic of nevirapine in haemodialysis. *Nephrol Dial Transplant.* 2001; **16**: 192–3.)

Nicardipine hydrochloride

CLINICAL USE

Calcium-channel blocker:
- Prophylaxis and treatment of angina
- Mild to moderate hypertension

DOSE IN NORMAL RENAL FUNCTION

20–40 mg 3 times daily
SR: 30–60 mg twice daily

PHARMACOKINETICS

Molecular weight (daltons)	516
% Protein binding	>99
% Excreted unchanged in urine	<1
Volume of distribution (L/kg)	0.8
Half-life – normal/ ESRF (hrs)	8.6/Unchanged

METABOLISM

Nicardipine is subject to saturable first-pass metabolism. It is extensively metabolised in the liver and excreted in the urine and faeces, mainly as inactive metabolites.

DOSE IN RENAL IMPAIRMENT GFR (mL/MIN)

20–50	Dose as in normal renal function.
10–20	Dose as in normal renal function. Start with small doses.
<10	Dose as in normal renal function. Start with small doses.

DOSE IN PATIENTS UNDERGOING RENAL REPLACEMENT THERAPIES

CAPD	Unlikely to be dialysed. Dose as in GFR<10 mL/min.
HD	Not dialysed. Dose as in GFR<10 mL/min.
HDF/High flux	Unknown dialysability. Dose as in GFR<10 mL/min.
CAV/ VVHD	Unknown dialysability. Dose as in GFR=10–20 mL/min.

IMPORTANT DRUG INTERACTIONS

Potentially hazardous interactions with other drugs
- Anaesthetics: enhanced hypotensive effect.
- Antibacterials: metabolism possibly accelerated by rifampicin; metabolism possibly inhibited by clarithromycin, erythromycin & telithromycin.
- Antidepressants: enhanced hypotensive effect with MAOIs.
- Anti-epileptics: effect reduced by carbamazepine, barbiturates, phenytoin and primidone.
- Antifungals: metabolism possibly inhibited by itraconazole and ketoconazole; negative inotropic effect possibly increased with itraconazole.
- Antihypertensives: enhanced hypotensive effect, increased risk of first dose hypotensive effect of post-synaptic alpha-blockers.
- Antivirals: concentration possibly increased by ritonavir; use telaprevir with caution.
- Cardiac glycosides: digoxin concentration increased.
- Ciclosporin: concentration of ciclosporin increased.
- Grapefruit juice: concentration increased – avoid concomitant use.
- Tacrolimus: may increase tacrolimus levels.
- Theophylline: possibly increased theophylline concentration.

ADMINISTRATION

RECONSTITUTION
–
ROUTE
- Oral
RATE OF ADMINISTRATION
–
COMMENTS
- Administration of nicardipine with food appears to reduce the bioavailability and delay the achievement of peak plasma concentrations.

OTHER INFORMATION

- Nicardipine blood levels may be elevated in some renally impaired patients. Therefore, start with a low dose and titrate to BP and response. The dose interval may also need to be extended to 12 hourly.

Nicorandil

CLINICAL USE

Prevention and treatment of chronic stable angina

DOSE IN NORMAL RENAL FUNCTION

5–30 mg twice daily

PHARMACOKINETICS

Molecular weight (daltons)	211.2
% Protein binding	Slightly
% Excreted unchanged in urine	1
Volume of distribution (L/kg)	No data
Half-life – normal/ ESRF (hrs)	1/Unchanged

METABOLISM

Metabolism of nicorandil is mainly by denitration of the molecule into the nicotinamide pathway.

About 20% of a dose is excreted in the urine, mainly as metabolites.

DOSE IN RENAL IMPAIRMENT GFR (mL/MIN)

20–50	Dose as in normal renal function.
10–20	Dose as in normal renal function.
<10	Dose as in normal renal function.

DOSE IN PATIENTS UNDERGOING RENAL REPLACEMENT THERAPIES

CAPD	Unknown dialysability. Dose as in normal renal function.
HD	Unknown dialysability. Dose as in normal renal function.
HDF/High flux	Unknown dialysability. Dose as in normal renal function.
CAV/ VVHD	Unknown dialysability. Dose as in normal renal function.

IMPORTANT DRUG INTERACTIONS

Potentially hazardous interactions with other drugs
- Sildenafil, tadalafil and vardenafil: enhanced hypotensive effect, avoid concomitant use.

ADMINISTRATION

RECONSTITUTION
–
ROUTE
- Oral
RATE OF ADMINISTRATION
–
COMMENTS
–

Nicotinic acid (unlicensed)

CLINICAL USE

Hyperlipidaemia

DOSE IN NORMAL RENAL FUNCTION

375 mg – 2 g daily at night
(only available from specials manufacturer)

PHARMACOKINETICS

Molecular weight (daltons)	123.1
% Protein binding	High
% Excreted unchanged in urine	12
Volume of distribution (L/kg)	Very high
Half-life – normal/ ESRF (hrs)	1–5/–

METABOLISM

The main route of metabolism is its conversion to N-methylnicotinamide and the 2-pyridone and 4-pyridone derivatives; nicotinuric acid is also formed. Small amounts of nicotinic acid are excreted unchanged in urine.

DOSE IN RENAL IMPAIRMENT GFR (mL/MIN)

30–50	50% of dose and increase according to response.
15–30	50% of dose and increase according to response.
<15	25% of dose and increase according to response.

DOSE IN PATIENTS UNDERGOING RENAL REPLACEMENT THERAPIES

CAPD	Dialysed. Dose as in GFR<15 mL/min.
HD	Dialysed. Dose as in GFR<15 mL/min.
HDF/High flux	Dialysed. Dose as in GFR<15 mL/min.
CAV/VVHD	Dialysed. Dose as in GFR=15–30 mL/min.

IMPORTANT DRUG INTERACTIONS

Potentially hazardous interactions with other drugs
- Lipid-regulating drugs: increased risk of myopathy when used in combination with statins.
- Aspirin: increased flushing.

ADMINISTRATION

RECONSTITUTION
–

ROUTE
- Oral

RATE OF ADMINISTRATION
–

COMMENTS
–

OTHER INFORMATION

- Doses from National Kidney Foundation Inc. *American Journal of Kidney Disease.* 2003; **41**(4) Suppl. 3: S1–S91 K/DOQI guidelines.
- Use with caution in renal failure due to increased risk of rhabdomyolysis.
- Toxic reactions are frequent in CKD 5.
- Nicotinic acid and its metabolites are renally excreted and the metabolites account for some of the side effects of nicotinic acid.
- One study showed that once daily nicotinic acid used in patients with a GFR<60 mL/min (average 61 mL/min) was safe and effective. (McGovern ME, Stanek E, Malott C, et al. Once-daily niacin extended-release is effective and safe for treatment of dyslipidaemia associated with chronic kidney disease. *J Am Coll Cardiol.* 2004; **43**(5) Suppl. 2: A487: 820–6.)

Nifedipine

CLINICAL USE

Calcium-channel blocker:
- Prophylaxis and treatment of angina
- Hypertension
- Raynaud's phenomenon

DOSE IN NORMAL RENAL FUNCTION

Capsules: 5–20 mg 3 times daily
Tablets: 20–40 mg twice daily
MR: 20–90 mg daily

PHARMACOKINETICS

Molecular weight (daltons)	346.3
% Protein binding	92–98
% Excreted unchanged in urine	<1
Volume of distribution (L/kg)	1.4
Half-life – normal/ ESRF (hrs)	1.4–11 (depends on preparation)/ Unchanged

METABOLISM

Nifedipine is metabolised in the gut wall and oxidised in the liver via the cytochrome P450 isoenzyme CYP3A4, to inactive metabolites.
  Excreted mainly as metabolites via the kidney.

DOSE IN RENAL IMPAIRMENT GFR (mL/MIN)

20–50	Dose as in normal renal function.
10–20	Dose as in normal renal function. Start with small doses.
<10	Dose as in normal renal function. Start with small doses.

DOSE IN PATIENTS UNDERGOING RENAL REPLACEMENT THERAPIES

CAPD	Not dialysed. Dose as in GFR<10 mL/min.
HD	Not dialysed. Dose as in GFR<10 mL/min.
HDF/High flux	Unknown dialysability. Dose as in GFR<10 mL/min.
CAV/ VVHD	Unknown dialysability. Dose as in GFR=10–20 mL/min.

IMPORTANT DRUG INTERACTIONS

Potentially hazardous interactions with other drugs
- Anaesthetics: enhanced hypotensive effect.
- Anti-arrhythmics: concentration of dronedarone increased.
- Antibacterials: metabolism accelerated by rifampicin; metabolism possibly inhibited by clarithromycin, erythromycin & telithromycin.
- Antidepressants: metabolism possibly inhibited by fluoxetine; concentration reduced by St John's wort; enhanced hypotensive effect with MAOIs.
- Anti-epileptics: effect reduced by carbamazepine, barbiturates, phenytoin and primidone.
- Antifungals: metabolism possibly inhibited by itraconazole and ketoconazole; concentration increased by micafungin; negative inotropic effect possibly increased with itraconazole.
- Antihypertensives: enhanced hypotensive effect, increased risk of first dose hypotensive effect of post-synaptic alpha-blockers; occasionally severe hypotension and heart failure with beta-blockers.
- Antivirals: concentration possibly increased by ritonavir; use telaprevir with caution.
- Cardiac glycosides: digoxin concentration possibly increased.
- Ciclosporin: may increase ciclosporin level, but not a problem in practice; nifedipine concentration may be increased.
- Cytotoxics: metabolism of vincristine possibly reduced.
- Grapefruit juice: concentration increased – avoid concomitant use.
- Magnesium salts: profound hypotension with IV magnesium.
- Tacrolimus: increased tacrolimus levels.
- Theophylline: possibly increased theophylline concentration.

ADMINISTRATION

RECONSTITUTION
–
ROUTE
- Oral
RATE OF ADMINISTRATION
–
COMMENTS
–

OTHER INFORMATION

- Protein binding decreased in severe renal impairment.
- Acute renal dysfunction reported.
- Increased incidence of side effects (headache, flushing, dizziness and peripheral oedema) in patients with ERF.
- For acute use, bite capsule then swallow contents with 10–50 mL water.

Nilotinib

CLINICAL USE

Tyrosine kinase inhibitors
● Treatment of chronic myelogenous leukaemia (CML)

DOSE IN NORMAL RENAL FUNCTION

● Newly diagnosed CML: 300 mg twice daily
● Chronic & accelerated phase CML: 400 mg twice daily
● Consult relevant local protocol

PHARMACOKINETICS

Molecular weight (daltons)	529.5 (584 as hydrochloride)
% Protein binding	98
% Excreted unchanged in urine	0
Volume of distribution (L/kg)	0.55–3.9[1]
Half-life – normal/ ESRF (hrs)	17/Unchanged

METABOLISM

Nilotinib is metabolised in the liver via oxidation and hydroxylation, in which cytochrome P450 isoenzyme CYP3A4 plays an important role. Most of an oral dose is eliminated unchanged in the faeces within 7 days.

DOSE IN RENAL IMPAIRMENT GFR (mL/MIN)

30–50	Dose as in normal renal function.
10–30	Dose as in normal renal function.
<10	Dose as in normal renal function.

DOSE IN PATIENTS UNDERGOING RENAL REPLACEMENT THERAPIES

CAPD	Not dialysed. Dose as in normal renal function.
HD	Not dialysed. Dose as in normal renal function.
HDF/High flux	Not dialysed. Dose as in normal renal function.
CAV/ VVHD	Not dialysed. Dose as in normal renal function.

IMPORTANT DRUG INTERACTIONS

Potentially hazardous interactions with other drugs
● Antibacterials: avoid concomitant use with clarithromycin, rifampicin (concentration reduced) & telithromycin.
● Antifungals: avoid concomitant use with itraconazole, ketoconazole (concentration increased) & voriconazole.
● Antipsychotics: avoid concomitant use with clozapine (increased risk of agranulocytosis).
● Antivirals: avoid concomitant use with ritonavir (concentration possibly increased) & boceprevir.
● Grapefruit juice: avoid concomitant administration.
● Avoid concomitant use with other inhibitors or inducers of CYP3A4. Dose alterations may be required.

ADMINISTRATION

RECONSTITUTION
–
ROUTE
● Oral
RATE OF ADMINISTRATION
–

OTHER INFORMATION

● Bioavailability is 30%.
● Clinical studies have not been performed in patients with impaired renal function but since nilotinib and its metabolites are not renally excreted, a decrease in total body clearance is not anticipated in patients with renal impairment.
● Prolongs QT interval.

Reference:
1. Binfeng Xia, Tycho Heimbach, Handan He, Tsu-han Lin. Nilotinib preclinical pharmacokinetics and practical application toward clinical projections of oral absorption and systemic availability. *Biopharm Drug Dispos.* 2012; **33**(9): 536–49.

Nimodipine

CLINICAL USE

Calcium-channel blocker:
- Prevention and treatment of ischaemic neurological deficits following subarachnoid haemorrhage

DOSE IN NORMAL RENAL FUNCTION

- Prevention: 60 mg orally every 4 hours
- Treatment via central catheter: 1 mg/hour initially, increased after 2 hours to 2 mg/hour. If BP unstable, weight <70 kg, start with 0.5 mg/hour or less if necessary.

PHARMACOKINETICS

Molecular weight (daltons)	418.4
% Protein binding	98
% Excreted unchanged in urine	<1
Volume of distribution (L/kg)	0.9–1.6
Half-life – normal/ESRF (hrs)	1.1–1.7/22

METABOLISM

Nimodipine is extensively metabolised in the liver via the cytochrome P450 isoenzyme CYP3A4. It is eliminated as metabolites, mainly by dehydrogenation of the dihydropyridine ring and oxidative O-demethylation. Oxidative ester cleavage, hydroxylation of the 2- and 6-methyl groups, and glucuronidation as a conjugation reaction are other important metabolic steps. The three primary metabolites occurring in plasma show no or only therapeutically negligible residual activity. The metabolites are excreted about 50% renally and 30% in faeces via the bile.

DOSE IN RENAL IMPAIRMENT GFR (mL/MIN)

20–50	Dose as in normal renal function.
10–20	Dose as in normal renal function.
<10	Dose as in normal renal function.

DOSE IN PATIENTS UNDERGOING RENAL REPLACEMENT THERAPIES

CAPD	Not dialysed. Dose as in normal renal function.
HD	Not dialysed. Dose as in normal renal function.
HDF/High flux	Unknown dialysability. Dose as in normal renal function.
CAV/ VVHD	Unknown dialysability. Dose as in normal renal function.

IMPORTANT DRUG INTERACTIONS

Potentially hazardous interactions with other drugs
- Anaesthetics: enhanced hypotensive effect.
- Antibacterials: metabolism accelerated by rifampicin; metabolism possibly inhibited by clarithromycin, erythromycin & telithromycin.
- Antidepressants: enhanced hypotensive effect with MAOIs.
- Anti-epileptics: effect reduced by carbamazepine, barbiturates, phenytoin and primidone.
- Antifungals: metabolism possibly inhibited by itraconazole and ketoconazole; negative inotropic effect possibly increased with itraconazole.
- Antihypertensives: enhanced hypotensive effect, increased risk of first dose hypotensive effect of post-synaptic alpha-blockers.
- Antivirals: concentration possibly increased by ritonavir; use telaprevir with caution.
- Grapefruit juice: concentration increased – avoid concomitant use.
- Theophylline: possibly increased theophylline concentration.

ADMINISTRATION

RECONSTITUTION
–

ROUTE
- Oral, IV

RATE OF ADMINISTRATION
- IV – First 2 hours: 1 mg (5 mL) nimodipine per hour.
- After 2 hours: Infuse 2 mg (10 mL) nimodipine per hour.

COMMENTS
- Nimodipine solution must not be added to an infusion bag or bottle and must not be mixed with other drugs.
- Nimodipine solution should be administered only via a bypass into a running drip (40 mL/hour) of either sodium chloride 0.9% or glucose 5%.
- In the event of nimodipine tablets and solution being administered sequentially, the total duration of treatment should not exceed 21 days.

OTHER INFORMATION

- Nimodipine solution reacts with PVC. Polyethylene tubes are supplied.
- Patients with known renal disease and/or receiving nephrotoxic drugs should have renal function monitored closely during IV treatment.

Nitrazepam

CLINICAL USE

Benzodiazepine:
- Hypnotic

DOSE IN NORMAL RENAL FUNCTION

5–10 mg at bedtime; elderly (or debilitated)
2.5–5 mg

PHARMACOKINETICS

Molecular weight (daltons)	281.3
% Protein binding	87
% Excreted unchanged in urine	<5
Volume of distribution (L/kg)	2
Half-life – normal/ ESRF (hrs)	24–30/Unchanged

METABOLISM

Metabolised in the liver, mainly by
nitroreduction followed by acetylation; none
of the metabolites possess significant activity.
   Excreted in the urine mainly as
metabolites.

DOSE IN RENAL IMPAIRMENT GFR (mL/MIN)

20–50	Dose as in normal renal function.
10–20	Dose as in normal renal function.
<10	Dose as in normal renal function. Start with small doses.

DOSE IN PATIENTS UNDERGOING RENAL REPLACEMENT THERAPIES

CAPD	Unlikely to be dialysed. Dose as in GFR<10 mL/min.
HD	Unlikely to be dialysed. Dose as in GFR<10 mL/min.
HDF/High flux	Unknown dialysability. Dose as in GFR<10 mL/min.
CAV/ VVHD	Unlikely to be dialysed. Dose as in normal renal function.

IMPORTANT DRUG INTERACTIONS

Potentially hazardous interactions with other
drugs
- Antibacterials: metabolism possibly increased by rifampicin.
- Antipsychotics: increased sedative effects; risk of serious adverse effects in combination with clozapine.
- Antivirals: concentration possibly increased by ritonavir.
- Disulfiram: metabolism of nitrazepam inhibited, increased sedative effects.
- Sodium oxybate: enhanced effects of sodium oxybate – avoid.

ADMINISTRATION

RECONSTITUTION
–
ROUTE
- Oral
RATE OF ADMINISTRATION
–
COMMENTS
–

OTHER INFORMATION

- Mild to moderate renal insufficiency does not alter the kinetics of nitrazepam.
- CKD 5 patients will be more susceptible to adverse effects (drowsiness, sedation, unsteadiness).

Nitrofurantoin

CLINICAL USE

Antibacterial agent

DOSE IN NORMAL RENAL FUNCTION

- Treatment: 50–100 mg every 6 hours
- Prophylaxis: 50–100 mg at night

PHARMACOKINETICS

Molecular weight (daltons)	238.2
% Protein binding	60–90
% Excreted unchanged in urine	30–40
Volume of distribution (L/kg)	0.3–0.7
Half-life – normal/ ESRF (hrs)	0.3–1/1

METABOLISM

Nitrofurantoin is metabolised in the liver and most body tissues, while about 30–40% of a dose is excreted rapidly in the urine as unchanged nitrofurantoin. Some tubular reabsorption may occur in acid urine.

DOSE IN RENAL IMPAIRMENT GFR (mL/MIN)

40–60	Dose as in normal renal function. Use with caution. See 'Other information'.
<40	Contraindicated. See 'Other information'.

DOSE IN PATIENTS UNDERGOING RENAL REPLACEMENT THERAPIES

CAPD	Dialysed. Avoid – contraindicated.
HD	Dialysed. Avoid – contraindicated.
HDF/High flux	Dialysed. Avoid – contraindicated.
CAV/ VVHD	Dialysed. Avoid – contraindicated.

IMPORTANT DRUG INTERACTIONS

Potentially hazardous interactions with other drugs
- None known

ADMINISTRATION

RECONSTITUTION

–

ROUTE

- Oral

RATE OF ADMINISTRATION

–

COMMENTS

- Urine may be coloured a dark yellow or brown.
- Macrocrystalline form has slower dissolution and absorption rates, produces lower serum concentration and takes longer to achieve peak concentration in the urine.

OTHER INFORMATION

- Anecdotally, nitrofurantoin may be used at GFR=40–60 mL/min but with increased risk of treatment failure and side effects.
- Toxic plasma concentrations can occur in moderate to severe renal impairment causing adverse effects, e.g. neuropathy, blood dyscrasias.
- Advice from MHRA advises to avoid nitrofurantoin if GFR<60 mL/min due to risk of treatment failure as the drug is ineffective due to inadequate urine concentration. (MHRA. *Drug Safety Update.* Nitrofurantoin: reminder on precautions for use, especially renal impairment in (elderly) patients. August 2013; 7(1).)
- An expert group from the MHRA has reconsidered nitrofurantoin. Their advice is for an amendment to the contraindication against use from CRCL <60 mL/min to eGFR <45 mL/min, with additional advice that nitrofurantoin may be used with caution in individual cases as short-course therapy only for the treatment of lower UTI with an eGFR between 30–44 mL/min to treat resistant pathogens, when the benefits may outweigh the risks of undesirable effects.
- Nitrofurantoin gives false positive urinary glucose (if testing for reducing substances).

Nizatidine

CLINICAL USE

H_2-receptor antagonist

DOSE IN NORMAL RENAL FUNCTION

Oral: 150–600 mg daily

PHARMACOKINETICS

Molecular weight (daltons)	331.5
% Protein binding	35
% Excreted unchanged in urine	60
Volume of distribution (L/kg)	0.8–1.3
Half-life – normal/ ESRF (hrs)	1–2/3.5–11

METABOLISM

A small amount of nizatidine is metabolised in the liver: nizatidine N-2-oxide, nizatidine S-oxide, and N-2-monodesmethylnizatidine have been identified, the latter having about 60% of the activity of nizatidine. More than 90% of a dose of nizatidine is excreted in the urine, in part by active tubular secretion, within 12 hours, about 60% as unchanged drug. Less than 6% is excreted in the faeces.

DOSE IN RENAL IMPAIRMENT GFR (mL/MIN)

20–50	150 mg every 12–48 hours
<20	150 mg every 24–72 hours.

DOSE IN PATIENTS UNDERGOING RENAL REPLACEMENT THERAPIES

CAPD	Not dialysed. Dose as in GFR<20 mL/min.
HD	Not dialysed. Dose as in GFR<20 mL/min.
HDF/High flux	Unknown dialysability. Dose as in GFR<20 mL/min.
CAV/ VVHD	Unknown dialysability. Dose as in GFR<20 mL/min.

IMPORTANT DRUG INTERACTIONS

Potentially hazardous interactions with other drugs

- Antifungals: absorption of itraconazole and ketoconazole reduced.
- Antivirals: concentration of atazanavir reduced; concentration of raltegravir possibly increased – avoid; avoid for 12 hours before and 4 hours after rilpivirine.
- Cytotoxics: avoid with erlotinib; possibly reduced absorption of pazopanib – give at least 2 hours before or 10 hours after nizatidine; possibly reduced absorption of lapatinib.
- Ulipristal: contraceptive effect possibly reduced – avoid with high dose ulipristal.

ADMINISTRATION

RECONSTITUTION

–

ROUTE

- Oral

RATE OF ADMINISTRATION

–

OTHER INFORMATION

- Frequency in renal failure depends on indication.
- The effect of haemodialysis is unproven. It is not expected to be efficient since nizatidine has a large volume of distribution.
- Oral bioavailability >70%.

Noradrenaline acid tartrate (norepinephrine bitartrate)

CLINICAL USE

- Hypotension
- Cardiac arrest (sympathomimetic)

DOSE IN NORMAL RENAL FUNCTION

(Doses expressed as noradrenaline base)
- Acute hypotension: 40 mcg/mL solution, initially 0.16–0.33 mL/minute; adjust according to response
- Cardiac arrest: 200 mcg/mL solution, 0.5–0.75 mL

PHARMACOKINETICS

Molecular weight (daltons)	337.3
% Protein binding	~50
% Excreted unchanged in urine	~16
Volume of distribution (L/kg)	0.09–0.4
Half-life – normal/ESRF (hrs)	1 minute/Unchanged

METABOLISM

Extensively metabolised by catechol-*O*-methyltransferase (COMT), and monoamine oxidase (MAO). Up to 16% of an intravenous dose is excreted unchanged in the urine with methylated and deaminated metabolites in free and conjugated forms.

DOSE IN RENAL IMPAIRMENT GFR (mL/MIN)

20–50	Dose as in normal renal function.
10–20	Dose as in normal renal function.
<10	Dose as in normal renal function.

DOSE IN PATIENTS UNDERGOING RENAL REPLACEMENT THERAPIES

CAPD	Not dialysed. Dose as in normal renal function.
HD	Not dialysed. Dose as in normal renal function.
HDF/High flux	Unknown dialysability. Dose as in normal renal function.
CAV/VVHD	Not dialysed. Dose as in normal renal function.

IMPORTANT DRUG INTERACTIONS

Potentially hazardous interactions with other drugs
- Adrenergic neurone blockers: antagonise hypotensive effect.
- Antidepressants: tricyclics may cause hypertension and arrhythmias; MAOIs and moclobemide may cause hypertensive crisis.
- Beta-blockers: can cause severe hypertension.
- Clonidine: possibly increased risk of hypertension.
- Dopaminergics: effects possibly increased by entacapone; avoid concomitant use with rasagiline.
- Sympathomimetics: effects possibly enhanced by dopexamine.

ADMINISTRATION

RECONSTITUTION
–
ROUTE
- IV
RATE OF ADMINISTRATION
- According to response
COMMENTS
- Preferably give centrally (low pH).
- Dilute 1–4 mg in 100 mL glucose 5%.
- Can be given undiluted.

OTHER INFORMATION

- Do not mix with alkaline drugs/solutions.
- The pharmacokinetics of noradrenaline are not significantly affected by renal or hepatic disease.
- 1 mg of noradrenaline base is equivalent to 2 mg noradrenaline acid tartrate.

Norethisterone

CLINICAL USE

Progestogen:
- Breast cancer, contraception, dysfunctional uterine bleeding, menorrhagia, dysmenorrhoea, endometriosis, premenstrual syndrome, postponement of menstruation

DOSE IN NORMAL RENAL FUNCTION

- Breast cancer: 40–60 mg daily
- Dysfunctional uterine bleeding, menorrhagia: 5 mg three times a day for 10 days to stop bleeding; to prevent bleeding 5 mg twice daily on days 19–26 of cycle
- Dysmenorrhoea: 5 mg three times daily from day 5–24 for 3–4 cycles
- Endometriosis: 10–15 mg daily beginning on day 5 of cycle, may be increased to 20–25 mg daily
- Premenstrual syndrome: 5 mg 2–3 times daily from day 19–26 of several cycles
- Postponement of menstruation: 5 mg three times daily starting 3 days before expected onset
- See product literature for more specific information.

PHARMACOKINETICS

Molecular weight (daltons)	298.4
% Protein binding	60
% Excreted unchanged in urine	50–80 (as metabolites)
Volume of distribution (L/kg)	3.1–5.7
Half-life – normal/ESRF (hrs)	5/–

METABOLISM

It is metabolised in the liver with 50–80% of a dose being excreted in the urine and up to 40% appearing in the faeces.

DOSE IN RENAL IMPAIRMENT GFR (mL/MIN)

20–50	Dose as in normal renal function.
10–20	Dose as in normal renal function.
<10	Dose as in normal renal function. Monitor carefully.

DOSE IN PATIENTS UNDERGOING RENAL REPLACEMENT THERAPIES

CAPD	Not dialysed. Dose as in GFR<10 mL/min.
HD	Unlikely to be dialysed. Dose as in GFR<10 mL/min.
HDF/High flux	Unlikely to be dialysed. Dose as in GFR<10 mL/min.
CAV/VVHD	Unlikely to be dialysed. Dose as in normal renal function.

IMPORTANT DRUG INTERACTIONS

Potentially hazardous interactions with other drugs
- Antibacterials: metabolism of progestogens accelerated by rifamycins (reduced contraceptive effect).
- Anticoagulants: progestogens antagonise anticoagulant effect of phenindione; may enhance or reduce anticoagulant effect of coumarins.
- Antidepressants: contraceptive effect reduced by St John's wort – avoid concomitant use.
- Anti-epileptics: metabolism accelerated by carbamazepine, eslicarbazepine, oxcarbazepine, phenobarbital, phenytoin, rufinamide and topiramate (reduced contraceptive effect); concentration reduced by high dose perampanel.
- Antivirals: contraceptive effect reduced by efavirenz; metabolism accelerated by nevirapine (reduced contraceptive effect); atazanavir increases norethisterone concentration.
- Aprepitant: possible contraceptive failure.
- Bosentan: possible contraceptive failure.
- Ciclosporin: progestogens inhibit metabolism of ciclosporin (increased plasma concentration).
- Cytotoxics: possibly reduced contraceptive effect with crizotinib and vemurafenib.
- Dopaminergics: concentration of selegiline increased – avoid concomitant use.
- Tacrolimus: tacrolimus levels are greatly increased – avoid concomitant use.
- Ulipristal: contraceptive effect of progestogens possibly reduced.

ADMINISTRATION

RECONSTITUTION
–
ROUTE
- Oral
RATE OF ADMINISTRATION
–
COMMENTS
–

OTHER INFORMATION

- Do not use in patients with porphyria.

Norfloxacin

CLINICAL USE

Antibacterial agent

DOSE IN NORMAL RENAL FUNCTION

400 mg twice daily, duration of course depends on indication

PHARMACOKINETICS

Molecular weight (daltons)	319.3
% Protein binding	14
% Excreted unchanged in urine	30
Volume of distribution (L/kg)	2.5–3.1
Half-life – normal/ ESRF (hrs)	3–4/6.5–8

METABOLISM

Some metabolism occurs, possibly in the liver. Norfloxacin is eliminated through metabolism, biliary excretion and renal excretion. Renal excretion occurs by both glomerular filtration and net tubular secretion. In the first 24 hours, 33–48% of the drug is recovered in the urine.

Norfloxacin exists in the urine as norfloxacin and six active metabolites of lesser antimicrobial potency. The parent compound accounts for over 70% of total excretion. About 30% of an oral dose appears in the faeces.

DOSE IN RENAL IMPAIRMENT GFR (mL/MIN)

30–50	Dose as in normal renal function.
10–30	400 mg every 12 to 24 hours.
<10	400 mg daily.

DOSE IN PATIENTS UNDERGOING RENAL REPLACEMENT THERAPIES

CAPD	Not dialysed. Dose as in GFR<10 mL/min.
HD	Not dialysed. Dose as in GFR<10 mL/min.
HDF/High flux	Unknown dialysability. Dose as in GFR<10 mL/min.
CAV/ VVHD	Not dialysed. Dose as in GFR=10–30 mL/min.

IMPORTANT DRUG INTERACTIONS

Potentially hazardous interactions with other drugs

- Analgesics: increased risk of convulsions with NSAIDs.
- Anticoagulants: anticoagulant effect of coumarins enhanced.
- Antimalarials: manufacturer of artemether with lumefantrine advises avoid concomitant use.
- Ciclosporin: increased risk of nephrotoxicity.
- Muscle relaxants: possibly increases tizanidine concentration.
- Theophylline: possibly increased risk of convulsion; increased levels of theophylline.

ADMINISTRATION

RECONSTITUTION

–

ROUTE

- Oral

RATE OF ADMINISTRATION

–

COMMENTS

–

Normal human immunoglobulin

CLINICAL USE

- Replacement therapy in primary and secondary immunodeficiency
- Idiopathic thrombocytopenic purpura
- Guillain–Barré syndrome
- Kawasaki disease
- Allogeneic bone marrow transplantation
- Treatment of infections and prophylaxis of graft versus host disease

DOSE IN NORMAL RENAL FUNCTION

Variable according to preparation and indication. See individual SPC.

PHARMACOKINETICS

Molecular weight (daltons)	150 000
% Protein binding	–
% Excreted unchanged in urine	–
Volume of distribution (L/kg)	–
Half-life – normal/ ESRF (hrs)	24–36 days/–

METABOLISM

IgG and IgG-complexes are broken down in the cells of the reticuloendothelial system.

DOSE IN RENAL IMPAIRMENT GFR (mL/MIN)

20–50	Dose as normal renal function.
10–20	Dose as normal renal function.
<10	Dose as normal renal function. See 'Other information'.

DOSE IN PATIENTS UNDERGOING RENAL REPLACEMENT THERAPIES

CAPD	Not dialysed. Dose as in normal renal function.
HD	Not dialysed. Dose as in normal renal function.
HDF/High flux	Probably not dialysed. Dose as in normal renal function.
CAV/ VVHD	Probably not dialysed. Dose as in normal renal function.

IMPORTANT DRUG INTERACTIONS

Potentially hazardous interactions with other drugs

- Immunoglobulin administration may impair (for a period of at least 6 weeks and up to 3 months) the efficacy of live attenuated virus vaccines such as measles, rubella, mumps and varicella.

ADMINISTRATION

RECONSTITUTION
–
ROUTE
- IV
RATE OF ADMINISTRATION
- Variable – see individual SPC.

OTHER INFORMATION

- Cases of acute kidney injury have been reported in patients receiving IVIg therapy. In most cases, risk factors have been identified, such as pre-existing renal insufficiency, diabetes mellitus, hypovolaemia, overweight, concomitant nephrotoxic medicinal products or, aged over 65. In all patients, IVIg administration requires:
  — adequate hydration prior to the initiation of the infusion of IVIg;
  — monitoring of urine output;
  — monitoring of serum creatinine levels;
  — avoidance of concomitant use of loop diuretics.
- In case of renal impairment, IVIg discontinuation should be considered. While reports of renal dysfunction and acute kidney injury have been associated with the use of many of the licensed IVIg products, those containing sucrose (compared to glycine, maltose or sorbitol) as a stabiliser accounted for a disproportionate share of the total number. In patients at risk, the use of IVIg products that do not contain sucrose may be considered. In addition, the product should be administered at the minimum concentration and infusion rate practicable.
- Overdose may lead to fluid overload and hyperviscosity, particularly in patients at risk, including elderly patients or patients with renal impairment.

- The MHRA has issued a Medical Device Alert relating to the following point of care and home-use blood glucose meters: Roche Accu-Chek and Glucotrend, Abbott Diabetes Care FreeStyle
  - There is a risk of overestimation of blood glucose results when these meters are used for samples from patients on treatments that contain (or are metabolised to) maltose, xylose or galactose. The MHRA advises that the affected meters should not be used to measure blood glucose in patients receiving such treatments. Treatments that are known to contain (or that are metabolised to) maltose, xylose or galactose include (Extraneal®) icodextrin (used in peritoneal dialysis, PD), and certain immunoglobulin preparations (including Octagam®).

Nortriptyline

CLINICAL USE

Tricyclic antidepressant

DOSE IN NORMAL RENAL FUNCTION

10–150 mg daily in single or divided doses

PHARMACOKINETICS

Molecular weight (daltons)	263.4 (299.8 as hydrochloride)
% Protein binding	95
% Excreted unchanged in urine	<5
Volume of distribution (L/kg)	15–23
Half-life – normal/ ESRF (hrs)	25–38/15–66

METABOLISM

Nortriptyline is the main active metabolite of amitriptyline. It has been reported to have a longer plasma half-life than amitriptyline.

Nortriptyline is subject to extensive first-pass metabolism in the liver to 10-hydroxynortriptyline, which is active.

DOSE IN RENAL IMPAIRMENT GFR (mL/MIN)

20–50	Dose as in normal renal function.
10–20	Dose as in normal renal function.
<10	Dose as in normal renal function. Start with small dose.

DOSE IN PATIENTS UNDERGOING RENAL REPLACEMENT THERAPIES

CAPD	Not dialysed. Dose as in GFR<10 mL/min.
HD	Not dialysed. Dose as in GFR<10 mL/min.
HDF/High flux	Unknown dialysability. Dose as in GFR<10 mL/min.
CAV/ VVHD	Not dialysed. Dose as in normal renal function.

IMPORTANT DRUG INTERACTIONS

Potentially hazardous interactions with other drugs

- Alcohol: increased sedative effect.
- Analgesics: increased risk of CNS toxicity with tramadol; possibly increased risk of side effects with nefopam; possibly increased sedative effects with opioids.
- Anti-arrhythmics: increased risk of ventricular arrhythmias with amiodarone – avoid concomitant use; increased risk of ventricular arrhythmias with disopyramide, flecainide or propafenone; avoid with dronedarone.
- Antibacterials: increased risk of ventricular arrhythmias with moxifloxacin and possibly telithromycin – avoid concomitant use with moxifloxacin.
- Anticoagulants: may alter anticoagulant effect of coumarins.
- Antidepressants: enhanced CNS excitation and hypertension with MAOIs and moclobemide – avoid concomitant use; concentration possibly increased with SSRIs.
- Anti-epileptics: convulsive threshold lowered; concentration reduced by carbamazepine, phenobarbital and possibly phenytoin.
- Antimalarials: avoid concomitant use with artemether/lumefantrine and piperaquine with artenimol.
- Antipsychotics: increased risk of ventricular arrhythmias especially with droperidol and pimozide – avoid; increased antimuscarinic effects with clozapine and phenothiazines; concentration increased by antipsychotics.
- Antivirals: increased risk of ventricular arrhythmias with saquinavir – avoid; concentration possibly increased with ritonavir.
- Atomoxetine: increased risk of ventricular arrhythmias and possibly convulsions.
- Beta-blockers: increased risk of ventricular arrhythmias with sotalol.
- Clonidine: tricyclics antagonise hypotensive effect; increased risk of hypertension on clonidine withdrawal.
- Dopaminergics: avoid use with entacapone; CNS toxicity reported with selegiline and rasagiline.
- Pentamidine: increased risk of ventricular arrhythmias.
- Sympathomimetics: increased risk of hypertension and arrhythmias with adrenaline and noradrenaline; metabolism possibly inhibited by methylphenidate.

ADMINISTRATION

RECONSTITUTION
–
ROUTE
• Oral
RATE OF ADMINISTRATION
–
COMMENTS
–

OTHER INFORMATION

• All metabolites are highly lipophilic.

Nystatin

CLINICAL USE

Antifungal agent

DOSE IN NORMAL RENAL FUNCTION

- Oral: 100 000–1 000 000 units (1–10 mL) every 6 hours
- Topical: Apply 2–4 times daily (depends on formulation)

PHARMACOKINETICS

Molecular weight (daltons)	926.1
% Protein binding	No data
% Excreted unchanged in urine	No data
Volume of distribution (L/kg)	No data
Half-life – normal/ ESRF (hrs)	No data

METABOLISM

No significant gastrointestinal absorption.

DOSE IN RENAL IMPAIRMENT GFR (mL/MIN)

20–50	Dose as in normal renal function.
10–20	Dose as in normal renal function.
<10	Dose as in normal renal function.

DOSE IN PATIENTS UNDERGOING RENAL REPLACEMENT THERAPIES

CAPD	Not dialysed. Dose as in normal renal function.
HD	Not dialysed. Dose as in normal renal function.
HDF/High flux	Not dialysed. Dose as in normal renal function.
CAV/ VVHD	Not dialysed. Dose as in normal renal function.

IMPORTANT DRUG INTERACTIONS

Potentially hazardous interactions with other drugs
- None known

ADMINISTRATION

RECONSTITUTION
–
ROUTE
- Oral, topical
RATE OF ADMINISTRATION
–
COMMENTS
–

OTHER INFORMATION

- Not absorbed from intact skin or mucous membranes.

Octreotide

CLINICAL USE

Relief of symptoms of gastro-
enteropancreatic endocrine tumours and
acromegaly

DOSE IN NORMAL RENAL FUNCTION

- 50 micrograms – 1.5 mg daily
- Long-acting preparation: 10–30 mg every
  4 weeks

PHARMACOKINETICS

Molecular weight (daltons)	1019.2 (as acetate)
% Protein binding	65
% Excreted unchanged in urine	32
Volume of distribution (L/kg)	0.27
Half-life – normal/ ESRF (hrs)	1.5/Increased

METABOLISM

Extensive hepatic metabolism.[1] About 32% of
a dose is excreted unchanged in the urine.

DOSE IN RENAL IMPAIRMENT GFR (mL/MIN)

20–50	Dose as in normal renal function.
10–20	Dose as in normal renal function.
<10	Dose as in normal renal function.

DOSE IN PATIENTS UNDERGOING RENAL REPLACEMENT THERAPIES

CAPD	Unknown dialysability. Dose as in normal renal function.
HD	Dialysed. Dose as in normal renal function.
HDF/High flux	Dialysed. Dose as in normal renal function.
CAV/ VVHD	Dialysed. Dose as in normal renal function.

IMPORTANT DRUG INTERACTIONS

Potentially hazardous interactions with other
drugs

- Ciclosporin: ciclosporin concentration
  reduced.

ADMINISTRATION

RECONSTITUTION

–

ROUTE

- SC, IV

RATE OF ADMINISTRATION

- IV bolus with ECG monitoring

COMMENTS

- IV: sodium chloride 0.9% to a ratio of not
  less than 1:1 and not more than 1:9

OTHER INFORMATION

- SC: to reduce local discomfort, warm to
  room temperature before injection.
- For multiple injections, use different sites.
- Patients with reduced renal function have
  been shown to have a reduced clearance
  of the drug (75 mL/minute vs. 175 mL/
  minute).

Reference:
1. Chanson P, Timsit J, Harris AG. Clinical
pharmacokinetics of octreotide. Therapeutic
applications in patients with pituitary
tumours. *Clin Pharmacokinet*. 1993 Nov;
25(5): 375–91.

Oestrogen, conjugated (unlicensed product)

CLINICAL USE

Second line haemostatic agent for uraemic bleeding

DOSE IN NORMAL RENAL FUNCTION

0.6 mg/kg/day for 5 days[1]

PHARMACOKINETICS

Molecular weight (daltons)	–
% Protein binding	–
% Excreted unchanged in urine	–
Volume of distribution (L/kg)	–
Half-life – normal/ ESRF (hrs)	–

METABOLISM

Conjugated oestrogens taken orally are hydrolysed by enzymes present in the intestine that remove the sulfate group and allow absorption of the unconjugated oestrogen. Metabolism occurs mainly in the liver; a variety of sulfate and glucuronide conjugates are formed, and these are excreted in the urine and the bile. Those excreted in the bile undergo enterohepatic recycling or are excreted in the faeces.

DOSE IN RENAL IMPAIRMENT GFR (mL/MIN)

20–50	Dose as in normal renal function.
10–20	Dose as in normal renal function.
<10	Dose as in normal renal function.

DOSE IN PATIENTS UNDERGOING RENAL REPLACEMENT THERAPIES

CAPD	Unknown dialysability. Dose as in normal renal function.
HD	Unknown dialysability. Dose as in normal renal function.
HDF/High flux	Unknown dialysability. Dose as in normal renal function.
CAV/ VVHD	Unknown dialysability. Dose as in normal renal function.

IMPORTANT DRUG INTERACTIONS

Potentially hazardous interactions with other drugs

- Ciclosporin: concentration of ciclosporin increased.
- Anticoagulants: antagonism of anticoagulant effect of coumarins and phenindione.
- Anti-epileptics: accelerate metabolism of oestrogens.

ADMINISTRATION

RECONSTITUTION
- To 50 mL with sodium chloride 0.9%
ROUTE
- IV
RATE OF ADMINISTRATION
- Over a minimum of 30–40 minutes
COMMENTS
–

OTHER INFORMATION

- Duration of effect about 14 days.
- Used in association with desmopressin (DDAVP) in intractable cases.
- Orally 10–20 mg daily for 5–7 days.
- Conjugated oestrogens are a mixture of sodium oestrone sulphate and sodium equilin sulphate and other oestrogenic substances of the type excreted by pregnant mares.

Reference:
1. Hedges SJ, Dehoney SB, Hooper JS, et al. Evidence-based treatment recommendations for uremic bleeding. www.nature.com/clinicalpractice/neph.

Ofatumumab

CLINICAL USE

Human monoclonal antibody (IgG1):
- Treatment of chronic lymphocytic leukaemia

DOSE IN NORMAL RENAL FUNCTION

300 mg for the first infusion and 2000 mg for all subsequent infusions.
Consult relevant local protocol.

PHARMACOKINETICS

Molecular weight (daltons)	149 000
% Protein binding	No data
% Excreted unchanged in urine	No data
Volume of distribution (L/kg)	1.7–5.1 litres
Half-life – normal/ ESRF (hrs)	1.3–14 days (depending on number of infusions)/–

METABOLISM

Ofatumumab is eliminated by proteolytic enzymes and via binding to B-cells.

DOSE IN RENAL IMPAIRMENT GFR (mL/MIN)

30–50	Dose as in normal renal impairment.
10–30	Dose as in normal renal impairment. Use with caution.
<10	Dose as in normal renal impairment. Use with caution.

DOSE IN PATIENTS UNDERGOING RENAL REPLACEMENT THERAPIES

CAPD	Unlikely to be dialysed. Dose as in GFR<10 mL/min.
HD	Unlikely to be dialysed. Dose as in GFR<10 mL/min.
HDF/High flux	Unlikely to be dialysed. Dose as in GFR<10 mL/min.
CAV/ VVHD	Unlikely to be dialysed. Dose as in GFR=10–30 mL/min.

IMPORTANT DRUG INTERACTIONS

Potentially hazardous interactions with other drugs
- Live vaccines: avoid concomitant use.

ADMINISTRATION

RECONSTITUTION
–
ROUTE
- IV infusion

RATE OF ADMINISTRATION
- 1st & 2nd infusion: initial rate: 12 mL/ hour. During infusion, the rate should be doubled every 30 minutes to a maximum of 200 mL/hour.
  If the 2nd infusion has been completed without severe infusion related adverse drug reactions, the remaining infusions can start at a rate of 25 mL/hour and doubled every 30 minutes up to a maximum of 400 mL/hour.

COMMENTS
- Further dilute to 1000 mL with sodium chloride 0.9%.
- The in-line filter must be used during the entire infusion.

OTHER INFORMATION

- No studies have been done in patients with GFR<30 mL/min although the pharmacokinetics do not appear to be altered in renal impairment down to 33 mL/min.
- Contains 34.8 mg sodium per 300 mg dose and 232 mg sodium per 2000 mg dose.

Ofloxacin

CLINICAL USE

Antibacterial agent

DOSE IN NORMAL RENAL FUNCTION

- Oral: 200–400 mg daily, increased if necessary to 400 mg twice daily
- IV: 200–400 mg twice daily

PHARMACOKINETICS

Molecular weight (daltons)	361.4
% Protein binding	25
% Excreted unchanged in urine	65–80
Volume of distribution (L/kg)	1.5–2.5
Half-life – normal/ ESRF (hrs)	4–6/15–60

METABOLISM

Ofloxacin undergoes limited metabolism to desmethyl and N-oxide metabolites; desmethylofloxacin has moderate antibacterial activity.

Excretion is by tubular secretion and glomerular filtration, and 65–80% of a dose is excreted unchanged in the urine over 24 to 48 hours, resulting in high urinary concentrations. Less than 5% is excreted in the urine as metabolites. From 4% to 8% of a dose may be excreted in the faeces.

DOSE IN RENAL IMPAIRMENT GFR (mL/MIN)

20–50	200–400 mg once daily
10–20	200–400 mg once daily[1,2]
<10	100–200 mg once daily[1,2]

DOSE IN PATIENTS UNDERGOING RENAL REPLACEMENT THERAPIES

CAPD	Not significantly dialysed. Dose as in GFR<10 mL/min.
HD	Dialysed. Dose as in GFR<10 mL/min.
HDF/High flux	Dialysed. Dose as in GFR<10 mL/min.
CAV/VVHD	Dialysed. Dose as in GFR=10–20 mL/min.

IMPORTANT DRUG INTERACTIONS

Potentially hazardous interactions with other drugs
- Analgesics: increased risk of convulsions with NSAIDs.
- Anticoagulants: anticoagulant effect of coumarins enhanced.
- Antimalarials: manufacturer of artemether with lumefantrine advises avoid concomitant use.
- Ciclosporin: increased risk of nephrotoxicity.
- Theophylline: possibly increased risk of convulsions.

ADMINISTRATION

RECONSTITUTION
–
ROUTE
- Oral, IV
RATE OF ADMINISTRATION
- 200 mg over 30 minutes
COMMENTS
–

OTHER INFORMATION

- Almost 100% oral bioavailability.

References:
1. www.thedrugmonitor.com/rdosing.html
2. Mojgan S. *Clinical Pharmacology in the ICU.* Section 1; 1994. p. 58.

Olanzapine

- Schizophrenia
- Moderate to severe mania

DOSE IN NORMAL RENAL FUNCTION

- Oral: 5–20 mg daily
- IM: 5–10 mg repeated after 2 hours if required; maximum 3 doses daily for 3 days
- Depot injection: 150–300 mg every 2 weeks or 300–405 mg every 4 weeks
- Maximum dose of combined routes: 20 mg per day

PHARMACOKINETICS

Molecular weight (daltons)	312.4
% Protein binding	93
% Excreted unchanged in urine	7 (57% as metabolites and unchanged drug)
Volume of distribution (L/kg)	10–20
Half-life – normal/ ESRF (hrs)	30–38/Unchanged

METABOLISM

Olanzapine is extensively metabolised in the liver, mainly by direct glucuronidation and by oxidation mediated through the cytochrome P450 isoenzymes CYP1A2, and, to a lesser extent, CYP2D6. The 2 major metabolites, 10-N-glucuronide and 4'-N-desmethyl olanzapine, appear to be inactive. About 57% of a dose is excreted in the urine, mainly as metabolites, and about 30% appears in the faeces.

DOSE IN RENAL IMPAIRMENT GFR (mL/MIN)

20–50	Initial dose: 5 mg daily; Depot: 150 mg every 4 weeks and titrate as necessary.
10–20	Initial dose: 5 mg daily; Depot: 150 mg every 4 weeks and titrate as necessary.
<10	Initial dose: 5 mg daily; Depot: 150 mg every 4 weeks and titrate as necessary.

DOSE IN PATIENTS UNDERGOING RENAL REPLACEMENT THERAPIES

CAPD	Not dialysed. Dose as in GFR<10 mL/min.
HD	Not dialysed. Dose as in GFR<10 mL/min.
HDF/High flux	Unknown dialysability. Dose as in GFR<10 mL/min.
CAV/ VVHD	Unknown dialysability. Dose as in GFR=10–20 mL/min.

IMPORTANT DRUG INTERACTIONS

Potentially hazardous interactions with other drugs

- Anaesthetics: enhanced hypotensive effect.
- Analgesics: increased risk of convulsions with tramadol; enhanced hypotensive and sedative effects with opioids.
- Antibacterials: concentration possibly increased by ciprofloxacin.
- Antidepressants: fluvoxamine increases concentration of olanzapine; increased concentration of tricyclics.
- Anti-epileptics: antagonism (convulsive threshold lowered); carbamazepine increases metabolism of olanzapine; increased risk of neutropenia with valproate.
- Antimalarials: avoid concomitant use with artemether/lumefantrine.
- Antivirals: concentration reduced by ritonavir – consider increasing olanzapine dose.
- Anxiolytics and hypnotics: increased sedative effects; increased risk of hypotension, bradycardia and respiratory depression with IM olanzapine and parenteral benzodiazepines.

ADMINISTRATION

RECONSTITUTION
- 2.1 mL water for injection

ROUTE
- Oral, IM

RATE OF ADMINISTRATION
–

COMMENTS
–

Olmesartan medoxomil

CLINICAL USE

Angiotensin-II receptor antagonist:
- Hypertension

DOSE IN NORMAL RENAL FUNCTION

10–40 mg once daily

PHARMACOKINETICS

Molecular weight (daltons)	558.6
% Protein binding	99.7
% Excreted unchanged in urine	35–50
Volume of distribution (L/kg)	0.24
Half-life – normal/ ESRF (hrs)	10–15/36

METABOLISM

Olmesartan medoxomil is an ester prodrug that is hydrolysed during absorption from the gastrointestinal tract to the active form olmesartan. It is excreted in the urine and the bile as olmesartan; about 35–50% of the absorbed dose is excreted in the urine and the remainder in the bile.

DOSE IN RENAL IMPAIRMENT GFR (mL/MIN)

20–50	Dose as in normal renal function.
10–20	Dose as in normal renal function. Start with low doses.
<10	Dose as in normal renal function. Initial dose 10 mg daily and gradually increase.

DOSE IN PATIENTS UNDERGOING RENAL REPLACEMENT THERAPIES

CAPD	Not dialysed. Dose as in GFR<10 mL/min.
HD	Not dialysed. Dose as in GFR<10 mL/min.
HDF/High flux	Unlikely to be dialysed. Dose as in GFR<10 mL/min.
CAV/ VVHD	Unknown dialysability. Dose as in GFR=10–20 mL/min.

IMPORTANT DRUG INTERACTIONS

Potentially hazardous interactions with other drugs
- Anaesthetics: enhanced hypotensive effect.
- Analgesics: antagonism of hypotensive effect and increased risk of renal impairment with NSAIDs; hyperkalaemia with ketorolac and other NSAIDs.
- Ciclosporin: increased risk of hyperkalaemia and nephrotoxicity.
- Diuretics: enhanced hypotensive effect; hyperkalaemia with potassium-sparing diuretics.
- ESAs: increased risk of hyperkalaemia; antagonism of hypotensive effect.
- Lithium: reduced excretion (possibility of enhanced lithium toxicity).
- Potassium salts: increased risk of hyperkalaemia.
- Tacrolimus: increased risk of hyperkalaemia and nephrotoxicity.

ADMINISTRATION

RECONSTITUTION
–
ROUTE
- Oral
RATE OF ADMINISTRATION
–
COMMENTS
–

OTHER INFORMATION

- Hyperkalaemia and other side effects are more common in patients with impaired renal function.
- Renal failure has been reported in association with angiotensin-II antagonists in patients with renal artery stenosis, post renal transplant, and in those with congestive heart failure.
- Close monitoring of renal function during therapy is necessary in those with renal insufficiency.
- In mild, moderate and severe renal failure, the AUC is increased by 62%, 82% and 179% respectively.

Olsalazine sodium

CLINICAL USE

Induction and maintenance of remission in ulcerative colitis

DOSE IN NORMAL RENAL FUNCTION

1–3 g daily
Maintenance: 500 mg twice daily

PHARMACOKINETICS

Molecular weight (daltons)	346.2
% Protein binding	>99
% Excreted unchanged in urine	1–2
Volume of distribution (L/kg)	6 litres
Half-life – normal/ ESRF (hrs)	1/Unchanged

METABOLISM

Olsalazine is broken down by the colonic bacterial flora into two molecules of 5-aminosalicylic acid (mesalazine).

The small amounts (1–2% of the dose or less) of intact olsalazine that are absorbed are excreted mainly in urine. Approximately 0.1% of an oral dose of olsalazine is hepatically metabolised to olsalazine-O-sulfate (olsalazine-S), which has a half-life of 7 days.

DOSE IN RENAL IMPAIRMENT GFR (mL/MIN)

20–50	Caution – use only if necessary; start with low dose and increase according to response.
10–20	Caution – use only if necessary; start with low dose and increase according to response.
<10	Caution – use only if necessary; start with low dose and increase according to response.

DOSE IN PATIENTS UNDERGOING RENAL REPLACEMENT THERAPIES

CAPD	Unlikely to be dialysed. Dose as in GFR<10 mL/min.
HD	Unlikely to be dialysed. Dose as in GFR<10 mL/min.
HDF/High flux	Unlikely to be dialysed. Dose as in GFR<10 mL/min.
CAV/ VVHD	Unknown dialysability. Dose as in GFR=10–20 mL/min.

IMPORTANT DRUG INTERACTIONS

Potentially hazardous interactions with other drugs
- None known

ADMINISTRATION

RECONSTITUTION
–
ROUTE
- Oral
RATE OF ADMINISTRATION
–
COMMENTS
–

OTHER INFORMATION

- Potential to be nephrotoxic due to 5-aminosalicylic acid (5-ASA) component. Both 5-ASA and its acetylated metabolite are rapidly excreted in the urine.
- Less than 3% of an oral dose is absorbed before the drug reaches the colon.
- Unlikely that renal dysfunction will have any important effect on the kinetics of the drug.
- UK SPC contraindicates the use of olsalazine in patients with significant renal impairment due to lack of experience of its use in this patient population.
- US SPC just advises close monitoring.

Omalizumab

CLINICAL USE

Monoclonal antibody:
- Add-on therapy to improve asthma control
- Treatment of chronic spontaneous urticaria (CSU).

DOSE IN NORMAL RENAL FUNCTION

- Usually 75–600 mg in 1 to 4 injections, dependent on baseline IgE levels and body weight every 2–4 weeks
- Maximum dose is 600 mg every 2 weeks
- See SPC for more information.
- CSU: 300 mg every 4 weeks

PHARMACOKINETICS

Molecular weight (daltons)	149 000
% Protein binding	0
% Excreted unchanged in urine	No data
Volume of distribution (L/kg)	0.046–0.11
Half-life – normal/ ESRF (hrs)	20–26 days/–

METABOLISM

Omalizumab is most likely metabolised by opsonisation via the reticuloendothelial system, and removed by IgG and IgE clearance processes in the liver. Liver elimination of IgG includes degradation in the liver reticuloendothelial system (RES) and endothelial cells. Intact IgG is also excreted in bile.

DOSE IN RENAL IMPAIRMENT GFR (mL/MIN)

20–50	Dose as in normal renal function.
10–20	Dose as in normal renal function. Use with caution.
<10	Dose as in normal renal function. Use with caution.

DOSE IN PATIENTS UNDERGOING RENAL REPLACEMENT THERAPIES

CAPD	Unlikely dialysability. Dose as in GFR<10 mL/min.
HD	Unlikely dialysability. Dose as in GFR<10 mL/min.
HDF/High flux	Unlikely dialysability. Dose as in GFR<10 mL/min.
CAV/ VVHD	Unlikely dialysability. Dose as in GFR=10–20 mL/min.

IMPORTANT DRUG INTERACTIONS

Potentially hazardous interactions with other drugs
- None known

ADMINISTRATION

RECONSTITUTION
- Water for injection

ROUTE
- SC

RATE OF ADMINISTRATION
–

COMMENTS
- Preferably administer in the deltoid region of arm; alternatively in the thigh.
- Do not give more than 150 mg at one injection site.
- After reconstitution, chemically and physically stable for 8 hours at 2–8°C and 4 hours at 30°C.

OTHER INFORMATION

- Has a bioavailability of 62%; peak concentrations occur after 7–8 days.
- UK SPC advises to use with caution in renal impairment due to lack of studies. Renal impairment does not appear to affect the pharmacokinetics, therefore suggest use with caution and monitor patients closely.

Omeprazole

CLINICAL USE

Gastric acid suppression

DOSE IN NORMAL RENAL FUNCTION

- Oral: 10–120 mg daily
- IV: 40–60 mg once daily for up to 5 days
- Patients with recent bleeding on endoscopy: 80 mg stat followed by 8 mg/hour for 72 hours (British Society of Gastroenterology)

PHARMACOKINETICS

Molecular weight (daltons)	345.4
% Protein binding	95
% Excreted unchanged in urine	Minimal
Volume of distribution (L/kg)	0.3
Half-life – normal/ ESRF (hrs)	0.5–3/Unchanged

METABOLISM

Omeprazole is completely metabolised in the liver by the cytochrome P450 system to form inactive metabolites which are excreted mostly in the urine and to a lesser extent in bile. CYP2C19 produces hydroxyomeprazole, the major metabolite, CYP3A4 produces omeprazole sulphone.

DOSE IN RENAL IMPAIRMENT GFR (mL/MIN)

20–50	Dose as in normal renal function.
10–20	Dose as in normal renal function.
<10	Dose as in normal renal function.

DOSE IN PATIENTS UNDERGOING RENAL REPLACEMENT THERAPIES

CAPD	Unlikely to be dialysed. Dose as in normal renal function.
HD	Not dialysed. Dose as in normal renal function.
HDF/High flux	Unknown dialysability. Dose as in normal renal function.
CAV/ VVHD	Unknown dialysability. Dose as in normal renal function.

IMPORTANT DRUG INTERACTIONS

Potentially hazardous interactions with other drugs

- Anticoagulants: effect of coumarins possibly enhanced.
- Anti-epileptics: effects of phenytoin possibly enhanced.
- Antifungals: absorption of itraconazole and ketoconazole reduced; avoid with posaconazole; concentration increased by voriconazole.
- Antivirals: reduced atazanavir concentration – avoid concomitant use; AUC of saquinavir increased by 82% (increased risk of toxicity) – avoid; concentration of raltegravir possibly increased – avoid; concentration of rilpivirine reduced – avoid; concentration of omeprazole reduced by tipranavir.
- Ciclosporin: variable response; mostly increase in ciclosporin level.
- Cilostazol: increased cilostazol concentration – reduce cilostazol dose.
- Clopidogrel: avoid concomitant use due to reduced efficacy of clopidogrel.
- Cytotoxics: possibly reduced excretion of methotrexate; avoid with erlotinib and vandetanib; possibly reduced lapatinib absorption; possibly reduced absorption of pazopanib.
- Tacrolimus: may increase tacrolimus concentration.
- Ulipristal: reduced contraceptive effect, avoid with high dose ulipristal.

ADMINISTRATION

RECONSTITUTION
- 5 mL solvent provided per 40 mg vial

ROUTE
- Oral, IV

RATE OF ADMINISTRATION
- Bolus: over 5 minutes
- Infusion: 40 mg over 20–30 minutes
- Continuous infusion: 8 mg/hour

COMMENTS
- Add to 100 mL sodium chloride 0.9% or glucose 5%.
- Once diluted stable for 12 hours in sodium chloride 0.9% and 3 hours in glucose 5%.
- Use oral as soon as possible.
- 200 mg in 50 mL for 8 mg/hour infusion. (UK Critical Care Group, *Minimum Infusion Volumes for Fluid Restricted Critically Ill Patients*, 3rd edition, 2006)

OTHER INFORMATION

- Omeprazole clearance is not limited by renal disease.

Ondansetron

CLINICAL USE

Anti-emetic

DOSE IN NORMAL RENAL FUNCTION

- Oral: 4–32 mg daily in 2–3 divided doses
- IV: 8–32 mg daily
- PR: 16 mg pre-chemotherapy

PHARMACOKINETICS

Molecular weight (daltons)	293.4
% Protein binding	70–76
% Excreted unchanged in urine	<5
Volume of distribution (L/kg)	2
Half-life – normal/ ESRF (hrs)	3–6/5.4

METABOLISM

Ondansetron is metabolised in the liver through multiple enzymatic pathways; it is a substrate for cytochrome P450 isoenzymes, primarily CYP3A4, but also CYP1A2 and CYP2D6. The metabolites do not contribute to the pharmacological activity of ondansetron. Less than 5% of a dose is excreted unchanged in the urine.

DOSE IN RENAL IMPAIRMENT GFR (mL/MIN)

20–50	Dose as in normal renal function.
10–20	Dose as in normal renal function.
<10	Dose as in normal renal function.

DOSE IN PATIENTS UNDERGOING RENAL REPLACEMENT THERAPIES

CAPD	Unlikely to be dialysed. Dose as in normal renal function.
HD	Not dialysed. Dose as in normal renal function.
HDF/High flux	Unknown dialysability. Dose as in normal renal function.
CAV/ VVHD	Unknown dialysability. Dose as in normal renal function.

IMPORTANT DRUG INTERACTIONS

Potentially hazardous interactions with other drugs
- Dopaminergics: possible increased risk of hypotension with apomorphine – avoid.

ADMINISTRATION

RECONSTITUTION
–
ROUTE
- Oral, IV, IM, rectal
RATE OF ADMINISTRATION
- IV bolus over 3–5 minutes
- IV infusion: over 15 minutes
- Continuous infusion: 1 mg/hour
COMMENTS
- Dilute in 50–100 mL of sodium chloride 0.9% or glucose 5%.
- Patients >65 years should always have the injection diluted for chemotherapy-induced nausea and vomiting.

OTHER INFORMATION

- Can be used to treat uraemic pruritis.
- Renal clearance of ondansetron is low.
- Due to risk of QT prolongation the MHRA has advised, patients >75 years should have an maximum IV dose of 8 mg for chemotherapy-induced nausea and vomiting, if less than 75 years, maximum single dose is 16 mg. All adults should receive doses at least 4 hours apart.
- Can cause a dose dependent QT interval prolongation.
- MHRA. *Drug Safety Update*. Ondansetron for intravenous use: dose-dependent QT interval prolongation—new posology. 2013 July; **6**(12).

Orlistat

CLINICAL USE

Adjunct in obesity

DOSE IN NORMAL RENAL FUNCTION

120 mg taken immediately before, during or up to 1 hour after each meal; maximum 360 mg daily

PHARMACOKINETICS

Molecular weight (daltons)	495.7
% Protein binding	>99
% Excreted unchanged in urine	0–4
Volume of distribution (L/kg)	No data
Half-life – normal/ ESRF (hrs)	1–2/Unchanged

METABOLISM

Orlistat is minimally absorbed and has no defined systemic pharmacokinetics. The metabolism of orlistat occurs mainly within the gastrointestinal wall to form two major inactive metabolites, M1 (4-member lactone ring hydrolysed) and M3 (M1 with N-formyl leucine moiety cleaved). Faecal excretion of the unabsorbed drug is the major route of elimination. Approximately 97% of the administered dose is excreted in faeces and 83% of that as unchanged orlistat.

DOSE IN RENAL IMPAIRMENT GFR (mL/MIN)

20–50	Dose as in normal renal function.
10–20	Dose as in normal renal function.
<10	Dose as in normal renal function.

DOSE IN PATIENTS UNDERGOING RENAL REPLACEMENT THERAPIES

CAPD	Unlikely to be dialysed. Dose as in normal renal function.
HD	Unlikely to be dialysed. Dose as in normal renal function.
HDF/High flux	Unlikely to be dialysed. Dose as in normal renal function.
CAV/ VVHD	Unlikely to be dialysed. Dose as in normal renal function.

IMPORTANT DRUG INTERACTIONS

Potentially hazardous interactions with other drugs

- Acarbose: avoid concomitant administration.
- Amiodarone: possibly slightly reduces absorption.[1]
- Anticoagulants: monitor INR more frequently (due to reduction in vitamin K absorption).[1]
- Anti-epileptics: possible increased risk of convulsions.
- Ciclosporin: possibly reduces absorption of ciclosporin.
- Tacrolimus: possibly reduces absorption of tacrolimus.[1]
- Thyroid hormones: possible increased risk of hypothyroidism with levothyroxine.
- Vitamins: may reduce the absorption of fat soluble vitamins.

ADMINISTRATION

RECONSTITUTION

–

ROUTE

- Oral

RATE OF ADMINISTRATION

–

COMMENTS

–

OTHER INFORMATION

- If the meal doesn't contain any fat, omit orlistat.
- Orlistat is poorly absorbed; bioavailability of less than 5%.
- Renal failure and fatal cases of hepatitis have been reported.

Reference:
1. Baxter K, Sharp J. Orlistat and possible drug interactions that can affect over-the-counter sales. *Pharm J.* 1 May 2010; **284**: 431.

Orphenadrine hydrochloride

CLINICAL USE

Anti-muscarinic:
- Parkinsonism
- Drug induced extra-pyramidal symptoms

DOSE IN NORMAL RENAL FUNCTION

150–400 mg daily in divided doses

PHARMACOKINETICS

Molecular weight (daltons)	305.8
% Protein binding	95
% Excreted unchanged in urine	8
Volume of distribution (L/kg)	No data
Half-life – normal/ ESRF (hrs)	14/–

METABOLISM

Orphenadrine is almost completely metabolised to at least eight metabolites in the liver. It is mainly excreted in the urine as metabolites and small amounts of unchanged drug.

DOSE IN RENAL IMPAIRMENT GFR (mL/MIN)

20–50	Dose as in normal renal function.
10–20	Dose as in normal renal function.
<10	Dose as in normal renal function.

DOSE IN PATIENTS UNDERGOING RENAL REPLACEMENT THERAPIES

CAPD	Unlikely dialysability. Dose as in normal renal function.
HD	Unlikely dialysability. Dose as in normal renal function.
HDF/High flux	Unlikely dialysability. Dose as in normal renal function.
CAV/ VVHD	Unlikely dialysability. Dose as in normal renal function.

IMPORTANT DRUG INTERACTIONS

Potentially hazardous interactions with other drugs
- None known.

ADMINISTRATION

RECONSTITUTION
–

ROUTE
- Oral

RATE OF ADMINISTRATION
–

COMMENTS
–

Oseltamivir

CLINICAL USE

Treatment and post-exposure prevention of influenza

DOSE IN NORMAL RENAL FUNCTION

- Treatment: 75 mg twice daily for 5 days
- Post-exposure prevention: 75 mg once daily for at least 10 days; up to 6 weeks if epidemic in community

PHARMACOKINETICS

Molecular weight (daltons)	410.4 (as phosphate)
% Protein binding	42 (3 as carboxylate)
% Excreted unchanged in urine	Negligible (99% excreted as carboxylate metabolite in urine)
Volume of distribution (L/kg)	0.3–0.4
Half-life – normal/ ESRF (hrs)	1–3, (6–10 as metabolite)/>20

METABOLISM

Oseltamivir is a prodrug; it is extensively metabolised by esterases in the liver to the active carboxylate metabolite. Oseltamivir carboxylate is not further metabolised and is eliminated entirely by renal excretion. Renal clearance exceeds glomerular filtration rate indicating that tubular secretion occurs in addition to glomerular filtration. Less than 20% of an oral radiolabelled dose is eliminated in faeces.

DOSE IN RENAL IMPAIRMENT GFR (mL/MIN)

30–50	Dose as in normal renal function.
10–30	Treatment: 75 mg once daily or 30 mg twice daily Prophylaxis: 75 mg every 48 hours or 30 mg once daily
<10	Treatment: 75 mg as a single dose Prophylaxis: 30 mg once a week[1] (2 doses). See 'Other information'.

DOSE IN PATIENTS UNDERGOING RENAL REPLACEMENT THERAPIES

CAPD	Dialysed. Treatment & Prophylaxis: 30 mg weekly (2 doses for prophylaxis).
HD	Dialysed. Treatment & Prophylaxis: 30 mg three times a week post dialysis.
HDF/High flux	Dialysed. Treatment & Prophylaxis: 75 mg three times a week post dialysis.
CAV/ VVHD	Dialysed. Dose as in GFR = 10–30 mL/min.

IMPORTANT DRUG INTERACTIONS

Potentially hazardous interactions with other drugs
- None known

ADMINISTRATION

RECONSTITUTION
–
ROUTE
- Oral
RATE OF ADMINISTRATION
–
COMMENTS
–

OTHER INFORMATION

- At least 75% of the oral dose reaches the systemic circulation as the carboxylate.
- All the active metabolite is excreted in the urine.
- A lower dose is required in severe renal disease due to the active metabolite accumulating.
- Due to shortages in availability of the 30 mg dosage size and after looking at the pharmacokinetics (low protein binding of the metabolite) and the good tolerability it would seem to be reasonable to suggest a dose of 75 mg post dialysis for high flux dialysis continuing for the length of time required, depending on whether it is treatment or prophylaxis.
- Anecdotally a dose of 75 mg after each dialysis session has been used in haemodialysis patients without any problems.
- More oseltamivir is removed by APD than CAPD.
- For patients in the Critical Care setting, many units are now prescribing double the usual dose for treatment:
  — GFR>30 mL/min: 150 mg twice daily
  — GFR=10–30 mL/min (including patients on CAVH/CVVH/CAVHD/ CVVHD): 75 mg twice daily

References:
1. Draft briefing and guidance for adult renal units in the UK during an influenza pandemic. Prepared for the Renal Association Clinical Affairs Board. 28/8/07.

2. Robson R, Buttimore A, Lynn K, *et al.* The pharmacokinetics and tolerability of oseltamivir suspension on haemodialysis and continuous ambulatory peritoneal dialysis. *Nephrol Dial Transplant.* 2006; **21**(9): 2556–62.

Oxaliplatin

CLINICAL USE

Antineoplastic platinum agent:
- Treatment of metastatic colorectal cancer in combination with fluorouracil and folinic acid and stage III colon cancer

DOSE IN NORMAL RENAL FUNCTION

$85 \, mg/m^2$; can be repeated at intervals of 2 weeks if toxicity permits.

PHARMACOKINETICS

Molecular weight (daltons)	397.3
% Protein binding	33[1]
% Excreted unchanged in urine	54
Volume of distribution (L/kg)	330 +/− 40.9 litres
Half-life – normal/ ESRF (hrs)	273/Increased

METABOLISM

Oxaliplatin is extensively metabolised by non-enzymatic biotransformation to both inactive and active compounds. There is no *in vitro* evidence of cytochrome P450 metabolism of the diaminocyclohexane (DACH) ring. Several cytotoxic biotransformation products including the monochloro-, dichloro- and diaquo-DACH platinum species have been identified in the systemic circulation together with a number of inactive conjugates. Platinum removal is mainly by renal excretion and tissue distribution; platinum metabolites mainly by renal excretion. By day 5, approximately 54% of the total dose was recovered in the urine and <3% in the faeces.

DOSE IN RENAL IMPAIRMENT GFR (mL/MIN)

30–50	Dose as in normal renal function.
10–30	$65 \, mg/m^2$, use with caution and monitor closely.
<10	$65 \, mg/m^2$, use with caution and monitor closely.

DOSE IN PATIENTS UNDERGOING RENAL REPLACEMENT THERAPIES

CAPD	Unlikely to be dialysed. Dose as in GFR<10 mL/min.
HD	Unlikely to be dialysed. Dose as in GFR<10 mL/min.
HDF/High flux	Dialysed. Dose as in GFR<10 mL/min.
CAV/ VVHD	Unlikely to be dialysed. Dose as in GFR=10–30 mL/min.

IMPORTANT DRUG INTERACTIONS

Potentially hazardous interactions with other drugs
- Aminoglycosides: increased risk of nephrotoxicity and possibly ototoxicity with aminoglycosides, capreomycin, polymyxins or vancomycin.
- Antipsychotics: avoid concomitant use with clozapine (increased risk of agranulocytosis).

ADMINISTRATION

RECONSTITUTION
- Glucose 5% or water for injection to give a concentration of 5 mg/mL
ROUTE
- IV infusion
RATE OF ADMINISTRATION
- 2–6 hours
COMMENTS
- Dilute with 250–500 mL glucose 5% to a concentration 0.2–0.7 mg/mL.

OTHER INFORMATION

- Contraindicated by manufacturer in UK SPC if GFR<30 mL/min due to lack of studies. Dose in severe renal impairment is from US SPC.
- No *in vitro* evidence of cytochrome P450 metabolism.
- Binds irreversibly to red blood cells, which can prolong the half-life of the drug.
- Reduced renal clearance and volume of distribution in renal impairment.
- There is a 38–44% reduction of platinum clearance in mild–moderate renal impairment (GFR=20–39 mL/min) but no increased incidence of side effects has been reported.[2]

References:
1. Massari C, Brienza S, Rotarski M, *et al*. Pharmacokinetics of oxaliplatin in patients with normal versus impaired renal function.

Cancer Chemother Pharmacol. 2000; **45**: 157–64.
2. Graham MA, Takimoto CH, Remick S, *et al.* A phase I study of oxaliplatin in cancer patients with impaired renal function.

Proceedings of the American Society of Clinical Oncology; 2001; **29**: 267. 37th Annual meeting of American Society of Clinical Oncology. 2001; 12–15 May; San Francisco, California.

Oxazepam

CLINICAL USE

Benzodiazepine:
- Anxiolytic
- Insomnia

DOSE IN NORMAL RENAL FUNCTION

- Anxiolytic: 15–30 mg 3 or 4 times a day
- Insomnia: 15–50 mg at night

PHARMACOKINETICS

Molecular weight (daltons)	286.7
% Protein binding	85–97
% Excreted unchanged in urine	<1
Volume of distribution (L/kg)	0.6–1.6
Half-life – normal/ ESRF (hrs)	3–21/25–90

METABOLISM

Oxazepam is the ultimate pharmacologically active metabolite of diazepam and is itself largely metabolised to the inactive glucuronide which is excreted in the urine.

DOSE IN RENAL IMPAIRMENT GFR (mL/MIN)

20–50	Dose as in normal renal function.
10–20	Dose as in normal renal function.
<10	Start at low dose and increase according to response.

DOSE IN PATIENTS UNDERGOING RENAL REPLACEMENT THERAPIES

CAPD	Not dialysed. Dose as in GFR<10 mL/min.
HD	Not dialysed. Dose as in GFR<10 mL/min.
HDF/High flux	Unknown dialysability. Dose as in GFR<10 mL/min.
CAV/ VVHD	Unknown dialysability. Dose as in normal renal function.

IMPORTANT DRUG INTERACTIONS

Potentially hazardous interactions with other drugs
- Antibacterials: metabolism possibly increased by rifampicin.
- Antipsychotics: enhanced sedative effects; risk of serious adverse effects in combination with clozapine.
- Antivirals: possibly increased concentration with ritonavir.
- Sodium oxybate: enhanced effects of sodium oxybate – avoid.
- Ulcer-healing drugs: metabolism inhibited by cimetidine.

ADMINISTRATION

RECONSTITUTION
–
ROUTE
- Oral
RATE OF ADMINISTRATION
–
COMMENTS
–

OTHER INFORMATION

- Protein binding decreased and volume of distribution increased in ERF.
- Inactive glucuronide metabolite accumulates in CKD 5; significance of this unknown.

Oxcarbazepine

CLINICAL USE

- Anti-epileptic agent
- Trigeminal neuralgia (unlicensed indication)

DOSE IN NORMAL RENAL FUNCTION

- Epilepsy: 600 mg–2.4 g daily in divided doses
- Trigeminal neuralgia: 400 mg–2.4 g in 2–4 divided doses

PHARMACOKINETICS

Molecular weight (daltons)	252.3
% Protein binding	40–60 (metabolite)
% Excreted unchanged in urine	<1
Volume of distribution (L/kg)	0.7–0.8
Half-life – normal/ ESRF (hrs)	1.3–2.3 (9 for metabolite)/ Unchanged (16–19 for metabolite)

METABOLISM

Oxcarbazepine is rapidly reduced by cytosolic enzymes in the liver to the active monohydroxy metabolite (licarbezine, or MHD). MHD is metabolised further by conjugation with glucuronic acid. Minor amounts (4% of the dose) are oxidised to a pharmacologically inactive metabolite. Oxcarbazepine is excreted in the urine mainly as metabolites; less than 1% is excreted as unchanged drug.

DOSE IN RENAL IMPAIRMENT GFR (mL/MIN)

30–50	Dose as in normal renal function.
10–30	Dose as in normal renal function. Start with 300 mg daily and titrate slowly.
<10	Dose as in normal renal function. Start with 300 mg daily and titrate slowly.

DOSE IN PATIENTS UNDERGOING RENAL REPLACEMENT THERAPIES

CAPD	Unknown dialysability. Dose as in GFR<10 mL/min.
HD	Unknown dialysability. Dose as in GFR<10 mL/min.
HDF/High flux	Unknown dialysability. Dose as in GFR<10 mL/min.
CAV/ VVHD	Unknown dialysability. Dose as in GFR=10–30 mL/min.

IMPORTANT DRUG INTERACTIONS

Potentially hazardous interactions with other drugs

- Antidepressants: antagonism of anticonvulsant effect; avoid concomitant use with St John's wort.
- Antimalarials: anticonvulsant effect antagonised by mefloquine.
- Antipsychotics: antagonism of anticonvulsant effect.
- Antivirals: concentration of rilpivirine reduced – avoid.
- Ciclosporin: metabolism accelerated (reduced ciclosporin concentration).
- Clopidogrel: possibly reduced anti-platelet effect.
- Cytotoxics: concentration of imatinib reduced – avoid.
- Oestrogens and progestogens: metabolism accelerated (reduced contraceptive effect).
- Orlistat: possible increased risk of convulsions.
- Tacrolimus: metabolism accelerated (reduced tacrolimus concentration).

ADMINISTRATION

RECONSTITUTION

–

ROUTE

- Oral

RATE OF ADMINISTRATION

–

COMMENTS

–

OTHER INFORMATION

- Hyponatraemia is more common with oxcarbazepine than carbamazepine, monitoring is recommended.
- Maximum plasma concentrations reached after about 1 hour.
- In severe renal impairment increase in at least weekly intervals.

Oxprenolol hydrochloride

CLINICAL USE

Beta-1 adrenoceptor blocker:
- Hypertension
- Angina
- Arrhythmias
- Anxiety

DOSE IN NORMAL RENAL FUNCTION

- Hypertension, angina: 80–160 mg daily in 2–3 divided doses; maximum 320 mg daily
- Arrhythmias: 40–240 mg daily in 2–3 divided doses
- Anxiety: 40–80 mg daily in 1–2 divided doses

PHARMACOKINETICS

Molecular weight (daltons)	301.8
% Protein binding	70–80
% Excreted unchanged in urine	<3
Volume of distribution (L/kg)	1.2
Half-life – normal/ ESRF (hrs)	1–2/Unchanged

METABOLISM

Oxprenolol is extensively metabolised in the liver, direct O-glucuronidation being the major metabolic pathway and oxidative reactions minor ones. Oxprenolol is excreted chiefly in the urine (almost exclusively in the form of inactive metabolites).

DOSE IN RENAL IMPAIRMENT GFR (mL/MIN)

20–50	Dose as in normal renal function.
10–20	Dose as in normal renal function.
<10	Dose as in normal renal function.

DOSE IN PATIENTS UNDERGOING RENAL REPLACEMENT THERAPIES

CAPD	Unlikely dialysability. Dose as in normal renal function.
HD	Unlikely dialysability. Dose as in normal renal function.
HDF/High flux	Unknown dialysability. Dose as in normal renal function.
CAV/ VVHD	Unknown dialysability. Dose as in normal renal function.

IMPORTANT DRUG INTERACTIONS

Potentially hazardous interactions with other drugs
- Anaesthetics: enhanced hypotensive effect.
- Analgesics: NSAIDs antagonise hypotensive effect.
- Anti-arrhythmics: increased risk of myocardial depression and bradycardia; increased risk of bradycardia, myocardial depression and AV block with amiodarone; increased risk of myocardial depression and bradycardia with flecainide.
- Antidepressants: enhanced hypotensive effect with MAOIs.
- Antihypertensives: enhanced hypotensive effect; increased risk of first dose hypotensive effect with post-synaptic alpha-blockers such as prazosin; increased risk of withdrawal hypertension with clonidine; increased risk of bradycardia and AV block with diltiazem; severe hypotension and heart failure occasionally with nifedipine; asystole, severe hypotension and heart failure with verapamil.
- Antimalarials: increased risk of bradycardia with mefloquine.
- Antipsychotics: enhanced hypotensive effect with phenothiazines.
- Cytotoxics: possible increased risk of bradycardia with crizotinib.
- Diuretics: enhanced hypotensive effect.
- Fingolimod: possibly increased risk of bradycardia.
- Moxisylyte: possibly severe postural hypotension.
- Sympathomimetics: severe hypertension with adrenaline and noradrenaline (especially with non-selective beta-blockers) and possibly with dopamine.

ADMINISTRATION

RECONSTITUTION
–
ROUTE
- Oral
RATE OF ADMINISTRATION
–
COMMENTS
–

OTHER INFORMATION

- Use with caution in patients with chronic obstructive airways disease, asthma or diabetes.
- Rhabdomyolysis with myoglobinuria has been reported in severe overdosage with oxprenolol.

Oxybutynin hydrochloride

CLINICAL USE

- Urinary frequency, urgency and incontinence
- Neurogenic bladder instability and nocturnal enuresis

DOSE IN NORMAL RENAL FUNCTION

- 2.5–5 mg 2 to 3 times a day; maximum 5 mg 4 times a day
- XL: 5–20 mg once daily
- Patches: 1 patch (36 mg) twice weekly

PHARMACOKINETICS

Molecular weight (daltons)	393.9
% Protein binding	83–85
% Excreted unchanged in urine	<0.1
Volume of distribution (L/kg)	193 litres
Half-life – normal/ ESRF (hrs)	1.1–3 (XL: 12–13)/–

METABOLISM

Oxybutynin undergoes extensive first-pass metabolism, particularly by the cytochrome P450 isoenzyme CYP3A4. One of the metabolites, N-desethyloxybutynin, is pharmacologically active. Oxybutynin and its metabolites are excreted in the urine and faeces.

DOSE IN RENAL IMPAIRMENT GFR (mL/MIN)

20–50	Dose as in normal renal function.
10–20	Dose as in normal renal function.
<10	Dose as in normal renal function.

DOSE IN PATIENTS UNDERGOING RENAL REPLACEMENT THERAPIES

CAPD	Dialysed. Dose as in normal renal function.
HD	Dialysed. Dose as in normal renal function.
HDF/High flux	Dialysed. Dose as in normal renal function.
CAV/ VVHD	Dialysed. Dose as in normal renal function.

IMPORTANT DRUG INTERACTIONS

Potentially hazardous interactions with other drugs
- Anti-arrhythmics: increased risk of antimuscarinic side effects with disopyramide.
- Other antimuscarinic agents: increased antimuscarinic effects.

ADMINISTRATION

RECONSTITUTION
–
ROUTE
- Oral, topical
RATE OF ADMINISTRATION
–
COMMENTS
–

OTHER INFORMATION

- Start with a low dose in elderly patients and those with renal impairment, and increase according to response.

Oxycodone hydrochloride

CLINICAL USE

Opioid analgesic for moderate to severe pain

DOSE IN NORMAL RENAL FUNCTION

- Oral: 5 mg 4–6 hourly; usual maximum dose 400 mg daily
- M/R: 10 mg 12 hourly; usual maximum dose 200 mg 12 hourly
- IV: 1–10 mg every 4 hours
- IV infusion: 2 mg/hour adjusted according to response
- SC: initially 5 mg every 4 hours
- SC infusion: initially 7.5 mg over 24 hours

PHARMACOKINETICS

Molecular weight (daltons)	351.8
% Protein binding	45
% Excreted unchanged in urine	<10
Volume of distribution (L/kg)	1.2–6.31
Half-life – normal/ESRF (hrs)	2–4 (4.5, M/R)/ 3–5 (5.5 M/R)

METABOLISM

Oxycodone is metabolised in the liver to produce noroxycodone via the CYP3A system, oxymorphone via the CYP2D6 system and various conjugated glucuronides. The analgesic effects of the metabolites are clinically insignificant. Both metabolites undergo glucuronidation and are excreted with unchanged drug in urine.

DOSE IN RENAL IMPAIRMENT GFR (mL/MIN)

20–50	Start with 75% of dose. Dose as in normal renal function.
10–20	Start with 75% of dose. Dose as in normal renal function.
<10	Start with small doses, e.g. 50% of dose. See 'Other information'.

DOSE IN PATIENTS UNDERGOING RENAL REPLACEMENT THERAPIES

CAPD	Unknown dialysability. Dose as in GFR<10 mL/min.
HD	Unknown dialysability. Dose as in GFR<10 mL/min.
HDF/High flux	Dialysed. Dose as in GFR<10 mL/min.
CAV/ VVHD	Unknown dialysability. Dose as in GFR=10–20 mL/min.

IMPORTANT DRUG INTERACTIONS

Potentially hazardous interactions with other drugs

- Antibacterials: metabolism possibly increased by rifampicin; metabolism inhibited by telithromycin.
- Antidepressants: CNS excitation or depression with MAOIs – avoid concomitant use; possible CNS excitation or depression with moclobemide; increased sedative effects with tricyclics.
- Antifungals: concentration increased by voriconazole.
- Antihistamines: increased sedative effects with sedating antihistamines.
- Antipsychotics: enhanced hypotensive and sedative effects.
- Antivirals: concentration possibly increased by ritonavir.
- Dopaminergics: avoid with selegiline.
- Sodium oxybate: enhanced effect of sodium oxybate – avoid concomitant use.

ADMINISTRATION

RECONSTITUTION
–
ROUTE
- Oral, IV, IM, SC
RATE OF ADMINISTRATION
- Infusion over 24 hours
COMMENTS
- Dilute to a concentration of 1 mg/mL with glucose 5% or sodium chloride 0.9%.

OTHER INFORMATION

- Has been used in CKD 5 patients; start with lowest dose and gradually increase dose according to response.
- Limited accumulation of metabolites in renal failure compared with morphine.
- Increased volume of distribution in renal failure. (Kirvela M, Lindgren L, Seppala T, et al. The pharmacokinetics of oxycodone in uremic patients undergoing renal transplantation. *J Clin Anes.* 1996; **8**: 13–18.)
- 2 mg of oral oxycodone is approximately equivalent to 1 mg of parenteral oxycodone.
- Doses in renal impairment are from *Drug Prescribing in Renal Failure*, 5th edition, by Aronoff et al.

Oxytetracycline

CLINICAL USE

Antibacterial agent

DOSE IN NORMAL RENAL FUNCTION

250–500 mg 4 times a day
Acne: 500 mg twice daily

PHARMACOKINETICS

Molecular weight (daltons)	460.4
% Protein binding	20–40
% Excreted unchanged in urine	10–35
Volume of distribution (L/kg)	1.5
Half-life – normal/ ESRF (hrs)	9/66

METABOLISM

Metabolism is negligible. The tetracyclines are excreted in the urine and in the faeces. Renal clearance is by glomerular filtration. Up to 60% of an intravenous dose of tetracycline, and up to 55% of an oral dose, is eliminated unchanged in the urine. The tetracyclines are excreted in the bile, where concentrations 5 to 25 times those in plasma can occur. There is some enterohepatic reabsorption and considerable quantities occur in the faeces after oral doses.

DOSE IN RENAL IMPAIRMENT GFR (mL/MIN)

20–50	Dose as in normal renal function.
10–20	Dose as in normal renal function.
<10	250 mg 4 times a day.

DOSE IN PATIENTS UNDERGOING RENAL REPLACEMENT THERAPIES

CAPD	Not dialysed. Dose as in GFR<10 mL/min.
HD	Not dialysed. Dose as in GFR<10 mL/min.
HDF/High flux	Unknown dialysability. Dose as in GFR<10 mL/min.
CAV/ VVHD	Unknown dialysability. Dose as in normal renal function.

IMPORTANT DRUG INTERACTIONS

Potentially hazardous interactions with other drugs
- Anticoagulants: possibly enhanced anticoagulant effect of coumarins and phenindione.
- Oestrogens: possibly reduced contraceptive effects of oestrogens (risk probably small).
- Retinoids: possible increased risk of benign intracranial hypertension with tetracyclines and retinoids – avoid concomitant use.

ADMINISTRATION

RECONSTITUTION

–

ROUTE

- Oral

RATE OF ADMINISTRATION

–

COMMENTS

–

OTHER INFORMATION

- Avoid if possible in renal impairment, due to potential nephrotoxicity and increased risk of azotaemia, hyperphosphataemia and acidosis.
- May cause an increase in blood urea which is dose related.
- Avoid in SLE.

Paclitaxel

CLINICAL USE

Antineoplastic agent:
- Ovarian and breast cancer
- Non-small cell lung carcinoma
- AIDS-related Kaposi's sarcoma

DOSE IN NORMAL RENAL FUNCTION

- 100–220 mg/m^2 every 3 weeks depending on condition being treated, local regime and duration of infusion
- Paclitaxel albumin: 260 mg/m^2 over 30 minutes every 3 weeks

PHARMACOKINETICS

Molecular weight (daltons)	853.9
% Protein binding	89–98
% Excreted unchanged in urine	1.3–12.6
Volume of distribution (L/kg)	198–688 litres/m^2
Half-life – normal/ ESRF (hrs)	3–52.7/–

METABOLISM

The distribution and metabolism of paclitaxel in humans has not been fully investigated. The cumulative excretion of unchanged paclitaxel in the urine has been between 1.3% and 12.6% of the dose on average, which is an indication of extensive non-renal clearance. Hepatic metabolism by the action of CYP450 enzyme and biliary clearance are possibly the principal mechanisms for elimination of paclitaxel. An average of 26% of the radioactively marked dose of paclitaxel was eliminated in the faeces as a 6α-hydroxypaclitaxel, 2% as 3'p-dihydroxypaclitaxel and 6% as 6α-3'p-dihydroxypaclitaxel.

DOSE IN RENAL IMPAIRMENT GFR (mL/MIN)

20–50	Dose as in normal renal function.
10–20	Dose as in normal renal function.
<10	Dose as in normal renal function.

DOSE IN PATIENTS UNDERGOING RENAL REPLACEMENT THERAPIES

CAPD	Not dialysed. Dose as in normal renal function.
HD	Not dialysed. Dose as in normal renal function.
HDF/High flux	Unlikely to be dialysed. Dose as in normal renal function.
CAV/ VVHD	Unknown dialysability. Dose as in normal renal function.

IMPORTANT DRUG INTERACTIONS

Potentially hazardous interactions with other drugs
- Antipsychotics: avoid concomitant use with clozapine (increased risk of agranulocytosis).
- Cytotoxics: increased risk of neutropenia with lapatinib.

ADMINISTRATION

RECONSTITUTION
–
ROUTE
- IV
RATE OF ADMINISTRATION
- 3 hours depending on regime
- 30 minutes for paclitaxel albumin
COMMENTS
- Dilute to a concentration of 0.3–1.2 mg/mL with sodium chloride 0.9% or glucose 5%.
- Stable for 27 hours at room temperature.

OTHER INFORMATION

- Administer through a 0.22 μm in-line filter.
- Use non-PVC infusion bags.
- Paclitaxel albumin manufacturer unable to advise on a dose in renal impairment due to lack of studies.

Paliperidone

CLINICAL USE

Atypical antipsychotic for schizophrenia

DOSE IN NORMAL RENAL FUNCTION

- Oral: 3–12 mg once daily
- IM: 25–150 mg monthly

PHARMACOKINETICS

Molecular weight (daltons)	426.5
% Protein binding	74
% Excreted unchanged in urine	59
Volume of distribution (L/kg)	487 litres
Half-life – normal/ESRF (hrs)	23/51

METABOLISM

Paliperidone is the active metabolite of risperidone.

Four metabolic pathways have been identified *in vivo*, none of which accounted for more than 6.5% of the dose: dealkylation, hydroxylation, dehydrogenation, and benzisoxazole scission. Following administration of ^{14}C-paliperidone, 59% of the dose was excreted unchanged into urine, indicating that paliperidone is not extensively metabolised in the liver. Approximately 80% of the administered radioactivity was recovered in urine and 11% in the faeces.

DOSE IN RENAL IMPAIRMENT GFR (mL/MIN)

50–80	Oral: 3 mg once daily and increase according to response. IM: Dose as in normal renal function for maintenance dose, reduce loading dose.
30–50	1.5 mg once daily, increasing to 3 mg daily according to response. IM: No experience.
10–30	1.5 mg daily, increasing to 3 mg daily according to response. IM: No experience.
<10	3 mg alternate days, increasing to 3 mg daily according to response. Use with caution. IM: No experience.

DOSE IN PATIENTS UNDERGOING RENAL REPLACEMENT THERAPIES

CAPD	Unknown dialysability. Dose as in GFR<10 mL/min.
HD	Unknown dialysability. Dose as in GFR<10 mL/min.
HDF/High flux	Unknown dialysability. Dose as in GFR<10 mL/min.
CAV/ VVHD	Unknown dialysability. Dose as in GFR=10–30 mL/min.

IMPORTANT DRUG INTERACTIONS

Potentially hazardous interactions with other drugs

- Anaesthetics: enhanced hypotensive effect.
- Analgesics: increased risk of convulsions with tramadol; enhanced hypotensive and sedative effects with opioids; increased risk of ventricular arrhythmias with methadone.
- Anti-arrhythmics: increased risk of ventricular arrhythmias when given with anti-arrhythmics that prolong the QT interval.
- Antidepressants: increases concentration of tricyclics (possibly increased risk of ventricular arrhythmias).
- Antimalarials: avoidance of antipsychotics advised by manufacturer of artemether/ lumefantrine.
- Antivirals: concentration possibly increased by ritonavir.
- Atomoxetine: increased risk of ventricular arrhythmias with atomoxetine.
- Anti-epileptics: antagonise anticonvulsant effect (convulsive threshold lowered); concentration reduced by carbamazepine.
- Antivirals: concentration possibly increased by ritonavir.
- Cytotoxics: increased risk of ventricular arrhythmias with arsenic trioxide.

ADMINISTRATION

RECONSTITUTION
–

ROUTE
- Oral

RATE OF ADMINISTRATION
–

COMMENTS
–

OTHER INFORMATION

- Clearance is reduced by 71% in ERF.
- Contraindicated (by manufacturer) in patients with GFR<10 mL/min, due to lack of experience.

Palonosetron

CLINICAL USE

Anti-emetic:
- For use with cancer chemotherapy

DOSE IN NORMAL RENAL FUNCTION

- IV: 250 mcg as a single dose approximately 30 minutes before chemotherapy.
- Oral: 500 mcg as a single dose approximately 60 minutes before chemotherapy.

PHARMACOKINETICS

Molecular weight (daltons)	332.9 (as hydrochloride)
% Protein binding	62
% Excreted unchanged in urine	40
Volume of distribution (L/kg)	6.9–7.9
Half-life – normal/ ESRF (hrs)	40/–

METABOLISM

Palonosetron is eliminated by a dual route, about 40% eliminated through the kidney and approximately 50% metabolised by CYP2D6, and to a lesser extent, CYP3A4 and CYP1A2 isoenzymes in the liver to form two primary metabolites, which have less than 1% of the 5HT$_3$ receptor antagonist activity of palonosetron. After a single intravenous dose of [^{14}C]-palonosetron, approximately 80% of the dose was recovered within 144 hours in the urine with unchanged palonosetron representing approximately 40% of the administered dose.

DOSE IN RENAL IMPAIRMENT GFR (mL/MIN)

20–50	Dose as in normal renal function.
10–20	Dose as in normal renal function.
<10	Dose as in normal renal function.

DOSE IN PATIENTS UNDERGOING RENAL REPLACEMENT THERAPIES

CAPD	Unlikely to be dialysed. Dose as in normal renal function.
HD	Unlikely to be dialysed. Dose as in normal renal function.
HDF/High flux	Unknown dialysability. Dose as in normal renal function.
CAV/ VVHD	Unlikely to be dialysed. Dose as in normal renal function.

IMPORTANT DRUG INTERACTIONS

Potentially hazardous interactions with other drugs
- None known

ADMINISTRATION

RECONSTITUTION
–
ROUTE
- IV bolus, Oral
RATE OF ADMINISTRATION
- 30 seconds
COMMENTS
–

OTHER INFORMATION

- Repeated doses within 7 days are not recommended.
- Use with caution in people at risk of QT prolongation.

Pancreatin

CLINICAL USE

Pancreatic enzyme replacement

DOSE IN NORMAL RENAL FUNCTION

1–10 capsules (depends on preparation) with meals, adjusted according to response (1–2 capsules with meals if using the strong preparation)

PHARMACOKINETICS

Molecular weight (daltons)	No data
% Protein binding	No data
% Excreted unchanged in urine	No data
Volume of distribution (L/kg)	No data
Half-life – normal/ ESRF (hrs)	No data

METABOLISM

Pharmacokinetic data are not available as the enzymes act locally in the gastrointestinal tract. After exerting their action, the enzymes are digested themselves in the intestine.

DOSE IN RENAL IMPAIRMENT GFR (mL/MIN)

20–50	Dose as in normal renal function.
10–20	Dose as in normal renal function.
<10	Dose as in normal renal function.

DOSE IN PATIENTS UNDERGOING RENAL REPLACEMENT THERAPIES

CAPD	Unlikely to be dialysed. Dose as in normal renal function.
HD	Unlikely to be dialysed. Dose as in normal renal function.
HDF/High flux	Unlikely to be dialysed. Dose as in normal renal function.
CAV/ VVHD	Unlikely to be dialysed. Dose as in normal renal function.

IMPORTANT DRUG INTERACTIONS

Potentially hazardous interactions with other drugs
- None known

ADMINISTRATION

RECONSTITUTION
–
ROUTE
- Oral
RATE OF ADMINISTRATION
–
COMMENTS
–

OTHER INFORMATION

- Not absorbed from GI tract.

Pancuronium bromide

CLINICAL USE

Non-depolarising muscle relaxant of long duration

DOSE IN NORMAL RENAL FUNCTION

- Initial dose: 50–100 micrograms/kg then
- Incremental dose: 10–20 micrograms/kg as required
- Intensive care: Initially 100 mcg/kg (optional) then 60 mcg/kg every 60–90 minutes

PHARMACOKINETICS

Molecular weight (daltons)	732.7
% Protein binding	80–90
% Excreted unchanged in urine	40–60
Volume of distribution (L/kg)	0.15–0.38
Half-life – normal/ ESRF (hrs)	2/4.3–8.2

METABOLISM

A small proportion of pancuronium is metabolised in the liver to metabolites with weak neuromuscular blocking activity. It is largely excreted in urine as unchanged drug and metabolites; a small amount is excreted in bile.

DOSE IN RENAL IMPAIRMENT GFR (mL/MIN)

20–50	Dose as in normal renal function.
10–20	Initial dose: 25–50 micrograms/kg Incremental dose: 5–10 micrograms/kg
<10	Initial dose: 10–25 micrograms/kg Incremental dose: 2.5–5 micrograms/kg

DOSE IN PATIENTS UNDERGOING RENAL REPLACEMENT THERAPIES

CAPD	Unknown dialysability. Dose as in GFR<10 mL/min.
HD	Unknown dialysability. Dose as in GFR<10 mL/min.
HDF/High flux	Unknown dialysability. Dose as in GFR<10 mL/min.
CAV/ VVHD	Unknown dialysability. Dose as in GFR=10–20 mL/min.

IMPORTANT DRUG INTERACTIONS

Potentially hazardous interactions with other drugs
- Anaesthetics: enhanced muscle relaxant effect.
- Anti-arrhythmics: procainamide enhances muscle relaxant effect.
- Antibacterials: effect enhanced by aminoglycosides, clindamycin, polymyxins and piperacillin.
- Anti-epileptics: muscle relaxant effects antagonised by carbamazepine; effects reduced by long-term use of phenytoin but might be increased by acute use.
- Botulinum toxin: neuromuscular block enhanced (risk of toxicity).

ADMINISTRATION

RECONSTITUTION
–
ROUTE
- IV
RATE OF ADMINISTRATION
- Bolus
COMMENTS
–

OTHER INFORMATION

- Active metabolites accumulate in CKD 5; duration of action prolonged.
- Dose in severe renal impairment estimated from evaluation of pharmacokinetic data.
- Pancuronium distributes rapidly into extracellular fluid and the initial neuromuscular blockade produced will depend upon the peak drug concentration in this fluid. Since extracellular fluid volume is increased in chronic renal failure such patients may require a larger initial dose of pancuronium and a 45% increase in dose requirement has been reported in patients with end-stage renal failure. (Gramstad L. Atracurium, vecuronium and pancuronium in end-stage renal failure. *Br J Anaesth.* 1987; **59**: 995–1003.)

Panitumumab

CLINICAL USE

Monoclonal antibody:
- Treatment of metastatic colorectal cancer

DOSE IN NORMAL RENAL FUNCTION

6 mg/kg every 2 weeks
Consult relevant local protocol.

PHARMACOKINETICS

Molecular weight (daltons)	147 000
% Protein binding	No data
% Excreted unchanged in urine	No data
Volume of distribution (L/kg)	0.042^1
Half-life – normal/ ESRF (hrs)	3.6–10.9 days/–

METABOLISM

Saturable elimination mediated
via reticuloendothelial system, and
internalisation and degradation of EGFR.

DOSE IN RENAL IMPAIRMENT GFR (mL/MIN)

20–50	Dose as in normal renal function. Use with caution.
10–20	Dose as in normal renal function. Use with caution.
<10	Dose as in normal renal function. Use with caution.

DOSE IN PATIENTS UNDERGOING RENAL REPLACEMENT THERAPIES

CAPD	Unlikely to be dialysed. Dose as in GFR<10 mL/min.
HD	Unlikely to be dialysed. Dose as in GFR<10 mL/min.
HDF/High flux	Unlikely to be dialysed. Dose as in GFR<10 mL/min.
CAV/ VVHD	Unlikely to be dialysed. Dose as in GFR=10–20 mL/min.

IMPORTANT DRUG INTERACTIONS

Potentially hazardous interactions with other drugs
- Live vaccines: avoid concomitant use.

ADMINISTRATION

RECONSTITUTION
–
ROUTE
- IV
RATE OF ADMINISTRATION
- Over 30–90 minutes depending on dose and tolerability
COMMENTS
- Dilute in sodium chloride 0.9% to 100 mL to not less than 10 mg/mL.
- Infuse through a 0.2 or 0.22 micron in-line filter.

OTHER INFORMATION

- Manufacturer is unable to provide a dose in renal impairment due to lack of studies although renal impairment did not affect the pharmacokinetics.

Reference:
1. www.bccancer.bc.ca/.../Panitumumabmon ograph_1October2011.pdf

Pantoprazole

CLINICAL USE

Gastric acid suppression

DOSE IN NORMAL RENAL FUNCTION

- Oral: 20–80 mg in the morning
- IV: 40–160 mg daily; doses >80 mg in 2 divided doses

PHARMACOKINETICS

Molecular weight (daltons)	383.4
% Protein binding	98
% Excreted unchanged in urine	80 (as metabolites)
Volume of distribution (L/kg)	0.15
Half-life – normal/ ESRF (hrs)	1/2–3

METABOLISM

Pantoprazole is extensively metabolised in the liver, primarily by the cytochrome P450 isoenzyme CYP2C19, to desmethylpantoprazole; small amounts are also metabolised by CYP3A4, CYP2D6, and CYP2C9.

Metabolites are excreted mainly (about 80%) in the urine, with the remainder being excreted in faeces via the bile.

DOSE IN RENAL IMPAIRMENT GFR (mL/MIN)

20–50	Dose as in normal renal function.
10–20	Dose as in normal renal function.
<10	Dose as in normal renal function.

DOSE IN PATIENTS UNDERGOING RENAL REPLACEMENT THERAPIES

CAPD	Not dialysed. Dose as in normal renal function.
HD	Not dialysed. Dose as in normal renal function.
HDF/High flux	Unknown dialysability. Dose as in normal renal function.
CAV/ VVHD	Unknown dialysability. Dose as in normal renal function.

IMPORTANT DRUG INTERACTIONS

Potentially hazardous interactions with other drugs

- Anticoagulants: effect of coumarins possibly enhanced.
- Antifungals: absorption of itraconazole and ketoconazole reduced; avoid with posaconazole.
- Antivirals: concentration of atazanavir and rilpivirine reduced – avoid concomitant use; concentration of raltegravir and saquinavir possibly increased – avoid.
- Clopidogrel: possibly reduced anti-platelet effect.
- Cytotoxics: possibly reduced excretion of methotrexate; avoid with erlotinib and vandetanib; possibly reduced lapatinib absorption; possibly reduced absorption of pazopanib.
- Ulipristal: reduced contraceptive effect, avoid with high dose ulipristal.

ADMINISTRATION

RECONSTITUTION
- 10 mL sodium chloride 0.9%

ROUTE
- Oral, IV

RATE OF ADMINISTRATION
- 2–15 minutes

COMMENTS
- Use within 12 hours of reconstitution.
- Dilute to 100 mL with sodium chloride 0.9% or glucose 5%.

Papaveretum

Opiate analgesia
(15.4 mg/mL) 1 mL contains 10 mg anhydrous morphine, 1.2 mg papaverine HCl, and 1.04 mg codeine HCl

DOSE IN NORMAL RENAL FUNCTION

- SC/IM: 0.5–1 mL (7.7–15.4 mg) every 4 hours
- IV: 25–50% of dose

PHARMACOKINETICS

	Papaverine HCl	Morphine HCl	Codeine HCl
Molecular weight (daltons)	375.8	375.8	371.9
% Protein binding	90	20–35	7
% Excreted unchanged in urine	<1	10	<5
Volume of distribution (L/kg)	0.99–1.52	3–5	3–4
Half-life – normal/ ESRF (hrs)	1.2–2.2/–	2–3/ Un- changed	2.5–4/–

METABOLISM

Papaverine: Mainly metabolised in the liver and excreted in the urine, almost entirely as glucuronide-conjugated phenolic metabolites.

DOSE IN RENAL IMPAIRMENT GFR (mL/MIN)

20–50	Dose as in normal renal function.
10–20	0.4–0.75 mL every 6–8 hours.
<10	0.25–0.5 mL every 6–8 hours. Avoid if possible.

DOSE IN PATIENTS UNDERGOING RENAL REPLACEMENT THERAPIES

CAPD	Unlikely to be dialysed. Dose as in GFR<10 mL/min.
HD	Unlikely to be dialysed. Dose as in GFR<10 mL/min.
HDF/High flux	Unlikely to be dialysed. Dose as in GFR<10 mL/min.
CAV/ VVHD	Unknown dialysability. Dose as in GFR=10–20 mL/min.

IMPORTANT DRUG INTERACTIONS

Potentially hazardous interactions with other drugs
- Anti-arrhythmics: delayed absorption of mexiletine.
- Antidepressants: possible CNS excitation or depression with MAOIs – avoid concomitant use; possible CNS excitation or depression with moclobemide; increased sedative effects with tricyclics.
- Antihistamines: increased sedative effects with sedating antihistamines.
- Antipsychotics: enhanced hypotensive and sedative effects.
- Dopaminergics: avoid with selegiline.
- Sodium oxybate: enhanced effect of sodium oxybate – avoid concomitant use.

ADMINISTRATION

RECONSTITUTION
–
ROUTE
- SC, IM, IV
RATE OF ADMINISTRATION
- IV bolus or continuous infusion (1 mg/mL)
COMMENTS
–

OTHER INFORMATION

- As with all opiates, use with extreme caution in patients with impaired renal function.
- May cause excessive sedation and respiratory depression.
- Papaveretum 15.4 mg =1 mL ≡ 10 mg morphine.

Paracetamol

CLINICAL USE

Analgesia and antipyretic

DOSE IN NORMAL RENAL FUNCTION

500 mg – 1 g every 4–6 hours, maximum 4 g daily
(IV: if <50 kg, dose is 15 mg/kg)

PHARMACOKINETICS

Molecular weight (daltons)	151.2
% Protein binding	20–30
% Excreted unchanged in urine	<5
Volume of distribution (L/kg)	1–2
Half-life – normal/ ESRF (hrs)	1–4/Unchanged

METABOLISM

Paracetamol is metabolised mainly in the liver and excreted in the urine mainly as the glucuronide and sulfate conjugates. Less than 5% is excreted as unchanged paracetamol. A minor hydroxylated metabolite (N-acetyl-p-benzoquinoneimine) is usually produced in very small amounts by cytochrome P450 isoenzymes (mainly CYP2E1 and CYP3A4) in the liver and kidney. It is usually detoxified by conjugation with glutathione but may accumulate after paracetamol overdosage and cause tissue damage.

DOSE IN RENAL IMPAIRMENT GFR (mL/MIN)

20–50	Dose as in normal renal function.
10–20	Dose as in normal renal function.
<10	500 mg – 1 g every 6–8 hours.

DOSE IN PATIENTS UNDERGOING RENAL REPLACEMENT THERAPIES

CAPD	Not dialysed. Dose as in GFR<10 mL/min.
HD	Dialysed. Dose as in GFR<10 mL/min.
HDF/High flux	Dialysed. Dose as in GFR<10 mL/min.
CAV/VVHD	Unknown dialysability. Dose as in normal renal function.

IMPORTANT DRUG INTERACTIONS

Potentially hazardous interactions with other drugs
• None known

ADMINISTRATION

RECONSTITUTION
–
ROUTE
• Oral, rectal, IV
RATE OF ADMINISTRATION
• 15 minutes
COMMENTS
–

OTHER INFORMATION

• Beware sodium content of soluble tablets (1 tablet ≡ 18.6 mmol sodium).
• Nephrotoxic in overdose due to a reactive alkylating metabolite.
• Metabolites may accumulate in CKD 5; normal doses are used in CKD 5.
• In smaller patients with CKD 5 a maximum oral dose of 3 g per day should be considered.
• IV preparation starts working within 5 to 10 minutes with peak activity after 60 minutes.

Parathyroid hormone

CLINICAL USE

Treatment of osteoporosis in postmenopausal women at increased risk of fractures

DOSE IN NORMAL RENAL FUNCTION

100 mcg daily

PHARMACOKINETICS

Molecular weight (daltons)	9420
% Protein binding	No data
% Excreted unchanged in urine	0 (all broken down into small fragments)
Volume of distribution (L/kg)	5.4 litres
Half-life – normal/ ESRF (hrs)	1.5/–

METABOLISM

Parathyroid hormone is metabolised in the liver and to a lesser degree in the kidney. Parathyroid hormone is not excreted from the body in its intact form. Circulating carboxy-terminal fragments are filtered by the kidney, but are subsequently broken to even smaller fragments during tubular reuptake.

Parathyroid hormone is efficiently removed from the blood by a receptor-mediated process in the liver and is broken down into smaller peptide fragments. The fragments derived from the amino-terminus are further degraded within the cell while the fragments derived from the carboxy-terminus are released back into the blood and cleared by the kidney. These carboxy-terminal fragments are thought to play a role in the regulation of parathyroid hormone activity.

DOSE IN RENAL IMPAIRMENT GFR (mL/MIN)

30–50	Dose as in normal renal function.
10–30	Avoid.
<10	Avoid.

DOSE IN PATIENTS UNDERGOING RENAL REPLACEMENT THERAPIES

CAPD	Unlikely to be dialysed. Dose as in GFR<10 mL/min.
HD	Unlikely to be dialysed. Dose as in GFR<10 mL/min.
HDF/High flux	Unlikely to be dialysed. Dose as in GFR<10 mL/min.
CAV/ VVHD	Unlikely to be dialysed. Dose as in GFR=10–30 mL/min.

IMPORTANT DRUG INTERACTIONS

Potentially hazardous interactions with other drugs
- None known.

ADMINISTRATION

RECONSTITUTION
–

ROUTE
- SC

RATE OF ADMINISTRATION
–

OTHER INFORMATION

- There is no data available in patients with severe renal impairment.
- Bioavailability is 55%.
- The overall exposure and C_{max} of parathyroid hormone were slightly increased (22% and 56%, respectively) in a group of 8 male and 8 female subjects with mild-to-moderate renal impairment (creatinine clearances of 30 to 80 mL/min) compared with a matched group of 16 subjects with normal renal function.

Parecoxib

CLINICAL USE

Cox 2 inhibitor:
- Short-term treatment of postoperative pain

DOSE IN NORMAL RENAL FUNCTION

- 40 mg initially then 20–40 mg every 6–12 hours if required; maximum dose 80 mg daily
- Elderly weighing <50 kg: 20–40 mg daily

PHARMACOKINETICS

Molecular weight (daltons)	392.4 (as sodium salt)
% Protein binding	98
% Excreted unchanged in urine	<5 (as valdecoxib)
Volume of distribution (L/kg)	55 litres
Half-life – normal/ESRF (hrs)	8 (as valdecoxib)/ Unchanged

METABOLISM

Parecoxib is rapidly and almost completely converted to valdecoxib and propionic acid. Elimination of valdecoxib is by extensive hepatic metabolism involving multiple pathways, including cytochrome P 450 (CYP) 3A4 and CYP2C9 isoenzymes and glucuronidation (about 20%) of the sulphonamide moiety. Excretion is mainly via the urine with about 70% of a dose appearing as inactive metabolites. Less than 5% of a dose appears as unchanged valdecoxib in the urine. No unchanged parecoxib is found in the urine with only trace amounts in the faeces.

DOSE IN RENAL IMPAIRMENT GFR (mL/MIN)

30–50	Dose as in normal renal function. Use with caution.
10–30	Dose as in normal renal function, but avoid if possible.
<10	Dose as in normal renal function, but only use if ERF on dialysis.

DOSE IN PATIENTS UNDERGOING RENAL REPLACEMENT THERAPIES

CAPD	Not dialysed. Dose as in GFR<10 mL/min.
HD	Not dialysed. Dose as in GFR<10 mL/min.
HDF/High flux	Not dialysed. Dose as in GFR<10 mL/min.
CAV/ VVHD	Not dialysed. Dose as in GFR=10–30 mL/min.

IMPORTANT DRUG INTERACTIONS

Potentially hazardous interactions with other drugs
- ACE inhibitors and angiotensin-II antagonists: antagonism of hypotensive effect; increased risk of nephrotoxicity and hyperkalaemia.
- Analgesics: avoid concomitant use of 2 or more NSAIDs, including aspirin (increased side effects); avoid with ketorolac (increased risk of side effects and haemorrhage).
- Antibacterials: possible increased risk of convulsions with quinolones.
- Anticoagulants: effects of coumarins and phenindione enhanced; possibly increased risk of bleeding with heparins and dabigatran.
- Antidepressants: increased risk of bleeding with SSRIs and venlafaxine.
- Antidiabetics: possibly enhanced effect of sulphonylureas.
- Anti-epileptics: possibly enhanced effect of phenytoin.
- Antifungals: if used with fluconazole reduce the dose of parecoxib.
- Antivirals: increased risk of haematological toxicity with zidovudine; concentration possibly increased by ritonavir.
- Ciclosporin: potential for increased risk of nephrotoxicity.
- Cytotoxic agents: reduced excretion of methotrexate (possible increased risk of toxicity); increased risk of bleeding with erlotinib.
- Diuretics: increased risk of nephrotoxicity; possible antagonism of diuretic effect; increased risk of hyperkalaemia with potassium-sparing diuretics.
- Lithium: reduced excretion of lithium (risk of toxicity).
- Pentoxifylline: possibly increased risk of bleeding.
- Tacrolimus: increased risk of nephrotoxicity.

ADMINISTRATION

RECONSTITUTION
- 2 mL sodium chloride 0.9%

ROUTE
- IV, IM

RATE OF ADMINISTRATION
–

OTHER INFORMATION

- Clinical trials have shown renal effects similar to those observed with comparative NSAIDs. Monitor patient for deterioration in renal function and fluid retention.
- Inhibition of renal prostaglandin synthesis by NSAIDs may interfere with renal function, especially in the presence of existing renal disease – avoid if possible; if not, check serum creatinine 48–72 hours after starting NSAID – if raised, discontinue NSAID therapy.
- Use normal doses in patients with ERF on dialysis.
- Use with caution in renal transplant recipients (can reduce intrarenal autocoid synthesis).
- Parecoxib should be used with caution in uraemic patients predisposed to gastrointestinal bleeding or uraemic coagulopathies.
- Works within 30 minutes.
- Contraindicated in patients with ischaemic heart disease or cerebrovascular disease and class II-IV NYHA congestive heart failure.

Paricalcitol

CLINICAL USE

Vitamin D analogue:
- Treatment and prevention of secondary hyperparathyroidism associated with chronic renal failure

DOSE IN NORMAL RENAL FUNCTION

- IV: Give dose every other day or post dialysis; dose is dependent on PTH levels. See SPC for details.
- Oral: 1–4 mcg either daily or 3×/week according to PTH levels.

PHARMACOKINETICS

Molecular weight (daltons)	416.6
% Protein binding	>99
% Excreted unchanged in urine	0 (16% as metabolites)
Volume of distribution (L/kg)	17–25 litres (6 litres in haemodialysis patients)
Half-life – normal/ ESRF (hrs)	15 (oral 5–7)/ Unchanged

METABOLISM

Extensively metabolised via hepatic and non-hepatic pathways to form two relatively inactive metabolites. After oral administration of ^{3}H-paricalcitol, only about 2% of the dose was eliminated unchanged in the faeces, and no parent drug found in the urine. Approximately 70% of the radioactivity was eliminated in the faeces and 18% was recovered in the urine. Most of the systemic exposure was from the parent drug.

DOSE IN RENAL IMPAIRMENT GFR (mL/MIN)

20–50	Dose as in normal renal function.
10–20	Dose as in normal renal function.
<10	Dose as in normal renal function.

DOSE IN PATIENTS UNDERGOING RENAL REPLACEMENT THERAPIES

CAPD	Not dialysed. Dose as in normal renal function.
HD	Not dialysed. Dose as in normal renal function.
HDF/High flux	Unknown dialysability. Dose as in normal renal function.
CAV/ VVHD	Not dialysed. Dose as in normal renal function.

IMPORTANT DRUG INTERACTIONS

Potentially hazardous interactions with other drugs
- None known

ADMINISTRATION

RECONSTITUTION
–
ROUTE
- IV, Oral
RATE OF ADMINISTRATION
- Not less than 30 seconds
COMMENTS
–

OTHER INFORMATION

- Monitor calcium and phosphate levels at least monthly, more frequently during dose titration.
- Paricalcitol solution for injection contains 30% v/v of propylene glycol as an excipient. Isolated cases of central nervous system depression, haemolysis, and lactic acidosis have been reported as toxic effects associated with propylene glycol administration at high doses. Although they are not expected to be found with paricalcitol administration (as propylene glycol is eliminated during the dialysis process), the risk of toxic effect in overdosing situations has to be taken into account.
- Paricalcitol injection contains 20% v/v of ethanol (alcohol). Each dose may contain up to 1.3 g ethanol. Harmful for those suffering from alcoholism.

Paroxetine

CLINICAL USE

Antidepressant:
- Panic disorders
- Obsessive compulsive disorder
- Social anxiety
- Post traumatic stress disorder

DOSE IN NORMAL RENAL FUNCTION

10–60 mg daily depending on indication

PHARMACOKINETICS

Molecular weight (daltons)	329.4
% Protein binding	95
% Excreted unchanged in urine	<2
Volume of distribution (L/kg)	13
Half-life – normal/ ESRF (hrs)	24/30

METABOLISM

Paroxetine is extensively metabolised in the liver to pharmacologically inactive metabolites. Urinary excretion of unchanged paroxetine is generally less than 2% of dose while that of metabolites is about 64% of dose. About 36% of the dose is excreted in faeces, probably via the bile, of which unchanged paroxetine represents less than 1% of the dose. Thus paroxetine is eliminated almost entirely by metabolism.

DOSE IN RENAL IMPAIRMENT GFR (mL/MIN)

30–50	Dose as in normal renal function.
10–30	20 mg daily and titrate slowly.
<10	20 mg daily and titrate slowly.

DOSE IN PATIENTS UNDERGOING RENAL REPLACEMENT THERAPIES

CAPD	Unlikely to be dialysed. Dose as in GFR<10 mL/min.
HD	Not dialysed. Dose as in GFR<10 mL/min.
HDF/High flux	Unknown dialysability. Dose as in GFR<10 mL/min.
CAV/ VVHD	Unknown dialysability. Dose as for GFR=10–30 mL/min.

IMPORTANT DRUG INTERACTIONS

Potentially hazardous interactions with other drugs
- Analgesics: increased risk of bleeding with aspirin and NSAIDs; risk of CNS toxicity increased with tramadol; concentration of methadone possibly increased.
- Anti-arrhythmics: possibly inhibits propafenone metabolism (increased risk of toxicity).
- Anticoagulants: effect of coumarins possibly enhanced; possibly increased risk of bleeding with dabigatran.
- Antidepressants: avoid concomitant use with MAOIs and moclobemide (increased risk of toxicity); avoid concomitant use with St John's wort; possibly enhanced serotonergic effects with duloxetine; can increase concentration of tricyclics; increased agitation and nausea with tryptophan.
- Anti-epileptics: antagonism (lowered convulsive threshold); concentration reduced by phenytoin and phenobarbital.
- Antimalarials: avoid concomitant use with artemether/lumefantrine and piperaquine with artenimol.
- Antipsychotics: concentration of clozapine and possibly risperidone increased; metabolism of perphenazine inhibited, reduce dose of perphenazine; possibly inhibits aripiprazole metabolism, reduce aripiprazole dose; concentration possibly increased by asenapine; increased risk of ventricular arrhythmias with pimozide – avoid.
- Antivirals: concentration possibly reduced by darunavir and ritonavir.
- Dopaminergics: increased risk of hypertension and CNS excitation with selegiline – avoid concomitant use; increased risk of CNS toxicity with rasagiline – avoid concomitant use.
- Hormone antagonists: metabolism of tamoxifen to active metabolite possibly reduced – avoid.
- $5HT_1$ agonist: risk of CNS toxicity increased by sumatriptan – avoid concomitant use; possibly increased risk of serotonergic effects with naratriptan.
- Lithium: increased risk of CNS effects – monitor levels.
- Methylthioninium: risk of CNS toxicity – avoid if possible.

ADMINISTRATION

RECONSTITUTION

–

ROUTE

● Oral

RATE OF ADMINISTRATION

–

COMMENTS

–

Pazopanib

CLINICAL USE

Tyrosine kinase inhibitor:
● Treatment of metastatic renal cell carcinoma & soft tissue sarcoma

DOSE IN NORMAL RENAL FUNCTION

800 mg once daily
Consult relevant local protocol

PHARMACOKINETICS

Molecular weight (daltons)	474 (as hydrochloride)
% Protein binding	>99
% Excreted unchanged in urine	<4
Volume of distribution (L/kg)	Large
Half-life – normal/ ESRF (hrs)	30.9/Unchanged

METABOLISM

Metabolism primarily by CYP3A4, with minor contributions from CYP1A2 and CYP2C8. The four principal pazopanib metabolites account for only 6% of the exposure in plasma. One of these metabolites inhibits the proliferation of VEGF-stimulated human umbilical vein endothelial cells with a similar potency to that of pazopanib, the others are 10- to 20-fold less active. Therefore, activity of pazopanib is mainly dependent on parent pazopanib exposure.

Elimination is mostly via the faeces with less than 4% in the urine.

DOSE IN RENAL IMPAIRMENT GFR (mL/MIN)

30–50	Dose as in normal renal function.
10–30	Dose as in normal renal function. Use with caution.
<10	Dose as in normal renal function. Use with caution.

DOSE IN PATIENTS UNDERGOING RENAL REPLACEMENT THERAPIES

CAPD	Not dialysed. Dose as in GFR<10 mL/min.
HD	Not dialysed. Dose as in GFR<10 mL/min.
HDF/High flux	Not dialysed. Dose as in GFR<10 mL/min.
CAV/ VVHD	Not dialysed. Dose as in GFR=10–30 mL/min.

IMPORTANT DRUG INTERACTIONS

Potentially hazardous interactions with other drugs
● Antibacterials: avoid concomitant use with clarithromycin, rifampicin & telithromycin.
● Antifungals: avoid concomitant use with itraconazole, ketoconazole & voriconazole.
● Antipsychotics: avoid concomitant use with clozapine (increased risk of agranulocytosis).
● Antivirals: avoid concomitant use with atazanavir, indinavir, ritonavir, saquinavir & boceprevir.
● Grapefruit juice: avoid concomitant administration.
● Avoid concomitant use with other inhibitors or inducers of CYP3A4. Dose alterations may be required.

ADMINISTRATION

RECONSTITUTION
–
ROUTE
● Oral
RATE OF ADMINISTRATION
–

OTHER INFORMATION

● Manufacturer advises to use pazopanib with caution if GFR<30 mL/min due to lack of studies but clearance is unlikely to be affected due to low renal excretion.
● LFTs should be measured before and regularly during treatment.

Pegfilgrastim

CLINICAL USE

Pegylated recombinant human granulocyte-colony stimulating factor (rhG-CSF):
- Reduction of duration of neutropenia (except in chronic myeloid leukaemia and myelodysplastic syndromes).

DOSE IN NORMAL RENAL FUNCTION

6 mg given approximately 24 hours post chemotherapy

PHARMACOKINETICS

Molecular weight (daltons)	39 000
% Protein binding	Very high (filgrastim)
% Excreted unchanged in urine	Minimal
Volume of distribution (L/kg)	0.15 (filgrastim)
Half-life – normal/ ESRF (hrs)	15–80/Unchanged

METABOLISM

Eliminated by neutrophil-mediated clearance.

DOSE IN RENAL IMPAIRMENT GFR (mL/MIN)

20–50	Dose as in normal renal function.
10–20	Dose as in normal renal function.
<10	Dose as in normal renal function.

DOSE IN PATIENTS UNDERGOING RENAL REPLACEMENT THERAPIES

CAPD	Not dialysed. Dose as in normal renal function.
HD	Not dialysed. Dose as in normal renal function.
HDF/High flux	Unlikely to be dialysed. Dose as in normal renal function.
CAV/ VVHD	Not dialysed. Dose as in normal renal function.

IMPORTANT DRUG INTERACTIONS

Potentially hazardous interactions with other drugs
- Cytotoxics: neutropenia possibly exacerbated if administered with fluorouracil.

ADMINISTRATION

RECONSTITUTION
–
ROUTE
- SC
RATE OF ADMINISTRATION
–
COMMENTS
- Incompatible with sodium chloride solutions.
- Discard after 72 hours if left at room temperature.

OTHER INFORMATION

- Pegfilgrastim is a sustained-release form of filgrastim.

Peginterferon alfa

CLINICAL USE

Treatment of chronic hepatitis B and C infection with or without ribavirin

DOSE IN NORMAL RENAL FUNCTION

- ViraferonPeg: 1.5 mcg/kg once weekly in combination with ribavirin
- Monotherapy: 0.5–1 mcg/kg once weekly
- Pegasys: 180 mcg weekly

PHARMACOKINETICS

Molecular weight (daltons)	40 000
% Protein binding	No data
% Excreted unchanged in urine	30
Volume of distribution (L/kg)	0.99
Half-life – normal/ ESRF (hrs)	40–80/Increased by about 25–45%

METABOLISM

The metabolism is not known. Clearance is via the kidneys.

DOSE IN RENAL IMPAIRMENT GFR (mL/MIN)

30–50	Pegasys: Dose as in normal renal function. ViraferonPeg: Reduce starting dose by 25%. See 'Other information'.
10–30	Pegasys: 135 mcg once weekly. ViraferonPeg: Reduce dose by 50%. See 'Other information'.
<10	Pegasys: 135 mcg once weekly. ViraferonPeg: Reduce dose and use with caution. See 'Other information'.

DOSE IN PATIENTS UNDERGOING RENAL REPLACEMENT THERAPIES

CAPD	Unlikely to be dialysed. Dose as in GFR<10 mL/min.
HD	Dialysed. Dose as in GFR<10 mL/min. See 'Other information'.
HDF/High flux	Dialysed. Dose as in GFR<10 mL/min. See 'Other information'.
CAV/ VVHD	Unknown dialysability. Dose as in GFR=10–30 mL/min.

IMPORTANT DRUG INTERACTIONS

Potentially hazardous interactions with other drugs

- Antivirals: use adefovir with caution; increased risk of peripheral neuropathy with telbivudine.
- Immunosuppressants: (e.g. ciclosporin, tacrolimus, sirolimus) may have an antagonistic effect.
- Theophylline: inhibits metabolism of theophylline (enhanced effect).

ADMINISTRATION

RECONSTITUTION
- 0.7 mL water for injection or pre-filled syringes

ROUTE
- SC

RATE OF ADMINISTRATION
-

COMMENTS
- Stable for 24 hours at 2–8°C after reconstitution.

OTHER INFORMATION

- Administer 12 hours after haemodialysis
- ViraferonPeg should be used with caution if GFR<10 mL/min due to lack of studies.
- If renal function deteriorates discontinue ViraferonPeg.
- US SPC suggests using 50% of the dose in haemodialysis patients and monitor carefully.
- In haemodialysis patients, 135 mcg Pegasys is equivalent to a 180 mcg dose in the general population. Reduce to 90 mcg if required due to adverse effects.
- In patients with CKD 5 undergoing haemodialysis there is a 25–45% reduction in clearance compared with patients with normal renal function.

Pemetrexed

CLINICAL USE

- Treatment of chemotherapy naive patients with unresectable malignant pleural mesothelioma in combination with cisplatin
- Monotherapy for non-small cell lung cancer

DOSE IN NORMAL RENAL FUNCTION

$500 \, mg/m^2$ on the first day of each 21 day cycle

PHARMACOKINETICS

Molecular weight (daltons)	471.4 (as disodium)
% Protein binding	81
% Excreted unchanged in urine	70–90
Volume of distribution (L/kg)	6–9 litres/m^2
Half-life – normal/ESRF (hrs)	2–4/Increased

METABOLISM

Pemetrexed undergoes minimal hepatic metabolism, and about 70–90% of a dose is eliminated unchanged in the urine within 24 hours. *In vitro* studies indicate that pemetrexed is actively secreted by OAT3 (organic anion transporter).

DOSE IN RENAL IMPAIRMENT GFR (mL/MIN)

45–50	Dose as in normal renal function.
20–45	Use with caution, at a lower dose. See 'Other information'.
<20	Use with caution, at a lower dose. See 'Other information'.

DOSE IN PATIENTS UNDERGOING RENAL REPLACEMENT THERAPIES

CAPD	Unlikely to be dialysed. Dose as in GFR<20 mL/min.
HD	Not dialysed.[1] Dose as in GFR<20 mL/min.
HDF/High flux	Unlikely to be dialysed. Dose as in GFR<20 mL/min.
CAV/ VVHD	Not dialysed.[1] Dose as in GFR=20–45 mL/min.

IMPORTANT DRUG INTERACTIONS

Potentially hazardous interactions with other drugs
- Antimalarials: antifolate effect increased by pyrimethamine.
- Antipsychotics: avoid with clozapine, increased risk of agranulocytosis.
- Nephrotoxic agents: may reduce clearance of pemetrexed – use with caution.
- Live vaccines: avoid use; YELLOW FEVER VACCINE ABSOLUTELY CONTRAINDICATED.

ADMINISTRATION

RECONSTITUTION
- 20 mL sodium chloride 0.9% per 500 mg vial

ROUTE
- IV infusion

RATE OF ADMINISTRATION
- Over 10 minutes

COMMENTS
- Dilute in 100 mL preservative-free sodium chloride 0.9%.
- Incompatible with calcium containing fluids.

OTHER INFORMATION

- Not recommended by manufacturer if GFR<45 mL/min due to lack of data.
- To reduce the incidence and severity of skin reactions, a steroid (equivalent to 4 mg of dexamethasone) should be given the day before, the day of, and the day after pemetrexed therapy. Patients should also take a vitamin preparation containing folic acid and IM vitamin B12.
- 25% of patients get reversible mild renal dysfunction.
- There has been a case report of a patient having severe rhabdomyolysis with pemetrexed in combination treatment with carboplatin. (Wan Y. Case report: severe rhabdomyolysis associated with pemetrexed. *Lancet Oncology*. 2006; 7(4): 353.)
- In one study, pemetrexed was discontinued in patients with a GFR<30 mL/min after a patient with a GFR=19 mL/min died due to drug related toxicities. (Mita C, Sweeney CJ, Baker SD, *et al*. Phase I and pharmacokinetic study of pemetrexed administered every 3 weeks to advanced cancer patients with normal and impaired renal function. *J Clin Oncol*. 2006; 24(4): 552–62.)

Reference:
1. Brandes JC, Grossman SA, Ahmad H. Alteration of pemetrexed excretion in the presence of acute renal failure and effusions: presentation of a case and review of the literature. *Cancer Invest*. 2006; 24(3): 283–7.

Penicillamine

CLINICAL USE

Rheumatoid arthritis, Wilson's disease, cystinuria
Lead poisoning, chronic active hepatitis

DOSE IN NORMAL RENAL FUNCTION

- Rheumatoid arthritis: 125–250 mg daily for first month; increase by same amount every 4–12 weeks until remission occurs. Maintenance dose: usually 500–750 mg daily in divided doses. Maximum 1.5 g daily
- Wilson's disease: 750–2000 mg daily in divided doses
- Cystinuria: Dissolution: 1–3 g daily in divided doses
  Prevention: 500–1000 mg on retiring
- Lead poisoning: 1–1.5 g daily in divided doses
- Chronic active hepatitis: 500–1250 mg daily in divided doses.

PHARMACOKINETICS

Molecular weight (daltons)	149.2
% Protein binding	80
% Excreted unchanged in urine	10–40
Volume of distribution (L/kg)	0.8
Half-life – normal/ ESRF (hrs)	1–3/Increased

METABOLISM

Penicillamine undergoes limited metabolism in the liver, to S-methyl penicillamine. It is mainly excreted in the urine as disulfides, along with some S-methyl penicillamine and unchanged drug; a small amount may be excreted in the faeces.

DOSE IN RENAL IMPAIRMENT GFR (mL/MIN)

20–50	Avoid if possible or reduce dose. 125 mg for first 12 weeks. Increase by same amount every 12 weeks.
10–20	Avoid – nephrotoxic.
<10	Avoid – nephrotoxic.

DOSE IN PATIENTS UNDERGOING RENAL REPLACEMENT THERAPIES

CAPD	Unknown dialysability. Avoid – nephrotoxic.
HD	Dialysed. 125–250 mg 3 times a week after HD.
HDF/High flux	Dialysed. 125–250 mg 3 times a week after HD.
CAV/ VVHD	Dialysed. Avoid – nephrotoxic.

IMPORTANT DRUG INTERACTIONS

Potentially hazardous interactions with other drugs
- Antipsychotics: avoid concomitant use with clozapine (increased risk of agranulocytosis).

ADMINISTRATION

RECONSTITUTION
–
ROUTE
- Oral
RATE OF ADMINISTRATION
–
COMMENTS
–

OTHER INFORMATION

- Proteinuria occurs frequently and is partially dose-related. In some patients it may progress to glomerulonephritis or nephrotic syndrome.
- Dose in haemodialysis is from *Drug Dosage in Renal Insufficiency* by Seyffart G and *Drug Prescribing in Renal Failure*, 5th edition, by Aronoff *et al.*
- Urinalysis should be carried out weekly for the first two months of treatment, after any change in dosage, and monthly thereafter. Increasing proteinuria may necessitate withdrawal of treatment.

Pentamidine isetionate

CLINICAL USE

Antibacterial agent:
- Pneumocystis treatment and prophylaxis
- Visceral leishmaniasis
- Cutaneous leishmaniasis
- Trypanosomiasis

DOSE IN NORMAL RENAL FUNCTION

- Pneumocystis:
  - Treatment: Nebuliser: 600 mg daily for 3 weeks;
  - IV: 4 mg/kg/day for at least 14 days
  - Prophylaxis: 300 mg monthly or 150 mg every 2 weeks
- Visceral leishmaniasis: 3–4 mg/kg on alternate days to a maximum of 10 doses (deep IM)
- Cutaneous leishmaniasis: 3–4 mg/kg once or twice weekly (deep IM)
- Trypanosomiasis: 4 mg/kg daily, or alternate days to a total of 7–10 doses (deep IM or IV)

PHARMACOKINETICS

Molecular weight (daltons)	592.7
% Protein binding	69
% Excreted unchanged in urine	<5
Volume of distribution (L/kg)	3–4
Half-life – normal/ ESRF (hrs)	6–9/9

METABOLISM

Extensively hepatically metabolised.
Renal clearance accounts for <5% of the plasma clearance of pentamidine.

DOSE IN RENAL IMPAIRMENT GFR (mL/MIN)

20–50	Dose as in normal renal function.
10–20	Dose as in normal renal function.
<10	Depending on severity of infection: 4 mg/kg/day IV for 7–10 days, then on alternate days to complete minimum 14 doses, OR, 4 mg/kg on alternate days to complete minimum 14 doses.

DOSE IN PATIENTS UNDERGOING RENAL REPLACEMENT THERAPIES

CAPD	Not dialysed. Dose as in GFR<10 mL/min.
HD	Not dialysed. Dose as in GFR<10 mL/min.
HDF/High flux	Unknown dialysability. Dose as in GFR<10 mL/min.
CAV/ VVHD	Unknown dialysability. Dose as in GFR=10–20 mL/min.

IMPORTANT DRUG INTERACTIONS

Potentially hazardous interactions with other drugs
- Anti-arrhythmics: increased risk of ventricular arrhythmias with amiodarone – avoid concomitant use; possible increased risk of ventricular arrhythmias with disopyramide.
- Antibacterials: increased risk of ventricular arrhythmias with moxifloxacin and parenteral erythromycin – avoid concomitant use with moxifloxacin; increased risk of ventricular arrhythmias with parenteral pentamidine and telithromycin.
- Antidepressants: increased risk of ventricular arrhythmias with tricyclics.
- Antimalarials: increased risk of ventricular arrhythmias with piperaquine with artenimol – avoid.
- Antipsychotics: increased risk of ventricular arrhythmias with amisulpride, droperidol and phenothiazines – avoid concomitant use with amisulpride and droperidol.
- Antivirals: increased risk of hypocalcaemia with parenteral pentamidine and foscarnet; increased risk of ventricular arrhythmias with saquinavir – avoid.
- Cytotoxics: increased risk of ventricular arrhythmias with vandetanib – avoid.
- Ivabradine: increased risk of ventricular arrhythmias.

ADMINISTRATION

RECONSTITUTION
- IV: 300 mg with 3–5 mL water for injection
- IM: 300 mg with 3 mL water for injection
- Inhalation: 600 mg with 6 mL water for injection

ROUTE
- IV, IM, nebulised

RATE OF ADMINISTRATION
- Over at least 1 hour

COMMENTS
- Dilute calculated dose in 50–250 mL sodium chloride 0.9% or glucose 5%.

OTHER INFORMATION

- Monitor patients closely.
- Patient must be lying down when drug is administered intravenously.
- If given by IV infusion, patient should be monitored closely: heart rate, blood pressure, blood glucose.

- IV prophylaxis (unlicensed): 4–5 mg/kg over a minimum of 1 hour every 4 weeks.
- Nebulise over 20 minutes using Respigard II or other suitable nebuliser, oxygen flow rate 6–10 L/minute.
- 5 mg nebulised salbutamol may be given prior to pentamidine nebulisation to reduce risk of bronchospasm. Do not mix together in nebuliser.
- May produce reversible impairment of renal function.

Pentostatin

Antineoplastic agent:
- Treatment of hairy cell leukaemia

DOSE IN NORMAL RENAL FUNCTION

$4\,mg/m^2$ every other week

PHARMACOKINETICS

Molecular weight (daltons)	268.3
% Protein binding	4
% Excreted unchanged in urine	50–96
Volume of distribution (L/kg)	36.1 litres
Half-life – normal/ ESRF (hrs)	2.6–10/18

METABOLISM

Only a small amount is metabolised via the liver.

It is primarily excreted unchanged by the kidneys (30–90% excreted by kidneys within 24 hours).

DOSE IN RENAL IMPAIRMENT GFR (mL/MIN)

50–60	50% of dose. See 'Other information'.
10–50	See 'Other information'.
<10	See 'Other information'.

DOSE IN PATIENTS UNDERGOING RENAL REPLACEMENT THERAPIES

CAPD	Unknown dialysability. Dose as in GFR<10 mL/min.
HD	Unknown dialysability. Dose as in GFR<10 mL/min.
HDF/High flux	Likely dialysability. Dose as in GFR<10 mL/min.
CAV/ VVHD	Unknown dialysability. Dose as in GFR=10–50 mL/min.

IMPORTANT DRUG INTERACTIONS

Potentially hazardous interactions with other drugs
- Antipsychotics: avoid concomitant use with clozapine (increased risk of agranulocytosis).
- Cytotoxics: increased risk of toxicity with high-dose cyclophosphamide – avoid concomitant use; increased pulmonary toxicity with fludarabine (unacceptably high incidence of fatalities).

ADMINISTRATION

RECONSTITUTION
- 5 mL water for injections
ROUTE
- IV bolus or infusion
RATE OF ADMINISTRATION
- 20–30 minutes
COMMENTS
- Add to 25–50 mL glucose 5% or sodium chloride 0.9% (final concentration 180–330 mcg/mL).

OTHER INFORMATION

- Patients with CKD are at a greater risk of toxicity with pentostatin.
- Contraindicated by manufacturer if GFR<60 mL/min due to lack of studies.
- One study used $3\,mg/m^2$ in patients with a GRF=41–60 mL/min and $2\,mg/m^2$ in patients with a GRF=21–40 mL/min without any problems. (Lathia C, Fleming GF, Meyer M, et al. Pentostatin pharmacokinetics and dosing recommendations in patients with mild renal impairment. *Cancer Chemother Pharmacol.* 2002 Aug; **50**(2): 121–6.)
- Another study used it in a haemodialysis patient at increasing doses of 1, 2, then $3\,mg/m^2$. Treatment was then continued at a dose of $2\,mg/m^2$. The patient was dialysed for 4 hours 1–2 hours after receiving the pentostatin to remove any remaining drug. The main complication was anorexia. Tumour lysis syndrome also occurred 4 days after the $3\,mg/m^2$ dose. (Arima N, Sugiyama T. Pentostatin treatment for a patient with chronic type adult T-cell leukaemia undergoing haemodialysis. *Rinsho Ketsueki.* 2005 Nov; **46**(11): 1191–5.)
- Hydration with 500–1000 mL of fluid is recommended before treatment and another 500 mL after treatment.
- Alternative schedule from Kintzel PE, Dorr RT. Anticancer drug renal toxicity and elimination: dosing guidelines for altered drug function. *Can Treat Rev.* 1995; **21**: 33–64:
  - GFR=60 mL/min, give 70% of dose.
  - GFR=45 mL/min, give 60% of dose.
  - GFR<30 mL/min, avoid.

Pentoxifylline (oxpentifylline)

CLINICAL USE

- Peripheral vascular disease
- Venous leg ulcers (unlicensed indication)

DOSE IN NORMAL RENAL FUNCTION

400 mg 2 to 3 times daily

PHARMACOKINETICS

Molecular weight (daltons)	278.3
% Protein binding	0
% Excreted unchanged in urine	0 (95% as active metabolites)
Volume of distribution (L/kg)	2.4–4.2
Half-life – normal/ ESRF (hrs)	0.4–1/Unchanged (see 'Other information')

METABOLISM

Pentoxifylline is hepatically metabolised to form active metabolites. In 24 hours most of a dose is excreted in the urine, mainly as metabolites, and less than 4% is recovered in the faeces.

DOSE IN RENAL IMPAIRMENT GFR (mL/MIN)

30–50	Dose as in normal renal function.
10–30	Reduce dose by 30–50% depending on individual tolerance (400 mg once or twice daily).
<10	Reduce dose by 30–50% depending on individual tolerance (400 mg once or twice daily).

DOSE IN PATIENTS UNDERGOING RENAL REPLACEMENT THERAPIES

CAPD	Not dialysed. 400 mg daily, slowly increasing if necessary.
HD	Not dialysed. 400 mg daily, slowly increasing if necessary.
HDF/High flux	Unknown dialysability. 400 mg daily, slowly increasing if necessary.
CAV/ VVHD	Not dialysed. Dose as in GFR=10–30 mL/min.

IMPORTANT DRUG INTERACTIONS

Potentially hazardous interactions with other drugs

- Analgesics: possibly increased risk of bleeding when administered in combination with NSAIDs; increased risk of bleeding with ketorolac – avoid concomitant use.

ADMINISTRATION

RECONSTITUTION

–

ROUTE

- Oral

RATE OF ADMINISTRATION

–

COMMENTS

–

OTHER INFORMATION

- May enhance hypoglycaemia.
- Avoid in porphyria.
- Active metabolites are renally excreted and have an extended half-life in renal impairment.

Perampanel

CLINICAL USE

Selective AMPA-type glutamate receptor antagonist:
- Anti-epileptic

DOSE IN NORMAL RENAL FUNCTION

2–12 mg daily before bedtime

PHARMACOKINETICS

Molecular weight (daltons)	349.4
% Protein binding	95
% Excreted unchanged in urine	22 (mainly as metabolites)
Volume of distribution (L/kg)	51–105 litres[1]
Half-life – normal/ ESRF (hrs)	105/Increased

METABOLISM

Extensively metabolised via primary oxidation via the cytochrome P450 isoenzyme CYP3A sub-family and sequential glucuronidation.

Perampanel is excreted in the urine and faeces mainly as oxidative and conjugated metabolites.

DOSE IN RENAL IMPAIRMENT GFR (mL/MIN)

30–50	Start with a low dose and titrate gradually.[1]
10–30	Start with a low dose and titrate gradually.
<10	Start with a low dose and titrate gradually.

DOSE IN PATIENTS UNDERGOING RENAL REPLACEMENT THERAPIES

CAPD	Not dialysed. Dose as in GFR<10 mL/min.
HD	Not dialysed. Dose as in GFR<10 mL/min.
HDF/High flux	Not dialysed. Dose as in GFR<10 mL/min.
CAV/ VVHD	Not dialysed. Dose as in GFR=10–30 mL/min.

IMPORTANT DRUG INTERACTIONS

Potentially hazardous interactions with other drugs
- Antidepressants: anticonvulsant effect antagonised; avoid concomitant use with St John's wort.
- Antimalarials: anticonvulsant effect antagonised by mefloquine.
- Antipsychotics: anticonvulsant effect antagonised.
- Orlistat: possibly increased risk of convulsions.
- Progestogens: high-dose perampanel reduces plasma concentration of progestogens (possibly reduced contraceptive effect).

ADMINISTRATION

RECONSTITUTION
–
ROUTE
- Oral
RATE OF ADMINISTRATION
–

OTHER INFORMATION

- Manufacturer advises to avoid in moderate to severe renal impairment due to lack of studies.
- Bioavailability is almost 100%.
- Results showed that perampanel apparent clearance was decreased by 27% in patients with mild renal impairment (creatinine clearance 50–80 mL/min) compared to patients with normal renal function (creatinine clearance >80 mL/min), with a corresponding 37% increase in AUC.[1]

Reference:
1. www.fda.gov/downloads/Drugs/.../ UCM332052.pdf

Perindopril

CLINICAL USE

Angiotensin-converting enzyme inhibitor:
- Hypertension
- Heart failure
- Following myocardial infarction or revascularisation

DOSE IN NORMAL RENAL FUNCTION

- Erbumine: 2–8 mg daily
- Arginine: 2.5–10 mg daily

PHARMACOKINETICS

Molecular weight (daltons)	441.6 (as Erbumine); 542.7 (as Arginine)
% Protein binding	60 (10–20 as perindoprilat)
% Excreted unchanged in urine	4–12
Volume of distribution (L/kg)	0.2
Half-life – normal/ ESRF (hrs)	1/27

METABOLISM

Perindopril is a prodrug. It is extensively metabolised, mainly in the liver, to the active perindoprilat and inactive metabolites including glucuronides. Perindopril is excreted mainly in the urine, as unchanged drug, as perindoprilat, and as other metabolites.

DOSE IN RENAL IMPAIRMENT GFR (mL/MIN)

30–60	Initially 2 mg (erbumine); 2.5 mg (arginine) daily, adjust according to response.
15–30	Initially 2 mg (erbumine); 2.5 mg (arginine) daily, adjust according to response.
<15	Initially 2 mg daily (erbumine); 2.5 mg (arginine) alternate days, adjust according to response.

DOSE IN PATIENTS UNDERGOING RENAL REPLACEMENT THERAPIES

CAPD	Unknown dialysability. Dose as in GFR<15 mL/min.
HD	Dialysed. Dose as in GFR<15 mL/min.
HDF/High flux	Dialysed. Dose as in GFR<15 mL/min.
CAV/ VVHD	Dialysed. Dose as in GFR=15–30 mL/min.

IMPORTANT DRUG INTERACTIONS

Potentially hazardous interactions with other drugs
- Anaesthetics: enhanced hypotensive effect.
- Analgesics: antagonism of hypotensive effect and increased risk of renal impairment with NSAIDs; hyperkalaemia with ketorolac and other NSAIDs.
- Ciclosporin: increased risk of hyperkalaemia and nephrotoxicity.
- Diuretics: enhanced hypotensive effect; hyperkalaemia with potassium-sparing diuretics.
- ESAs: increased risk of hyperkalaemia; antagonism of hypotensive effect.
- Gold: flushing and hypotension with sodium aurothiomalate.
- Lithium: reduced excretion (possibility of enhanced lithium toxicity).
- Potassium salts: increased risk of hyperkalaemia.
- Tacrolimus: increased risk of hyperkalaemia and nephrotoxicity.

ADMINISTRATION

RECONSTITUTION
–
ROUTE
- Oral
RATE OF ADMINISTRATION
–
COMMENTS
–

OTHER INFORMATION

- Active metabolite perindoprilat has a half-life of 25–30 hours.
- Titrate dose according to response; normal doses have been used in CKD 5.
- Small volume of distribution due to low lipophilicity.
- Close monitoring of renal function during therapy is necessary in those with renal insufficiency.
- Renal failure has been reported in association with ACE inhibitors in patients with renal artery stenosis, post renal transplant and those with severe congestive heart failure.
- High incidence of anaphylactoid reactions has been reported in patients dialysed with

high-flux polyacrylonitrile membranes and treated concomitantly with an ACE inhibitor – this combination should therefore be avoided.

- Hyperkalaemia and other side-effects are more common in patients with renal impairment.

Pethidine hydrochloride

CLINICAL USE

Opiate analgesia

DOSE IN NORMAL RENAL FUNCTION

- IV: 25–50 mg every 4 hours
- Oral: 50–150 mg every 4 hours
- S/C, IM: 25–100 mg every 4 hours

PHARMACOKINETICS

Molecular weight (daltons)	283.8
% Protein binding	60–80
% Excreted unchanged in urine	5
Volume of distribution (L/kg)	4.17
Half-life – normal/ESRF (hrs)	3–6/7–32

METABOLISM

Pethidine is metabolised in the liver by hydrolysis to pethidinic acid or by demethylation to norpethidine (active metabolite) and hydrolysis to norpethidinic acid, followed by conjugation with glucoronic acid. Norpethidine is pharmacologically active and its accumulation may result in toxicity. Pethidine has a half-life of about 3–6 hours; norpethidine is eliminated more slowly, with a half-life reported to be up to about 20 hours.

DOSE IN RENAL IMPAIRMENT GFR (mL/MIN)

20–50	Dose as in normal renal function.
10–20	Use small doses – increase dosing interval to 6 hours and decrease dose by 25%.
<10	Avoid if possible. If not, use small doses: increase dosing interval to 8 hours and decrease dose by 50%.

DOSE IN PATIENTS UNDERGOING RENAL REPLACEMENT THERAPIES

CAPD	Unknown dialysability. Dose as in GFR<10 mL/min.
HD	Not dialysed. Dose as in GFR<10 mL/min.
HDF/High flux	Unknown dialysability. Dose as in GFR<10 mL/min.
CAV/ VVHD	Unlikely dialysability. Dose as in GFR=10–20 mL/min.

IMPORTANT DRUG INTERACTIONS

Potentially hazardous interactions with other drugs
- Anti-arrhythmics: delayed absorption of mexiletine.
- Antidepressants: possible CNS excitation or depression with MAOIs and moclobemide – avoid concomitant use; possibly increased serotonergic effects with duloxetine; increased sedative effects with tricyclics.
- Antihistamines: increased sedative effects with sedating antihistamines.
- Antipsychotics: enhanced sedative and hypotensive effect.
- Antivirals: concentration reduced by ritonavir but concentration of toxic pethidine metabolite increased – avoid concomitant use.
- Dopaminergics: risk of CNS toxicity with rasagiline – avoid concomitant use; hyperpyrexia and CNS toxicity reported with selegiline – avoid concomitant use.
- Sodium oxybate: enhanced effect of sodium oxybate – avoid concomitant use.

ADMINISTRATION

RECONSTITUTION
–

ROUTE
- IV, Oral, SC, IM

RATE OF ADMINISTRATION
- IV: Bolus 3–4 minutes

COMMENTS
–

OTHER INFORMATION

- Risk of CNS and respiratory depression or convulsions, particularly in ERF patients receiving regular doses, due to accumulation of active metabolite, norpethidine. Norpethidine levels can be measured.

Phenelzine

CLINICAL USE

MAOI antidepressant

DOSE IN NORMAL RENAL FUNCTION

15 mg 3 times daily; maximum: 30 mg 3 times daily

PHARMACOKINETICS

Molecular weight (daltons)	136 (234.3 as sulphate)
% Protein binding	No data
% Excreted unchanged in urine	0.25–1.1
Volume of distribution (L/kg)	No data
Half-life – normal/ ESRF (hrs)	1.2/–

METABOLISM

Phenelzine is metabolised in the liver by oxidation via monoamine oxidase, and is excreted in the urine almost entirely in the form of metabolites.

DOSE IN RENAL IMPAIRMENT GFR (mL/MIN)

20–50	Dose as in normal renal function.
10–20	Dose as in normal renal function.
<10	Dose as in normal renal function.

DOSE IN PATIENTS UNDERGOING RENAL REPLACEMENT THERAPIES

CAPD	Possibly dialysed. Dose as in normal renal function.
HD	Possibly dialysed. Dose as in normal renal function.
HDF/High flux	Possibly dialysed. Dose as in normal renal function.
CAV/ VVHD	Unknown dialysability. Dose as in normal renal function.

IMPORTANT DRUG INTERACTIONS

Potentially hazardous interactions with other drugs

- Alcohol: some alcoholic and dealcoholised drinks contain tyramine which can cause hypertensive crisis.
- Alpha-blockers: avoid concomitant use with indoramin; enhanced hypotensive effect.
- Analgesics: CNS excitation or depression with pethidine, other opioids and nefopam – avoid concomitant use; increased risk of serotonergic effects and convulsions with tramadol – avoid.
- Antidepressants: enhancement of CNS effects and toxicity. Care with all antidepressants including drug free periods when changing therapies.
- Anti-epileptics: antagonism of anticonvulsant effect; avoid carbamazepine with or within 2 weeks of MAOIs.
- Antimalarials: avoid concomitant use with artemether/lumefantrine and piperaquine with artenimol.
- Antipsychotics: effects enhanced by clozapine.
- Atomoxetine: avoid concomitant use and for 2 weeks after use.
- Bupropion: avoid with or for 2 weeks after MAOIs.
- Dopaminergics: avoid concomitant use with entacapone and tolcapone; hypertensive crisis with levodopa and rasagiline – avoid for at least 2 weeks after stopping MAOI; hypotension with selegiline.
- $5HT_1$ agonist: risk of CNS toxicity with sumatriptan, rizatriptan and zolmitriptan – avoid sumatriptan and rizatriptan for 2 weeks after MAOI.
- Methyldopa: avoid concomitant use.
- Sympathomimetics: hypertensive crisis with sympathomimetics – avoid with methylphenidate.
- Tetrabenazine: risk of CNS excitation and hypertension avoid.

ADMINISTRATION

RECONSTITUTION

–

ROUTE

- Oral

RATE OF ADMINISTRATION

–

COMMENTS

–

Phenindione

CLINICAL USE

Anticoagulant

DOSE IN NORMAL RENAL FUNCTION

- Day 1: 200 mg
- Day 2: 100 mg
- Maintenance dose: 50–150 mg daily according to INR

PHARMACOKINETICS

Molecular weight (daltons)	222.2
% Protein binding	>97
% Excreted unchanged in urine	No data
Volume of distribution (L/kg)	No data
Half-life – normal/ ESRF (hrs)	5–6/–

METABOLISM

Hepatically metabolised. Metabolites of phenindione often colour the urine pink or orange.

DOSE IN RENAL IMPAIRMENT GFR (mL/MIN)

20–50	Dose as in normal renal function.
10–20	Dose as in normal renal function.
<10	Dose as in normal renal function.

DOSE IN PATIENTS UNDERGOING RENAL REPLACEMENT THERAPIES

CAPD	Unknown dialysability. Dose as in normal renal function.
HD	Unknown dialysability. Dose as in normal renal function.
HDF/High flux	Unknown dialysability. Dose as in normal renal function.
CAV/ VVHD	Unknown dialysability. Dose as in normal renal function.

IMPORTANT DRUG INTERACTIONS

Potentially hazardous interactions with other drugs

There are many significant interactions with coumarins.

Prescribe with care with regard to the following:

- Anticoagulant effect enhanced by: alcohol, amiodarone, anabolic steroids, aspirin, aztreonam, bicalutamide, cephalosporins, chloramphenicol, cimetidine, ciprofloxacin, fibrates, clopidogrel, cranberry juice, danazol, dipyridamole, disulfiram, fibrates, grapefruit juice, levofloxacin, macrolides, metronidazole, nalidixic acid, neomycin, norfloxacin, NSAIDs, ofloxacin, paracetamol, penicillins, ritonavir, rosuvastatin, sulphonamides, thyroid hormones, testosterone, tetracyclines, tigecycline, tramadol, trimethoprim.
- Anticoagulant effect decreased by: oral contraceptives, rifamycins, vitamin K.
- Anticoagulant effects enhanced/reduced by: anion exchange resins, corticosteroids, dietary changes.
- Analgesics: increased risk of bleeding with IV diclofenac and ketorolac – avoid concomitant use.
- Anticoagulants: increased risk of haemorrhage with apixaban, dabigatran and rivaroxaban – avoid concomitant use.
- Ciclosporin: there have been a few reports of altered anticoagulant effect; decreased ciclosporin levels have been seen rarely.

ADMINISTRATION

RECONSTITUTION

–

ROUTE

- Oral

RATE OF ADMINISTRATION

–

COMMENTS

–

OTHER INFORMATION

- Contraindicated by manufacturer in severe renal impairment.
- Titrate dose to INR.
- Enhanced anticoagulant effect in renal impairment, due to reduced protein binding.

Phenobarbital (phenobarbitone)

CLINICAL USE

Anti-epileptic agent

DOSE IN NORMAL RENAL FUNCTION

- Oral: 60–180 mg at night
- Status epilepticus: 10 mg/kg, max 1 g IV

PHARMACOKINETICS

Molecular weight (daltons)	232.2 (254.2 as sodium salt)
% Protein binding	45–60
% Excreted unchanged in urine	25
Volume of distribution (L/kg)	1
Half-life – normal/ ESRF (hrs)	75–120/Unchanged

METABOLISM

Partly metabolised in the liver.

Some 25% of a dose is excreted in the urine unchanged at normal urinary pH.

DOSE IN RENAL IMPAIRMENT GFR (mL/MIN)

20–50	Dose as in normal renal function.
10–20	Dose as in normal renal function, but avoid very large doses.
<10	Reduce dose by 25–50% and avoid very large single doses.

DOSE IN PATIENTS UNDERGOING RENAL REPLACEMENT THERAPIES

CAPD	Dialysed. Dose as in GFR<10 mL/min.
HD	Dialysed. Dose as in GFR<10 mL/min.
HDF/High flux	Dialysed. Dose as in GFR<10 mL/min.
CAV/VVHD	Not dialysed. Dose as in GFR=10–20 mL/min.

IMPORTANT DRUG INTERACTIONS

Potentially hazardous interactions with other drugs

- Anti-arrhythmics: reduced concentration of disopyramide; possibly reduced concentration of dronedarone – avoid.
- Antibacterials: reduced concentration of chloramphenicol, doxycycline, metronidazole, telithromycin and rifampicin – avoid with telithromycin.
- Anticoagulants: increased metabolism of coumarins (reduced effect).
- Antidepressants: antagonise anticonvulsant effect; reduces concentration of paroxetine, reboxetine, mianserin and tricyclics; concentration reduced by St John's wort – avoid concomitant use.
- Antiepileptics: concentration increased by oxcarbazepine, phenytoin, stiripentol and valproate and possibly carbamazepine, also active metabolite of oxcarbazepine reduced and valproate concentration reduced, concentration of phenytoin usually reduced but can also be increased; concentration of ethosuximide, rufinamide and topiramate possibly reduced; concentration of lamotrigine, tiagabine and zonisamide reduced.
- Antifungals: possibly reduced concentration of itraconazole, posaconazole and voriconazole – avoid concomitant use with voriconazole; reduced absorption of griseofulvin (reduced effect).
- Antimalarials: avoid with piperaquine with artenimol; anticonvulsant effect antagonised by mefloquine
- Antipsychotics: antagonise anticonvulsant effect; metabolism of haloperidol increased; possibly reduces aripiprazole concentration – increase aripiprazole dose; concentration of both drugs reduced with chlorpromazine; possibly reduces clozapine concentration.
- Antivirals: concentration of abacavir, boceprevir, darunavir, fosamprenavir, indinavir, lopinavir, rilpivirine and saquinavir possibly reduced; avoid with boceprevir and rilpivirine; avoid with etravirine and telaprevir.
- Calcium-channel blockers: effects of calcium-channel blockers probably reduced – avoid with isradipine and nimodipine.
- Ciclosporin: reduced ciclosporin levels.
- Corticosteroids: metabolism of corticosteroids accelerated, reduced effect.
- Cytotoxics: possibly reduced concentration of axitinib, increase axitinib dose; possibly reduced concentration of crizotinib and

vandetanib – avoid; avoid with cabazitaxel and gefitinib; concentration of irinotecan and its active metabolite and possibly etoposide reduced.

- Diuretics: concentration of eplerenone reduced – avoid concomitant use; increased risk of osteomalacia with carbonic anhydrase inhibitors.
- Oestrogens and progestogens: metabolism accelerated, reduced contraceptive effect.
- **Orlistat: possibly increased risk of convulsions.**
- Sodium oxybate: enhanced effects of sodium oxybate – avoid.
- Tacrolimus: concentration of tacrolimus reduced.
- Theophylline: metabolism of theophylline increased, reduced effect.
- Ulipristal: contraceptive effect reduced – avoid.

ADMINISTRATION

RECONSTITUTION
–

ROUTE
- IV, Oral

RATE OF ADMINISTRATION
- Not more than 100 mg/minute

COMMENTS
- For IV administration, dilute 1 in 10 with water for injection.

OTHER INFORMATION

- Aim for plasma concentration of 15–40 mg/L (65–170 μmol/L) for optimum response.
- Contraindicated by manufacturer in severe renal impairment in UK. The SPC for the US just advises to reduce dose in renal impairment.
- Dose in renal impairment is from *Drug Dosage in Renal Insufficiency* by Seyffart G.
- May cause excessive sedation and increased osteomalacia in ERF.
- Charcoal haemoperfusion and haemodialysis more effective than peritoneal dialysis for poisoning.
- Up to 50% unchanged drug excreted in urine with alkaline diuresis.

Phenoxybenzamine hydrochloride

CLINICAL USE

Non-competitive long acting-adrenergic receptor antagonist:
- Hypertensive episodes in phaeochromocytoma

DOSE IN NORMAL RENAL FUNCTION

- IV: 1 mg/kg daily, do not repeat within 24 hours
- Oral: 10 mg daily, increased by 10 mg daily to usual dose of 1–2 mg/kg in 2 divided doses.

PHARMACOKINETICS

Molecular weight (daltons)	340.3
% Protein binding	No data
% Excreted unchanged in urine	No data
Volume of distribution (L/kg)	No data
Half-life – normal/ ESRF (hrs)	24 (IV)/–

METABOLISM

Metabolised in the liver and excreted in the urine and bile, but small amounts remain in the body for several days.

DOSE IN RENAL IMPAIRMENT GFR (mL/MIN)

20–50	Dose as in normal renal function.
10–20	Dose as in normal renal function. Use with caution.
<10	Dose as in normal renal function. Use with caution.

DOSE IN PATIENTS UNDERGOING RENAL REPLACEMENT THERAPIES

CAPD	Unknown dialysability. Dose as in GFR<10 mL/min.
HD	Unknown dialysability. Dose as in GFR<10 mL/min.
HDF/High flux	Unknown dialysability. Dose as in GFR<10 mL/min.
CAV/ VVHD	Unknown dialysability. Dose as in GFR=10–20 mL/min.

IMPORTANT DRUG INTERACTIONS

Potentially hazardous interactions with other drugs
- Anaesthetics: enhanced hypotensive effect.
- Antidepressants: enhanced hypotensive effect with MAOIs, avoid concomitant use.
- Beta-blockers: enhanced hypotensive effect.
- Calcium-channel blockers: enhanced hypotensive effect.
- Diuretics: enhanced hypotensive effect.
- Moxisylyte: possibly severe postural hypotension when used in combination.
- Vardenafil, sildenafil and tadalafil: enhanced hypotensive effect, avoid concomitant use.

ADMINISTRATION

RECONSTITUTION
–
ROUTE
- IV, Oral
RATE OF ADMINISTRATION
- At least 2 hours
COMMENTS
- Dilute in 200–500 mL of sodium chloride 0.9%

OTHER INFORMATION

- Phenoxybenzamine is incompletely and variably absorbed from the gastrointestinal tract.

Phenoxymethylpenicillin (penicillin V)

CLINICAL USE

Antibacterial agent

DOSE IN NORMAL RENAL FUNCTION

500–1000 mg every 6 hours

PHARMACOKINETICS

Molecular weight (daltons)	350.4
% Protein binding	80
% Excreted unchanged in urine	60–90
Volume of distribution (L/kg)	0.5
Half-life – normal/ ESRF (hrs)	0.5–1/4

METABOLISM

Penicillin V is metabolised in the liver to form several metabolites, including penicilloic acid. The unchanged drug and metabolites are excreted rapidly in the urine. Only small amounts are excreted in the bile.

DOSE IN RENAL IMPAIRMENT GFR (mL/MIN)

20–50	Dose as in normal renal function.
10–20	Dose as in normal renal function.
<10	Dose as in normal renal function.

DOSE IN PATIENTS UNDERGOING RENAL REPLACEMENT THERAPIES

CAPD	Not dialysed. Dose as normal renal function.
HD	Dialysed. Dose as in normal renal function.
HDF/High flux	Dialysed. Dose as in normal renal function.
CAV/ VVHD	Dialysed. Dose as in normal renal function.

IMPORTANT DRUG INTERACTIONS

Potentially hazardous interactions with other drugs
- Reduces excretion of methotrexate

ADMINISTRATION

RECONSTITUTION
–
ROUTE
- Oral
RATE OF ADMINISTRATION
–
COMMENTS
–

OTHER INFORMATION

- Renal failure prolongs half-life of phenoxymethylpenicillin, but as it has a wide therapeutic index no dose adjustment is necessary.
- UK SPC advises to reduce dose in severe renal impairment but not the US version.
- Doses in renal impairment are from *Drug Prescribing in Renal Failure*, 5th edition, by Aronoff *et al.*

Phentolamine mesilate

CLINICAL USE

Alpha-adrenoceptor blocker:
- Hypertensive crisis

DOSE IN NORMAL RENAL FUNCTION

2–5 mg repeated if necessary

PHARMACOKINETICS

Molecular weight (daltons)	377.5
% Protein binding	54
% Excreted unchanged in urine	13
Volume of distribution (L/kg)	No data
Half-life – normal/ ESRF (hrs)	19 minutes/–

METABOLISM

Phentolamine is extensively metabolised. Only about 10–13% of an intravenous dose is excreted unchanged in the urine, and the fate of the remainder of the drug is unknown.

DOSE IN RENAL IMPAIRMENT GFR (mL/MIN)

20–50	Dose as in normal renal function.
10–20	Dose as in normal renal function.
<10	Dose as in normal renal function. Titrate dose to end point, i.e. lower BP.

DOSE IN PATIENTS UNDERGOING RENAL REPLACEMENT THERAPIES

CAPD	Unknown dialysability. Dose as in normal renal function.
HD	Unknown dialysability. Dose as in normal renal function.
HDF/High flux	Unknown dialysability. Dose as in normal renal function.
CAV/ VVHD	Unknown dialysability. Dose as in normal renal function.

IMPORTANT DRUG INTERACTIONS

Potentially hazardous interactions with other drugs
- Anaesthetics: enhanced hypotensive effect.
- Antidepressants: additive hypotensive effect with MAOIs – avoid concomitant use.
- Antihypertensives: enhanced hypotensive effect.
- Diuretics: enhanced hypotensive effect.
- Linezolid: additive hypotensive effect.
- Moxisylyte: possibly severe postural hypotension.
- Vardenafil, sildenafil and tadalafil: enhanced hypotensive effect – avoid concomitant use.

ADMINISTRATION

RECONSTITUTION
–
ROUTE
- IV
RATE OF ADMINISTRATION
–
COMMENTS
–

OTHER INFORMATION

- Titrate according to response.
- Manufacturer advises to use with caution due to lack of studies in UK SPC only. No dose reduction recommended in US data sheet.

Phenytoin

CLINICAL USE

- Anti-epileptic agent
- Diabetic neuropathy
- Trigeminal neuralgia

DOSE IN NORMAL RENAL FUNCTION

- Oral: 150–500 mg/day or 3–4 mg/kg/day in 1–2 divided doses; higher doses can be used in exceptional cases.
- Status epilepticus (IV): 20 mg/kg (max 2 g, at a rate of no more than 1 mg/kg/minute) (with BP and ECG monitoring) then 100 mg every 6–8 hours according to levels

PHARMACOKINETICS

Molecular weight (daltons)	252.3 (274.2 as sodium salt)
% Protein binding	90
% Excreted unchanged in urine	up to 5
Volume of distribution (L/kg)	0.52–1.19
Half-life – normal/ ESRF (hrs)	7–42/Unchanged

METABOLISM

Phenytoin is hydroxylated in the liver to inactive metabolites chiefly 5-(4-hydroxyphenyl)-5-phenylhydantoin by an enzyme system which is saturable. Phenytoin undergoes enterohepatic recycling and is excreted in the urine, mainly as its hydroxylated metabolite, in either free or conjugated form.

DOSE IN RENAL IMPAIRMENT GFR (mL/MIN)

20–50	Dose as in normal renal function.
10–20	Dose as in normal renal function.
<10	Dose as in normal renal function.

DOSE IN PATIENTS UNDERGOING RENAL REPLACEMENT THERAPIES

CAPD	Not dialysed. Dose as in normal renal function.
HD	Not dialysed. Dose as in normal renal function.
HDF/High flux	Dialysed. Dose as in normal renal function.
CAV/ VVHD	Unknown dialysability. Dose as in normal renal function.

IMPORTANT DRUG INTERACTIONS

Potentially hazardous interactions with other drugs

- Analgesics: enhanced effect with NSAIDs; metabolism of methadone accelerated.
- Anti-arrhythmics: increased concentration with amiodarone; concentration of disopyramide and mexiletine and possibly dronedarone reduced – avoid with dronedarone.
- Antibacterials: level increased by clarithromycin, chloramphenicol, isoniazid, metronidazole, sulfonamides and trimethoprim (+ antifolate effect); concentration increased or decreased by ciprofloxacin; concentration of doxycycline and telithromycin reduced – avoid with telithromycin; concentration reduced by rifamycins.
- Anticoagulants: increased metabolism of coumarins (reduced effect but also reports of enhancement); possibly reduced dabigatran concentration – avoid.
- Antidepressants: antagonise anticonvulsant effect, concentration increased by fluoxetine and fluvoxamine and possibly sertraline; concentration of mianserin, mirtazapine and paroxetine and possibly tricyclics reduced; concentration reduced by St John's wort – avoid.
- Anti-epileptics: concentration of both drugs reduced with carbamazepine, concentration may also be increased by carbamazepine, eslicarbazepine, ethosuximide, oxcarbazepine, stiripentol and topiramate; concentration of ethosuximide, active oxcarbazepine metabolite, retigabine, rufinamide (concentration of phenytoin possibly increased), topiramate and valproate possibly reduced; concentration of eslicarbazepine, ethosuximide, lamotrigine, perampanel, tiagabine and zonisamide reduced; concentration of phenobarbital often increased; phenobarbital and valproate may alter concentration; concentration reduced by vigabatrin.
- Antifungals: concentration of ketoconazole, itraconazole, posaconazole, voriconazole and possibly caspofungin reduced – avoid with itraconazole, increase voriconazole dose and possibly caspofungin; levels increased by fluconazole, miconazole and voriconazole.
- Antimalarials: avoid with piperaquine with artenimol; mefloquine and pyrimethamine antagonise anticonvulsant effect; increased antifolate effect with pyrimethamine.

- Antipsychotics: antagonise anticonvulsant effect; possibly reduced aripiprazole concentration – increase aripiprazole dose; metabolism of clozapine, haloperidol, quetiapine and sertindole increased; concentration increased or decreased with chlorpromazine.
- Antivirals: possibly reduced concentration of abacavir, darunavir, indinavir, lopinavir, ritonavir and saquinavir; concentration of boceprevir and rilpivirine reduced – avoid; concentration possibly increased by indinavir and ritonavir; concentration increased or decreased with zidovudine; avoid with etravirine and telaprevir
- Calcium-channel blockers: levels increased by diltiazem; concentration of diltiazem, felodipine, isradipine, nimodipine and verapamil reduced; avoid with isradipine and nimodipine.
- Ciclosporin: reduced ciclosporin levels.
- Corticosteroids: metabolism accelerated (effect reduced).
- Cytotoxics: metabolism possibly inhibited by fluorouracil; increased antifolate effect with methotrexate; concentration of busulfan, eribulin, etoposide and imatinib reduced – avoid with imatinib; concentration possibly reduced by cisplatin; possibly reduced concentration of axitinib, increase axitinib dose; possibly reduced concentration of crizotinib – avoid; avoid with cabazitaxel, gefitinib, lapatinib and vemurafenib; concentration of irinotecan and its active metabolite reduced.
- Disulfiram: levels of phenytoin increased.
- Diuretics: concentration increased by acetazolamide; concentration of eplerenone reduced – avoid concomitant use; increased risk of osteomalacia with carbonic anhydrase inhibitors; antagonises effect of furosemide.
- Muscle relaxants: long-term use of phenytoin reduces effects of non-depolarising muscle relaxants, but acute use may enhance effects.
- Oestrogens and progestogens: metabolism increased (reduced contraceptive effect).
- Orlistat: possibly increased risk of convulsions.
- Sulfinpyrazone: concentration increased by sulfinpyrazone.
- Theophylline: concentration of both drugs reduced.
- Ulcer-healing drugs: metabolism inhibited by cimetidine; absorption reduced by sucralfate; enhanced effect with esomeprazole and omeprazole.
- Ulipristal: contraceptive effect possibly reduced – avoid.

ADMINISTRATION

RECONSTITUTION
–
ROUTE
- IV, Oral
RATE OF ADMINISTRATION
- IV infusion and bolus: not greater than 50 mg/minute
COMMENTS
- Infusion: dilute in 50–100 mL sodium chloride 0.9%; final concentration not exceeding 10 mg/mL
- An in-line filter (0.22–0.50 microns) should be used due to high risk of precipitation, e.g. via a separate filter attached to giving set or giving sets like those used for taxol.
- Give by slow IV injection into large vein followed by sodium chloride 0.9% flush, to avoid irritation. Cardiac monitoring recommended.

OTHER INFORMATION

- Aim for phenytoin levels of 10–20 mg/L (40–80 micromol/L).
- Total phenytoin levels must be adjusted for hypoalbuminaemia and uraemia (levels of 5–12 mcg/mL may be enough).
- Decreased protein binding and volume of distribution in renal failure.
- Free fraction of phenytoin is increased in uraemia to approximately 0.2.
- Request free phenytoin serum levels, if possible.
- Loading dose 15 mg/kg IV or oral, then 5 mg/kg/day. Steady state reached in 3–5 days if loading dose given.
- Increase dose gradually (25–50 mg/day at weekly intervals); demonstrates saturation kinetics.
- Phenytoin absorption is markedly reduced by concurrent nasogastric enteral nutrition administration. Avoid concomitant administration with divalent cations.
- May cause folate deficiency.
- A useful equation:
To correct a phenytoin level for low albumin: from Winter ME. *Basic Clinical Pharmacokinetics*, 3rd ed. Philadelphia PA. Lippincott Williams & Wilkins; 1994.

$$C_{normal} = \frac{C_{observed}}{[(0.48) \times (1-0.1) \times \frac{albumin}{4.4(g/dl)}] + 0.1}$$

Phosphate supplements

CLINICAL USE

Hypophosphataemia

DOSE IN NORMAL RENAL FUNCTION

- Oral: 4–6 tablets daily
- IV: 9–50 mmol/day (maximum 500 micromols/kg in critically ill patients)
- See 'Other information'.

PHARMACOKINETICS

Molecular weight (daltons)	94–97 (Phosphate)
% Protein binding	No data
% Excreted unchanged in urine	High
Volume of distribution (L/kg)	No data
Half-life – normal/ ESRF (hrs)	No data

METABOLISM

Approximately two thirds of ingested phosphate is absorbed from the gastro-intestinal tract; most of the absorbed phosphate is then filtered by the glomeruli and subsequently undergoes reabsorption.

DOSE IN RENAL IMPAIRMENT GFR (mL/MIN)

20–50	Dose as in normal renal function.
10–20	Dose as in normal renal function.
<10	Dose as in normal renal function.

DOSE IN PATIENTS UNDERGOING RENAL REPLACEMENT THERAPIES

CAPD	Dialysed. Dose as in normal renal function.
HD	Dialysed. Dose as in normal renal function.
HDF/High flux	Dialysed. Dose as in normal renal function.
CAV/ VVHD	Dialysed. Dose as in normal renal function.

IMPORTANT DRUG INTERACTIONS

Potentially hazardous interactions with other drugs
- Avoid insoluble incompatibilities, e.g. calcium salts.

ADMINISTRATION

RECONSTITUTION

–

ROUTE
- IV, oral

RATE OF ADMINISTRATION
- Usually over 6–12 hours

COMMENTS
- Phosphate polyfusor: give undiluted over 24 hours, peripherally.
- Addiphos: peripherally – give each vial (20 mL) diluted to 250–500 mL with glucose 5% over 6–12 hours; centrally – 20 mL vial made up to 60 mL with glucose 5% over 6–8 hours via syringe driver.

OTHER INFORMATION

- Oral dosing: Phosphate Sandoz – 16.1 mmol phosphate, 20.4 mmol sodium, 3.1 mmol potassium per tablet.
- IV dosing: (i) Phosphate Polyfusor (500 mL) containing: 50 mmol phosphate, 81 mmol sodium, 9.5 mmol potassium. (ii) Addiphos (20 mL) containing: 40 mmol phosphate, 30 mmol sodium, 30 mmol potassium.
- Some units use a phosphate polyfuser before and after dialysis for low phosphate.
- Fleet phosphate enema can also be added to dialysate for hypophosphataemia in haemodialysis patients. (Su WS, Lekas P, Carlisle EJ, *et al.* Management of hypophosphatemia in nocturnal hemodialysis with phosphate containing enema: A technical study. *Hemodial Int.* 2011; **15**: 219–25.)
- HD patients usually need 15–20 mmol/day in TPN.
- CAV/VVHD patients usually need 30–40 mmol/day.
- During IV phosphate replacement, serum calcium, potassium and phosphate should be monitored 6–12 hourly. Repeat the dose within 24 hours if an adequate level has not been achieved. Urinary output should also be monitored.
- There is experience giving 15 mmol over 2 hours up to 3 times a day.
- Excessive doses of phosphate may cause hypocalcaemia and metastatic calcification.

Phytomenadione (vitamin K)

CLINICAL USE

- Vitamin K deficiency
- Antidote to oral anticoagulants

DOSE IN NORMAL RENAL FUNCTION

- Menadiol: Oral: 10–40 mg daily
- Konakion: IV: 5–40 mg daily in divided doses

PHARMACOKINETICS

Molecular weight (daltons)	450.7
% Protein binding	90
% Excreted unchanged in urine	<10
Volume of distribution (L/kg)	0.05–0.13
Half-life – normal/ ESRF (hrs)	1.5–3/Unchanged

METABOLISM

Phytomenadione is rapidly metabolised to more polar metabolites and is excreted in bile and urine as glucuronide and sulphate conjugates.

DOSE IN RENAL IMPAIRMENT GFR (mL/MIN)

20–50	Dose as in normal renal function.
10–20	Dose as in normal renal function.
<10	Dose as in normal renal function.

DOSE IN PATIENTS UNDERGOING RENAL REPLACEMENT THERAPIES

CAPD	Unlikely to be dialysed. Dose as in normal renal function.
HD	Unlikely to be dialysed. Dose as in normal renal function.
HDF/High flux	Dialysed. Dose as in normal renal function.
CAV/ VVHD	Unlikely to be dialysed. Dose as in normal renal function.

IMPORTANT DRUG INTERACTIONS

Potentially hazardous interactions with other drugs
- Antagonises effect of coumarins and phenindione.

ADMINISTRATION

RECONSTITUTION

–

ROUTE
- IV, IM, oral

RATE OF ADMINISTRATION
- Konakion® – very slow injection (1 mg/min)
  Konakion MM® – dilute each 10 mg with 55 mL of glucose 5% and give by slow infusion over 15–30 minutes.

COMMENTS
- Risk of anaphylaxis if IV injected too rapidly.
- Protect infusion from light.
- Konakion® should not be diluted (non-micellar).
- Only Konakion MM Paediatric® can be given IM or orally.

OTHER INFORMATION

- Konakion MM® recommended for severe haemorrhage.
- Anticoagulation antidote: re-test prothrombin time 8–12 hours after Konakion®, 3 hours after Konakion MM® – repeat dose if inadequate.
- Patients with obstructive jaundice requiring oral vitamin K should be prescribed the water-soluble preparation menadiol sodium diphosphate – dosage range is similar.

Pimozide

CLINICAL USE

Antipsychotic

DOSE IN NORMAL RENAL FUNCTION

2–20 mg daily

PHARMACOKINETICS

Molecular weight (daltons)	461.5
% Protein binding	99
% Excreted unchanged in urine	<1
Volume of distribution (L/kg)	No data
Half-life – normal/ESRF (hrs)	55–150/–

METABOLISM

Pimozide is metabolised in the liver via the cytochrome P450 isoenzyme CYP3A4 and to a lesser extent by CYP2D6 mainly by N-dealkylation and excreted in the urine and faeces in the form of metabolites and unchanged drug.

DOSE IN RENAL IMPAIRMENT GFR (mL/MIN)

20–50	Dose as in normal renal function.
10–20	Dose as in normal renal function.
<10	Start with low dose and increase according to response.

DOSE IN PATIENTS UNDERGOING RENAL REPLACEMENT THERAPIES

CAPD	Unknown dialysability. Dose as in GFR<10 mL/min.
HD	Unknown dialysability. Dose as in GFR<10 mL/min.
HDF/High flux	Unknown dialysability. Dose as in GFR<10 mL/min.
CAV/ VVHD	Unknown dialysability. Dose as in normal renal function.

IMPORTANT DRUG INTERACTIONS

Potentially hazardous interactions with other drugs
- Anaesthetics: enhanced hypotensive effect.
- Analgesics: increased risk of convulsions with tramadol; enhanced hypotensive and sedative effects with opioids; increased risk of ventricular arrhythmias with methadone.
- Anti-arrhythmics: increased risk of ventricular arrhythmias with anti-arrhythmics that prolong the QT interval – avoid concomitant use with amiodarone and disopyramide (risk of ventricular arrhythmias).
- Antibacterials: avoid concomitant use with macrolides and moxifloxacin (increased risk of ventricular arrhythmias).
- Antidepressants: concentration increased by SSRIs – avoid concomitant use; increased risk of ventricular arrhythmias with tricyclics – avoid concomitant use.
- Anti-epileptics: antagonises anticonvulsant effect.
- Antifungals: avoid concomitant use with imidazoles and triazoles.
- Antimalarials: avoid concomitant use with artemether/lumefantrine and piperaquine with artenimol; increased risk of ventricular arrhythmias with mefloquine and quinine – avoid concomitant use.
- Antipsychotics: increased risk of ventricular arrhythmias with droperidol, phenothiazines or sulpiride – avoid concomitant use.
- Antivirals: concentration increased by atazanavir, boceprevir, efavirenz, fosamprenavir, indinavir, ritonavir, saquinavir and telaprevir, increased risk of ventricular arrhythmias – avoid concomitant use.
- Anxiolytics and hypnotics: increased sedative effects.
- Aprepitant: avoid concomitant use.
- Atomoxetine: increased risk of ventricular arrhythmias.
- Beta-blockers: increased risk of ventricular arrhythmias with sotalol.
- Cytotoxics: use crizotinib with caution; avoid with lapatinib; increased risk of ventricular arrhythmias with vandetanib – avoid; increased risk of ventricular arrhythmias with arsenic trioxide.
- Diuretics increased risk of ventricular arrhythmias due to hypokalaemia.
- Ivabradine: increased risk of ventricular arrhythmias.

ADMINISTRATION

RECONSTITUTION

–

ROUTE
- Oral

RATE OF ADMINISTRATION

–

COMMENTS

–

OTHER INFORMATION

- ECG required before treatment. To be repeated annually.

Pindolol

CLINICAL USE

Beta-blocker:
- Hypertension
- Angina

DOSE IN NORMAL RENAL FUNCTION

- Hypertension: 15–45 mg daily in divided doses (15 mg can be given as a single dose.)
- Angina: 2.5–5 mg up to 3 times daily

PHARMACOKINETICS

Molecular weight (daltons)	248.3
% Protein binding	40–60
% Excreted unchanged in urine	30–40
Volume of distribution (L/kg)	2–3
Half-life – normal/ ESRF (hrs)	3–4/Increased

METABOLISM

Pindolol undergoes minimal hepatic metabolism to form inactive metabolites, and is excreted in the urine both unchanged and in the form of metabolites.

DOSE IN RENAL IMPAIRMENT GFR (mL/MIN)

20–50	Dose as in normal renal function.
10–20	Dose as in normal renal function.
<10	Dose as in normal renal function.

DOSE IN PATIENTS UNDERGOING RENAL REPLACEMENT THERAPIES

CAPD	Not dialysed. Dose as in normal renal function.
HD	Not dialysed. Dose as in normal renal function.
HDF/High flux	Unknown dialysability. Dose as in normal renal function.
CAV/ VVHD	Not dialysed. Dose as in normal renal function.

IMPORTANT DRUG INTERACTIONS

Potentially hazardous interactions with other drugs
- Anaesthetics: enhanced hypotensive effect.
- Analgesics: NSAIDs antagonise hypotensive effect.
- Anti-arrhythmics: increased risk of myocardial depression and bradycardia; increased risk of bradycardia, myocardial depression and AV block with amiodarone; increased risk of myocardial depression and bradycardia with flecainide.
- Antidepressants: enhanced hypotensive effect with MAOIs.
- Antihypertensives; enhanced hypotensive effect; increased risk of withdrawal hypertension with clonidine; increased risk of first dose hypotensive effect with post-synaptic alpha-blockers such as prazosin.
- Antimalarials: increased risk of bradycardia with mefloquine.
- Antipsychotics: enhanced hypotensive effect with phenothiazines.
- Calcium-channel blockers: increased risk of bradycardia and AV block with diltiazem; hypotension and heart failure possible with nifedipine and nisoldipine; asystole, severe hypotension and heart failure with verapamil.
- Cytotoxics: possible increased risk of bradycardia with crizotinib.
- Diuretics: enhanced hypotensive effect.
- Fingolimod: possibly increased risk of bradycardia.
- Moxisylyte: possible severe postural hypotension.
- Sympathomimetics: severe hypertension with adrenaline and noradrenaline and possibly with dobutamine.

ADMINISTRATION

RECONSTITUTION
–
ROUTE
- Oral
RATE OF ADMINISTRATION
–
COMMENTS
–

Pioglitazone

CLINICAL USE

Treatment of type 2 diabetes mellitus

DOSE IN NORMAL RENAL FUNCTION

15–45 mg once daily

PHARMACOKINETICS

Molecular weight (daltons)	392.9 (as hydrochloride)
% Protein binding	>99
% Excreted unchanged in urine	<1
Volume of distribution (L/kg)	0.25
Half-life – normal/ ESRF (hrs)	5–6 (active metabolites: 16–23)/ Unchanged

METABOLISM

Pioglitazone undergoes extensive hepatic metabolism by hydroxylation mainly via cytochrome P450 2C8 to form active and inactive metabolites. Three of the six identified metabolites are active (M-II, M-III, and M-IV). Following oral administration of radiolabelled pioglitazone to man, recovered label was mainly in faeces (55%) and a lesser amount in urine (45%).

DOSE IN RENAL IMPAIRMENT GFR (mL/MIN)

20–50	Dose as in normal renal function.
10–20	Dose as in normal renal function.
<10	Dose as in normal renal function.

DOSE IN PATIENTS UNDERGOING RENAL REPLACEMENT THERAPIES

CAPD	Unlikely to be dialysed. Dose as in normal renal function and monitor carefully.
HD	Unlikely to be dialysed. Dose as in normal renal function and monitor carefully.
HDF/High flux	Unlikely to be dialysed. Dose as in normal renal function and monitor carefully.
CAV/ VVHD	Unlikely to be dialysed. Dose as in normal renal function and monitor carefully.

IMPORTANT DRUG INTERACTIONS

Potentially hazardous interactions with other drugs
- None known

ADMINISTRATION

RECONSTITUTION
–

ROUTE
- Oral

RATE OF ADMINISTRATION
–

COMMENTS
–

OTHER INFORMATION

- Manufacturer doesn't advise using in dialysis patients due to lack of studies.
- There has been a case report of rhabdomyolysis 6 months after starting therapy in a patient. (Slim R, Salem CB, Zami M, Brour M. Pioglitazone-induced acute rhabdomyolysis. *Diabetes Care.* 2009; **32**(7): 84.)
- Liver function tests should be measured prior to initiation of therapy and then every 2 months for the first 12 months, and thereafter at regular intervals.
- Pioglitazone should not be used in patients with heart failure or history of heart failure; incidence of heart failure is increased when pioglitazone is combined with insulin. Patients should be closely monitored for signs of heart failure.

Piperazine

CLINICAL USE

Treatment of threadworm and roundworm infections

DOSE IN NORMAL RENAL FUNCTION

- Threadworm: 4 g sachet stirred into a glass of milk or water and drunk immediately; repeat after 14 days.
- Roundworms: 4 g sachet stirred into a glass of milk or water and drunk immediately; repeat at monthly intervals for up to 3 months if re-infection risk.

PHARMACOKINETICS

Molecular weight (daltons)	86.14 (202.1 as phosphate); (642.7 as citrate)
% Protein binding	No data
% Excreted unchanged in urine	5–30
Volume of distribution (L/kg)	No data
Half-life – normal/ ESRF (hrs)	No data

METABOLISM

About 25% is metabolised in the liver. Piperazine is nitrosated to form N-mononitrosopiperazine (MNPz) in gastric juice, which is then metabolised to N-nitroso-3-hydroxypyrrolidine (NHPYR). It is excreted in the urine mainly as metabolites.

DOSE IN RENAL IMPAIRMENT GFR (mL/MIN)

20–50	Dose as in normal renal function.
10–20	Dose as in normal renal function.
<10	Dose as in normal renal function but avoid repeated administration.

DOSE IN PATIENTS UNDERGOING RENAL REPLACEMENT THERAPIES

CAPD	Unknown dialysability. Dose as in GFR<10 mL/min.
HD	Unknown dialysability. Dose as in GFR<10 mL/min.
HDF/High flux	Unknown dialysability. Dose as in GFR<10 mL/min.
CAV/ VVHD	Unknown dialysability. Dose as in normal renal function.

IMPORTANT DRUG INTERACTIONS

Potentially hazardous interactions with other drugs
- Pyrantel: antagonises effect of piperazine

ADMINISTRATION

RECONSTITUTION
–
ROUTE
- Oral
RATE OF ADMINISTRATION
–
COMMENTS
–

OTHER INFORMATION

- May accumulate in severe renal impairment causing neurotoxicity.
- Acts within the lumen of the gastrointestinal tract which is independent of any systemic absorption.

Piracetam

CLINICAL USE

Myoclonus

DOSE IN NORMAL RENAL FUNCTION

7.2 g daily in 2–3 divided doses titrated to a maximum of 24 g daily

PHARMACOKINETICS

Molecular weight (daltons)	142.2
% Protein binding	15
% Excreted unchanged in urine	>90
Volume of distribution (L/kg)	0.7
Half-life – normal/ ESRF (hrs)	5/Increased

METABOLISM

Up to now, no metabolite of piracetam has been found. Piracetam is excreted almost completely in urine and the fraction of the dose excreted in urine is independent of the dose given.

DOSE IN RENAL IMPAIRMENT GFR (mL/MIN)

50–80	4.8 g in 2–3 divided doses
30–50	1.2 g twice daily
20–30	1.2 g daily
<20	Contraindicated.

DOSE IN PATIENTS UNDERGOING RENAL REPLACEMENT THERAPIES

CAPD	Likely dialysability. Avoid. Contraindicated.
HD	Dialysed. Avoid. Contraindicated.
HDF/High flux	Dialysed. Avoid. Contraindicated.
CAV/ VVHD	Dialysed. Dose as in GFR=20– 30 mL/min.

IMPORTANT DRUG INTERACTIONS

Potentially hazardous interactions with other drugs
● None known

ADMINISTRATION

RECONSTITUTION
–

ROUTE
● Oral

RATE OF ADMINISTRATION
–

COMMENTS
–

Piroxicam

CLINICAL USE

NSAID and analgesic

DOSE IN NORMAL RENAL FUNCTION

20 mg once daily

PHARMACOKINETICS

Molecular weight (daltons)	331.3
% Protein binding	99
% Excreted unchanged in urine	<5
Volume of distribution (L/kg)	0.14
Half-life – normal/ ESRF (hrs)	50/Unchanged

METABOLISM

Piroxicam metabolism is mainly via cytochrome P450 CYP 2C9 in the liver by hydroxylation of the pyridyl ring of the piroxicam side-chain, followed by conjugation with glucuronic acid. It is excreted mainly in the urine with smaller amounts in the faeces. Enterohepatic recycling occurs. Less than 5% of the dose is excreted unchanged in the urine and faeces.

DOSE IN RENAL IMPAIRMENT GFR (mL/MIN)

20–50	Dose as in normal renal function, but avoid if possible.
10–20	Dose as in normal renal function, but avoid if possible.
<10	Dose as in normal renal function, but only use if on dialysis.

DOSE IN PATIENTS UNDERGOING RENAL REPLACEMENT THERAPIES

CAPD	Not dialysed. Dose as in GFR<10 mL/min. See 'Other information'.
HD	Not dialysed. Dose as in GFR<10 mL/min. See 'Other information'.
HDF/High flux	Unknown dialysability. Dose as in GFR<10 mL/min. See 'Other information'.
CAV/ VVHD	Not dialysed. Dose as in GFR=10–20 mL/min.

IMPORTANT DRUG INTERACTIONS

Potentially hazardous interactions with other drugs

- ACE inhibitors and angiotensin-II antagonists: antagonism of hypotensive effect; increased risk of nephrotoxicity and hyperkalaemia.
- Analgesics: avoid concomitant use of 2 or more NSAIDs, including aspirin (increased side effects); avoid with ketorolac (increased risk of side effects and haemorrhage).
- Antibacterials: possibly increased risk of convulsions with quinolones.
- Anticoagulants: effects of coumarins and phenindione enhanced; possibly increased risk of bleeding with heparins and dabigatran.
- Antidepressants: increased risk of bleeding with SSRIs and venlafaxine.
- Antidiabetic agents: effects of sulphonylureas enhanced.
- Anti-epileptics: possibly increased phenytoin concentration.
- Antivirals: increased risk of haematological toxicity with zidovudine; concentration increased by ritonavir.
- Ciclosporin: may potentiate nephrotoxicity.
- Cytotoxic agents: reduced excretion of methotrexate; increased risk of bleeding with erlotinib.
- Diuretics: increased risk of nephrotoxicity; antagonism of diuretic effect; hyperkalaemia with potassium-sparing diuretics.
- Lithium: excretion decreased.
- Pentoxifylline: increased risk of bleeding.
- Tacrolimus: increased risk of nephrotoxicity.

ADMINISTRATION

RECONSTITUTION

–

ROUTE

- Oral, topical

RATE OF ADMINISTRATION

–

COMMENTS

–

OTHER INFORMATION

- Inhibition of renal prostaglandin synthesis by NSAIDs may interfere with renal function, especially in the presence of existing renal disease – avoid if possible; if not, check serum creatinine 48–72 hours after starting NSAID – if serum creatinine is increased, stop NSAID.

- Use normal doses in patients with CKD 5 if on dialysis and do not pass any urine.
- Use with caution in renal transplant recipients – can reduce intrarenal autocoid synthesis.
- Water soluble inactive metabolites may be removed by HD and CAPD.

Pivmecillinam hydrochloride

CLINICAL USE

Antibacterial agent

DOSE IN NORMAL RENAL FUNCTION

- Acute uncomplicated cystitis: 400 mg initially, then 200 mg 3 times a day
- Chronic or recurrent bacteriuria: 400 mg every 6–8 hours
- Enteric fever (typhoid): 1.2–2.4 g daily for 14 days

PHARMACOKINETICS

Molecular weight (daltons)	476
% Protein binding	5–10
% Excreted unchanged in urine	45–50 (as mecillinam)
Volume of distribution (L/kg)	0.2–0.4 (as mecillinam)
Half-life – normal/ ESRF (hrs)	1.2/Increased

METABOLISM

Pivmecillinam is rapidly hydrolysed to mecillinam which is the active drug, plus pivalic acid and formaldehyde. About 45% of a dose may be excreted in the urine as mecillinam, mainly within the first 6 hours. Mecillinam is partly excreted with bile, giving rise to biliary concentrations about 3 times the serum levels.

DOSE IN RENAL IMPAIRMENT GFR (mL/MIN)

20–50	Dose as in normal renal function.
10–20	Dose as in normal renal function.
<10	Dose as in normal renal function. See 'Other information'.

DOSE IN PATIENTS UNDERGOING RENAL REPLACEMENT THERAPIES

CAPD	Likely dialysability. Dose as in GFR<10 mL/min.
HD	Dialysed. Dose as in GFR<10 mL/ min.
HDF/High flux	Dialysed. Dose as in GFR<10 mL/ min.
CAV/ VVHD	Dialysed. Dose as in normal renal function.

IMPORTANT DRUG INTERACTIONS

Potentially hazardous interactions with other drugs
- Anti-epileptics: avoid concomitant use with valproate.
- Methotrexate: penicillins can reduce the excretion of methotrexate (increased risk of toxicity).
- Probenecid: reduces excretion of penicillins.

ADMINISTRATION

RECONSTITUTION

–

ROUTE
- Oral

RATE OF ADMINISTRATION

–

COMMENTS
- Take with food

OTHER INFORMATION

- Contraindicated in carnitine deficiency as it can cause carnitine deficiency.
- Can cause oesophageal injury; take with water and food while standing up.
- Can cause porphyria.
- Can be crushed and administered with water down a PEG tube.
- Accumulation may occur in patients with severe renal impairment, so use the lower dose if using for extended periods of time.
- Unlikely to work in people with little residual kidney function as works by renal excretion into the bladder, where its site of action is.

Pizotifen

CLINICAL USE

Prophylactic treatment of vascular headaches including migraine

DOSE IN NORMAL RENAL FUNCTION

- 1.5 mg at night or 500 mcg 3 times a day adjusted according to response
- Maximum single dose: 3 mg
- Maximum daily dose: 4.5 mg

PHARMACOKINETICS

Molecular weight (daltons)	429.5 (as malate)
% Protein binding	>90
% Excreted unchanged in urine	<1 (55% as metabolites)
Volume of distribution (L/kg)	6–8
Half-life – normal/ ESRF (hrs)	1 (metabolite 23 hours)/–

METABOLISM

Pizotifen undergoes extensive metabolism. Over half of a dose is excreted in the urine, chiefly as metabolites; a significant proportion is excreted in the faeces. The primary metabolite of pizotifen (N-glucuronide conjugate) has a long elimination half-life of about 23 hours.

DOSE IN RENAL IMPAIRMENT GFR (mL/MIN)

20–50	Dose as in normal renal function.
10–20	Dose as in normal renal function.
<10	Dose reduction may be required. Monitor for drowsiness.

DOSE IN PATIENTS UNDERGOING RENAL REPLACEMENT THERAPIES

CAPD	Unlikely to be dialysed. Dose as in GFR<10 mL/min.
HD	Unlikely to be dialysed. Dose as in GFR<10 mL/min.
HDF/High flux	Unknown dialysability. Dose as in GFR<10 mL/min.
CAV/ VVHD	Unlikely to be dialysed. Dose as in normal renal function.

IMPORTANT DRUG INTERACTIONS

Potentially hazardous interactions with other drugs
- Adrenergic neurone blockers: pizotifen antagonises hypotensive effect.

ADMINISTRATION

RECONSTITUTION
–
ROUTE
- Oral
RATE OF ADMINISTRATION
–
COMMENTS
–

OTHER INFORMATION

- Use with caution in people with a predisposition for urinary retention or closed angle glaucoma.
- Pizotifen has appetite stimulating properties.

Plerixafor

CLINICAL USE

Chemokine receptor antagonist:
- To enhance mobilisation of haematopoietic stem cells to the peripheral blood for collection and subsequent autologous transplantation in patients with lymphoma and multiple myeloma whose cells mobilise poorly

DOSE IN NORMAL RENAL FUNCTION

240 mcg/kg/day in combination with G-CSF
Maximum dose 40 mg daily

PHARMACOKINETICS

Molecular weight (daltons)	502.8
% Protein binding	58
% Excreted unchanged in urine	70
Volume of distribution (L/kg)	0.3
Half-life – normal/ ESRF (hrs)	3–5/Increased

METABOLISM

Not metabolised.
   About 70% of a dose is eliminated in the urine within 24 hours.

DOSE IN RENAL IMPAIRMENT GFR (mL/MIN)

20–50	0.16 mg/kg/day. Maximum 27 mg daily.
10–20	0.16 mg/kg/day. Maximum 27 mg daily.
<10	0.16 mg/kg/day. Maximum 27 mg daily.

DOSE IN PATIENTS UNDERGOING RENAL REPLACEMENT THERAPIES

CAPD	Dialysed. Dose as in GFR<10 mL/min.
HD	Dialysed. Dose as in GFR<10 mL/min.
HDF/High flux	Dialysed. Dose as in GFR<10 mL/min.
CAV/VVHD	Dialysed. Dose as in GFR=10–20 mL/min.

IMPORTANT DRUG INTERACTIONS

Potentially hazardous interactions with other drugs
- None known

ADMINISTRATION

RECONSTITUTION
–
ROUTE
- SC
RATE OF ADMINISTRATION
–

OTHER INFORMATION

- In UK data sheet manufacturer has no dose for GFR<20 mL/min due to lack of experience but in the data sheet for the USA they advise dose as in GFR<50 mL/min.
- Following a single dose of 0.24 mg/kg, clearance was reduced in people with varying degrees of renal impairment and was positively correlated with creatinine clearance (CRCL). The mean AUC_{0-24h} in people with mild (CRCL 51–80 mL/min), moderate (CRCL 31–50 mL/min), and severe (CRCL <31 mL/min) renal impairment was 7%, 32%, and 39% higher than healthy subjects with normal renal function. Renal impairment had no effect on C_{max}.

Posaconazole

CLINICAL USE

Triazole antifungal agent

DOSE IN NORMAL RENAL FUNCTION

- 400 mg twice daily with food or 240 mL of a nutritional supplement
- Or 200 mg 4 times a day without food
- Oropharyngeal candidiasis severe infection or in immunocompromised patients: Loading dose of 200 mg once a day on the first day, then 100 mg once a day for 13 days.
- Prophylaxis of invasive fungal infections: 200 mg 3 times a day

PHARMACOKINETICS

Molecular weight (daltons)	700.8
% Protein binding	>98
% Excreted unchanged in urine	<0.2
Volume of distribution (L/kg)	1774 litres
Half-life – normal/ESRF (hrs)	20–66 (average 35)/ Unchanged

METABOLISM

Limited metabolism, most circulating metabolites are glucuronide conjugates with only small amounts of oxidative metabolites. The main elimination route of posaconazole is via the faeces (77%) where 66% of a dose is excreted unchanged. About 14% of a dose is excreted in the urine with only trace amounts excreted unchanged.

DOSE IN RENAL IMPAIRMENT GFR (mL/MIN)

20–50	Dose as in normal renal function.
10–20	Dose as in normal renal function.
<10	Dose as in normal renal function.

DOSE IN PATIENTS UNDERGOING RENAL REPLACEMENT THERAPIES

CAPD	Not dialysed. Dose as in normal renal function.
HD	Not dialysed. Dose as in normal renal function.
HDF/High flux	Not dialysed. Dose as in normal renal function.
CAV/ VVHD	Not dialysed. Dose as in normal renal function.

IMPORTANT DRUG INTERACTIONS

Potentially hazardous interactions with other drugs

- Analgesics: concentration of fentanyl possibly increased.
- Anti-arrhythmics: avoid concomitant use with dronedarone.
- Antibacterials: rifamycins may reduce posaconazole concentration; avoid concomitant administration unless benefit outweighs risk; rifabutin concentration increased.
- Anticoagulants: avoid with apixaban and rivaroxaban.
- Antidepressants: avoid concomitant use with reboxetine.
- Antidiabetics: posaconazole can decrease glucose concentrations, monitor glucose levels in diabetic patients. Possibly enhances hypoglycaemic effect of glipizide.
- Anti-epileptics: phenytoin, carbamazepine and phenobarbital may reduce posaconazole concentration – avoid concomitant administration unless benefit outweighs risk.
- Antimalarials: avoid concomitant administration with artemether/ lumefantrine and piperaquine with artenimol.
- Antipsychotics: increased risk of ventricular arrhythmias with pimozide – avoid concomitant use; possibly increase quetiapine levels – reduce dose of quetiapine.
- Antivirals: concentration of atazanavir increased; concentration reduced by efavirenz and possibly fosamprenavir; possibly increases saquinavir levels; increased risk of ventricular arrhythmias with telaprevir.
- Anxiolytics and hypnotics: increases midazolam levels.
- Ciclosporin: increases posaconazole concentration. Posaconazole can increase ciclosporin concentration – dose reduction may be required.
- Cytotoxics: possibly increase everolimus concentration – avoid; avoid with lapatinib; reduce dose of ruxolitinib; possibly inhibits metabolism of vinblastine & vincristine, increased risk of neurotoxicity.
- Ergot alkaloids: may increase ergot alkaloid concentration leading to ergotism – avoid concomitant administration.

- Lipid-lowering drugs: possibly increased risk of myopathy with atorvastatin or simvastatin. Avoid concomitant use.[1]
- Ranolazine: possibly increased ranolazine concentration – avoid.
- Sirolimus: may increase concentration of sirolimus – adjust sirolimus dose as required according to levels.
- Tacrolimus: increases C_{max} and AUC of tacrolimus by 121% and 358% respectively – reduce tacrolimus dose to about a third of current dose and adjust as required.
- Ulcer-healing drugs: cimetidine may reduce posaconazole concentration by 39% – avoid concomitant administration unless benefit outweighs risk; avoid with histamine H_2-antagonists and proton pump inhibitors.

ADMINISTRATION

RECONSTITUTION
–
ROUTE
- Oral
RATE OF ADMINISTRATION
–
COMMENTS
–

OTHER INFORMATION

- Use with caution in people with arrhythmias, electrolyte disturbances, QT prolongation, sinus bradycardia and cardiomyopathy.
- Contains 7 g of glucose per 800 mg daily dose.
- Measure liver function tests as moderate increases have been noted.

Reference:
1. MHRA. *Drug Safety Update*. Statins: interactions and updated advice. August 2012; **6**(1): 2–4.

Potassium chloride

CLINICAL USE

Hypokalaemia

DOSE IN NORMAL RENAL FUNCTION

2–4 g (25–50 mmol) daily

PHARMACOKINETICS

Molecular weight (daltons)	74.6
% Protein binding	N/A
% Excreted unchanged in urine	N/A
Volume of distribution (L/kg)	N/A
Half-life – normal/ ESRF (hrs)	N/A

METABOLISM

Potassium is excreted mainly by the kidneys; it is secreted in the distal tubules in exchange for sodium or hydrogen ions. Some potassium is excreted in the faeces and small amounts may also be excreted in sweat.

DOSE IN RENAL IMPAIRMENT GFR (mL/MIN)

20–50	According to response.
10–20	According to response.
<10	According to response.

DOSE IN PATIENTS UNDERGOING RENAL REPLACEMENT THERAPIES

CAPD	Dialysed. Dose according to response.
HD	Dialysed. Dose according to response.
HDF/High flux	Dialysed. Dose according to response.
CAV/ VVHD	Dialysed. Dose according to response.

IMPORTANT DRUG INTERACTIONS

Potentially hazardous interactions with other drugs
- ACE inhibitors and angiotensin-II antagonists: increased risk of hyperkalaemia.
- Ciclosporin: increased risk of hyperkalaemia.
- Potassium-sparing diuretics: increased risk of hyperkalaemia.
- Tacrolimus: increased risk of hyperkalaemia.

ADMINISTRATION

RECONSTITUTION
–
ROUTE
- Oral, IV
RATE OF ADMINISTRATION
- Infusion up to 20 mmol potassium per hour except in extreme hypokalaemic emergency where some units give up to 40 mmol/hour with cardiac monitoring.
COMMENTS
- Give IV solution well diluted (not exceeding 40 mmol/500 mL) for peripheral administration.
- Mix IV solutions thoroughly to avoid layering effect.
- Some units give more concentrated solution centrally: 100–200 mmol/100 mL sodium chloride 0.9% or glucose 5%, but at a rate not more than 20 mmol/hour.
- Cardiac monitoring mandatory.

OTHER INFORMATION

- Potassium chloride injection MUST NOT be injected undiluted.
- Monitor serum potassium levels.
- Sando K: 12 mmol potassium per tablet.
- Slow K: 8 mmol potassium per tablet.
- Kay-Cee-L Syrup: 1 mmol potassium per mL.
- Potassium chloride strong 15% injection: 20 mmol potassium/10 mL.
- Potassium levels cannot be corrected until magnesium levels are normal.

Pramipexole

CLINICAL USE

- Parkinson's disease
- Symptomatic treatment of restless legs

DOSE IN NORMAL RENAL FUNCTION

- Parkinson's disease: 88–1100 mcg 3 times a day
- Prolonged release: 0.26–3.15 mg daily
- Restless legs: 88–540 mcg taken 2–3 hours before bedtime

(Doses expressed as base)

PHARMACOKINETICS

Molecular weight (daltons)	302.3 (as hydrochloride)
% Protein binding	<20
% Excreted unchanged in urine	<90
Volume of distribution (L/kg)	400–500 litres
Half-life – normal/ ESRF (hrs)	8–14/36

METABOLISM

Pramipexole undergoes <10% metabolism to inactive metabolites. More than 90% of a dose is excreted via renal tubular secretion unchanged into the urine.

DOSE IN RENAL IMPAIRMENT GFR (mL/MIN)

20–50	Initially 88 mcg twice daily and titrate slowly. Maximum 1.57 mg daily.
10–20	Initially 88 mcg once daily and titrate slowly. Maximum 1.1 mg daily.
<10	Initially 88 mcg once daily and titrate slowly. Maximum 1.1 mg daily.

DOSE IN PATIENTS UNDERGOING RENAL REPLACEMENT THERAPIES

CAPD	Not dialysed. Dose as in GFR<10 mL/min.
HD	Not dialysed. Dose as in GFR<10 mL/min.
HDF/High flux	Unknown dialysability. Dose as in GFR<10 mL/min.
CAV/ VVHD	Not dialysed. Dose as in GFR=10–20 mL/min.

IMPORTANT DRUG INTERACTIONS

Potentially hazardous interactions with other drugs
- Avoid concomitant use with antipsychotics.

ADMINISTRATION

RECONSTITUTION
–

ROUTE
- Oral

RATE OF ADMINISTRATION
–

COMMENTS
–

OTHER INFORMATION

- 88 mcg of base ≡ 125 mcg of salt, 180 mcg ≡ 250 mcg, 350 mcg ≡ 500 mcg, 700 mcg ≡ 1 mg, 1.1 mg ≡ 1.5 mg.
- Less than 9% of dose is removed by haemodialysis.
- Drowsiness is a common side effect especially at higher doses.
- For restless legs, dose as in normal renal function.

Prasugrel

CLINICAL USE

Anti-platelet agent

DOSE IN NORMAL RENAL FUNCTION

60 mg loading dose followed by 10 mg daily
(5 mg daily if weight<60 kg or aged >75 years)

PHARMACOKINETICS

Molecular weight (daltons)	409.9 (as hydrochloride)
% Protein binding	98 (active metabolite)
% Excreted unchanged in urine	0 (68% as active metabolite)
Volume of distribution (L/kg)	44–68 litres
Half-life – normal/ ESRF (hrs)	2–15 (active metabolite)/ Unchanged

METABOLISM

Prasugrel is a prodrug and is rapidly
metabolised in the liver by various
cytochrome P450 enzymes to an active
metabolite and inactive metabolites. The
active metabolite is further metabolised to
two inactive compounds which are excreted
in the urine and faeces; about 68% of a dose
is excreted in urine and about 27% in faeces.

DOSE IN RENAL IMPAIRMENT GFR (mL/MIN)

20–50	Dose as in normal renal function. Use with caution.
10–20	Dose as in normal renal function. Use with caution.
<10	Dose as in normal renal function. Use with caution.

DOSE IN PATIENTS UNDERGOING RENAL REPLACEMENT THERAPIES

CAPD	Unlikely to be dialysed. Dose as in GFR<10 mL/min.
HD	Unlikely to be dialysed. Dose as in GFR<10 mL/min.
HDF/High flux	Unlikely to be dialysed. Dose as in GFR<10 mL/min.
CAV/ VVHD	Unlikely to be dialysed. Dose as in GFR=10–20 mL/min.

IMPORTANT DRUG INTERACTIONS

Potentially hazardous interactions with other
drugs
* Anticoagulants: enhanced anticoagulant
  effect with coumarins and phenindione.

ADMINISTRATION

RECONSTITUTION

–

ROUTE

* Oral

RATE OF ADMINISTRATION

–

OTHER INFORMATION

* Use with caution in renal impairment
  due to limited use and increased risk of
  bleeding complications.
* C_{max} and AUC of the active metabolite
  decreased by 51% and 42%, respectively, in
  CKD 5 patients.

Pravastatin sodium

CLINICAL USE

HMG CoA reductase inhibitor:
- Hypercholesterolaemia

DOSE IN NORMAL RENAL FUNCTION

10–40 mg daily at night

PHARMACOKINETICS

Molecular weight (daltons)	446.5
% Protein binding	Approx 50
% Excreted unchanged in urine	20
Volume of distribution (L/kg)	0.5
Half-life – normal/ ESRF (hrs)	1.5–2/Unchanged

METABOLISM

Pravastatin undergoes extensive hepatic metabolism to a relatively inactive metabolite. About 70% of an oral dose of pravastatin is excreted in the faeces, as unabsorbed drug and via the bile, and about 20% is excreted in the urine.

DOSE IN RENAL IMPAIRMENT GFR (mL/MIN)

20–50	Dose as in normal renal function.
10–20	Dose as in normal renal function.
<10	Dose as in normal renal function.

DOSE IN PATIENTS UNDERGOING RENAL REPLACEMENT THERAPIES

CAPD	Unlikely to be dialysed. Dose as in normal renal function.
HD	Not dialysed. Dose as in normal renal function.
HDF/High flux	Unknown dialysability. Dose as in normal renal function.
CAV/ VVHD	Unlikely to be dialysed. Dose as in normal renal function.

IMPORTANT DRUG INTERACTIONS

Potentially hazardous interactions with other drugs
- Antibacterials: increased risk of myopathy with daptomycin, fusidic acid (avoid concomitant use) and telithromycin; concentration increased by clarithromycin and erythromycin.
- Antivirals: increased risk of myopathy with atazanavir and boceprevir; concentration possibly increased by darunavir; concentration reduced by efavirenz.
- Ciclosporin: increased risk of myopathy.
- Colchicine: possible increased risk of myopathy.
- Lipid lowering agents: increased risk of myopathy with fibrates, gemfibrozil (avoid) and nicotinic acid.

ADMINISTRATION

RECONSTITUTION
–
ROUTE
- Oral
RATE OF ADMINISTRATION
–
COMMENTS
–

OTHER INFORMATION

- Rhabdomyolysis with acute renal failure, secondary to statin-induced myoglobinaemia, has been reported.
- Inactive polar metabolite accumulates but is readily removed by haemodialysis.

Praziquantel (unlicensed product)

CLINICAL USE

- Treatment of tapeworm
- *Hymenolepis nana*
- *Schistosoma haematobium* worms
- *S. japonicum* infections

DOSE IN NORMAL RENAL FUNCTION

- Tapeworm: 5–10 mg/kg after a light breakfast
- *Hymenolepis nana*: 15–25 mg/kg
- *Schistosomiasis*: 20 mg/kg repeated after 4–6 hours
- *S. japonicum*: 60 mg/kg in 3 divided doses on 1 day.

PHARMACOKINETICS

Molecular weight (daltons)	312.4
% Protein binding	80
% Excreted unchanged in urine	80% as metabolites
Volume of distribution (L/kg)	No data
Half-life – normal/ ESRF (hrs)	1–1.5 (metabolites 4 hours)/Slightly increased

METABOLISM

Praziquantel undergoes rapid and extensive metabolism in the liver, mainly via the cytochrome P450 isoenzymes CYP2B1 and CYP3A4, being hydroxylated to metabolites that are thought to be inactive. It is excreted in the urine, mainly as metabolites, about 80% of the dose being eliminated within 4 days and more than 90% of this in the first 24 hours.

DOSE IN RENAL IMPAIRMENT GFR (mL/MIN)

20–50	Dose as in normal renal function.
10–20	Dose as in normal renal function.
<10	Dose as in normal renal function.

DOSE IN PATIENTS UNDERGOING RENAL REPLACEMENT THERAPIES

CAPD	Not dialysed. Dose as in GFR<10 mL/min.
HD	Not dialysed. Dose as in GFR<10 mL/min.
HDF/High flux	Unknown dialysability. Dose as in GFR<10 mL/min.
CAV/ VVHD	Not dialysed. Dose as in normal renal function.

IMPORTANT DRUG INTERACTIONS

Potentially hazardous interactions with other drugs

- Carbamazepine, phenytoin, chloroquine: reduce bioavailability of praziquantel.
- Cimetidine and albendazole: increase bioavailability.

ADMINISTRATION

RECONSTITUTION

–

ROUTE

- Oral

RATE OF ADMINISTRATION

–

COMMENTS

–

OTHER INFORMATION

- Available on a named patient basis from Merck (Cysticide).
- One study did not show any adverse effects in a haemodialysis patient.

Prazosin

CLINICAL USE

Alpha-adrenoceptor blocker:
- Hypertension
- Congestive heart failure
- Raynaud's syndrome
- Benign prostatic hyperplasia (BPH)

DOSE IN NORMAL RENAL FUNCTION

- 0.5–20 mg daily in 2–3 divided doses
- Raynaud's syndrome, BPH: 0.5–2 mg twice daily

PHARMACOKINETICS

Molecular weight (daltons)	419.9
% Protein binding	97
% Excreted unchanged in urine	<10
Volume of distribution (L/kg)	1.2–1.5
Half-life – normal/ ESRF (hrs)	2–4/Unchanged

METABOLISM

Prazosin is extensively metabolised in the liver, mainly by demethylation and conjugation; some of the metabolites have antihypertensive activity. It is excreted as metabolites and 5–11% as unchanged prazosin mainly in the faeces via the bile. Less than 10% is excreted in the urine.

DOSE IN RENAL IMPAIRMENT GFR (mL/MIN)

20–50	Dose as in normal renal function.
10–20	Dose as in normal renal function.
<10	Dose as in normal renal function.

DOSE IN PATIENTS UNDERGOING RENAL REPLACEMENT THERAPIES

CAPD	Not dialysed. Dose as in normal renal function.
HD	Not dialysed. Dose as in normal renal function.
HDF/High flux	Unknown dialysability. Dose as in normal renal function.
CAV/ VVHD	Not dialysed. Dose as in normal renal function.

IMPORTANT DRUG INTERACTIONS

Potentially hazardous interactions with other drugs
- Anaesthetics: enhanced hypotensive effect.
- Antidepressants: enhanced hypotensive effect with MAOIs.
- Beta-blockers: enhanced hypotensive effect, increased risk of first dose hypotensive effect.
- Calcium-channel blockers: enhanced hypotensive effect, increased risk of first dose hypotensive effect.
- Diuretics: enhanced hypotensive effect, increased risk of first dose hypotensive effect.
- Moxisylyte: possibly severe postural hypotension when used in combination.
- Vardenafil, sildenafil and tadalafil: enhanced hypotensive effect – avoid concomitant use.

ADMINISTRATION

RECONSTITUTION
–
ROUTE
- Oral
RATE OF ADMINISTRATION
–
COMMENTS
–

Prednisolone

CLINICAL USE

Corticosteroid:
- Immunosuppression
- Anti-inflammatory

DOSE IN NORMAL RENAL FUNCTION

- Oral: variable.
- IM: 25–100 mg once or twice weekly (as prednisolone acetate)

PHARMACOKINETICS

Molecular weight (daltons)	360.4
% Protein binding	70–95 saturable
% Excreted unchanged in urine	11–30
Volume of distribution (L/kg)	1.3–1.7
Half-life – normal/ ESRF (hrs)	2–4/Increased

METABOLISM

Prednisolone is hepatically metabolised and excreted in the urine as sulphate and glucuronide conjugates, with an appreciable proportion of unchanged prednisolone.

DOSE IN RENAL IMPAIRMENT GFR (mL/MIN)

20–50	Dose as in normal renal function.
10–20	Dose as in normal renal function.
<10	Dose as in normal renal function.

DOSE IN PATIENTS UNDERGOING RENAL REPLACEMENT THERAPIES

CAPD	Not dialysed. Dose as in normal renal function.
HD	Not dialysed. Dose as in normal renal function.
HDF/High flux	Not dialysed. Dose as in normal renal function.
CAV/ VVHD	Unknown dialysability. Dose as in normal renal function.

IMPORTANT DRUG INTERACTIONS

Potentially hazardous interactions with other drugs
- Aldesleukin: avoid concomitant use.
- Antibacterials: metabolism accelerated by rifampicin; metabolism possibly inhibited by erythromycin; concentration of isoniazid possibly reduced.
- Anticoagulants: efficacy of coumarins and phenindione may be altered.
- Anti-epileptics: metabolism accelerated by carbamazepine, phenobarbital and phenytoin.
- Antifungals: increased risk of hypokalaemia with amphotericin – avoid concomitant use; metabolism possibly inhibited by itraconazole and ketoconazole.
- Antivirals: concentration possibly increased by ritonavir.
- Ciclosporin: rare reports of convulsions in patients on ciclosporin and high-dose corticosteroids; increased levels of prednisolone; increased ciclosporin levels reported with prednisolone.
- Diuretics: enhanced hypokalaemic effects of acetazolamide, loop diuretics and thiazide diuretics.
- Vaccines: high dose corticosteroids can impair immune response to vaccines – avoid concomitant use with live vaccines.

ADMINISTRATION

RECONSTITUTION
–
ROUTE
- Oral, IM, rectal
RATE OF ADMINISTRATION
–
COMMENTS
–

OTHER INFORMATION

- Evidence of unpredictable bioavailability from enteric coated tablets – avoid if possible.

Pregabalin

CLINICAL USE

- Anti-epileptic agent
- Neuropathic pain
- Generalised anxiety disorder

DOSE IN NORMAL RENAL FUNCTION

150–600 mg daily in 2 or 3 divided doses

PHARMACOKINETICS

Molecular weight (daltons)	159.2
% Protein binding	0
% Excreted unchanged in urine	92–99
Volume of distribution (L/kg)	0.56
Half-life – normal/ ESRF (hrs)	5–6.5/Increased

METABOLISM

Pregabalin undergoes negligible metabolism, and about 98% of a dose is excreted in the urine as unchanged drug.

DOSE IN RENAL IMPAIRMENT GFR (mL/MIN)

30–60	Initial dose 75 mg daily and titrate according to tolerability and response.
15–30	Initial dose 25–50 mg daily and titrate according to tolerability and response.
<15	Initial dose 25 mg daily and titrate according to tolerability and response.

DOSE IN PATIENTS UNDERGOING RENAL REPLACEMENT THERAPIES

CAPD	Dialysed. Dose as in GFR<15 mL/min.
HD	Dialysed. Dose as in GFR<15 mL/min.
HDF/High flux	Dialysed. Dose as in GFR<15 mL/min.
CAV/VVHD	Dialysed. Dose as in GFR=15–30 mL/min.

IMPORTANT DRUG INTERACTIONS

Potentially hazardous interactions with other drugs
- None known

ADMINISTRATION

RECONSTITUTION
–
ROUTE
- Oral
RATE OF ADMINISTRATION
–
COMMENTS
–

OTHER INFORMATION

- Oral bioavailability >90%.
- 50% of dose is removed after a 4 hour haemodialysis session.
- Use with caution in people with severe congestive heart failure.
- May cause reversible deterioration in renal function.

Primaquine phosphate

CLINICAL USE

- Treatment of malaria (*Plasmodium vivax* and *Plasmodium ovale*), in combination with chloroquine
- Treatment of *Pneumocystis jiroveci* pneumonia (PCP), in combination with clindamycin

DOSE IN NORMAL RENAL FUNCTION

- Malaria: 15–30 mg once daily for 14 days
- PCP: 30 mg once daily

PHARMACOKINETICS

Molecular weight (daltons)	455.3
% Protein binding	No data
% Excreted unchanged in urine	<1
Volume of distribution (L/kg)	3–4
Half-life – normal/ ESRF (hrs)	3–6/Unknown

METABOLISM

Rapidly metabolised in the liver. Its major metabolite carboxyprimaquine accumulates in the plasma on repeated dosage but possesses less antimalarial activity than the parent compound. Little unchanged drug is excreted in the urine.

DOSE IN RENAL IMPAIRMENT GFR (mL/MIN)

20–50	Dose as in normal renal function.
10–20	Dose as in normal renal function.
<10	Dose as in normal renal function.

DOSE IN PATIENTS UNDERGOING RENAL REPLACEMENT THERAPIES

CAPD	Unknown dialysability. Dose as in normal renal function.
HD	Not dialysed. Dose as in normal renal function.
HDF/High flux	Unknown dialysability. Dose as in normal renal function.
CAV/ VVHD	Unknown dialysability. Dose as in normal renal function.

IMPORTANT DRUG INTERACTIONS

Potentially hazardous interactions with other drugs
- Antimalarials: avoid concomitant use with artemether/lumefantrine.

ADMINISTRATION

RECONSTITUTION
–

ROUTE
- Oral

RATE OF ADMINISTRATION
–

COMMENTS
–

OTHER INFORMATION

- Primaquine base 7.5 mg is approximately equivalent to 13.2 mg primaquine phosphate.
- Contraindicated in acutely ill patients with rheumatoid arthritis or SLE – increased risk of developing granulocytopenia.
- Risk of haemolytic anaemia in patients with G-6-PD deficiency; haemolysis generally appears 2–3 days after primaquine administration.
- Risk of methaemoglobinaemia at high doses.

Primaxin (imipenem/cilastatin)

CLINICAL USE

Antibacterial agent

DOSE IN NORMAL RENAL FUNCTION

- IV: 500 mg every 6 hours or 1 g every 6–8 hours (as Imipenem)
- IM, mild-moderate infections: 500–750 mg every 12 hours

PHARMACOKINETICS

Molecular weight (daltons)	Imipenem: 317.4; Cilastatin: 380.4
% Protein binding	Imipenem: 20; Cilastatin: 40
% Excreted unchanged in urine	Imipenem: 20–70; Cilastatin: 75
Volume of distribution (L/kg)	Imipenem: 0.23; Cilastatin: 0.22
Half-life – normal/ ESRF (hrs)	Imipenem: 1/4; Cilastatin: 1/12

METABOLISM

When administered alone, imipenem is metabolised in the kidneys by dehydropeptidase-I, an enzyme in the brush border of the renal tubules, to inactive, nephrotoxic metabolites, with only about 5% to 40% or 45% of a dose excreted in the urine as unchanged active drug. Cilastin inhibits the metabolism of imipenem. When given with cilastatin about 70% of an intravenous dose of imipenem is recovered unchanged in the urine within 10 hours. Cilastatin is also excreted mainly in the urine, the majority as unchanged drug and about 12% as N-acetyl cilastatin. Less than 1% of imipenem is excreted via the bile in the faeces.

DOSE IN RENAL IMPAIRMENT GFR (mL/MIN)

41–70	500 mg every 6–8 hours or 750 mg every 8 hours
21–40	250 mg every 6 hours or 500 mg every 6–8 hours
<20	250–500 mg (or 3.5 mg/kg whichever is lower) every 12 hours

DOSE IN PATIENTS UNDERGOING RENAL REPLACEMENT THERAPIES

CAPD	Dialysed. Dose as in GFR<20 mL/min.
HD	Dialysed. Dose as in GFR<20 mL/min.
HDF/High flux	Dialysed. Dose as in GFR<20 mL/min.
CAV/VVH	Dialysed. 250 mg every 6 hours or 500 mg every 8 hours.[1]
CVVHD/ HDF	Dialysed. 250 mg every 6 hours or 500 mg every 6–8 hours.[1]

IMPORTANT DRUG INTERACTIONS

Potentially hazardous interactions with other drugs

- Anti-epileptics: reduced valproate concentration – avoid concomitant use.
- Ciclosporin: variable reports of increase/ no change in ciclosporin levels, and of neurotoxicity.
- Convulsions reported with concomitant administration of ganciclovir.

ADMINISTRATION

RECONSTITUTION
- 250 mg with 50 mL, 500 mg with 100 mL sodium chloride 0.9% (in some units 500 mg with 50 mL)
- IM: 2 mL lidocaine 1%
ROUTE
- IM, IV peripherally or centrally (500 mg/50 mL – given centrally)
RATE OF ADMINISTRATION
- 250 or 500 mg dose over 20–30 minutes
- 1 g over 40–60 minutes
COMMENTS
–

OTHER INFORMATION

- Risk of adverse neurological effects, e.g. convulsions. Extreme caution required in patients with history of CNS disease.
- Cilastatin can accumulate in patients with impaired renal function.
- Sodium content 1.72 mmol/500 mg vial.
- Imipenem is administered with cilastatin to prevent metabolism of imipenem within the kidney.
- Non-renal clearance in acute renal failure is less than in chronic renal failure.
- Patients with GFR<5 mL/min should not receive drug unless HD is started within 48 hours.

Reference:
1. Trotman RL, Williamson JC, Shoemaker DM. Antibiotic dosing in critically ill adult patients receiving continuous renal replacement therapy. *Clin Infect Dis.* 2005 Oct 15; **41**: 1159–66.

Primidone

CLINICAL USE

- Anti-epileptic agent
- Also used for essential tremor

DOSE IN NORMAL RENAL FUNCTION

- Epilepsy: 500 mg–1.5 g daily in 2 divided doses
- Essential tremor: 50–750 mg daily

PHARMACOKINETICS

Molecular weight (daltons)	218.3
% Protein binding	20
% Excreted unchanged in urine	40
Volume of distribution (L/kg)	0.4–1
Half-life – normal/ESRF (hrs)	10–15/ Unchanged

METABOLISM

Partially metabolised to phenobarbital and phenylethylmalonamide in the liver, both of which are active and have longer half-lives compared to primidone (metabolites may accumulate in renal impairment). It is excreted in urine as unchanged drug (40%) and metabolites.

DOSE IN RENAL IMPAIRMENT GFR (mL/MIN)

20–50	Dose as in normal renal function.
10–20	Dose as in normal renal function, but avoid very large doses.
<10	Reduce dose by 25–50% initially, and avoid very large single doses.

DOSE IN PATIENTS UNDERGOING RENAL REPLACEMENT THERAPIES

CAPD	Unknown dialysability. Dose as in GFR<10 mL/min.
HD	Dialysed. Dose as in GFR<10 mL/ min.
HDF/High flux	Dialysed. Dose as in GFR<10 mL/ min.
CAV/ VVHD	Dialysed. Dose as in GFR=10– 20 mL/min.

IMPORTANT DRUG INTERACTIONS

Potentially hazardous interactions with other drugs

- Anti-arrhythmics: reduced concentration of disopyramide; possibly reduced concentration of dronedarone – avoid.
- Antibacterials: reduced concentration of chloramphenicol, doxycycline, metronidazole, telithromycin and rifampicin – avoid with telithromycin.
- Anticoagulants: increased metabolism of coumarins (reduced effect).
- Antidepressants: antagonise anticonvulsant effect; reduces concentration of paroxetine, reboxetine, mianserin and tricyclics; concentration reduced by St John's wort – avoid concomitant use.
- Anti-epileptics: concentration increased by oxcarbazepine, phenytoin, stiripentol and valproate and possibly carbamazepine, also active metabolite of oxcarbazepine reduced and valproate concentration reduced, concentration of phenytoin usually reduced but can also be increased; concentration of ethosuximide, rufinamide and topiramate possibly reduced; concentration of lamotrigine, tiagabine and zonisamide reduced.
- Antifungals: possibly reduced concentration of itraconazole, posaconazole and voriconazole – avoid concomitant use with voriconazole; reduced absorption of griseofulvin (reduced effect).
- Antimalarials: avoid with piperaquine with artenimol; anticonvulsant effect antagonised by mefloquine.
- Antipsychotics: antagonise anticonvulsant effect; metabolism of haloperidol increased; possibly reduces aripiprazole concentration – increase aripiprazole dose; concentration of both drugs reduced with chlorpromazine; possibly reduces clozapine concentration.
- Antivirals: concentration of abacavir, boceprevir, darunavir, fosamprenavir, indinavir, lopinavir, rilpivirine and saquinavir possibly reduced; avoid with boceprevir and rilpivirine; avoid with etravirine and telaprevir.
- Calcium-channel blockers: effects of calcium-channel blockers probably reduced – avoid with isradipine and nimodipine.
- Ciclosporin: reduced ciclosporin levels.
- Corticosteroids: metabolism of corticosteroids accelerated, reduced effect.
- Cytotoxics: possibly reduced concentration of axitinib, increase axitinib dose; possibly reduced concentration of crizotinib and vandetanib – avoid; avoid with

cabazitaxel and gefitinib; concentration of irinotecan and its active metabolite and possibly etoposide reduced.

- Diuretics: concentration of eplerenone reduced – avoid concomitant use; increased risk of osteomalacia with carbonic anhydrase inhibitors.
- Oestrogens and progestogens: metabolism accelerated, reduced contraceptive effect.
- Orlistat: possibly increased risk of convulsions.
- Sodium oxybate: enhanced effects of sodium oxybate – avoid.
- Tacrolimus: concentration of tacrolimus reduced.
- Theophylline: metabolism of theophylline increased, reduced effect.
- Ulipristal: contraceptive effect reduced – avoid.

ADMINISTRATION

RECONSTITUTION

–

ROUTE

- Oral

RATE OF ADMINISTRATION

–

COMMENTS

–

OTHER INFORMATION

- Plasma concentrations of 5–12 mcg/L (23–55 μmol/L) have been loosely correlated with optimum response.
- May cause excessive sedation and osteomalacia.

Procainamide hydrochloride (unlicensed)

CLINICAL USE

Anti-arrhythmic agent:
- Treatment of ventricular arrhythmias, especially after myocardial infarction
- Atrial tachycardia

DOSE IN NORMAL RENAL FUNCTION

- Slow IV injection: 50 mg/min (100 mg with ECG monitoring), repeated at 5-minute intervals until arrhythmia is controlled; max dose 1 g
- Infusion: 500–600 mg over 25–30 minutes with ECG monitoring, then maintenance of 2–6 mg/minute. If required start oral anti-arrhythmics 3–4 hours after infusion.

PHARMACOKINETICS

Molecular weight (daltons)	271.8
% Protein binding	15–20
% Excreted unchanged in urine	30–70
Volume of distribution (L/kg)	1.48–4.3
Half-life – normal/ESRF (hrs)	2.5–5/9.6–11.3

METABOLISM

Hepatically metabolised to form the active metabolite, N-acetyl-procainamide (NAPA) which is 80% renally excreted.

DOSE IN RENAL IMPAIRMENT GFR (mL/MIN)

20–50	Dose as in normal renal function.
10–20	Dose as in normal renal function.
<10	Normal loading dose. Maintenance dose according to response, lower doses or longer dosage intervals may be required.

DOSE IN PATIENTS UNDERGOING RENAL REPLACEMENT THERAPIES

CAPD	Dialysed. Dose as in GFR<10 mL/min.
HD	Dialysed. Dose as in GFR<10 mL/min.
HDF/High flux	Dialysed. Dose as in GFR<10 mL/min.
CAV/VVHD	Dialysed. Dose as in normal renal function.

IMPORTANT DRUG INTERACTIONS

Potentially hazardous interactions with other drugs
- Anti-arrhythmics: amiodarone increases procainamide levels, increased risk of ventricular arrhythmias – avoid concomitant use; increased myocardial depression with other anti-arrhythmics.
- Antibacterials: increased risk of ventricular arrhythmias with moxifloxacin – avoid concomitant use; concentration increased by trimethoprim.
- Antidepressants: increased risk of ventricular arrhythmias with tricyclics.
- Antihistamines: increased risk of ventricular arrhythmias with mizolastine – avoid concomitant use.
- Antimalarials: increased risk of ventricular arrhythmias with artemether/lumefantrine – avoid concomitant use.
- Antipsychotics: increased risk of ventricular arrhythmias with phenothiazines and any antipsychotics that prolong the QT interval; avoid with amisulpride, pimozide and sertindole.
- Atomoxetine: increased risk of ventricular arrhythmias.
- Beta-blockers: increased myocardial depression; increased risk of ventricular arrhythmias with sotalol – avoid concomitant use.
- Fingolimod: possible increased risk of bradycardia.
- Muscle relaxants: enhanced effect of muscle relaxants.
- Ulcer-healing drugs: levels increased by cimetidine.

ADMINISTRATION

RECONSTITUTION
–

ROUTE
- IV bolus, IV infusion, IM

RATE OF ADMINISTRATION
- Bolus: 50–100 mg/minute
- Infusion: 2–6 mg/minute

COMMENTS
- Stable in glucose 5%.
- Dilute to a concentration of 2 mg/mL and give at a rate of 1–3 mL/minute, or to a

concentration of 4 mg/mL and give at a rate of 0.5–1.5 mL/minute.

- Stability of solution can be improved by adding sodium bicarbonate to glucose solution.

OTHER INFORMATION

- For optimum response, plasma concentration should be 3–10 mcg/L; severe toxicity has been noted at concentrations above 12 mcg/L.
- Haemofiltration can be used in cases of procainamide poisoning.

- Half-life depends on acetylator status of patient.
- Can cause systemic lupus erythematosus in up to 30% of patients with long-term use.
- CAPD removes 19% of procainamide and 24% of NAPA.
- Available from 'special order' manufacturers.

Procarbazine

CLINICAL USE

Antineoplastic agent:
- Main indication is Hodgkin's disease

DOSE IN NORMAL RENAL FUNCTION

250–300 mg daily in divided doses; begin with small doses.
- Maintenance: 50–150 mg daily.

PHARMACOKINETICS

Molecular weight (daltons)	257.8 (as hydrochloride)
% Protein binding	No data
% Excreted unchanged in urine	5
Volume of distribution (L/kg)	No data
Half-life – normal/ ESRF (hrs)	10 minutes/Increased

METABOLISM

Procarbazine is metabolised to an active alkylating agent by microsomal enzymes in the liver and kidneys and only about 5% is excreted unchanged in the urine. The remainder is oxidised to N-isopropylterephthalamic acid and excreted in the urine, with up to 70% of a dose recovered in the urine after 24 hours.

DOSE IN RENAL IMPAIRMENT GFR (mL/MIN)

20–50	50–100% of dose.
10–20	50–100% of dose. Use with caution.
<10	50–100% of dose. Use with caution.

DOSE IN PATIENTS UNDERGOING RENAL REPLACEMENT THERAPIES

CAPD	Unknown dialysability. Dose as in GFR<10 mL/min.
HD	Unlikely to be dialysed. Dose as in GFR<10 mL/min.
HDF/High flux	Unknown dialysability. Dose as in GFR<10 mL/min.
CAV/ VVHD	Unknown dialysability. Dose as in GFR=10–20 mL/min.

IMPORTANT DRUG INTERACTIONS

Potentially hazardous interactions with other drugs
- Alcohol: may produce a disulfiram reaction.
- Antipsychotics: avoid concomitant use with clozapine (increased risk of agranulocytosis).

ADMINISTRATION

RECONSTITUTION
–
ROUTE
- Oral
RATE OF ADMINISTRATION
–
COMMENTS
–

OTHER INFORMATION

- Contraindicated by manufacturer in severe renal impairment in UK SPC only.
- After oral absorption, the drug appears to be rapidly and completely absorbed.
- Nadir for bone-marrow depression is 4 weeks with recovery within 6 weeks.
- For 48 hours after dose, wear protective clothing to handle urine.
- Increased toxicity reported in patients with renal impairment.
- Doses from Kintzel PE, Dorr RT. Anticancer drug renal toxicity and elimination: dosing guidelines for altered renal function. *Can Treat Rev.* 1995; **21**: 33–64.

Prochlorperazine

CLINICAL USE

- Nausea and vomiting
- Labyrinthine disorders
- Psychoses
- Severe anxiety

DOSE IN NORMAL RENAL FUNCTION

- Oral: 5–10 mg 2–3 times daily
- Buccal: 1–2 tablets twice daily
- IM/IV: 12.5 mg (unlicensed IV)
- Psychoses: Oral: 75–100 mg daily, IM: 12.5–25 mg 2–3 times daily
- Severe anxiety: 15–20 mg daily by mouth, in divided doses; maximum 40 mg daily

PHARMACOKINETICS

Molecular weight (daltons)	373.9
% Protein binding	96
% Excreted unchanged in urine	Minimal
Volume of distribution (L/kg)	23
Half-life – normal/ ESRF (hrs)	6–9/–

METABOLISM

Prochlorperazine undergoes extensive first pass metabolism in the gut wall. It is also extensively metabolised in the liver and is excreted in the urine and bile. The metabolites are inactive.

DOSE IN RENAL IMPAIRMENT GFR (mL/MIN)

20–50	Dose as in normal renal function.
10–20	Dose as in normal renal function.
<10	Dose as in normal renal function.

DOSE IN PATIENTS UNDERGOING RENAL REPLACEMENT THERAPIES

CAPD	Unlikely to be dialysed. Dose as in normal renal function.
HD	Unlikely to be dialysed. Dose as in normal renal function.
HDF/High flux	Unknown dialysability. Dose as in normal renal function.
CAV/ VVHD	Unlikely to be dialysed. Dose as in normal renal function.

IMPORTANT DRUG INTERACTIONS

Potentially hazardous interactions with other drugs

- Anaesthetics: enhanced hypotensive effect.
- Analgesics: increased risk of convulsions with tramadol; enhanced hypotensive and sedative effects with opioids.
- Anti-arrhythmics increased risk of ventricular arrhythmias with anti-arrhythmics that prolong the QT interval, e.g. procainamide, disopyramide, dronedarone and amiodarone – avoid concomitant use with amiodarone and dronedarone.
- Antibacterials: increased risk of ventricular arrhythmias with moxifloxacin – avoid concomitant use.
- Antidepressants: increase concentrations and additive antimuscarinic effects, notably with tricyclics.
- Anti-epileptics: antagonised (convulsive threshold lowered).
- Antimalarials: avoid concomitant use with artemether/lumefantrine and piperaquine with artenimol.
- Antipsychotics: increased risk of ventricular arrhythmias with droperidol and pimozide – avoid concomitant use.
- Antivirals: concentration possibly increased with ritonavir.
- Anxiolytics and hypnotics: increased sedative effects.
- Atomoxetine: increased risk of ventricular arrhythmias.
- Beta-blockers: enhanced hypotensive effect; increased risk of ventricular arrhythmias with sotalol.
- Cytotoxics: increased risk of ventricular arrhythmias with arsenic trioxide.
- Desferrioxamine: avoid concomitant use.
- Diuretics: enhanced hypotensive effect.
- Lithium: increased risk of extrapyramidal side effects and possibly neurotoxicity.
- Pentamidine: increased risk of ventricular arrhythmias.

ADMINISTRATION

RECONSTITUTION

–

ROUTE
- IM, IV (unlicensed), oral, buccal

RATE OF ADMINISTRATION
- IM or IV over 3–4 minutes

COMMENTS
- Unlicensed IV administration methods:

- Either: dilute with water for injection to 5 times its own volume, and administer slowly over not less than 5 minutes,
- Or dilute to 1 mg/mL and administer at rate not greater than 1 mg/minute.

- Increased CNS sensitivity in severe renal impairment.
- Doses estimated from evaluation of pharmacokinetic data.

Procyclidine hydrochloride

CLINICAL USE

- Control of extrapyramidal symptoms
- Acute dystonias

DOSE IN NORMAL RENAL FUNCTION

- Oral: 2.5–10 mg 3 times a day; maximum 60 mg daily
- Acute dystonias: IM/IV: 5–10 mg

PHARMACOKINETICS

Molecular weight (daltons)	323.9
% Protein binding	No data
% Excreted unchanged in urine	<5
Volume of distribution (L/kg)	1
Half-life – normal/ ESRF (hrs)	12/–

METABOLISM

When given orally about one fifth of the dose is known to be metabolised in the liver, principally by cytochrome P450 and then conjugated with glucuronic acid. Metabolites have been found in the urine.

DOSE IN RENAL IMPAIRMENT GFR (mL/MIN)

20–50	Dose as in normal renal function.
10–20	Dose as in normal renal function.
<10	Dose as in normal renal function.

DOSE IN PATIENTS UNDERGOING RENAL REPLACEMENT THERAPIES

CAPD	Unknown dialysability. Dose as in normal renal function.
HD	Not dialysed. Dose as in normal renal function.
HDF/High flux	Unknown dialysability. Dose as in normal renal function.
CAV/ VVHD	Unknown dialysability. Dose as in normal renal function.

IMPORTANT DRUG INTERACTIONS

Potentially hazardous interactions with other drugs
- None known

ADMINISTRATION

RECONSTITUTION
–
ROUTE
- IV, IM, Oral
RATE OF ADMINISTRATION
- Bolus over 3–5 minutes
COMMENTS
–

OTHER INFORMATION

- Oral bioavailability is 75%.

Proguanil hydrochloride

CLINICAL USE

Malaria chemoprophylaxis

DOSE IN NORMAL RENAL FUNCTION

200 mg daily

PHARMACOKINETICS

Molecular weight (daltons)	290.2
% Protein binding	75
% Excreted unchanged in urine	60
Volume of distribution (L/kg)	No data
Half-life – normal/ ESRF (hrs)	20/–

METABOLISM

Proguanil is metabolised in the liver to the active metabolite, cycloguanil, and to *p*-chlorophenylbiguanide which is inactive, mainly by cytochrome P450, CYP 2C19 and slightly by CYP 3A4. Unlike proguanil and *p*-chlorophenylbiguanide, cycloguanil is not concentrated in erythrocytes so concentrations of cycloguanil in plasma and whole blood are similar. About 40–60% of a dose of proguanil is excreted in the urine, 60% of this as the unchanged drug, 30% as cycloguanil, and 8% as *p*-chlorophenylbiguanide. About 10% of a dose is excreted in the faeces.

DOSE IN RENAL IMPAIRMENT GFR (mL/MIN)

20–60	100 mg daily
10–20	50 mg every 48 hours
<10	50 mg weekly

DOSE IN PATIENTS UNDERGOING RENAL REPLACEMENT THERAPIES

CAPD	Unlikely to be dialysed. Dose as in GFR<10 mL/min.
HD	Not dialysed. Dose as in GFR<10 mL/min.
HDF/High flux	Unknown dialysability. Dose as in GFR<10 mL/min.
CAV/ VVHD	Unknown dialysability. Dose as in GFR=10–20 mL/min.

IMPORTANT DRUG INTERACTIONS

Potentially hazardous interactions with other drugs
- Anticoagulants: effect of warfarin possibly enhanced.
- Antimalarials: avoid concomitant use with artemether/lumefantrine; increased antifolate effect with pyrimethamine.

ADMINISTRATION

RECONSTITUTION
–
ROUTE
- Oral
RATE OF ADMINISTRATION
–
COMMENTS
–

OTHER INFORMATION

- Rare reports of haematological changes (e.g. megaloblastic anaemia and pancytopenia) in patients with severe renal impairment.

Promazine hydrochloride

CLINICAL USE

Antipsychotic for agitation and restlessness

DOSE IN NORMAL RENAL FUNCTION

- Psychomotor agitation: 100–200 mg 4 times a day
- Agitation and restlessness in elderly: 25–50 mg 4 times a day

PHARMACOKINETICS

As for chlorpromazine[1]

Molecular weight (daltons)	320.9
% Protein binding	95–98
% Excreted unchanged in urine	<1
Volume of distribution (L/kg)	7–20
Half-life – normal/ESRF (hrs)	23–37/ Unchanged

METABOLISM

Promazine undergoes considerable first-pass metabolism in the gut wall. It is also extensively metabolised in the liver and is excreted in the urine and faeces in the form of numerous active and inactive metabolites.

DOSE IN RENAL IMPAIRMENT GFR (mL/MIN)

20–50	Dose as in normal renal function.
10–20	Dose as in normal renal function.
<10	Start with low doses and titrate slowly.

DOSE IN PATIENTS UNDERGOING RENAL REPLACEMENT THERAPIES

CAPD	Unlikely to be dialysed. Dose as in GFR<10 mL/min.
HD	Unlikely to be dialysed. Dose as in GFR<10 mL/min.
HDF/High flux	Unknown dialysability. Dose as in GFR<10 mL/min.
CAV/ VVHD	Unknown dialysability. Dose as in normal renal function.

IMPORTANT DRUG INTERACTIONS

Potentially hazardous interactions with other drugs
- Anaesthetics: enhanced hypotensive effect.
- Analgesics: increased risk of convulsions with tramadol; enhanced hypotensive and sedative effects with opioids; increased risk of ventricular arrhythmias with methadone.
- Anti-arrhythmics: increased risk of ventricular arrhythmias with anti-arrhythmics that prolong the QT interval – avoid concomitant use with amiodarone, disopyramide and dronedarone.
- Antibacterials: increased risk of ventricular arrhythmias with moxifloxacin – avoid concomitant use.
- Antidepressants: increased level of tricyclics (possibly increased risk of ventricular arrhythmias and antimuscarinic side effects).
- Anticonvulsant: antagonises anticonvulsant effect.
- Antimalarials: avoid concomitant use with artemether/lumefantrine and piperaquine with artenimol.
- Antipsychotics: increased risk of ventricular arrhythmias with droperidol and pimozide – avoid concomitant use.
- Antivirals: concentration possibly increased with ritonavir.
- Anxiolytics and hypnotics: increased sedative effects.
- Atomoxetine: increased risk of ventricular arrhythmias.
- Beta-blockers: enhanced hypotensive effect; increased risk of ventricular arrhythmias with sotalol.
- Cytotoxics: increased risk of ventricular arrhythmias with arsenic trioxide.
- Diuretics: enhanced hypotensive effect.
- Lithium: increased risk of extrapyramidal side effects and possibly neurotoxicity.
- Pentamidine: increased risk of ventricular arrhythmias.

ADMINISTRATION

RECONSTITUTION
–

ROUTE
- Oral

RATE OF ADMINISTRATION
–

COMMENTS
–

Reference:
1. Ereshefsky L. Pharmacokinetics and drug interactions: update for new antipsychotics. *J Clin Psychiatry*. 1996; **57**(Suppl. 11): 12–25.

Promethazine hydrochloride

CLINICAL USE

Antihistamine

DOSE IN NORMAL RENAL FUNCTION

- Oral: 25 mg at night increased to twice daily, or 10–20 mg 2–3 times a day
- Slow IV/IM: 25–100 mg

PHARMACOKINETICS

Molecular weight (daltons)	320.9
% Protein binding	76–93
% Excreted unchanged in urine	0
Volume of distribution (L/kg)	13.5
Half-life – normal/ ESRF (hrs)	5–14/–

METABOLISM

Extensively hepatically metabolised, mainly to promethazine sulfoxide, and also to N-desmethylpromethazine.

It is excreted slowly via the urine and bile, mainly as metabolites.

DOSE IN RENAL IMPAIRMENT GFR (mL/MIN)

20–50	Dose as in normal renal function.
10–20	Dose as in normal renal function.
<10	Dose as in normal renal function.

DOSE IN PATIENTS UNDERGOING RENAL REPLACEMENT THERAPIES

CAPD	Unknown dialysability. Dose as in normal renal function.
HD	Not dialysed. Dose as in normal renal function.
HDF/High flux	Unknown dialysability. Dose as in normal renal function.
CAV/ VVHD	Unknown dialysability. Dose as in normal renal function.

IMPORTANT DRUG INTERACTIONS

Potentially hazardous interactions with other drugs
- None known

ADMINISTRATION

RECONSTITUTION

–

ROUTE
- IV, IM, oral

RATE OF ADMINISTRATION
- Bolus over 3–5 minutes

COMMENTS
- Administer in 10 mL water for injection for slow IV injection (2.5 mg/mL).

OTHER INFORMATION

- Excessive sedation may occur in CKD 5.

Propafenone hydrochloride

CLINICAL USE

Anti-arrhythmic agent:
- Ventricular arrhythmias
- Paroxysmal supraventricular tachyarrhythmias (including paroxysmal atrial flutter or fibrillation, and paroxysmal re-entrant tachycardias involving the AV node or accessory pathway) where standard therapy has failed or is unsuitable

DOSE IN NORMAL RENAL FUNCTION

>70 kg: 150–300 mg 3 times daily.
If <70 kg start with a lower dose.

PHARMACOKINETICS

Molecular weight (daltons)	377.9
% Protein binding	>95
% Excreted unchanged in urine	<1
Volume of distribution (L/kg)	1.9–3
Half-life – normal/ ESRF (hrs)	2–10 (10–32 hours in slow metabolisers)/ Unchanged

METABOLISM

Propafenone is hepatically metabolised mainly by CYP2D6 isoenzyme but also to a small extent by CYP1A2 and CYP3A4. This forms 2 active metabolites, 5-hydroxypropafenone and N-depropylpropafenone and some inactive ones. Propafenone and its metabolites also undergo glucuronidation.

The extent of metabolism is genetically determined.

Propafenone is excreted in the urine and faeces mainly in the form of conjugated metabolites.

DOSE IN RENAL IMPAIRMENT GFR (mL/MIN)

20–50	Dose as in normal renal function.
10–20	Dose as in normal renal function.
<10	Dose as in normal renal function. Use with caution.

DOSE IN PATIENTS UNDERGOING RENAL REPLACEMENT THERAPIES

CAPD	Not dialysed. Dose as in GFR<10 mL/min.
HD	Not dialysed. Dose as in GFR<10 mL/min.
HDF/High flux	Unknown dialysability. Dose as in GFR<10 mL/min.
CAV/ VVHD	Not dialysed. Dose as in normal renal function.

IMPORTANT DRUG INTERACTIONS

Potentially hazardous interactions with other drugs
- Anti-arrhythmics: increased myocardial depression with other anti-arrhythmics.
- Antibacterials: increased metabolism with rifampicin (reduced effect).
- Anticoagulants: enhanced anticoagulant effect of coumarins.
- Antidepressants: increased risk of arrhythmias with tricyclics; metabolism of propafenone possibly inhibited by paroxetine (increased risk of toxicity).
- Antihistamines: increased risk of ventricular arrhythmias with mizolastine – avoid concomitant use.
- Antipsychotics: increased risk of ventricular arrhythmias with antipsychotics that prolong the QT interval.
- Antivirals: concentration of propafenone increased by saquinavir and ritonavir and possibly by fosamprenavir, increased risk of ventricular arrhythmias – avoid concomitant use; use with caution with telaprevir.
- Beta-blockers: increased myocardial depression; increased concentration of metoprolol and propranolol.
- Cardiac glycosides: increased digoxin concentration – halve digoxin dose.
- Ciclosporin: possibly increased ciclosporin concentration.
- Ulcer-healing drugs: levels increased by cimetidine.

ADMINISTRATION

RECONSTITUTION
–

ROUTE
● Oral

RATE OF ADMINISTRATION
–

COMMENTS
–

OTHER INFORMATION

● Half-life depends on acetylator status of patient.
● Ensure that electrolyte disturbances are corrected before commencing treatment.
● Therapeutic plasma concentrations are 150–1500 ng/mL.

Propiverine hydrochloride

CLINICAL USE

- Treatment of urinary frequency, urgency and incontinence
- Neurogenic bladder instability

DOSE IN NORMAL RENAL FUNCTION

15 mg 1–4 times a day
XL: 30 mg once daily

PHARMACOKINETICS

Molecular weight (daltons)	403.9
% Protein binding	90–95
% Excreted unchanged in urine	<1
Volume of distribution (L/kg)	125–473 litres (Average: 279 litres)
Half-life – normal/ ESRF (hrs)	20/–

METABOLISM

Propiverine is extensively metabolised by intestinal and hepatic enzymes. Four metabolites were identified in urine; two of them are pharmacologically active and may contribute to the therapeutic efficacy. Propiverine and its metabolites are excreted in the urine, bile, and faeces.

DOSE IN RENAL IMPAIRMENT GFR (mL/MIN)

30–50	Dose as in normal renal function.
10–30	Dose as in normal renal function. Maximum 30 mg daily.
<10	Dose as in normal renal function. Maximum 30 mg daily.

DOSE IN PATIENTS UNDERGOING RENAL REPLACEMENT THERAPIES

CAPD	Unknown dialysability. Dose as in GFR<10 mL/min.
HD	Unknown dialysability. Dose as in GFR<10 mL/min.
HDF/High flux	Unknown dialysability. Dose as in GFR<10 mL/min.
CAV/ VVHD	Unknown dialysability. Dose as in GFR=10–30 mL/min.

IMPORTANT DRUG INTERACTIONS

Potentially hazardous interactions with other drugs
- Anti-arrhythmics: increased risk of antimuscarinic side effects with disopyramide.

ADMINISTRATION

RECONSTITUTION
–

ROUTE
- Oral

RATE OF ADMINISTRATION
–

COMMENTS
–

Propofol

CLINICAL USE

- Induction and maintenance of general anaesthesia
- Sedation of ventilated patients for up to 3 days

DOSE IN NORMAL RENAL FUNCTION

- Induction: 1.5–2.5 mg/kg at a rate of 20–40 mg every 10 seconds
- If >55 years or debilitated: 1–1.5 mg/kg at a rate of 20 mg every 10 seconds
- Maintenance: 25–50 mg repeated according to response or 4–12 mg/kg/hour (3–6 mg/kg/hour in elderly or debilitated)
- Sedation: 0.3–4 mg/kg/hour
- Sedation for surgical and diagnostic procedures: 0.5–1 mg/kg over 1–5 minutes then maintenance: 1.5–4.5 mg/kg/hour or 10–20 mg/kg

PHARMACOKINETICS

Molecular weight (daltons)	178.3
% Protein binding	>95
% Excreted unchanged in urine	<0.3
Volume of distribution (L/kg)	8–19
Half-life – normal/ ESRF (hrs)	3–12/Unchanged

METABOLISM

Clearance of propofol occurs by metabolic processes, mainly in the liver where it is blood flow dependent, to form inactive conjugates of propofol and its corresponding quinol, which are excreted in urine.

DOSE IN RENAL IMPAIRMENT GFR (mL/MIN)

20–50	Dose as in normal renal function.
10–20	Dose as in normal renal function.
<10	Dose as in normal renal function.

DOSE IN PATIENTS UNDERGOING RENAL REPLACEMENT THERAPIES

CAPD	Unlikely to be dialysed. Dose as in normal renal function.
HD	Unlikely to be dialysed. Dose as in normal renal function.
HDF/High flux	Unlikely to be dialysed. Dose as in normal renal function.
CAV/ VVHD	Unknown dialysability. Dose as in normal renal function.

IMPORTANT DRUG INTERACTIONS

Potentially hazardous interactions with other drugs

- Adrenergic-neurone blockers: enhanced hypotensive effect.
- Antihypertensives: enhanced hypotensive effect.
- Antidepressants: avoid MAOIs for 2 weeks before surgery; increased risk of arrhythmias and hypotension with tricyclics.
- Antipsychotics: enhanced hypotensive effect.
- Muscle relaxants: increased risk of myocardial depression and bradycardia with suxamethonium.

ADMINISTRATION

RECONSTITUTION

–

ROUTE

- IV

RATE OF ADMINISTRATION

- See local protocols.

COMMENTS

–

Propranolol hydrochloride

CLINICAL USE

Beta-adrenoceptor blocker:
- Hypertension
- Phaeochromocytoma
- Angina
- Arrhythmias
- Anxiety
- Migraine prophylaxis

DOSE IN NORMAL RENAL FUNCTION

- Hypertension: 40–160 mg twice daily
- Prophylaxis of variceal bleeding in portal hypertension: 40–160 mg twice daily
- Phaeochromocytoma: 60 mg daily for 3 days before surgery, or 30 mg daily if unsuitable for surgery
- Angina: 120–240 mg daily in divided doses
- Arrhythmias, anxiety, hypertrophic cardiomyopathy, thyrotoxicosis: 10–40 mg 3–4 times daily
- Anxiety with symptoms, e.g. palpitations: 40 mg 1–3 times daily
- Prophylaxis after an MI: 40 mg 4 times daily then 80 mg twice daily
- Essential tremor: 80–240 mg daily
- Migraine: 80–240 mg daily in divided doses
- IV: 1 mg over 1 minute repeated after 2 minutes to a maximum of 10 mg (5 mg with anaesthesia)

PHARMACOKINETICS

Molecular weight (daltons)	295.8
% Protein binding	80–95
% Excreted unchanged in urine	<5
Volume of distribution (L/kg)	4
Half-life – normal/ ESRF (hrs)	2–6/Unchanged

METABOLISM

Propranolol is subject to considerable hepatic-tissue binding and first-pass metabolism. It is metabolised in the liver to an active metabolite (4-hydroxypropranolol) and several inactive ones. The metabolites and small amounts of unchanged drug are excreted in the urine.

DOSE IN RENAL IMPAIRMENT GFR (mL/MIN)

20–50	Dose as in normal renal function.
10–20	Start with small doses and increase according to response.
<10	Start with small doses and increase according to response.

DOSE IN PATIENTS UNDERGOING RENAL REPLACEMENT THERAPIES

CAPD	Not dialysed. Dose as in GFR<10 mL/min.
HD	Not dialysed. Dose as in GFR<10 mL/min.
HDF/High flux	Unknown dialysability. Dose as in GFR<10 mL/min.
CAV/ VVHD	Unknown dialysability. Dose as in GFR=10–20 mL/min.

IMPORTANT DRUG INTERACTIONS

Potentially hazardous interactions with other drugs
- Anaesthetics: enhanced hypotensive effect; risk of bupivacaine toxicity increased.
- Analgesics: NSAIDs antagonise hypotensive effect.
- Anti-arrhythmics: increased risk of myocardial depression and bradycardia; increased risk of bradycardia, myocardial depression and AV block with amiodarone; concentration increased by propafenone and possibly dronedarone; increased risk of myocardial depression and bradycardia with flecainide; increased risk of lidocaine toxicity.
- Antibacterials: metabolism increased by rifampicin.
- Antidepressants: enhanced hypotensive effect with MAOIs; concentration increased by fluvoxamine; concentration of imipramine increased.
- Antihypertensives; enhanced hypotensive effect; increased risk of withdrawal hypertension with clonidine; increased risk of first dose hypotensive effect with post-synaptic alpha-blockers such as prazosin.
- Antimalarials: increased risk of bradycardia with mefloquine.
- Antipsychotics: enhanced hypotensive effect with phenothiazines; concentration

of both drugs increased with chlorpromazine.
- Calcium-channel blockers: increased risk of bradycardia and AV block with diltiazem; hypotension and heart failure possible with nifedipine and nisoldipine; asystole, severe hypotension and heart failure with verapamil.
- Cytotoxics: possible increased risk of bradycardia with crizotinib.
- Diuretics: enhanced hypotensive effect.
- Fingolimod: possibly increased risk of bradycardia.
- Moxisylyte: possible severe postural hypotension.
- Sympathomimetics: severe hypertension with adrenaline and noradrenaline and possibly with dobutamine.

ADMINISTRATION

RECONSTITUTION
–
ROUTE
- Oral, IV
RATE OF ADMINISTRATION
–
COMMENTS
–

OTHER INFORMATION

- Non-selective active metabolites accumulate in renal impairment. Consider metoprolol or atenolol.
- May reduce renal blood flow in severe renal impairment.

Propylthiouracil

CLINICAL USE

Hyperthyroidism

DOSE IN NORMAL RENAL FUNCTION

- Initially: 200–400 mg daily
- Maintenance dose: 50–150 mg daily

PHARMACOKINETICS

Molecular weight (daltons)	170.2
% Protein binding	80
% Excreted unchanged in urine	<2
Volume of distribution (L/kg)	0.3–0.4
Half-life – normal/ ESRF (hrs)	1–2/8.5

METABOLISM

Propylthiouracil undergoes rapid first-pass metabolism in the liver, and is mainly excreted in the urine as the glucuronic acid conjugate, with very little excreted as unchanged drug.

DOSE IN RENAL IMPAIRMENT GFR (mL/MIN)

20–50	Dose as in normal renal function.
10–20	75% of normal dose and titrate to response. See 'Other information'.
<10	50% of normal dose and titrate to response. See 'Other information'.

DOSE IN PATIENTS UNDERGOING RENAL REPLACEMENT THERAPIES

CAPD	Unknown dialysability. Dose as in GFR<10 mL/min.
HD	Not dialysed. Dose as in GFR<10 mL/min.
HDF/High flux	Unknown dialysability. Dose as in GFR<10 mL/min.
CAV/ VVHD	Unknown dialysability. Dose as in GFR=10–20 mL/min.

IMPORTANT DRUG INTERACTIONS

Potentially hazardous interactions with other drugs
- None known

ADMINISTRATION

RECONSTITUTION

–

ROUTE

- Oral

RATE OF ADMINISTRATION

–

COMMENTS

–

OTHER INFORMATION

- Renally impaired patients are at a greater risk of cardiotoxicity and leucopenia.
- UK manufacturer advises a dose reduction if GFR<50 mL/min but not in the US SPC.
- *Drug Prescribing in Renal Failure*, 5th edition, by Aronoff *et al.* advises to use 100% of dose.

Protamine sulphate

CLINICAL USE
Counteract anticoagulant effect of heparin

DOSE IN NORMAL RENAL FUNCTION
Depends on time since stopping IV/
subcutaneous heparin and dose of heparin
given.

PHARMACOKINETICS

Molecular weight (daltons)	Approx 4500
% Protein binding	1
% Excreted unchanged in urine	No data
Volume of distribution (L/kg)	12.3 litres
Half-life – normal/ ESRF (hrs)	7.4 minutes/–

METABOLISM
The metabolism of the heparin-protamine
complex has not been elucidated, it has
been postulated that it may be partially
metabolised or may be attacked by
fibrinolysin, thus freeing heparin.

DOSE IN RENAL IMPAIRMENT GFR (mL/MIN)

20–50	Dose as in normal renal function.
10–20	Dose as in normal renal function.
<10	Dose as in normal renal function.

DOSE IN PATIENTS UNDERGOING RENAL REPLACEMENT THERAPIES

CAPD	Unknown dialysability. Dose as in normal renal function.
HD	Unknown dialysability. Dose as in normal renal function.
HDF/High flux	Unknown dialysability. Dose as in normal renal function.
CAV/ VVHD	Unknown dialysability. Dose as in normal renal function.

IMPORTANT DRUG INTERACTIONS
Potentially hazardous interactions with other
drugs
* None known

ADMINISTRATION
RECONSTITUTION
–
ROUTE
–
RATE OF ADMINISTRATION
* 5 mg/minute
COMMENTS
–

OTHER INFORMATION
* Counteracting the anticoagulant effect of
heparin during extra-corporeal treatments
requires approximately 1.5 mg protamine
per 100 IU heparin.
* Most clinicians recommend a dose of
1–1.5 mg protamine sulphate for each
100 units heparin given depending
on the length of time since heparin
administration.
* May be used topically to stop bleeding
fistulae.

Pseudoephedrine hydrochloride

CLINICAL USE

Nasal decongestant

DOSE IN NORMAL RENAL FUNCTION

60 mg 4 times a day

PHARMACOKINETICS

Molecular weight (daltons)	201.7
% Protein binding	No data
% Excreted unchanged in urine	90–98
Volume of distribution (L/kg)	2–3
Half-life – normal/ ESRF (hrs)	5.5 (depends on pH of urine)/–

METABOLISM

A small amount of pseudoephedrine is hepatically metabolised by N-demethylation. It is excreted largely unchanged in the urine with small amounts of its hepatic metabolite.

DOSE IN RENAL IMPAIRMENT GFR (mL/MIN)

20–50	Dose as in normal renal function.
10–20	Dose as in normal renal function. Use with caution.
<10	Dose as in normal renal function. Use with caution.

DOSE IN PATIENTS UNDERGOING RENAL REPLACEMENT THERAPIES

CAPD	Unlikely dialysability. Dose as in normal renal function.
HD	Not dialysed. Dose as in normal renal function.
HDF/High flux	Unknown dialysability. Dose as in normal renal function.
CAV/ VVHD	Unknown dialysability. Dose as in normal renal function.

IMPORTANT DRUG INTERACTIONS

Potentially hazardous interactions with other drugs

- Adrenergic neurone blockers: antagonise hypotensive effect of adrenergic neurone blockers.
- Antibacterials: risk of hypertensive crisis with linezolid.
- Antidepressants: risk of hypertensive crisis with MAOIs and moclobemide.
- Dopaminergics: avoid concomitant use with selegiline and rasagiline.

ADMINISTRATION

RECONSTITUTION

–

ROUTE

- Oral

RATE OF ADMINISTRATION

–

COMMENTS

–

OTHER INFORMATION

- Between 5% and 20% is removed by haemodialysis.
- Increased risk of developing hypertension in patients with GFR<20 mL/min.
- Not recommended in severe renal impairment in UK SPC.

Pyrazinamide (unlicensed product)

CLINICAL USE

Antimicrobial agent for tuberculosis

DOSE IN NORMAL RENAL FUNCTION

<50 kg: 1.5 g per day or 2 g three times a week
>50 kg: 2 g per day or 2.5 g three times a week

PHARMACOKINETICS

Molecular weight (daltons)	123.1
% Protein binding	10
% Excreted unchanged in urine	4
Volume of distribution (L/kg)	0.75–1.3
Half-life – normal/ ESRF (hrs)	9–10/26

METABOLISM

Pyrazinamide is metabolised mainly in the liver by hydrolysis to the major active metabolite pyrazinoic acid, which is subsequently hydroxylated to the major excretory product 5-hydroxypyrazinoic acid.

It is excreted via the kidneys mainly by glomerular filtration. About 70% of a dose appears in the urine within 24 hours mainly as metabolites and about 4% as unchanged drug.

DOSE IN RENAL IMPAIRMENT GFR (mL/MIN)

20–50	Dose as in normal renal function.
10–20	Dose as in normal renal function. See 'Other information'.
<10	Use 50–100% of dose. See 'Other information'.

DOSE IN PATIENTS UNDERGOING RENAL REPLACEMENT THERAPIES

CAPD	Not dialysed. Dose as in GFR<10 mL/min.
HD	50–100% dialysed. Dose as in GFR<10 mL/min or 25–30 mg/kg post dialysis.[1]
HDF/High flux	Dialysed. Dose as in GFR<10 mL/min or 25–30 mg/kg post dialysis.[1]
CAV/ VVHD	Dialysed. Dose as in normal renal function.

IMPORTANT DRUG INTERACTIONS

Potentially hazardous interactions with other drugs
- Ciclosporin: on limited evidence, pyrazinamide appears to reduce ciclosporin levels.

ADMINISTRATION

RECONSTITUTION
–
ROUTE
- Oral
RATE OF ADMINISTRATION
–
COMMENTS
–

OTHER INFORMATION

- Available from IDIS on a named patient basis.
- Can precipitate gout as impairs urate excretion.
- Doses in renal impairment are from *Drug Prescribing in Renal Failure*, 5th edition, by Aronoff *et al.*
- WHO recommends a dose of 25 mg/kg three times a week in CKD 4 & 5. (Treatment of tuberculosis: guidelines, 4th edition. Geneva: WHO, 2010. Available at: http://whqlibdoc.who.int/publications/2010/9789241547833_eng.pdf)

Reference:
1. Lacroix C, Heimelin A, Guiberteau R, *et al.* Haemodialysis of pyrazinamide in uraemic patients. *Eur J Clin Pharmacol.* 1989; 37: 309–11.

Pyridostigmine bromide

CLINICAL USE

Myasthenia gravis

DOSE IN NORMAL RENAL FUNCTION

0.3–1.2 g per day in divided doses

PHARMACOKINETICS

Molecular weight (daltons)	261.1
% Protein binding	No data
% Excreted unchanged in urine	80–90
Volume of distribution (L/kg)	0.8–1.4
Half-life – normal/ ESRF (hrs)	3–4/6

METABOLISM

Pyridostigmine undergoes hydrolysis by cholinesterases and is also metabolised in the liver. It appears that 75% of the plasma clearance of pyridostigmine depends on renal function. 3-Hydroxy-N-methylpyridinium has been identified as one of the three metabolites isolated from the urine. Pyridostigmine is excreted mainly in the urine as unchanged drug and metabolites.

DOSE IN RENAL IMPAIRMENT GFR (mL/MIN)

20–50	35% of daily dose
10–20	35% of daily dose
<10	20% of daily dose

DOSE IN PATIENTS UNDERGOING RENAL REPLACEMENT THERAPIES

CAPD	Unknown dialysability. Dose as in GFR<10 mL/min.
HD	Unknown dialysability. Dose as in GFR<10 mL/min.
HDF/High flux	Unknown dialysability. Dose as in GFR<10 mL/min.
CAV/ VVHD	Unknown dialysability. Dose as in GFR=10–20 mL/min.

IMPORTANT DRUG INTERACTIONS

Potentially hazardous interactions with other drugs
- Aminoglycosides, clindamycin and polymyxins antagonise effects of pyridostigmine.

ADMINISTRATION

RECONSTITUTION

–

ROUTE
- Oral

RATE OF ADMINISTRATION

–

COMMENTS

–

OTHER INFORMATION

- Doses in renal impairment are from *Drug Prescribing in Renal Failure*, 5th edition, by Aronoff *et al.*

Pyridoxine hydrochloride

CLINICAL USE

Vitamin B$_6$

DOSE IN NORMAL RENAL FUNCTION

- Deficiency: 20–50 mg up to 3 times daily
- Prophylaxis against isoniazid neuropathy: 10–20 mg daily; 50 mg 3 times daily for treatment
- Idiopathic sideroblastic anaemia: 100–400 mg daily in divided doses
- Penicillamine induced nephropathy, prophylaxis in Wilson's disease (unlicensed): 20 mg daily
- Premenstrual syndrome: 50–100 mg daily

PHARMACOKINETICS

Molecular weight (daltons)	205.6
% Protein binding	High (as pyridoxal and pyridoxal phosphate)
% Excreted unchanged in urine	No data
Volume of distribution (L/kg)	No data
Half-life – normal/ ESRF (hrs)	15–20 days/–

METABOLISM

Pyridoxine is metabolised to its active form pyridoxamine phosphate. It is stored mainly in the liver where there is oxidation to 4-pyridoxic acid and other inactive metabolites which are excreted in the urine.

DOSE IN RENAL IMPAIRMENT GFR (mL/MIN)

20–50	Dose as in normal renal function.
10–20	Dose as in normal renal function.
<10	Dose as in normal renal function.

DOSE IN PATIENTS UNDERGOING RENAL REPLACEMENT THERAPIES

CAPD	Unknown dialysability. Dose as in normal renal function
HD	Dialysed. Dose as in normal renal function.
HDF/High flux	Dialysed. Dose as in normal renal function.
CAV/ VVHD	Dialysed. Dose as in normal renal function.

IMPORTANT DRUG INTERACTIONS

Potentially hazardous interactions with other drugs
- None known

ADMINISTRATION

RECONSTITUTION
–

ROUTE
- Oral

RATE OF ADMINISTRATION
–

COMMENTS
–

OTHER INFORMATION

- Long-term use of pyridoxine in doses greater than 200 mg daily has been associated with neuropathy.

Pyrimethamine

CLINICAL USE

Antiprotozoal agent:
- Malaria
- Toxoplasmosis

DOSE IN NORMAL RENAL FUNCTION

- Malaria: used in dual drug combinations
- Malaria prophylaxis: 25 mg weekly
- Toxoplasmosis: 100–200 mg daily for 2–3 days then 25–100 mg daily for 2–6 weeks (in combination with sulfadiazine)

PHARMACOKINETICS

Molecular weight (daltons)	248.7
% Protein binding	80–90
% Excreted unchanged in urine	15–30
Volume of distribution (L/kg)	2
Half-life – normal/ ESRF (hrs)	35–175/Unchanged

METABOLISM

Pyrimethamine is metabolised in the liver and slowly excreted via the kidney, with up to 30% recovered in the urine as parent compound over a period of several weeks. Several metabolites have also been detected in the urine, although data are lacking on the nature of these metabolites, their route, rate of formation and elimination, and any pharmacological activity, particularly after prolonged daily dosing.

DOSE IN RENAL IMPAIRMENT GFR (mL/MIN)

20–50	Dose as in normal renal function.
10–20	Dose as in normal renal function.
<10	Dose as in normal renal function.

DOSE IN PATIENTS UNDERGOING RENAL REPLACEMENT THERAPIES

CAPD	Not dialysed. Dose as in normal renal function.
HD	Not dialysed. Dose as in normal renal function.
HDF/High flux	Unknown dialysability. Dose as in normal renal function.
CAV/ VVHD	Not dialysed. Dose as in normal renal function.

IMPORTANT DRUG INTERACTIONS

Potentially hazardous interactions with other drugs
- Increased antifolate effect with sulphonamides, trimethoprim, methotrexate and pemetrexed.
- Anti-epileptics: anticonvulsant effect of phenytoin antagonised; increased antifolate effect with phenytoin.
- Antimalarials: avoid concomitant use with artemether/lumefantrine; increased antifolate effect with proguanil.

ADMINISTRATION

RECONSTITUTION

–

ROUTE
- Oral

RATE OF ADMINISTRATION

–

COMMENTS

–

OTHER INFORMATION

- Pyrimethamine should always be administered with a folate supplement to reduce the risk of bone marrow depression.

Quetiapine

CLINICAL USE

- Schizophrenia
- Mania in bipolar disorder
- Depression in bipolar disorder

DOSE IN NORMAL RENAL FUNCTION

- Schizophrenia: 50–750 mg daily in 2 divided doses.
- Mania/mania & depression in bipolar disorder: 50–400 mg twice daily
- Depression in bipolar disorder: 50–600 mg once daily
- XL: Schizophrenia/mania/mania & depression: 300–800 mg once daily
- Depression in bipolar disorder: 50–600 mg once daily

PHARMACOKINETICS

Molecular weight (daltons)	883.1 (as fumarate)
% Protein binding	83
% Excreted unchanged in urine	<5
Volume of distribution (L/kg)	6–14
Half-life – normal/ ESRF (hrs)	6–7/Unchanged

METABOLISM

Quetiapine is extensively metabolised in the liver by sulfoxidation mediated mainly by the cytochrome P450 isoenzyme CYP3A4 and by oxidation. The primary metabolite is norquetiapine, which is also eliminated by CYP3A4. Following the administration of radiolabelled quetiapine, the parent compound accounted for less than 5% of unchanged drug-related material in the urine or faeces. Approximately 73% of the radioactivity is excreted in the urine and 21% in the faeces, mainly as inactive metabolites.

DOSE IN RENAL IMPAIRMENT GFR (mL/MIN)

20–50   Dose as in normal renal function. Initial dose 25 mg/day and increase in increments of 25–50 mg/day according to response.

10–20   Dose as in normal renal function. Initial dose 25 mg/day and increase in increments of 25–50 mg/day according to response.

<10   Dose as in normal renal function. Initial dose 25 mg/day and increase in increments of 25–50 mg/day according to response.

DOSE IN PATIENTS UNDERGOING RENAL REPLACEMENT THERAPIES

CAPD	Unknown dialysability. Dose as in GFR<10 mL/min.
HD	Unknown dialysability. Dose as in GFR<10 mL/min.
HDF/High flux	Unknown dialysability. Dose as in GFR<10 mL/min.
CAV/ VVHD	Unknown dialysability. Dose as in GFR=10–20 mL/min.

IMPORTANT DRUG INTERACTIONS

Potentially hazardous interactions with other drugs

- Anaesthetics: enhanced hypotensive effect.
- Analgesics: increased risk of convulsions with tramadol; enhanced hypotensive and sedative effects with opioids; increased risk of ventricular arrhythmias with methadone.
- Antibacterials: concentration possibly increased by macrolides – avoid.
- Antidepressants: concentration of tricyclics possibly increased.
- Anti-epileptics: antagonism of convulsive threshold; metabolism accelerated by carbamazepine and phenytoin; concentration possibly increased by valproate.
- Antifungals: concentration possibly increased by imidazoles and triazoles – avoid.
- Antimalarials: manufacturer advises avoid use with artemether and lumefantrine.
- Antivirals: concentration possibly increased by atazanavir, boceprevir, darunavir, fosamprenavir, indinavir, lopinavir, ritonavir, saquinavir, telaprevir and tipranavir – avoid concomitant use.
- Anxiolytics and hypnotics: enhanced sedative effects.
- Atomoxetine: increased risk of ventricular arrhythmias.
- Cytotoxics: increased risk of ventricular arrhythmias with arsenic trioxide.
- Grapefruit juice: concentration of quetiapine possibly increased – avoid.

ADMINISTRATION

RECONSTITUTION

–

ROUTE

● Oral

RATE OF ADMINISTRATION

–

COMMENTS

–

OTHER INFORMATION

● Plasma clearance is reduced by 25% in severe renal impairment.
● Absorption is increased by food so it should be taken consistently either with or without food.

Quinagolide

CLINICAL USE

Hyperprolactinaemia

DOSE IN NORMAL RENAL FUNCTION

75–150 micrograms daily

PHARMACOKINETICS

Molecular weight (daltons)	432 (as hydrochloride)
% Protein binding	90
% Excreted unchanged in urine	Very little
Volume of distribution (L/kg)	100 litres
Half-life – normal/ ESRF (hrs)	17

METABOLISM

Quinagolide is extensively metabolised. Quinagolide and its N-desethyl analogue are the biologically active but minor components. Their inactive sulphate or glucuronide conjugates represent the major circulating metabolites. Studies performed with ^{3}H-labelled quinagolide revealed that more than 95% of the drug is excreted as metabolites. About equal amounts of total radioactivity are found in faeces and urine.

DOSE IN RENAL IMPAIRMENT GFR (mL/MIN)

20–50	Use with caution. Start with low dose and titrate according to response.
10–20	Use with caution. Start with low dose and titrate according to response.
<10	Use with caution. Start with low dose and titrate according to response.

DOSE IN PATIENTS UNDERGOING RENAL REPLACEMENT THERAPIES

CAPD	Unknown dialysability. Dose as in GFR<10 mL/min.
HD	Unknown dialysability. Dose as in GFR<10 mL/min.
HDF/High flux	Unknown dialysability. Dose as in GFR<10 mL/min.
CAV/ VVHD	Unknown dialysability. Dose as in GFR=10–20 mL/min.

IMPORTANT DRUG INTERACTIONS

Potentially hazardous interactions with other drugs
• None known

ADMINISTRATION

RECONSTITUTION
–
ROUTE
• Oral
RATE OF ADMINISTRATION
–
COMMENTS
–

OTHER INFORMATION

• Manufacturer advises to avoid use in renal impairment due to lack of data.

Quinapril

CLINICAL USE

Angiotensin converting enzyme inhibitor:
- Hypertension
- Congestive heart failure

DOSE IN NORMAL RENAL FUNCTION

- Hypertension: 2.5–80 mg daily in 1–2 divided doses
- Congestive heart failure: 2.5–40 mg daily in 1–2 divided doses

PHARMACOKINETICS

Molecular weight (daltons)	475 (as hydrochloride)
% Protein binding	97
% Excreted unchanged in urine	30
Volume of distribution (L/kg)	1.5
Half-life – normal/ ESRF (hrs)	1/12–14

METABOLISM

Quinapril is a prodrug which is metabolised in the liver to its active form, quinaprilat, and to minor inactive metabolites. Quinaprilat is eliminated primarily by renal excretion.

DOSE IN RENAL IMPAIRMENT GFR (mL/MIN)

20–50	Start with low dose, adjust according to response.
10–20	Start with low dose, adjust according to response.
<10	Start with low dose, adjust according to response.

DOSE IN PATIENTS UNDERGOING RENAL REPLACEMENT THERAPIES

CAPD	Not dialysed. Dose as in GFR<10 mL/min.
HD	25% dialysed. Dose as in GFR<10 mL/min.
HDF/High flux	Dialysed. Dose as in GFR<10 mL/min.
CAV/ VVHD	Unknown dialysability. Dose as in GFR=10–20 mL/min.

IMPORTANT DRUG INTERACTIONS

Potentially hazardous interactions with other drugs
- Anaesthetics: enhanced hypotensive effect.
- Analgesics: antagonism of hypotensive effect and increased risk of renal impairment with NSAIDs; hyperkalaemia with ketorolac and other NSAIDs.
- Ciclosporin: increased risk of hyperkalaemia and nephrotoxicity.
- Diuretics: enhanced hypotensive effect; hyperkalaemia with potassium-sparing diuretics.
- ESAs: increased risk of hyperkalaemia; antagonism of hypotensive effect.
- Gold: flushing and hypotension with sodium aurothiomalate.
- Lithium: reduced excretion (possibility of enhanced lithium toxicity).
- Potassium salts: increased risk of hyperkalaemia.
- Tacrolimus: increased risk of hyperkalaemia and nephrotoxicity.

ADMINISTRATION

RECONSTITUTION
–
ROUTE
- Oral
RATE OF ADMINISTRATION
–
COMMENTS
–

OTHER INFORMATION

- Renal failure has been reported with ACE inhibitors: mainly in patients with renal artery stenosis, post renal transplant and those with severe congestive heart failure.
- A high incidence of anaphylactoid reactions has been reported in patients dialysed with high-flux polyacrylonitrile membranes and treated concomitantly with an ACE inhibitor – this combination should be avoided.
- Hyperkalaemia and other side effects more common in patients with renal impairment.
- Close monitoring of renal function during therapy is necessary in those patients with known renal insufficiency.

Quinine

CLINICAL USE

- Severe and complicated falciparum malaria
- Nocturnal cramp

DOSE IN NORMAL RENAL FUNCTION

- IV: Quinine dihydrochloride: Loading dose 20 mg/kg to maximum 1.4 g, then after 8 hours, maintenance 10 mg/kg (up to maximum 700 mg) 8 hourly, reduced to 5–7 mg/kg if parenteral treatment required for more than 48 hours
- Oral: Quinine sulphate 600 mg every 8 hours for 5–7 days
- Nocturnal cramp: Quinine sulphate 200–300 mg at night

PHARMACOKINETICS

Molecular weight (daltons)	324.4 (397.3 as dihydrochloride); (782.9 as sulphate)
% Protein binding	70–90
% Excreted unchanged in urine	5–20
Volume of distribution (L/kg)	2.5–7.1
Half-life – normal/ ESRF (hrs)	11 (healthy), 18 (malaria)/26

METABOLISM

Quinine is extensively metabolised in the liver and rapidly excreted mainly in the urine. Excretion is increased in acid urine.

DOSE IN RENAL IMPAIRMENT GFR (mL/MIN)

20–50	Malaria: 5–7 mg/kg every 8 hours Cramp: dose as in normal renal function.
10–20	Malaria: 5–7 mg/kg every 8–12 hours Cramp: dose as in normal renal function.
<10	Malaria: 5–7 mg/kg every 24 hours Cramp: dose as in normal renal function.

DOSE IN PATIENTS UNDERGOING RENAL REPLACEMENT THERAPIES

CAPD	Dialysed. Dose as in GFR<10 mL/min.
HD	Dialysed. Dose as in GFR<10 mL/min.
HDF/High flux	Dialysed. Dose as in GFR<10 mL/min.
CAV/VVHD	Not dialysed. Dose as in GFR=10–20 mL/min.

IMPORTANT DRUG INTERACTIONS

Potentially hazardous interactions with other drugs

- Anti-arrhythmics: flecainide levels increased; increased risk of ventricular arrhythmias with amiodarone – avoid concomitant use.
- Antibacterials: increased risk of ventricular arrhythmias with moxifloxacin – avoid concomitant use; concentration reduced by rifampicin.
- Antimalarials: increased risk of convulsions with mefloquine; avoid concomitant use with artemether/lumefantrine.
- Antipsychotics: increased risk of ventricular arrhythmias with droperidol, pimozide and possibly haloperidol – avoid concomitant use.
- Antivirals: concentration possibly increased by atazanavir, darunavir, fosamprenavir, indinavir and tipranavir; concentration increased by ritonavir; increased risk of ventricular arrhythmias with saquinavir – avoid.
- Cardiac glycosides: levels of digoxin increased (halve maintenance dose).
- Ciclosporin: decreased ciclosporin levels reported.
- Cimetidine: may increase plasma levels of quinine.

ADMINISTRATION

RECONSTITUTION
–

ROUTE
- IV infusion, Oral, IM (quinine dihydrochloride)

RATE OF ADMINISTRATION
- 4 hours

COMMENTS
- Add to sodium chloride 0.9% or glucose 5% for infusion.
- Loading dose of 20 mg/kg may be required in some cases (refer to specialist treatment). Not to be given if patient has had quinine or mefloquine in previous 12–24 hours.

OTHER INFORMATION

- Quinine dihydrochloride injection is available as a special order.
- Monitor for signs of cardiotoxicity.
- Give doses after haemodialysis on dialysis days.
- Monitor quinine levels if patient exhibits any symptoms of toxicity.
- Doses in renal impairment are from *Drug Prescribing in Renal Failure*, 5th edition, by Aronoff *et al.*

Rabeprazole sodium

CLINICAL USE

Gastric acid suppression

DOSE IN NORMAL RENAL FUNCTION

10–120 mg daily, doses >100 mg in 2 divided doses

PHARMACOKINETICS

Molecular weight (daltons)	381.4
% Protein binding	97
% Excreted unchanged in urine	0 (90 as metabolites)
Volume of distribution (L/kg)	0.34
Half-life – normal/ ESRF (hrs)	0.7–1.5/Unchanged

METABOLISM

Rabeprazole is mainly metabolised via nonenzymatic reduction and, to a lesser extent, via the cytochrome P450 isoenzymes CYP2C19 and CYP3A4.

Metabolites are excreted principally in the urine (about 90%) with the remainder in the faeces.

DOSE IN RENAL IMPAIRMENT GFR (mL/MIN)

20–50	Dose as in normal renal function.
10–20	Dose as in normal renal function.
<10	Dose as in normal renal function.

DOSE IN PATIENTS UNDERGOING RENAL REPLACEMENT THERAPIES

CAPD	Unlikely to be dialysed. Dose as in normal renal function.
HD	Not dialysed. Dose as in normal renal function.
HDF/High flux	Unlikely to be dialysed. Dose as in normal renal function.
CAV/ VVHD	Unlikely to be dialysed. Dose as in normal renal function.

IMPORTANT DRUG INTERACTIONS

Potentially hazardous interactions with other drugs

- Antifungals: absorption of itraconazole and ketoconazole reduced; avoid with posaconazole.
- Antivirals: concentration of atazanavir and rilpivirine reduced – avoid concomitant use; concentration of raltegravir and saquinavir possibly increased – avoid.
- Clopidogrel: possibly reduced anti-platelet effect.
- Cytotoxics: possibly reduced excretion of methotrexate; avoid with erlotinib and vandetanib; possibly reduced lapatinib absorption; possibly reduced absorption of pazopanib.
- Ulipristal: reduced contraceptive effect, avoid with high dose ulipristal.

ADMINISTRATION

RECONSTITUTION

–

ROUTE

- Oral

RATE OF ADMINISTRATION

–

COMMENTS

–

OTHER INFORMATION

- Interstitial nephritis has been reported with rabeprazole.
- Oral bioavailability is 52%.

Racecadotril

CLINICAL USE

Treatment of acute diarrhoea

DOSE IN NORMAL RENAL FUNCTION

100 mg followed by 100 mg three times a day preferably before main meals

PHARMACOKINETICS

Molecular weight (daltons)	385.5
% Protein binding	90 (active metabolite – mainly to albumin)
% Excreted unchanged in urine	81.4 (as active and inactive metabolites)
Volume of distribution (L/kg)	66.4
Half-life – normal/ ESRF (hrs)	3/Increased

METABOLISM

Quickly metabolised by hydrolysis to active metabolite, thiorphan.

Racecadotril is eliminated as active and inactive metabolites. Elimination is mainly via the renal route (81.4%), and to a much lesser extent via the faecal route (around 8%). The pulmonary route is not significant (less than 1% of the dose).

DOSE IN RENAL IMPAIRMENT GFR (mL/MIN)

20–50	Dose as in normal renal function. Use with caution.
10–20	Dose as in normal renal function. Use with caution.
<10	Dose as in normal renal function. Use with caution.

DOSE IN PATIENTS UNDERGOING RENAL REPLACEMENT THERAPIES

CAPD	Unknown dialysability. Dose as in GFR<10 mL/min.
HD	Unknown dialysability. Dose as in GFR<10 mL/min.
HDF/High flux	Unknown dialysability. Dose as in GFR<10 mL/min.
CAV/ VVHD	Unknown dialysability. Dose as in GFR<10 mL/min.

IMPORTANT DRUG INTERACTIONS

Potentially hazardous interactions with other drugs
● None known

ADMINISTRATION

RECONSTITUTION
–
ROUTE
● Oral
RATE OF ADMINISTRATION
–

OTHER INFORMATION

● In patients with severe renal failure (creatinine clearance 11–39 mL/min), the kinetic profile of the active metabolite of racecadotril showed smaller C_{max} (−49%) and greater AUC (+16%) and half-life as compared to healthy volunteers (creatinine clearance >70 mL/min).

Raloxifene hydrochloride

CLINICAL USE

Treatment and prevention of osteoporosis in post menopausal women

DOSE IN NORMAL RENAL FUNCTION

60 mg daily

PHARMACOKINETICS

Molecular weight (daltons)	510
% Protein binding	98–99
% Excreted unchanged in urine	<0.2
Volume of distribution (L/kg)	2348
Half-life – normal/ ESRF (hrs)	27.7/Unchanged

METABOLISM

Raloxifene undergoes extensive first-pass metabolism to the glucuronide conjugates: raloxifene-4'-glucuronide, raloxifene-6-glucuronide, and raloxifene-6, 4'-diglucuronide. Raloxifene undergoes enterohepatic recycling, and is excreted almost entirely in the faeces.

Less than 6% of dose is excreted in the urine.

DOSE IN RENAL IMPAIRMENT GFR (mL/MIN)

20–50	Dose as in normal renal function.
10–20	Dose as in normal renal function.
<10	Dose as in normal renal function.

DOSE IN PATIENTS UNDERGOING RENAL REPLACEMENT THERAPIES

CAPD	Unlikely to be dialysed. Dose as in normal renal function.
HD	Unlikely to be dialysed. Dose as in normal renal function.
HDF/High flux	Unknown dialysability. Dose as in normal renal function.
CAV/ VVHD	Unlikely to be dialysed. Dose as in normal renal function.

IMPORTANT DRUG INTERACTIONS

Potentially hazardous interactions with other drugs
- Anticoagulants: antagonism of anticoagulant effect of coumarins.
- Cholestyramine: reduced absorption of raloxifene – avoid concomitant use.

ADMINISTRATION

RECONSTITUTION

–

ROUTE
- Oral

RATE OF ADMINISTRATION

–

COMMENTS

–

OTHER INFORMATION

- There are case reports of it being beneficial in females on haemodialysis and also a benefit to the lipid profile. (Hernandez E, Valera R, Alonzo E, et al. Effects of raloxifene on bone metabolism and serum lipids in postmenopausal women on chronic haemodialysis. *Kidney Int.* 2003; **63**(6): 2269–74.)
- This study showed that raloxifene could reduce vertebral fractures although they were more likely to suffer from side effects. (Ishani A, Blackwell T, Jamal SA, et al. The effect of raloxifene treatment in postmenopausal women with CKD. *J Am Soc Nephrol.* 2008; **19**: 1430–8.)
- UK SPC advises use is contraindicated in severe renal impairment due to lack of data rather than known toxicity. The US data sheet advises to use with caution.

Raltegravir

Integrase inhibitor:
- Treatment of HIV infection, in combination with other antiretroviral medication

DOSE IN NORMAL RENAL FUNCTION

400 mg twice daily

PHARMACOKINETICS

Molecular weight (daltons)	444.4 (482.5 as potassium)
% Protein binding	83
% Excreted unchanged in urine	7–14[1]
Volume of distribution (L/kg)	No data
Half-life – normal/ ESRF (hrs)	9/Unchanged

METABOLISM

Metabolised via glucuronidation, catalysed by the enzyme uridine diphosphate glucuronosyltransferase.

Raltegravir is excreted in both urine and faeces as unchanged drug and metabolites.

DOSE IN RENAL IMPAIRMENT GFR (mL/MIN)

20–50	Dose as in normal renal function.
10–20	Dose as in normal renal function.
<10	Dose as in normal renal function.

DOSE IN PATIENTS UNDERGOING RENAL REPLACEMENT THERAPIES

CAPD	Unlikely to be dialysed. Dose as in normal renal function.
HD	Minimal dialysability.[2] Dose as in normal renal function.
HDF/High flux	Dialysed. Dose as in normal renal function.
CAV/ VVHD	Unknown dialysability. Dose as in normal renal function.

IMPORTANT DRUG INTERACTIONS

Potentially hazardous interactions with other drugs
- Antibacterials: concentration reduced by rifampicin, consider increasing raltegravir dose.
- Antivirals: avoid with fosamprenavir.
- Ulcer-healing drugs: concentration increased by omeprazole and possibly by H_2-antagonists and other proton pump inhibitors – avoid concomitant use.

ADMINISTRATION

RECONSTITUTION
–
ROUTE
- Oral
RATE OF ADMINISTRATION
–

OTHER INFORMATION

References:
1. Iwamoto M, Wenning LA, Petry AS, et al. Safety, tolerability, and pharmacokinetics of raltegravir after single and multiple doses in healthy subjects. Clin Pharmacol Ther. 2008; 83(2): 293–9.
2. Malto J, Sanz Moreno J, Valle M, et al. Effect of haemodialysis on raltegravir clearance in HIV-infected patients with end stage renal disease. Pharmacology presentations at 11th International Workshop on Clinical Pharmacology of HIV Therapy. Sorrento, April 2010.

Raltitrexed

CLINICAL USE

Treatment of colorectal cancer when fluorouracil and folinic acid cannot be used

DOSE IN NORMAL RENAL FUNCTION

$3 \, mg/m^2$ every 3 weeks

PHARMACOKINETICS

Molecular weight (daltons)	458.5
% Protein binding	93
% Excreted unchanged in urine	40–50
Volume of distribution (L/kg)	548 litres
Half-life – normal/ ESRF (hrs)	198/Increased

METABOLISM

Raltitrexed is actively transported into cells and metabolised to active polyglutamate forms. The remainder of a dose is not metabolised and is excreted unchanged, about 50% of a dose appearing in the urine, and about 15% in the faeces.

DOSE IN RENAL IMPAIRMENT GFR (mL/MIN)

55–65	Use 75% of the dose ($2.25 \, mg/m^2$) every 4 weeks.
25–54	Use 50% of the dose ($1.5 \, mg/m^2$) every 4 weeks.
<25	Avoid. See 'Other information'.

DOSE IN PATIENTS UNDERGOING RENAL REPLACEMENT THERAPIES

CAPD	Unlikely to be dialysed. Dose as in GFR<25 mL/min.
HD	Unlikely to be dialysed. Dose as in GFR<25 mL/min.
HDF/High flux	Unknown dialysability. Dose as in GFR<25 mL/min.
CAV/ VVHD	Unlikely to be dialysed. Dose as in GFR<25 mL/min.

IMPORTANT DRUG INTERACTIONS

Potentially hazardous interactions with other drugs
- Antipsychotics: avoid with clozapine, increased risk of agranulocytosis.
- Folic and folinic acid: impairs cytotoxic action – avoid concomitant use.

ADMINISTRATION

RECONSTITUTION
- 4 mL water for injection
ROUTE
- IV infusion
RATE OF ADMINISTRATION
- Over 15 minutes
COMMENTS
- Dilute in 50–250 mL sodium chloride 0.9% or glucose 5%.
- Stable for 24 hours at 2–8°C.

OTHER INFORMATION

- Doses above $3 \, mg/m^2$ have an increased incidence of life-threatening/fatal toxicity.
- Increased risk of treatment-related toxicity if CRCL<65 mL/min.
- Anecdotal reports of using 30–40% of the dose every 4 weeks in patients with severe renal impairment and closely monitoring haematological parameters. Risk of severe and prolonged side effects – use if risk of not treating the patient outweighs the risk of adverse effects.

Ramipril

CLINICAL USE

Angiotensin-converting enzyme inhibitor:
- Hypertension
- Secondary prevention of myocardial infarction (MI), stroke or cardiovascular death
- Heart failure
- Diabetic nephropathy

DOSE IN NORMAL RENAL FUNCTION

- 1.25–10 mg once a day
- Prophylaxis after a MI: 2.5–5 mg twice daily
- Diabetic nephropathy: 1.25–5 mg once daily

PHARMACOKINETICS

Molecular weight (daltons)	416.5
% Protein binding	56 (as ramiprilat)
% Excreted unchanged in urine	<2
Volume of distribution (L/kg)	1.2
Half-life – normal/ESRF (hrs)	13–17/Increased (as ramiprilat)

METABOLISM

Ramipril is metabolised in the liver to its active metabolite, ramiprilat, and other inactive metabolites. It is excreted mainly in the urine, as ramiprilat, other metabolites, and some unchanged drug. About 40% of an oral dose appears in the faeces; this may represent both biliary excretion and unabsorbed drug.

DOSE IN RENAL IMPAIRMENT GFR (mL/MIN)

20–50	Dose as in normal renal function.
10–20	Initial dose 1.25 mg daily and increase according to response.
<10	Initial dose 1.25 mg daily and increase according to response.

DOSE IN PATIENTS UNDERGOING RENAL REPLACEMENT THERAPIES

CAPD	Unknown dialysability. Dose as in GFR<10 mL/min.
HD	Not dialysed. Dose as in GFR<10 mL/min.
HDF/High flux	Dialysed. Dose as in GFR<10 mL/min.
CAV/ VVHD	Dialysed. Dose as in GFR=10–20 mL/min.

IMPORTANT DRUG INTERACTIONS

Potentially hazardous interactions with other drugs
- Anaesthetics: enhanced hypotensive effect.
- Analgesics: antagonism of hypotensive effect and increased risk of renal impairment with NSAIDs; hyperkalaemia with ketorolac and other NSAIDs.
- Ciclosporin: increased risk of hyperkalaemia and nephrotoxicity.
- Diuretics: enhanced hypotensive effect; hyperkalaemia with potassium-sparing diuretics.
- ESAs: increased risk of hyperkalaemia; antagonism of hypotensive effect.
- Gold: flushing and hypotension with sodium aurothiomalate.
- Lithium: reduced excretion (possibility of enhanced lithium toxicity).
- Potassium salts: increased risk of hyperkalaemia.
- Tacrolimus: increased risk of hyperkalaemia and nephrotoxicity.

ADMINISTRATION

RECONSTITUTION
–
ROUTE
- Oral
RATE OF ADMINISTRATION
–
COMMENTS
–

OTHER INFORMATION

- Renal failure has been reported in association with ACE inhibitors in patients with renal artery stenosis, post renal transplant, and those with congestive heart failure.
- A high incidence of anaphylactoid reactions has been reported in patients dialysed with high-flux polyacrylonitrile membranes and treated concomitantly with an ACE inhibitor – this combination should therefore be avoided.
- Hyperkalaemia and other side effects more common in patients with impaired renal function.
- Close monitoring of renal function during therapy is necessary in those patients with known renal insufficiency.
- Normal doses have been used in CKD 5.

Ranitidine

CLINICAL USE

H$_2$ antagonist:
* Conditions associated with hyperacidity

DOSE IN NORMAL RENAL FUNCTION

* Oral: 150–300 mg once or twice daily
* Zollinger Ellison: 150 mg 3 times daily up to 6 g/day
* IM/Slow IV injection: 50 mg every 6–8 hours
* IV infusion: 25 mg/hour for 2 hours, 6–8 hourly; or for stress ulceration prophylaxis 125–250 mcg/kg/hour

PHARMACOKINETICS

Molecular weight (daltons)	314.4
% Protein binding	15
% Excreted unchanged in urine	Oral: 30–35; IV: 80
Volume of distribution (L/kg)	1.4
Half-life – normal/ESRF (hrs)	2–3/6–9

METABOLISM

Ranitidine is not extensively metabolised. A small proportion of ranitidine is metabolised in the liver to the N-oxide, the S-oxide, and desmethylranitidine; the N-oxide is the major metabolite but accounts for only about 4–6% of a dose. The fraction of the dose recovered as metabolites is similar after both oral and IV dosing; and includes 6% of the dose in urine as the N-oxide, 2% as the S-oxide, 2% as desmethylranitidine and 1–2% as the furoic acid analogue. There is also some excretion in the faeces.

DOSE IN RENAL IMPAIRMENT GFR (mL/MIN)

20–50	Dose as in normal renal function.
10–20	Dose as in normal renal function.
<10	50–100% of normal dose.

DOSE IN PATIENTS UNDERGOING RENAL REPLACEMENT THERAPIES

CAPD	Not dialysed. Dose as in GFR<10 mL/min.
HD	Dialysed. Dose as in GFR<10 mL/min.
HDF/High flux	Dialysed. Dose as in GFR<10 mL/min.
CAV/ VVHD	Dialysed. IV: 50 mg every 8–12 hours.[1] Oral: Dose as in normal renal function.

IMPORTANT DRUG INTERACTIONS

Potentially hazardous interactions with other drugs
* Alpha-blockers: effects of tolazoline antagonised.
* Antifungals: absorption of itraconazole and ketoconazole reduced; concentration of posaconazole possibly reduced – avoid.
* Antivirals: concentration of atazanavir reduced; concentration of raltegravir possibly increased – avoid; avoid for 12 hours before and 4 hours after rilpivirine.
* Ciclosporin: may increase or not change ciclosporin levels; nephrotoxicity, additive hepatotoxicity and thrombocytopenia reported.
* Cytotoxics: reduced gefitinib concentration; reduces concentration of erlotinib, give at least 2 hours before or 10 hours after ranitidine; possibly reduced absorption of pazopanib – give at least 2 hours before or 10 hours after ranitidine; possibly reduced absorption of lapatinib.
* Ulipristal: contraceptive effect possibly reduced – avoid with high dose ulipristal.

ADMINISTRATION

RECONSTITUTION
–
ROUTE
* Oral, IV, IM (undiluted)
RATE OF ADMINISTRATION
* Bolus: 50 mg made up to 20 mL, over at least 2 minutes
* Intermittent infusion: 50 mg to 100 mL of appropriate intravenous solution run over 2 hours
* Continuous infusion: required dose in 250 mL of intravenous fluid over 24 hours
COMMENTS
* Compatible with sodium chloride 0.9%, glucose 5% and other fluids.
* Admixtures stable for 24 hours.
* Minimum volume: can be used undiluted as a bolus over at least 2 minutes. (UK Critical Care Group, *Minimum Infusion Volumes for Fluid Restricted Critically Ill Patients*, 3rd edition, 2006)

OTHER INFORMATION

- In CKD 5 usually twice daily for IV preparation and normal dose for oral.

Reference:
1. Dose from CVVH Initial Drug Dosing Guidelines on www.thedrugmonitor.com.

Ranolazine

CLINICAL USE

Add on therapy for angina

DOSE IN NORMAL RENAL FUNCTION

375–750 mg twice daily

PHARMACOKINETICS

Molecular weight (daltons)	427.5
% Protein binding	62
% Excreted unchanged in urine	<5 (75% as metabolites)
Volume of distribution (L/kg)	180 litres
Half-life – normal/ ESRF (hrs)	7/Increased

METABOLISM

Extensively metabolised in the gastrointestinal tract and liver. Four main metabolites have been identified.

Approximately 75% of a dose is excreted in the urine with the remainder in the faeces, with less than 5% as unchanged drug.

DOSE IN RENAL IMPAIRMENT GFR (mL/MIN)

30–50	Dose as in normal renal function. Titrate slowly.
10–30	Use lower dose with caution. See 'Other information'.
<30	Use lower dose with caution. See 'Other information'.

DOSE IN PATIENTS UNDERGOING RENAL REPLACEMENT THERAPIES

CAPD	Unlikely to be dialysed. Dose as in GFR<10 mL/min.
HD	Unlikely to be dialysed. Dose as in GFR<10 mL/min.
HDF/High flux	Unknown dialysability. Dose as in GFR<10 mL/min.
CAV/ VVHD	Unknown dialysability. Dose as in GFR=10–30 mL/min.

IMPORTANT DRUG INTERACTIONS

Potentially hazardous interactions with other drugs
- Anti-arrhythmics: avoid concomitant use with disopyramide.
- Antibacterials: concentration possibly increased by clarithromycin and telithromycin – avoid concomitant use; concentration reduced by rifampicin – avoid concomitant use.
- Antifungals: concentration increased by ketoconazole and possibly itraconazole, posaconazole and voriconazole – avoid concomitant use.
- Antivirals: concentration possibly increased by atazanavir, darunavir, fosamprenavir, indinavir, lopinavir, ritonavir, saquinavir and tipranavir – avoid concomitant use.
- Beta-blockers: avoid concomitant use with sotalol.
- Ciclosporin: concentration of both drugs possibly increased.
- Grapefruit juice: concentration of ranolazine possibly increased – avoid concomitant use.
- Statins: concentration of simvastatin increased – maximum dose of simvastatin is 20 mg.
- Tacrolimus: concentration of tacrolimus increased.

ADMINISTRATION

RECONSTITUTION
–

ROUTE
- Oral

RATE OF ADMINISTRATION
–

OTHER INFORMATION

- Contraindicated by manufacturer in UK SPC in severe renal impairment (GFR<30 mL/min).
- Bioavailability is 35–50%.
- May cause an increase in QT interval.
- May increase blood pressure in patients with severe renal impairment.
- Steady state occurs within 3 days.
- In patients with renal impairment there may be an increased incidence of side effects.
- The AUC of ranolazine was on average 1.7 to 2-fold higher in subjects with mild, moderate, and severe renal impairment compared with subjects with normal renal function. The AUC of metabolites increased with decreased renal function. The AUC of one pharmacologically active ranolazine metabolite was 5-fold increased in patients with severe renal impairment.

- Case report of use in a HDF patient who didn't tolerate 375 mg twice daily due to intolerable side effects but tolerated once daily.

Rasagiline

CLINICAL USE

Treatment of Parkinson's disease

DOSE IN NORMAL RENAL FUNCTION

1 mg daily

PHARMACOKINETICS

Molecular weight (daltons)	267.3 (as mesilate)
% Protein binding	60–70
% Excreted unchanged in urine	<1
Volume of distribution (L/kg)	243 litres
Half-life – normal/ ESRF (hrs)	0.6–2/Unchanged

METABOLISM

Rasagiline is extensively metabolised in the liver by N-dealkylation and hydroxylation, via the cytochrome P450 isoenzyme CYP1A2, and conjugation. 1-Aminoindan is a major metabolite and is stated to be active although it is not a monoamine oxidase B inhibitor.

The metabolites are excreted mainly in the urine and partly in the faeces; less than 1% of a dose is excreted as unchanged drug in the urine.

DOSE IN RENAL IMPAIRMENT GFR (mL/MIN)

20–50	Dose as in normal renal function.
10–20	Dose as in normal renal function.
<10	Dose as in normal renal function.

DOSE IN PATIENTS UNDERGOING RENAL REPLACEMENT THERAPIES

CAPD	Unknown dialysability. Dose as in normal renal function.
HD	Unknown dialysability. Dose as in normal renal function.
HDF/High flux	Likely to be dialysed. Dose as in normal renal function.
CAV/ VVHD	Unknown dialysability. Dose as in normal renal function.

IMPORTANT DRUG INTERACTIONS

Potentially hazardous interactions with other drugs

- Analgesics: avoid concomitant use with dextromethorphan; avoid concomitant use with pethidine (risk of serious adverse reactions) – allow at least 14 days before starting pethidine.
- Antidepressants: avoid concomitant use with other MAOIs (can lead to hypertensive crisis) – allow at least 14 days before starting a MAOI; avoid concomitant use with fluoxetine and fluvoxamine; allow 5 weeks between stopping fluoxetine and starting rasagiline; allow 14 days between stopping rasagiline and starting fluoxetine or fluvoxamine; increased CNS toxicity with SSRIs and tricyclics.
- Sympathomimetics: concomitant use is not recommended.

ADMINISTRATION

RECONSTITUTION
–
ROUTE
- Oral
RATE OF ADMINISTRATION
–
COMMENTS
–

OTHER INFORMATION

- Rasagiline is an irreversible selective inhibitor of monoamine oxidase type B.
- Bioavailability is 36%.

Rasburicase

CLINICAL USE

Prophylaxis and treatment of acute hyperuricaemia with initial chemotherapy for haematological malignancy

DOSE IN NORMAL RENAL FUNCTION

200 mcg/kg once daily for up to 7 days

PHARMACOKINETICS

Molecular weight (daltons)	34 000
% Protein binding	0
% Excreted unchanged in urine	0
Volume of distribution (L/kg)	0.11–0.127
Half-life – normal/ ESRF (hrs)	19/–

METABOLISM

Rasburicase is a protein; it is expected that metabolic degradation will follow the pathways of other proteins, i.e. peptide hydrolysis.

DOSE IN RENAL IMPAIRMENT GFR (mL/MIN)

20–50	Dose as in normal renal function.
10–20	Dose as in normal renal function.
<10	Dose as in normal renal function.

DOSE IN PATIENTS UNDERGOING RENAL REPLACEMENT THERAPIES

CAPD	Unlikely to be dialysed. Dose as in normal renal function.
HD	Unlikely to be dialysed. Dose as in normal renal function.
HDF/High flux	Unlikely to be dialysed. Dose as in normal renal function.
CAV/ VVHD	Unlikely to be dialysed. Dose as in normal renal function.

IMPORTANT DRUG INTERACTIONS

Potentially hazardous interactions with other drugs
● None known

ADMINISTRATION

RECONSTITUTION
● With solvent provided
ROUTE
● IV
RATE OF ADMINISTRATION
● Over 30 minutes
COMMENTS
● Add appropriate volume to 50 mL sodium chloride 0.9%

OTHER INFORMATION

● Renal elimination of rasburicase is considered to be a minor pathway for rasburicase clearance.
● After infusion of rasburicase at a dose of 0.2 mg/kg/day, steady state is achieved at day 2–3.

Reboxetine

CLINICAL USE

Antidepressant

DOSE IN NORMAL RENAL FUNCTION

4–5 mg twice daily; maximum 12 mg daily

PHARMACOKINETICS

Molecular weight (daltons)	409.5 (as mesilate)
% Protein binding	97 (92% in elderly)
% Excreted unchanged in urine	10
Volume of distribution (L/kg)	26–63 litres
Half-life – normal/ ESRF (hrs)	13/26

METABOLISM

Reboxetine is predominantly metabolised *in vitro* via cytochrome P4503A (CYP3A4); the main metabolic pathways identified are dealkylation, hydroxylation, and oxidation followed by glucuronide or sulfate conjugation. Elimination is mainly via urine (78%) with 10% excreted as unchanged drug.

DOSE IN RENAL IMPAIRMENT GFR (mL/MIN)

20–50	Dose as in normal renal function.
10–20	2 mg twice daily and adjust according to response.
<10	2 mg twice daily and adjust according to response.

DOSE IN PATIENTS UNDERGOING RENAL REPLACEMENT THERAPIES

CAPD	Unknown dialysability. Dose as in GFR<10 mL/min.
HD	Unknown dialysability. Dose as in GFR<10 mL/min.
HDF/High flux	Unknown dialysability. Dose as in GFR<10 mL/min.
CAV/ VVHD	Unknown dialysability. Dose as in GFR=10–20 mL/min.

IMPORTANT DRUG INTERACTIONS

Potentially hazardous interactions with other drugs
- Antibacterials: avoid concomitant use with macrolides and linezolid.
- Antidepressants: risk of increased toxicity with MAOIs – avoid; avoid concomitant use with fluvoxamine.
- Antifungals: avoid concomitant use with imidazoles and triazoles.
- Antimalarials: avoid concomitant use with artemether with lumefantrine and piperaquine with artenimol.
- Ciclosporin: use with caution as high concentrations of reboxetine inhibit CYP3A4 and CYP2D6.

ADMINISTRATION

RECONSTITUTION
–
ROUTE
- Oral
RATE OF ADMINISTRATION
–
COMMENTS
–

OTHER INFORMATION

–

Remifentanil

CLINICAL USE

- Analgesic
- Induction of anaesthesia

DOSE IN NORMAL RENAL FUNCTION

- Induction: 0.5–1 microgram/kg/min
- Maintenance:
  - Ventilated patients: 0.05–2 mcg/kg/min
  - Spontaneous respiration:
    25–100 nanograms/kg/min
- Analgesia and sedation in ventilated, intensive care patients: 6–740 nanograms/ kg/minute
- Additional analgesia during painful procedures in ventilated, intensive care patients: 100–750 nanograms/kg/minute

PHARMACOKINETICS

Molecular weight (daltons)	412.9 (as hydrochloride
% Protein binding	70
% Excreted unchanged in urine	95 (as metabolites)
Volume of distribution (L/kg)	0.35
Half-life – normal/ ESRF (hrs)	3–10 minutes (biological activity)/ unchanged Terminal elimination 10–20 minutes

METABOLISM

Remifentanil is an esterase metabolised opioid that is susceptible to metabolism by non-specific blood and tissue esterases. The metabolism of remifentanil results in the formation of an essentially inactive carboxylic acid metabolite (1/4600th as potent as remifentanil). About 95% of a dose of remifentanil is excreted in the urine as the metabolite.

DOSE IN RENAL IMPAIRMENT GFR (mL/MIN)

20–50	Dose as in normal renal function.
10–20	Dose as in normal renal function.
<10	Dose as in normal renal function.

DOSE IN PATIENTS UNDERGOING RENAL REPLACEMENT THERAPIES

CAPD	Unlikely to be dialysed. Dose as in normal renal function.
HD	Not dialysed. Dose as in normal renal function.
HDF/High flux	Unlikely to be dialysed. Dose as in normal renal function.
CAV/ VVHD	Unknown dialysability. Dose as in normal renal function.

IMPORTANT DRUG INTERACTIONS

Potentially hazardous interactions with other drugs

- Anti-arrhythmics: delayed absorption of mexiletine.
- Antidepressants: possible CNS excitation or depression (hypertension or hypotension) in patients also receiving MAOIs (including moclobemide) – avoid concomitant use; possibly increased sedative effects with tricyclics.
- Antihistamines: sedative effects possibly increased with sedating antihistamines.
- Antipsychotics: enhanced sedative and hypotensive effect.
- Antivirals: concentration possibly increased by ritonavir (risk of toxicity) – avoid.
- Dopaminergics: avoid with selegiline. Sodium oxybate: enhanced effect of sodium oxybate – avoid concomitant use.

ADMINISTRATION

RECONSTITUTION
- To 1 mg/mL with infusion fluid
ROUTE
- IV
RATE OF ADMINISTRATION
- Dependent on indication
COMMENTS
- Dilute to 20–250 mcg/mL with glucose 5%, sodium chloride 0.9% or water for injection; usually 50 micrograms/mL for general anaesthesia.

OTHER INFORMATION

- Half-life of metabolite is increased to 30 hours in renal failure compared with 90 minutes in patients with normal renal function.
- Remifentanil would be expected to be metabolised before patient needs to be dialysed.
- 25–35% of metabolites are removed by dialysis.

Repaglinide

CLINICAL USE

Type 2 Diabetes mellitus

DOSE IN NORMAL RENAL FUNCTION

0.5–16 mg daily, doses given 15–30 minutes before a meal; doses up to 4 mg can be given as a single dose

PHARMACOKINETICS

Molecular weight (daltons)	452.6
% Protein binding	>98
% Excreted unchanged in urine	<8 (mainly as metabolites)
Volume of distribution (L/kg)	30 litres
Half-life – normal/ ESRF (hrs)	1/2

METABOLISM

Repaglinide appears to be a substrate for active hepatic uptake by the organic anion transporting protein OATP1B1, and undergoes almost complete hepatic metabolism involving the cytochrome P450 isoenzymes CYP2C8 and CYP3A4. The glucuronidation of repaglinide is thought to involve uridine diphosphate glucuronosyltransferase (UGT) enzymes, particularly UGT1A1. The metabolites, which are inactive, are excreted in the bile.

DOSE IN RENAL IMPAIRMENT GFR (mL/MIN)

20–50	Dose as in normal renal function.
10–20	Start at a low dose and gradually increase according to response.
<10	Start at a low dose and gradually increase according to response.

DOSE IN PATIENTS UNDERGOING RENAL REPLACEMENT THERAPIES

CAPD	Unlikely to be dialysed. Dose as in GFR<10 mL/min.
HD	Not dialysed. Dose as in GFR<10 mL/min.
HDF/High flux	Not dialysed. Dose as in GFR<10 mL/min.
CAV/ VVHD	Not dialysed. Dose as in GFR=10–20 mL/min.

IMPORTANT DRUG INTERACTIONS

Potentially hazardous interactions with other drugs

- Antibacterials: effects enhanced by clarithromycin and possibly trimethoprim – avoid with trimethoprim; hypoglycaemic effect antagonised by rifampicin.
- Antifungals: effect possibly enhanced by itraconazole.
- Ciclosporin: may increase repaglinide concentration, possibly enhanced hypoglycaemic effect.
- Cytotoxics: avoid with lapatinib.
- Lipid-lowering agents: increased risk of severe hypoglycaemia with gemfibrozil – avoid concomitant use.

ADMINISTRATION

RECONSTITUTION

–

ROUTE

- Oral

RATE OF ADMINISTRATION

–

COMMENTS

–

OTHER INFORMATION

–

Reteplase

CLINICAL USE

Thrombolytic, used for acute myocardial infarction

DOSE IN NORMAL RENAL FUNCTION

10 units over 2 minutes; second dose of 10 units given 30 minutes later

PHARMACOKINETICS

Molecular weight (daltons)	39571.1
% Protein binding	No data
% Excreted unchanged in urine	Negligible
Volume of distribution (L/kg)	6–6.5 litres
Half-life – normal/ ESRF (hrs)	Fibrinolytic half-life is 1.6 hours/Increased Dominant (α) half-life is 14.6 +/− 6.7 minutes. Terminal (β) half-life is 1.6 hours +/− 39 minutes.

METABOLISM

Cleared primarily by liver and kidneys.

DOSE IN RENAL IMPAIRMENT GFR (mL/MIN)

20–50	Dose as in normal renal function.
10–20	Dose as in normal renal function.
<10	Dose as in normal renal function. Use with caution.

DOSE IN PATIENTS UNDERGOING RENAL REPLACEMENT THERAPIES

CAPD	Unknown dialysability. Dose as in GFR<10 mL/min.
HD	Unknown dialysability. Dose as in GFR<10 mL/min.
HDF/High flux	Unknown dialysability. Dose as in GFR<10 mL/min.
CAV/ VVHD	Unknown dialysability. Dose as in normal renal function.

IMPORTANT DRUG INTERACTIONS

Potentially hazardous interactions with other drugs
- Antiplatelets, heparin, vitamin K antagonists: increased risk of bleeding.

ADMINISTRATION

RECONSTITUTION
- With diluent provided

ROUTE
- Slow IV

RATE OF ADMINISTRATION
- Over not more than 2 minutes

COMMENTS
- Use immediately once reconstituted.
- Do not mix with heparin in the same line.

OTHER INFORMATION

- Heparin and aspirin should be given before and after reteplase therapy to reduce the risk of re-thrombosis but may increase the risk of bleeding.
- Half-life is increased in severe renal failure in animal models.
- Possible increased risk of bleeding complications in severe renal impairment.
- Contraindicated in severe renal impairment in UK SPC but only use with caution in US data sheet due to increased risk of bleeding.

Retigabine

CLINICAL USE

Anti-epileptic agent

DOSE IN NORMAL RENAL FUNCTION

100 mg three times daily, maximum 1200 mg daily

PHARMACOKINETICS

Molecular weight (daltons)	303.3
% Protein binding	80
% Excreted unchanged in urine	36 (84% including metabolites)
Volume of distribution (L/kg)	2–3
Half-life – normal/ ESRF (hrs)	6–10/–

METABOLISM

Extensively metabolised to inactive N-glucuronides (majority) and to an N-acetyl metabolite (NAMR) that is also then glucuronidated. NAMR has antiepileptic activity, but is less potent than retigabine.

Eight-five per cent excreted in the urine (36% as unchanged drug, 18% as NAMR) and 14% via the faeces (3% as unchanged drug).

DOSE IN RENAL IMPAIRMENT GFR (mL/MIN)

20–50	Reduce dose by 50% and increase according to response, max 600 mg daily
10–20	Reduce dose by 50% and increase according to response, max 600 mg daily
<10	Reduce dose by 50% and increase according to response, max 600 mg daily.

DOSE IN PATIENTS UNDERGOING RENAL REPLACEMENT THERAPIES

CAPD	Dialysed. Dose as in GFR<10 mL/min.
HD	Dialysed. Dose as in GFR<10 mL/min.
HDF/High flux	Dialysed. Dose as in GFR<10 mL/min.
CAV/ VVHD	Dialysed. Dose as in GFR=10–20 mL/min.

IMPORTANT DRUG INTERACTIONS

Potentially hazardous interactions with other drugs
- Antidepressants: convulsive threshold lowered; avoid concomitant use with St John's wort.
- Antimalarials: anticonvulsant effect antagonised by mefloquine.
- Antipsychotics: anticonvulsant effect antagonised.
- Orlistat: possibly increased risk of convulsions.

ADMINISTRATION

RECONSTITUTION
–
ROUTE
- Oral
RATE OF ADMINISTRATION
–

OTHER INFORMATION

- May prolong QT interval.
- Bioavailability is 60%.
- In a single dose study, retigabine AUC was increased by approximately 30% in volunteers with creatinine clearance 50 to 80 mL/min and by approximately 100% in volunteers with creatinine clearance <50 mL/min, compared to healthy volunteers.
- 50% of retigabine and NAMR are removed by haemodialysis.

Ribavirin (tribavirin)

CLINICAL USE

Antiviral agent:
Chronic Hepatitis C in combination with
interferon α or peginterferon α

DOSE IN NORMAL RENAL FUNCTION

Rebetol:
- <65 kg: 400 mg twice daily
- 65–80 kg: 400 mg in the morning and
  600 mg at 6pm
- 81–105 kg: 600 mg twice daily
- >105 kg: 600 mg in the morning and
  800 mg at 6pm

Copegus:
- <75 kg: 400 mg in the morning and 600 mg
  at 6 pm
- >75 kg: 600 mg twice daily
- Dose depends on genotype, see SPC

PHARMACOKINETICS

Molecular weight (daltons)	244.2
% Protein binding	0
% Excreted unchanged in urine	10–40
Volume of distribution (L/kg)	5000 litres
Half-life – normal/ ESRF (hrs)	Oral: 79/Increased

METABOLISM

Ribavirin is metabolised by reversible
phosphorylation and a degradative pathway
involving deribosylation and amide
hydrolysis to produce an active triazole
carboxyacid metabolite. Ribavirin is mainly
excreted in the urine as unchanged drug and
metabolites.

DOSE IN RENAL IMPAIRMENT GFR (mL/MIN)

20–50	Avoid. See 'Other information'.
10–20	Avoid. See 'Other information'.
<10	Avoid. See 'Other information'.

DOSE IN PATIENTS UNDERGOING RENAL REPLACEMENT THERAPIES

CAPD	Unlikely to be dialysed. Dose as in GFR<10 mL/min.
HD	Not dialysed. Dose as in GFR<10 mL/min.
HDF/High flux	Unknown dialysability. Dose as in GFR<10 mL/min.
CAV/ VVHD	Unknown dialysability. Dose as in GFR=10–20 mL/min.

IMPORTANT DRUG INTERACTIONS

Potentially hazardous interactions with other
drugs
- Antivirals: effects possibly reduced by
  abacavir; increased risk of toxicity with
  stavudine; increased side effects with
  didanosine – avoid; increased risk of
  anaemia with zidovudine – avoid.
- Azathioprine: possibly enhances
  myelosuppressive effects of azathioprine.

ADMINISTRATION

RECONSTITUTION
- Dissolve contents of one vial in water for
  injection.
ROUTE
- Oral, IV
RATE OF ADMINISTRATION
- IV: over 10–15 minutes
COMMENTS
–

OTHER INFORMATION

- Oral: Administer ribavirin with
  interferon α 3 MIU 3 times a week or
  peginterferon α 1.5 mcg/kg/week.
- Contraindicated by the manufacturer
  of Rebetol, use with great caution by
  manufacturer of Copegus due to reduced
  clearance leading to increased side effects.
- There are two studies using ribavirin
  (200–400 mg daily) in combination
  with interferon in haemodialysis and
  peritoneal dialysis patients. Anaemia was
  one of the main problems, resulting in
  either increased doses of erythropoietin
  or discontinuation of ribavirin therapy.
  Most patients were stabilised on a dose
  of 200 mg daily or 200 mg 3 times a week.
  A dose of 200 mg daily gave troughs
  comparable to those in patients with
  normal renal function taking 1200 mg
  daily. (Bruchfeld A, Stahle L, Andrsson J, *et
  al*. Ribavirin treatment in dialysis patients
  with chronic hepatitis C virus infection – a
  pilot study. *J Viral Hepat*. 2001 Jul 8: 287–
  92 and Tan AC, Brouwer JT, Glue P, *et al*.
  Safety of interferon and ribavirin therapy

in haemodialysis patients with chronic hepatitis C: results of a pilot study. *Nephrol Dial Transplant*. 2001; **16**: 193–5.)

- After stopping therapy the half-life was approximately 298 hours, due to slow elimination from non-plasma compartments.
- Ribavirin is also available (on named patient basis) as an intravenous infusion, from ICN Pharmaceuticals.
- Recommended IV dosing schedule in patients with normal renal function is:
  — Initial loading dose: 33 mg/kg
  — Six hours after the initial dose: 16 mg/kg every 6 hours for 4 days (16 doses)
  — Eight hours following the last of these doses: 8 mg/kg every 8 hours for 3 days (9 doses).
- Patients with impaired renal function should be carefully monitored during therapy with ribavirin for signs and symptoms of toxicity, such as haemolytic anaemia.
  — Available clinical experience suggests that patients with renal insufficiency and creatinine clearance of 50–80 mL/min tolerate the usual dosage regimen of ribavirin.
  — Individuals with moderate to severe renal insufficiency (creatinine clearance 30–50 mL/min) have tolerated, without reports of complications, a dose regimen with an initial loading dose of 20–25 mg/kg, followed by single daily doses of 10 mg/kg for 9–10 consecutive days.
  — There is no experience in patients with end-stage renal disease.
- See SPC for further information.

Rifabutin

CLINICAL USE

Antibacterial agent:
- Tuberculosis
- Mycobacterial infection

DOSE IN NORMAL RENAL FUNCTION

- Prophylaxis of *Mycobacterium avium* in patients with low CD4 count: 300 mg daily
- Treatment of non-tuberculous mycobacterial disease, in combination with other drugs 450–600 mg daily
- Treatment of pulmonary tuberculosis, in combination with other drugs 150–450 mg daily

PHARMACOKINETICS

Molecular weight (daltons)	847
% Protein binding	70
% Excreted unchanged in urine	5
Volume of distribution (L/kg)	8–9
Half-life – normal/ESRF (hrs)	35–40/ Unchanged

METABOLISM

Rifabutin is rapidly metabolised in the liver by the cytochrome P450 isoenzyme CYP3A4 mainly to active 25-O-deacetyl and 31-hydroxy metabolites.

Rifabutin induces its own metabolism resulting in a lower area under the curve after 4 weeks of continuous treatment than after the first few doses. About 53% of a dose is found in the urine, mainly as metabolites, and about 30% of a dose is excreted in the faeces.

DOSE IN RENAL IMPAIRMENT GFR (mL/MIN)

30–50	Dose as in normal renal function.
10–30	Maximum 300 mg daily. (Dose reduction of 50%).
<10	Maximum 300 mg daily. (Dose reduction of 50%).

DOSE IN PATIENTS UNDERGOING RENAL REPLACEMENT THERAPIES

CAPD	Unlikely to be dialysed. Dose as in GFR<10 mL/min.
HD	Not dialysed. Dose as in GFR<10 mL/min.
HDF/High flux	Not dialysed. Dose as in GFR<10 mL/min.
CAV/ VVHD	Unknown dialysability. Dose as in GFR=10–30 mL/min.

IMPORTANT DRUG INTERACTIONS

Potentially hazardous interactions with other drugs
- Anti-arrhythmics: metabolism of disopyramide, and propafenone accelerated; concentration of dronedarone reduced.
- Antibacterials: increased risk of side effects with azithromycin; clarithromycin and other macrolides increase concentration of rifabutin, resulting in increased risk of uveitis – reduce rifabutin dose; reduced concentration of dapsone and clarithromycin.
- Anticoagulants: reduced anticoagulant effect of coumarins.
- Antidiabetics: reduced antidiabetic effect of tolbutamide; possibly reduced antidiabetic effect with sulphonylureas.
- Anti-epileptics: reduced concentration of phenytoin and carbamazepine.
- Antifungals: fluconazole, triazoles, posaconazole and voriconazole increase the concentration of rifabutin resulting in increased risk of uveitis – reduce rifabutin dose; rifabutin reduces concentration of posaconazole, voriconazole and itraconazole – increase voriconazole dose, avoid with itraconazole.
- Antipsychotics: possibly reduced aripiprazole concentration – increase dose of aripiprazole.
- Antivirals: atazanavir darunavir, fosamprenavir, saquinavir and tipranavir and possibly nevirapine increase concentration of rifabutin – halve or reduce dose of rifabutin; efavirenz reduces the concentration of rifabutin – increase dose of rifabutin; concentration of both drugs reduced with etravirine; indinavir increases rifabutin concentration – avoid; concentration of indinavir reduced – increase indinavir dose; concentration of rilpivirine reduced – increase rilpivirine dose to 50 mg once daily; ritonavir increases the concentration of rifabutin resulting in increased risk of uveitis – reduce rifabutin dose; concentration of saquinavir reduced – avoid concomitant use unless another protease inhibitor is also given; avoid with telaprevir.

- Atovaquone: concentration of atovaquone reduced (possible therapeutic failure of atovaquone).
- Ciclosporin: possibly reduced ciclosporin levels.
- Corticosteroids: reduced level of corticosteroids – double steroid dose. Give as twice daily dosage.
- Cytotoxics: possibly reduced concentration of axitinib (increase axitinib dose), cabazitaxel, crizotinib, lapatinib and vemurafenib – avoid.
- Oestrogens and progestogens: reduced contraceptive effect due to increased metabolism.
- Sirolimus: reduced sirolimus concentration – avoid.
- Tacrolimus: possibly reduced tacrolimus trough concentration.

ADMINISTRATION

RECONSTITUTION

–

ROUTE

- Oral

RATE OF ADMINISTRATION

–

COMMENTS

–

OTHER INFORMATION

- Can cause an orange-tan skin pigmentation as well as discoloured urine.
- Can cause abnormal LFTs and hepatitis.
- Can cause uveitis especially in combination with clarithromycin and fluconazole.
- Rifabutin is a less potent CYP4503A enzyme inducer than rifampicin but similar interactions may occur.
- *Drug Prescribing in Renal Failure*, 5th edition, by Aronoff *et al.* recommends a dose of 300 mg daily in renal impairment.

Rifampicin

CLINICAL USE

Antibacterial agent:
- Tuberculosis
- Staphylococcal infection

DOSE IN NORMAL RENAL FUNCTION

600–1200 mg daily in 2–4 divided doses

PHARMACOKINETICS

Molecular weight (daltons)	822.9
% Protein binding	80
% Excreted unchanged in urine	15–30
Volume of distribution (L/kg)	0.64–0.66
Half-life – normal/ESRF (hrs)	2–5/1.8–11

METABOLISM

Rifampicin is rapidly metabolised in the liver mainly to active 25-O-deacetylrifampicin and excreted in the bile. Deacetylation diminishes intestinal reabsorption and increases faecal excretion, although significant enterohepatic circulation still takes place. About 60% of a dose eventually appears in the faeces. The amount excreted in the urine increases with increasing doses and up to 30% of a dose may be excreted in the urine, about half of it being unchanged drug. The metabolite formylrifampicin is also excreted in the urine.

DOSE IN RENAL IMPAIRMENT GFR (mL/MIN)

20–50	Dose as in normal renal function.
10–20	Dose as in normal renal function.
<10	50–100% of normal dose.

DOSE IN PATIENTS UNDERGOING RENAL REPLACEMENT THERAPIES

CAPD	Not dialysed. Dose as in GFR<10 mL/min.
HD	Not dialysed. Dose as in GFR<10 mL/min.
HDF/High flux	Not dialysed. Dose as in GFR<10 mL/min.
CAV/VVHD	Unknown dialysability. Dose as in normal renal function.

IMPORTANT DRUG INTERACTIONS

Potentially hazardous interactions with other drugs

- Anti-arrhythmics: metabolism of disopyramide, and propafenone accelerated; concentration of dronedarone reduced.
- Antibacterials: reduced concentration of chloramphenicol, clarithromycin, dapsone, doxycycline, linezolid, trimethoprim and telithromycin and possibly tinidazole – avoid with telithromycin; concentration increased by clarithromycin and other macrolides.
- Anticoagulants: reduced anticoagulant effect of coumarins; reduced concentration of apixaban and rivaroxaban; avoid with dabigatran.
- Antidiabetics: reduced antidiabetic effect of linagliptin and tolbutamide; concentration of nateglinide and repaglinide reduced; possibly reduced antidiabetic effect with sulphonylureas.
- Anti-epileptics: reduced concentration of phenytoin and lamotrigine; concentration possibly reduced by phenobarbital.
- Antifungals: concentration of both drugs may be reduced with ketoconazole; reduced concentration of fluconazole, itraconazole, posaconazole and terbinafine; concentration of voriconazole reduced – avoid concomitant use; initially increases then reduces caspofungin concentration.
- Antimalarials: avoid concomitant use with piperaquine with artenimol; concentration of mefloquine reduced – avoid, concentration of quinine reduced.
- Antipsychotics: reduced concentration of haloperidol, aripiprazole and clozapine – increase dose of aripiprazole.
- Antivirals: concentration of abacavir, ritonavir and tipranavir possibly reduced – avoid with tipranavir; concentration of atazanavir, boceprevir, darunavir, etravirine, fosamprenavir, indinavir, lopinavir, maraviroc, nevirapine, raltegravir, rilpivirine, saquinavir and telaprevir reduced – avoid; concentration of efavirenz reduced – increase dose of efavirenz; avoid with zidovudine.
- Atovaquone: concentration of atovaquone reduced (possible therapeutic failure of atovaquone); concentration of rifampicin increased.

- Bosentan: reduced bosentan concentration – avoid.
- Calcium-channel blockers: metabolism of diltiazem, verapamil, isradipine, nicardipine, nifedipine and nimodipine accelerated.
- Ciclosporin: markedly reduced levels (danger of transplant rejection); ciclosporin dose may need increasing 5-fold or more.
- Corticosteroids: reduced level of corticosteroids – double steroid dose. Give as twice daily dosage.
- Cytotoxics: reduced concentration of axitinib, brentuximab, cabazitaxel, crizotinib, dasatinib, eribulin, erlotinib, everolimus, gefitinib, imatinib, lapatinib, nilotinib, pazopanib, ruxolitinib, sorafenib, sunitinib, vandetanib, vemurafenib and vinflunine – avoid; active metabolite of temsirolimus reduced.
- Diuretics: concentration of eplerenone reduced – avoid.
- Mycophenolate: concentration of active mycophenolate metabolite reduced.
- Oestrogens and progestogens: reduced contraceptive effect due to increased metabolism.
- Ranolazine: concentration of ranolazine reduced – avoid.
- Sirolimus: reduced sirolimus concentration.
- Tacrolimus: reduced tacrolimus concentration.
- Tadalafil: concentration of tadalafil reduced – avoid.
- Ticagrelor: concentration of ticagrelor reduced.
- Ulipristal: contraceptive effect possibly reduced – avoid.

ADMINISTRATION

RECONSTITUTION
- Use solvent provided.

ROUTE
- Oral, IV

RATE OF ADMINISTRATION
- 2–3 hours

COMMENTS
- Dilute in 500 mL glucose 5% or sodium chloride 0.9%.
- For central administration, 600 mg in 100 mL glucose 5% over 0.5–2 hours has been used (unlicensed).
- Stable for up to 24 hours at room temperature.

OTHER INFORMATION

- Some units give dose in concentrations up to 60 mg/mL (in its own solvent) over 10 minutes, on prescriber's responsibility.
- May cause acute interstitial nephritis, potassium wasting or renal tubular defects.
- Reduce dose if LFTs are abnormal or patient <45 kg.
- Absorption from gastrointestinal tract can be reduced by up to 80% by the presence of food in the gastrointestinal tract.
- CAPD exit site infections: 300 mg twice daily for 4 weeks has been used.
- Rifampicin is excreted into CAPD fluid causing an orange/yellow colour.
- Monitor rifampicin levels if necessary.
- In severe renal impairment there is no increase in half-life at doses less than 600 mg daily.

Rifaximin

CLINICAL USE

Antibacterial agent:
- Treatment of traveller's diarrhoea
- Reduction of recurrence of hepatic encephalopathy

DOSE IN NORMAL RENAL FUNCTION

- Traveller's diarrhoea: 200 mg every 8 hours for 3 days
- Hepatic encephalopathy: 550 mg twice daily

PHARMACOKINETICS

Molecular weight (daltons)	785.9
% Protein binding	67.5
% Excreted unchanged in urine	0.03
Volume of distribution (L/kg)	No data
Half-life – normal/ ESRF (hrs)	5.85/–

METABOLISM

Not greatly absorbed. Systemically available rifaximin is believed to be metabolised in the liver, similarly to other rifamycin derivatives.
   Excreted mainly in faeces (97%) as unchanged drug.

DOSE IN RENAL IMPAIRMENT GFR (mL/MIN)

20–50   Dose as in normal renal function.
10–20   Dose as in normal renal function.
<10   Dose as in normal renal function.

DOSE IN PATIENTS UNDERGOING RENAL REPLACEMENT THERAPIES

CAPD	Unlikely to be dialysed. Dose as in normal renal function.
HD	Unlikely to be dialysed. Dose as in normal renal function.
HDF/High flux	Unlikely to be dialysed. Dose as in normal renal function.
CAV/ VVHD	Unlikely to be dialysed. Dose as in normal renal function.

IMPORTANT DRUG INTERACTIONS

Potentially hazardous interactions with other drugs
- None known

ADMINISTRATION

RECONSTITUTION
–
ROUTE
- Oral
RATE OF ADMINISTRATION
–

OTHER INFORMATION

- Not effective for diarrhoea caused by invasive enteric pathogens, e.g. *Shigella, Campylobacter*.
- Bioavailability <0.4%.
- Use higher dose for encephalopathy with caution in renal impairment.

Rilpivirine

CLINICAL USE

Non-nucleoside reverse transcriptase
inhibitor:
- Treatment of progressive or advanced HIV
  infection in combination with at least two
  other antivirals

DOSE IN NORMAL RENAL FUNCTION

25 mg once daily
(50 mg daily in combination with rifabutin)

PHARMACOKINETICS

Molecular weight (daltons)	366.4 (402.9 as hydrochloride)
% Protein binding	99.7
% Excreted unchanged in urine	<1
Volume of distribution (L/kg)	No data
Half-life – normal/ ESRF (hrs)	45/–

METABOLISM

Primarily undergoes oxidative metabolism
mediated by the cytochrome P450 (CYP) 3A
system.
   Eighty-five per cent is excreted via the
faeces (25% as unchanged drug) and 6% via
the urine (<1% as unchanged drug).

DOSE IN RENAL IMPAIRMENT GFR (mL/MIN)

20–50	Dose as in normal renal function.
10–20	Dose as in normal renal function.
<10	Dose as in normal renal function. Use with caution.

DOSE IN PATIENTS UNDERGOING RENAL REPLACEMENT THERAPIES

CAPD	Not dialysed. Dose as in GFR<10 mL/min.
HD	Not dialysed. Dose as in GFR<10 mL/min.
HDF/High flux	Not dialysed. Dose as in GFR<10 mL/min.
CAV/ VVHD	Unlikely to be dialysed. Dose as in normal renal function.

IMPORTANT DRUG INTERACTIONS

Potentially hazardous interactions with other
drugs
- Antibacterials: avoid concomitant use
  with clarithromycin & erythromycin
  – concentration possibly increased;
  concentration decreased by rifampicin &
  rifabutin – avoid with rifampicin, increase
  dose of rilpivirine to 50 mg daily.
- Antidepressants: concentration possibly
  reduced by St John's wort – avoid
  concomitant use.
- Antiepileptics: concentration possibly
  reduced by carbamazepine, oxcarbazepine,
  phenobarbital & phenytoin – avoid
  concomitant use.
- Corticosteroids: avoid concomitant use
  with dexamethasone (except as a single
  dose).
- Ulcer-healing drugs: concentration
  possibly reduced by esomeprazole,
  lansoprazole, omeprazole, pantoprazole
  & rabeprazole – avoid concomitant
  use; avoid histamine H2-antagonists
  for 12 hours before and 4 hours after
  rilpivirine.

ADMINISTRATION

RECONSTITUTION
–
ROUTE
- Oral
RATE OF ADMINISTRATION
–
COMMENTS
–

OTHER INFORMATION

- Use with caution in severe renal
  impairment and ESRD due to lack of
  studies.

Risedronate sodium

CLINICAL USE

Bisphosphonate:
- Treatment and prevention of osteoporosis (including corticosteroid induced)
- Paget's disease

DOSE IN NORMAL RENAL FUNCTION

- Osteoporosis: 5 mg daily or 35 mg weekly
- Paget's disease: 30 mg daily for 2 months

PHARMACOKINETICS

Molecular weight (daltons)	305.1
% Protein binding	24
% Excreted unchanged in urine	50
Volume of distribution (L/kg)	6.3
Half-life – normal/ ESRF (hrs)	480/Increased

METABOLISM

The mean bioavailability of risedronate is 0.63% in the fasting state, and there is no evidence of systemic metabolism of risedronate sodium. About half of the absorbed portion is excreted in the urine within 24 hours; the remainder is sequestered to bone for a prolonged period. Unabsorbed drug is eliminated unchanged in the faeces.

DOSE IN RENAL IMPAIRMENT GFR (mL/MIN)

30–50	Dose as in normal renal function.
10–30	See 'Other information'.
<10	See 'Other information'.

DOSE IN PATIENTS UNDERGOING RENAL REPLACEMENT THERAPIES

CAPD	Unknown dialysability. Dose as in GFR<10 mL/min.
HD	Unknown dialysability. Dose as in GFR<10 mL/min.
HDF/High flux	Unknown dialysability. Dose as in GFR<10 mL/min.
CAV/ VVHD	Unknown dialysability. Dose as in GFR=10–30 mL/min.

IMPORTANT DRUG INTERACTIONS

Potentially hazardous interactions with other drugs
- Calcium-containing substances: avoid for 2 hours before and after administration.

ADMINISTRATION

RECONSTITUTION
–
ROUTE
- Oral
RATE OF ADMINISTRATION
–
COMMENTS
–

OTHER INFORMATION

- Swallow whole with a glass of water 30 minutes before food. Sit or stand upright for 30 minutes after administration.
- Renal clearance is decreased by 70% in patients with creatinine clearance <30 mL/min.
- No data, but one paper suggests using a decreased dose when GFR<20 mL/min. (Mitchell DY, St Peter JV, Eusebio RA, *et al*. Effect of renal function on risedronate pharmacokinetics after a single oral dose. *Br J Clin Pharmacol*. 2000; **49**(3): 215–22.)
- One paper reviewed all the information available and concluded that 50% of the recommended dose may be possible in ESRF, but more trials are required, and osteomalacia and adynamic bone disease must first be excluded. (Miller PD. Treatment of osteoporosis in chronic kidney disease and end-stage renal disease. *Curr Osteoporos Rep*. 2005; **3**: 5–12.)
- Examples of use in other units in HD patients: Normal doses; 5 mg once weekly.
- If used in patients with ESRD ensure the patient has an adequate PTH, e.g. at least 3 times the upper limit of normal.

Risperidone

CLINICAL USE

- Schizophrenia
- Psychoses
- Mania

DOSE IN NORMAL RENAL FUNCTION

- Oral: 2–16 mg daily in divided doses
- IM: 25–50 mg every 2 weeks

PHARMACOKINETICS

Molecular weight (daltons)	410.5
% Protein binding	90
% Excreted unchanged in urine	70
Volume of distribution (L/kg)	1–2
Half-life – normal/ESRF (hrs)	19.5/Increased

METABOLISM

Risperidone is metabolised in the liver by CYP 2D6 to its main active metabolite, 9-hydroxy-risperidone (paliperidone), which has a similar pharmacological activity as risperidone. This hydroxylation is subject to genetic polymorphism. Oxidative N-dealkylation is a minor metabolic pathway. Excretion is mainly in the urine and, to a lesser extent, in the faeces.

DOSE IN RENAL IMPAIRMENT GFR (mL/MIN)

20–50	Initially 50% of dose, increases should also be 50% less and at a slower rate. Use with caution. See 'Other information' for IM dosing.
20–50	Initially 50% of dose, increases should also be 50% less and at a slower rate. Use with caution. See 'Other information' for IM dosing.
<10	Initially 50% of dose, increases should also be 50% less and at a slower rate. Use with caution. See 'Other information' for IM dosing.

DOSE IN PATIENTS UNDERGOING RENAL REPLACEMENT THERAPIES

CAPD	Unlikely to be dialysed. Dose as in GFR<10 mL/min.
HD	Dialysed. Dose as in GFR<10 mL/min.
HDF/High flux	Dialysed. Dose as in GFR<10 mL/min.
CAV/ VVHD	Dialysed. Dose as in GFR=10–20 mL/min.

IMPORTANT DRUG INTERACTIONS

Potentially hazardous interactions with other drugs

- Anaesthetics: enhanced hypotensive effect.
- Analgesics: increased risk of convulsions with tramadol; enhanced hypotensive and sedative effects with opioids; increased risk of ventricular arrhythmias with methadone – avoid.
- Antidepressants: concentration increased by fluoxetine and possibly paroxetine; concentration of tricyclics possibly increased.
- Anti-epileptics: antagonism, convulsive threshold may be lowered; metabolism accelerated by carbamazepine.
- Antimalarials: avoid concomitant use with artemether with lumefantrine.
- Antipsychotics: avoid concomitant use of depot formulations with clozapine (cannot be withdrawn quickly if neutropenia occurs).
- Antivirals: ritonavir may increase concentration of risperidone.
- Anxiolytics and hypnotics: enhanced sedative effects.
- Atomoxetine: increased risk of ventricular arrhythmias.
- Cytotoxics: increased risk of ventricular arrhythmias with arsenic trioxide.

ADMINISTRATION

RECONSTITUTION
- With solvent provided
ROUTE
- Oral, deep IM
RATE OF ADMINISTRATION
-
COMMENTS
-

OTHER INFORMATION

- At a dose of 3 mg twice daily, 1.5 mg (i.e. 25%) of risperidone is removed after a 5 hour dialysis session with a dialysate flow of 500 mL/min.
- In overdose, rare cases of QT prolongation have been reported.
- Clearance of risperidone and active metabolites decreased by 60% in severe renal impairment.
- If a dose of 2 mg daily orally is tolerated then a dose of 25 mg (IM) every 2 weeks can be used initially in renal impairment.

Ritonavir

CLINICAL USE

Protease inhibitor:
- Treatment of HIV-1 infection in combination with other antiretrovirals

DOSE IN NORMAL RENAL FUNCTION

- 600 mg twice daily
- As low dose booster with other protease inhibitors: 100–200 mg once or twice daily

PHARMACOKINETICS

Molecular weight (daltons)	720.9
% Protein binding	98–99
% Excreted unchanged in urine	3.5
Volume of distribution (L/kg)	0.4
Half-life – normal/ESRF (hrs)	3–5/ Unchanged

METABOLISM

Ritonavir is extensively metabolised in the liver mainly by cytochrome P450 isoenzymes CYP3A4 and to a lesser extent by CYP2D6. Five metabolites have been identified and the major metabolite has antiviral activity, but concentrations in plasma are low.

About 86% of a dose is eliminated through the faeces (both as unchanged drug and as metabolites) and about 11% is excreted in the urine.

DOSE IN RENAL IMPAIRMENT GFR (mL/MIN)

20–50	Dose as in normal renal function.
10–20	Dose as in normal renal function.
<10	Dose as in normal renal function.

DOSE IN PATIENTS UNDERGOING RENAL REPLACEMENT THERAPIES

CAPD	Not dialysed. Dose as in normal renal function.
HD	Not dialysed. Dose as in normal renal function.
HDF/High flux	Not dialysed. Dose as in normal renal function.
CAV/ VVHD	Unlikely to be dialysed. Dose as in normal renal function.

IMPORTANT DRUG INTERACTIONS

Potentially hazardous interactions with other drugs
- Alfuzosin: avoid concomitant use.
- Analgesics: buprenorphine and NSAID levels may be increased (risk of toxicity) – avoid dextropropoxyphene and piroxicam; methadone, pethidine and possibly morphine concentration reduced; increased alfentanil, fentanyl and toxic pethidine metabolite concentration – avoid with pethidine.
- Anti-arrhythmics: increased concentration of amiodarone, flecainide and propafenone (increased risk of ventricular arrhythmias) – avoid concomitant use; possible increased risk of arrhythmias with disopyramide; avoid with dronedarone.
- Antibacterials: rifabutin concentration increased (risk of uveitis) – reduce rifabutin dose; concentration of clarithromycin and other macrolides increased – reduce dose of clarithromycin in renal impairment; concentration possibly reduced by rifampicin; concentration of both drugs may be increased in combination with fusidic acid; avoid with telithromycin in renal and hepatic failure.
- Anticoagulants: anticoagulant effect of coumarins and phenindione possibly increased; effect of warfarin may be enhanced or reduced; avoid with apixaban; concentration of rivaroxaban increased – avoid.
- Antidepressants: SSRIs and tricyclic concentrations possibly increased; concentration reduced by St John's wort – avoid; possibly reduced paroxetine concentration; increased side effects with trazodone.
- Anti-epileptics: carbamazepine and phenytoin concentration may be increased; concentration reduced by phenytoin; concentration of lamotrigine reduced and valproate reduced.
- Antifungals: in combination with itraconazole or ketoconazole concentration of both drugs may be increased; concentration increased by fluconazole; voriconazole concentration reduced – avoid.
- Antimalarials: use artemether/ lumefantrine with caution; concentration of quinine increased.
- Antipsychotics: concentration of pimozide, quetiapine, clozapine and possibly other antipsychotics may be increased (risk of toxicity) – avoid concomitant use; possibly inhibits metabolism of aripiprazole

- reduce aripiprazole dose; olanzapine concentration reduced.
- Antivirals: concentration of both drugs reduced with boceprevir; indinavir, maraviroc and saquinavir levels increased; increased risk of toxicity with efavirenz – monitor LFTs; possibly reduces telaprevir concentration.
- Anxiolytics and hypnotics: levels of many of them increased (risk of extreme sedation and respiratory depression) – avoid alprazolam, diazepam, flurazepam, midazolam, zolpidem; concentration of buspirone increased.
- Bosentan: increases bosentan concentration.
- Calcium-channel blockers: levels of blockers possibly increased – avoid with lercanidipine.
- Ciclosporin: levels possibly increased by ritonavir.
- Colchicine: possibly increases risk of colchicine toxicity, avoid in hepatic or renal impairment.
- Corticosteroids: possibly increased corticosteroid concentration; increased concentration of inhaled/intranasal budesonide and fluticasone.
- Cytotoxics: possibly increases concentration of axitinib, reduce dose of axitinib; possibly increases concentration of crizotinib, everolimus, nilotinib and vinflunine – avoid; avoid with cabazitaxel, lapatinib and pazopanib; reduce dose of ruxolitinib.
- Diuretics: eplerenone concentration increased – avoid concomitant use.
- Ergot alkaloids: risk of ergotism – avoid.
- Ivabradine: ivabradine concentration possibly increased – avoid concomitant use.

- Lipid-lowering drugs: increased risk of myopathy with rosuvastatin and simvastatin – avoid; possibly increased risk of myopathy with atorvastatin.
- Oestrogens and progestogens: metabolism accelerated (contraceptive effect reduced).
- 5HT$_1$ agonists: concentration of eletriptan increased – avoid.
- Ranolazine: possibly increases ranolazine concentration – avoid.
- Sildenafil: concentrations of sildenafil significantly increased – avoid.
- Tacrolimus: levels possibly increased by ritonavir.
- Tadalafil: concentrations of tadalafil increased – avoid.
- Theophylline: metabolism accelerated, theophylline levels reduced.
- Ticagrelor: possibly increases concentration of ticagrelor – avoid.
- Ulipristal: contraceptive effect reduced – avoid.
- Vardenafil: possibly increased vardenafil concentration – avoid concomitant use.

ADMINISTRATION

RECONSTITUTION
-
ROUTE
- Oral
RATE OF ADMINISTRATION
-
COMMENTS
-

OTHER INFORMATION

- Administer with food.

Rituximab

CLINICAL USE

Monoclonal antibody:
- Lymphomas
- Diffuse large B-cell non-Hodgkin's lymphoma in combination with other chemotherapy
- Rheumatoid arthritis
- Severe, active granulomatosis with polyangiitis (Wegener's) (GPA) and microscopic polyangiitis (MPA)
- Lupus nephritis (unlicensed)

DOSE IN NORMAL RENAL FUNCTION

- 375 mg/m^2 weekly for 4 weeks
- Follicular lymphoma: 375 mg/m^2 once every 2–3 months for up to 2 years
- Rheumatoid arthritis: two 1 g doses 2 weeks apart
- GPA/MPA: 375 mg/m^2 once weekly for 4 weeks
- Lupus nephritis: 375 mg/m^2 for 1–2 doses, two weeks apart

PHARMACOKINETICS

Molecular weight (daltons)	144 000
% Protein binding	No data
% Excreted unchanged in urine	No data
Volume of distribution (L/kg)	No data
Half-life – normal/ ESRF (hrs)	76.3 (after 1st infusion)/– 205.8 (after 4th infusion)/–

METABOLISM

The mechanisms involved in the metabolism and elimination of rituximab are not fully understood; it is postulated that rituximab is most likely removed by opsonisation via the reticuloendothelial system when bound to B lymphocytes, or by human antimurine antibody production. It is then degraded nonspecifically in the liver and excreted in the urine.

DOSE IN RENAL IMPAIRMENT GFR (mL/MIN)

20–50	Dose as in normal renal function. Use with caution.
10–20	Dose as in normal renal function. Use with caution.
<10	Dose as in normal renal function. Use with caution.

DOSE IN PATIENTS UNDERGOING RENAL REPLACEMENT THERAPIES

CAPD	Unlikely to be dialysed. Use with caution.
HD	Not dialysed. Use with caution.
HDF/High flux	Unlikely to be dialysed. Use with caution.
CAV/ VVHD	Unlikely to be dialysed. Use with caution.

IMPORTANT DRUG INTERACTIONS

Potentially hazardous interactions with other drugs
- None known

ADMINISTRATION

RECONSTITUTION

–

ROUTE
- IV infusion

RATE OF ADMINISTRATION
- 1st dose: 50 mg/hour then increase the rate every 30 minutes by 50 mg/hour to achieve a maximum rate of 400 mg/hour.
- Further doses: 100 mg/hour, increasing by 100 mg/hour every 30 minutes to achieve a maximum rate of 400 mg/hour.

COMMENTS
- Add to sodium chloride 0.9% or glucose 5% to achieve a concentration of 1–4 mg/mL, and gently invert to prevent foaming.
- Use immediately after dilution. Infusion solution is stable for 12 hours at room temperature.
- Prepared solution has 24 hours chemical stability at 2–8°C.

OTHER INFORMATION

- Always give a premedication of methylprednisolone 125 mg, paracetamol and an antihistamine before infusion.
- Mean serum half-life increases with dose and repeated dosing (76.3 hours after 1st infusion and 205.8 hours after 4th infusion). Detectable in body for 3–6 months.
- Alternative regime for vasculitis (anecdotal): 1 g/m^2 on days 1 and 14, repeated at relapse or after 6 months.
- Patients with high tumour burden or malignant cells >50 000 mm^3 may be at risk of severe cytokine release syndrome which may be associated with acute renal failure – treat with caution.
- Rituximab has been used to reduce alloreactive antibodies pre-transplant, to treat focal segmental glomerulosclerosis, mixed essential cryoglobulinaemia, SLE, primary systemic vasculitis, PRCA, HUS, and PTLD. (Salama AD, Pusey CD. Drug insight: rituximab in renal disease and transplantation. *Nat Clin Pract Nephrol.* 2006; **2**(4): 221–30.)
- There is a case report of it being used in a haemodialysis patient at 375 mg/m^2; the main problem was life-threatening hyperkalaemia due to probable tumour lysis syndrome. (Jillella AP, Dainer PM, Kallab AM, Ustun C. Treatment of a patient with end-stage renal disease with Rituximab: pharmacokinetic evaluation suggests Rituximab is not eliminated by hemodialysis. *Am J Hematol.* 2002 Nov; **71**(3): 219–22.)

Rivaroxaban

CLINICAL USE

Factor Xa inhibitor:
- Prevention of venous thromboembolism in adult patients undergoing elective hip or knee replacement surgery
- Treatment of DVT or PE
- Prophylaxis of stroke in AF

DOSE IN NORMAL RENAL FUNCTION

- Surgery: 10 mg daily
- Treatment of DVT or PE: 15 mg twice daily for 21 days then 20 mg once daily
- AF: 20 mg once daily

PHARMACOKINETICS

Molecular weight (daltons)	435.9
% Protein binding	92–95
% Excreted unchanged in urine	36
Volume of distribution (L/kg)	50 litres
Half-life – normal/ESRF (hrs)	7–11/ Increased

METABOLISM

Metabolised by the cytochrome P450 isoenzymes CYP3A4 and CYP2J2 and by other mechanisms. About two-thirds of an oral dose is metabolised, with the metabolites excreted equally in the urine and faeces; the remaining third is excreted unchanged in the urine, mainly by active renal secretion.

DOSE IN RENAL IMPAIRMENT GFR (mL/MIN)

30–50	Dose as in normal renal function.
15–29	Use with caution.
<15	Avoid.

DOSE IN PATIENTS UNDERGOING RENAL REPLACEMENT THERAPIES

CAPD	Not dialysed. Avoid.
HD	Not dialysed. Avoid.
HDF/High flux	Not dialysed. Avoid.
CAV/ VVHD	Not dialysed. Dose as in GFR=15–29 mL/min.

IMPORTANT DRUG INTERACTIONS

Potentially hazardous interactions with other drugs
- Analgesics: increased risk of haemorrhage with IV diclofenac and ketorolac – avoid concomitant use.
- Anticoagulants: increased risk of haemorrhage with other anticoagulants – avoid.
- Antifungals: concentration increased by ketoconazole – avoid concomitant use; avoid concomitant use with itraconazole, posaconazole and voriconazole.
- Antivirals: avoid concomitant use with atazanavir, darunavir, fosamprenavir, indinavir, lopinavir, saquinavir and tipranavir; concentration increased by ritonavir – avoid concomitant use.

ADMINISTRATION

RECONSTITUTION
–
ROUTE
- Oral
RATE OF ADMINISTRATION
–

OTHER INFORMATION

- Bioavailability is 80–100%.
- AUC increased 1.5 and 1.6 fold in GFR=30–49 and 15–29 mL/min respectively leading to an increased risk of bleeding
- Protamine and vitamin K are not expected to affect the anticoagulant activity of rivaroxaban.

Rivastigmine

CLINICAL USE

- Mild–moderate dementia in Alzheimer's disease
- Idiopathic Parkinson's disease

DOSE IN NORMAL RENAL FUNCTION

- 3–6 mg twice daily (initially 1.5 mg twice daily)
- Transdermal: 4.6–13.3 mg/hour

PHARMACOKINETICS

Molecular weight (daltons)	250.3 (400.4 as hydrogen tartrate)
% Protein binding	40
% Excreted unchanged in urine	0 (>90 as pharmacologically inactive metabolites)
Volume of distribution (L/kg)	1.8–2.7
Half-life – normal/ ESRF (hrs)	1/–

METABOLISM

Rivastigmine is rapidly and extensively metabolised, primarily via cholinesterase-mediated hydrolysis to the weakly active decarbamylated metabolite. After oral use, more than 90% of a dose is excreted in the urine within 24 hours; no unchanged rivastigmine is detected in the urine. Less than 1% of a dose appears in the faeces.

DOSE IN RENAL IMPAIRMENT GFR (mL/MIN)

20–50	Start at a low dose and gradually increase.
10–20	Start at a low dose and gradually increase.
<10	Start at a low dose and gradually increase.

DOSE IN PATIENTS UNDERGOING RENAL REPLACEMENT THERAPIES

CAPD	Likely dialysability. Dose as in GFR<10 mL/min.
HD	Likely dialysability. Dose as in GFR<10 mL/min.
HDF/High flux	Likely dialysability. Dose as in GFR<10 mL/min.
CAV/ VVHD	Likely dialysability. Dose as in GFR=10–20 mL/min.

IMPORTANT DRUG INTERACTIONS

Potentially hazardous interactions with other drugs
- Muscle relaxants: enhances effect of suxamethonium; antagonises effect of non-depolarising muscle relaxants.

ADMINISTRATION

RECONSTITUTION
–
ROUTE
- Oral, transdermal
RATE OF ADMINISTRATION
–
COMMENTS
–

OTHER INFORMATION

- Administer with food. Swallow whole.

Rizatriptan

CLINICAL USE

$5HT_1$ receptor agonist:
Acute treatment of migraine

DOSE IN NORMAL RENAL FUNCTION

10 mg, repeated after 2 hours if required;
maximum of 2 doses in 24 hours

PHARMACOKINETICS

Molecular weight (daltons)	391.5 (as benzoate)
% Protein binding	14
% Excreted unchanged in urine	14
Volume of distribution (L/kg)	110 litres (females), 140 litres (males)
Half-life – normal/ ESRF (hrs)	2–3/Unchanged

METABOLISM

The main route of rizatriptan metabolism
is via oxidative deamination by monoamine
oxidase-A (MAO-A) to the indole acetic acid
metabolite, which is not pharmacologically
active. N-monodesmethyl-rizatriptan, a
metabolite with activity similar to that of
parent compound, is formed to a minor
degree, but does not contribute significantly
to the pharmacodynamic activity of
rizatriptan. Less than 1% is excreted in the
urine as active N-monodesmethyl metabolite.

DOSE IN RENAL IMPAIRMENT GFR (mL/MIN)

20–50	Dose as in normal renal function.
10–20	Dose as in normal renal function.
<10	Use with caution. 5 mg, repeated after 2 hours; maximum 15 mg daily.

DOSE IN PATIENTS UNDERGOING RENAL REPLACEMENT THERAPIES

CAPD	Unknown dialysability. Dose as in GFR<10 mL/min.
HD	Unknown dialysability. Dose as in GFR<10 mL/min.
HDF/High flux	Unknown dialysability. Dose as in GFR<10 mL/min.
CAV/ VVHD	Unknown dialysability. Dose as in GR=10–20 mL/min.

IMPORTANT DRUG INTERACTIONS

Potentially hazardous interactions with other
drugs
- Antidepressants: increased risk of CNS
  excitation with citalopram – avoid; risk of
  CNS toxicity with MAOIs, moclobemide
  and linezolid – avoid for 2 weeks after
  discontinuation of MAOI & moclobemide;
  possibly increased serotonergic effects
  with duloxetine and venlafaxine; increased
  serotonergic effects with St John's wort –
  avoid concomitant use.
- Ergot alkaloids: increased risk of
  vasospasm – avoid concomitant use.
- Propranolol: rizatriptan levels increased,
  reduce dose of rizatriptan to 5 mg (max
  10 mg in 24 hours).

ADMINISTRATION

RECONSTITUTION
–
ROUTE
- Oral
RATE OF ADMINISTRATION
–
COMMENTS
–

OTHER INFORMATION

- Contraindicated in severe renal
  impairment by manufacturer in UK SPC
  only.
- Bioavailability is 40–45%.
- Administration with food delays
  absorption by approximately 1 hour.
- AUC increases by 44% in haemodialysis
  patients.
- Doses in renal impairment from Baillie
  G, Johnson CA, Mason NA, St Peter
  WL. (Nephrology Pharmacy Associates).
  Triptans for migraine treatment: dosing
  considerations in CKD. *Medfacts*. 2002.
  4(5).

Rocuronium bromide

CLINICAL USE

Muscle relaxant in general anaesthesia, medium duration

DOSE IN NORMAL RENAL FUNCTION

- IV injection: intubation dose: 0.6 mg/kg; maintenance: 0.075–0.15 mg/kg
- IV infusion: 0.6 mg/kg loading dose, followed by 0.3–0.6 mg/kg/hour

PHARMACOKINETICS

Molecular weight (daltons)	609.7
% Protein binding	25–30
% Excreted unchanged in urine	40
Volume of distribution (L/kg)	0.2
Half-life – normal/ ESRF (hrs)	1.2–1.4/Unchanged

METABOLISM

Rocuronium is metabolised by the liver to a less active metabolite, 17-desacetylrocuronium, which is reported to have weak neuromuscular blocking effect.

Up to 40% of a dose may be excreted in the urine within 24 hours; rocuronium is also excreted in the bile. After injection of a radiolabelled dose of rocuronium bromide, excretion of the radiolabel is on average 47% in urine and 43% in faeces after 9 days. Approximately 50% is recovered as the parent compound. No metabolites are detected in plasma.

DOSE IN RENAL IMPAIRMENT GFR (mL/MIN)

20–50	Dose as in normal renal function.
10–20	Normal loading dose; maintenance to 0.075–0.1 mg/kg; infusion: 0.3–0.4 mg/kg/hr. See 'Other information'.
<10	Normal loading dose; maintenance to 0.075–0.1 mg/kg; infusion: 0.3–0.4 mg/kg/hr. See 'Other information'.

DOSE IN PATIENTS UNDERGOING RENAL REPLACEMENT THERAPIES

CAPD	Unknown dialysability. Dose as in GFR<10 mL/min.
HD	Unknown dialysability. Dose as in GFR<10 mL/min.
HDF/High flux	Unknown dialysability. Dose as in GFR<10 mL/min.
CAV/ VVHD	Unknown dialysability. Dose as in GFR=10–20 mL/min.

IMPORTANT DRUG INTERACTIONS

Potentially hazardous interactions with other drugs

- Anaesthetics: enhanced muscle relaxant effect.
- Anti-arrhythmics: procainamide enhances muscle relaxant effect.
- Antibacterials: effect enhanced by aminoglycosides, clindamycin, polymyxins and piperacillin.
- Anti-epileptics: muscle relaxant effects antagonised by carbamazepine; effects reduced by long-term use of phenytoin but might be increased by acute use.
- Botulinum toxin: neuromuscular block enhanced (risk of toxicity).

ADMINISTRATION

RECONSTITUTION

–

ROUTE

- IV

RATE OF ADMINISTRATION

- Slow bolus or continuous infusion

COMMENTS

- Compatible with sodium chloride 0.9% and glucose 5%

OTHER INFORMATION

- Use with caution in renal failure: variable duration of action (range: 22–90 minutes).
- Use the lowest possible dose in patients with GFR<20 mL/min, as at risk of prolonged paralysis.

Ropinirole

CLINICAL USE

- Anti-Parkinson agent
- Restless legs syndrome

DOSE IN NORMAL RENAL FUNCTION

- Parkinson's disease (PD): 9–24 mg daily in divided doses
- MR: 8–24 mg once daily
- Restless legs syndrome (RLS): 0.25 mg daily initially, increasing to a maximum of 4 mg daily

PHARMACOKINETICS

Molecular weight (daltons)	260.4 (296.8 as hydrochloride)
% Protein binding	10–40
% Excreted unchanged in urine	<10
Volume of distribution (L/kg)	8
Half-life – normal/ ESRF (hrs)	6/–

METABOLISM

Ropinirole is hepatically metabolised by the cytochrome P450 enzyme, CYP1A2, and excreted in the urine as inactive metabolites; less than 10% of an oral dose is excreted as unchanged drug.

DOSE IN RENAL IMPAIRMENT GFR (mL/MIN)

30–50	Dose as in normal renal function.
10–30	Dose as in normal renal function. Use with caution.
<10	Dose as in normal renal function. Use with caution.

DOSE IN PATIENTS UNDERGOING RENAL REPLACEMENT THERAPIES

CAPD	Unlikely to be dialysed. Dose as in GFR<10 mL/min.
HD	Unlikely dialysability. RLS: 0.25–3 mg daily; PD: 0.75–18 mg daily in divided doses; MR: 2–18 mg daily.
HDF/High flux	Unlikely to be dialysed. RLS: 0.25–2 mg daily; PD: 0.75–18 mg daily in divided doses; MR: 2–18 mg daily.
CAV/VVHD	Unlikely dialysability. Dose as in GFR=10–30 mL/min.

IMPORTANT DRUG INTERACTIONS

Potentially hazardous interactions with other drugs
- Antipsychotics: antagonism of anti-Parkinsonian effect – avoid concomitant use.
- Metoclopramide: antagonism of anti-Parkinsonian effect – avoid concomitant use.
- Oestrogens: concentration increased.

ADMINISTRATION

RECONSTITUTION
-
ROUTE
- Oral
RATE OF ADMINISTRATION
-
COMMENTS
-

OTHER INFORMATION

- If administered with L-dopa, decrease the dose of L-dopa by 20%.
- Take with meals to improve GI tolerance, but T_{max} increases by 2.6 hours.
- Manufacturer has not studied patients with a GFR<30 mL/min who are not on haemodialysis so does not supply dosage information for this group.
- For use in restless legs syndrome in CKD 5, start with a low dose and increase according to tolerability.

Rosuvastatin

CLINICAL USE

HMG CoA reductase inhibitor:
- Hyperlipidaemia

DOSE IN NORMAL RENAL FUNCTION

- 5–40 mg daily
- Asians, elderly, people at increased risk of myopathy, and in combination with fibrates: 5–20 mg daily

PHARMACOKINETICS

Molecular weight (daltons)	1001.1 (as calcium salt)
% Protein binding	90
% Excreted unchanged in urine	5
Volume of distribution (L/kg)	134 litres
Half-life – normal/ ESRF (hrs)	19/Increased

METABOLISM

Rosuvastatin undergoes limited metabolism in the liver mainly by the cytochrome P450 isoenzyme CYP2C9 (approximately 10%).

Approximately 90% of the rosuvastatin dose is excreted unchanged in the faeces (consisting of absorbed and non-absorbed active substance) and the remaining part is excreted in urine.

DOSE IN RENAL IMPAIRMENT GFR (mL/MIN)

30–60	5–20 mg daily.
10–30	5–10 mg daily. Use with caution.
<10	5–10 mg daily. Use with caution.

DOSE IN PATIENTS UNDERGOING RENAL REPLACEMENT THERAPIES

CAPD	Unlikely dialysability. Dose as in GFR<10 mL/min.
HD	Not dialysed. Dose as in GFR<10 mL/min.
HDF/High flux	Unknown dialysability. Dose as in GFR<10 mL/min.
CAV/ VVHD	Unknown dialysability. Dose as in GFR=10–30 mL/min.

IMPORTANT DRUG INTERACTIONS

Potentially hazardous interactions with other drugs
- Anti-arrhythmics: concentration possibly increased by dronedarone.
- Antibacterials: erythromycin reduces concentration of rosuvastatin; increased risk of myopathy with daptomycin and fusidic acid – avoid.
- Anticoagulants: effect of coumarins and phenindione enhanced.
- Antivirals: increased risk of myopathy with atazanavir, darunavir, fosamprenavir, indinavir, lopinavir, ritonavir, saquinavir and tipranavir – avoid;
- Ciclosporin: increased risk of myopathy – avoid concomitant use.
- Colchicine: possible increased risk of myopathy.
- Eltrombopag: increased rosuvastatin concentration – reduce dose of rosuvastatin.
- Lipid-lowering agents: increased risk of myopathy with fibrates, gemfibrozil (avoid) and nicotinic acid.

ADMINISTRATION

RECONSTITUTION
–
ROUTE
- Oral
RATE OF ADMINISTRATION
–
COMMENTS
–

OTHER INFORMATION

- Contraindicated in UK SPC in severe renal impairment due to a 3-fold increase in plasma concentration and 9-fold increase in metabolite concentration. Dose recommendations taken from US data sheet.
- In renal impairment, doses above 20 mg should not be used due to risk of myopathy.
- Always start at a dose of 5 mg.
- The 40 mg dose should only be used under specialist supervision.
- Increased risk of proteinuria with doses above 40 mg.
- Case studies from Glasgow have shown that statins in combination with fusidic acid have an increased risk of causing myopathy in diabetic patients.

Rotigotine

CLINICAL USE

Treatment of Parkinson's disease
Restless legs syndrome

DOSE IN NORMAL RENAL FUNCTION

- 2–8 mg every 24 hours
- With levodopa: max 16 mg every 24 hours
- Restless legs syndrome: 1–3 mg every 24 hours

PHARMACOKINETICS

Molecular weight (daltons)	315.5
% Protein binding	92
% Excreted unchanged in urine	71
Volume of distribution (L/kg)	84
Half-life – normal/ESRF (hrs)	5–7/Unchanged

METABOLISM

Rotigotine is metabolised in the gut wall and liver by N-dealkylation as well as direct and secondary conjugation. Main metabolites are sulfates and glucuronide conjugates of the parent compound as well as N-desalkyl-metabolites, which are biologically inactive.

Approximately 71% of the rotigotine dose is excreted in urine and a smaller part of about 23% is excreted in faeces.

DOSE IN RENAL IMPAIRMENT GFR (mL/MIN)

20–50	Dose as in normal renal function.
10–20	Dose as in normal renal function.
<10	Dose as in normal renal function.

DOSE IN PATIENTS UNDERGOING RENAL REPLACEMENT THERAPIES

CAPD	Unlikely to be dialysed. Dose as in normal renal function.
HD	Not dialysed. Dose as in normal renal function.
HDF/High flux	Unlikely to be dialysed. Dose as in normal renal function.
CAV/VVHD	Unlikely to be dialysed. Dose as in normal renal function.

IMPORTANT DRUG INTERACTIONS

Potentially hazardous interactions with other drugs
- Antipsychotics: avoid concomitant use (antagonism of effect).
- Metoclopramide: avoid concomitant use (antagonism of effect).

ADMINISTRATION

RECONSTITUTION
–
ROUTE
- Topical
RATE OF ADMINISTRATION
–
COMMENTS
–

OTHER INFORMATION

- Discontinue gradually at a rate of 2 mg/24 hours, every other day.
- Apply to intact skin on the abdomen, thigh, hip, flank, shoulder or upper arm.
- If a patch falls off replace with a new one.
- Backing layer contains aluminium and should be removed prior to MRIs or cardioversion.

Rufinamide

CLINICAL USE

Adjunctive treatment of seizures in Lennox-Gastaut syndrome

DOSE IN NORMAL RENAL FUNCTION

200 mg twice daily increasing to a maximum dose of:
- Weight 30–50 kg: 900 mg twice daily
- Weight 50–70 kg: 1.2 g twice daily
- Weight >70 kg: 1.6 g twice daily

PHARMACOKINETICS

Molecular weight (daltons)	238.2
% Protein binding	34
% Excreted unchanged in urine	<2
Volume of distribution (L/kg)	50 litres (dose dependant)
Half-life – normal/ ESRF (hrs)	6–10/Unchanged

METABOLISM

Almost exclusively eliminated by metabolism via hydrolysis of the carboxylamide group to the pharmacologically inactive acid derivative CGP 47292. Cytochrome P450-mediated metabolism is very minor. The formation of small amounts of glutathione conjugates cannot be completely excluded.

Some 84.7% was excreted by the renal route.

DOSE IN RENAL IMPAIRMENT GFR (mL/MIN)

20–50	Dose as in normal renal function.
10–20	Dose as in normal renal function.
<10	Dose as in normal renal function.

DOSE IN PATIENTS UNDERGOING RENAL REPLACEMENT THERAPIES

CAPD	Dialysed. Dose as in normal renal function.
HD	Dialysed. Dose as in normal renal function.
HDF/High flux	Dialysed. Dose as in normal renal function.
CAV/ VVHD	Dialysed. Dose as in normal renal function.

IMPORTANT DRUG INTERACTIONS

Potentially hazardous interactions with other drugs
- Antidepressants: antagonism of anticonvulsant effect (convulsive threshold lowered); avoid concomitant use with St John's wort.
- Antimalarials: mefloquine antagonises anticonvulsant effect.
- Antipsychotics: antagonism of anticonvulsant effect (convulsive threshold lowered).
- Oestrogens & progestogens: metabolism accelerated by rufinamide.
- Orlistat: possibly increased risk of convulsions with orlistat.

ADMINISTRATION

RECONSTITUTION
–
ROUTE
- Oral
RATE OF ADMINISTRATION
–

OTHER INFORMATION

30% is removed by haemodialysis.

Rupatadine

CLINICAL USE

Antihistamine

DOSE IN NORMAL RENAL FUNCTION

10 mg once daily

PHARMACOKINETICS

Molecular weight (daltons)	416
% Protein binding	98.5–99
% Excreted unchanged in urine	Insignificant
Volume of distribution (L/kg)	3–7[1]
Half-life – normal/ ESRF (hrs)	5.9/–

METABOLISM

Mainly metabolised by the cytochrome P450 (CYP 3A4) enzyme pathway. The amounts of unaltered active substance found in urine and faeces were insignificant. This means that rupatadine is almost completely metabolised.

DOSE IN RENAL IMPAIRMENT GFR (mL/MIN)

20–50	Dose as in normal renal function.
10–20	Dose as in normal renal function.
<10	Dose as in normal renal function. Use with caution.

DOSE IN PATIENTS UNDERGOING RENAL REPLACEMENT THERAPIES

CAPD	Unlikely to be dialysed. Dose as in GFR<10 mL/min.
HD	Unlikely to be dialysed. Dose as in GFR<10 mL/min.
HDF/High flux	Unknown dialysability. Dose as in GFR<10 mL/min.
CAV/ VVHD	Unknown dialysability. Dose as in GFR=10–20 mL/min.

IMPORTANT DRUG INTERACTIONS

Potentially hazardous interactions with other drugs
- Antibacterials: concentration increased by erythromycin.
- Antifungals: concentration increased by ketoconazole.
- Antivirals: concentration possibly increased by ritonavir.
- Grapefruit juice: concentration increased – avoid concomitant administration.

ADMINISTRATION

RECONSTITUTION
–
ROUTE
- Oral
RATE OF ADMINISTRATION
–

OTHER INFORMATION

- Manufacturer contraindicates use due to lack of experience.

Reference:
1. www.tga.gov.au/pdf/auspar/auspar-rupafin.pdf

Ruxolitinib

CLINICAL USE

Tyrosine kinase inhibitor:
- Treatment of disease related splenomegaly or symptoms in patients with primary myelofibrosis, post polycythaemia vera myelofibrosis or post-essential thrombocythaemia myelofibrosis

DOSE IN NORMAL RENAL FUNCTION

5–25 mg twice daily
Dose depends on platelet count

PHARMACOKINETICS

Molecular weight (daltons)	404.4 (as phosphate)
% Protein binding	97 (mostly to albumin)
% Excreted unchanged in urine	<1
Volume of distribution (L/kg)	53–65 litres
Half-life – normal/ESRF (hrs)	3 (metabolites 5.8 hours)/–

METABOLISM

Ruxolitinib is mainly metabolised by CYP3A4 (>50%), with additional contribution from CYP2C9 to produce 2 major and active metabolites.

About 74% of a dose is excreted in the urine and about 22% via the faeces.

DOSE IN RENAL IMPAIRMENT GFR (mL/MIN)

30–50	Dose as in normal renal function.
15–30	Reduce dose by approximately 50% and give twice daily; platelet count between 100 000/mm³ and 200 000/mm³: 15 mg stat. Avoid if platelet counts <100 000/mm³.
<15	Reduce dose by approximately 50% and give twice daily; platelet count between 100 000/mm³ and 200 000/mm³: 15 mg stat. Avoid if platelet counts <100 000/mm³. Use with caution.

DOSE IN PATIENTS UNDERGOING RENAL REPLACEMENT THERAPIES

CAPD	Not dialysed. Use with caution.
HD	Not dialysed. 15–20 mg post dialysis or 10 mg 12 hourly on dialysis days only, given after dialysis. See 'Other information'.
HDF/High flux	Not dialysed. 15–20 mg post dialysis or 10 mg 12 hourly on dialysis days only, given after dialysis. See 'Other information'.
CAV/VVHD	Not dialysed. Dose as in GFR=15–30 mL/min. Use with caution.

IMPORTANT DRUG INTERACTIONS

Potentially hazardous interactions with other drugs
- Antibacterials: concentration increased by clarithromycin and telithromycin, reduced dose of ruxolitinib; concentration reduced by rifampicin.
- Antifungals: reduce dose of ruxolitinib with fluconazole, itraconazole, ketoconazole, posaconazole and voriconazole.
- Antipsychotics: avoid concomitant use with clozapine, risk of agranulocytosis.
- Antivirals: reduce dose of ruxolitinib with boceprevir, indinavir, lopinavir, ritonavir, saquinavir and telaprevir.

ADMINISTRATION

RECONSTITUTION
–
ROUTE
- Oral
RATE OF ADMINISTRATION
–

OTHER INFORMATION

- Treatment of patients on dialysis: The dosing recommended is from limited data. Other dosing regimens may be more suitable from an efficacy perspective. However, due to increased metabolite exposure and lack of knowledge on the potential safety consequences of these exposures, dose modification should be followed by careful monitoring of safety and efficacy in individual patients.
- No data is available for dosing patients who are undergoing peritoneal dialysis or continuous venovenous haemofiltration.
- Following a single ruxolitinib dose of 25 mg, the exposure of ruxolitinib was similar in subjects with various degrees of renal impairment and in those with normal renal function. However, plasma AUC values of ruxolitinib metabolites tended to increase with increasing severity of renal impairment, and were most markedly increased in the subjects with severe renal impairment. It is unknown

whether the increased metabolite exposure is of safety concern. A dose modification is recommended in patients with severe renal impairment and end-stage renal disease. Dosing only on dialysis days reduces the metabolite exposure, but also the pharmacodynamic effect, especially on the days between dialysis.

Salbutamol

CLINICAL USE

Beta2-adrenoceptor agonist:
- Reversible airways disease

DOSE IN NORMAL RENAL FUNCTION

- Oral: 2–4 mg 3–4 times daily
- SC/IM: 500 micrograms, repeated 4 hourly if necessary
- IV: 250 micrograms slow bolus, repeated if required. Infusion: start with 5 micrograms/minute, adjust according to response, usually 3–20 micrograms/minute
- Aerosol: 100–200 micrograms (1–2 puffs) 4 times daily
- Powder: 200–400 micrograms 4 times daily
- Nebulisation: 2.5–5 mg 4 times daily, or more frequently

PHARMACOKINETICS

Molecular weight (daltons)	239.3
% Protein binding	10
% Excreted unchanged in urine	51–64
Volume of distribution (L/kg)	2–2.5
Half-life – normal/ ESRF (hrs)	4–6/Unchanged

METABOLISM

Salbutamol is subject to first-pass metabolism in the liver and possibly in the gut wall but does not appear to be metabolised in the lung; the main metabolite is the inactive sulphate conjugate.

Salbutamol is rapidly excreted, mainly in the urine, as metabolites and unchanged drug; a smaller proportion is excreted in the faeces.

DOSE IN RENAL IMPAIRMENT GFR (mL/MIN)

20–50	Dose as in normal renal function.
10–20	Dose as in normal renal function.
<10	Dose as in normal renal function.

DOSE IN PATIENTS UNDERGOING RENAL REPLACEMENT THERAPIES

CAPD	Unknown dialysability. Dose as in normal renal function.
HD	Unknown dialysability. Dose as in normal renal function.
HDF/High flux	Unknown dialysability. Dose as in normal renal function.
CAV/ VVHD	Unknown dialysability. Dose as in normal renal function.

IMPORTANT DRUG INTERACTIONS

Potentially hazardous interactions with other drugs
- Increased risk of hypokalaemia when diuretics, theophylline or large doses of corticosteroids are given with high doses of salbutamol.
- Antihypertensives: acute hypotension with IV infusion of salbutamol and methyldopa.

ADMINISTRATION

RECONSTITUTION
–
ROUTE
- IV, SC, IM, oral, inhaled, nebulised
RATE OF ADMINISTRATION
- IV slow bolus; IV infusion 3–20 micrograms/minute
COMMENTS
- Infusion: dilute 10 mL (10 mg) to 500 mL with sodium chloride 0.9% or glucose 5% (20 micrograms/mL).
- Via syringe pump: dilute 10 mL (10 mg) to 50 mL with sodium chloride 0.9% or glucose 5% (200 micrograms/mL).

OTHER INFORMATION

- Monitor ECG/BP/pulse.
- Nebulised salbutamol may be prescribed for hypokalaemic effect in acute hyperkalaemia (unlicensed).

Saquinavir

CLINICAL USE

Protease inhibitor:
- Treatment of HIV infection in combination with other antiviral drugs

DOSE IN NORMAL RENAL FUNCTION

- Previously treated with antiretrovirals, with low dose ritonavir: 1 g twice daily
- Previously not treated with antiretrovirals, with low dose ritonavir: initially 500 mg twice daily then 1 g twice daily

PHARMACOKINETICS

Molecular weight (daltons)	670.8
% Protein binding	98
% Excreted unchanged in urine	<4
Volume of distribution (L/kg)	10
Half-life – normal/ ESRF (hrs)	13.2/–

METABOLISM

Saquinavir is absorbed to a limited extent (about 30%) after oral doses of the mesilate and undergoes extensive first-pass hepatic metabolism via cytochrome P450 isoenzyme, CYP3A4 to form a range of mono- and di-hydroxylated inactive compounds. It is excreted mainly in the faeces.

DOSE IN RENAL IMPAIRMENT GFR (mL/MIN)

20–50	Dose as in normal renal function.
10–20	Dose as in normal renal function.
<10	Dose as in normal renal function.

DOSE IN PATIENTS UNDERGOING RENAL REPLACEMENT THERAPIES

CAPD	Unlikely to be dialysed. Dose as in normal renal function.
HD	Unlikely to be dialysed. Dose as in normal renal function.
HDF/High flux	Not dialysed. Dose as in normal renal function.
CAV/ VVHD	Unknown dialysability. Dose as in normal renal function.

IMPORTANT DRUG INTERACTIONS

Potentially hazardous interactions with other drugs

- Analgesics: increased risk of ventricular arrhythmias with alfentanil, fentanyl and methadone – avoid.
- Anti-arrhythmics: increased risk of ventricular arrhythmias with amiodarone, disopyramide, dronedarone, flecainide, lidocaine or propafenone – avoid.
- Antibacterials: increased risk of ventricular arrhythmias with clarithromycin, dapsone, erythromycin, moxifloxacin or telithromycin – avoid; concentration of rifabutin increased; rifampicin and rifabutin can reduce saquinavir levels by 80% and 40% respectively (metabolism accelerated); increased hepatoxicity with rifampicin – avoid; concentration of both drugs increased with fusidic acid.
- Antidepressants: increased risk of ventricular arrhythmias with trazodone or tricyclics – avoid; concentration reduced by St John's wort – avoid.
- Anti-epileptics: carbamazepine, phenobarbital, and phenytoin can reduce saquinavir levels.
- Antihistamines: increased risk of ventricular arrhythmias with mizolastine – avoid.
- Antimalarials: avoid concomitant use with piperaquine with artenimol; use artemether/lumefantrine with caution; increased risk of ventricular arrhythmias with quinine – avoid.
- Antipsychotics: increased risk of ventricular arrhythmias with clozapine, haloperidol or phenothiazines – avoid; possibly increased risk of ventricular arrhythmias with pimozide and quetiapine – avoid concomitant use; possibly inhibits aripiprazole metabolism – reduce aripiprazole dose.
- Antivirals: tipranavir and efavirenz can reduce saquinavir levels; increased risk of ventricular arrhythmias with atazanavir or lopinavir; concentration increased by indinavir and ritonavir; reduced darunavir concentration; concentration of maraviroc increased, consider reducing dose of maraviroc.
- Anxiolytics and hypnotics: midazolam concentration possibly increased (prolonged sedation) – avoid with oral midazolam.

- Beta-blockers: increased risk of ventricular arrhythmias with sotalol – avoid.
- Ciclosporin: concentration of both drugs increased.
- Cytotoxics: possibly increases concentration of axitinib, reduce dose of axitinib; possibly increases concentration of crizotinib and everolimus – avoid; avoid with cabazitaxel, lapatinib and pazopanib; reduce dose of ruxolitinib.
- Ergot alkaloids: risk of ergotism – avoid.
- Lipid-lowering drugs: increased risk of myopathy with rosuvastatin and simvastatin – avoid; possibly increased myopathy with atorvastatin.
- Pentamidine: increased risk of ventricular arrhythmias – avoid.
- Ranolazine: possibly increases ranolazine concentration – avoid.
- Sildenafil, tadalafil, vardenafil: increased risk of ventricular arrhythmias – avoid.
- Tacrolimus: possibly increased tacrolimus concentration – may need to reduce dose.
- Ulcer-healing drugs: concentration increased by cimetidine; possibly increased by esomeprazole, lansoprazole, pantoprazole and rabeprazole – avoid; omeprazole increases AUC of saquinavir by 82% (increased risk of toxicity) – avoid.

ADMINISTRATION

RECONSTITUTION

–

ROUTE
- Oral

RATE OF ADMINISTRATION

–

COMMENTS
- Administer within 2 hours after meal.

OTHER INFORMATION

- Therapeutic drug monitoring is available from HIV Focus Roche Products UK and the University of Liverpool, but this service is not available to all patients.
- Manufacturer advises to use with caution in severe renal impairment due to lack of studies but saquinavir has minimal renal clearance.

Saxagliptin

CLINICAL USE

Dipeptidyl peptidase 4 inhibitor:
- Treatment of type 2 diabetes

DOSE IN NORMAL RENAL FUNCTION

5 mg daily

PHARMACOKINETICS

Molecular weight (daltons)	315.4 (351.9 as hydrochloride)
% Protein binding	Negligible
% Excreted unchanged in urine	24
Volume of distribution (L/kg)	1.3–5.2[1]
Half-life – normal/ ESRF (hrs)	2.5 (3.1 for metabolite)/–

METABOLISM

Metabolism is mainly by cytochrome P450 3A4/5. The major metabolite of saxagliptin is also a selective, reversible, competitive DPP 4 inhibitor, half as potent as saxagliptin.

Saxagliptin and 5-hydroxy saxagliptin are excreted in the urine; there may be some active renal excretion of unchanged saxagliptin. There is also some elimination via the faeces.

DOSE IN RENAL IMPAIRMENT GFR (mL/MIN)

20–50	2.5 mg daily
10–20	2.5 mg daily
<10	2.5 mg daily

DOSE IN PATIENTS UNDERGOING RENAL REPLACEMENT THERAPIES

CAPD	Dialysed. Dose as in GFR<10 mL/min.
HD	Dialysed. Dose as in GFR<10 mL/min.
HDF/High flux	Dialysed. Dose as in GFR<10 mL/min.
CAV/ VVHD	Dialysed. Dose as in GFR=10–20 mL/min.

IMPORTANT DRUG INTERACTIONS

Potentially hazardous interactions with other drugs
- None known

ADMINISTRATION

RECONSTITUTION
–

ROUTE
- Oral

RATE OF ADMINISTRATION
–

OTHER INFORMATION

- UK manufacturer advises to use with caution in moderate to severe renal impairment due to lack of studies.
- Saxagliptin and its major metabolite can be removed by haemodialysis (23% of dose over 4 hours).
- In subjects with moderate or severe renal impairment, the AUC values of saxagliptin and its active metabolite were up to 2.1- and 4.5-fold higher, respectively, than AUC values in subjects with normal renal function.

Reference:
1. Fura A, Khanna A, Vyas V, et al. Pharmacokinetics of the dipeptidyl peptidase 4 inhibitor saxagliptin in rats, dogs, and monkeys and clinical projections. *Drug Metab Dispos.* 2009 Jun; **37**(6): 1164–71.

Selegiline hydrochloride

CLINICAL USE

Monoamine-oxidase-B inhibitor:
- Treatment of Parkinson's disease

DOSE IN NORMAL RENAL FUNCTION

- Oral: 5–10 mg daily in the morning
- Oral lyophilisate: 1.25 mg daily before breakfast

PHARMACOKINETICS

Molecular weight (daltons)	223.7
% Protein binding	75–85
% Excreted unchanged in urine	Mainly as metabolites
Volume of distribution (L/kg)	500 litres
Half-life – normal/ ESRF (hrs)	1.5–3.5/Unchanged

METABOLISM

Extensive first-pass metabolism in the liver to produce at least 5 metabolites, including desmethylselegiline (norselegiline), N-methylamfetamine, and amfetamine. Plasma concentrations of selegiline metabolites are greatly reduced after doses of the oral lyophilisate preparation, the majority of which undergoes absorption through the buccal mucosa.

Selegiline is excreted as metabolites mainly in the urine and about 15% appears in the faeces.

DOSE IN RENAL IMPAIRMENT GFR (mL/MIN)

20–50	Dose as in normal renal function.
10–20	Dose as in normal renal function.
<10	Dose as in normal renal function.

DOSE IN PATIENTS UNDERGOING RENAL REPLACEMENT THERAPIES

CAPD	Unknown dialysability. Dose as in normal renal function.
HD	Unknown dialysability. Dose as in normal renal function.
HDF/High flux	Likely to be dialysed. Dose as in normal renal function.
CAV/ VVHD	Unknown dialysability. Dose as in normal renal function.

IMPORTANT DRUG INTERACTIONS

Potentially hazardous interactions with other drugs
- Analgesics: hyperpyrexia and CNS toxicity reported with pethidine – avoid; avoid with opioid analgesics.
- Antidepressants: avoid with citalopram and escitalopram; increased risk of hypertension and CNS excitation with fluvoxamine, sertraline or venlafaxine, do not start selegiline until 1 week after stopping them, avoid for 2 weeks after stopping selegiline; increased risk of hypertension and CNS excitation with paroxetine, do not start selegiline until 2 week after stopping paroxetine, avoid for 2 weeks after stopping selegiline, avoid concomitant use with other MAOIs and moclobemide (can lead to hypertensive crisis) – allow at least 14 days before starting a MAOI; avoid concomitant use with fluoxetine, allow 5 weeks between stopping fluoxetine and starting selegiline; allow 14 days between stopping selegiline and starting fluoxetine; increased CNS toxicity with tricyclics.
- Oestrogens & progestogens: concentration of selegiline increased – avoid.
- Sympathomimetics: concomitant use is not recommended; risk of hypertensive crisis with dopamine.

ADMINISTRATION

RECONSTITUTION
–
ROUTE
- Oral
RATE OF ADMINISTRATION
–
COMMENTS
–

OTHER INFORMATION

- 1.25 mg oral lyophilisate is equivalent to a 10 mg tablet
- Bioavailability is 10%.

Senna

CLINICAL USE

Constipation

DOSE IN NORMAL RENAL FUNCTION

- Tablets: 15–30 mg (2–4 tablets) at night
- Granules: 5–10 mL with at least 150 mL water, juice, milk or a warm drink at night
- Syrup: 10–20 mL at night

PHARMACOKINETICS

Molecular weight (daltons)	862.7
% Protein binding	Systemic bioavailability less than 5%
% Excreted unchanged in urine	No data
Volume of distribution (L/kg)	No data
Half-life – normal/ ESRF (hrs)	No data

METABOLISM

Absorbed senna is metabolised in the liver. Unabsorbed senna is hydrolysed in the colon by bacteria to release the active free anthraquinones.

DOSE IN RENAL IMPAIRMENT GFR (mL/MIN)

20–50	Dose as in normal renal function.
10–20	Dose as in normal renal function.
<10	Dose as in normal renal function.

DOSE IN PATIENTS UNDERGOING RENAL REPLACEMENT THERAPIES

CAPD	Unknown dialysability. Dose as in normal renal function.
HD	Unknown dialysability. Dose as in normal renal function.
HDF/High flux	Unknown dialysability. Dose as in normal renal function.
CAV/ VVHD	Unknown dialysability. Dose as in normal renal function.

IMPORTANT DRUG INTERACTIONS

Potentially hazardous interactions with other drugs
- None known

ADMINISTRATION

RECONSTITUTION

–

ROUTE
- Oral

RATE OF ADMINISTRATION

–

COMMENTS

–

OTHER INFORMATION

- Acts in 8–12 hours.
- Syrup available, 5 mL ≡ 1 tablet.
- Granules available, 1×5 mL spoonful ≡ 2 tablets.
- Diabetic patients should use the tablets as these have negligible sugar content.

Sertraline

CLINICAL USE

SSRI:
- Antidepressant
- Post-traumatic stress disorder
- Obsessive compulsive disorder

DOSE IN NORMAL RENAL FUNCTION

25–200 mg daily depending on indication

PHARMACOKINETICS

Molecular weight (daltons)	342.7 (as hydrochloride)
% Protein binding	>98
% Excreted unchanged in urine	0
Volume of distribution (L/kg)	25
Half-life – normal/ESRF (hrs)	26/Probably unchanged

METABOLISM

Sertraline undergoes extensive first-pass metabolism in the liver. The main pathway is demethylation to inactive N-desmethylsertraline, a process that appears to involve multiple cytochrome P450 isoenzymes; further metabolism and glucuronide conjugation occurs. Sertraline is excreted in about equal amounts in the urine and faeces, mainly as metabolites.

DOSE IN RENAL IMPAIRMENT GFR (mL/MIN)

20–50	Dose as in normal renal function.
10–20	Dose as in normal renal function.
<10	Dose as in normal renal function.

DOSE IN PATIENTS UNDERGOING RENAL REPLACEMENT THERAPIES

CAPD	Unlikely to be dialysed. Dose as in normal renal function.
HD	Not dialysed. Dose as in normal renal function.
HDF/High flux	Unknown dialysability. Dose as in normal renal function.
CAV/ VVHD	Unknown dialysability. Dose as in normal renal function.

IMPORTANT DRUG INTERACTIONS

Potentially hazardous interactions with other drugs
- Analgesics: increased risk of bleeding with aspirin and NSAIDs; risk of CNS toxicity increased with tramadol; concentration of methadone possibly increased.
- Anticoagulants: effect of coumarins possibly enhanced; possibly increased risk of bleeding with dabigatran.
- Antidepressants: increased risk of toxic CNS effects of MAOIs and moclobemide; sertraline and MAOIs should not be prescribed within a 2 week period of each other; avoid concomitant use with St John's wort; possibly enhanced serotonergic effects with duloxetine; can increase tricyclics antidepressant concentration; increased agitation and nausea with tryptophan.
- Anti-epileptics: antagonism (lowered convulsive threshold); concentration possibly reduced by phenytoin, also concentration of phenytoin possibly increased.
- Antimalarials: avoid concomitant use with artemether/lumefantrine and piperaquine with artenimol.
- Antipsychotics: concentration of clozapine increased; increased risk of ventricular arrhythmias with droperidol and possibly pimozide – avoid.
- Antivirals: concentration possibly reduced by darunavir; possibly increased concentration with ritonavir.
- Ciclosporin: may increase serotonin syndrome.
- Dopaminergics: increased risk of hypertension and CNS excitation with selegiline – avoid concomitant use; increased risk of CNS toxicity with rasagiline – avoid concomitant use.
- 5HT$_1$ agonist: increased risk of CNS toxicity with sumatriptan – avoid concomitant use; possibly increased risk of serotonergic effects with naratriptan.
- Linezolid: use with caution.
- Lithium: increased risk of CNS effects; lithium toxicity reported.
- Methylthioninium: risk of CNS toxicity – avoid if possible.

ADMINISTRATION

RECONSTITUTION

–

ROUTE
- Oral

RATE OF ADMINISTRATION

–

COMMENTS

–

Sevelamer

Phosphate-binding agent

DOSE IN NORMAL RENAL FUNCTION

- 1–5 tablets (average: 3–5) 3 times a day with meals; adjust according to serum phosphate level
- Renvela sachets: 2.4 g three times a day with meals

PHARMACOKINETICS

Molecular weight (daltons)	Large
% Protein binding	No data
% Excreted unchanged in urine	No data
Volume of distribution (L/kg)	No data
Half-life – normal/ ESRF (hrs)	No data

METABOLISM

Sevelamer is not systemically absorbed.

DOSE IN RENAL IMPAIRMENT GFR (mL/MIN)

20–50	Dose as in normal renal function.
10–20	Dose as in normal renal function.
<10	Dose as in normal renal function.

DOSE IN PATIENTS UNDERGOING RENAL REPLACEMENT THERAPIES

CAPD	Unlikely to be dialysed. Dose as in normal renal function.
HD	Unlikely to be dialysed. Dose as in normal renal function.
HDF/High flux	Unlikely to be dialysed. Dose as in normal renal function.
CAV/ VVHD	Unlikely to be dialysed. Dose as in normal renal function.

IMPORTANT DRUG INTERACTIONS

Potentially hazardous interactions with other drugs

- Antibacterials: reduces bioavailability of ciprofloxacin.
- Ciclosporin: possibly reduces ciclosporin concentration.
- Calcitriol: absorption may be impaired by sevelamer.
- Mycophenolate: may reduce mycophenolate levels.
- Tacrolimus: possibly reduces tacrolimus concentration.
- Thyroid hormones: possibly reduces levothyroxine concentration.

ADMINISTRATION

RECONSTITUTION

–

ROUTE

- Oral

RATE OF ADMINISTRATION

–

COMMENTS

–

OTHER INFORMATION

- Do not use if the patient has swallowing disorders or untreated or severe gastroparesis.
- Available as hydrochloride (Renagel®) and carbonate (Renvela®).
- One tablet = 800 mg of poly(allylamine hydrochloride or carbonate) polymer.
- Renagel tablets can be dispersed in 10 mL sodium bicarbonate 8.4% injection if patient is unable to take the tablets. (Info from the Royal Hospital for Sick Children, Yorkhill, Glasgow).
- Sachets should be dispersed in 60 mL of water.

Sildenafil

CLINICAL USE

- Treatment of erectile dysfunction (ED)
- To increase exercise ability in pulmonary arterial hypertension

DOSE IN NORMAL RENAL FUNCTION

- ED: 25–100 mg 0.5–4 hours before sexual intercourse (ideally, about 1 hour); no more than 1 dose per day.
- Pulmonary arterial hypertension:
  - Oral: 20 mg 3 times daily
  - IV: 10 mg 3 times daily

PHARMACOKINETICS

Molecular weight (daltons)	666.7 (as citrate)
% Protein binding	96
% Excreted unchanged in urine	<2
Volume of distribution (L/kg)	1–2
Half-life – normal/ ESRF (hrs)	4/Increased

METABOLISM

Sildenafil is metabolised in the liver mainly by cytochrome P450 isoenzymes CYP3A4 (the major route) and CYP2C9. The major metabolite, N-desmethylsildenafil, also has some activity.

Sildenafil is excreted as metabolites, mainly in the faeces, and to a lesser extent the urine.

DOSE IN RENAL IMPAIRMENT GFR (mL/MIN)

30–50	Dose as in normal renal function.
10–30	Dose as in normal renal function. ED: Initial dose 25 mg and increase if required.
<10	Dose as in normal renal function. See 'Other information'. ED: Initial dose 25 mg and increase if required. See 'Other information'.

DOSE IN PATIENTS UNDERGOING RENAL REPLACEMENT THERAPIES

CAPD	Unlikely to be dialysed. Dose as in GFR<10 mL/min.
HD	Unlikely to be dialysed. Dose as in GFR<10 mL/min.
HDF/High flux	Not dialysed. Dose as in GFR<10 mL/min.
CAV/ VVHD	Unlikely to be dialysed. Dose as in GFR=10–20 mL/min.

IMPORTANT DRUG INTERACTIONS

Potentially hazardous interactions with other drugs

- Alpha-blockers: enhanced hypotensive effect – avoid for 4 hours after sildenafil.
- Antivirals: ritonavir significantly increases sildenafil concentration – avoid concomitant use; concentration possibly increased by saquinavir, fosamprenavir and indinavir – reduce dose of sildenafil; concentration reduced by etravirine and possibly reduced by atazanavir; side effects possibly increased by atazanavir; increased risk of ventricular arrhythmias with saquinavir – avoid; avoid with telaprevir.
- Nicorandil: enhanced hypotensive effect – avoid concomitant use.
- Nitrates: enhanced hypotensive effect – absolutely contraindicated.

ADMINISTRATION

RECONSTITUTION

–

ROUTE

- Oral, IV bolus

RATE OF ADMINISTRATION

–

COMMENTS

–

OTHER INFORMATION

- Oral bioavailability is 40%.
- For pulmonary arterial hypertension, the dose can be reduced to twice daily if there are problems with tolerability.
- Dialysis is not expected to increase clearance as sildenafil is highly protein bound.
- Patients should seek prompt medical advice if their erections last for more than 4 hours.
- Recommend use on non-dialysis days due to hypotension. In peritoneal dialysis, treatment with sildenafil is well tolerated.
- Anecdotally it has been used at Guy's Hospital, London for diabetic gastroparesis at a dose of 25 mg 3 times a day.
- The use of sildenafil is potentially hazardous in patients with active coronary ischaemia, those with congestive heart

failure, and those with complicated multi-drug antihypertensive therapy regimens.

- In 9 patients on maintenance haemodialysis, sildenafil 50 mg appeared to produce firmer erections and greater sexual satisfaction, but the effects were prolonged for up to 48 hours after administration.

Simple linctus

CLINICAL USE

Relief of dry, irritating coughs

DOSE IN NORMAL RENAL FUNCTION

5 mL 3–4 times daily

PHARMACOKINETICS

Molecular weight (daltons)	210.1 (Citric acid monohydrate)
% Protein binding	No data
% Excreted unchanged in urine	No data
Volume of distribution (L/kg)	No data
Half-life – normal/ ESRF (hrs)	No data

METABOLISM

No data

DOSE IN RENAL IMPAIRMENT GFR (mL/MIN)

20–50	Dose as in normal renal function.
10–20	Dose as in normal renal function.
<10	Dose as in normal renal function.

DOSE IN PATIENTS UNDERGOING RENAL REPLACEMENT THERAPIES

CAPD	Unknown dialysability. Dose as in normal renal function.
HD	Unknown dialysability. Dose as in normal renal function.
HDF/High flux	Unknown dialysability. Dose as in normal renal function.
CAV/ VVHD	Unknown dialysability. Dose as in normal renal function.

IMPORTANT DRUG INTERACTIONS

Potentially hazardous interactions with other drugs
- None known

ADMINISTRATION

RECONSTITUTION

–

ROUTE

- Oral

RATE OF ADMINISTRATION

–

COMMENTS

–

OTHER INFORMATION

- Sugar content has not been found to alter diabetics' insulin requirements. Use diabetic cough preparations whenever possible.

Simvastatin

HMG CoA reductase inhibitor:
- Primary hypercholesterolaemia

DOSE IN NORMAL RENAL FUNCTION

5–80 mg at night

PHARMACOKINETICS

Molecular weight (daltons)	418.6
% Protein binding	>95
% Excreted unchanged in urine	13
Volume of distribution (L/kg)	54
Half-life – normal/ESRF (hrs)	1.9/–

METABOLISM

Simvastatin is absorbed from the gastrointestinal tract and must be hydrolysed to its active β-hydroxyacid form. Other active metabolites have been detected and several inactive metabolites are also formed. Simvastatin is a substrate for the cytochrome P450 isoenzyme CYP3A4 and undergoes extensive first-pass metabolism in the liver, its primary site of action. Less than 5% of an oral dose has been reported to reach the circulation as active metabolites. Simvastatin is mainly excreted in the faeces via the bile as metabolites. About 10–15% is recovered in the urine, mainly in inactive forms.

DOSE IN RENAL IMPAIRMENT GFR (mL/MIN)

30–50	Dose as in normal renal function.
10–30	Dose as in normal renal function.
<10	Doses above 10 mg should be used with caution (doses up to 40 mg have been used).

DOSE IN PATIENTS UNDERGOING RENAL REPLACEMENT THERAPIES

CAPD	Unlikely to be dialysed. Dose as in GFR<10 mL/min.
HD	Unlikely to be dialysed. Dose as in GFR<10 mL/min.
HDF/High flux	Unknown dialysability. Dose as in GFR<10 mL/min.
CAV/ VVHD	Unknown dialysability. Dose as in GFR=10–30 mL/min.

IMPORTANT DRUG INTERACTIONS

Potentially hazardous interactions with other drugs
- Anti-arrhythmics: increased risk of myopathy with amiodarone – do not exceed 20 mg of simvastatin;[1] increased risk of myopathy with dronedarone.
- Antibacterials: increased risk of myopathy with clarithromycin, daptomycin, telithromycin, erythromycin and fusidic acid – avoid concomitant use; concentration possibly reduced by rifampicin.
- Anticoagulants: effects of coumarins enhanced.
- Anti-epileptics: concentration reduced by carbamazepine and eslicarbazepine.
- Antifungals: increased risk of myopathy with itraconazole, posaconazole or ketoconazole and possibly miconazole – avoid concomitant use; possibly increased risk of myopathy with imidazoles and triazoles.
- Antivirals: increased risk of myopathy with atazanavir, indinavir, ritonavir or saquinavir and possibly fosamprenavir, lopinavir or tipranavir – avoid concomitant use; concentration reduced by efavirenz; avoid concomitant use with boceprevir and telaprevir.
- Calcium-channel blockers: increased risk of myopathy with verapamil, diltiazem and amlodipine – do not exceed 20 mg of simvastatin.[1]
- Ciclosporin: increased risk of myopathy – avoid concomitant use.[1]
- Colchicine: possible increased risk of myopathy.
- Danazol: avoid concomitant use.
- Grapefruit: increased risk of myopathy – avoid concomitant use.
- Hormone antagonists: possibly increased risk of myopathy with danazol – avoid concomitant use.[1]
- Lipid-lowering agents: increased risk of myopathy with fibrates – do not exceed 10 mg of simvastatin except with fenofibrate;[1] gemfibrozil – avoid; increased risk of myopathy with nicotinic acid.
- Ticagrelor: concentration of simvastatin increased; maximum dose of simvastatin is 40 mg.

ADMINISTRATION

RECONSTITUTION
–

ROUTE
● Oral

RATE OF ADMINISTRATION
–

COMMENTS
–

OTHER INFORMATION

● *Drug Prescribing in Renal Failure*, 5th edition, by Aronoff *et al.* suggests that doses up to 40 mg are acceptable.

Reference:
1. MHRA. *Drug Safety Update*. Statins: interactions and updated advice. August 2012; **6**(1): 2–4.

Sirolimus

CLINICAL USE

Immunosuppressant:
- Prophylaxis of transplant allograft rejection

DOSE IN NORMAL RENAL FUNCTION

6 mg loading dose followed by 2 mg daily, adjusted according to levels – See 'Other information'.

PHARMACOKINETICS

Molecular weight (daltons)	914.2
% Protein binding	92
% Excreted unchanged in urine	2.2
Volume of distribution (L/kg)	4–20
Half-life – normal/ ESRF (hrs)	48–78/Unchanged

METABOLISM

Sirolimus is metabolised by the cytochrome P450 isoenzyme CYP3A4. Metabolism occurs by demethylation or hydroxylation, and the majority of a dose is excreted via the faeces, with only about 2% excreted in the urine.

DOSE IN RENAL IMPAIRMENT GFR (mL/MIN)

20–50	Dose as in normal renal function.
10–20	Dose as in normal renal function.
<10	Dose as in normal renal function.

DOSE IN PATIENTS UNDERGOING RENAL REPLACEMENT THERAPIES

CAPD	Unlikely to be dialysed. Dose as in normal renal function.
HD	Not dialysed. Dose as in normal renal function.
HDF/High flux	Unknown dialysability. Dose as in normal renal function.
CAV/ VVHD	Unlikely to be dialysed. Dose as in normal renal function.

IMPORTANT DRUG INTERACTIONS

Potentially hazardous interactions with other drugs
- Antibacterials: concentration increased by clarithromycin and telithromycin – avoid; concentration of both drugs increased with erythromycin; concentration reduced by rifampicin and rifabutin – avoid.
- Antifungals: concentration increased by itraconazole, fluconazole, ketoconazole, micafungin, miconazole, posaconazole and voriconazole – avoid with itraconazole, ketoconazole and voriconazole.
- Antivirals: concentration possibly increased by atazanavir, boceprevir and lopinavir; concentration of both drugs increased with telaprevir, reduce dose of sirolimus.
- Calcium-channel blockers: concentration increased by diltiazem; concentration of both drugs increased with verapamil.
- Ciclosporin: increased absorption of sirolimus – give sirolimus 4 hours after ciclosporin; sirolimus concentration increased; long term concomitant administration may be associated with deterioration in renal function.
- Cytotoxics: use crizotinib with caution.
- Grapefruit juice: concentration of sirolimus increased – avoid concomitant use.
- Mycophenolate: concomitant use of mycophenolate and sirolimus increases plasma levels of both sirolimus and mycophenolic acid.

ADMINISTRATION

RECONSTITUTION
–
ROUTE
- Oral
RATE OF ADMINISTRATION
–
COMMENTS
–

OTHER INFORMATION

- Aim for trough levels of 4–12 ng/mL where sirolimus is used in combination with low dose ciclosporin.
- In cases of delayed graft function or where a calcineurin inhibitor is not tolerated or contraindicated, sirolimus may be used with steroids alone. A loading dose of 10–15 mg may be given, followed by maintenance dose of 3–6 mg daily and adjust according to levels. Aim for trough levels of 8–20 ng/mL.
- May be used in combination with MMF, but can lead to delayed wound healing post surgery. Sirolimus can increase levels

- of mycophenolate mofetil leading to anaemia.
- Some centres successfully using level-controlled sirolimus in conjunction with low dose tacrolimus.
- Anecdotally, has been used for encapsulating sclerosing peritonitis in a CAPD patient at Guy's Hospital, London. Acts by interfering with various growth factors and their effect on impairing wound healing.
- Pneumonitis appears to be more common with sirolimus than initially thought, especially if the trough levels are on the high side. (Glare J. Adverse effect report – pneumonitis with sirolimus. *Ann Intern Med.* 2006; **144**: 505–9.)
- If changing from tablets to solution, give the same dose and monitor trough levels 1–2 weeks later.
- Tablet has a 27% increased bioavailability compared with the solution.
- Sirolimus has been associated with anaphylactic/anaphylactoid reactions, angioedema and hypersensitivity vasculitis.

Sitagliptin

CLINICAL USE

Treatment of type 2 diabetes in combination
with metformin or a thiazolidinedione.

DOSE IN NORMAL RENAL FUNCTION

100 mg once daily

PHARMACOKINETICS

Molecular weight (daltons)	523.3 (as phosphate)
% Protein binding	38
% Excreted unchanged in urine	79
Volume of distribution (L/kg)	198 litres
Half-life – normal/ ESRF (hrs)	12.4/Probably increased

METABOLISM

Sitagliptin undergoes minimal metabolism,
mainly by the cytochrome P450 isoenzyme
CYP3A4, and to a lesser extent by CYP2C8.
About 79% of a dose is excreted unchanged
in the urine. Renal excretion of sitagliptin
involves active tubular secretion; it is a
substrate for organic anion transporter-3 and
P-glycoprotein.

DOSE IN RENAL IMPAIRMENT GFR (mL/MIN)

30–50	50 mg once daily
<30	25 mg once daily

DOSE IN PATIENTS UNDERGOING RENAL REPLACEMENT THERAPIES

CAPD	Not dialysed. Dose as in GFR<30 mL/min.
HD	Not dialysed. Dose as in GFR<30 mL/min.
HDF/High flux	Dialysed. Dose as in GFR<30 mL/min.
CAV/ VVHD	Unknown dialysability. Dose as in GFR<30 mL/min.

IMPORTANT DRUG INTERACTIONS

Potentially hazardous interactions with other
drugs
- None known

ADMINISTRATION

RECONSTITUTION
–
ROUTE
- Oral
RATE OF ADMINISTRATION
–

COMMENTS
–

OTHER INFORMATION

- 13.5% of dose is removed during a
  3–4 hour haemodialysis session.
- In severe renal impairment (GFR<30 mL/
  min) the AUC was increased 4-fold.

Sodium aurothiomalate

CLINICAL USE

Active progressive rheumatoid arthritis in adults

DOSE IN NORMAL RENAL FUNCTION

10 mg as a test dose followed by 50–100 mg weekly, frequency is altered according to duration and response. See product literature for more information.

PHARMACOKINETICS

Molecular weight (daltons)	368.1
% Protein binding	85–95
% Excreted unchanged in urine	Majority
Volume of distribution (L/kg)	No data
Half-life – normal/ ESRF (hrs)	5–6 days/–

METABOLISM

Mainly excreted in the urine with smaller amounts in the faeces.

DOSE IN RENAL IMPAIRMENT GFR (mL/MIN)

20–50	Avoid
10–20	Avoid
<10	Avoid

DOSE IN PATIENTS UNDERGOING RENAL REPLACEMENT THERAPIES

CAPD	Unknown dialysability. Dose as in GFR<10 mL/min.
HD	Not dialysed. Dose as in GFR<10 mL/min.
HDF/High flux	Unknown dialysability. Dose as in GFR<10 mL/min.
CAV/ VVHD	Not dialysed. Dose as in GFR=10–20 mL/min.

IMPORTANT DRUG INTERACTIONS

Potentially hazardous interactions with other drugs
- ACE-inhibitors: flushing and hypotension reported in combination.
- Penicillamine: increased risk of toxicity – avoid.

ADMINISTRATION

RECONSTITUTION
–
ROUTE
- Deep IM
RATE OF ADMINISTRATION
–
COMMENTS
–

OTHER INFORMATION

- Warn patients to tell the doctor immediately if any of the following develop: sore throat, mouth ulcers, bruising, fever, malaise, rash, diarrhoea or non-specific illness.
- Blood tests should be carried out monthly, and treatment should be withdrawn if the platelets fall below 100 000/mm^3, or if signs and symptoms suggestive of thrombocytopenia appear.
- Gold can produce nephrotic syndrome or less severe glomerular disease with proteinuria and haematuria, which are usually mild and transient. If persistent or clinically significant proteinuria develops, treatment with gold should be discontinued. Minor transient changes in renal function may also occur.
- Urine tests should be carried out pre-treatment and before each injection to test for proteinuria and haematuria.
- Gold may be found in the urine for up to 1 year or more owing to its presence in deep body compartments.

Sodium bicarbonate

CLINICAL USE

- Metabolic acidosis
- Alkalinisation of urine
- Renoprotection against contrast media

DOSE IN NORMAL RENAL FUNCTION

- Oral: 0.5–1.5 g 3 times daily (or more may be required)
- IV: 8.4%, 60–120 mL per hour; 4.2%, up to 120 mL per hour; 1.26% or 1.4% – See 'Other information'

PHARMACOKINETICS

Molecular weight (daltons)	84
% Protein binding	0
% Excreted unchanged in urine	<1
Volume of distribution (L/kg)	Dependent on the physical state of the patient at the time.
Half-life – normal/ ESRF (hrs)	No data

METABOLISM

Oral bicarbonate, such as sodium bicarbonate, neutralises gastric acid with the production of carbon dioxide. Bicarbonate not involved in that reaction is absorbed and in the absence of a deficit of bicarbonate in the plasma, bicarbonate ions are excreted in the urine, which is rendered alkaline, and there is an accompanying diuresis.

DOSE IN RENAL IMPAIRMENT GFR (mL/MIN)

20–50	Dose as in normal renal function.
10–20	Dose as in normal renal function.
<10	Dose as in normal renal function.

DOSE IN PATIENTS UNDERGOING RENAL REPLACEMENT THERAPIES

CAPD	Dialysed. Dose as in normal renal function.
HD	Dialysed. Dose as in normal renal function.
HDF/High flux	Dialysed. Dose as in normal renal function.
CAV/ VVHD	Dialysed. Dose as in normal renal function.

IMPORTANT DRUG INTERACTIONS

Potentially hazardous interactions with other drugs
Increases lithium excretion.

ADMINISTRATION

RECONSTITUTION
–

ROUTE
- Oral, IV, central administration for undiluted 8.4% infusion

RATE OF ADMINISTRATION
–

COMMENTS
–

OTHER INFORMATION

- Caution – may result in sodium retention and oedema.
- Sodium bicarbonate 1.26% or 1.4% may be given IV to prevent the nephrotoxicity associated with scans or procedures involving radiological contrast media. A typical hydration regimen is 3 mL/kg/hour for 1 hour prior to the procedure, followed by 1 mL/kg/hour for 6 hours afterwards.
- 8.4% ≡ 1 mmol bicarbonate + 1 mmol sodium per mL.
- 500 mg sodium bicarbonate tablet ≡ 6 mmol sodium + 6 mmol bicarbonate.
- Sodium bicarbonate reduces serum potassium concentrations by inducing a shift of potassium ions into the cell.
- A sugar free raspberry flavoured oral solution of 8.4% sodium bicarbonate is available from Martindale.

Sodium chloride

CLINICAL USE

Treatment and prophylaxis of sodium
chloride deficiency

DOSE IN NORMAL RENAL FUNCTION

- Oral prophylaxis: 40–80 mmol sodium
  daily, up to a maximum of 200 mmol
  sodium daily
- IV: in severe deficiency 2–3 litres over
  2–3 hours then reduce

PHARMACOKINETICS

Molecular weight (daltons)	58.4
% Protein binding	0
% Excreted unchanged in urine	No data
Volume of distribution (L/kg)	Dependent on the physiological state of the patient at the time
Half-life – normal/ ESRF (hrs)	No data

METABOLISM

Excess sodium is mainly excreted by the
kidney, and small amounts are lost in the
faeces and sweat.

DOSE IN RENAL IMPAIRMENT GFR (mL/MIN)

20–50	Dose as in normal renal function.
10–20	Dose as in normal renal function.
<10	Dose as in normal renal function.

DOSE IN PATIENTS UNDERGOING RENAL REPLACEMENT THERAPIES

CAPD	Dialysed. Dose as in normal renal function.
HD	Dialysed. Dose as in normal renal function.
HDF/High flux	Dialysed. Dose as in normal renal function.
CAV/ VVHD	Dialysed. Dose as in normal renal function.

IMPORTANT DRUG INTERACTIONS

Potentially hazardous interactions with other
drugs
- May impair the efficacy of
  antihypertensive drugs in chronic renal
  failure.

ADMINISTRATION

RECONSTITUTION
–
ROUTE
- Oral, IV
RATE OF ADMINISTRATION
–
COMMENTS
–

OTHER INFORMATION

- Other regimens: for acute muscular
  cramps post haemodialysis, 10 mL sodium
  chloride 30% injection diluted in 100 mL
  sodium chloride 0.9%, and infused over
  30 minutes or in dialysis washback.
- Sodium salts should be administered with
  caution to patients with congestive heart
  failure, peripheral or pulmonary oedema,
  or impaired renal function.
- Slow Sodium® 600 mg tablet =
  approximately 10 mmol sodium and
  10 mmol chloride.

Sodium clodronate

CLINICAL USE

Bisphosphonate:
Management of osteolytic lesions,
hypercalcaemia and bone pain associated
with skeletal metastases in patients with
breast cancer or multiple myeloma

DOSE IN NORMAL RENAL FUNCTION

- 1.6–3.2 g daily in single or 2 divided doses
- Loron-520: 2–4 tablets daily

PHARMACOKINETICS

Molecular weight (daltons)	360.9 (as disodium salt)
% Protein binding	36
% Excreted unchanged in urine	>70
Volume of distribution (L/kg)	0.3
Half-life – normal/ ESRF (hrs)	1st phase: 2; 2nd phase: 13/51

METABOLISM

Clodronate is not metabolised. Over 70% of
an intravenous dose is excreted unchanged
in the urine within 24 hours, the remainder
being sequestered to bone tissue. The
substance which is bound to bone is excreted
more slowly, and the renal clearance is about
75% of the plasma clearance.

DOSE IN RENAL IMPAIRMENT GFR (mL/MIN)

30–50	Dose as in normal renal function.
10–30	50% of normal dose.
<10	Avoid.

DOSE IN PATIENTS UNDERGOING RENAL REPLACEMENT THERAPIES

CAPD	Not dialysed. Dose as in GFR<10 mL/min.
HD	Dialysed. Dose as in GFR<10 mL/min.
HDF/High flux	Dialysed. Dose as in GFR<10 mL/min.
CAV/ VVHD	Unknown dialysability. Dose as in GFR=10–30 mL/min.

IMPORTANT DRUG INTERACTIONS

Potentially hazardous interactions with other
drugs
- Cytotoxics: concentration of estramustine
  increased.

ADMINISTRATION

RECONSTITUTION
–
ROUTE
- Oral

OTHER INFORMATION

- Reversible elevations of creatinine have
  been reported. Renal function should be
  monitored during treatment.
- Orally: avoid food for one hour before
  and after treatment, particularly calcium-
  containing products; also avoid iron,
  mineral supplements and antacids.

Sodium fusidate

Antibacterial agent

DOSE IN NORMAL RENAL FUNCTION

- Oral: 0.5–1 g (as sodium fusidate) every 8 hours
- Suspension: 750 mg every 8 hours (as fusidic acid)

PHARMACOKINETICS

Molecular weight (daltons)	538.7
% Protein binding	95
% Excreted unchanged in urine	<1
Volume of distribution (L/kg)	0.2
Half-life – normal/ ESRF (hrs)	10–15/Unchanged

METABOLISM

Fusidic acid is excreted in the bile, almost entirely as metabolites, some of which have weak antimicrobial activity.

Approximately 2% appears unchanged in the faeces.

DOSE IN RENAL IMPAIRMENT GFR (mL/MIN)

20–50	Dose as in normal renal function.
10–20	Dose as in normal renal function.
<10	Dose as in normal renal function.

DOSE IN PATIENTS UNDERGOING RENAL REPLACEMENT THERAPIES

CAPD	Not dialysed. Dose as in normal renal function.
HD	Not dialysed. Dose as in normal renal function.
HDF/High flux	Unknown dialysability. Dose as in normal renal function.
CAV/ VVHD	Not dialysed. Dose as in normal renal function.

IMPORTANT DRUG INTERACTIONS

Potentially hazardous interactions with other drugs

- Antivirals: concentration of both drugs increased in combination with ritonavir and saquinavir – avoid with ritonavir.
- Statins: increased risk of myopathy with simvastatin and atorvastatin especially in diabetics. Avoid concomitant use with simvastatin and for 7 days after last dose.[1]

ADMINISTRATION

RECONSTITUTION

–

ROUTE

- Oral

RATE OF ADMINISTRATION

–

COMMENTS

–

OTHER INFORMATION

Reference:
1. MHRA. *Drug Safety Update*. Statins: interactions and updated advice. August 2012; **6**(1): 2–4.

Sodium nitroprusside

CLINICAL USE

- Hypertensive crisis
- Heart failure
- Controlled hypotension in surgery

DOSE IN NORMAL RENAL FUNCTION

- Hypertensive emergencies: 0.3–8 mcg/kg/minute
- Maintenance of blood pressure: 20–400 mcg/minute
- Heart failure: 10–200 mcg/minute
- Controlled blood pressure in surgery: maximum 1.5 mcg/kg/minute

PHARMACOKINETICS

Molecular weight (daltons)	297.9
% Protein binding	0
% Excreted unchanged in urine	<10
Volume of distribution (L/kg)	0.2
Half-life – normal/ ESRF (hrs)	2–10 minutes/ Unchanged

METABOLISM

Sodium nitroprusside is rapidly metabolised to cyanide in erythrocytes and smooth muscle, and this is then followed by the release of nitric oxide, the active metabolite. Cyanide is further metabolised in the liver to thiocyanate, which is slowly excreted in the urine.

DOSE IN RENAL IMPAIRMENT GFR (mL/MIN)

20–50	Dose as in normal renal function.
10–20	Dose as in normal renal function. Avoid prolonged use.
<10	Dose as in normal renal function. Avoid prolonged use.

DOSE IN PATIENTS UNDERGOING RENAL REPLACEMENT THERAPIES

CAPD	Dialysed. Dose as in GFR<10 mL/min.
HD	Dialysed. Dose as in GFR<10 mL/min.
HDF/High flux	Dialysed. Dose as in GFR<10 mL/min.
CAV/VVHD	Dialysed. Dose as in GFR=10–20 mL/min.

IMPORTANT DRUG INTERACTIONS

Potentially hazardous interactions with other drugs
- Anaesthetics: enhanced hypotensive effect.

ADMINISTRATION

RECONSTITUTION
- 2–3 mL glucose 5%

ROUTE
- IV

RATE OF ADMINISTRATION
- 10–400 micrograms/minute, adjusted according to response

COMMENTS
- Dilute 50 mg in 250–1000 mL glucose 5% to give a concentration of 50–200 mcg/mL.
- Minimum volume is 1 mg/mL via central line. (UK Critical Care Group, *Minimum Infusion Volumes for Fluid Restricted Critically Ill Patients*, 3rd edition, 2006)
- Wrap syringes and lines in foil to protect from light.

OTHER INFORMATION

- Avoid prolonged use in renal impairment because accumulation of thiocyanate (which is dialysable) may cause seizures or a coma.
- Monitor thiocyanate and cyanide levels.
- Do not stop infusion abruptly – tail off over 10–30 minutes.

Sodium stibogluconate

CLINICAL USE

Treatment of leishmaniasis.

DOSE IN NORMAL RENAL FUNCTION

20 mg/kg daily. Maximum dose 850 mg

PHARMACOKINETICS

Molecular weight (daltons)	910.9
% Protein binding	No data
% Excreted unchanged in urine	0.8[1]
Volume of distribution (L/kg)	0.21[2]
Half-life – normal/ ESRF (hrs)	Initial phase: 2; slower terminal phase: 33–7/–

METABOLISM

No data on possible metabolic pathways.
Elimination occurs in two phases; a rapid initial phase, in which the majority of a dose is excreted via the kidneys within 12 hours, and a slower phase, possibly reflecting reduction to trivalent antimony.

DOSE IN RENAL IMPAIRMENT GFR (mL/MIN)

20–50	Avoid
10–20	Avoid
<10	Avoid

DOSE IN PATIENTS UNDERGOING RENAL REPLACEMENT THERAPIES

CAPD	Unknown dialysability. Avoid.
HD	Unknown dialysability. Avoid.
HDF/High flux	Unknown dialysability. Avoid.
CAV/ VVHD	Unknown dialysability. Avoid.

IMPORTANT DRUG INTERACTIONS

Potentially hazardous interactions with other drugs
• None known

ADMINISTRATION

RECONSTITUTION
–
ROUTE
• IM, IV
RATE OF ADMINISTRATION
• Over 5 minutes
COMMENTS
• Due to the presence of particulates (size range 20 to 300 microns) the solution should be drawn up through a filter immediately prior to administration.

OTHER INFORMATION

• Has caused acute renal failure and accumulates in renal impairment therefore avoid use.

References:
1. May Al laser MA, El-Yazigi A, Croft SL. Pharmacokinetics of antimony in patients treated with sodium stibogluconate for cutaneous leishmaniasis. *Pharmaceut Res.* January 1995; **12**(1): 113–16.
2. Nieto J, Alvar J, Mullen A, *et al.* Pharmacokinetics, toxicities, and efficacies of sodium stibogluconate formulations after intravenous administration in animals. http://pure.strath.ac.uk/portal/en/journals/antimicrobial-agents-and-chemotherapy(0366207a-5f0b-4910-ae8c-8520b5887a0d).html

Sodium valproate

CLINICAL USE

All forms of epilepsy
Migraine prophylaxis (unlicensed)

DOSE IN NORMAL RENAL FUNCTION

- Oral: 600 mg – 2.5 g daily in divided doses.
- IV: For continuation of existing oral therapy, IV and oral doses are equivalent, give the same dose.
- For initiation of new therapy: give a loading dose of 400–800 mg (up to 10 mg/kg), followed by either a constant infusion or intermittent doses up to a cumulative daily dose of 2.5 g.
- Migraine prophylaxis: 200 mg twice daily increasing to 1.2–1.5 g daily in divided doses if necessary.

PHARMACOKINETICS

Molecular weight (daltons)	166.2
% Protein binding	90–95
% Excreted unchanged in urine	3–7
Volume of distribution (L/kg)	0.1–0.4[1]
Half-life – normal/ ESRF (hrs)	6–15/Unchanged

METABOLISM

Valproic acid is extensively metabolised in the liver, a large part by glucuronidation (up to 60%) and the rest by a variety of complex pathways (up to 45%). It is excreted in the urine almost entirely in the form of its metabolites; small amounts are excreted in faeces and expired air.

DOSE IN RENAL IMPAIRMENT GFR (mL/MIN)

20–50	Dose as in normal renal function.
10–20	Dose as in normal renal function.
<10	Dose as in normal renal function.

DOSE IN PATIENTS UNDERGOING RENAL REPLACEMENT THERAPIES

CAPD	Not dialysed. Dose as in normal renal function.
HD	Not dialysed. Dose as in normal renal function.
HDF/High flux	Dialysed. Dose as in normal renal function.
CAV/ VVHD	Dialysed. Dose as in normal renal function.

IMPORTANT DRUG INTERACTIONS

Potentially hazardous interactions with other drugs
- Antibacterials: metabolism possibly inhibited by erythromycin; avoid with pivmecillinam; concentration reduced by carbapenems – avoid.
- Antidepressants: antagonise anticonvulsant effect; avoid with St John's wort.
- Anti-epileptics: concentration reduced by carbamazepine; concentration of active carbamazepine metabolite increased; increased concentration of lamotrigine, phenobarbital, rufinamide and possibly ethosuximide; sometimes reduces concentration of active metabolite of oxcarbazepine; alters phenytoin concentration; phenytoin and phenobarbital reduce valproate concentration; hyperammonaemia and CNS toxicity with topiramate.
- Antimalarials: mefloquine antagonises anticonvulsant effect.
- Antipsychotics: antagonise anticonvulsant effect; increased neutropenia with olanzapine; possibly increases or decreases concentration of clozapine; possibly increases quetiapine concentration.
- Ciclosporin: variable ciclosporin blood level response.
- Orlistat: possibly increased risk of convulsions.
- Ulcer-healing drugs: metabolism inhibited by cimetidine, increased concentration.

ADMINISTRATION

RECONSTITUTION
- Use solvent provided
ROUTE
- IV, oral, PR (unlicensed)
RATE OF ADMINISTRATION
- 3–5 minutes bolus, or continuous infusion
COMMENTS
–

OTHER INFORMATION

- Increases ketones in urine. May give false positive urine tests for ketones.
- Sodium valproate serum levels do not correlate with anti-epileptic activity.

- Monitor serum levels to ensure not greater than 100 micrograms/mL, or if non-compliance is suspected.
- Suppositories are available on a named patient basis.

Reference:
1. Faught E. Pharmacokinetic considerations in prescribing anti-epileptic drugs. *Epilepsia*. 2001; **42**(Suppl. 4): 19–23.

Solifenacin succinate

CLINICAL USE

Selective M_3 antimuscarinic
- Symptomatic treatment of urge incontinence and/or increased urinary frequency and urgency

DOSE IN NORMAL RENAL FUNCTION

5–10 mg once daily

PHARMACOKINETICS

Molecular weight (daltons)	480.6
% Protein binding	98
% Excreted unchanged in urine	11
Volume of distribution (L/kg)	600 litres
Half-life – normal/ ESRF (hrs)	45–68/Increased by 60%

METABOLISM

Extensively metabolised in the liver, mainly by the cytochrome P450 isoenzyme CYP3A4 and is excreted mainly as metabolites in urine and faeces.

DOSE IN RENAL IMPAIRMENT GFR (mL/MIN)

30–50	Dose as in normal renal function.
10–30	5 mg once daily.
<10	5 mg once daily.

DOSE IN PATIENTS UNDERGOING RENAL REPLACEMENT THERAPIES

CAPD	Unlikely to be dialysed. Dose as in GFR<10 mL/min. Use with caution.
HD	Unlikely to be dialysed. Dose as in GFR<10 mL/min. Use with caution.
HDF/High flux	Unknown dialysability. Dose as in GFR<10 mL/min. Use with caution.
CAV/ VVHD	Unknown dialysability. Dose as in GFR=10–30 mL/min. Use with caution.

IMPORTANT DRUG INTERACTIONS

Potentially hazardous interactions with other drugs
- Avoid if GFR<30 mL/min if also taking itraconazole, ketoconazole or ritonavir.
- Anti-arrhythmics: increased risk of antimuscarinic side effects with disopyramide.

ADMINISTRATION

RECONSTITUTION
–
ROUTE
- Oral
RATE OF ADMINISTRATION
–

OTHER INFORMATION

- Contraindicated by manufacturer in haemodialysis due to lack of data
- Bioavailability is 90%.
- In patients with severe renal impairment (creatinine clearance ≤30 mL/min), exposure to solifenacin was significantly greater than in the controls, with increases in C_{max} of about 30%, AUC of more than 100% and t½ of more than 60%. A statistically significant relationship was observed between creatinine clearance and solifenacin clearance.

Sorafenib

CLINICAL USE

Protein kinase inhibitor:
- Treatment of advanced renal cell carcinoma
- Treatment of hepatocellular carcinoma

DOSE IN NORMAL RENAL FUNCTION

400 mg twice daily

PHARMACOKINETICS

Molecular weight (daltons)	464.8 (637 as tosylate)
% Protein binding	99.5
% Excreted unchanged in urine	0
Volume of distribution (L/kg)	No data
Half-life – normal/ ESRF (hrs)	25–48/–

METABOLISM

Sorafenib is metabolised primarily in the liver and undergoes oxidative metabolism mediated by CYP3A4, as well as glucuronidation mediated by UGT1A9.

Eight metabolites have been identified, during *in vitro* studies; one has been shown to have equal activity to sorafenib. About 96% of a dose is excreted within 14 days, with 77%, mostly as unchanged drug, recovered in the faeces, and 19% in the urine as glucuronidated metabolites.

DOSE IN RENAL IMPAIRMENT GFR (mL/MIN)

30–50	Dose as in normal renal function.
10–30	Dose as in normal renal function.
<10	Dose as in normal renal function.

DOSE IN PATIENTS UNDERGOING RENAL REPLACEMENT THERAPIES

CAPD	Unlikely to be dialysed. Dose as in GFR<10 mL/min.
HD	Unlikely to be dialysed. Dose as in GFR<10 mL/min.
HDF/High flux	Unlikely to be dialysed. Dose as in GFR<10 mL/min.
CAV/ VVHD	Unlikely to be dialysed. Dose as in GFR=10–30 mL/min.

IMPORTANT DRUG INTERACTIONS

Potentially hazardous interactions with other drugs
- Anticoagulants: may enhance effect of coumarins.
- Antipsychotics: avoid concomitant use with clozapine (increased risk of agranulocytosis).
- Antivirals: avoid with boceprevir.

ADMINISTRATION

RECONSTITUTION
–

ROUTE
- Oral

RATE OF ADMINISTRATION
–

COMMENTS
- Administer preferably without food.

OTHER INFORMATION

- Increased amylase and lipase and hypophosphataemia are common.
- Most common side effects are diarrhoea and dermatological effects.
- A case report of interstitial nephritis has been reported in a patient with CRF due to FSGS. (Izzedine H. Interstitial nephritis in a patient taking sorafenib. *Nephrol Dial Transplant.* 2007; **22**: 2411.)

Sotalol hydrochloride

CLINICAL USE

Beta-adrenoceptor blocker:
- Treatment of life-threatening ventricular arrhythmias
- Prophylaxis of SVT

DOSE IN NORMAL RENAL FUNCTION

- Oral: 80–640 mg per day in single or divided doses (480–640 mg under specialist supervision)
- IV: 20–120 mg every 6 hours

PHARMACOKINETICS

Molecular weight (daltons)	308.8
% Protein binding	0
% Excreted unchanged in urine	>90
Volume of distribution (L/kg)	1.6–2.4
Half-life – normal/ESRF (hrs)	10–20/56

METABOLISM

Metabolism of sotalol is negligible, and it is excreted unchanged in the urine.

DOSE IN RENAL IMPAIRMENT GFR (mL/MIN)

30–60	50% of normal dose.
10–30	25% of normal dose.
<10	25% of normal dose and increase dosage interval. Use with caution.

DOSE IN PATIENTS UNDERGOING RENAL REPLACEMENT THERAPIES

CAPD	Unlikely to be dialysed. Dose as in GFR<10 mL/min.
HD	Dialysed. Dose as in GFR<10 mL/min.
HDF/High flux	Dialysed. Dose as in GFR<10 mL/min.
CAV/VVHD	Dialysed. Dose as in GFR=10–30 mL/min.

IMPORTANT DRUG INTERACTIONS

Potentially hazardous interactions with other drugs
- Anaesthetics: enhanced hypotensive effect.
- Analgesics: NSAIDs antagonise hypotensive effect.
- Anti-arrhythmics: increased risk of myocardial depression and bradycardia; increased risk of bradycardia, myocardial depression and AV block with amiodarone; increased risk of ventricular arrhythmias with amiodarone, dronedarone, disopyramide or procainamide – avoid; increased risk of myocardial depression and bradycardia with flecainide.
- Antibacterials: increased risk of ventricular arrhythmias with moxifloxacin – avoid.
- Antidepressants: enhanced hypotensive effect with MAOIs; increased risk of ventricular arrhythmias with tricyclics.
- Antihistamines: increased risk of ventricular arrhythmias with mizolastine – avoid.
- Antihypertensives: enhanced hypotensive effect; increased risk of withdrawal hypertension with clonidine; increased risk of first dose hypotensive effect with post-synaptic alpha-blockers such as prazosin.
- Antimalarials: increased risk of bradycardia with mefloquine; avoid with artemether and lumefantrine and piperaquine with artenimol – increased risk of ventricular arrhythmias.
- Antimuscarinics: increased risk of ventricular arrhythmias with tolterodine.
- Antipsychotics: enhanced hypotensive effect with phenothiazines; increased risk of ventricular arrhythmias with amisulpride, droperidol, haloperidol, phenothiazines, pimozide or zuclopenthixol – avoid concomitant use with droperidol and zuclopenthixol.
- Antivirals: increased risk of ventricular arrhythmias with saquinavir or telaprevir – avoid.
- Atomoxetine: increased risk of ventricular arrhythmias.
- Calcium-channel blockers: increased risk of bradycardia and AV block with diltiazem; hypotension and heart failure possible with nifedipine and nisoldipine; asystole, severe hypotension and heart failure with verapamil.
- Cytotoxics: possible increased risk of bradycardia with crizotinib; increased risk of ventricular arrhythmias with vandetanib – avoid; increased risk of ventricular arrhythmias with arsenic trioxide.
- Diuretics: enhanced hypotensive effect; increased risk of ventricular arrhythmias due to hypokalaemia.

- Fingolimod: possibly increased risk of bradycardia.
- Ivabradine: increased risk of ventricular arrhythmias.
- Moxisylyte: possible severe postural hypotension.
- Ranolazine: avoid concomitant use.
- Sympathomimetics: severe hypertension with adrenaline and noradrenaline and possibly with dobutamine.

ADMINISTRATION

RECONSTITUTION

–

ROUTE
- IV, oral

RATE OF ADMINISTRATION
- Slow IV bolus with ECG monitoring
- Over 10 minutes

COMMENTS

–

OTHER INFORMATION

- Oral bioavailability is >90%.
- Contraindicated in UK SPC but use with caution in US data sheet.
- Sotalol prolongs the QT interval, which predisposes to the development of *torsades de pointes*.
- If used in haemodialysis, give lowest possible dose, after dialysis.

Spironolactone

CLINICAL USE

Aldosterone antagonist, diuretic:
- Oedema
- Heart failure
- Ascites in liver and malignant cirrhosis
- Resistant hypertension (unlicensed)
- Treatment of primary hyperaldosteronism

DOSE IN NORMAL RENAL FUNCTION

25–400 mg daily, dose varies according to indication

PHARMACOKINETICS

Molecular weight (daltons)	416.6
% Protein binding	90
% Excreted unchanged in urine	0 (47–57 as metabolites)
Volume of distribution (L/kg)	No data
Half-life – normal/ESRF (hrs)	1.3–1.4/ Unchanged

METABOLISM

Spironolactone is metabolised extensively to several metabolites including canrenone and 7α-thiomethylspirolactone, both of which are pharmacologically active. The major metabolite may be 7α-thiomethylspirolactone, although it is uncertain to what extent the actions of spironolactone are dependent on the parent compound or its metabolites. Spironolactone is excreted mainly in the urine and also in the faeces, in the form of metabolites.

DOSE IN RENAL IMPAIRMENT GFR (mL/MIN)

20–50	50% of normal dose[1]
10–20	50% of normal dose[1]
<10	Use with caution. See 'Other information'.

DOSE IN PATIENTS UNDERGOING RENAL REPLACEMENT THERAPIES

CAPD	Not dialysed. Dose as in GFR<10 mL/min.
HD	Not dialysed. Dose as in GFR<10 mL/min.
HDF/High flux	Unknown dialysability. Dose as in GFR<10 mL/min.
CAV/ VVHD	Not dialysed. Dose as in GFR=10–20 mL/min.

IMPORTANT DRUG INTERACTIONS

Potentially hazardous interactions with other drugs
- ACE inhibitors or angiotensin-II antagonists: enhanced hypotensive effect; risk of severe hyperkalaemia.
- Antibacterials: avoid concomitant use with lymecycline.
- Antidepressants: increased risk of postural hypotension with tricyclics.
- Antihypertensives: enhanced hypotensive effect; increased risk of first dose hypotensive effect with post-synaptic alpha-blockers.
- Cardiac glycosides: increased digoxin concentration.
- Ciclosporin: increased risk of hyperkalaemia.
- Cytotoxics: avoid concomitant use with mitotane; increased risk of nephrotoxicity and ototoxicity with platinum compounds.
- Lithium: reduced lithium excretion.
- NSAIDs: increased risk of hyperkalaemia (especially with indomethacin); increased risk of nephrotoxicity; diuretic effect of spironolactone antagonised by aspirin.
- Potassium salts: increased risk of hyperkalaemia.
- Tacrolimus: increased risk of hyperkalaemia.

ADMINISTRATION

RECONSTITUTION
–

ROUTE
- Oral

RATE OF ADMINISTRATION
–

COMMENTS
–

OTHER INFORMATION

- Contraindicated by manufacturer in severe renal impairment.
- It can be used in renal patients but they are at an increased risk of hyperkalaemia and therefore spironolactone should be used with caution. It has active metabolites with long half-lives.
- Small studies have shown that doses of 25 mg of spironolactone 3 times a week can be safely used in haemodialysis patients although unknown whether that dose would be therapeutic – potassium levels should be monitored closely. (Sauden P, Mach F, Perneger T, et al. Safety

of low-dose spironolactone administration in chronic haemodialysis patients. *Nephrol Dial Transplant.* 2003 Nov; **18**(11): 2359–63.)

- Another small study used 25 mg daily but the potassium was monitored 3 times a week. (Hussain S, Dreyfuss, DE, Marcus RJ, *et al.* Is spironolactone safe for dialysis patients? *Nephrol Dial Transplant.* 2003 Nov; **18**(11): 2364–8.)

Reference:

1. Sani M. *Clinical Pharmacology in the ICU.* 1994. Section 1, p. 66.

Stavudine

CLINICAL USE

Nucleoside reverse transcriptase inhibitor:
- Treatment of HIV in combination with other antiretroviral drugs

DOSE IN NORMAL RENAL FUNCTION

<60 kg: 30 mg twice daily
>60 kg: 40 mg twice daily

PHARMACOKINETICS

Molecular weight (daltons)	224.2
% Protein binding	<1
% Excreted unchanged in urine	40
Volume of distribution (L/kg)	0.5
Half-life – normal/ ESRF (hrs)	1–1.5/5.5–8

METABOLISM

Stavudine is metabolised intracellularly to the active antiviral triphosphate. Following an oral 80-mg dose of ^{14}C-stavudine to healthy subjects, approximately 95% and 3% of the total radioactivity was recovered in urine and faeces, respectively. Approximately 70% of the orally administered stavudine dose was excreted as an unchanged drug in urine. However, in HIV-infected patients, 42% (range: 13–87%) of the dose is excreted unchanged in the urine, by active tubular secretion and glomerular filtration.

DOSE IN RENAL IMPAIRMENT GFR (mL/MIN)

26–50	<60 kg: 15 mg twice daily >60 kg: 20 mg twice daily
<25	<60 kg: 15 mg daily >60 kg: 20 mg daily

DOSE IN PATIENTS UNDERGOING RENAL REPLACEMENT THERAPIES

CAPD	Unknown dialysability. Dose as in GFR<25 mL/min.
HD	Dialysed. Dose as in GFR<25 mL/min.
HDF/High flux	Dialysed. Dose as in GFR<25 mL/min.
CAV/VVHD	Dialysed. Dose as in GFR=26–50 mL/min.

IMPORTANT DRUG INTERACTIONS

Potentially hazardous interactions with other drugs
- Antivirals: zidovudine may inhibit intracellular activation – avoid concomitant use; increased risk of side effects with didanosine; increased risk of toxicity with ribavirin.
- Cytotoxics: effects possibly inhibited by doxorubicin; increased risk of toxicity with hydroxycarbamide – avoid concomitant use.

ADMINISTRATION

RECONSTITUTION
–
ROUTE
- Oral
RATE OF ADMINISTRATION
–
COMMENTS
- Administer at least an hour before food.

OTHER INFORMATION

- Oral bioavailability is 86%.
- Clearance by haemodialysis is 120 mL/min.
- Lactic acidosis, sometimes fatal, has been reported with the use of nucleoside analogues.
- Patients with ESRF are more likely to develop peripheral neuropathy.

Streptokinase

CLINICAL USE

Fibrinolytic:
- Thrombolysis in DVT, PE, acute arterial thromboembolism, acute MI, thrombosed A-V shunts

DOSE IN NORMAL RENAL FUNCTION

- Loading dose: 250 000 IU followed by 100 000 IU/hour for 12–72 hours (refer to SPC)
- Myocardial Infarction: 1.5 MIU followed by aspirin
- Thrombosed HD shunts: 10–25 000 IU sealed in shunt and repeated after 30–45 minutes

PHARMACOKINETICS

Molecular weight (daltons)	47 408
% Protein binding	No data
% Excreted unchanged in urine	0
Volume of distribution (L/kg)	0.02–0.08
Half-life – normal/ ESRF (hrs)	18 minutes/–

METABOLISM

A small proportion of the dose is bound to anti-streptokinase antibodies and metabolised with a half-life of 18 minutes, while most of it forms the streptokinase-plasminogen activator complex and is biotransformed with a half-life of about 80 minutes.

DOSE IN RENAL IMPAIRMENT GFR (mL/MIN)

20–50	Dose as in normal renal function.
10–20	Dose as in normal renal function.
<10	Dose as in normal renal function.

DOSE IN PATIENTS UNDERGOING RENAL REPLACEMENT THERAPIES

CAPD	Not dialysed. Dose as in normal renal function.
HD	Not dialysed. Dose as in normal renal function.
HDF/High flux	Unlikely to be dialysed. Dose as in normal renal function.
CAV/ VVHD	Not dialysed. Dose as in normal renal function.

IMPORTANT DRUG INTERACTIONS

Potentially hazardous interactions with other drugs
- Anticoagulants should not be given with streptokinase.
- Heparin infusions should be stopped 4 hours before streptokinase infusion. If this is not possible, protamine sulphate should be used to neutralise the heparin; heparin infusions can be restarted 4 hours post streptokinase infusion followed by oral anticoagulants.

ADMINISTRATION

RECONSTITUTION
- See manufacturer's literature.

ROUTE
- IV

RATE OF ADMINISTRATION
- Give loading dose of 250 000 IU in 100 mL fluid over 30 minutes, followed by an appropriate volume for the maintenance dose.
- Give 1.5 MIU for acute MI in 50–200 mL fluid over 1 hour.

COMMENTS
- For occluded HD shunts, add 100 000 IU to 100 mL sodium chloride 0.9% and put 10–25 mL into the clotted portion of the shunt.

OTHER INFORMATION

- There are no significant changes in pharmacokinetics in patients with renal insufficiency. Dosage reduction is therefore not necessary.
- Manufacturer advises to use in severe renal impairment only if benefit outweighs the risks.

Streptomycin (unlicensed)

CLINICAL USE

Antibacterial agent:
- Tuberculosis, in combination with other drugs
- Adjunct to doxycycline in brucellosis
- Enterococcal endocarditis
- Streptococcal endocarditis

DOSE IN NORMAL RENAL FUNCTION

- TB: <40 years and weight >50 kg: 15 mg/kg (maximum 1 g) daily or 3 times a week
- TB: >40 years OR weight <50 kg: 500–750 mg daily or 750 mg 3 times a week
- Doses of 25–30 mg/kg up to a maximum of 1.5 g twice weekly may be used
- Non-tuberculosis infections: 1–2 g daily in divided doses
- Enterococcal endocarditis: 1 g twice daily for 2 weeks, then 500 mg twice daily for a further 4 weeks, in combination with penicillin
- Streptococcal endocarditis: 1 g twice daily for 1 week, then 500 mg twice daily for 1 week, in combination with penicillin. If >60 years, 500 mg twice daily for 2 weeks.
- Adjust doses according to levels

PHARMACOKINETICS

Molecular weight (daltons)	581.6 (1457.4 as sulphate)
% Protein binding	34–35
% Excreted unchanged in urine	29–89
Volume of distribution (L/kg)	0.26
Half-life – normal/ESRF (hrs)	2.5/100

METABOLISM

It is rapidly excreted by glomerular filtration and the concentration of streptomycin in the urine is often very high, with about 30–90% of a dose usually being excreted within 24 hours.

DOSE IN RENAL IMPAIRMENT GFR (mL/MIN)

50–80	1 g loading dose then 7.5 mg/kg every 24 hours. Dose according to levels.
10–49	1 g loading dose then 7.5 mg/kg every 24–72 hours. Dose according to levels.
<10	7.5 mg/kg every 72–96 hours. Dose according to levels.

DOSE IN PATIENTS UNDERGOING RENAL REPLACEMENT THERAPIES

CAPD	Dialysed. Dose as in GFR<10 mL/min.
HD	Dialysed. 50–75% of loading dose after each dialysis.
HDF/High flux	Dialysed. 50–75% of loading dose after each dialysis.
CAV/VVHD	Dialysed. Dose as in GFR=10–20 mL/min.

IMPORTANT DRUG INTERACTIONS

Potentially hazardous interactions with other drugs
- Antibacterials: increased risk of nephrotoxicity with colistimethate or polymyxins and possibly cephalosporins; increased risk of ototoxicity and nephrotoxicity with capreomycin or vancomycin.
- Ciclosporin: increased risk of nephrotoxicity.
- Cytotoxics: increased risk of nephrotoxicity and ototoxicity with platinum compounds.
- Loop diuretics: increased risk of ototoxicity.
- Muscle relaxants: enhanced effects of non-depolarising muscle relaxants and suxamethonium.
- Parasympathomimetics: neostigmine and pyridostigmine antagonised by aminoglycosides.
- Tacrolimus: increased risk of nephrotoxicity.

ADMINISTRATION

RECONSTITUTION
- Dissolve 1 g in 2 or 3 mL water for injection.

ROUTE
- IM, IV

RATE OF ADMINISTRATION
- In 100 mL sodium chloride 0.9% or glucose 5% over 30 minutes

COMMENTS
- In patients who experience tingling sensations or dizziness during administration, increase the infusion time to 60 minutes.

OTHER INFORMATION

- Available on a named patient basis from Pfizer.
- Peak level taken 1 hour post dose and should be in the range 15–40 mg/litre; trough level (taken pre dose) should be <5 mg/litre, or <1 mg/litre in renal impairment or those over 50 years of age.
- May be less nephrotoxic than other aminoglycosides.
- PD peritonitis dose is 20–40 mg/litre/day.
- Risk of side effects increases after a cumulative dose of 100 g.
- A study in 4 patients used IV streptomycin at a dose of 7–15 mg/kg over 30–60 minutes without any problems, although IV administration did increase risk of toxicity.
- Due to the efficacy of twice weekly therapy, it is recommended that tuberculosis patients with severe renal impairment be given a dose of 750 mg 2–3 times a week for the first 2 months of treatment; trough levels should not exceed 4 mg/L. (Ellard GA. Cerebrospinal fluid drug concentrations and the treatment of tuberculous meningitis. *Am Rev Respir Dis.* 1993; **148**: 650–5.)
- Peak serum concentrations in individuals with renal impairment should not exceed 20–25 mcg/mL.
- Risk of severe neurotoxicity, irreversible vestibular damage and cochlear reactions are greatly increased in patients with impaired renal function; optic nerve dysfunction, peripheral neuritis, arachnoiditis and encephalopathy may also occur.

Reference:

1. www.uphs.upenn.edu/bugdrug/antibiotic_manual/renal.htm

Strontium ranelate

CLINICAL USE

Treatment of post menopausal osteoporosis and men at high risk of fractures.

DOSE IN NORMAL RENAL FUNCTION

2 g once daily

PHARMACOKINETICS

Molecular weight (daltons)	513.5
% Protein binding	25
% Excreted unchanged in urine	66
Volume of distribution (L/kg)	1
Half-life – normal/ ESRF (hrs)	60/Increased

METABOLISM

Strontium ranelate has a high affinity for bone tissue. It is not metabolised, and excretion occurs via the kidneys and gastrointestinal tract.

DOSE IN RENAL IMPAIRMENT GFR (mL/MIN)

30–50	Dose as in normal renal function.
10–30	See 'Other information'.
<10	See 'Other information'.

DOSE IN PATIENTS UNDERGOING RENAL REPLACEMENT THERAPIES

CAPD	Unknown dialysability. Dose as in GFR<10 mL/min
HD	Unknown dialysability. Dose as in GFR<10 mL/min.
HDF/High flux	Unknown dialysability. Dose as in GFR<10 mL/min.
CAV/ VVHD	Unknown dialysability. Dose as in GFR=10–30 mL/min.

IMPORTANT DRUG INTERACTIONS

Potentially hazardous interactions with other drugs
- Calcium-containing compounds: separate administration by at least 2 hours.
- Antacids: separate administration by at least 2 hours.
- Antibiotics: strontium can reduce absorption of oral tetracycline and quinolones – suspend strontium therapy during treatment.

ADMINISTRATION

RECONSTITUTION
- Glass of water
ROUTE
- Oral
RATE OF ADMINISTRATION
–

COMMENTS
–

OTHER INFORMATION

- Manufacturer advises to use with caution in severe renal impairment due to lack of bone safety studies.
- Give between meals as the absorption of strontium is reduced by food and milk products.
- Interferes with colorimetric methods of blood and urinary calcium concentrations.
- Give with calcium and vitamin D supplements.
- Steady state strontium levels are approximately 50% higher in patients with a GFR<25 mL/min compared to patients with normal renal function. No specific treatment effect was detected in patients with renal impairment (Cohen-Solal ME et al. Fluoride and strontium accumulation in bone does not correlate with osteoid tissue in dialysis patients. Nephrol Dial Transplant. 2002; 17: 449–54.)
- Another study found that haemodialysis patients with osteomalacia developed high bone-strontium levels. (D'Haese PC et al. Increased bone strontium levels in hemodialysis patients with osteomalacia. Kidney Int. 2000 Mar; 57: 1107–14.)
- There is no evidence of high levels of bone strontium in dialysis patients being related to osteomalacia (Data from Servier. Meunier PJ et al. The effects of strontium ranelate on the risk of vertebral fracture in women with postmenopausal osteoporosis. NEJM. 2004; 350(5): 459–68.)
- Oral bioavailability is about 25%.
- An increased incidence of nervous system disorders has been seen in patients with severe renal impairment (GFR<25 mL/min). Steady state strontium

concentrations are increased by 50% in severe renal impairment. Prescribing should be balanced against the risks and benefits of using the medication. (UKMI. Is strontium ranelate safe to use for patients with renal impairment? *Clinical Pharmacist.* September 2013. **5**(7): 204.)

Sucralfate (aluminium sucrose sulphate)

CLINICAL USE

- Treatment of peptic ulcer and chronic gastritis
- Prophylaxis of stress ulceration in seriously ill patients

DOSE IN NORMAL RENAL FUNCTION

- 4 g daily in 2–4 divided doses
- Prophylaxis of stress ulceration: 1 g 6 times daily
- Maximum 8 g daily

PHARMACOKINETICS

Molecular weight (daltons)	2086.7
% Protein binding	No data
% Excreted unchanged in urine	3.5
Volume of distribution (L/kg)	No data
Half-life – normal/ESRF (hrs)	No data

METABOLISM

Sucralfate is only slightly absorbed from the gastrointestinal tract after oral doses. However, there can be some release of aluminium ions and of sucrose sulphate; small quantities of sucrose sulphate may then be absorbed and excreted, mainly in the urine; some absorption of aluminium may also occur.

DOSE IN RENAL IMPAIRMENT GFR (mL/MIN)

20–50	4 g daily
10–20	2–4 g daily
<10	2–4 g daily

DOSE IN PATIENTS UNDERGOING RENAL REPLACEMENT THERAPIES

CAPD	Not dialysed. Dose as in GFR<10 mL/min.
HD	Not dialysed. Dose as in GFR<10 mL/min.
HDF/High flux	Not dialysed. Dose as in GFR<10 mL/min.
CAV/ VVHD	Not dialysed. Dose as in GFR=10–20 mL/min.

IMPORTANT DRUG INTERACTIONS

Potentially hazardous interactions with other drugs
- Reduced absorption of digoxin, tetracyclines, quinolones, coumarins and phenytoin – give 2 hours after sucralfate.

ADMINISTRATION

RECONSTITUTION
-
ROUTE
- Oral
RATE OF ADMINISTRATION
-
COMMENTS
- Sucralfate exerts its action at the site of the ulcer, and is minimally absorbed (3–5%) from the GI tract as sucrose sulphate.
- In normal renal function, any aluminium which is absorbed is excreted in the urine.
- Tablets may be dispersed in 10–15 mL of water.

OTHER INFORMATION

- Sucralfate should be used with caution in renal impairment as aluminium may be absorbed and accumulate.
- In severe renal impairment and patients receiving dialysis, sucralfate should be used with extreme caution and only for short periods.
- Absorbed aluminium is bound to plasma proteins and is not dialysable.
- Use of other aluminium-containing products with sucralfate can increase the total body burden of aluminium.

Sulfadiazine

CLINICAL USE

Antimicrobial agent:
- Toxoplasmosis in AIDS patients (unlicensed indication)
- Prevention of rheumatic fever

DOSE IN NORMAL RENAL FUNCTION

- Loading dose: 2–4 g
- Maintenance dose: up to 4 g daily in divided doses

PHARMACOKINETICS

Molecular weight (daltons)	250.3; 272.3 (as sodium salt)
% Protein binding	20–55
% Excreted unchanged in urine	80
Volume of distribution (L/kg)	0.29
Half-life – normal/ ESRF (hrs)	17/Prolonged

METABOLISM

Sulfadiazine is metabolised in the liver to the acetylated form, with elimination predominantly via the kidneys.

Urinary excretion of sulfadiazine and its acetyl derivative is dependent on pH; when the urine is acidic about 30% is excreted unchanged in both fast and slow acetylators, whereas when the urine is alkaline about 75% is excreted unchanged by slow acetylators.

DOSE IN RENAL IMPAIRMENT GFR (mL/MIN)

20–50	Dose as in normal renal function.
10–20	Use 50% of dose and monitor levels.
<10	Use 25% of dose and monitor levels.

DOSE IN PATIENTS UNDERGOING RENAL REPLACEMENT THERAPIES

CAPD	Unknown dialysability. Dose as in GFR<10 mL/min.
HD	Dialysed. Dose as in GFR<10 mL/min.
HDF/High flux	Dialysed. Dose as in GFR<10 mL/min.
CAV/ VVHD	Dialysed. Dose as in GFR=10–20 mL/min.

IMPORTANT DRUG INTERACTIONS

Potentially hazardous interactions with other drugs
- Antibacterials: increased risk of crystalluria with methenamine.
- Anticoagulants: effect of coumarins enhanced; metabolism of phenindione possibly inhibited.
- Anti-epileptics: antifolate effect and concentration of phenytoin increased.
- Antimalarials: increased risk of antifolate effect with pyrimethamine.
- Antipsychotics: avoid concomitant use with clozapine (increased risk of agranulocytosis).
- Ciclosporin: reduced levels of ciclosporin; increased risk of nephrotoxicity.
- Cytotoxics: increase risk of methotrexate toxicity.

ADMINISTRATION

RECONSTITUTION
–

ROUTE
- Oral

RATE OF ADMINISTRATION
–

COMMENTS
–

OTHER INFORMATION

- Contraindicated by manufacturer in severe renal impairment.
- Doses estimated from evaluation of pharmacokinetic data.
- Penetrates into the CSF within 4 hours of oral administration to produce therapeutic concentrations which may be more than half those in the blood.
- Crystalluria may be avoided by adequate hydration and alkalinising the urine to a pH >7.15.
- Blood concentrations of 100–150 micrograms/mL are desirable.
- For treatment of toxoplasmosis, use sulfadiazine in conjunction with pyrimethamine 25–100 mg daily.

Sulfasalazine (sulphasalazine)

CLINICAL USE

- Ulcerative colitis
- Crohn's disease
- Rheumatoid arthritis

DOSE IN NORMAL RENAL FUNCTION

- Oral: 1–2 g 4 times daily, reduced to 0.5 g 4 times daily
- Suppositories: 0.5–1 g twice daily
- Rheumatoid arthritis: 0.5 g daily, increased to 1.5 g twice daily

PHARMACOKINETICS

Molecular weight (daltons)	398.4
% Protein binding	95–99
% Excreted unchanged in urine	10–15
Volume of distribution (L/kg)	5.9–9.1
Half-life – normal/ ESRF (hrs)	18/–

METABOLISM

After cleavage of the sulfasalazine molecule about 60–80% of available sulfapyridine is absorbed, and undergoes extensive metabolism in the liver by acetylation, hydroxylation, and glucuronidation.

Most of a dose of sulfasalazine is excreted in the urine. Unchanged sulfasalazine accounts for 15% of the original dose, sulfapyridine and its metabolites 60%, and 5-ASA and its metabolites 20–33%.

DOSE IN RENAL IMPAIRMENT GFR (mL/MIN)

20–50	Dose as in normal renal function. Use with caution.
10–20	Dose as in normal renal function. Use with caution.
<10	Start at very low dose and monitor. Use with caution.

DOSE IN PATIENTS UNDERGOING RENAL REPLACEMENT THERAPIES

CAPD	Unlikely to be dialysed. Dose as in GFR<10 mL/min.
HD	Unlikely to be dialysed. Dose as in GFR<10 mL/min.
HDF/High flux	Unlikely to be dialysed. Dose as in GFR<10 mL/min.
CAV/ VVHD	Unknown dialysability. Dose as in GFR=10–20 mL/min.

IMPORTANT DRUG INTERACTIONS

Potentially hazardous interactions with other drugs
- Ciclosporin: may reduce ciclosporin levels.

ADMINISTRATION

RECONSTITUTION
–
ROUTE
- Oral, rectal
RATE OF ADMINISTRATION
–
COMMENTS
–

OTHER INFORMATION

- 15% of a dose of sulfasalazine is absorbed in the small intestine and becomes highly bound to plasma proteins. The remainder is split into sulfapyridine and 5-ASA by colonic bacteria. Sulfapyridine is rapidly absorbed from the colon, whereas 5-ASA is poorly absorbed.
- Unabsorbed drug is excreted in the faeces.
- In patients with moderate to severe renal impairment, toxicity includes increased risk of crystalluria – ensure high fluid intake.

Sulfinpyrazone

CLINICAL USE

- Gout prophylaxis
- Hyperuricaemia

DOSE IN NORMAL RENAL FUNCTION

100–200 mg daily with food (or milk); maximum dose 600–800 mg

PHARMACOKINETICS

Molecular weight (daltons)	404.5
% Protein binding	98
% Excreted unchanged in urine	22–42
Volume of distribution (L/kg)	0.06
Half-life – normal/ ESRF (hrs)	2–4/Unchanged

METABOLISM

Sulfinpyrazone is partly metabolised in the liver and some of the metabolites are active. On long-term therapy, sulfinpyrazone induces its own metabolism. Unchanged drug and metabolites are mainly excreted in the urine.

DOSE IN RENAL IMPAIRMENT GFR (mL/MIN)

20–50	Initially 50% of dose. Use lower dose range.
10–20	Initially 50% of dose. Use lower dose range.
<10	Avoid.

DOSE IN PATIENTS UNDERGOING RENAL REPLACEMENT THERAPIES

CAPD	Not dialysed. Avoid. See 'Other information'.
HD	Not dialysed. Avoid. See 'Other information'.
HDF/High flux	Unknown dialysability. Avoid. See 'Other information'.
CAV/ VVHD	Not dialysed. Dose as in GFR=10–20 mL/min.

IMPORTANT DRUG INTERACTIONS

Potentially hazardous interactions with other drugs

- Anticoagulants: increased risk of bleeding with apixaban; enhances anticoagulant effect of coumarins; possibly increased risk of bleeding with dabigatran.
- Antidiabetics: enhances effect of sulphonylureas.
- Anti-epileptics: increases concentration of phenytoin.
- Ciclosporin: may reduce ciclosporin levels.

ADMINISTRATION

RECONSTITUTION
–
ROUTE
- Oral
RATE OF ADMINISTRATION
–
COMMENTS
–

OTHER INFORMATION

- An adequate fluid intake of 2–3 litres daily should be taken to reduce risk of uric acid renal calculi.
- Uricosuric effects are lost when GFR<10 mL/min.
- Reversible acute renal failure may occur especially with high initial doses.
- Can cause salt and water retention.
- In combination with aspirin, has been shown to improve vascular access thrombosis in haemodialysis patients, but there was an increased occurrence of gastrointestinal bleeding (Domoto DT, Bauman JE, Joist JH. Combined aspirin and sulfinpyrazone in the prevention of recurrent hemodialysis vascular access thrombosis. *Throm Res.* 1991 Jun 15; **62**(6): 737–43.)
- Doses in renal impairment are from *Drug Prescribing in Renal Failure*, 5th edition, by Aronoff *et al.*

Sulindac

CLINICAL USE

NSAID and analgesic

DOSE IN NORMAL RENAL FUNCTION

200 mg twice daily

PHARMACOKINETICS

Molecular weight (daltons)	356.4
% Protein binding	95
% Excreted unchanged in urine	7
Volume of distribution (L/kg)	No data
Half-life – normal/ ESRF (hrs)	7.8/16.4 (metabolite)/ Unchanged

METABOLISM

Sulindac is metabolised by reversible reduction to the sulfide metabolite, which appears to be the active form, and by irreversible oxidation to the sulfone metabolite. About 50% is excreted in the urine mainly as the sulfone metabolite and its glucuronide conjugate, with smaller amounts of sulindac and its glucuronide conjugate; about 25% appears in the faeces, primarily as sulfone and sulfide metabolites. Sulindac and its metabolites are also excreted in bile and undergo extensive enterohepatic circulation.

DOSE IN RENAL IMPAIRMENT GFR (mL/MIN)

20–50	Dose as in normal renal function. Avoid if possible.
10–20	Give 50–100% of normal dose. Avoid if possible.
<10	Give 50–100% of normal dose. Avoid if possible.

DOSE IN PATIENTS UNDERGOING RENAL REPLACEMENT THERAPIES

CAPD	Unlikely to be dialysed. Dose as in GFR<10 mL/min.
HD	Not dialysed. Dose as in GFR<10 mL/min.
HDF/High flux	Unknown dialysability. Dose as in GFR<10 mL/min.
CAV/ VVHD	Unknown dialysability. Dose as in GFR=10–20 mL/min.

IMPORTANT DRUG INTERACTIONS

Potentially hazardous interactions with other drugs

- ACE inhibitors and angiotensin-II antagonists: antagonism of hypotensive effect; increased risk of nephrotoxicity and hyperkalaemia.
- Analgesics: avoid concomitant use of 2 or more NSAIDs, including aspirin (increased side effects); avoid with ketorolac (increased risk of side effects and haemorrhage).
- Antibacterials: possibly increased risk of convulsions with quinolones.
- Anticoagulants: effects of coumarins and phenindione enhanced; possibly increased risk of bleeding with heparins and dabigatran.
- Antidepressants: increased risk of bleeding with SSRIs and venlafaxine.
- Antidiabetic agents: effects of sulphonylureas enhanced.
- Anti-epileptics: possibly increased phenytoin concentration.
- Antivirals: increased risk of haematological toxicity with zidovudine; concentration possibly increased by ritonavir.
- Ciclosporin: may potentiate nephrotoxicity.
- Cytotoxic agents: reduced excretion of methotrexate; increased risk of bleeding with erlotinib.
- Dimethyl sulfoxide: avoid concomitant use.
- Diuretics: increased risk of nephrotoxicity; antagonism of diuretic effect; hyperkalaemia with potassium-sparing diuretics.
- Lithium: excretion decreased.
- Pentoxifylline: increased risk of bleeding.
- Tacrolimus: increased risk of nephrotoxicity.

ADMINISTRATION

RECONSTITUTION

–

ROUTE

- Oral

RATE OF ADMINISTRATION

–

COMMENTS

–

OTHER INFORMATION

- Sulindac has become the NSAID of choice in some centres for patients with renal impairment because of reports of its renal sparing effects. There is evidence that this sparing effect is dose-related and is lost if doses above 100 mg twice daily are used.
- Inhibition of renal prostaglandin synthesis by NSAIDs may interfere with renal function, especially in the presence of existing renal disease – avoid NSAIDs if possible; if not, check serum creatinine 48–72 hours after starting NSAID – if increased, discontinue therapy.
- Use normal doses in patients with CKD 5 on dialysis if they do not pass any urine.
- Use with caution in renal transplant recipients (can reduce intrarenal autocoid synthesis).

Sulpiride

CLINICAL USE

Antipsychotic:
- Acute and chronic schizophrenia

DOSE IN NORMAL RENAL FUNCTION

200–400 mg twice daily increasing to maximum 2.4 g daily

PHARMACOKINETICS

Molecular weight (daltons)	341.4
% Protein binding	40
% Excreted unchanged in urine	90–95
Volume of distribution (L/kg)	1.2–1.7
Half-life – normal/ ESRF (hrs)	8–9/26

METABOLISM

Sulpiride undergoes little metabolism; 95% of a dose is excreted in the urine and faeces, mainly as unchanged drug.

DOSE IN RENAL IMPAIRMENT GFR (mL/MIN)

20–50	Give 66% of normal dose, or increase dosing interval by factor of 1.5.
10–20	Give 50% of normal dose, or increase dosing interval by factor of 2.
<10	Give 30% of normal dose, or increase dosing interval by factor of 3.

DOSE IN PATIENTS UNDERGOING RENAL REPLACEMENT THERAPIES

CAPD	Unlikely to be dialysed. Dose as in GFR<10 mL/min.
HD	Partly dialysed. Dose as in GFR<10 mL/min.
HDF/High flux	Unknown dialysability. Dose as in GFR<10 mL/min.
CAV/ VVHD	Unknown dialysability. Dose as in GFR=10–20 mL/min.

IMPORTANT DRUG INTERACTIONS

Potentially hazardous interactions with other drugs
- Anaesthetics: enhanced hypotensive effect.
- Analgesics: increased risk of convulsions with tramadol; enhanced hypotensive and sedative effects with opioids; increased risk of ventricular arrhythmias with methadone.
- Anti-arrhythmics increased risk of ventricular arrhythmias with anti-arrhythmics that prolong the QT interval, e.g. procainamide, disopyramide and amiodarone – avoid concomitant use with amiodarone.
- Antibacterials: increased risk of ventricular arrhythmias with moxifloxacin and parenteral erythromycin – avoid concomitant use with moxifloxacin.
- Antidepressants: increased concentration of tricyclics; possibly increased risk of ventricular arrhythmias and antimuscarinic side effects.
- Anti-epileptics: antagonism (convulsive threshold lowered).
- Antimalarials: avoid concomitant use with artemether/lumefantrine.
- Antipsychotics: increased risk of ventricular arrhythmias with droperidol, haloperidol and pimozide – avoid concomitant use.
- Antivirals: concentration possibly increased by ritonavir.
- Anxiolytics and hypnotics: increased sedative effects.
- Atomoxetine: increased risk of ventricular arrhythmias.
- Beta-blockers: enhanced hypotensive effect; increased risk of ventricular arrhythmias with sotalol.
- Cytotoxics: increased risk of ventricular arrhythmias with vandetanib – avoid; increased risk of ventricular arrhythmias with arsenic trioxide.
- Diuretics: enhanced hypotensive effect.
- Lithium: increased risk of extrapyramidal side effects and possibly neurotoxicity.
- Pentamidine: increased risk of ventricular arrhythmias.

ADMINISTRATION

RECONSTITUTION
–
ROUTE
- Oral
RATE OF ADMINISTRATION
–
COMMENTS
–

OTHER INFORMATION

- Administer with caution and decrease the dose in renal impairment.

Sumatriptan

CLINICAL USE

5HT$_1$ receptor agonist:
- Acute relief of migraine

DOSE IN NORMAL RENAL FUNCTION

- Oral: 50–100 mg; maximum 300 mg in 24 hours
- SC: 6 mg; maximum 12 mg in 24 hours
- Intranasally: 10–20 mg; maximum 40 mg in 24 hours

PHARMACOKINETICS

Molecular weight (daltons)	295.4; 413.5 (as succinate)
% Protein binding	14–21
% Excreted unchanged in urine	<20
Volume of distribution (L/kg)	170 litres
Half-life – normal/ ESRF (hrs)	2/Probably unchanged

METABOLISM

Sumatriptan is extensively metabolised in the liver mainly by monoamine oxidase type A and is excreted mainly in the urine as the inactive indoleacetic acid derivative and its glucuronide. Non-renal clearance accounts for about 80% of the total clearance. The remaining 20% is excreted in urine, mainly as metabolites, by active renal tubular secretion

Sumatriptan and its metabolites also appear in the faeces.

DOSE IN RENAL IMPAIRMENT GFR (mL/MIN)

20–50	Dose as in normal renal function.
10–20	Dose as in normal renal function, use with caution.
<10	Dose as in normal renal function, use with caution.

DOSE IN PATIENTS UNDERGOING RENAL REPLACEMENT THERAPIES

CAPD	Unknown dialysability. Dose as in GFR<10 mL/min.
HD	Unknown dialysability. Dose as in GFR<10 mL/min.
HDF/High flux	Unknown dialysability. Dose as in GFR<10 mL/min.
CAV/VVHD	Unknown dialysability. Dose as in GFR=10–20 mL/min.

IMPORTANT DRUG INTERACTIONS

Potentially hazardous interactions with other drugs
- Antidepressants: increased risk of CNS toxicity with citalopram – avoid; risk of CNS toxicity with MAOIs, moclobemide, SSRIs, sertraline, St John's wort – avoid concomitant use; possibly increased serotonergic effects with duloxetine and venlafaxine.
- Ergot alkaloids: increased risk of vasospasm – avoid concomitant use.

ADMINISTRATION

RECONSTITUTION
- Injection is pre-filled into syringes ready for administration.

ROUTE
- Oral, SC, nasal

RATE OF ADMINISTRATION
–

COMMENTS
–

OTHER INFORMATION

- Oral bioavailability is 14%.

Sunitinib

CLINICAL USE

Tyrosine kinase inhibitors
● Treatment of metastatic renal cell carcinoma (MRCC), gastrointestinal stromal tumours (GIST) & pancreatic neuroendocrine tumours (pNET)

DOSE IN NORMAL RENAL FUNCTION

● MRCC & GIST: 25–75 mg daily with a 2 week treatment free period within 6 week cycle.
● pNET: 37.5–50 mg daily.
Consult relevant local protocol.

PHARMACOKINETICS

Molecular weight (daltons)	532.6 (as malate)
% Protein binding	95
% Excreted unchanged in urine	16 (unchanged drug + metabolites)
Volume of distribution (L/kg)	2230 litres
Half-life – normal/ ESRF (hrs)	40–60/Unchanged

METABOLISM

Metabolised mainly via the cytochrome P450 isoenzyme CYP3A4 to its primary active metabolite, which itself is then further metabolised via CYP3A4.

Elimination is primarily via faeces. In a human mass balance study of [^{14}C]sunitinib, 61% of the dose was eliminated in faeces and 16% by the renal route.

DOSE IN RENAL IMPAIRMENT GFR (mL/MIN)

20–50	Dose as in normal renal function.
10–20	Dose as in normal renal function.
<10	Dose as in normal renal function.

DOSE IN PATIENTS UNDERGOING RENAL REPLACEMENT THERAPIES

CAPD	Not dialysed. Dose as in normal renal function.
HD	Not dialysed. Dose as in normal renal function.
HDF/High flux	Not dialysed. Dose as in normal renal function.
CAV/ VVHD	Not dialysed. Dose as in normal renal function.

IMPORTANT DRUG INTERACTIONS

Potentially hazardous interactions with other drugs
● Antipsychotics: avoid concomitant use with clozapine (increased risk of agranulocytosis).
● Antivirals: avoid concomitant use with boceprevir.
● Avoid concomitant use with other inhibitors or inducers of CYP3A4. Dose alterations may be required.

ADMINISTRATION

RECONSTITUTION
–
ROUTE
● Oral
RATE OF ADMINISTRATION
–

OTHER INFORMATION

● Systemic exposures after a single dose of sunitinib were similar in subjects with severe renal impairment (CRCL<30 mL/min) compared to subjects with normal renal function (CRCL>80 mL/min). Although sunitinib and its primary metabolite were not eliminated through haemodialysis in subjects with ESRD, the total systemic exposures were lower by 47% for sunitinib and 31% for its primary metabolite compared to subjects with normal renal function.

Suxamethonium chloride

CLINICAL USE

Depolarising muscle relaxant used in short procedures and ECT

DOSE IN NORMAL RENAL FUNCTION

- IV injection: 1–1.5 mg/kg
- IV infusion: 2–5 mg/minute; maximum 500 mg/hour
- IM: 2.5 mg/kg, to a maximum of 150 mg Dose depends on preparation

PHARMACOKINETICS

Molecular weight (daltons)	397.3
% Protein binding	70
% Excreted unchanged in urine	<10
Volume of distribution (L/kg)	No data
Half-life – normal/ ESRF (hrs)	2–3 minutes/–

METABOLISM

Suxamethonium is rapidly hydrolysed to succinylmonocholine a weak neuromuscular blocking drug. This is metabolised to succinic acid with only a small amount excreted in the urine.

DOSE IN RENAL IMPAIRMENT GFR (mL/MIN)

20–50	Dose as in normal renal function.
10–20	Dose as in normal renal function.
<10	Dose as in normal renal function. Use with caution. See 'Other information'.

DOSE IN PATIENTS UNDERGOING RENAL REPLACEMENT THERAPIES

CAPD	Unknown dialysability. Dose as in GFR<10 mL/min.
HD	Unknown dialysability. Dose as in GFR<10 mL/min.
HDF/High flux	Unknown dialysability. Dose as in GFR<10 mL/min.
CAV/ VVHD	Unknown dialysability. Dose as in normal renal function.

IMPORTANT DRUG INTERACTIONS

Potentially hazardous interactions with other drugs

- Anaesthetics: increased risk of myocardial depression and bradycardia with propofol; enhanced effect with volatile liquid general anaesthetics.
- Anti-arrhythmics: lidocaine and procainamide enhance muscle relaxant effect.
- Antibacterials: effect enhanced by aminoglycosides, clindamycin, polymyxins, vancomycin and piperacillin.
- Cardiac glycosides: increased risk of ventricular arrhythmias.

ADMINISTRATION

RECONSTITUTION

–

ROUTE

- IV

RATE OF ADMINISTRATION

- Over 10–30 seconds
- Infusion: 2.5–4 mg/minute, maximum 500 mg/hour

COMMENTS

- For continuous infusion add 10 mL to 500 mL glucose 5% or sodium chloride 0.9% = 0.1% solution.

OTHER INFORMATION

- Suxamethonium is predominantly excreted in the urine as active and inactive metabolites. Patients on dialysis may require a dose at the lower end of the range due to reduced plasma cholinesterase activity.
- Use with caution in hyperkalaemia as potassium is released from depolarised muscle.
- Hyperkalaemia may occur when suxamethonium is used in CKD 5.

Tacrolimus

CLINICAL USE

Immunosuppressive agent:
- Prophylaxis and treatment of acute rejection in liver, heart and kidney transplantation
- Treatment of moderate to severe atopic eczema

DOSE IN NORMAL RENAL FUNCTION

Oral: Initially:
- Liver transplantation: 100–200 mcg/kg/day in 2 divided doses
- Kidney transplantation: 200–300 mcg/kg/day in 2 divided doses
- Heart transplantation: 75 mcg/kg/day in 2 divided doses

Advagraf:
- Liver transplant: 100–200 mcg/kg once daily
- Renal transplant: 200–300 mcg/kg once daily

IV:
- Liver transplantation: 10–50 mcg/kg as a continuous 24 hour infusion, starting 6 hours post surgery
- Kidney transplantation: 50–100 mcg/kg as a continuous 24 hour infusion, starting within 24 hours of surgery
- Heart transplantation: 10–20 mcg/kg as a continuous 24 hour infusion

PHARMACOKINETICS

Molecular weight (daltons)	822
% Protein binding	>98
% Excreted unchanged in urine	<1
Volume of distribution (L/kg)	1300
Half-life – normal/ ESRF (hrs)	12–16/Probably unchanged

METABOLISM

Tacrolimus is extensively bound to erythrocytes in the blood, and variations in red cell binding account for much of the variability in pharmacokinetics. It is extensively metabolised in the liver, mainly by cytochrome P450 isoenzyme CYP3A4, and excreted, primarily in bile, almost entirely as metabolites. Considerable metabolism also occurs in the intestinal wall.

There are several metabolites identified. Only one of these has been shown *in vitro* to have immunosuppressive activity similar to that of tacrolimus. The other metabolites have only weak or no immunosuppressive activity. In systemic circulation only one of the inactive metabolites is present at low concentrations. Therefore, metabolites do not contribute to pharmacological activity of tacrolimus.

DOSE IN RENAL IMPAIRMENT GFR (mL/MIN)

20–50	Dose as in normal renal function.
10–20	Dose as in normal renal function.
<10	Dose as in normal renal function.

DOSE IN PATIENTS UNDERGOING RENAL REPLACEMENT THERAPIES

CAPD	Not dialysed. Dose as in normal renal function.
HD	Not dialysed. Dose as in normal renal function.
HDF/High flux	Unknown dialysability. Dose as in normal renal function.
CAV/ VVHD	Not dialysed. Dose as in normal renal function.

IMPORTANT DRUG INTERACTIONS

Potentially hazardous interactions with other drugs
- Ciclosporin: may increase the half-life of ciclosporin and exacerbate any toxic effects. The two should not be prescribed concomitantly. Care should be taken when converting from ciclosporin to tacrolimus.
- Tacrolimus levels increased by: atazanavir, basiliximab, boceprevir, bromocriptine, chloramphenicol, cimetidine, cortisone, danazol, dapsone, diltiazem, ergotamine, ethinyl oestradiol, felodipine, fosamprenavir, gestodene, grapefruit juice, imidazole and triazole antifungals, lidocaine, felodipine, lansoprazole, possibly levofloxacin, macrolides, midazolam, nicardipine, nifedipine, omeprazole, pantoprazole, ritonavir, saquinavir, tamoxifen, telaprevir (concentration of both drugs increased), theophylline, verapamil and voriconazole.
- Tacrolimus levels decreased by: carbamazepine, caspofungin, isoniazid, phenobarbital, phenytoin (phenytoin levels possibly increased), rifampicin, possibly rifabutin and St John's wort.

- Increased nephrotoxicity with: aciclovir, aminoglycosides, amphotericin, ganciclovir, NSAIDs and vancomycin.
- Increased risk of hyperkalaemia with: potassium-sparing-diuretics and potassium salts.
- Anticoagulants: possibly increases concentration of dabigatran – avoid.
- Antipsychotics: avoid with droperidol.
- Antivirals: concentration affected by efavirenz.
- Clotrimazole: more than doubles the bioavailability of tacrolimus (US-based researchers report that concomitant clotrimazole substantially increases the relative oral bioavailability of tacrolimus in renal transplant recipients. *Inpharma.* 2005 Dec 10; **1517**: 15).
- Cytotoxics: use crizotinib with caution.

ADMINISTRATION

RECONSTITUTION
–

ROUTE
- IV, oral, topical
RATE OF ADMINISTRATION
- Continuous infusion over 24 hours
COMMENTS
- Dilute in glucose 5% or sodium chloride 0.9% to a concentration of 4–100 micrograms/mL, i.e. 5 mg in 50–1000 mL.
- Incompatible with PVC.
- Use infusion fluids in polyethylene or glass containers.
- Use giving sets as used for the administration of taxol.
- Contains polyethoxylated castor oil which has been associated with anaphylaxis.

OTHER INFORMATION

- When converting from oral to IV, give one fifth of the total daily dose over 24 hours and monitor levels. Since administration is as a 24-hour infusion, a true 12 hour trough level will not be measured. Levels will therefore be expected to be slightly above the quoted ranges for oral tacrolimus.
- The different brands of oral tacrolimus are not interchangeable. Patients should ONLY be switched between brands under the close supervision of a transplant/renal unit and monitored appropriately.
- Approximate ranges:
  — Initially: liver: 5–10 ng/mL, renal: 8–15 ng/mL
  — Maintenance: 5–15 ng/mL
- Oral bioavailability is 20–25%.
- Also available as a 0.03% and 0.1% ointment for eczema and anal Crohn's disease.

Tadalafil

CLINICAL USE

Treatment of erectile dysfunction (ED)
Benign prostate hyperplasia (BPH)
Pulmonary arterial hypertension (PAH)

DOSE IN NORMAL RENAL FUNCTION

- ED: 10–20 mg, 30 minutes to 12 hours before sexual activity
- BPH: 5 mg once daily
- PAH: 40 mg once daily

PHARMACOKINETICS

Molecular weight (daltons)	389.4
% Protein binding	94
% Excreted unchanged in urine	36
Volume of distribution (L/kg)	63 litres
Half-life – normal/ESRF (hrs)	17.5/Increased

METABOLISM

Tadalafil is metabolised in the liver mainly by the cytochrome P450 isoenzyme CYP3A4. The major metabolite, the methylcatechol glucuronide, is inactive. Tadalafil is excreted, mainly as metabolites, in the faeces (61% of the dose), and to a lesser extent the urine (36% of the dose).

DOSE IN RENAL IMPAIRMENT GFR (mL/MIN)

30–50	ED: Dose as in normal renal function. BPH/PAH: 2.5–5 mg daily.
10–30	ED: 5–10 mg not more than every 72 hours and use with caution. BPH/PAH: Avoid.
<10	ED: 5–10 mg not more than every 72 hours and use with caution. BPH/PAH: Avoid.

DOSE IN PATIENTS UNDERGOING RENAL REPLACEMENT THERAPIES

CAPD	Unlikely to be dialysed. Dose as in GFR<10 mL/min.
HD	Not dialysed. Dose as in GFR<10 mL/min.
HDF/High flux	Unlikely to be dialysed. Dose as in GFR<10 mL/min.
CAV/VVHD	Unlikely to be dialysed. Dose as in GFR=10–30 mL/min.

IMPORTANT DRUG INTERACTIONS

Potentially hazardous interactions with other drugs

- Alpha-blockers: enhanced hypotensive effect – avoid concomitant use.
- Antibacterials: concentration possibly increased by clarithromycin and erythromycin; concentration reduced by rifampicin – avoid.
- Antifungals: concentration increased by ketoconazole – avoid; concentration possibly increased by itraconazole.
- Antivirals: concentration possibly increased by fosamprenavir and indinavir; increased by ritonavir – avoid; increased risk of ventricular arrhythmias with saquinavir – avoid; avoid high doses of tadalafil with telaprevir.
- Nicorandil: possibly enhanced hypotensive effect – avoid concomitant use.
- Nitrates: enhanced hypotensive effect – avoid concomitant use.

ADMINISTRATION

RECONSTITUTION

–

ROUTE

- Oral

RATE OF ADMINISTRATION

–

COMMENTS

–

OTHER INFORMATION

- Due to lack of trial data, manufacturer recommends a maximum on-demand dose for ED of 10 mg in severe renal impairment; in practice a higher dose may be used with caution.
- Manufacturer contraindicates use in severe renal impairment for BPH and PAH due to lack of studies and increased AUC.
- Protein binding is not affected by renal impairment.

Tamoxifen

CLINICAL USE

- Treatment of breast cancer
- Anovulatory infertility

DOSE IN NORMAL RENAL FUNCTION

- Breast cancer: 20 mg daily
- Anovulatory infertility: 20–80 mg daily on days 2–5 of menstrual cycle

PHARMACOKINETICS

Molecular weight (daltons)	371.5; (563.6 as citrate)
% Protein binding	>99
% Excreted unchanged in urine	0
Volume of distribution (L/kg)	20
Half-life – normal/ ESRF (hrs)	7 days/Probably unchanged

METABOLISM

Tamoxifen is extensively metabolised by cytochrome P450 isoenzymes, to active metabolites that include N-desmethyltamoxifen, 4-hydroxytamoxifen, and 4-hydroxy-N-desmethyltamoxifen (endoxifen). Metabolism is by hydroxylation, demethylation and conjugation.

In vitro studies suggest that both N-desmethyltamoxifen and 4-hydroxytamoxifen are further metabolised to endoxifen.

Elimination occurs, chiefly as conjugates with practically no unchanged drug, principally through the faeces and to a lesser extent through the kidneys.

DOSE IN RENAL IMPAIRMENT GFR (mL/MIN)

20–50	Dose as in normal renal function.
10–20	Dose as in normal renal function.
<10	Dose as in normal renal function.

DOSE IN PATIENTS UNDERGOING RENAL REPLACEMENT THERAPIES

CAPD	Unknown dialysability. Dose as in normal renal function.
HD	Unknown dialysability. Dose as in normal renal function.
HDF/High flux	Unknown dialysability. Dose as in normal renal function.
CAV/ VVHD	Unknown dialysability. Dose as in normal renal function.

IMPORTANT DRUG INTERACTIONS

Potentially hazardous interactions with other drugs

- Anticoagulants: effects of coumarins enhanced.
- Antidepressants: metabolism of tamoxifen to active metabolite possibly inhibited by fluoxetine and paroxetine – avoid.
- Antipsychotics: increased risk of ventricular arrhythmias with droperidol – avoid.
- Bupropion: metabolism of tamoxifen to active metabolite possibly inhibited – avoid.
- Cinacalcet: metabolism of tamoxifen to active metabolite possibly inhibited – avoid.

ADMINISTRATION

RECONSTITUTION

–

ROUTE

- Oral

RATE OF ADMINISTRATION

–

COMMENTS

–

OTHER INFORMATION

- Tamoxifen has been used for the treatment of sclerosing encapsulating peritonitis, at a dose of 20 mg daily (Eltoum MA. Four consecutive cases of peritoneal dialysis-related encapsulating peritoneal sclerosis treated successfully with tamoxifen. *Perit Dial Int.* 2006 Mar-Apr; **26**(2): 183–4.)

Tamsulosin hydrochloride

CLINICAL USE

Treatment of benign prostatic hyperplasia

DOSE IN NORMAL RENAL FUNCTION

400 mcg in the morning after breakfast

PHARMACOKINETICS

Molecular weight (daltons)	445
% Protein binding	99
% Excreted unchanged in urine	9
Volume of distribution (L/kg)	0.2
Half-life – normal/ ESRF (hrs)	4– 5.5 (M/R: 10–15)/ Increased

METABOLISM

Tamsulosin is metabolised slowly in the liver primarily by the cytochrome P450 isoenzymes CYP2D6 and CYP3A4; it is excreted mainly in the urine as metabolites and some unchanged drug.

DOSE IN RENAL IMPAIRMENT GFR (mL/MIN)

20–50	Dose as in normal renal function.
10–20	Dose as in normal renal function.
<10	Dose as in normal renal function. Use with caution.

DOSE IN PATIENTS UNDERGOING RENAL REPLACEMENT THERAPIES

CAPD	Not dialysed. Dose as in GFR<10 mL/min.
HD	Not dialysed. Dose as in GFR<10 mL/min.
HDF/High flux	Unknown dialysability. Dose as in GFR<10 mL/min.
CAV/ VVHD	Not dialysed. Dose as in normal renal function.

IMPORTANT DRUG INTERACTIONS

Potentially hazardous interactions with other drugs
- Anaesthetics: enhanced hypotensive effect.
- Antidepressants: enhanced hypotensive effect with MAOIs.
- Beta-blockers: enhanced hypotensive effect; increased risk of first dose hypotensive effect.
- Calcium-channel blockers: enhanced hypotensive effect; increased risk of first dose hypotensive effect.
- Diuretics: enhanced hypotensive effect; increased risk of first dose hypotensive effect.
- Moxisylyte: possibly severe postural hypotension.
- Vardenafil, sildenafil and tadalafil: enhanced hypotensive effect, avoid concomitant use.

ADMINISTRATION

RECONSTITUTION

–

ROUTE

- Oral

RATE OF ADMINISTRATION

–

COMMENTS

–

OTHER INFORMATION

- Manufacturer advises to use with caution if GFR<10 mL/min due to lack of studies.
- Swallow whole with 150 mL of water while sitting or standing.
- Protein binding is increased in renal impairment.

Tapentadol hydrochloride

CLINICAL USE

μ-opioid receptor agonist with additional noradrenaline reuptake inhibition properties:
- Treatment of moderate to severe acute pain

DOSE IN NORMAL RENAL FUNCTION

- 50 mg every 4–6 hours, maximum dose 600 mg daily (700 mg on 1st day)
- SR: Initially 50 mg twice daily, maximum 500 mg daily

PHARMACOKINETICS

Molecular weight (daltons)	257.8
% Protein binding	20
% Excreted unchanged in urine	3
Volume of distribution (L/kg)	442–638 litres
Half-life – normal/ ESRF (hrs)	4 (SR: 5–6)/Probably increased

METABOLISM

Approximately 97% of the parent compound is metabolised by conjugation with glucuronic acid to produce glucuronides. It is also metabolised, to a lesser extent, via the cytochrome P450 isoenzymes CYP2C9, CYP2C19, and CYP2D6, before further conjugation.

None of the metabolites have analgesic activity.

Approximately 70% of the dose is excreted in the urine in the conjugated form and 3% as unchanged drug.

DOSE IN RENAL IMPAIRMENT GFR (mL/MIN)

20–50	Dose as in normal renal function.
10–20	Dose as in normal renal function.
<10	Use small doses, extended dosing intervals. Titrate according to response.

DOSE IN PATIENTS UNDERGOING RENAL REPLACEMENT THERAPIES

CAPD	Probably dialysed. Dose as in GFR<10 mL/min.
HD	Probably dialysed. Dose as in GFR<10 mL/min.
HDF/High flux	Probably dialysed. Dose as in GFR<10 mL/min.
CAV/ VVHD	Probably dialysed. Dose as in GFR=10–20 mL/min.

IMPORTANT DRUG INTERACTIONS

Potentially hazardous interactions with other drugs
- Antidepressants: possible CNS excitation or depression with MAOIs – avoid concomitant use, and for 2 weeks after stopping MAOI; possible CNS excitation or depression with moclobemide; increased sedative effects with tricyclics.
- Antihistamines: increased sedative effects with sedating antihistamines.
- Antipsychotics: enhanced hypotensive and sedative effects.
- Dopaminergics: avoid with selegiline.
- Sodium oxybate: enhanced effect of sodium oxybate – avoid concomitant use.

ADMINISTRATION

RECONSTITUTION
–
ROUTE
- Oral
RATE OF ADMINISTRATION
–

OTHER INFORMATION

- Not recommended by manufacturer in severe renal impairment due to lack of studies.
- Extreme caution with all opiates in patients with impaired renal function.
- Bioavailability is 32%.
- AUC and C_{max} of tapentadol were comparable in subjects with varying degrees of renal function (from normal to severely impaired). In people with mild, moderate, and severe renal impairment, the AUC of tapentadol-O-glucuronide are 1.5-, 2.5-, and 5.5-fold higher compared with normal renal function, respectively.

Tazocin (piperacillin/tazobactam)

CLINICAL USE

Antibacterial agent

DOSE IN NORMAL RENAL FUNCTION

4.5 g every 6–8 hours

PHARMACOKINETICS

Molecular weight (daltons)	Piperacillin: 539.5, Tazobactam: 322.3 (as sodium)
% Protein binding	Piperacillin: 20–30, Tazobactam: 20–30
% Excreted unchanged in urine	Piperacillin: 60–80, Tazobactam: 80
Volume of distribution (L/kg)	Piperacillin: 0.18–0.3, Tazobactam: 0.18–0.33[1]
Half-life – normal/ ESRF (hrs)	Piperacillin: 1/4–6, Tazobactam: 1/7

METABOLISM

Piperacillin is metabolised to a minor microbiologically active desethyl metabolite. Tazobactam is metabolised to a single metabolite that has been found to be microbiologically inactive.

Piperacillin and tazobactam are eliminated via the kidney by glomerular filtration and tubular secretion. Piperacillin, tazobactam, and desethyl piperacillin are also secreted into the bile.

DOSE IN RENAL IMPAIRMENT GFR (mL/MIN)

40–50	Dose as in normal renal function
20–40	4.5 g every 8 hours.
<20	4.5 g every 12 hours.

DOSE IN PATIENTS UNDERGOING RENAL REPLACEMENT THERAPIES

CAPD	Not dialysed. Dose as in GFR<20 mL/minute.
HD	Dialysed. Dose as in GFR<20 mL/minute.
HDF/High flux	Dialysed. Dose as in GFR<20 mL/minute.
CAV/VVH	Dialysed. Dose as in GFR=20–40 mL/minute, or 2.25 g every 6 hours,[1] or 4.5 g every 12 hours.
CVVHD/ HDF	Dialysed: 2.25–3.375 g every 6 hours,[1] or 4.5 g every 8 hours.

IMPORTANT DRUG INTERACTIONS

Potentially hazardous interactions with other drugs
- Reduced excretion of methotrexate – monitor methotrexate levels during concomitant treatment.
- Enhanced action of vecuronium and similar neuromuscular blocking agents.

ADMINISTRATION

RECONSTITUTION
- Reconstitute each 4.5 g with 20 mL sterile water for injection or sodium chloride 0.9%.
ROUTE
- IV
RATE OF ADMINISTRATION
- IV bolus over 3–5 minutes (unlicensed)
- IV infusion over 30 minutes
COMMENTS
- May be given as an infusion in glucose 5% or sodium chloride 0.9%.

OTHER INFORMATION

- Change in administration was due to pharmacokinetic data showing an improved MIC with the infusion, not due to safety issues. (Personal communication with Pfizer, January 2014)
- Sodium content is 2.79 mmol/g of injection.
- Has been used intraperitoneally for treatment of PD peritonitis at a concentration of 250 mg/L.
- Patients with renal impairment are at a greater risk of neuromuscular excitability or convulsions that are associated with overdose.
- May cause *in vitro* inactivation of aminoglycosides.
- 6–21% is removed by peritoneal dialysis and 30–50% by haemodialysis plus an extra 5% as the metabolite.

Reference:
1. Trotman RL. Antibiotic dosing in critically ill adult patients receiving continuous renal replacement therapy. *Clin Infect Dis*. 2005 Oct 15; **41**: 1159–66.

Tegafur with uracil

CLINICAL USE

Antineoplastic agent
- Metastatic colorectal cancer

DOSE IN NORMAL RENAL FUNCTION

Tegafur: 300 mg/m^2 with uracil: 672 mg/m^2 daily in 3 divided doses for 28 days then nothing for 7 days. Consult relevant local protocol.

PHARMACOKINETICS

Molecular weight (daltons)	Tegafur/Uracil 200.2/112.1
% Protein binding	52/Negligible
% Excreted unchanged in urine	<20
Volume of distribution (L/kg)	59/474 litres
Half-life – normal/ESRF (hrs)	11/20–40 minutes/ Unchanged

METABOLISM

Tegafur is an oral prodrug of 5-FU and uracil reversibly inhibits DPD, the primary catabolic enzyme for 5-FU. Metabolism occurs in the liver. Conversion of tegafur to 5-FU occurs via C-5' oxidation (microsomal enzymes) and C-2' hydrolysis (cytosolic enzymes). Microsomal oxidation of tegafur is partially mediated by CYP2A6. The cytosolic enzymes responsible for the metabolism of tegafur are not known. Other metabolic products of tegafur include 3'-hydroxy tegafur, 4'-hydroxy tegafur, and dihydro tegafur which are all significantly less cytotoxic than 5-FU. The metabolism of 5-FU formed from tegafur follows the intrinsic *de novo* pathways for the naturally occurring pyrimidine, uracil.

DOSE IN RENAL IMPAIRMENT GFR (mL/MIN)

20–50	Dose as in normal renal function.
10–20	Dose as in normal renal function.
<10	Dose as in normal renal function.

DOSE IN PATIENTS UNDERGOING RENAL REPLACEMENT THERAPIES

CAPD	Unknown dialysability. Dose as in normal renal function.
HD	Dialysed. Dose as in normal renal function.
HDF/High flux	Dialysed. Dose as in normal renal function.
CAV/VVHD	Dialysed. Dose as in normal renal function.

IMPORTANT DRUG INTERACTIONS

Potentially hazardous interactions with other drugs
- Anticoagulants: possibly enhances effect of coumarins.
- Antipsychotics: avoid concomitant use with clozapine, increased risk of agranulocytosis.
- Metronidazole and cimetidine inhibit metabolism (increased toxicity).

ADMINISTRATION

RECONSTITUTION
–
ROUTE
- Oral

OTHER INFORMATION

- Tegafur with uracil has not been studied in renal impairment but due to low renal clearance no dose adjustment is recommended. Use with care.

Teicoplanin

CLINICAL USE

Antibacterial agent.

DOSE IN NORMAL RENAL FUNCTION

- Loading dose: IM/IV: 400 mg every 12 hours for 3 doses, then 200–400 mg daily, or 3–6 mg/kg/day
- (up to 12 mg/kg/day in some reports) in life threatening infections.
- *Clostridium difficile* infections: Oral: 200 mg twice daily

PHARMACOKINETICS

Molecular weight (daltons)	1875–1891
% Protein binding	90–95
% Excreted unchanged in urine	>97
Volume of distribution (L/kg)	0.94–1.4
Half-life – normal/ESRF (hrs)	150/62–230

METABOLISM

Teicoplanin is excreted almost entirely by glomerular filtration in the urine, as unchanged drug. No metabolites have been identified.

DOSE IN RENAL IMPAIRMENT GFR (mL/MIN)

40–60	Dose as in normal renal function, then reduce dose after 4th day to 200 mg daily or 400 mg every 48 hours.
<40	Dose as in normal renal function, then reduce dose after 4th day to 30% of the dose daily or 400 mg every 72 hours.

DOSE IN PATIENTS UNDERGOING RENAL REPLACEMENT THERAPIES

CAPD	Not dialysed. Dose as in GFR<40 mL/min.
HD	Not dialysed. Dose as in GFR<40 mL/min.
HDF/High flux	Dialysed.[1] Dose as in GFR<40 mL/min.
CAV/VVHD	Unknown dialysability. Dose as in GFR<40 mL/min.

IMPORTANT DRUG INTERACTIONS

Potentially hazardous interactions with other drugs
- None known

ADMINISTRATION

RECONSTITUTION
- Use water for injection provided.

ROUTE
- IV, IM

RATE OF ADMINISTRATION
- IV bolus: 2–3 minutes; IV infusion: 30 minutes

COMMENTS
- USE IN CAPD
- Give 400 mg IV stat dose, then 20 mg/L/bag IP for 7 days, then 20 mg/L/alternate-bag for 7 days, then 20 mg/L/night-bag only for 7 days.

OTHER INFORMATION

- TDM optimises therapy, but not essential. Troughs not less than 10 mg/L. Peaks 1 hour after dose: 20–50 mg/L.
- Relationship between blood level and toxicity not established.
- Long-term concurrent use of gentamicin and teicoplanin causes additive ototoxicity.
- Injection can be used to prepare oral solution.
- Has been used at a dose of 200 mg daily in GFR<10 mL/min safely from personal experience.

Reference:
1. Thalhammer TF. Single-dose pharmacokinetics of teicoplanin during haemodialysis therapy using high-flux polysulfone membranes. *Wien Klin Wochenschr*. 1997 May 23; **109**(10): 362–5.

Telaprevir

CLINICAL USE

HCV-protease inhibitor:
- Treatment of hepatitis C with compensated liver disease

DOSE IN NORMAL RENAL FUNCTION

750 mg every 8 hours or 1.125 mg twice daily with food

PHARMACOKINETICS

Molecular weight (daltons)	679.8
% Protein binding	59–76
% Excreted unchanged in urine	1
Volume of distribution (L/kg)	252 litres
Half-life – normal/ ESRF (hrs)	9–11/–

METABOLISM

Extensively metabolised in the liver, involving hydrolysis, oxidation, and reduction.
   Multiple metabolites were detected in faeces, plasma, and urine.

DOSE IN RENAL IMPAIRMENT GFR (mL/MIN)

20–50	Dose as in normal renal function.
10–20	Dose as in normal renal function.
<10	Dose as in normal renal function.

DOSE IN PATIENTS UNDERGOING RENAL REPLACEMENT THERAPIES

CAPD	Possibly dialysed. Dose as in normal renal function.
HD	Possibly dialysed. Dose as in normal renal function.
HDF/High flux	Possibly dialysed. Dose as in normal renal function.
CAV/ VVHD	Possibly dialysed. Dose as in normal renal function.

IMPORTANT DRUG INTERACTIONS

Potentially hazardous interactions with other drugs
- Alpha-blockers: avoid concomitant use with alfuzosin.
- Analgesics: risk of ventricular arrhythmias with methadone.
- Anti-arrhythmics: risk of ventricular arrhythmias with amiodarone & disopyramide – avoid concomitant use; risk of ventricular arrhythmias with flecainide & propafenone – use with caution; use IV lidocaine with caution.
- Antibacterials: concentration of both drugs increased with clarithromycin, erythromycin & telithromycin, increased risk of ventricular arrhythmias; avoid concomitant use with rifabutin & rifampicin (concentration significantly reduced by rifampicin).
- Anticoagulants: concentration of warfarin possibly affected; avoid with apixaban; possibly increased dabigatran concentration.
- Antidepressants: possibly increased trazodone concentration; avoid concomitant use with St John's wort.
- Antiepileptics; avoid concomitant use with carbamazepine, phenobarbital & phenytoin.
- Antifungals: concentration of both drugs possibly increased with ketoconazole, increased risk of ventricular arrhythmias; possibly increased itraconazole concentration; possibly increased posaconazole concentration – increased risk of ventricular arrhythmias; possibly altered voriconazole concentration – increased risk of ventricular arrhythmias.
- Antipsychotics: avoid concomitant use with pimozide; possibly increases quetiapine concentration – avoid.
- Antivirals: concentration possibly reduced by atazanavir; concentration of atazanavir possibly increased; avoid concomitant use with darunavir, fosamprenavir & lopinavir; concentration reduced by efavirenz – increase telaprevir dose; concentration possibly reduced by ritonavir; concentration of tenofovir possibly increased.
- Anxiolytics & hypnotics: possibly increased midazolam concentration – risk of prolonged sedation, avoid concomitant use with oral midazolam.
- Beta-blockers: risk of ventricular arrhythmias with sotalol – avoid concomitant use.
- Ciclosporin: concentration of both drugs increased, reduce ciclosporin dose.
- Colchicine: possibly increased risk of colchicine toxicity – suspend or reduce

colchicine dose, avoid concomitant use in hepatic or renal impairment.
- Cytotoxics: reduce dose of ruxolitinib.
- Domperidone: possibly increased domperidone concentration – avoid concomitant use.
- Ergot alkaloids: avoid concomitant use.
- Lipid-regulating drugs: avoid concomitant use with simvastatin & atorvastatin.
- Oestrogens: possibly reduced ethinylestradiol concentration & contraceptive effect.
- Sildenafil: avoid concomitant use.
- Sirolimus: concentration of both drugs increased, reduce sirolimus dose.
- Beta2-sympathomimetics: avoid concomitant use with salmeterol – risk of ventricular arrhythmias.
- Tacrolimus: concentration of both drugs increased, reduce tacrolimus dose.
- Tadalafil: avoid concomitant use with high dose tadalafil.
- Vardenafil: avoid concomitant use.

ADMINISTRATION

RECONSTITUTION

–

ROUTE
- Oral

RATE OF ADMINISTRATION

–

OTHER INFORMATION

- The pharmacokinetics of telaprevir were assessed after administration of a single dose of 750 mg to HCV-negative subjects with severe renal impairment (CRCL <30 mL/min). The mean telaprevir C_{max} and AUC were 10% and 21% greater, respectively, compared to healthy subjects.

Telbivudine

CLINICAL USE

Treatment of chronic hepatitis B infection

DOSE IN NORMAL RENAL FUNCTION

600 mg daily

PHARMACOKINETICS

Molecular weight (daltons)	242.2
% Protein binding	3.3
% Excreted unchanged in urine	42
Volume of distribution (L/kg)	No data
Half-life – normal/ ESRF (hrs)	30–53.6/Increased

METABOLISM

Telbivudine is not metabolised. It is eliminated primarily by urinary excretion of unchanged substance.

DOSE IN RENAL IMPAIRMENT GFR (mL/MIN)

30–50	Tablet: 600 mg every 48 hours; oral solution: 400 mg daily
<30	Tablet: 600 mg every 72 hours; oral solution: 200 mg daily

DOSE IN PATIENTS UNDERGOING RENAL REPLACEMENT THERAPIES

CAPD	Dialysed. Tablet: 600 mg every 96 hours; oral solution: 120 mg daily.
HD	Dialysed. 600 mg every 96 hours; oral solution: 120 mg daily.
HDF/High flux	Dialysed. 600 mg every 96 hours; oral solution: 120 mg daily.
CAV/ VVHD	Dialysed. Dose as in GFR<30 mL/ oral solution: 120 mg daily min.

IMPORTANT DRUG INTERACTIONS

Potentially hazardous interactions with other drugs

- Interferons: increased risk of peripheral neuropathy.

ADMINISTRATION

RECONSTITUTION

–

ROUTE

- Oral

RATE OF ADMINISTRATION

–

COMMENTS

–

OTHER INFORMATION

- Dosage guidelines are from the company and have not been tested so adjust the dose according to virological response and monitor for side effects.
- Has been associated with myopathy and myalgia.
- 4 hours of haemodialysis removes 23% of the dose.

Telithromycin

CLINICAL USE

Antibacterial agent

DOSE IN NORMAL RENAL FUNCTION

800 mg daily

PHARMACOKINETICS

Molecular weight (daltons)	812
% Protein binding	60–70
% Excreted unchanged in urine	12
Volume of distribution (L/kg)	1.9–3.9
Half-life – normal/ ESRF (hrs)	2–3/14.64

METABOLISM

About two-thirds of a dose is metabolised in the liver to inactive metabolites and the remaining third is eliminated unchanged in the urine and faeces. Metabolism is mediated both by cytochrome P450 isoenzymes (mainly CYP3A4) and non-cytochrome P450 enzymes. The pharmacokinetics of telithromycin are triphasic with a biphasic elimination phase.

DOSE IN RENAL IMPAIRMENT GFR (mL/MIN)

30–50	Dose as in normal renal function.
10–30	600 mg daily (Given as 800 mg/400 mg alternating days).
<10	600 mg daily (Given as 800 mg/400 mg alternating days).

DOSE IN PATIENTS UNDERGOING RENAL REPLACEMENT THERAPIES

CAPD	Unknown dialysability. Dose as in GFR<10 mL/min.
HD	Dialysed. Dose as in GFR<10 mL/min. (Give 800 mg dose after dialysis session.)
HDF/High flux	Dialysed. Dose as in GFR<10 mL/min. (Give 800 mg dose after dialysis session.)
CAV/ VVHD	Dialysed. Dose as in GFR=10–30 mL/min.

IMPORTANT DRUG INTERACTIONS

Potentially hazardous interactions with other drugs

- Analgesics: possible increased risk of ventricular arrhythmias with methadone; metabolism of oxycodone inhibited.
- Anti-arrhythmics: increased risk of ventricular arrhythmias with amiodarone and disopyramide; increased risk of ventricular arrhythmias with dronedarone – avoid.
- Antibacterials: possible increased risk of ventricular arrhythmias with moxifloxacin; concentration reduced by rifampicin – avoid during and for 2 weeks after rifampicin therapy.
- Antidepressants: increased risk of ventricular arrhythmias with citalopram and tricyclics; concentration reduced by St John's wort – avoid during and for 2 weeks after St John's wort therapy.
- Anti-epileptics: concentration reduced by carbamazepine, phenytoin and phenobarbital – avoid during and for 2 weeks after treatment.
- Antifungals: avoid in combination with ketoconazole in severe renal and hepatic impairment.
- Antipsychotics: possibly increased risk of ventricular arrhythmias with chlorpromazine; increased risk of ventricular arrhythmias with pimozide – avoid concomitant use; possibly increased quetiapine concentration.
- Antivirals: avoid concomitant use with atazanavir, fosamprenavir, indinavir, lopinavir, ritonavir and tipranavir in severe renal and hepatic impairment; possibly increased maraviroc concentration, consider reducing maraviroc dose; increased risk of ventricular arrhythmias with saquinavir – avoid; concentration of both drugs possibly increased with telaprevir, increased risk of ventricular arrhythmias.
- Anxiolytics and hypnotics: inhibits metabolism of midazolam (increased sedation).
- Calcium-channel blockers: possibly inhibits metabolism of calcium-channel blockers.
- Ciclosporin: possibly increased ciclosporin levels.
- Colchicine: increased risk of colchicine toxicity – suspend or reduce dose of

colchicine, avoid in hepatic or renal impairment.

- Cytotoxics: concentration of axitinib possibly increased – reduce axitinib dose; concentration of crizotinib and everolimus possibly increased – avoid; avoid with cabazitaxel, lapatinib, nilotinib and pazopanib; reduce dose of ruxolitinib.
- Diuretics: increased eplerenone concentration – avoid concomitant use.
- Telithromycin and ergot derivatives should not be co-administered due to possibility of ergotism.
- Ivabradine: possibly increased ivabradine concentration – avoid concomitant use.
- Lipid-regulating drugs: possibly increased risk of myopathy with pravastatin; increased risk of myopathy with atorvastatin and simvastatin – avoid concomitant use.[1]
- Pentamidine: possibly increased risk of ventricular arrhythmias with IV pentamidine.
- Ranolazine: concentration of ranolazine possibly increased – avoid.
- Sirolimus: increased sirolimus levels – avoid concomitant use.
- Tacrolimus: possibly increased tacrolimus levels.

ADMINISTRATION

RECONSTITUTION

–

ROUTE

- Oral

RATE OF ADMINISTRATION

–

COMMENTS

–

OTHER INFORMATION

- Do not give to people at risk of QT interval prolongation due to its potential to prolong the QT interval.
- Oral bioavailability is approximately 57% after a single dose of 800 mg.
- The 800 mg dose should be given on haemodialysis days after dialysis.
- In patients with both renal and hepatic impairment the dose should be reduced to 400 mg daily.
- Monitor for signs of liver toxicity.
- AUC increased 2-fold if GFR<30 mL/min.

Reference:

1. MHRA. *Drug Safety Update*. Statins: interactions and updated advice. August 2012; **6**(1): 2–4.

Telmisartan

CLINICAL USE

Angiotensin-II antagonist:
- Hypertension
- Prevention of cardiovascular events

DOSE IN NORMAL RENAL FUNCTION

- Hypertension: 20–80 mg daily
- Prevention of cardiovascular events: 80 mg daily

PHARMACOKINETICS

Molecular weight (daltons)	514.6
% Protein binding	>99.5
% Excreted unchanged in urine	>1
Volume of distribution (L/kg)	500 litres
Half-life – normal/ ESRF (hrs)	24/Unchanged

METABOLISM

Telmisartan is metabolised by conjugation to the glucuronide of the parent compound. No pharmacological activity has been shown for the conjugate.

Telmisartan is excreted almost entirely in the faeces via bile, mainly as unchanged drug.

DOSE IN RENAL IMPAIRMENT GFR (mL/MIN)

20–50	Dose as in normal renal function.
10–20	Dose as in normal renal function.
<10	Start with 20 mg and adjust according to response.

DOSE IN PATIENTS UNDERGOING RENAL REPLACEMENT THERAPIES

CAPD	Not dialysed. Dose as in GFR<10 mL/min.
HD	Not dialysed. Dose as in GFR<10 mL/min.
HDF/High flux	Unknown dialysability. Dose as in GFR<10 mL/min.
CAV/ VVHD	Unlikely to be dialysed. Dose as in normal renal function.

IMPORTANT DRUG INTERACTIONS

Potentially hazardous interactions with other drugs
- Anaesthetics: enhanced hypotensive effect.
- Analgesics: antagonism of hypotensive effect and increased risk of renal impairment with NSAIDs; hyperkalaemia with ketorolac and other NSAIDs.
- Cardiac glycosides: concentration of digoxin increased.
- Ciclosporin: increased risk of hyperkalaemia and nephrotoxicity.
- Diuretics: enhanced hypotensive effect; hyperkalaemia with potassium-sparing diuretics.
- ESAs: increased risk of hyperkalaemia; antagonism of hypotensive effect.
- Lithium: reduced excretion (possibility of enhanced lithium toxicity).
- Potassium salts: increased risk of hyperkalaemia.
- Tacrolimus: increased risk of hyperkalaemia and nephrotoxicity.

ADMINISTRATION

RECONSTITUTION
–
ROUTE
- Oral
RATE OF ADMINISTRATION
–
COMMENTS
–

OTHER INFORMATION

- Hyperkalaemia and other side effects are more common in patients with impaired renal function.
- Close monitoring of renal function required during therapy in patients with renal insufficiency.
- Renal failure has been reported in association with angiotensin-II inhibitors in patients with renal artery stenosis, post renal transplant, and those with congestive heart failure.
- Oral bioavailability is 42–58% depending on dose.

Temazepam

CLINICAL USE

Benzodiazepine:
- Insomnia (short term use)
- Pre-med anxiolytic prior to minor procedures

DOSE IN NORMAL RENAL FUNCTION

- 10–40 mg at night
- Premedication: 20–40 mg, 60 minutes prior to procedure

PHARMACOKINETICS

Molecular weight (daltons)	300.7
% Protein binding	96
% Excreted unchanged in urine	<2
Volume of distribution (L/kg)	1.3–1.5
Half-life – normal/ ESRF (hrs)	7–11/Unchanged

METABOLISM

Temazepam is metabolised mainly in the liver.

It is excreted mainly in the urine in the form of its inactive glucuronide conjugate together with small amounts of the demethylated derivative, oxazepam, also in conjugated form.

DOSE IN RENAL IMPAIRMENT GFR (mL/MIN)

20–50	Dose as in normal renal function.
10–20	Dose as in normal renal function. Start with small doses.
<10	Dose as in normal renal function. Start with small doses.

DOSE IN PATIENTS UNDERGOING RENAL REPLACEMENT THERAPIES

CAPD	Dose as in normal renal function. Start with small doses.
HD	Not dialysed. Dose as in GFR<10 mL/min.
HDF/High flux	Unknown dialysability. Dose as in GFR<10 mL/min.
CAV/ VVHD	Not dialysed. Dose as in GFR=10–20 mL/min.

IMPORTANT DRUG INTERACTIONS

Potentially hazardous interactions with other drugs
- Antibacterials: metabolism possibly increased by rifampicin.
- Antipsychotics: increased sedative effects; risk serious adverse effects in combination with clozapine.
- Antivirals: concentration possibly increased by ritonavir.
- Disulfiram: metabolism of temazepam inhibited (increased toxicity).
- Sodium oxybate: enhanced effects of sodium oxybate – avoid.

ADMINISTRATION

RECONSTITUTION
–
ROUTE
- Oral
RATE OF ADMINISTRATION
–
COMMENTS
–

OTHER INFORMATION

- Increased CNS sensitivity in renal impairment.
- Long-term use may lead to dependence and withdrawal symptoms in certain patients.
- 80% of metabolites excreted in the urine.

Temocillin

CLINICAL USE

Antibacterial agent

DOSE IN NORMAL RENAL FUNCTION

- 1–2 g every 12 hours
- Acute uncomplicated UTIs: 1 g daily in a single or divided doses

PHARMACOKINETICS

Molecular weight (daltons)	458.4 (as sodium salt)
% Protein binding	75–85
% Excreted unchanged in urine	90
Volume of distribution (L/kg)	0.23
Half-life – normal/ ESRF (hrs)	3.1–5.4/28.2

METABOLISM

Temocillin is excreted unchanged mainly in the kidney.

DOSE IN RENAL IMPAIRMENT GFR (mL/MIN)

30–60	1 g every 12 hours. See 'Other information'.
10–30	1 g daily. See 'Other information'.
<10	1 g every 48 hours or 500 mg daily. See 'Other information'.

DOSE IN PATIENTS UNDERGOING RENAL REPLACEMENT THERAPIES

CAPD	Not dialysed. Dose as in GFR<10 mL/min.
HD	Dialysed. Dose as in GFR<10 mL/min.
HDF/High flux	Dialysed. Dose as in GFR<10 mL/min.
CAV/ VVHD	Dialysed. Dose as in GFR=10–30 mL/min.

IMPORTANT DRUG INTERACTIONS

Potentially hazardous interactions with other drugs
- Temocillin can reduce the excretion of methotrexate (increased risk of toxicity).

ADMINISTRATION

RECONSTITUTION
- IV: Dissolve in 20 mL water for injection.
- IV infusion: Dilute in 50–100 mL sodium chloride 0.9%.
- IM: Dissolve in 2 mL water for injection or lidocaine 0.5–1% (volume 2.7 mL).
ROUTE
- IV, IM
RATE OF ADMINISTRATION
- Slow IV bolus over 3–4 minutes
- Infusion over 30–40 minutes
COMMENTS
- Incompatible with proteins, blood products, lipid emulsions and aminoglycosides.

OTHER INFORMATION

- Bleeding has occurred in some patients (more likely in those with renal impairment).
- 20% is removed by haemodialysis and 17–26% by peritoneal dialysis.
- A study in Dundee looked at the safety and effectiveness of temocillin for urinary sepsis in patients with renal impairment and found it a safe and effective treatment. (Oliver S, Kennedy H, Nathwan D, Bell S. Presented at the SRA, 12 November 2011, Glasgow.)
- An alternative dosing regimen used by some units is:

GFR (mL/min)	Dose
30–60	Dose as in normal renal function.
10–30	1–2 g daily
<10	1–2 g every 48 hours

Temozolomide

CLINICAL USE

Antineoplastic agent:
- Glioblastoma multiforme
- Malignant glioma

DOSE IN NORMAL RENAL FUNCTION

- 75 mg/m² daily for 42 days with radiotherapy
- Adjuvant phase/monotherapy: 150–200 mg/m² once daily for 5 days
- Or according to local policy

PHARMACOKINETICS

Molecular weight (daltons)	194.2
% Protein binding	10–20
% Excreted unchanged in urine	5–10
Volume of distribution (L/kg)	0.3–0.5 (IV) (15–18 L/ m² oral)
Half-life – normal/ ESRF (hrs)	1.8/Unchanged

METABOLISM

Temozolomide undergoes spontaneous hydrolysis to its active metabolite 5-(3-methyl-triazen-1-yl)-imidazole-4-carboxamide (MTIC), which is then further hydrolysed to 5-amino-imidazole-4-carboxamide (AIC) and methylhydrazine.

Temozolomide is largely eliminated by the kidneys, about 5–10% as unchanged drug.

DOSE IN RENAL IMPAIRMENT GFR (mL/MIN)

20–50	Dose as in normal renal function.
10–20	Dose as in normal renal function.
<10	Dose as in normal renal function. Use with caution.

DOSE IN PATIENTS UNDERGOING RENAL REPLACEMENT THERAPIES

CAPD	Unknown dialysability. Dose as in GFR<10 mL/min.
HD	Unknown dialysability. Dose as in GFR<10 mL/min.
HDF/High flux	Unknown dialysability. Dose as in GFR<10 mL/min.
CAV/ VVHD	Unknown dialysability. Dose as in normal renal function.

IMPORTANT DRUG INTERACTIONS

Potentially hazardous interactions with other drugs
- Antipsychotics: avoid concomitant use with clozapine, increased risk of agranulocytosis.

ADMINISTRATION

RECONSTITUTION
–

ROUTE
- Oral

RATE OF ADMINISTRATION
–

COMMENTS
- Do not administer with food.

OTHER INFORMATION

- Nadir for white cell count usually occurs 21–28 days after a dose, with recovery within 1–2 weeks.
- Rapidly and completely absorbed with 100% bioavailability and has extensive tissue distribution.
- Manufacturer advises to use with caution in severe renal failure due to lack of data but pharmacokinetics indicate that no dose change should be required.

Temsirolimus

Protein kinase inhibitor
- Treatment of advanced renal cell carcinoma
- Treatment of mantle cell lymphoma

DOSE IN NORMAL RENAL FUNCTION

- Renal cell carcinoma: 25 mg once weekly
- Mantle cell lymphoma: 175 mg once weekly for 3 weeks then weekly doses of 75 mg

PHARMACOKINETICS

Molecular weight (daltons)	1030.3
% Protein binding	87
% Excreted unchanged in urine	4.6
Volume of distribution (L/kg)	172
Half-life – normal/ ESRF (hrs)	17.7/–

METABOLISM

Mainly metabolised by cytochrome P450 isoenzyme CYP3A4 to 5 metabolites; sirolimus is the main active metabolite, there is increased exposure to sirolimus compared with temsirolimus due to longer half-life of sirolimus.

Elimination is mainly in faeces; about 5% is recovered in the urine.

DOSE IN RENAL IMPAIRMENT GFR (mL/MIN)

20–50	Dose as in normal renal function.
10–20	Dose as in normal renal function. Use with caution.
<10	Use with caution.

DOSE IN PATIENTS UNDERGOING RENAL REPLACEMENT THERAPIES

CAPD	Not dialysed. Dose as in GFR<10 mL/min.
HD	Not dialysed. Dose as in GFR<10 mL/min.
HDF/High flux	Not dialysed. Dose as in GFR<10 mL/min.
CAV/ VVHD	Not dialysed. Dose as in GFR=10–20 mL/min.

IMPORTANT DRUG INTERACTIONS

Potentially hazardous interactions with other drugs
- Antibacterials: concentration increased by clarithromycin and telithromycin – avoid; concentration of both drugs increased with erythromycin; concentration reduced by rifampicin and rifabutin – avoid.
- Antifungals: concentration increased of active metabolite increased by ketoconazole – avoid; concentration increased by fluconazole, miconazole, micafungin, posaconazole and voriconazole.
- Antipsychotics: increased risk of agranulocytosis with clozapine – avoid concomitant use.
- Antivirals: concentration possibly increased by atazanavir, boceprevir and lopinavir; concentration of both drugs increased with telaprevir.
- Calcium-channel blockers: concentration increased by diltiazem; concentration of both drugs increased with verapamil.
- Ciclosporin: increased absorption of temsirolimus – give temsirolimus 4 hours after ciclosporin; temsirolimus concentration increased; long term concomitant administration may be associated with deterioration in renal function.
- Cytotoxics: use crizotinib with caution.
- Grapefruit juice: concentration of temsirolimus increased – avoid concomitant use.
- Mycophenolate: concomitant use of mycophenolate and sirolimus increases plasma levels of both temsirolimus and mycophenolic acid.

ADMINISTRATION

RECONSTITUTION
- 1.8 mL of diluent

ROUTE
- IV

RATE OF ADMINISTRATION
- 30–60 minutes

COMMENTS
- Add to 250 mL sodium chloride 0.9% after dilution with diluent.
- Protect from light. Avoid PVC equipment.
- Administer through an infusion set with an in-line filter with a maximum pore size of 5 microns within 6 hours of being added to sodium chloride 0.9%.

OTHER INFORMATION

- Use with caution as limited clinical experience of temsirolimus in renal impairment.
- Approximately 30 minutes before each dose patients should receive 25–50 mg of IV diphenhydramine or similar anti-histamine.
- Associated with abnormal wound healing.
- May increase blood glucose levels.
- May commonly increase creatinine levels.

Tenecteplase

CLINICAL USE

Thrombolytic:
- Acute myocardial infarction

DOSE IN NORMAL RENAL FUNCTION

30–50 mg depending on patient weight
(500–600 micrograms/kg)

PHARMACOKINETICS

Molecular weight (daltons)	70 000
% Protein binding	No data
% Excreted unchanged in urine	Minimal
Volume of distribution (L/kg)	6.1–9.1 litres[1] (weight and dose related)
Half-life – normal/ ESRF (hrs)	90–130 minutes/ Unchanged

METABOLISM

Tenecteplase is cleared from circulation
by binding to specific receptors in the liver
followed by catabolism to small peptides.

DOSE IN RENAL IMPAIRMENT GFR (mL/MIN)

20–50	Dose as in normal renal function.
10–20	Dose as in normal renal function.
<10	Dose as in normal renal function.

DOSE IN PATIENTS UNDERGOING RENAL REPLACEMENT THERAPIES

CAPD	Unlikely to be dialysed. Dose as in normal renal function.
HD	Unlikely to be dialysed. Dose as in normal renal function.
HDF/High flux	Unknown dialysability. Dose as in normal renal function.
CAV/ VVHD	Unknown dialysability. Dose as in normal renal function.

IMPORTANT DRUG INTERACTIONS

Potentially hazardous interactions with other
drugs
- Drugs that affect coagulation or platelet
  function: increased risk of bleeding.

ADMINISTRATION

RECONSTITUTION
- Water for injection
ROUTE
- IV
RATE OF ADMINISTRATION
- Over 10 seconds
COMMENTS
- Incompatible with dextrose

OTHER INFORMATION

- It has an initial half-life of 20–24 minutes.
- Cleared mainly by hepatic metabolism.
- Re-administration is not recommended
  due to lack of experience.

Reference:
1. Tanswell P. Pharmacokinetics and
pharmacodynamics of tenecteplase in
fibrinolytic therapy of acute myocardial
infarction. *Clin Pharmacokinet*. 2002; **41**(15):
1229–45.

Tenofovir disoproxil

CLINICAL USE

Nucleoside reverse transcriptase inhibitor
- Treatment of HIV in combination with other antiretroviral drugs
- Treatment of hepatitis B in compensated liver disease

DOSE IN NORMAL RENAL FUNCTION

245 mg once daily.

PHARMACOKINETICS

Molecular weight (daltons)	635.5 (as disoproxil fumarate)
% Protein binding	0.7–7.2
% Excreted unchanged in urine	IV: 70–80; Oral: 32
Volume of distribution (L/kg)	0.8
Half-life – normal/ ESRF (hrs)	12–18/Increased

METABOLISM

Tenofovir is excreted mainly in the urine by both active tubular secretion and glomerular filtration.

DOSE IN RENAL IMPAIRMENT GFR (mL/MIN)

30–50	245 mg every 48 hours or 132 mg (4 scoops) once daily.
20–30	245 mg every 72–96 hours or 65 mg (2 scoops) once daily.
10–20	245 mg every 72–96 hours or 33 mg (1 scoop) once daily.
<10	245 mg every 72–96 hours or 33 mg (1 scoop) once daily. Use with caution.[1,2]

DOSE IN PATIENTS UNDERGOING RENAL REPLACEMENT THERAPIES

CAPD	Unknown dialysability. 245 mg every 7 days or 16.5 mg (0.5 of a scoop) once daily.
HD	Dialysed. 245 mg every 7 days or after a total of 12 hours dialysis or 16.5 mg (0.5 of a scoop) once daily.
HDF/High flux	Dialysed. 245 mg every 7 days or after a total of 12 hours dialysis or 16.5 mg (0.5 of a scoop) once daily.
CAV/ VVHD	Dialysed. Dose as in GFR=20–30 mL/min.

IMPORTANT DRUG INTERACTIONS

Potentially hazardous interactions with other drugs
- Antivirals: avoid with adefovir and cidofovir; reduces concentration of atazanavir, also concentration of tenofovir possibly increased; increased didanosine concentration resulting in increased toxicity (e.g. pancreatitis and lactic acidosis) – avoid concomitant use; concentration increased by lopinavir and telaprevir.
- Co-administration with other drugs that are actively secreted via the tubular anionic transporter.

ADMINISTRATION

RECONSTITUTION
–
ROUTE
- Oral
RATE OF ADMINISTRATION
–
COMMENTS
–

OTHER INFORMATION

- Manufacturer has no studies on the use of tenofovir in non-haemodialysis patients with GFR<10 mL/min. Use with caution as doses are based on limited data and may not be optimal.
- Lactic acidosis, sometimes fatal, and usually associated with severe hepatomegaly and steatosis, has been reported in patients receiving nucleoside reverse transcriptase inhibitors.
- Following a single 300 mg dose of tenofovir, subjects with a calculated creatinine clearance <50 mL/min, and those with ESRF requiring dialysis, had substantial reductions in renal elimination of tenofovir, resulting in high systemic exposures necessitating an adjustment in dose.
- A 4 hour high-flux haemodialysis session was found to remove 10% of tenofovir from plasma.
- Renal impairment, which may include hypophosphataemia, has been reported with the use of tenofovir. The majority of these cases occurred in patients with underlying systemic or renal disease, or

in patients taking nephrotoxic agents
– monitor creatinine clearance and
phosphate levels.

References:
1. Kearney BP, Yale K, Shah J, *et
al.* Pharmacokinetics and dosing
recommendations of tenofovir disoproxil
fumarate in hepatic or renal impairment.
Clin Pharmacokinet. 2006; **45**(11): 1115–24.
2. http://depts.washington.edu/madclin/
pharmacy/renal/impairment.pdf

Tenoxicam

CLINICAL USE

NSAID and analgesic

DOSE IN NORMAL RENAL FUNCTION

20 mg once daily

PHARMACOKINETICS

Molecular weight (daltons)	337.4
% Protein binding	99
% Excreted unchanged in urine	<1 (67% as metabolites and unchanged drug)
Volume of distribution (L/kg)	10–12 litres
Half-life – normal/ ESRF (hrs)	72/–

METABOLISM

Metabolised in the liver via cytochrome P450 2C9 to several pharmacologically inactive metabolites (mainly 5'-hydroxy-tenoxicam).

Metabolites are excreted mainly in the urine; there is some biliary excretion of glucuronide conjugates of the metabolites.

DOSE IN RENAL IMPAIRMENT GFR (mL/MIN)

20–50	Dose as in normal renal function, but avoid if possible.
10–20	Dose as in normal renal function, but avoid if possible.
<10	Dose as in normal renal function, but only use if on dialysis.

DOSE IN PATIENTS UNDERGOING RENAL REPLACEMENT THERAPIES

CAPD	Unlikely to be dialysed. Dose as in GFR<10 mL/min. See 'Other information'.
HD	Unlikely to be dialysed. Dose as in GFR<10 mL/min. See 'Other information'.
HDF/High flux	Unlikely to be dialysed. Dose as in GFR<10 mL/min. See 'Other information'.
CAV/ VVHD	Unlikely to be dialysed. Dose as in GFR=10–20 mL/min.

IMPORTANT DRUG INTERACTIONS

Potentially hazardous interactions with other drugs

- ACE inhibitors and angiotensin-II antagonists: antagonism of hypotensive effect; increased risk of nephrotoxicity and hyperkalaemia.
- Analgesics: avoid concomitant use of 2 or more NSAIDs, including aspirin (increased side effects); avoid with ketorolac (increased risk of side effects and haemorrhage).
- Antibacterials: possibly increased risk of convulsions with quinolones.
- Anticoagulants: effects of coumarins and phenindione enhanced; possibly increased risk of bleeding with heparins and dabigatran.
- Antidepressants: increased risk of bleeding with SSRIs and venlafaxine.
- Antidiabetic agents: effects of sulphonylureas enhanced.
- Anti-epileptics: possibly increased phenytoin concentration.
- Antivirals: increased risk of haematological toxicity with zidovudine; concentration possibly increased by ritonavir.
- Ciclosporin: may potentiate nephrotoxicity.
- Cytotoxic agents: reduced excretion of methotrexate; increased risk of bleeding with erlotinib.
- Diuretics: increased risk of nephrotoxicity; antagonism of diuretic effect; hyperkalaemia with potassium-sparing diuretics.
- Lithium: excretion decreased.
- Pentoxifylline: increased risk of bleeding.
- Tacrolimus: increased risk of nephrotoxicity.

ADMINISTRATION

RECONSTITUTION

–

ROUTE

- Oral, (IV, IM – unlicensed)

RATE OF ADMINISTRATION

–

COMMENTS

–

OTHER INFORMATION

- Inhibition of renal prostaglandin synthesis by NSAIDs may interfere with renal function, especially in the presence of existing renal disease – avoid if possible; if not, check serum creatinine 48–72 hours after starting NSAID – if serum creatinine is increased, stop NSAID.

- Use normal doses in patients with CKD 5 if on dialysis and do not pass any urine.
- Use with caution in renal transplant recipients – can reduce intrarenal autocoid synthesis.

Terazosin

CLINICAL USE

Alpha-adrenoceptor blocker:
- Hypertension
- Benign prostatic hyperplasia (BPH)

DOSE IN NORMAL RENAL FUNCTION

- Hypertension: 1–20 mg once daily
- BPH: 1–10 mg once daily

PHARMACOKINETICS

Molecular weight (daltons)	459.9
% Protein binding	90–94
% Excreted unchanged in urine	10
Volume of distribution (L/kg)	0.5–0.9
Half-life – normal/ ESRF (hrs)	9–12/Unchanged

METABOLISM

Terazosin is metabolised in the liver; one of the metabolites has antihypertensive activity.

Terazosin is excreted in faeces via the bile, and in the urine, as unchanged drug and metabolites.

DOSE IN RENAL IMPAIRMENT GFR (mL/MIN)

20–50	Dose as in normal renal function.
10–20	Dose as in normal renal function.
<10	Dose as in normal renal function.

DOSE IN PATIENTS UNDERGOING RENAL REPLACEMENT THERAPIES

CAPD	Not dialysed. Dose as in normal renal function.
HD	Not dialysed. Dose as in normal renal function.
HDF/High flux	Unknown dialysability. Dose as in normal renal function.
CAV/ VVHD	Unknown dialysability. Dose as in normal renal function.

IMPORTANT DRUG INTERACTIONS

Potentially hazardous interactions with other drugs
- Anaesthetics: enhanced hypotensive effect.
- Antidepressants: enhanced hypotensive effect with MAOIs.
- Beta-blockers: enhanced hypotensive effect; increased risk of first dose hypotensive effect.
- Calcium-channel blockers: enhanced hypotensive effect; increased risk of first dose hypotensive effect.
- Diuretics: enhanced hypotensive effect; increased risk of first dose hypotensive effect.
- Moxisylyte: possibly severe postural hypotension when used in combination.
- Vardenafil, sildenafil and tadalafil: enhanced hypotensive effect – avoid concomitant use.

ADMINISTRATION

RECONSTITUTION
–

ROUTE
- Oral

RATE OF ADMINISTRATION
–

COMMENTS
–

OTHER INFORMATION

- Therapy should be initiated with a single dose of 1 mg given at bedtime.

Terbinafine

CLINICAL USE

Antifungal agent:
- Fungal infections of the skin and nails

DOSE IN NORMAL RENAL FUNCTION

- 250 mg daily
- Topical: apply once or twice daily

PHARMACOKINETICS

Molecular weight (daltons)	291.4; (327.9 as hydrochloride)
% Protein binding	99
% Excreted unchanged in urine	0
Volume of distribution (L/kg)	6–11[1,2]
Half-life – normal/ ESRF (hrs)	17–36/Increased

METABOLISM

Terbinafine undergoes extensive first-pass loss. It is hepatically metabolised to two major inactive metabolites, 80% of which are renally excreted.

DOSE IN RENAL IMPAIRMENT GFR (mL/MIN)

20–50	100% on alternate days.
10–20	100% on alternate days.
<10	100% on alternate days.

DOSE IN PATIENTS UNDERGOING RENAL REPLACEMENT THERAPIES

CAPD	Unlikely to be dialysed. Dose as in GFR<10 mL/min.
HD	Unlikely to be dialysed. Dose as in GFR<10 mL/min.
HDF/High flux	Unknown dialysability. Dose as in GFR<10 mL/min.
CAV/ VVHD	Unknown dialysability. Dose as in GFR=10–20 mL/min.

IMPORTANT DRUG INTERACTIONS

Potentially hazardous interactions with other drugs
- Antibacterials: concentration reduced by rifampicin.

ADMINISTRATION

RECONSTITUTION
–

ROUTE
- Oral, Topical

RATE OF ADMINISTRATION
–

COMMENTS
–

OTHER INFORMATION

- Oral bioavailability is 40%.
- Manufacturer contraindicates use in severe renal impairment due to lack of studies in UK SPC but not US data sheet.
- Clearance is reduced by 50% if GFR<50 mL/min.
- Dosage recommendations in renal impairment are from New Zealand data sheet. (www.medsafe.govt.nz/profs/ datasheet/a/arrowterbinafinetab.pdf)
- In CKD 5 use with caution and monitor for side effects.

References:
1. Hosseini-Yeganeh M. Physiologically based pharmacokinetic model for terbinafine in rats and humans. *Antimicrob Agents Chemother.* 2002 Jul; **46**(7): 2219–28.
2. Hosseini-Yeganeh M. Tissue distribution of terbinafine in rats. *J Pharm Sci.* 2006; **90**(11): 1817–28.

Terbutaline sulphate

CLINICAL USE

Beta$_2$-adrenoceptor agonist:
- Reversible airways obstruction

DOSE IN NORMAL RENAL FUNCTION

- Oral: 2.5–5 mg 3 times daily
- SC/IM/IV: 250–500 micrograms up to 4 times daily
- IV infusion: 90–300 micrograms/hour
- Turbohaler: 500 micrograms (1 inhalation) up to 4 times daily
- Nebulisation: 5–10 mg 2–4 times daily, or more frequently

PHARMACOKINETICS

Molecular weight (daltons)	548.6
% Protein binding	15–25
% Excreted unchanged in urine	55–60
Volume of distribution (L/kg)	0.9–1.5
Half-life – normal/ ESRF (hrs)	16–20/–

METABOLISM

Terbutaline undergoes extensive first-pass metabolism by sulphate (and some glucuronide) conjugation in the liver and the gut wall. It is excreted in the urine and faeces partly as the inactive sulphate conjugate and partly as unchanged terbutaline, the ratio depending upon the route by which it is given.

DOSE IN RENAL IMPAIRMENT GFR (mL/MIN)

20–50	Dose as in normal renal function.
10–20	Dose as in normal renal function.
<10	Dose as in normal renal function.

DOSE IN PATIENTS UNDERGOING RENAL REPLACEMENT THERAPIES

CAPD	Likely dialysability. Dose as in normal renal function.
HD	Likely dialysability. Dose as in normal renal function.
HDF/High flux	Likely dialysability. Dose as in normal renal function.
CAV/ VVHD	Likely dialysability. Dose as in normal renal function.

IMPORTANT DRUG INTERACTIONS

Potentially hazardous interactions with other drugs
- Effect may be diminished by beta-blockers.
- Theophylline: increased risk of hypokalaemia.

ADMINISTRATION

RECONSTITUTION
–
ROUTE
- IV, SC, IM, oral, inhaled, nebulised
RATE OF ADMINISTRATION
- 1.5–5 mcg/minute
COMMENTS
- For IV infusion, add 1.5–2.5 mg to 500 mL glucose 5% or sodium chloride 0.9% (3–5 micrograms/mL).

OTHER INFORMATION

–

Teriparatide

CLINICAL USE

Active fragment (1–34) of endogenous
human parathyroid hormone:
- Treatment of osteoporosis in
  postmenopausal women and men at
  increased risk of fractures
- Treatment of corticosteroid-induced
  osteoporosis

DOSE IN NORMAL RENAL FUNCTION

20 mcg daily

PHARMACOKINETICS

Molecular weight (daltons)	4117.8
% Protein binding	No data
% Excreted unchanged in urine	As metabolites
Volume of distribution (L/kg)	1.7
Half-life – normal/ ESRF (hrs)	1/Increased by 77%

METABOLISM

No metabolism or excretion studies have
been performed. Peripheral metabolism of
PTH is believed to occur by non-specific
enzymatic mechanisms in the liver followed
by excretion via the kidneys. The 24-hour
urine excretion of calcium was reduced by a
clinically unimportant amount (15%).

DOSE IN RENAL IMPAIRMENT GFR (mL/MIN)

30–50	Dose as in normal renal function.
10–30	Dose as in normal renal function. Use with caution.
<10	Use with caution.

DOSE IN PATIENTS UNDERGOING RENAL REPLACEMENT THERAPIES

CAPD	Unlikely to be dialysed. Dose as in GFR<10 mL/min.
HD	Unlikely to be dialysed. Dose as in GFR<10 mL/min.
HDF/High flux	Unlikely to be dialysed. Dose as in GFR<10 mL/min.
CAV/ VVHD	Unlikely to be dialysed. Dose as in GFR=10–30 mL/min.

IMPORTANT DRUG INTERACTIONS

Potentially hazardous interactions with other
drugs
- None known

ADMINISTRATION

RECONSTITUTION
–
ROUTE
- SC
RATE OF ADMINISTRATION
–

OTHER INFORMATION

- Contraindicated by UK manufacturer in
  severe renal impairment.
- Use with caution advised in New Zealand
  data sheet due to patients with renal
  impairment having reduced calcaemic and
  calciuric responses to teriparatide.
- Bioavailability is 95%.
- No pharmacokinetic differences were
  identified in 11 patients with mild or
  moderate renal impairment (creatinine
  clearance 30 to 72 mL/min) administered
  a single dose of teriparatide. In 5 patients
  with severe renal impairment (CRCL
  <30 mL/min), the AUC and half-life of
  teriparatide were increased by 73% and
  77%, respectively. Maximum serum
  concentration of teriparatide was
  not increased. No studies have been
  performed in patients undergoing dialysis.

Terlipressin

CLINICAL USE

Treatment of bleeding oesophageal varices

DOSE IN NORMAL RENAL FUNCTION

- 2 mg stat dose followed by 1–2 mg every 4–6 hours when required (until bleeding is controlled) for up to 72 hours
- Doses are expressed as acetate

PHARMACOKINETICS

Molecular weight (daltons)	1227.4 (1437.6 as acetate)
% Protein binding	≈30
% Excreted unchanged in urine	<2
Volume of distribution (L/kg)	0.6–0.9
Half-life – normal/ ESRF (hrs)	50–70 minutes/–

METABOLISM

Terlipressin is metabolised by tissue peptidases resulting in the slow release of lypressin. Terlipressin is almost completely metabolised in the kidneys and liver, with less than 1% of terlipressin and less than 0.1% of lypressin excreted in the urine.

DOSE IN RENAL IMPAIRMENT GFR (mL/MIN)

20–50	Dose as in normal renal function.
10–20	Dose as in normal renal function. Use with caution.
<10	Dose as in normal renal function. Use with caution.

DOSE IN PATIENTS UNDERGOING RENAL REPLACEMENT THERAPIES

CAPD	Unknown dialysability. Dose as in GFR<10 mL/min.
HD	Unlikely to be dialysed. Dose as in GFR<10 mL/min.
HDF/High flux	Unknown dialysability. Dose as in GFR<10 mL/min.
CAV/ VVHD	Unknown dialysability. Dose as in GFR=10–20 mL/min.

IMPORTANT DRUG INTERACTIONS

Potentially hazardous interactions with other drugs
- None known

ADMINISTRATION

RECONSTITUTION
- With solvent provided

ROUTE
- IV

RATE OF ADMINISTRATION
-

COMMENTS
- Store reconstituted solution in the fridge and discard after 12 hours.

OTHER INFORMATION

- 1 mg of terlipressin acetate is equivalent to about 0.85 mg of terlipressin.
- Maximum plasma levels are reached after 1–2 hours with a duration of action of 4–6 hours.
- Initial response within 25–40 minutes, duration 2–10 hours.
- Information from Martindale; some studies have found it can be used to improve renal function in hepatorenal syndrome, 1 mg every 6 hours, if the creatinine hasn't reduced by 30% after 3 days then the dose can be increased to 2 mg every 6 hours providing there is no cardiovascular disease.
- May cause hypertension.
- There is a case report of rhabdomyolysis.

Tetracycline

CLINICAL USE

Antibacterial agent

DOSE IN NORMAL RENAL FUNCTION

- 250–500 mg 4 times a day
- Acne: 500 mg twice daily

PHARMACOKINETICS

Molecular weight (daltons)	444.44
% Protein binding	20–65
% Excreted unchanged in urine	55–60
Volume of distribution (L/kg)	>0.7
Half-life – normal/ ESRF (hrs)	6–12/57–120

METABOLISM

Tetracycline is excreted in the urine and in the faeces. Renal clearance is by glomerular filtration. Up to 60% of an intravenous dose of tetracycline, and up to 55% of an oral dose, is eliminated unchanged in the urine. The tetracyclines are excreted in the bile, where concentrations 5 to 25 times those in plasma can occur. There is some enterohepatic reabsorption and considerable quantities occur in the faeces after oral doses.

DOSE IN RENAL IMPAIRMENT GFR (mL/MIN)

20–50	Dose as in normal renal function.
10–20	Dose as in normal renal function.
<10	250 mg 4 times a day

DOSE IN PATIENTS UNDERGOING RENAL REPLACEMENT THERAPIES

CAPD	Not dialysed. Dose as in GFR<10 mL/min
HD	Not dialysed. Dose as in GFR<10 mL/min
HDF/High flux	Unknown dialysability. Dose as in GFR<10 mL/min.
CAV/ VVHD	Unlikely to be dialysed. Dose as in GFR=10–20 mL/min.

IMPORTANT DRUG INTERACTIONS

Potentially hazardous interactions with other drugs

- Anticoagulants: possibly enhance anticoagulant effect of coumarins and phenindione.
- Oestrogens: possibly reduce contraceptive effects of oestrogens (risk probably small).
- Retinoids: possible increased risk of benign intracranial hypertension with retinoids – avoid concomitant use.

ADMINISTRATION

RECONSTITUTION

–

ROUTE

- Oral

RATE OF ADMINISTRATION

–

COMMENTS

–

OTHER INFORMATION

- 10% is removed by haemodialysis and 7% by peritoneal dialysis.
- Avoid if possible in renal impairment due to its potential nephrotoxicity and increased risk of azotaemia, hyperphosphataemia and acidosis.
- May cause an increase in blood urea which is dose related.
- Avoid in SLE.

Thalidomide

CLINICAL USE

- Untreated multiple myeloma in patients >65 or who are ineligible for high dose chemotherapy, in combination with either melphalan and prednisone, or cyclophosphamide and dexamethasone. (Unlicensed indications):
- Erythema nodusum leprosum
- Lupus erythematosus, aphthous ulceration, stomatitis, graft-versus-host disease, AIDS-associated waste syndrome, rheumatoid arthritis and other acute inflammatory conditions.

DOSE IN NORMAL RENAL FUNCTION

- 200 mg daily
- Unlicensed dose: 50–800 mg daily

PHARMACOKINETICS

Molecular weight (daltons)	258.2
% Protein binding	55–66
% Excreted unchanged in urine	<0.7
Volume of distribution (L/kg)	166 litres
Half-life – normal/ ESRF (hrs)	5–7/Unchanged

METABOLISM

Thalidomide is metabolised almost exclusively by non-enzymatic hydrolysis. In plasma, unchanged thalidomide represents 80% of the circulatory components. Unchanged thalidomide was a minor component (<3% of the dose) in urine. In addition to thalidomide, hydrolytic products N-(o-carboxybenzoyl) glutarimide and phthaloyl isoglutamine formed via non-enzymatic processes are also present in plasma and in urine.

DOSE IN RENAL IMPAIRMENT GFR (mL/MIN)

20–50	Dose as in normal renal function.
10–20	Dose as in normal renal function.
<10	Dose as in normal renal function.

DOSE IN PATIENTS UNDERGOING RENAL REPLACEMENT THERAPIES

CAPD	Unlikely to be dialysed. Dose as in normal renal function.
HD	Unlikely to be dialysed. Dose as in normal renal function.
HDF/High flux	Not dialysed. Dose as in normal renal function.
CAV/ VVHD	Unknown dialysability. Dose as in normal renal function.

IMPORTANT DRUG INTERACTIONS

Potentially hazardous interactions with other drugs
- Thalidomide enhances the effects of barbiturates, alcohol, chlorpromazine and reserpine.
- Use with caution with other drugs that can cause peripheral neuropathy.

ADMINISTRATION

RECONSTITUTION
–
ROUTE
- Oral
RATE OF ADMINISTRATION
–
COMMENTS
–

OTHER INFORMATION

- Major route of elimination is non-renal therefore normal doses may be given in renal failure.
- Manufacturer advises to monitor patients closely due to lack of studies.
- Has been used to treat uraemic pruritis in haemodialysis patients unresponsive to other therapy. (Silva SR. Thalidomide for the treatment of uraemic pruritis: a crossover randomised double-blind trial. *Nephron*. 1994; **67**(3): 270–3.)
- Can cause unexplained hyperkalaemia. (Harris E *et al.* Use of thalidomide in patients with myeloma and renal failure may be associated with unexplained hyperkalaemia. *Br J Haematol*. 2003 Jul; **122**(1): 160–1.)

Theophylline

CLINICAL USE

- Reversible airways obstruction
- Acute severe asthma

DOSE IN NORMAL RENAL FUNCTION

Depends on preparation used

PHARMACOKINETICS

Molecular weight (daltons)	180.2
% Protein binding	35–60
% Excreted unchanged in urine	10
Volume of distribution (L/kg)	0.3–0.7
Half-life – normal/ ESRF (hrs)	3–12/Unchanged

METABOLISM

Theophylline is metabolised in the liver to 1,3-dimethyluric acid, 1-methyluric acid, and 3-methylxanthine. Demethylation to 3-methylxanthine (and possibly to 1-methylxanthine) is catalysed by the cytochrome P450 isoenzyme CYP1A2; hydroxylation to 1, 3-dimethyluric acid is catalysed by CYP2E1 and CYP3A3. Both the demethylation and hydroxylation pathways of theophylline metabolism are capacity-limited, resulting in non-linear elimination. The metabolites are excreted in the urine. In adults, about 10% of a dose of theophylline is excreted unchanged in the urine.

DOSE IN RENAL IMPAIRMENT GFR (mL/MIN)

20–50	Dose as in normal renal function.
10–20	Dose as in normal renal function.
<10	Dose as in normal renal function. See 'Other information'.

DOSE IN PATIENTS UNDERGOING RENAL REPLACEMENT THERAPIES

CAPD	Not dialysed. Dose as in GFR<10 mL/min.
HD	Dialysed. Dose as in GFR<10 mL/ min.
HDF/High flux	Dialysed. Dose as in GFR<10 mL/ min.
CAV/ VVHD	Dialysed. Dose as in normal renal function.

IMPORTANT DRUG INTERACTIONS

Potentially hazardous interactions with other drugs

- Antibacterials: increased concentration with azithromycin, clarithromycin, erythromycin, ciprofloxacin, norfloxacin and isoniazid; decreased plasma levels of erythromycin if erythromycin taken orally; increased risk of convulsions if given with quinolones; rifampicin accelerates metabolism of theophylline.
- Antidepressants: concentration increased by fluvoxamine – avoid concomitant use or halve theophylline dose and monitor levels; concentration reduced by St John's wort – avoid concomitant use.
- Anti-epileptics: metabolism increased by carbamazepine and phenobarbital; concentration of both drugs increased with phenytoin.
- Antifungals: concentration increased by fluconazole and ketoconazole.
- Antivirals: metabolism of theophylline increased by ritonavir; concentration possibly increased by aciclovir.
- Calcium-channel blockers: concentration increased by diltiazem and verapamil and possibly other calcium-channel blockers.
- Deferasirox: concentration of theophylline increased.
- Febuxostat: use with caution.
- Interferons: reduced metabolism of theophylline.
- Tacrolimus: may increase tacrolimus levels.
- Ulcer-healing drugs: metabolism inhibited by cimetidine; absorption possibly reduced by sucralfate.

ADMINISTRATION

RECONSTITUTION
–
ROUTE
- Oral
RATE OF ADMINISTRATION
–
COMMENTS
–

OTHER INFORMATION

- Therapeutic levels should be in the range 10–20 mg/litre (55–110 micromoles/litre).
- 50% of dose is removed by haemodialysis.
- Studies have used it to protect against contrast nephropathy, with conflicting results.

Thiotepa

CLINICAL USE

Alkylating antineoplastic agent

DOSE IN NORMAL RENAL FUNCTION

- IM, bladder and intracavitary instillations: 60 mg in single or divided doses
- Intrathecal: maximum 10 mg
- Other doses depend on indication or local protocol.

PHARMACOKINETICS

Molecular weight (daltons)	189.2
% Protein binding	10–40
% Excreted unchanged in urine	<2
Volume of distribution (L/kg)	0.3–1.6
Half-life – normal/ ESRF (hrs)	2.4/–

METABOLISM

Thiotepa is extensively metabolised to triethylenephosphoramide (TEPA), the primary metabolite, and some of the other metabolites have cytotoxic activity and are eliminated more slowly than the parent compound. It is excreted in the urine: less than 2% of a dose is reported to be present as unchanged drug or its primary metabolite.

DOSE IN RENAL IMPAIRMENT GFR (mL/MIN)

20–50	IM: Use a reduced dose with caution.
10–20	IM: Use a reduced dose with caution.
<10	IM: Use a reduced dose with caution.

DOSE IN PATIENTS UNDERGOING RENAL REPLACEMENT THERAPIES

CAPD	Unknown dialysability. Dose as in GFR<10 mL/min.
HD	Dialysed. Dose as in GFR<10 mL/min.
HDF/High flux	Dialysed. Dose as in GFR<10 mL/min.
CAV/ VVHD	Dialysed. Dose as in GFR=10–20 mL/min.

IMPORTANT DRUG INTERACTIONS

Potentially hazardous interactions with other drugs
- Antipsychotics: avoid concomitant use with clozapine.
- Avoid concomitant use with other myelosuppressive agents.

ADMINISTRATION

RECONSTITUTION
- 1.5 mL water for injection
ROUTE
- IV, IM, intrathecal (can be administered directly into pleural, pericardial or peritoneal cavities and as a bladder instillation)
RATE OF ADMINISTRATION
–
COMMENTS
–

OTHER INFORMATION

- Manufacturer advises to use with caution due to lack of pharmacokinetic studies in renal impairment.
- Haemorrhagic cystitis has been reported.

Tiagabine

CLINICAL USE

Anti-epileptic agent

DOSE IN NORMAL RENAL FUNCTION

15–45 mg daily in 3 divided doses if dose
>30 mg

PHARMACOKINETICS

Molecular weight (daltons)	412
% Protein binding	96
% Excreted unchanged in urine	<2
Volume of distribution (L/kg)	1
Half-life – normal/ ESRF (hrs)	7–9 (2–3 in patients on enzyme inducing drugs)/–

METABOLISM

Tiagabine has negligible renal clearance.
Hepatic metabolism is the principal route
for elimination of tiagabine. Less than 2%
of the dose is excreted unchanged in urine
and faeces. No active metabolites have been
identified.

DOSE IN RENAL IMPAIRMENT GFR (mL/MIN)

20–50	Dose as in normal renal function.
10–20	Dose as in normal renal function.
<10	Dose as in normal renal function.

DOSE IN PATIENTS UNDERGOING RENAL REPLACEMENT THERAPIES

CAPD	Unknown dialysability. Dose as in normal renal function.
HD	Not dialysed. Dose as in normal renal function.
HDF/High flux	Unknown dialysability. Dose as in normal renal function.
CAV/ VVHD	Unknown dialysability. Dose as in normal renal function.

IMPORTANT DRUG INTERACTIONS

Potentially hazardous interactions with other
drugs
- Antidepressants: antagonism of
  anticonvulsant effect (convulsive threshold
  lowered); avoid with St John's wort.
- Anti-epileptics: concentration reduced
  by phenytoin, carbamazepine and
  phenobarbital.
- Antimalarials: mefloquine antagonises
  anticonvulsant.
- Antipsychotics: anticonvulsant effect
  antagonised.
- Orlistat: possibly increased risk of
  convulsions.

ADMINISTRATION

RECONSTITUTION
–
ROUTE
- Oral
RATE OF ADMINISTRATION
–
COMMENTS
–

OTHER INFORMATION

- Although there is no evidence of
  withdrawal seizures, it is recommended
  to taper off treatment over a period of
  2–3 weeks.
- Oral bioavailability is 89%.

Tiaprofenic acid

CLINICAL USE

NSAID and analgesic

DOSE IN NORMAL RENAL FUNCTION

- 300 mg twice daily
- or 200 mg three times a day

PHARMACOKINETICS

Molecular weight (daltons)	260.3
% Protein binding	97–98
% Excreted unchanged in urine	50 (10% as metabolites)
Volume of distribution (L/kg)	5.4–6.7
Half-life – normal/ ESRF (hrs)	1.5–2/–

METABOLISM

Sparingly metabolised in the liver to two inactive metabolites.

Excretion of tiaprofenic acid and its metabolites are mainly in the urine in the form of acyl glucuronides; some is excreted in the bile.

DOSE IN RENAL IMPAIRMENT GFR (mL/MIN)

20–50	Dose as in normal renal function, but avoid if possible.
10–20	Dose as in normal renal function, but avoid if possible.
<10	Dose as in normal renal function, but only use if on dialysis.

DOSE IN PATIENTS UNDERGOING RENAL REPLACEMENT THERAPIES

CAPD	Unlikely to be dialysed. Dose as in GFR<10 mL/min. See 'Other information'.
HD	Unlikely to be dialysed. Dose as in GFR<10 mL/min. See 'Other information'.
HDF/High flux	Unlikely to be dialysed. Dose as in GFR<10 mL/min. See 'Other information'.
CAV/ VVHD	Unlikely to be dialysed. Dose as in GFR=10–20 mL/min.

IMPORTANT DRUG INTERACTIONS

Potentially hazardous interactions with other drugs

- ACE inhibitors and angiotensin-II antagonists: antagonism of hypotensive effect; increased risk of nephrotoxicity and hyperkalaemia.
- Analgesics: avoid concomitant use of 2 or more NSAIDs, including aspirin (increased side effects); avoid with ketorolac (increased risk of side effects and haemorrhage).
- Antibacterials: possibly increased risk of convulsions with quinolones.
- Anticoagulants: effects of coumarins and phenindione enhanced; possibly increased risk of bleeding with heparins and dabigatran.
- Antidepressants: increased risk of bleeding with SSRIs and venlafaxine.
- Antidiabetic agents: effects of sulphonylureas enhanced.
- Anti-epileptics: possibly increased phenytoin concentration.
- Antivirals: increased risk of haematological toxicity with zidovudine; concentration increased by ritonavir.
- Ciclosporin: may potentiate nephrotoxicity.
- Cytotoxic agents: reduced excretion of methotrexate; increased risk of bleeding with erlotinib.
- Diuretics: increased risk of nephrotoxicity; antagonism of diuretic effect; hyperkalaemia with potassium-sparing diuretics.
- Lithium: excretion decreased.
- Pentoxifylline: increased risk of bleeding.
- Tacrolimus: increased risk of nephrotoxicity.

ADMINISTRATION

RECONSTITUTION

–

ROUTE

- Oral

RATE OF ADMINISTRATION

–

COMMENTS

–

OTHER INFORMATION

- Inhibition of renal prostaglandin synthesis by NSAIDs may interfere with renal function, especially in the presence of existing renal disease – avoid if possible; if not, check serum creatinine 48–72 hours after starting NSAID – if serum creatinine is increased, stop NSAID.
- Use normal doses in patients with CKD 5 if on dialysis and do not pass any urine.
- Use with caution in renal transplant recipients – can reduce intrarenal autocoid synthesis.

Ticagrelor

CLINICAL USE

Anti-platelet agent

DOSE IN NORMAL RENAL FUNCTION

180 mg loading dose followed by 90 mg twice daily in combination with aspirin

PHARMACOKINETICS

Molecular weight (daltons)	522.6
% Protein binding	>99
% Excreted unchanged in urine	<1
Volume of distribution (L/kg)	87.5 litres
Half-life – normal/ ESRF (hrs)	7/–

METABOLISM

CYP3A4 is the major enzyme responsible for ticagrelor metabolism and the formation of the active metabolite and their interactions with other CYP3A substrates ranges from activation through to inhibition.

The systemic exposure to the active metabolite is approximately 30–40% of that obtained for ticagrelor.

The primary route of ticagrelor elimination is via hepatic metabolism. The primary route of elimination for the active metabolite is most likely via biliary secretion.

DOSE IN RENAL IMPAIRMENT GFR (mL/MIN)

20–50	Dose as in normal renal function.
10–20	Dose as in normal renal function.
<10	Dose as in normal renal function.

DOSE IN PATIENTS UNDERGOING RENAL REPLACEMENT THERAPIES

CAPD	Not dialysed. Dose as in normal renal function.
HD	Not dialysed. Dose as in normal renal function.
HDF/High flux	Unlikely to be dialysed. Dose as in normal renal function.
CAV/ VVHD	Unlikely to be dialysed. Dose as in normal renal function.

IMPORTANT DRUG INTERACTIONS

Potentially hazardous interactions with other drugs

- Antibacterials: concentration possibly increased by clarithromycin – avoid concomitant use; concentration possibly increased by erythromycin; concentration reduced by rifampicin.
- Antifungals: concentration increased by ketoconazole – avoid concomitant use.
- Antivirals: concentration possibly increased by atazanavir and ritonavir – avoid concomitant use.
- Cardiac glycosides: concentration of digoxin increased.
- Ciclosporin: possibly increases ciclosporin concentration.
- Ergot alkaloids: concentration of ergot alkaloids possibly increased.
- Lipid-regulating drugs: concentration of simvastatin increased – increased risk of toxicity.

ADMINISTRATION

RECONSTITUTION

–

ROUTE

- Oral

RATE OF ADMINISTRATION

–

OTHER INFORMATION

- Manufacturer doesn't recommend use in dialysis patients due to lack of data.
- Oral bioavailability is 36%.

Tigecycline

CLINICAL USE

Antibacterial agent

DOSE IN NORMAL RENAL FUNCTION

Loading dose of 100 mg, then 50 mg twice daily

PHARMACOKINETICS

Molecular weight (daltons)	585.6
% Protein binding	71–89
% Excreted unchanged in urine	22
Volume of distribution (L/kg)	7–9
Half-life – normal/ ESRF (hrs)	42/Probably unchanged

METABOLISM

Tigecycline is not thought to be extensively metabolised, although some trace metabolites have been identified including a glucuronide, an N-acetyl metabolite, and a tigecycline epimer. Tigecycline is primarily eliminated (about 60%) via biliary excretion of unchanged drug and some metabolites.

DOSE IN RENAL IMPAIRMENT GFR (mL/MIN)

20–50	Dose as in normal renal function.
10–20	Dose as in normal renal function.
<10	Dose as in normal renal function.

DOSE IN PATIENTS UNDERGOING RENAL REPLACEMENT THERAPIES

CAPD	Not dialysed. Dose as in normal renal function.
HD	Not dialysed. Dose as in normal renal function.
HDF/High flux	Unknown dialysability. Dose as in normal renal function.
CAV/ VVHD	Unknown dialysability. Dose as in normal renal function.

IMPORTANT DRUG INTERACTIONS

Potentially hazardous interactions with other drugs
- Anticoagulants: possibly enhanced anticoagulant effect of coumarins.
- Oestrogens: possibly reduced contraceptive effects of oestrogens (risk probably small).

ADMINISTRATION

RECONSTITUTION
- 5.3 mL of sodium chloride 0.9% or glucose 5% (gently swirl to reconstitute)

ROUTE
- IV infusion

RATE OF ADMINISTRATION
- 30–60 minutes

COMMENTS
- Add required dose to 100 mL of sodium chloride 0.9% or glucose 5%.

OTHER INFORMATION

- AUC increased by 30% in CKD 5.

Timentin (ticarcillin/clavulanic acid)

CLINICAL USE

Antibacterial agent

DOSE IN NORMAL RENAL FUNCTION

3.2 g every 6–8 hours, increased to every 4 hours in severe infections

PHARMACOKINETICS

Molecular weight (daltons)	Ticarcillin (as Na) 428.4, Clavulanic acid 199.2
% Protein binding	Ticarcillin 50, Clavulanic acid 25
% Excreted unchanged in urine	Ticarcillin 85–90, Clavulanic acid 40
Volume of distribution (L/kg)	Ticarcillin 0.14–0.21, Clavulanic acid 0.3
Half-life – normal/ ESRF (hrs)	Ticarcillin 1.2/15, Clavulanic acid 1/3–4

METABOLISM

The major route of elimination for ticarcillin is in the urine via glomerular filtration and tubular secretion. Ticarcillin is also metabolised to a limited extent. Up to 90% of a dose is excreted unchanged in the urine, mostly within 6 hours after a dose. Plasma concentrations are enhanced by probenecid. Clavulanate is also excreted via the kidneys.

DOSE IN RENAL IMPAIRMENT GFR (mL/MIN)

>30	3.2 g every 8 hours
10–30	1.6 g every 8 hours
<10	1.6 g every 12 hours

DOSE IN PATIENTS UNDERGOING RENAL REPLACEMENT THERAPIES

CAPD	Dialysed. Dose as in GFR<10 mL/min.
HD	Dialysed. Dose as in GFR<10 mL/min.
HDF/High flux	Dialysed. Dose as in GFR<10 mL/min.
CAV/VVH	Unknown dialysability. Dose as in GFR=10–30 mL/min or 2.4 g every 6–8 hours.[1]
CVVHD/HDF	Dialysed. 3.2 g every 6 hours.[1]

IMPORTANT DRUG INTERACTIONS

Potentially hazardous interactions with other drugs
- Anticoagulants: effects of coumarins are potentially enhanced.
- Oral contraceptives: potentially reduced efficacy.
- Methotrexate: reduced excretion thereby increasing risk of toxicity.

ADMINISTRATION

RECONSTITUTION
- With 10 mL water for injection and add to 100 mL glucose 5%
ROUTE
- IV
RATE OF ADMINISTRATION
- 30–40 minutes
COMMENTS
- Each 3.2 g of ticarcillin/clavulanic acid contains 16 mmol of sodium and 1 mmol of potassium.

OTHER INFORMATION

- CSM has advised that cholestatic jaundice may occur if treatment exceeds a period of 14 days and can present up to 6 weeks after treatment has been stopped. The incidence of cholestatic jaundice occurring with timentin is higher in males than in females and is particularly prevalent in men over the age of 65 years.

Reference:
1. Trotman RL. Antibiotic dosing in critically ill adult patients receiving continuous renal replacement therapy. *Clinical Infectious Diseases*. 2005 Oct 15; **41**: 1159–66.

Timolol maleate

CLINICAL USE

Beta-adrenoceptor blocker
- Hypertension
- Angina
- Glaucoma
- Migraine prophylaxis

DOSE IN NORMAL RENAL FUNCTION

- Hypertension: 10–60 mg daily, doses >30 mg in divided doses
- Angina: 5–30 mg twice daily
- Post MI: 5–10 mg twice daily
- Migraine: 10–20 mg daily in 1–2 divided doses

PHARMACOKINETICS

Molecular weight (daltons)	432.5
% Protein binding	10
% Excreted unchanged in urine	5
Volume of distribution (L/kg)	1.7
Half-life – normal/ESRF (hrs)	4/Unchanged

METABOLISM

Timolol undergoes significant hepatic metabolism, but first pass metabolism is low. The metabolites are excreted in the urine with some unchanged timolol.

DOSE IN RENAL IMPAIRMENT GFR (mL/MIN)

20–50	Dose as in normal renal function.
10–20	Dose as in normal renal function. Start with lowest dose and titrate according to response.
<10	Dose as in normal renal function. Start with lowest dose and titrate according to response.

DOSE IN PATIENTS UNDERGOING RENAL REPLACEMENT THERAPIES

CAPD	Not dialysed. Dose as in GFR<10 mL/min.
HD	Not dialysed. Dose as in GFR<10 mL/min.
HDF/High flux	Unknown dialysability. Dose as in GFR<10 mL/min.
CAV/ VVHD	Unknown dialysability. Dose as in GFR=10–20 mL/min.

IMPORTANT DRUG INTERACTIONS

Potentially hazardous interactions with other drugs
- Anaesthetics: enhanced hypotensive effect.
- Analgesics: NSAIDs antagonise hypotensive effect.
- Anti-arrhythmics: increased risk of myocardial depression and bradycardia; increased risk of bradycardia, myocardial depression and AV block with amiodarone; increased risk of myocardial depression and bradycardia with flecainide.
- Antidepressants: enhanced hypotensive effect with MAOIs.
- Antihypertensives; enhanced hypotensive effect; increased risk of withdrawal hypertension with clonidine; increased risk of first dose hypotensive effect with post-synaptic alpha-blockers such as prazosin.
- Antimalarials: increased risk of bradycardia with mefloquine.
- Antipsychotics: enhanced hypotensive effect with phenothiazines.
- Calcium-channel blockers: increased risk of bradycardia and AV block with diltiazem; hypotension and heart failure possible with nifedipine and nisoldipine; asystole, severe hypotension and heart failure with verapamil.
- Cytotoxics: possible increased risk of bradycardia with crizotinib.
- Diuretics: enhanced hypotensive effect.
- Fingolimod: possibly increased risk of bradycardia.
- Moxisylyte: possible severe postural hypotension.
- Sympathomimetics: severe hypertension with adrenaline and noradrenaline and possibly with dobutamine.

ADMINISTRATION

RECONSTITUTION
–

ROUTE
- Oral, topical

RATE OF ADMINISTRATION
–

COMMENTS
–

OTHER INFORMATION

- Timolol is more hydrophilic than lipophilic.

Tinidazole

CLINICAL USE

Antibacterial agent

DOSE IN NORMAL RENAL FUNCTION

1–2 g daily

PHARMACOKINETICS

Molecular weight (daltons)	247.3
% Protein binding	8–12[1]
% Excreted unchanged in urine	20–25
Volume of distribution (L/kg)	0.61–0.67[1]
Half-life – normal/ ESRF (hrs)	12–14/Unchanged

METABOLISM

Tinidazole is excreted by the liver (up to 5%) and kidneys as unchanged drug and metabolites. An active hydroxy metabolite has been identified.

DOSE IN RENAL IMPAIRMENT GFR (mL/MIN)

20–50	Dose as in normal renal function.
10–20	Dose as in normal renal function.
<10	Dose as in normal renal function.

DOSE IN PATIENTS UNDERGOING RENAL REPLACEMENT THERAPIES

CAPD	Unknown dialysability, but likely to be dialysed. Dose as in normal renal function.
HD	Dialysed. Dose as in normal renal function.
HDF/High flux	Dialysed. Dose as in normal renal function.
CAV/ VVHD	Dialysed. Dose as in normal renal function.

IMPORTANT DRUG INTERACTIONS

Potentially hazardous interactions with other drugs
- Alcohol: disulfiram-like reaction.

ADMINISTRATION

RECONSTITUTION
–

ROUTE
- Oral

RATE OF ADMINISTRATION
–

COMMENTS
–

OTHER INFORMATION

- Dosage adjustment in renal failure is not necessary as a decrease in renal clearance is compensated for by increased faecal excretion of tinidazole.
- 43% can be removed during a 6 hour haemodialysis session.[1]

Reference:
1. Flouvat BL. Imbert C, Temperville BP, et al. Pharmacokinetics of tinidazole in chronic renal failure and in patients on haemodialysis. Br J Clin Pharmacol. 1983 Jun; 15(6): 735–41.

Tinzaparin sodium (LMWH)

CLINICAL USE

- Peri- and postoperative surgical thromboprophylaxis
- Treatment of DVT and pulmonary embolism
- Prevention of thrombus formation in extracorporeal circulation during HD

DOSE IN NORMAL RENAL FUNCTION

- General surgery: (low-moderate risk) 3500 IU daily
- Orthopaedic surgery: (high risk) 50 IU/kg or 4500 IU daily
- DVT and PE: 175 IU/kg bodyweight once daily for at least 6 days and until adequate oral anticoagulation is established

PHARMACOKINETICS

Molecular weight (daltons)	5500–7500 (average 6500)
% Protein binding	14
% Excreted unchanged in urine	80–90
Volume of distribution (L/kg)	3.1–5
Half-life – normal/ ESRF (hrs)	1.5/5.2 (detectable anti-Factor Xa activity persists for 24 hours)

METABOLISM

Low molecular weight heparins are partially metabolised by desulphation and depolymerisation. The kidneys are the major site of tinzaparin excretion (approximately 70% based on animal studies).

DOSE IN RENAL IMPAIRMENT GFR (mL/MIN)

20–50	Dose as in normal renal function. See 'Other information'.
<20	Consider a dose reduction. See 'Other information'.

DOSE IN PATIENTS UNDERGOING RENAL REPLACEMENT THERAPIES

CAPD	Not dialysed. Dose as in GFR<20 mL/min.
HD	Not dialysed. Dose as in GFR<20 mL/min.
HDF/High flux	Dialysed. Dose as in GFR<20 mL/min.
CAV/ VVHD	Not dialysed. Dose as in GFR=20–50 mL/min

IMPORTANT DRUG INTERACTIONS

Potentially hazardous interactions with other drugs

- Analgesics: increased risk of bleeding with NSAIDs – avoid concomitant use with IV diclofenac; increased risk of haemorrhage with ketorolac – avoid concomitant use.
- Nitrates: anticoagulant effect reduced by infusions of glyceryl trinitrate.
- Use with care in patients receiving oral anticoagulants, platelet aggregation inhibitors, aspirin or dextran.

ADMINISTRATION

RECONSTITUTION

–

ROUTE

- SC injection
- IV bolus/infusion

RATE OF ADMINISTRATION

- See 'Other information'.

COMMENTS

–

OTHER INFORMATION

- Tinzaparin is also indicated for prevention of clotting in the extracorporeal circulation during haemodialysis.
  - Dose for >4 hour session: IV bolus (into arterial side of the dialyser or intravenously) of 3500–4500 IU
  - Dose for <4 hour session: IV bolus of 2500 IU.
- Additional tinzaparin (500–1000 IU) may be given if concentrated RBCs or blood transfusions are given during dialysis, or additional treatment beyond the normal dialysis duration is employed.
- Determination of plasma anti-Xa levels may be used to monitor the tinzaparin dose during haemodialysis; plasma anti-Xa levels, one hour after dosing should be within the range 0.4–0.5 IU/mL.
- Additional doses may be required if using LMWHs for anticoagulation in intermittent HDF.
- Heparin can suppress adrenal secretion of aldosterone leading to hyperkalaemia particularly in patients with chronic renal impairment and diabetes mellitus.

- Low molecular weight heparins are renally excreted and hence accumulate in severe renal impairment. While the doses recommended for prophylaxis against DVT and prevention of thrombus formation in extracorporeal circuits are well tolerated in patients with CKD 5, the doses recommended for treatment of DVT and PE have not yet been verified as safe. LMWHs have been associated with severe, sometimes fatal, bleeding episodes in such patients. Hence the use of unfractionated heparin would be preferable in these instances.
- Information from Leo Pharma states that tinzaparin can safely be used in elderly patients with a GFR>20 mL/min for 10 days without any accumulation.

(Nagge J. Is impaired renal function a contraindication to the use of low-molecular weight heparin? *Arch Intern Med.* 2002; **162**: 2605–9.)
(Siguret V. Elderly patients treated with tinzaparin (Innohep) administered once daily (175 anti-Xa IU/kg): anti-Xa and anti-IIa activities over 10 days. *Thromb Haemostat.* 2000; **84**: 800–4.)

- Some units routinely use a dose of 125 anti Xa IU/kg in patients with GFR<20 mL/min who require full anticoagulation.
- Use 1 mg of protamine for every 100 anti-Xa IU to neutralise the effects of tinzaparin. If prothrombin time is still raised 2–4 hours later, give 0.5 mg/kg infusion of protamine.

Tioguanine

CLINICAL USE

Antineoplastic agent (antimetabolite)
● Acute leukaemia
● Chronic granulocytic leukaemia

DOSE IN NORMAL RENAL FUNCTION

100–200 mg/m² daily

PHARMACOKINETICS

Molecular weight (daltons)	167.2
% Protein binding	Probably low
% Excreted unchanged in urine	40
Volume of distribution (L/kg)	0.148
Half-life – normal/ ESRF (hrs)	80 minutes/–

METABOLISM

Tioguanine undergoes extensive metabolism in the liver and other tissues to several active and inactive metabolites. Tioguanine is inactivated mainly by methylation to aminomethylthiopurine; small amounts are deaminated to thioxanthine, and may go on to be oxidised by xanthine oxidase to thiouric acid, but inactivation is essentially independent of xanthine oxidase and is not affected by inhibition of the enzyme. Some 24–46% of the dose is excreted in the urine within 24 hours. It is excreted in the urine almost entirely as metabolites.

DOSE IN RENAL IMPAIRMENT GFR (mL/MIN)

20–50	Dose as in normal renal function, use with care. See 'Other information'.
10–20	Dose as in normal renal function, use with care. See 'Other information'.
<10	Dose as in normal renal function, use with care. See 'Other information'.

DOSE IN PATIENTS UNDERGOING RENAL REPLACEMENT THERAPIES

CAPD	Unknown dialysability. Dose as in GFR<10 mL/min.
HD	Not dialysed. Dose as in GFR<10 mL/min.
HDF/High flux	Unknown dialysability. Dose as in GFR<10 mL/min.
CAV/ VVHD	Unknown dialysability. Dose as in GFR=10–20 mL/min.

IMPORTANT DRUG INTERACTIONS

Potentially hazardous interactions with other drugs
● Antipsychotics: avoid concomitant use with clozapine (increased risk of agranulocytosis).

ADMINISTRATION

RECONSTITUTION
–
ROUTE
● Oral
RATE OF ADMINISTRATION
–
COMMENTS
–

OTHER INFORMATION

● Variable and incomplete oral absorption with 14–46% bioavailability.
● *Drug Prescribing in Renal Failure*, 5th edition, by Aronoff *et al.* suggests using 100% of dose as tioguanine is hepatically metabolised.

Reference:
1. Kintzel PE, Dorr RT. Anticancer drug renal toxicity and elimination: dosing guidelines for altered renal function. *Cancer Treat Rev.* 1995; **21**: 33–64.

Tiotropium

CLINICAL USE

Maintenance treatment of chronic obstructive pulmonary disease

DOSE IN NORMAL RENAL FUNCTION

- 18 micrograms once daily
- Respimat: 5 micrograms once daily

PHARMACOKINETICS

Molecular weight (daltons)	472.4 (as bromide)
% Protein binding	72
% Excreted unchanged in urine	14 (of inhaled dose)
Volume of distribution (L/kg)	32
Half-life – normal/ ESRF (hrs)	5–6 days/Increased

METABOLISM

Tiotropium is excreted largely unchanged in the urine, although it may undergo some metabolism by non-enzymatic cleavage and by the cytochrome P450 isoenzymes CYP2D6 and CYP3A4.

DOSE IN RENAL IMPAIRMENT GFR (mL/MIN)

20–50	Dose as in normal renal function.
10–20	Dose as in normal renal function. Use with caution.
<10	Dose as in normal renal function. Use with caution.

DOSE IN PATIENTS UNDERGOING RENAL REPLACEMENT THERAPIES

CAPD	Unknown dialysability. Dose as in normal renal function. Use with caution.
HD	Unknown dialysability. Dose as in normal renal function. Use with caution.
HDF/High flux	Unknown dialysability. Dose as in normal renal function. Use with caution.
CAV/VVHD	Unknown dialysability. Dose as in normal renal function. Use with caution.

IMPORTANT DRUG INTERACTIONS

Potentially hazardous interactions with other drugs

- Avoid administration with other anticholinergic drugs.
- Anti-arrhythmics: increased risk of antimuscarinic side effects with disopyramide.

ADMINISTRATION

RECONSTITUTION
–
ROUTE
- Inhalation
RATE OF ADMINISTRATION
–
COMMENTS
–

OTHER INFORMATION

- Manufacturer advises to use with caution due to reduced renal clearance. In practice used in normal doses in renal impairment.
- Not to be used for acute episodes of bronchospasm.

Tipranavir

CLINICAL USE

Protease inhibitor:
- Treatment of HIV infected patients in combination with ritonavir and other antiretroviral agents

DOSE IN NORMAL RENAL FUNCTION

500 mg twice daily in combination with ritonavir 200 mg twice daily

PHARMACOKINETICS

Molecular weight (daltons)	602.7
% Protein binding	>99.9
% Excreted unchanged in urine	0.5
Volume of distribution (L/kg)	7.7–10.2
Half-life – normal/ ESRF (hrs)	5.5–6/Unchanged

METABOLISM

Tipranavir is metabolised by the cytochrome P450 system (mainly the isoenzyme CYP3A4), although when given with ritonavir metabolism is minimal with the majority of tipranavir being excreted unchanged in the faeces.

DOSE IN RENAL IMPAIRMENT GFR (mL/MIN)

20–50	Dose as in normal renal function.
10–20	Dose as in normal renal function.
<10	Dose as in normal renal function.

DOSE IN PATIENTS UNDERGOING RENAL REPLACEMENT THERAPIES

CAPD	Not dialysed. Dose as in normal renal function.
HD	Not dialysed. Dose as in normal renal function.
HDF/High flux	Not dialysed. Dose as in normal renal function.
CAV/ VVHD	Not dialysed. Dose as in normal renal function.

IMPORTANT DRUG INTERACTIONS

Potentially hazardous interactions with other drugs
- Antacids: avoid giving for 2 hours after tipranavir administration.
- Antibacterials: plasma concentration of clarithromycin and other macrolides increased – reduce dose of clarithromycin in renal impairment; concentration increased by clarithromycin; rifabutin concentration increased (risk of uveitis) – reduce dose; concentration possibly reduced by rifampicin – avoid concomitant use; avoid concomitant use with telithromycin in severe renal and hepatic failure.
- Antidepressants: concentration possibly reduced by St John's wort – avoid concomitant use.
- Antimalarials: use artemether/ lumefantrine with caution; concentration of quinine increased.
- Antipsychotics: possibly increases quetiapine concentration – avoid.
- Antivirals: reduces concentration of abacavir, didanosine, fosamprenavir, lopinavir, saquinavir and zidovudine; concentration increased by atazanavir, also concentration of atazanavir reduced; concentration reduced by etravirine, also concentration of tipranavir increased – avoid.
- Beta-blockers: avoid concomitant use with metoprolol for heart failure.
- Ciclosporin: levels possibly altered by tipranavir.
- Lipid-lowering drugs: increased risk of myopathy with atorvastatin, max dose 10 mg; concentration of rosuvastatin and simvastatin increased – avoid concomitant use.[1]
- Ranolazine: possibly increases ranolazine concentration – avoid.
- Sirolimus: levels possibly altered by tipranavir.
- Tacrolimus: levels possibly altered by tipranavir.
- Ulcer-healing drugs: concentration of esomeprazole and omeprazole reduced.

ADMINISTRATION

RECONSTITUTION
–
ROUTE
- Oral
RATE OF ADMINISTRATION
–
COMMENTS
–

OTHER INFORMATION

- Administer with food; enhanced bioavailability with high fat meals.

Reference:

1. MHRA. *Drug Safety Update*. Statins: interactions and updated advice. August 2012; **6**(1): 2–4.

Tirofiban

CLINICAL USE

Antiplatelet agent
- Prevention of early myocardial infarction in patients with unstable angina or non-ST segment elevation myocardial infarction, and with last episode of chest pain within 12 hours

DOSE IN NORMAL RENAL FUNCTION

- Angiography planned for 4–48 hours after diagnosis: Initially 0.4 mcg/kg/minute for 30 minutes then 0.1 mcg/kg/minute for at least 48 hours.
- Angiography within 4 hours of diagnosis: 25 mcg/kg over 3 minutes then 0.15 mcg/kg/minute for 18–24 hours. Max 48 hours.

PHARMACOKINETICS

Molecular weight (daltons)	495.1
% Protein binding	65
% Excreted unchanged in urine	66
Volume of distribution (L/kg)	22–42 litres
Half-life – normal/ ESRF (hrs)	1.5–2/Increased

METABOLISM

Tirofiban is eliminated largely unchanged in the urine, with some biliary excretion in the faeces.

DOSE IN RENAL IMPAIRMENT GFR (mL/MIN)

30–50	Dose as in normal renal function.
10–30	Give 50% of dose.
<10	Give 50% of dose.

DOSE IN PATIENTS UNDERGOING RENAL REPLACEMENT THERAPIES

CAPD	Unknown dialysability. Dose as in GFR<10 mL/min.
HD	Dialysed. Dose as in GFR<10 mL/min.
HDF/High flux	Dialysed. Dose as in GFR<10 mL/min.
CAV/ VVHD	Unknown dialysability. Dose as in GFR=10–30 mL/min.

IMPORTANT DRUG INTERACTIONS

Potentially hazardous interactions with other drugs
- Iloprost: increased risk of bleeding.
- Heparin: increased risk of bleeding.

ADMINISTRATION

RECONSTITUTION
–
ROUTE
- IV infusion
RATE OF ADMINISTRATION
- 0.1–0.4 mcg/kg/minute
COMMENTS
- Add 50 mL of the concentrate (250 mcg/mL) to 250 mL sodium chloride 0.9% or glucose 5%, to give a final concentration of 50 mcg/mL (remove 50 mL from bag first).

OTHER INFORMATION

- Antiplatelet effect lasts for about 4–8 hours after stopping infusion.
- Main side effect is bleeding.
- Increased risk of bleeding once renal function falls to a GFR<60 mL/min – monitor carefully.

Tizanidine

CLINICAL USE

Spasticity associated with multiple sclerosis or spinal cord injury/disease.

DOSE IN NORMAL RENAL FUNCTION

2–24 mg daily in up to 3–4 divided doses (depending on response)
Max 36 mg daily

PHARMACOKINETICS

Molecular weight (daltons)	290.2 (as hydrochloride)
% Protein binding	30
% Excreted unchanged in urine	<1[1]
Volume of distribution (L/kg)	2.4
Half-life – normal/ ESRF (hrs)	2.4/Increased

METABOLISM

Tizanidine undergoes rapid and extensive first-pass metabolism in the liver mainly via the cytochrome P450 isoenzyme CYP1A2. The metabolites (mainly inactive) constitute 70% of the administered dose and are excreted via the renal route.

DOSE IN RENAL IMPAIRMENT GFR (mL/MIN)

25–50	Dose as in normal renal function.
<25	Initial dose 2 mg once daily and slowly increase by 2 mg increments. Increase daily dose before increasing frequency of administration.

DOSE IN PATIENTS UNDERGOING RENAL REPLACEMENT THERAPIES

CAPD	Unknown dialysability. Dose as in GFR<25 mL/min.
HD	Unknown dialysability. Dose as in GFR<25 mL/min.
HDF/High flux	Unknown dialysability. Dose as in GFR<25 mL/min.
CAV/ VVHD	Unknown dialysability. Dose as in GFR=25–50 mL/min.

IMPORTANT DRUG INTERACTIONS

Potentially hazardous interactions with other drugs

- Anti-arrhythmics: enhanced muscle relaxant effect with procainamide.
- Antibacterials: concentration increased by ciprofloxacin – avoid concomitant use; concentration possibly increased by norfloxacin; concentration possibly reduced by rifampicin.
- Antidepressants: concentration increased by fluvoxamine – avoid.
- Antihypertensives: enhanced hypotensive effect.
- Oral contraceptives: clearance of tizanidine reduced by 50%.

ADMINISTRATION

RECONSTITUTION
–
ROUTE
- Oral
RATE OF ADMINISTRATION
–
COMMENTS
–

OTHER INFORMATION

- Pharmacokinetic data suggest that renal clearance in the elderly may be decreased by up to 3-fold.
- May induce hypotension; therefore may potentiate the effect of antihypertensive drugs, including diuretics – exercise caution.
- With beta-blockers or digoxin, may potentiate hypotension or bradycardia.
- LFTs should be monitored monthly for the first 4 months.

Reference:
1. Shellenberger MK. A controlled pharmacokinetic evaluation of tizanidine and baclofen at steady state. *Drug Metab Dispos*. 1999; **27**(2): 201–4.

Tobramycin

CLINICAL USE

Antibacterial agent

DOSE IN NORMAL RENAL FUNCTION

- IM/IV: 3 mg/kg/day in 3 divided doses; maximum 5 mg/kg/day in 3–4 divided doses
- Urinary tract infections: 2–3 mg/kg daily as a single dose (IM)

PHARMACOKINETICS

Molecular weight (daltons)	467.5
% Protein binding	<5
% Excreted unchanged in urine	90
Volume of distribution (L/kg)	0.25
Half-life – normal/ ESRF (hrs)	2–3/5–70

METABOLISM

Tobramycin is almost completely eliminated by the kidneys and the drug is eliminated unchanged almost entirely by glomerular filtration.

DOSE IN RENAL IMPAIRMENT GFR (mL/MIN)

20–50	Give 1–2 mg/kg then dose according to serum levels.
10–20	Give 1 mg/kg then dose according to serum levels.
<10	Give 1 mg/kg then dose according to serum levels.

DOSE IN PATIENTS UNDERGOING RENAL REPLACEMENT THERAPIES

CAPD	Dialysed. Dose as in GFR<10 mL/min.
HD	Dialysed. Dose as in GFR<10 mL/min.
HDF/High flux	Dialysed. Dose as in GFR<10 mL/min.
CAV/VVHD	Dialysed. 1.5–2 mg/kg every 24 hours and monitor levels.[1]

IMPORTANT DRUG INTERACTIONS

Potentially hazardous interactions with other drugs
- Antibacterials: increased risk of nephrotoxicity with colistimethate or polymyxins and possibly cephalosporins; increased risk of ototoxicity and nephrotoxicity with capreomycin or vancomycin.
- Ciclosporin: increased risk of nephrotoxicity.
- Cytotoxics: increased risk of nephrotoxicity and possibly of ototoxicity with platinum compounds.
- Diuretics: increased risk of ototoxicity with loop diuretics.
- Muscle relaxants: enhanced effect of non-depolarising muscle relaxants and suxamethonium.
- Parasympathomimetics: antagonism of effect of neostigmine and pyridostigmine.
- Tacrolimus: increased risk of nephrotoxicity.

ADMINISTRATION

RECONSTITUTION
- Add to 50–100 mL sodium chloride 0.9% or glucose 5% for IV infusion.
ROUTE
- IV, IM, IP, nebulised
RATE OF ADMINISTRATION
- 20–60 minutes
COMMENTS
- Plasma concentrations should be measured frequently; trough ≤2 mg/L, peak 60 minutes post dose ≤10 mg/L; avoid prolonged peaks above 12 mg/L.

OTHER INFORMATION

- 25–70% can be removed by haemodialysis.
- Used via nebuliser for chronic pulmonary *Pseudomonas aeruginosa* infection in cystic fibrosis: 300 mg every 12 hours for 28 days, repeat after 28 days.
- Can be used for peritonitis at doses of 6 mg/L intraperitoneally.

Reference:
1. Dose from CVVH Initial Drug Dosing Guidelines on www.thedrugmonitor.com.

Tocilizumab

CLINICAL USE

Interleukin inhibitor
- Treatment of rheumatoid arthritis in combination with methotrexate

DOSE IN NORMAL RENAL FUNCTION

8 mg/kg every 4 weeks
(maximum dose: 800 mg)

PHARMACOKINETICS

Molecular weight (daltons)	148 000
% Protein binding	Not applicable
% Excreted unchanged in urine	No data
Volume of distribution (L/kg)	6.4 litres
Half-life – normal/ ESRF (hrs)	11–13 days (concentration dependent)/–

METABOLISM

Tocilizumab undergoes biphasic elimination from the circulation.

DOSE IN RENAL IMPAIRMENT GFR (mL/MIN)

20–50	Dose as in normal renal function. Use with caution.
10–20	Dose as in normal renal function. Use with caution.
<10	Dose as in normal renal function. Use with caution.

DOSE IN PATIENTS UNDERGOING RENAL REPLACEMENT THERAPIES

CAPD	Unknown dialysability. Dose as in normal renal function. Use with caution.
HD	Unknown dialysability. Dose as in normal renal function. Use with caution.
HDF/High flux	Unknown dialysability. Dose as in normal renal function. Use with caution.
CAV/ VVHD	Unknown dialysability. Dose as in normal renal function. Use with caution.

IMPORTANT DRUG INTERACTIONS

Potentially hazardous interactions with other drugs
- Live vaccines: avoid concomitant administration.

ADMINISTRATION

RECONSTITUTION
–
ROUTE
- IV
RATE OF ADMINISTRATION
- Over 60 minutes
COMMENTS
- Add to 100 mL sodium chloride 0.9%

OTHER INFORMATION

- There have been no studies in moderate to severe renal impairment. Manufacturer advises to monitor renal function closely.
- Contains 1.17 mmol (26.55 mg) sodium per 1200 mg.
- There is a case report of tocilizumab being used safely and effectively in a patient with eGFR of 26 mL/min. (Kato T, Koni I, Inoue R, et al. A case of active rheumatoid arthritis with renal dysfunction treated effectively with tocilizumab monotherapy. Mod Rheumatol. 2010; 20: 316–18.)

Tolbutamide

CLINICAL USE

Hypoglycaemic agent for non-insulin dependent diabetes

DOSE IN NORMAL RENAL FUNCTION

0.5–2 g daily in divided doses

PHARMACOKINETICS

Molecular weight (daltons)	270.3
% Protein binding	95–97
% Excreted unchanged in urine	0
Volume of distribution (L/kg)	0.1–0.15
Half-life – normal/ ESRF (hrs)	4–7/Unchanged

METABOLISM

Tolbutamide is metabolised in the liver by hydroxylation mediated by the cytochrome P450 isoenzyme CYP2C9.

It is excreted in the urine chiefly as inactive metabolites.

DOSE IN RENAL IMPAIRMENT GFR (mL/MIN)

20–50	Dose as in normal renal function. Use with caution.
10–20	Dose as in normal renal function. Use with caution.
<10	Dose as in normal renal function. Use with caution.

DOSE IN PATIENTS UNDERGOING RENAL REPLACEMENT THERAPIES

CAPD	Unlikely to be dialysed. Dose as in GFR<10 mL/min.
HD	Not dialysed. Dose as in GFR<10 mL/min.
HDF/High flux	Unlikely to be dialysed. Dose as in GFR<10 mL/min.
CAV/ VVHD	Not dialysed. Dose as in GFR=10–20 mL/min.

IMPORTANT DRUG INTERACTIONS

Potentially hazardous interactions with other drugs

- Analgesics: effects enhanced by NSAIDs – avoid with azapropazone.
- Antibacterials: effects enhanced by chloramphenicol, sulphonamides, tetracyclines and trimethoprim; effect reduced by rifamycins.
- Anticoagulants: effect possibly enhanced by coumarins; also possibly changes to INR.
- Antifungals: concentration increased by fluconazole and miconazole, and possibly voriconazole.
- Lipid-regulating drugs: possibly additive hypoglycaemic effect with fibrates.
- Sulfinpyrazone: enhanced effect of sulphonylureas.

ADMINISTRATION

RECONSTITUTION
–
ROUTE
- Oral
RATE OF ADMINISTRATION
–
COMMENTS
–

OTHER INFORMATION

- Tolbutamide is not removed by dialysis. It is contraindicated in severe renal impairment, and should be started with a lower dose in mild to moderate renal impairment because of risk of hypoglycaemia.
- *Drug Prescribing in Renal Failure*, 5th edition, by Aronoff *et al.* suggest that 100% of dose can be used.

Tolcapone

CLINICAL USE

Catechol-o-methyltransferase inhibitor:
- Treatment of Parkinson's disease

DOSE IN NORMAL RENAL FUNCTION

- 100 mg three times daily, leave 6 hours between each dose
- In exceptional circumstances can be increased to 200 mg three times daily

PHARMACOKINETICS

Molecular weight (daltons)	273.2
% Protein binding	>99.9
% Excreted unchanged in urine	0.5
Volume of distribution (L/kg)	9 litres
Half-life – normal/ ESRF (hrs)	2–3/Unchanged

METABOLISM

Extensively metabolised, mainly by conjugation to the inactive glucuronide, but methylation by catechol-O-methyltransferase to 3-O-methyltolcapone and metabolism by cytochrome P450 isoenzymes CYP3A4 and CYP2A6 also occurs.

Approximately 60% of a dose is excreted in the urine with the remainder appearing in the faeces.

DOSE IN RENAL IMPAIRMENT GFR (mL/MIN)

20–50	Dose as in normal renal function.
10–20	Use with caution.
<10	Use with caution.

DOSE IN PATIENTS UNDERGOING RENAL REPLACEMENT THERAPIES

CAPD	Unlikely to be dialysed. Dose as GFR<10 mL/min.
HD	Unlikely to be dialysed. Dose as GFR<10 mL/min.
HDF/High flux	Unlikely to be dialysed. Dose as GFR<10 mL/min.
CAV/ VVHD	Unlikely to be dialysed. Dose as GFR=10–30 mL/min.

IMPORTANT DRUG INTERACTIONS

Potentially hazardous interactions with other drugs
- Antidepressants: avoid with MAOIs.

ADMINISTRATION

ROUTE
- Oral

RATE OF ADMINISTRATION
–

OTHER INFORMATION

- Bioavailability is 65%.
- Use with caution due to lack of data, although the pharmacokinetics are relatively unchanged in renal impairment.

Tolfenamic acid

CLINICAL USE

NSAID:
- Treatment of migraine

DOSE IN NORMAL RENAL FUNCTION

200 mg when first symptoms appear; repeat once after 1–2 hours if satisfactory response is not obtained.

PHARMACOKINETICS

Molecular weight (daltons)	261.7
% Protein binding	>99
% Excreted unchanged in urine	8 (90% as metabolites)
Volume of distribution (L/kg)	0.16
Half-life – normal/ ESRF (hrs)	2.5/–

METABOLISM

Tolfenamic acid is metabolised in the liver; the metabolites and unchanged drug are conjugated with glucuronic acid.

About 90% of an ingested dose is excreted in the urine and the remainder in the faeces.

DOSE IN RENAL IMPAIRMENT GFR (mL/MIN)

20–50	Dose as in normal renal function.
10–20	Use with caution and monitor renal function.
<10	Avoid.

DOSE IN PATIENTS UNDERGOING RENAL REPLACEMENT THERAPIES

CAPD	Removal unlikely. Use with caution.
HD	Not dialysed. Use with caution.
HDF/High flux	Unknown dialysability. Use with caution.
CAV/ VVHD	Unlikely to be dialysed. Avoid.

IMPORTANT DRUG INTERACTIONS

Potentially hazardous interactions with other drugs
- ACE inhibitors and angiotensin-II antagonists: antagonism of hypotensive effect; increased risk of nephrotoxicity and hyperkalaemia.
- Analgesics: avoid concomitant use of 2 or more NSAIDs, including aspirin (increased side effects); avoid with ketorolac (increased risk of side effects and haemorrhage).
- Antibacterials: possibly increased risk of convulsions with quinolones.
- Anticoagulants: effects of coumarins and phenindione enhanced; possibly increased risk of bleeding with heparins and dabigatran.
- Antidepressants: increased risk of bleeding with SSRIs and venlafaxine.
- Antidiabetic agents: effects of sulphonylureas enhanced.
- Anti-epileptics: possibly increased phenytoin concentration.
- Antivirals: increased risk of haematological toxicity with zidovudine; concentration possibly increased by ritonavir.
- Ciclosporin: may potentiate nephrotoxicity.
- Cytotoxic agents: reduced excretion of methotrexate; increased risk of bleeding with erlotinib.
- Diuretics: increased risk of nephrotoxicity; antagonism of diuretic effect; hyperkalaemia with potassium-sparing diuretics.
- Lithium: excretion decreased.
- Pentoxifylline: increased risk of bleeding.
- Tacrolimus: increased risk of nephrotoxicity.

ADMINISTRATION

RECONSTITUTION
–

ROUTE
- Oral

RATE OF ADMINISTRATION
–

COMMENTS
–

OTHER INFORMATION

- Contraindicated in significantly impaired kidney or liver function.
- The urine may become a little more lemon-coloured due to coloured metabolites.
- Use only with extreme caution (or not at all) in haemodialysis patients with some degree of urine output, especially if other risk factors are present, e.g.

nephrotic syndrome or diabetes mellitus or treatment with loop diuretics.

- Use normal doses in patients with CKD 5 on dialysis as long as they no longer pass any urine.
- Inhibition of renal prostaglandin synthesis by NSAIDs may interfere with renal function, especially in the presence of existing renal disease – avoid NSAIDs if possible; if not, check serum creatinine 48–72 hours after starting NSAID – if increased, discontinue therapy.
- Use with caution in renal transplant recipients as can reduce intrarenal autocoid synthesis.

Tolterodine tartrate

CLINICAL USE

Treatment of urinary frequency, urgency and incontinence

DOSE IN NORMAL RENAL FUNCTION

- 1–2 mg twice daily
- M/R: 4 mg daily

PHARMACOKINETICS

Molecular weight (daltons)	475.6
% Protein binding	96
% Excreted unchanged in urine	<1
Volume of distribution (L/kg)	0.9–1.6
Half-life – normal/ ESRF (hrs)	2–3 (10 hours in poor metabolisers)/– MR: 6/–

METABOLISM

Tolterodine is mainly metabolised in the liver by the cytochrome P450 isoenzyme CYP2D6 to the active 5-hydroxymethyl derivative; in a minority of poor metabolisers tolterodine is metabolised by CYP3A4 isoenzymes to its inactive N-dealkylated derivative. Tolterodine is excreted primarily in the urine with about 17% appearing in the faeces; less than 1% of a dose is excreted as unchanged drug.

DOSE IN RENAL IMPAIRMENT GFR (mL/MIN)

30–50	Dose as in normal renal function. Use with caution.
10–30	1 mg twice daily. Use with caution.
<10	1 mg twice daily. Use with caution.

DOSE IN PATIENTS UNDERGOING RENAL REPLACEMENT THERAPIES

CAPD	Unlikely to be dialysed. Dose as in GFR<10 mL/min.
HD	Unlikely to be dialysed. Dose as in GFR<10 mL/min.
HDF/High flux	Unlikely to be dialysed. Dose as in GFR<10 mL/min.
CAV/ VVHD	Unlikely to be dialysed. Dose as in GFR<10 mL/min. Unlikely to be dialysed. Dose as in GFR=10– 30 mL/min.

IMPORTANT DRUG INTERACTIONS

Potentially hazardous interactions with other drugs

- Anti-arrhythmics: increased risk of ventricular arrhythmias with amiodarone, disopyramide and flecainide; increased risk of antimuscarinic side effects with disopyramide.
- Antifungals: avoid concomitant use with itraconazole and ketoconazole.
- Antivirals: avoid concomitant use with fosamprenavir, indinavir, lopinavir, ritonavir and saquinavir.
- Beta-blockers: increased risk of ventricular arrhythmias with sotalol.

ADMINISTRATION

RECONSTITUTION
–

ROUTE
- Oral

RATE OF ADMINISTRATION
–

COMMENTS
–

OTHER INFORMATION

- Active metabolites may accumulate in renal failure.
- Bioavailability is 17%.
- Use with caution in patients at risk of QT elongation.

Tolvaptan

CLINICAL USE

Selective vasopressin V_2-receptor antagonist.
- Treatment of hyponatraemia secondary to SIADH
- To slow the progression of adult polycystic kidney disease (unlicensed)

DOSE IN NORMAL RENAL FUNCTION

SIADH: 15–60 mg once daily

PHARMACOKINETICS

Molecular weight (daltons)	448.9
% Protein binding	98
% Excreted unchanged in urine	<1
Volume of distribution (L/kg)	3
Half-life – normal/ ESRF (hrs)	12/–

METABOLISM

Metabolised mainly by the cytochrome P450 isoenzyme CYP3A4.
Eliminated mainly by the faecal route.

DOSE IN RENAL IMPAIRMENT GFR (mL/MIN)

20–50	Dose as in normal renal function.
10–20	Dose as in normal renal function.
<10	Use with care. See 'Other information'.

DOSE IN PATIENTS UNDERGOING RENAL REPLACEMENT THERAPIES

CAPD	Unlikely to be dialysed. Dose as in GFR<10 mL/min.
HD	Unlikely to be dialysed. Dose as in GFR<10 mL/min.
HDF/High flux	Unlikely to be dialysed. Dose as in GFR<10 mL/min.
CAV/ VVHD	Unlikely to be dialysed. Dose as in normal renal function.

IMPORTANT DRUG INTERACTIONS

Potentially hazardous interactions with other drugs
- Grapefruit juice: avoid concomitant administration, exposure increased by a factor of 1.8.

ADMINISTRATION

RECONSTITUTION
–
ROUTE
- Oral
RATE OF ADMINISTRATION
–

OTHER INFORMATION

- Contraindicated in anuric patients. Not recommended in severe renal impairment due to lack of studies.
- If fluid restricted patients are treated with tolvaptan, care should be taken to ensure that patients do not become overly dehydrated.
- Tolvaptan may cause a rapid increase in sodium levels.
- Bioavailability is 56%.
- Cases of severe hepatic failure have been seen in trials for the treatment of adult polycystic kidney disease where higher doses are used.

Topiramate

CLINICAL USE

- Anti-epileptic agent
- Prophylactic treatment of migraine

DOSE IN NORMAL RENAL FUNCTION

- Monotherapy: Epilepsy: 50–500 mg daily in 2 divided doses
- Adjunctive treatment: 200–400 mg daily in 2 divided doses
- Migraine: Initially, 25 mg at night. Maintenance, 50–200 mg daily in 2 divided doses

PHARMACOKINETICS

Molecular weight (daltons)	339.4
% Protein binding	9–17
% Excreted unchanged in urine	81 (as unchanged drug and metabolites)
Volume of distribution (L/kg)	0.55–0.8
Half-life – normal/ ESRF (hrs)	20–30/48–60 (12–15 hours if used with another enzyme-inducing anti-epileptic drug)

METABOLISM

Topiramate is not extensively metabolised (~20%) in healthy volunteers. It is metabolised up to 50% in patients receiving enzyme-inducing drugs. Six metabolites formed through hydroxylation, hydrolysis and glucuronidation have been identified but have little activity. It is eliminated chiefly in urine, as unchanged drug and metabolites.

DOSE IN RENAL IMPAIRMENT GFR (mL/MIN)

20–50	Dose as in normal renal function.
10–20	Initially 50% of normal dose and increase according to response.
<10	Initially 50% of normal dose and increase according to response.

DOSE IN PATIENTS UNDERGOING RENAL REPLACEMENT THERAPIES

CAPD	Unknown dialysability. Dose as for GFR<10 mL/min.
HD	Dialysed. Dose as for GFR<10 mL/min.
HDF/High flux	Dialysed. Dose as for GFR<10 mL/min.
CAV/ VVHD	Dialysed. Dose as for GFR=10–20 mL/min.

IMPORTANT DRUG INTERACTIONS

Potentially hazardous interactions with other drugs

- Antidepressants: antagonism of anticonvulsant effect; avoid with St John's wort.
- Anti-epileptics: concentration reduced by phenytoin and carbamazepine and possibly phenobarbital; increases phenytoin concentration; reduces concentration of perampanel; hyperammonaemia and CNS toxicity reported with valproate.
- Antimalarials: mefloquine antagonises anticonvulsant effect.
- Antipsychotics: anticonvulsant effect antagonised.
- Oestrogens and progestogens: reduced contraceptive effect.
- Orlistat: possibly increased risk of convulsions.

ADMINISTRATION

RECONSTITUTION

–

ROUTE

- Oral

RATE OF ADMINISTRATION

–

COMMENTS

–

OTHER INFORMATION

- Patients with moderate to severe renal impairment may take 10–15 days to reach steady state, compared to 4–8 days in patients with normal renal function.
- A higher frequency of renal stones has been noted in topiramate treated patients, although the risk is not related to dose or duration of therapy. Adequate hydration is recommended to reduce this risk.

Topotecan

CAV/   Dialysed. Dose as in GFR=20–
VVHD   39 mL/min.

CLINICAL USE

Antineoplastic agent:
- Treatment of metastatic ovarian, cervical and small cell lung cancer

DOSE IN NORMAL RENAL FUNCTION

- IV: 0.75–1.5 mg/m^2 for 5 days, repeated every 3 weeks
- Oral: 2.3 mg/m^2 for 5 days, repeated every 3 weeks

PHARMACOKINETICS

Molecular weight (daltons)	457.9 (as hydrochloride)
% Protein binding	35
% Excreted unchanged in urine	51
Volume of distribution (L/kg)	132 litres +/– 57
Half-life – normal/ ESRF (hrs)	2–3/4.9 (in moderate renal failure)

METABOLISM

Topotecan undergoes reversible, pH-dependent hydrolysis of the active lactone moiety to the inactive hydroxyacid (carboxylate) form. A relatively small amount of topotecan is metabolised by hepatic microsomal enzymes to an active metabolite, N-demethyltopotecan; the clinical significance of this metabolite is not known. Excretion is via biliary and renal routes with 20–60% excreted in the urine as topotecan or the open ring form.

DOSE IN RENAL IMPAIRMENT GFR (mL/MIN)

40–59	Dose as in normal renal function. See 'Other information'.
20–39	IV: 50% of dose. See 'Other information'.
<20	IV: 25% of dose. Use with caution. See 'Other information'.

DOSE IN PATIENTS UNDERGOING RENAL REPLACEMENT THERAPIES

CAPD	Unknown dialysability. Dose as in GFR<20 mL/min.
HD	Dialysed. Dose as in GFR<20 mL/min.
HDF/High flux	Dialysed. Dose as in GFR<20 mL/min.

IMPORTANT DRUG INTERACTIONS

Potentially hazardous interactions with other drugs
- None known

ADMINISTRATION

RECONSTITUTION
- Add 4 mL of water for injection to each 4 mg vial.

ROUTE
- Oral, IV infusion

RATE OF ADMINISTRATION
- Over 30 minutes

COMMENTS
- Dilute further in sodium chloride 0.9% or glucose 5% to obtain a concentration of 25–50 mcg/mL.
- Once reconstituted use within 12 hours if stored at room temperature, and 24 hours if stored at 2–8˚C if made under aseptic conditions.

OTHER INFORMATION

- If the patient has received extensive prior therapy it has been suggested that 1 mg/m^2/day can be used in mild renal impairment and 0.5 mg/m^2/day in moderate renal impairment. (Ormrod D, Spencer CM. Topotecan: a review of its efficacy in small cell lung cancer. *Drugs.* 1999 Sep; **58**(3): 533–51.)
- In renal failure there is an increased risk of haematological toxicity (even at low doses, e.g. 0.5 mg/m^2/day), therefore if it is to be used in severe renal failure, start at doses less than 0.5 mg/m^2/day and monitor closely.
- No data for oral therapy in GFR<30 mL/ min. Advice from SPC gives a dose of 1.9 mg/m^2/day increasing to 2.3 mg/m^2 if tolerated for GFR=30–49 mL/min.
- An alternative dosing schedule (Kintzel PE, Dorr RT. Anticancer drug renal toxicity and elimination: dosing guidelines for altered renal function. *Cancer Treat Rev.* 1995; **21**: 33–64):
  — CRCL 60 mL/min: 80% of dose
  — CRCL 45 mL/min: 75% of dose
  — CRCL 30 mL/min: 70% of dose
- *Drug Prescribing in Renal Failure*, 5th edition, by Aronoff *et al.* suggests:
  — GFR>50 mL/min: 75% of dose
  — GFR=10–50 mL/min: 50% of dose
  — GFR<10 mL/min: 25% of dose

Torasemide

CLINICAL USE

Loop diuretic:
- Hypertension
- Oedema

DOSE IN NORMAL RENAL FUNCTION

- 2.5–40 mg once daily (varies according to indication)
- Maximum dose: 200 mg daily in resistant oedema in renal patients

PHARMACOKINETICS

Molecular weight (daltons)	348.4
% Protein binding	>99
% Excreted unchanged in urine	25
Volume of distribution (L/kg)	0.09–0.33[1]
Half-life – normal/ ESRF (hrs)	3–4/Unchanged

METABOLISM

Torasemide is metabolised by the cytochrome P450 isoenzyme CYP2C9 to three inactive metabolites, M1, M3 and M5 by stepwise oxidation, hydroxylation or ring hydroxylation. The inactive metabolites are excreted in the urine.

DOSE IN RENAL IMPAIRMENT GFR (mL/MIN)

20–50	Dose as in normal renal function.
10–20	Dose as in normal renal function.
<10	Dose as in normal renal function.

DOSE IN PATIENTS UNDERGOING RENAL REPLACEMENT THERAPIES

CAPD	Unlikely to be dialysed. Dose as in normal renal function.
HD	Not dialysed. Dose as in normal renal function.
HDF/High flux	Unlikely to be dialysed. Dose as in normal renal function.
CAV/ VVHD	Not dialysed. Dose as in normal renal function.

IMPORTANT DRUG INTERACTIONS

Potentially hazardous interactions with other drugs
- Analgesics: increased risk of nephrotoxicity with NSAIDs; antagonism of diuretic effect with NSAIDs.
- Anti-arrhythmics: risk of cardiac toxicity with anti-arrhythmics if hypokalaemia occurs; effects of lidocaine and mexiletine antagonised.
- Antibacterials: increased risk of ototoxicity with aminoglycosides, polymyxins and vancomycin; avoid concomitant use with lymecycline.
- Antidepressants: increased risk of hypokalaemia with reboxetine; enhanced hypotensive effect with MAOIs; increased risk of postural hypotension with tricyclics.
- Anti-epileptics: increased risk of hyponatraemia with carbamazepine.
- Antifungals: increased risk of hypokalaemia with amphotericin.
- Antihypertensives: enhanced hypotensive effect; increased risk of first dose hypotensive effect with alpha-blockers; increased risk of ventricular arrhythmias with sotalol if hypokalaemia occurs.
- Antipsychotics: increased risk of ventricular arrhythmias with amisulpride or pimozide (avoid with pimozide) if hypokalaemia occurs; enhanced hypotensive effect with phenothiazines.
- Atomoxetine: hypokalaemia increases risk of ventricular arrhythmias.
- Cardiac glycosides: increased toxicity if hypokalaemia occurs.
- Cytotoxics: increased risk of ventricular arrhythmias due to hypokalaemia with arsenic trioxide; increased risk of nephrotoxicity and ototoxicity with platinum compounds.
- Lithium: risk of toxicity.

ADMINISTRATION

RECONSTITUTION
–

ROUTE
- Oral

RATE OF ADMINISTRATION
–

COMMENTS
–

OTHER INFORMATION

- Torasemide 10 mg is equivalent to furosemide 20–40 mg.
- In patients with renal failure, the renal clearance is reduced but total plasma clearance is not significantly altered.
- Approximately 80% of dose is excreted renally as parent drug and metabolites.

Reference:
1. Dunn CJ, Fitton A, Brogden RN. Torasemide. An update of its pharmacological properties and therapeutic efficacy. *Drugs*. 1995; **49**(1): 121–42.

Toremifene

CLINICAL USE

Hormone dependent metastatic breast cancer in post menopausal women

DOSE IN NORMAL RENAL FUNCTION

60 mg daily

PHARMACOKINETICS

Molecular weight (daltons)	406
% Protein binding	>99.5
% Excreted unchanged in urine	10% as metabolites
Volume of distribution (L/kg)	580 litres
Half-life – normal/ ESRF (hrs)	5 days/Unchanged

METABOLISM

Toremifene is metabolised mainly by the cytochrome P450 isoenzyme CYP3A4. The main metabolite is N-demethyltoremifene and has similar anti-oestrogenic activity but weaker anti-tumour activity than toremifene.

Toremifene is eliminated mainly as metabolites in the faeces.

DOSE IN RENAL IMPAIRMENT GFR (mL/MIN)

20–50	Dose as in normal renal function.
10–20	Dose as in normal renal function.
<10	Dose as in normal renal function.

DOSE IN PATIENTS UNDERGOING RENAL REPLACEMENT THERAPIES

CAPD	Unlikely to be dialysed. See 'Other information'.
HD	Unlikely to be dialysed. See 'Other information'.
HDF/High flux	Unknown dialysability. See 'Other information'.
CAV/ VVHD	Unlikely to be dialysed. Dose as in GFR=10–20 mL/min.

IMPORTANT DRUG INTERACTIONS

Potentially hazardous interactions with other drugs
- Anticoagulants: enhanced anticoagulant effect of coumarins.
- Cytotoxics: possible increased risk of ventricular arrhythmias with vandetanib – avoid.

ADMINISTRATION

RECONSTITUTION
–
ROUTE
- Oral
RATE OF ADMINISTRATION
–

COMMENTS
–

OTHER INFORMATION

- As it is not renally excreted, it may be possible to prescribe the normal dose in dialysis patients, although it has not previously been used in this population.

Trabectedin

CLINICAL USE

Antineoplastic agent:
- Advanced soft tissue sarcoma
- Ovarian cancer

DOSE IN NORMAL RENAL FUNCTION

- Soft tissue sarcoma: 1.5 mg/m²
- Ovarian cancer: 1.1 mg/m²
- Administered at 3 weekly intervals

PHARMACOKINETICS

Molecular weight (daltons)	761.8
% Protein binding	94–98
% Excreted unchanged in urine	<1
Volume of distribution (L/kg)	>5000 litres
Half-life – normal/ ESRF (hrs)	180/Probably unchanged

METABOLISM

Metabolised in the liver, mainly by cytochrome P450 isoenzyme CYP3A4. Excreted mainly via the faeces.

DOSE IN RENAL IMPAIRMENT GFR (mL/MIN)

30–60	Dose as in normal renal function with monotherapy. Avoid with combination therapy.
<30	Avoid. See 'Other information'.

DOSE IN PATIENTS UNDERGOING RENAL REPLACEMENT THERAPIES

CAPD	Not dialysed. Dose as in GFR<30 mL/min.
HD	Not dialysed. Dose as in GFR<30 mL/min.
HDF/High flux	Not dialysed. Dose as in GFR<30 mL/min.
CAV/ VVHD	Not dialysed. Dose as in GFR<30 mL/min.

IMPORTANT DRUG INTERACTIONS

Potentially hazardous interactions with other drugs
- Antipsychotics: avoid with clozapine, increased risk of agranulocytosis.

ADMINISTRATION

RECONSTITUTION
–
ROUTE
- IV infusion
RATE OF ADMINISTRATION
- 3–24 hours, rate depends on indication
COMMENTS
- Dilute to 50 mL for central access and at least 1 litre for peripheral access.

OTHER INFORMATION

- UK manufacturer advises to avoid if GFR<30 mL/min in monotherapy due to lack of studies although pharmacokinetics for mild to moderate renal impairment are unchanged compared to those with normal renal function.
- Corticosteroids should be administered 30 minutes before treatment to reduce hepatotoxicity and nausea.

Tramadol hydrochloride

CLINICAL USE

Analgesic

DOSE IN NORMAL RENAL FUNCTION

- Oral: 50–100 mg up to 4 hourly; maximum 400 mg daily
- IM/IV: 50–100 mg every 4–6 hours; total daily dose 600 mg
- MR: 50–200 mg twice daily
- XL: 100–400 mg once daily

PHARMACOKINETICS

Molecular weight (daltons)	299.8
% Protein binding	20
% Excreted unchanged in urine	90
Volume of distribution (L/kg)	163–243 litres
Half-life – normal/ ESRF (hrs)	6/11

METABOLISM

Tramadol is metabolised by N- and O-demethylation via the cytochrome P450 isoenzymes CYP3A4 and CYP2D6 and glucuronidation or sulphation in the liver. Only O-desmethyl-tramadol is pharmacologically active. Tramadol and its metabolites are almost completely excreted renally.

DOSE IN RENAL IMPAIRMENT GFR (mL/MIN)

20–50	Dose as in normal renal function
10–20	50–100 mg every 8 hours initially and titrate dose as tolerated.
<10	50 mg every 8 hours initially and titrate dose as tolerated.

DOSE IN PATIENTS UNDERGOING RENAL REPLACEMENT THERAPIES

CAPD	Unknown dialysability. Dose as in GFR<10 mL/min.
HD	Dialysed. Dose as in GFR<10 mL/min.
HDF/High flux	Dialysed. Dose as in GFR<10 mL/min.
CAV/ VVHD	Dialysed. Dose as in GFR=10–20 mL/min.

IMPORTANT DRUG INTERACTIONS

Potentially hazardous interactions with other drugs
- Anticoagulants: enhances effect of coumarins.
- Antidepressants: possibly increased serotonergic effects with duloxetine, mirtazapine or venlafaxine; possible CNS excitation or depression with MAOIs and moclobemide – avoid concomitant use with MAOIs as increased risk of serotonergic effects and convulsions; increased risk of CNS toxicity with SSRIs or tricyclics.
- Anti-epileptics: effect reduced by carbamazepine.
- Antihistamines: increased sedative effects with sedating antihistamines.
- Antipsychotics: enhanced hypotensive and sedative effects; increased risk of convulsions.
- Atomoxetine: increased risk of convulsions.
- Dopaminergics: avoid with selegiline.
- Sodium oxybate: enhanced effect of sodium oxybate – avoid concomitant use.

ADMINISTRATION

RECONSTITUTION
–
ROUTE
- IV, IM, oral
RATE OF ADMINISTRATION
- Slow bolus or continuous IV infusion/PCA
COMMENTS
–

OTHER INFORMATION

- Tramadol is a centrally acting opioid agonist which also acts on inhibitory pain pathways.
- Bioavailability is 60–95%.

Trandolapril

CLINICAL USE

Angiotensin converting enzyme inhibitor:
- Hypertension
- Heart failure
- After myocardial infarction

DOSE IN NORMAL RENAL FUNCTION

0.5–4 mg once daily

PHARMACOKINETICS

Molecular weight (daltons)	430.5
% Protein binding	>80 (as trandolaprilat)
% Excreted unchanged in urine	10–15
Volume of distribution (L/kg)	18 litres
Half-life – normal/ ESRF (hrs)	16–24/– (as trandolaprilat)

METABOLISM

Trandolapril is metabolised in the liver to the active trandolaprilat and to some inactive metabolites. About 33% of an oral dose of trandolapril is excreted in the urine, mainly as trandolaprilat; the rest is excreted in the faeces.

DOSE IN RENAL IMPAIRMENT GFR (mL/MIN)

20–50	Dose as in normal renal function.
10–20	Dose as in normal renal function.
<10	Initial dose 500 mcg once daily, and increase according to response.

DOSE IN PATIENTS UNDERGOING RENAL REPLACEMENT THERAPIES

CAPD	Unknown dialysability. Dose as in GFR<10 mL/min.
HD	Dialysed. Dose as in GFR<10 mL/min.
HDF/High flux	Dialysed. Dose as in GFR<10 mL/min.
CAV/ VVHD	Dialysed. Dose as in GFR=10–20 mL/min.

IMPORTANT DRUG INTERACTIONS

Potentially hazardous interactions with other drugs
- Anaesthetics: enhanced hypotensive effect.
- Analgesics: antagonism of hypotensive effect and increased risk of renal impairment with NSAIDs; hyperkalaemia with ketorolac and other NSAIDs.
- Ciclosporin: increased risk of hyperkalaemia and nephrotoxicity.
- Diuretics: enhanced hypotensive effect; hyperkalaemia with potassium-sparing diuretics.
- ESAs: increased risk of hyperkalaemia; antagonism of hypotensive effect.
- Gold: flushing and hypotension with sodium aurothiomalate.
- Lithium: reduced excretion (possibility of enhanced lithium toxicity).
- Potassium salts: increased risk of hyperkalaemia.
- Tacrolimus: increased risk of hyperkalaemia and nephrotoxicity.

ADMINISTRATION

RECONSTITUTION
–
ROUTE
- Oral
RATE OF ADMINISTRATION
–
COMMENTS
–

OTHER INFORMATION

- Hyperkalaemia and other side effects are more common in patients with impaired renal function.
- Close monitoring of renal function required during therapy in patients with renal insufficiency.
- Renal failure has been reported in association with ACE inhibitors in patients with renal artery stenosis, post renal transplant, and those with congestive heart failure.
- High incidence of anaphylactoid reactions has been reported in patients dialysed with high-flux polyacrylonitrile membranes and treated concomitantly with an ACE inhibitor – this combination should therefore be avoided.
- Normal doses can be used in CKD 5.

Tranexamic acid

CLINICAL USE

Haemostatic agent

DOSE IN NORMAL RENAL FUNCTION

- Oral: 1–1.5 g every 8–12 hours (15–25 mg/kg every 8–12 hours)
- IV: 0.5–1 g every 8 hours (25–50 mg/kg daily in divided doses)
- Dose depends on indication

PHARMACOKINETICS

Molecular weight (daltons)	157.2
% Protein binding	3
% Excreted unchanged in urine	90
Volume of distribution (L/kg)	1
Half-life – normal/ ESRF (hrs)	2/–

METABOLISM

Tranexamic acid is excreted as unchanged drug mainly by urinary excretion via glomerular filtration.

DOSE IN RENAL IMPAIRMENT GFR (mL/MIN)

20–50	IV: 10 mg/kg 12 hourly. Oral: 25 mg/kg 12 hourly.
10–20	IV: 10 mg/kg 24 hourly. Oral: 25 mg/kg 12–24 hourly.
<10	IV: 5 mg/kg 24 hourly. Oral: 12.5 mg/kg 24 hourly.

DOSE IN PATIENTS UNDERGOING RENAL REPLACEMENT THERAPIES

CAPD	Unknown dialysability. Dose as in GFR<10 mL/min.
HD	Unknown dialysability. Dose as in GFR<10 mL/min.
HDF/High flux	Unknown dialysability. Dose as in GFR<10 mL/min.
CAV/VVHD	Unknown dialysability. Dose as in GFR=10–20 mL/min.

IMPORTANT DRUG INTERACTIONS

Potentially hazardous interactions with other drugs
- None known

ADMINISTRATION

RECONSTITUTION
–
ROUTE
- IV, Oral
RATE OF ADMINISTRATION
- Slow bolus =100 mg/minute or continuous IV infusion in glucose 5% or sodium chloride 0.9%
COMMENTS
–

OTHER INFORMATION

- Contraindicated by one manufacturer in the UK in severe renal impairment due to accumulation and increased risk of thrombus formation.
- A 5% topical solution can be made up using the IV preparation, mixed with water for injection. This can be used as a mouthwash to stop bleeding after dental surgery, or placed on a swab to reduce bleeding at fistula or other bleeding sites if conventional measures have not worked (anecdotal).
- Bioavailability is 45%.

Trastuzumab

CLINICAL USE

Antineoplastic agent:
- HER2-expressing breast cancer
- Metastatic gastric cancer

DOSE IN NORMAL RENAL FUNCTION

- 4 mg/kg then 2 mg/kg weekly
- Or 8 mg/kg initially then 6 mg/kg every 3 weeks
- Breast cancer only (SC): 600 mg every 3 weeks
- Or according to local policy

PHARMACOKINETICS

Molecular weight (daltons)	148 000–185 000
% Protein binding	No data
% Excreted unchanged in urine	No data
Volume of distribution (L/kg)	0.044
Half-life – normal/ ESRF (hrs)	1.7–28.5 days/ Probably unchanged

METABOLISM

Trastuzumab is most likely removed by opsonisation via the reticuloendothelial system.

DOSE IN RENAL IMPAIRMENT GFR (mL/MIN)

20–50	Dose as in normal renal function.
10–20	Dose as in normal renal function. Use with caution.
<10	Dose as in normal renal function. Use with caution.

DOSE IN PATIENTS UNDERGOING RENAL REPLACEMENT THERAPIES

CAPD	Unlikely to be dialysed. Dose as in GFR<10 mL/min.
HD	Unlikely to be dialysed. Dose as in GFR<10 mL/min.
HDF/High flux	Unlikely to be dialysed. Dose as in GFR<10 mL/min.
CAV/ VVHD	Unknown dialysability. Dose as in GFR=10–20 mL/min.

IMPORTANT DRUG INTERACTIONS

Potentially hazardous interactions with other drugs
- None known

ADMINISTRATION

RECONSTITUTION
- 7.2 mL water for injection per 150 mg vial

ROUTE
- IV infusion, SC

RATE OF ADMINISTRATION
- 4 mg/kg over 90 minutes
- 2 mg/kg over 30 minutes
- SC: 2–5 minutes

COMMENTS
- Allow to stand for 5 minutes after reconstitution.
- Dilute dose in 250 mL sodium chloride 0.9%.

OTHER INFORMATION

- Manufacturer has not done any studies in renal impairment but no dose reduction is probably required as trastuzumab doesn't require hepatic or renal metabolism for elimination.
- Distributes to normal cells, tumour cells and serum where HER2 antigens are found.
- Nadir for bone-marrow depression is 4 weeks with recovery within 6 weeks.
- Associated with cardiotoxicity.
- May remain in circulation for up to 24 weeks.

Trazodone hydrochloride

CLINICAL USE

Tricyclic-related antidepressant

DOSE IN NORMAL RENAL FUNCTION

- Depression: 100–300 mg daily; maximum 600 mg daily in divided doses for hospital patients
- Anxiety: 75–300 mg daily

PHARMACOKINETICS

Molecular weight (daltons)	408.3
% Protein binding	89–95
% Excreted unchanged in urine	<5
Volume of distribution (L/kg)	1–2
Half-life – normal/ ESRF (hrs)	5–13/–

METABOLISM

Trazodone is hepatically metabolised via the cytochrome P450 isoenzyme CYP3A4 by n-oxidation and hydroxylation. The metabolite m-chlorophenylpiperazine is active.

Trazodone is excreted in the urine almost entirely in the form of its metabolites.

DOSE IN RENAL IMPAIRMENT GFR (mL/MIN)

20–50	Dose as in normal renal function.
10–20	Dose as in normal renal function. Start with small doses and increase gradually.
<10	Start with small doses and increase gradually.

DOSE IN PATIENTS UNDERGOING RENAL REPLACEMENT THERAPIES

CAPD	Unlikely to be dialysed. Dose as in GFR<10 mL/min.
HD	Unlikely to be dialysed. Dose as in GFR<10 mL/min.
HDF/High flux	Unknown dialysability. Dose as in GFR<10 mL/min.
CAV/VVHD	Unknown dialysability. Dose as in GFR=10–20 mL/min.

IMPORTANT DRUG INTERACTIONS

Potentially hazardous interactions with other drugs

- Alcohol: increased sedative effects.
- Antidepressants: avoid concomitant use with MAOIs and moclobemide.
- Anti-epileptics: antagonism of anticonvulsant effect; concentration reduced by carbamazepine.
- Antimalarials: manufacturer advises avoid concomitant use with artemether and lumefantrine and piperaquine with artenimol.
- Antivirals: concentration increased by ritonavir; increased risk of ventricular arrhythmias with saquinavir – avoid; concentration possibly increased by telaprevir.

ADMINISTRATION

RECONSTITUTION

–

ROUTE

- Oral

RATE OF ADMINISTRATION

–

COMMENTS

–

OTHER INFORMATION

- Use lower doses in elderly patients.

Treosulfan

CLINICAL USE

Alkylating agent for ovarian cancer

DOSE IN NORMAL RENAL FUNCTION

- IV: $3-8\,g/m^2$ every 1–3 weeks; doses $>3\,g/m^2$ should be given as an infusion.
- Doses up to $1.5\,g/m^2$ have been given IP.
- Oral: 1 g daily in 4 divided doses for 2–4 weeks or 1.5 g daily in 3 divided doses for 1 week.
- Or according to local protocol.

PHARMACOKINETICS

Molecular weight (daltons)	278.3
% Protein binding	No data
% Excreted unchanged in urine	22–30
Volume of distribution (L/kg)	44–88 litres
Half-life – normal/ ESRF (hrs)	1.5–1.94/–

METABOLISM

Treosulfan is a prodrug of a bifunctional alkylating agent, converted *in vivo* to epoxide compounds. Approximately 30% of the substance is excreted unchanged in the urine within 24 hours, nearly 90% of which is within the first 6 hours after administration.

DOSE IN RENAL IMPAIRMENT GFR (mL/MIN)

20–50	Use a reduced dose. See 'Other information'.
10–20	Use a reduced dose. See 'Other information'.
<10	Use a reduced dose. See 'Other information'.

DOSE IN PATIENTS UNDERGOING RENAL REPLACEMENT THERAPIES

CAPD	Unknown dialysability. Dose as in GFR<10 mL/min.
HD	Dialysed. Dose as in GFR<10 mL/min.
HDF/High flux	Dialysed. Dose as in GFR<10 mL/min.
CAV/ VVHD	Dialysed. Dose as in GFR=10–20 mL/min.

IMPORTANT DRUG INTERACTIONS

Potentially hazardous interactions with other drugs
- None known

ADMINISTRATION

RECONSTITUTION
- 20 or 100 mL water for injection for 1 g and 5 g vials respectively

ROUTE
- Oral, IV, IP

RATE OF ADMINISTRATION
- $3\,g/m^2$ every 5–10 minutes ($8\,g/m^2$ over 30 minutes)

COMMENTS
- Powder reconstitutes easier if water heated to 25–30°C

OTHER INFORMATION

- A dose reduction of 60% has been suggested for a GFR<30 mL/min. www.avon.nhs.uk/aswcs-chemo/STCP/Gynae/ASWCS11GYN015_Treosulfan_Final_120106.pdf.
- Haemorrhagic cystitis has occurred after intravesical or intravenous administration.

Tretinoin

CLINICAL USE

Retinoid:
- Induction of remission in promyelocytic leukaemia (APL)
- Acne
- Photo-damage

DOSE IN NORMAL RENAL FUNCTION

APL: 45 mg/m^2 in 2 divided doses

PHARMACOKINETICS

Molecular weight (daltons)	300.4
% Protein binding	>95
% Excreted unchanged in urine	60 (excreted as metabolites)
Volume of distribution (L/kg)	No data
Half-life – normal/ ESRF (hrs)	0.5–2/–

METABOLISM

Metabolised in the liver by the cytochrome P450 isoenzyme system to form isotretinoin, 4-oxo-trans-retinoic acid, and 4-oxo-cis-retinoic acid.

Tretinoin is excreted in the bile and the urine.

DOSE IN RENAL IMPAIRMENT GFR (mL/MIN)

20–50	25 mg/m^2 daily.
10–20	25 mg/m^2 daily.
<10	25 mg/m^2 daily.

DOSE IN PATIENTS UNDERGOING RENAL REPLACEMENT THERAPIES

CAPD	Unlikely to be dialysed. Dose as in GFR<10 mL/min.
HD	Not dialysed. Dose as in GFR<10 mL/min.
HDF/High flux	Unlikely to be dialysed. Dose as in GFR<10 mL/min.
CAV/ VVHD	Unknown dialysability. Dose as in GFR=10–20 mL/min.

IMPORTANT DRUG INTERACTIONS

Potentially hazardous interactions with other drugs
- Antibacterials: possibly increased risk of benign intracranial hypertension with tetracyclines – avoid concomitant use.
- Vitamin A: risk of hypervitaminosis – avoid concomitant use.

ADMINISTRATION

RECONSTITUTION
–
ROUTE
- Oral, topical
RATE OF ADMINISTRATION
–
COMMENTS
–

OTHER INFORMATION

- Manufacturer recommends a reduced dose in renal impairment due to lack of data.
- Oral bioavailability is 50%.
- Monitor for signs of vitamin A toxicity.
- There is a report of 2 patients who required dialysis during tretinoin treatment for acute promyelocytic leukaemia and who achieved remission; one was given a dose of 20 mg/m^2 daily in 2 divided doses and the other received 35 mg/m^2 daily in 3 divided doses. (Takitani K, *et al.* Pharmacokinetics of all-trans retinoic acid in acute promyelocytic leukemia patients on dialysis. *Am J Hematol.* 2003; **74**: 147–8.)

Triamcinolone

CLINICAL USE

Corticosteroid

DOSE IN NORMAL RENAL FUNCTION

- IM: 40 mg of acetonide; maximum single dose 100 mg
- Intra-articular: 2.5–40 mg of acetonide, total max 80 mg
- Intra-dermal: 2–3 mg, maximum 5 mg at any one site, total maximum 30 mg

PHARMACOKINETICS

Molecular weight (daltons)	394.4 (434.5 as acetonide)
% Protein binding	Low
% Excreted unchanged in urine	<1
Volume of distribution (L/kg)	1.4–2.1
Half-life – normal/ ESRF (hrs)	2–5/Unchanged

METABOLISM

Triamcinolone is metabolised largely hepatically but also by the kidney and is excreted in urine. The main metabolic route is 6-beta-hydroxylation; no significant hydrolytic cleavage of the acetonide occurs.

DOSE IN RENAL IMPAIRMENT GFR (mL/MIN)

20–50	Dose as in normal renal function.
10–20	Dose as in normal renal function.
<10	Dose as in normal renal function.

DOSE IN PATIENTS UNDERGOING RENAL REPLACEMENT THERAPIES

CAPD	Unknown dialysability. Dose as in normal renal function.
HD	Unknown dialysability. Dose as in normal renal function.
HDF/High flux	Unknown dialysability. Dose as in normal renal function.
CAV/ VVHD	Unknown dialysability. Dose as in normal renal function.

IMPORTANT DRUG INTERACTIONS

Potentially hazardous interactions with other drugs

- Aldesleukin: avoid concomitant use.
- Antibacterials: metabolism accelerated by rifampicin; metabolism possibly inhibited by erythromycin; concentration of isoniazid possibly reduced.
- Anticoagulants: efficacy of coumarins and phenindione may be altered.
- Anti-epileptics: metabolism accelerated by carbamazepine, phenobarbital and phenytoin.
- Antifungals: increased risk of hypokalaemia with amphotericin – avoid concomitant use; metabolism possibly inhibited by itraconazole and ketoconazole.
- Antivirals: concentration possibly increased by ritonavir.
- Ciclosporin: rare reports of convulsions in patients on ciclosporin and high-dose corticosteroids.
- Diuretics: enhanced hypokalaemic effects of acetazolamide, loop diuretics and thiazide diuretics.
- Vaccines: high dose corticosteroids can impair immune response to vaccines; avoid concomitant use with live vaccines.

ADMINISTRATION

RECONSTITUTION

–

ROUTE

- IM, intra-articular, topical, nasal, intradermal

RATE OF ADMINISTRATION

–

COMMENTS

–

OTHER INFORMATION

- Use with caution in severe renal impairment as sodium and water retention may occur.
- 4 mg is equivalent to 5 mg of prednisolone.

Triamterene

CLINICAL USE

Diuretic (potassium-sparing)

DOSE IN NORMAL RENAL FUNCTION

150–250 mg daily in divided doses; reduce to alternate days after 1 week.

PHARMACOKINETICS

Molecular weight (daltons)	253
% Protein binding	60
% Excreted unchanged in urine	5–10
Volume of distribution (L/kg)	2.2–3.7
Half-life – normal/ ESRF (hrs)	2/10

METABOLISM

Triamterene is extensively metabolised apparently via the cytochrome P450 isoenzyme CYP1A2.

It is mainly excreted in the urine in the form of metabolites with some unchanged triamterene; variable amounts are also excreted in the bile.

DOSE IN RENAL IMPAIRMENT GFR (mL/MIN)

20–50	Dose as in normal renal function.
10–20	Avoid. See 'Other information'.
<10	Avoid. See 'Other information'.

DOSE IN PATIENTS UNDERGOING RENAL REPLACEMENT THERAPIES

CAPD	Unknown dialysability. Avoid.
HD	Unknown dialysability. Avoid.
HDF/High flux	Unknown dialysability. Avoid.
CAV/ VVHD	Unknown dialysability. Avoid.

IMPORTANT DRUG INTERACTIONS

Potentially hazardous interactions with other drugs

- ACE inhibitors and angiotensin-II antagonists: enhanced hypotensive effect (risk of severe hyperkalaemia).
- Analgesics: increased risk of nephrotoxicity with NSAIDs; increased risk of hyperkalaemia, especially with indomethacin; antagonism of hypotensive effect.
- Antibacterials: avoid concomitant use with lymecycline.
- Antidepressants: enhanced hypotensive effect with MAOIs; increased risk of postural hypotension with tricyclics.
- Antipsychotics: enhanced hypotensive effect with phenothiazines.
- Antihypertensives: enhanced hypotensive effect; increased risk of first dose hypotensive effect of post-synaptic alpha-blockers, e.g. prazosin.
- Ciclosporin: increased risk of hyperkalaemia.
- Cytotoxics: increased risk of nephrotoxicity and ototoxicity with platinum compounds.
- Lithium: reduced excretion of lithium (risk of lithium toxicity).
- Potassium salts: increased risk of hyperkalaemia.
- Tacrolimus: increased risk of hyperkalaemia.

ADMINISTRATION

RECONSTITUTION
–
ROUTE
- Oral
RATE OF ADMINISTRATION
–
COMMENTS
–

OTHER INFORMATION

- Hyperkalaemia is common when GFR<30 mL/min. May cause acute kidney injury.
- Potassium-sparing diuretics are weak diuretics and are ineffective in moderate to severe renal failure.
- Bioavailability is 50%.

Trifluoperazine

CLINICAL USE

- Schizophrenia and other psychoses
- Anxiety
- Severe nausea and vomiting

DOSE IN NORMAL RENAL FUNCTION

- Schizophrenia: initially 5 mg twice daily, increased by 5 mg after 1 week, then at intervals of 3 days according to response.
- Anxiolytic and anti-emetic: 2–4 mg daily in divided doses; maximum 6 mg

PHARMACOKINETICS

Molecular weight (daltons)	407.5
% Protein binding	>99
% Excreted unchanged in urine	<1
Volume of distribution (L/kg)	160
Half-life – normal/ ESRF (hrs)	22/–

METABOLISM

Trifluoperazine undergoes extensive first-pass metabolism. The major metabolite is the possibly active N-oxide; other metabolites include the sulfoxide and the 7-hydroxy derivative.

Elimination occurs in the bile and urine.

DOSE IN RENAL IMPAIRMENT GFR (mL/MIN)

20–50	Dose as in normal renal function. Start with low dose.
10–20	Dose as in normal renal function. Start with low dose.
<10	Dose as in normal renal function. Start with low dose.

DOSE IN PATIENTS UNDERGOING RENAL REPLACEMENT THERAPIES

CAPD	Not dialysed. Dose as in GFR<10 mL/min.
HD	Not dialysed. Dose as in GFR<10 mL/min.
HDF/High flux	Unknown dialysability. Dose as in GFR<10 mL/min.
CAV/ VVHD	Unlikely to be dialysed. Dose as in GFR=10–20 mL/min.

IMPORTANT DRUG INTERACTIONS

Potentially hazardous interactions with other drugs

- Anaesthetics: enhanced hypotensive effect.
- Analgesics: increased risk of convulsions with tramadol; enhanced hypotensive and sedative effects with opioids.
- Anti-arrhythmics: increased risk of ventricular arrhythmias with anti-arrhythmics that prolong the QT interval, e.g. procainamide, disopyramide, dronedarone and amiodarone – avoid concomitant use with amiodarone and dronedarone.
- Antibacterials: increased risk of ventricular arrhythmias with moxifloxacin – avoid concomitant use.
- Antidepressants: increased level of tricyclics; possibly increased risk of antimuscarinic side effects.
- Anti-epileptics: antagonism (convulsive threshold lowered).
- Antimalarials: avoid concomitant use with artemether/lumefantrine and piperaquine with artenimol.
- Antipsychotics: increased risk of ventricular arrhythmias with pimozide – avoid concomitant use.
- Antivirals: concentration possibly increased with ritonavir.
- Anxiolytics and hypnotics: increased sedative effects.
- Beta-blockers: enhanced hypotensive effect; increased risk of ventricular arrhythmias with sotalol.
- Diuretics: enhanced hypotensive effect.
- Lithium: increased risk of extrapyramidal side effects and possibly neurotoxicity.
- Pentamidine: increased risk of ventricular arrhythmias.

ADMINISTRATION

RECONSTITUTION

–

ROUTE

- Oral

RATE OF ADMINISTRATION

–

COMMENTS

–

OTHER INFORMATION

- Reduce starting dose in elderly or frail patients by at least half.

Trimethoprim

CLINICAL USE

Antibacterial agent

DOSE IN NORMAL RENAL FUNCTION

- Treatment: 200 mg every 12 hours
- Prophylaxis: 100 mg at night

PHARMACOKINETICS

Molecular weight (daltons)	290.3
% Protein binding	45
% Excreted unchanged in urine	40–60
Volume of distribution (L/kg)	1–2.2
Half-life – normal/ ESRF (hrs)	8–10/20–49

METABOLISM

About 10–20% of trimethoprim is metabolised in the liver and small amounts are excreted in the faeces via the bile, but most, about 40–60% of a dose, is excreted in urine, mainly as unchanged drug.

Trimethoprim is excreted mainly by the kidneys through glomerular filtration and tubular secretion.

DOSE IN RENAL IMPAIRMENT GFR (mL/MIN)

>25	Dose as in normal renal function.
15–25	Dose as in normal renal function.
<15	50–100% of dose.

DOSE IN PATIENTS UNDERGOING RENAL REPLACEMENT THERAPIES

CAPD	Not dialysed. Dose as in GFR<15 mL/min.
HD	Dialysed. Dose as in GFR<15 mL/min.
HDF/High flux	Dialysed. Dose as in GFR<15 mL/min.
CAV/ VVHD	Probably dialysed. Dose as in normal renal function.

IMPORTANT DRUG INTERACTIONS

Potentially hazardous interactions with other drugs

- Anti-arrhythmics: increased risk of ventricular arrhythmias with amiodarone – avoid concomitant use; concentration of procainamide increased.
- Anti-epileptics: antifolate effect and concentration of phenytoin increased.
- Antimalarials: increased risk of antifolate effect with pyrimethamine.
- Ciclosporin: increased risk of nephrotoxicity; concentration of ciclosporin reduced by IV trimethoprim.
- Cytotoxics: increased risk of haematological toxicity with azathioprine, methotrexate and mercaptopurine; antifolate effect of methotrexate increased.

ADMINISTRATION

RECONSTITUTION

–

ROUTE

- Oral

RATE OF ADMINISTRATION

–

COMMENTS

–

OTHER INFORMATION

- Serum creatinine may rise due to competition for renal secretion.
- Hyperkalaemia is common in CKD 5 and transplant patients.
- New Zealand data sheet advises to use with caution if GFR<10 mL/min and monitor potassium.
- Short-term folic acid supplementation may be prescribed in patients with CKD 4–5 to cover antifolate effects of treatment dose.

Trimipramine

CLINICAL USE

Tricyclic antidepressant

DOSE IN NORMAL RENAL FUNCTION

- 50–300 mg daily in divided doses
- Elderly: 10–25 mg 3 times daily; half the dose should be sufficient for maintenance

PHARMACOKINETICS

Molecular weight (daltons)	410.5 (as maleate)
% Protein binding	95
% Excreted unchanged in urine	0
Volume of distribution (L/kg)	31
Half-life – normal/ESRF (hrs)	23/–

METABOLISM

Trimipramine is metabolised in the liver to its major metabolite desmethyltrimipramine, which is active. Trimipramine is excreted in the urine mainly in the form of its metabolites.

DOSE IN RENAL IMPAIRMENT GFR (mL/MIN)

20–50	Dose as in normal renal function.
10–20	Dose as in normal renal function.
<10	Dose as in normal renal function.

DOSE IN PATIENTS UNDERGOING RENAL REPLACEMENT THERAPIES

CAPD	Not dialysed. Dose as in normal renal function.
HD	Not dialysed. Dose as in normal renal function.
HDF/High flux	Unknown dialysability. Dose as in normal renal function.
CAV/ VVHD	Unknown dialysability. Dose as in normal renal function.

IMPORTANT DRUG INTERACTIONS

Potentially hazardous interactions with other drugs

- Alcohol: increased sedative effect.
- Analgesics: increased risk of CNS toxicity with tramadol; possibly increased risk of side effects with nefopam; possibly increased sedative effects with opioids.
- Anti-arrhythmics: increased risk of ventricular arrhythmias with amiodarone – avoid concomitant use; increased risk of ventricular arrhythmias with disopyramide, flecainide or propafenone; avoid with dronedarone.
- Antibacterials: increased risk of ventricular arrhythmias with moxifloxacin and possibly telithromycin – avoid concomitant use with moxifloxacin.
- Anticoagulants: may alter anticoagulant effect of coumarins.
- Antidepressants: enhanced CNS excitation and hypertension with MAOIs and moclobemide – avoid concomitant use; concentration possibly increased with SSRIs.
- Anti-epileptics: convulsive threshold lowered; concentration reduced by carbamazepine, phenobarbital and possibly phenytoin.
- Antimalarials: avoid concomitant use with artemether/lumefantrine and piperaquine with artenimol.
- Antipsychotics: increased risk of ventricular arrhythmias especially with droperidol and pimozide – avoid; increased antimuscarinic effects with clozapine and phenothiazines; concentration increased by antipsychotics.
- Antivirals: increased risk of ventricular arrhythmias with saquinavir – avoid; concentration possibly increased with ritonavir.
- Atomoxetine: increased risk of ventricular arrhythmias and possibly convulsions.
- Beta-blockers: increased risk of ventricular arrhythmias with sotalol.
- Clonidine: tricyclics antagonise hypotensive effect; increased risk of hypertension on clonidine withdrawal.
- Dopaminergics: avoid use with entacapone; CNS toxicity reported with selegiline and rasagiline.
- Pentamidine: increased risk of ventricular arrhythmias.
- Sympathomimetics: increased risk of hypertension and arrhythmias with adrenaline and noradrenaline; metabolism possibly inhibited by methylphenidate.

ADMINISTRATION

RECONSTITUTION

–

ROUTE

- Oral

RATE OF ADMINISTRATION

–

COMMENTS

–

Triptorelin

CLINICAL USE

- Advanced prostate cancer
- Endometriosis
- Precocious puberty
- Uterine fibroids prior to surgery

DOSE IN NORMAL RENAL FUNCTION

3–3.75 mg every 4 weeks; depends on preparation
11.25 mg every 3 months

PHARMACOKINETICS

Molecular weight (daltons)	1311.4
% Protein binding	No data
% Excreted unchanged in urine	3–14
Volume of distribution (L/kg)	92.4–115.8 litres
Half-life – normal/ ESRF (hrs)	7.5/Unchanged

METABOLISM

The metabolism of triptorelin in humans is unknown, but it is thought to be hydrolysed in the plasma and excreted in the urine as inactive metabolites.

DOSE IN RENAL IMPAIRMENT GFR (mL/MIN)

20–50	Dose as in normal renal function.
10–20	Dose as in normal renal function, but monitor carefully.
<10	Dose as in normal renal function, but monitor carefully.

DOSE IN PATIENTS UNDERGOING RENAL REPLACEMENT THERAPIES

CAPD	Unlikely to be dialysed. Dose as in GFR<10 mL/min.
HD	Unlikely to be dialysed. Dose as in GFR<10 mL/min.
HDF/High flux	Unknown dialysability. Dose as in GFR<10 mL/min
CAV/ VVHD	Unknown dialysability. Dose as in GFR=10–20 mL/min

IMPORTANT DRUG INTERACTIONS

Potentially hazardous interactions with other drugs
- None known

ADMINISTRATION

RECONSTITUTION
- With 2 mL diluent provided
ROUTE
- SC, IM
RATE OF ADMINISTRATION
–
COMMENTS
–

OTHER INFORMATION

–

Trospium chloride

CLINICAL USE

Antimuscarinic:
- Symptomatic treatment of urinary incontinence, frequency or urgency

DOSE IN NORMAL RENAL FUNCTION

20 mg twice daily
XL: 60 mg once daily

PHARMACOKINETICS

Molecular weight (daltons)	428
% Protein binding	50–80
% Excreted unchanged in urine	5.8
Volume of distribution (L/kg)	395 litres/XL: >600 litres
Half-life – normal/ ESRF (hrs)	10–20 (XL: 38.5)/ 20–40 (XL: 77)

METABOLISM

The metabolic pathway of trospium in humans has not been fully defined. Of the 10% of the dose absorbed, metabolites account for approximately 40% of the excreted dose following oral administration. The major metabolic pathway is hypothesised as ester hydrolysis with subsequent conjugation of benzylic acid to form azoniaspironortropanol with glucuronic acid.

The mean renal clearance for trospium (29 L/hour) is 4-fold higher than average glomerular filtration rate, indicating that active tubular secretion is a major route of elimination for trospium. There may be competition for elimination with other compounds that are also renally eliminated.

DOSE IN RENAL IMPAIRMENT GFR (mL/MIN)

30–50	Dose as in normal renal function.
10–30	20 mg daily or on alternate days. See 'Other information'.
<10	20 mg daily or on alternate days. See 'Other information'.

DOSE IN PATIENTS UNDERGOING RENAL REPLACEMENT THERAPIES

CAPD	Probably dialysed. Dose as in GFR<10 mL/min.
HD	Probably dialysed. Dose as in GFR<10 mL/min.
HDF/High flux	Probably dialysed. Dose as in GFR<10 mL/min.
CAV/ VVHD	Probably dialysed. Dose as in GFR=10–30 mL/min.

IMPORTANT DRUG INTERACTIONS

Potentially hazardous interactions with other drugs
- Anti-arrhythmics: increased risk of antimuscarinic side effects with disopyramide.

ADMINISTRATION

RECONSTITUTION
–

ROUTE
- Oral

RATE OF ADMINISTRATION
–

OTHER INFORMATION

- Oral bioavailability is <10%.
- In a study conducted on patients with creatinine clearance=8–32 mL/min the average AUC was increased 4-fold and the C_{max} 2-fold.
- Avoid XL preparation patients with GFR<30 mL/min due to lack of data for dosage adjustments.

Tryptophan

CLINICAL USE

Antidepressant

DOSE IN NORMAL RENAL FUNCTION

1–2 g 3 times daily

PHARMACOKINETICS

Molecular weight (daltons)	204.2
% Protein binding	80
% Excreted unchanged in urine	10–20
Volume of distribution (L/kg)	0.34–0.7
Half-life – normal/ ESRF (hrs)	1–3/–

METABOLISM

Tryptophan is metabolised in the liver by tryptophan pyrrolase and tryptophan hydroxylase. Metabolites include hydroxytryptophan, which is then converted to serotonin, and kynurenine derivatives. Some tryptophan is converted to nicotinic acid and nicotinamide. Pyridoxine and ascorbic acid are cofactors in the decarboxylation and hydroxylation, respectively, of tryptophan; pyridoxine apparently prevents the accumulation of the kynurenine metabolites.

DOSE IN RENAL IMPAIRMENT GFR (mL/MIN)

20–50	Dose as in normal renal function.
10–20	Dose as in normal renal function.
<10	Use lower doses initially.

DOSE IN PATIENTS UNDERGOING RENAL REPLACEMENT THERAPIES

CAPD	Unknown dialysability. Dose as in GFR<10 mL/min.
HD	Not dialysed. Dose as in GFR<10 mL/min.
HDF/High flux	Not dialysed. Dose as in GFR<10 mL/min.
CAV/VVHD	Unknown dialysability. Dose as in normal renal function.

IMPORTANT DRUG INTERACTIONS

Potentially hazardous interactions with other drugs
- Antidepressants: possible increased serotonergic effects with duloxetine; CNS excitation and confusion with MAOIs – reduce dose of tryptophan; agitation and nausea with SSRIs; CNS toxicity reported with fluoxetine.
- Antimalarials: avoid concomitant administration with artemether/lumefantrine and piperaquine with artenimol.

ADMINISTRATION

RECONSTITUTION

–

ROUTE

- Oral

RATE OF ADMINISTRATION

–

COMMENTS

–

OTHER INFORMATION

- Associated with eosinophilia-myalgia syndrome, therefore not first line therapy.

Urokinase

CLINICAL USE

Fibrinolytic agent:
- Thrombosed arteriovenous shunts and intravenous cannulas
- Treatment of thromboembolic occlusive vascular disease, e.g. DVT, PE, peripheral vascular occlusion

DOSE IN NORMAL RENAL FUNCTION

- Lock: 5000–250000 IU for 30 minutes – 2 hours
- Infusion: 5000–250000 IU over 30 minutes – 48 hours, depending on local protocol
- Treatment of thromboembolic occlusive vascular disease: dose varies according to preparation and location of thrombus
- Consult product literature for more information

PHARMACOKINETICS

Molecular weight (daltons)	33 000–54 000
% Protein binding	No data
% Excreted unchanged in urine	Low
Volume of distribution (L/kg)	No data
Half-life – normal/ ESRF (hrs)	20 minutes/Increased

METABOLISM

Urokinase is eliminated rapidly from the circulation by the liver.

The inactive degradation products are excreted mainly via the kidneys and also the bile.

DOSE IN RENAL IMPAIRMENT GFR (mL/MIN)

20–50	Dose as in normal renal function.
10–20	Dose as in normal renal function.
<10	Dose as in normal renal function.

DOSE IN PATIENTS UNDERGOING RENAL REPLACEMENT THERAPIES

CAPD	Not dialysed. Dose as in normal renal function.
HD	Not dialysed. Dose as in normal renal function.
HDF/High flux	Unknown dialysability. Dose as in normal renal function.
CAV/ VVHD	Not dialysed. Dose as in normal renal function.

IMPORTANT DRUG INTERACTIONS

Potentially hazardous interactions with other drugs
- None known

ADMINISTRATION

RECONSTITUTION
- 2 mL of sodium chloride 0.9%

ROUTE
–

RATE OF ADMINISTRATION
- Various

COMMENTS
–

OTHER INFORMATION

- Doses from Kumwenda M, Cornall A, Corner L, et al. Urokinase for dysfunctional haemodialysis catheters. *Br J Renal Med*. 2005, **10**(3): 10–11.
- Can also be administered during dialysis.
- Care in patients with uraemic coagulopathies or bleeding diatheses.
- Some units mix 5000 IU of urokinase with 1.5 mL heparin 1000 u/mL.

Ursodeoxycholic acid

CLINICAL USE

- Dissolution of gallstones
- Primary biliary cirrhosis

DOSE IN NORMAL RENAL FUNCTION

- Dissolution of gallstones: 8–12 mg/kg/day in 1–2 divided doses
- Primary biliary cirrhosis: 12–16 mg/kg in 3 divided doses

PHARMACOKINETICS

Molecular weight (daltons)	392.6
% Protein binding	96–98
% Excreted unchanged in urine	0
Volume of distribution (L/kg)	No data
Half-life – normal/ ESRF (hrs)	No data

METABOLISM

Ursodeoxycholic acid is absorbed from the gastrointestinal tract and undergoes enterohepatic recycling. It is partly conjugated in the liver before being excreted into the bile. Under the influence of intestinal bacteria the free and conjugated forms undergo 7α-dehydroxylation to lithocholic acid, some of which is excreted directly in the faeces and the rest absorbed and mainly conjugated and sulphated by the liver before excretion in the faeces.

DOSE IN RENAL IMPAIRMENT GFR (mL/MIN)

20–50	Dose as in normal renal function.
10–20	Dose as in normal renal function.
<10	Dose as in normal renal function.

DOSE IN PATIENTS UNDERGOING RENAL REPLACEMENT THERAPIES

CAPD	Unknown dialysability. Dose as in normal renal function.
HD	Unknown dialysability. Dose as in normal renal function.
HDF/High flux	Unknown dialysability. Dose as in normal renal function.
CAV/ VVHD	Unknown dialysability. Dose as in normal renal function.

IMPORTANT DRUG INTERACTIONS

Potentially hazardous interactions with other drugs
- Ciclosporin: unpredictably increases the absorption of ciclosporin in some patients.

ADMINISTRATION

RECONSTITUTION

–

ROUTE

- Oral

RATE OF ADMINISTRATION

–

COMMENTS

–

OTHER INFORMATION

–

Valaciclovir

CLINICAL USE

Antiviral:
- Herpes zoster and simplex
- Prevention of cytomegalovirus (CMV) disease after renal transplantation

DOSE IN NORMAL RENAL FUNCTION

- Herpes simplex (HSV): 500 mg twice daily for 5–10 days
- Herpes zoster: 1 g 3 times a day for 7 days
- Herpes simplex suppression: 500 mg daily in 1–2 divided doses (500 mg twice daily in the immunocompromised)
- Prevention of CMV disease: 2 g 4 times a day for 90 days

PHARMACOKINETICS

Molecular weight (daltons)	360.8 (as hydrochloride)
% Protein binding	15
% Excreted unchanged in urine	<1
Volume of distribution (L/kg)	0.7
Half-life – normal/ ESRF (hrs)	3/14

METABOLISM

Valaciclovir is readily absorbed from the gastrointestinal tract after oral doses, and is rapidly and almost completely converted to aciclovir and valine by first-pass intestinal or hepatic metabolism.

Aciclovir is converted to a small extent to the metabolites 9(carboxymethoxy) methylguanine (CMMG) by alcohol and aldehyde dehydrogenase and to 8-hydroxy-aciclovir (8-OH-ACV) by aldehyde oxidase. Approximately 88% of the total combined plasma exposure is attributable to aciclovir, 11% to CMMG and 1% to 8-OH-ACV. Valaciclovir is eliminated mainly as aciclovir and its metabolite 9-CMMG; less than 1% of a dose of valaciclovir is excreted unchanged in the urine.

DOSE IN RENAL IMPAIRMENT GFR (mL/MIN)

For HSV & Herpes zoster
50–75	Dose as in normal renal function.
30–50	HSV (treatment & suppression): Dose as in normal renal function. Herpes zoster: 1 g every 12 hours
10–30	HSV treatment: 500 mg daily. HSV treatment (immunocompromised): 1 g daily HSV suppression: 250 mg daily HSV suppression (immunocompromised): 500 mg daily or 250 mg every 12 hours Herpes zoster: 1 g daily
<10	HSV treatment: 500 mg daily HSV treatment (immunocompromised): 1 g daily HSV suppression: 250 mg daily HSV suppression (immunocompromised): 500 mg daily or 250 mg every 12 hours Herpes zoster: 500 mg daily

For CMV prophylaxis:
50–75	1.5 g every 6 hours
25–50	1.5 g every 8 hours
10–25	1.5 g every 12 hours
<10	1.5 g once daily

DOSE IN PATIENTS UNDERGOING RENAL REPLACEMENT THERAPIES

CAPD	Likely dialysability. Dose as in GFR<10 mL/min.
HD	Dialysed. Dose as in GFR<10 mL/min post dialysis.
HDF/High flux	Dialysed. Dose as in GFR<10 mL/min post dialysis.
CAV/ VVHD	Likely dialysability. Dose as in GFR=10–30 mL/min.

IMPORTANT DRUG INTERACTIONS

Potentially hazardous interactions with other drugs
- Ciclosporin: may alter ciclosporin levels; possibly increased risk of nephrotoxicity.
- Mycophenolate: higher concentrations of both aciclovir and mycophenolic acid on concomitant administration.
- Tacrolimus: possibly increased risk of nephrotoxicity.

ADMINISTRATION

RECONSTITUTION
–

ROUTE
- Oral

RATE OF ADMINISTRATION
–

COMMENTS
–

OTHER INFORMATION

- Bioavailability of aciclovir from 1 g oral dose of valaciclovir is 54%.
- Mean peak aciclovir concentrations occur 1.5 hours post dose; peak plasma concentrations of valaciclovir are 4% of aciclovir levels, occur at a median of 30–60 minutes post dose, and are at or below the limit of quantification 3 hours post dose.
- The dose quoted in the literature for CMV prophylaxis in transplant recipients is 2 g 4 times a day. However, in practice this results in severe aciclovir toxicity, especially in patients with poorly functioning grafts.

Valganciclovir

CLINICAL USE

- Induction and maintenance treatment of CMV retinitis in AIDS patients
- Treatment and prophylaxis of CMV disease in transplant patients

DOSE IN NORMAL RENAL FUNCTION

- Induction/Treatment: 900 mg twice daily for 21 days
- Maintenance/Prophylaxis: 900 mg once daily

PHARMACOKINETICS

Molecular weight (daltons)	390.8 (as hydrochloride)
% Protein binding	<2 (as ganciclovir)
% Excreted unchanged in urine	84.6–94.6 (as ganciclovir)
Volume of distribution (L/kg)	0.519–0.841
Half-life – normal/ ESRF (hrs)	4.1/67.5

METABOLISM

Valganciclovir is well absorbed from the gastrointestinal tract and rapidly and extensively metabolised in the intestinal wall and liver to ganciclovir. Valganciclovir is eliminated in the urine as unchanged ganciclovir, mainly by glomerular filtration and also active tubular secretion.

DOSE IN RENAL IMPAIRMENT GFR (mL/MIN)

40–59	Treatment: 450 mg twice daily Prophylaxis: 450 mg daily
25–39	Treatment: 450 mg daily Prophylaxis: 225 mg daily or 450 mg every 48 hours
10–24	Treatment: 225 mg daily or 450 mg every 48 hours Prophylaxis: 125 mg daily or 450 mg twice weekly
<10	Treatment: 200 mg 3 times a week or 450 mg 2–3 times a week Prophylaxis: 100 mg 3 times a week or 450 mg 1–2 times a week See 'Other information'.

DOSE IN PATIENTS UNDERGOING RENAL REPLACEMENT THERAPIES

CAPD	Dialysed. See 'Other information'.
HD	Dialysed. See 'Other information'.
HDF/High flux	Dialysed. See 'Other information'.
CAV/ VVHD	Dialysed. Dose as in GFR=10–24 mL/min.

IMPORTANT DRUG INTERACTIONS

Potentially hazardous interactions with other drugs
- Antibacterials: increased risk of convulsions with imipenem-cilastatin.
- Antivirals: possibly increased didanosine concentration; profound myelosuppression with zidovudine – avoid if possible.
- Mycophenolate: possibly increased concentrations of both mycophenolic acid and ganciclovir.
- Increased risk of myelosuppression with other myelosuppressive drugs.

ADMINISTRATION

RECONSTITUTION
-
ROUTE
- Oral
RATE OF ADMINISTRATION
-
COMMENTS
-

OTHER INFORMATION

- 900 mg valganciclovir twice daily is therapeutically equivalent to 5 mg/kg intravenous ganciclovir twice daily.
- Valganciclovir is a prodrug of ganciclovir.
- Take with food if possible.
- It is recommended that complete blood counts and platelet counts be monitored during therapy especially in patients with renal impairment.
- Approximately 50% of ganciclovir is removed by haemodialysis.
- An alternative treatment regimen used in some units is:

GFR (mL/min)	Dose
>50	900 mg twice daily
25–50	450 mg twice daily
10–25	450 mg once daily
<10	450 mg 3 times a week

Valproate semisodium

CLINICAL USE

- Treatment of manic episodes associated with bipolar disorder
- Migraine prophylaxis (unlicensed)

DOSE IN NORMAL RENAL FUNCTION

- 750 mg–2 g daily in 2–3 divided doses
- Migraine prophylaxis: 250 mg twice daily increased to 1 g daily in divided doses if required

PHARMACOKINETICS

Molecular weight (daltons)	310.4
% Protein binding	85–94
% Excreted unchanged in urine	<3
Volume of distribution (L/kg)	0.1–0.4
Half-life – normal/ ESRF (hrs)	14/Increased

METABOLISM

Valproic acid is extensively metabolised in the liver, a large part by glucuronidation (up to 60%) and the rest by a variety of complex pathways (up to 45%). It is excreted in the urine almost entirely in the form of its metabolites; small amounts are excreted in faeces and expired air.

DOSE IN RENAL IMPAIRMENT GFR (mL/MIN)

20–50	Dose as in normal renal function.
10–20	Dose as in normal renal function.
<10	Start with a low dose, adjust according to response.

DOSE IN PATIENTS UNDERGOING RENAL REPLACEMENT THERAPIES

CAPD	Not dialysed. Dose as in GFR<10 mL/min.
HD	Dialysed. Dose as in GFR<10 mL/min.
HDF/High flux	Dialysed. Dose as in GFR<10 mL/min.
CAV/ VVHD	Dialysed. Dose as in normal renal function.

IMPORTANT DRUG INTERACTIONS

Potentially hazardous interactions with other drugs

- Antibacterials: metabolism possibly inhibited by erythromycin; avoid with pivmecillinam; concentration reduced by carbapenems – avoid.
- Antidepressants: avoid with St John's wort.
- Anti-epileptics: concentration reduced by carbamazepine; concentration of active carbamazepine metabolite increased; increased concentration of lamotrigine, phenobarbital, rufinamide and possibly ethosuximide; sometimes reduces concentration of active metabolite of oxcarbazepine; alters phenytoin concentration; phenytoin and phenobarbital reduce valproate concentration; hyperammonaemia and CNS toxicity with topiramate.
- Antipsychotics: increased neutropenia with olanzapine; possibly increases or decreases concentration of clozapine; possibly increases quetiapine concentration.
- Ciclosporin: variable ciclosporin blood level response.
- Ulcer-healing drugs: metabolism inhibited by cimetidine, increased concentration.

ADMINISTRATION

RECONSTITUTION

–

ROUTE

- Oral

RATE OF ADMINISTRATION

–

COMMENTS

–

OTHER INFORMATION

- May cause carnitine deficiency.
- Dialysis removes about 20% of dose.
- Tablets can be crushed but may result in increased gastrointestinal side effects.

Valsartan

CLINICAL USE

Angiotensin-II antagonist:
- Hypertension
- Heart failure
- Myocardial infarction with left ventricular failure

DOSE IN NORMAL RENAL FUNCTION

- Hypertension: 40–320 mg daily in divided doses
- Heart failure: 40–160 mg twice daily
- Myocardial infarction: 20–160 mg twice daily

PHARMACOKINETICS

Molecular weight (daltons)	435.5
% Protein binding	94–97
% Excreted unchanged in urine	13
Volume of distribution (L/kg)	17
Half-life – normal/ ESRF (hrs)	5–9/Unchanged

METABOLISM

Valsartan is not highly metabolised as only about 20% of dose is recovered as metabolites. A hydroxy metabolite has been identified in plasma at low concentrations (less than 10% of the valsartan AUC). This metabolite is pharmacologically inactive.

Valsartan is mainly eliminated by biliary excretion in faeces (about 83% of dose) and renally in urine (about 13% of dose), mainly as unchanged drug.

DOSE IN RENAL IMPAIRMENT GFR (mL/MIN)

20–50	Dose as in normal renal function.
10–20	Initial dose 40 mg; titrate according to response.
<10	Initial dose 40 mg; titrate according to response.

DOSE IN PATIENTS UNDERGOING RENAL REPLACEMENT THERAPIES

CAPD	Not dialysed. Dose as in GFR<10 mL/min.
HD	Not dialysed. Dose as in GFR<10 mL/min.
HDF/High flux	Unknown dialysability. Dose as in GFR<10 mL/min.
CAV/ VVHD	Unlikely to be dialysed. Dose as in GFR=10–20 mL/min.

IMPORTANT DRUG INTERACTIONS

Potentially hazardous interactions with other drugs
- Anaesthetics: enhanced hypotensive effect.
- Analgesics: antagonism of hypotensive effect and increased risk of renal impairment with NSAIDs; hyperkalaemia with ketorolac and other NSAIDs.
- Ciclosporin: increased risk of hyperkalaemia and nephrotoxicity.
- Diuretics: enhanced hypotensive effect; hyperkalaemia with potassium-sparing diuretics.
- ESAs: increased risk of hyperkalaemia; antagonism of hypotensive effect.
- Lithium: reduced excretion (possibility of enhanced lithium toxicity).
- Potassium salts: increased risk of hyperkalaemia.
- Tacrolimus: increased risk of hyperkalaemia and nephrotoxicity.

ADMINISTRATION

RECONSTITUTION
–
ROUTE
- Oral
RATE OF ADMINISTRATION
–
COMMENTS
—

OTHER INFORMATION

- Bioavailability is 23%.
- Side effects (e.g. hyperkalaemia, metabolic acidosis) are more common in patients with impaired renal function.
- Close monitoring of renal function during therapy is necessary in those with renal insufficiency.
- Renal failure has been reported in association with angiotensin-II antagonists in patients with renal artery stenosis, post renal transplant, and in those with severe congestive heart failure.

Vancomycin

CLINICAL USE

Antibacterial agent

DOSE IN NORMAL RENAL FUNCTION

- IV: 1–1.5 g every 12 hours
- Oral: 125 mg up to 500 mg 4 times daily
- (Higher dose for resistant cases of *Clostridium difficile*)

PHARMACOKINETICS

Molecular weight (daltons)	1449.3; (1485.7 as hydrochloride)
% Protein binding	10–50 (19 CKD 5)
% Excreted unchanged in urine	80–90
Volume of distribution (L/kg)	0.47–1.1 (0.88 CKD 5)
Half-life – normal/ ESRF (hrs)	6/120–216

METABOLISM

Little or no metabolism of vancomycin is thought to take place. It is excreted unchanged by the kidneys, mostly by glomerular filtration. There is a small amount of non-renal clearance, although the mechanism for this has not been determined.

DOSE IN RENAL IMPAIRMENT GFR (mL/MIN)

See 'Other information' for alternative method in moderate and severe renal impairment.

20–50	IV: 0.5–1 g every 12–24 hours Oral: Dose as in normal renal function.
10–20	IV: 0.5–1 g every 24–48 hours Oral: Dose as in normal renal function.
<10	IV: 0.5–1 g every 48–96 hours Oral: Dose as in normal renal function.

DOSE IN PATIENTS UNDERGOING RENAL REPLACEMENT THERAPIES

CAPD	Not dialysed. Dose as in GFR<10 mL/min.
HD	Not dialysed. Dose as in GFR<10 mL/min.
HDF/High flux	Dialysed. See 'Other information'.
CAV/ VVHD	Dialysed. 1 g every 48 hours.[1]
CVVHD/ HDF	Dialysed. 1 g daily and see 'Other information'.[1]

IMPORTANT DRUG INTERACTIONS

Potentially hazardous interactions with other drugs

- Antibacterials: increased risk of nephrotoxicity and ototoxicity with aminoglycosides, capreomycin or colistimethate sodium; increased risk of nephrotoxicity with polymyxins.
- Ciclosporin: variable response; increased risk of nephrotoxicity.
- Diuretics: increased risk of ototoxicity with loop diuretics.
- Muscle relaxants: enhanced effects of suxamethonium.
- Tacrolimus: possible increased risk of nephrotoxicity.

ADMINISTRATION

RECONSTITUTION
- 10 mL water for injection per 500 mg vial, then dilute 1 g to 250 mL with sodium chloride 0.9% (50 mL if giving centrally).

ROUTE
- IV, oral

RATE OF ADMINISTRATION
- Not faster than 10 mg/minute

COMMENTS
- Usual dilution is 10–20 mg/mL. (UK Critical Care Group, *Minimum Infusion Volumes for Fluid Restricted Critically Ill Patients*, 3rd edition, 2006.)

USE IN CAPD PERITONITIS:
- 12.5–25 mg/L per bag (See local protocol.)
- Various other regimens used in PD ranging from IV dosing to high dose stat IP use.
- Some units use the following:
  — Patient weight >60 kg: stat dose of 2 g IP on days 1, 7 and 14 with a 6 hour dwell
  — Patient weight <60 kg: 1.5 g IP on days 1, 7 and 14.

OTHER INFORMATION

- Second line to metronidazole in treatment of pseudomembranous colitis.
- Not absorbed via oral route at low doses but monitor plasma levels at higher doses.
- Injection solution may be given orally; however, oral capsules available.

- Alternative dosage adjustment in moderate and severe renal impairment:
  — Give 1 g loading dose and monitor serum levels at 24 hour intervals. When level <10 mg/L give another 1 g dose. Peak levels, 2 hours after dose, should be in range 18–26 mg/L. Some units use a 500 mg loading dose.
- Anephric/dialysis patients usually need 1 g once or twice weekly.
- In HDF higher doses are required; possible doses are 1 g initially followed by 500 mg every dialysis for 3 dialysis sessions. (Ariano RE, Fine A, Sitar DS. Adequacy of a vancomycin dosing regimen in patients receiving high-flux haemodialysis. *Am J Kidney Dis.* 2005; **46**(4): 681–7.)

- 25 mg/kg once weekly in anuric patients. (Foote EF, Dreitlein WB, Steward CA, *et al.* Pharmacokinetics of vancomycin when administered during high flux hemodialysis. *Clin Nephrol.* 1998; **50**(1): 51–5.)
- For CVVHDF: 450–750 mg every 12 hours has been suggested. (Deldot ME, Lipman J, Tett SE. Vancomycin pharmacokinetics in critically ill patients receiving continuous venovenous haemodiafiltration. *Br J Clin Pharmacol.* 2004; **58**(3): 259–68.)

Reference:
1. Trotman RL, Williamson JC, Shoemaker DM, *et al.* Antibiotic dosing in critically ill adult patients receiving continuous renal replacement therapy. *Clin Infect Dis.* 2005 Oct 15; **41**: 1159–66.

Vandetanib

CLINICAL USE

Tyrosine kinase inhibitor:
- Treatment of aggressive and symptomatic medullary thyroid cancer

DOSE IN NORMAL RENAL FUNCTION

300 mg once daily

PHARMACOKINETICS

Molecular weight (daltons)	475.4
% Protein binding	Approximately 90
% Excreted unchanged in urine	25
Volume of distribution (L/kg)	7450 litres
Half-life – normal/ ESRF (hrs)	19 days/Increased

METABOLISM

N-desmethyl-vandetanib is primarily produced by CYP3A4, and vandetanib-N-oxide is primarily produced by flavin-containing monooxygenase enzymes FMO1 and FMO3.

Unchanged vandetanib and metabolites vandetanib N-oxide and N-desmethyl vandetanib were detected in plasma, urine (25%) and faeces (44%).

DOSE IN RENAL IMPAIRMENT GFR (mL/MIN)

30–50	Initially 200 mg daily. See 'Other information'.
10–30	Initially 200 mg daily. See 'Other information'.
<10	Initially 200 mg daily. See 'Other information'.

DOSE IN PATIENTS UNDERGOING RENAL REPLACEMENT THERAPIES

CAPD	Unlikely to be dialysed. Dose as in GFR<10 mL/min. Use with caution.
HD	Unlikely to be dialysed. Dose as in GFR<10 mL/min. Use with caution.
HDF/High flux	Unlikely to be dialysed. Dose as in GFR<10 mL/min. Use with caution.
CAV/ VVHD	Unlikely to be dialysed. Dose as in GFR=10–30 mL/min. Use with caution.

IMPORTANT DRUG INTERACTIONS

Potentially hazardous interactions with other drugs
- Analgesics: possibly increased risk of ventricular arrhythmias with methadone – avoid.
- Anti-arrhythmics: possibly increased risk of ventricular arrhythmias with amiodarone or disopyramide – avoid.
- Antibacterials: possibly increased risk of ventricular arrhythmias with parenteral erythromycin and moxifloxacin – avoid; concentration reduced by rifampicin – avoid.
- Antihistamines: possibly increased risk of ventricular arrhythmias with mizolastine – avoid.
- Antimalarials: possibly increased risk of ventricular arrhythmias with artemether with lumefantrine – avoid.
- Antipsychotics: possibly increased risk of ventricular arrhythmias with amisulpride, chlorpromazine, haloperidol, pimozide, sulpiride and zuclopenthixol – avoid; avoid concomitant use with clozapine, risk of agranulocytosis.
- Beta-blockers: possibly increased risk of ventricular arrhythmias with sotalol – avoid.
- Cytotoxics: possibly increased risk of ventricular arrhythmias with arsenic trioxide – avoid.
- Hormone antagonist: possibly increased risk of ventricular arrhythmias with toremifene – avoid.
- $5HT_3$-receptor antagonists: possibly increased risk of ventricular arrhythmias with ondansetron – avoid.
- Pentamidine: possibly increased risk of ventricular arrhythmias – avoid.

ADMINISTRATION

RECONSTITUTION

–

ROUTE
- Oral

RATE OF ADMINISTRATION

–

OTHER INFORMATION

- Although an initial dose of 200 mg has been recommended by the UK manufacturer in moderate renal impairment there is little safety or efficacy data for this dose. Not recommended in severe renal impairment due to lack of data.

- Dosage in severe renal impairment from US data sheet.
- Vandetanib can prolong the Q-T interval so is contraindicated for use in patients with serious cardiac complications such as congenital long QT syndrome and uncompensated heart failure.
- A pharmacokinetic study in volunteers with mild, moderate and severe renal impairment (GFR<30 mL/min) shows that exposure to vandetanib after a single dose is increased up to 1.5, 1.6 and 2-fold respectively.

Vardenafil

CLINICAL USE

Treatment of erectile dysfunction

DOSE IN NORMAL RENAL FUNCTION

- 5–20 mg approximately 25–60 minutes before sexual activity
- Dose depends on preparation

PHARMACOKINETICS

Molecular weight (daltons)	488.6
% Protein binding	95
% Excreted unchanged in urine	2–6
Volume of distribution (L/kg)	208
Half-life – normal/ ESRF (hrs)	4–5

METABOLISM

Vardenafil is metabolised in the liver primarily by cytochrome P450 isoenzymes CYP3A4 (the major route) as well as CYP3A5 and CYP2C isoforms. The major metabolite produced by desethylation of vardenafil also has some activity.

Vardenafil is excreted as metabolites mainly in the faeces (91–95%), and to a lesser extent in the urine.

DOSE IN RENAL IMPAIRMENT GFR (mL/MIN)

30–50	Dose as in normal renal function.
10–30	Initial dose 5 mg and adjust accordingly.
<10	Initial dose 5 mg and adjust accordingly.

DOSE IN PATIENTS UNDERGOING RENAL REPLACEMENT THERAPIES

CAPD	Not dialysed. Dose as in GFR<10 mL/min. Use with caution.
HD	Not dialysed. Dose as in GFR<10 mL/min. Use with caution.
HDF/High flux	Unknown dialysability. Dose as in GFR<10 mL/min. Use with caution.
CAV/ VVHD	Not dialysed. Dose as in GFR=10–30 mL/min.

IMPORTANT DRUG INTERACTIONS

Potentially hazardous interactions with other drugs

- Alpha-blockers: enhanced hypotensive effect – avoid for 6 hours after alpha-blockers (max dose 5 mg).
- Antifungals: concentration increased by ketoconazole, and itraconazole – avoid concomitant use.
- Antivirals: concentration increased by fosamprenavir, indinavir and ritonavir – avoid with indinavir and ritonavir; increased risk of ventricular arrhythmias with saquinavir – avoid; avoid with telaprevir, use tipranavir with caution.
- Grapefruit juice: concentration possibly increased – avoid concomitant use.
- Nicorandil: possibly enhanced hypotensive effect – avoid concomitant use.
- Nitrates: possibly enhanced hypotensive effect – avoid concomitant use.

ADMINISTRATION

RECONSTITUTION

–

ROUTE

- Oral

RATE OF ADMINISTRATION

–

COMMENTS

–

OTHER INFORMATION

- Contraindicated in dialysis patients due to lack of information, therefore suggest use with caution.
- Bioavailability is 15%.

Varenicline

CLINICAL USE

Aid to smoking cessation

DOSE IN NORMAL RENAL FUNCTION

0.5 mg once daily for 3 days, 0.5 mg twice daily for 4 days, then 0.5–1 mg twice daily

PHARMACOKINETICS

Molecular weight (daltons)	361.3 (as tartrate)
% Protein binding	<20
% Excreted unchanged in urine	92
Volume of distribution (L/kg)	415
Half-life – normal/ ESRF (hrs)	24/Increased

METABOLISM

Varenicline undergoes minimal metabolism with less than 10% excreted as metabolites. About 92% of a dose is excreted unchanged in the urine.

Minor metabolites in urine include varenicline N-carbamoylglucuronide, N-glucosylvarenicline and hydroxyvarenicline. In circulation, varenicline comprises 91% of drug-related material.

DOSE IN RENAL IMPAIRMENT GFR (mL/MIN)

Initial doses as for normal renal function, then maintenance doses of:
30–50 1 mg once or twice daily.
10–30 0.5–1 mg daily.
<10   0.5–1 mg daily.

DOSE IN PATIENTS UNDERGOING RENAL REPLACEMENT THERAPIES

CAPD	Unknown dialysability. 0.5 mg once daily.
HD	Dialysed. 0.5 mg once daily.
HDF/High flux	Dialysed. 0.5 mg once daily.
CAV/ VVHD	Dialysed. Dose as in GFR=10–30 mL/min.

IMPORTANT DRUG INTERACTIONS

Potentially hazardous interactions with other drugs
• None known

ADMINISTRATION

RECONSTITUTION
–
ROUTE
• Oral
RATE OF ADMINISTRATION
–
COMMENTS
–

OTHER INFORMATION

• Contraindicated by manufacturer in end-stage renal disease in UK SPC, US data sheet advises a maximum dose of 0.5 mg once daily.

Vecuronium bromide

CLINICAL USE

Non-depolarising muscle relaxant

DOSE IN NORMAL RENAL FUNCTION

- Intubation: 80–100 micrograms/kg, with maintenance of 20–30 micrograms/kg
- IV infusion: 0.8–1.4 micrograms/kg/minute adjusted according to response

PHARMACOKINETICS

Molecular weight (daltons)	637.7
% Protein binding	30
% Excreted unchanged in urine	25
Volume of distribution (L/kg)	0.18–0.27
Half-life – normal/ESRF (hrs)	0.5–1.3/Unchanged

METABOLISM

Vecuronium partly metabolised by the liver; the metabolites have some neuromuscular blocking activity. It is excreted mainly in bile as unchanged drug and metabolites; some is also excreted in the urine.

DOSE IN RENAL IMPAIRMENT GFR (mL/MIN)

20–50	Dose as in normal renal function.
10–20	Dose as in normal renal function.
<10	Dose as in normal renal function.

DOSE IN PATIENTS UNDERGOING RENAL REPLACEMENT THERAPIES

CAPD	Unlikely to be dialysed. Dose as in normal renal function.
HD	Unlikely to be dialysed. Dose as in normal renal function.
HDF/High flux	Unknown dialysability. Dose as in normal renal function.
CAV/VVHD	Unknown dialysability. Dose as in normal renal function.

IMPORTANT DRUG INTERACTIONS

Potentially hazardous interactions with other drugs
- Anaesthetics: enhanced muscle relaxant effect.
- Anti-arrhythmics: procainamide enhances muscle relaxant effect.
- Antibacterials: effect enhanced by aminoglycosides, clindamycin, polymyxins and piperacillin.
- Anti-epileptics: muscle relaxant effects antagonised by carbamazepine; effects reduced by long-term use of phenytoin but might be increased by acute use.
- Botulinum toxin: neuromuscular block enhanced (risk of toxicity).

ADMINISTRATION

RECONSTITUTION
- 5 mL water for injection to reconstitute 10 mg vial; up to 10 mL sodium chloride 0.9% or glucose 5% may be used.

ROUTE
- IV

RATE OF ADMINISTRATION
- See dose.

COMMENTS
- May be added to sodium chloride 0.9%, glucose 5% or Ringer's solution to give a final concentration of 40 mg/L.

OTHER INFORMATION

- Use normal doses with caution in renal failure as has active metabolites which may accumulate.

Vemurafenib

CLINICAL USE

BRAF kinase inhibitor:
- Treatment of metastatic melanoma

DOSE IN NORMAL RENAL FUNCTION

960 mg twice daily (doses 12 hours apart)

PHARMACOKINETICS

Molecular weight (daltons)	489.9
% Protein binding	>99
% Excreted unchanged in urine	1
Volume of distribution (L/kg)	91–106 litres
Half-life – normal/ ESRF (hrs)	51.6/–

METABOLISM

Only 5% of a dose of vemurafenib is metabolised.

Some 94% of the dose is excreted in the faeces and 1% in the urine.

DOSE IN RENAL IMPAIRMENT GFR (mL/MIN)

40–50	Dose as in normal renal function.
10–40	Use with caution.
<10	Use with caution.

DOSE IN PATIENTS UNDERGOING RENAL REPLACEMENT THERAPIES

CAPD	Unlikely to be dialysed. Use with caution.
HD	Unlikely to be dialysed. Use with caution.
HDF/High flux	Unlikely to be dialysed. Use with caution.
CAV/ VVHD	Unlikely to be dialysed. Use with caution.

IMPORTANT DRUG INTERACTIONS

Potentially hazardous interactions with other drugs
- Anticoagulants: possibly enhances anticoagulant effect of warfarin.
- Antipsychotics: avoid concomitant use with clozapine, risk of agranulocytosis.
- Oestrogens & progestogens: contraceptive effect possibly reduced.

ADMINISTRATION

RECONSTITUTION
–
ROUTE
- Oral
RATE OF ADMINISTRATION
–

OTHER INFORMATION

- Manufacturer advises to use with caution in severe renal impairment due to lack of data.
- Accumulation may occur in patients with renal impairment although there was no difference in clearance down to a GFR<40 mL/min.
- May cause exposure dependent QT prolongation in which case the dose should be reduced.

Venlafaxine

CLINICAL USE

Antidepressant:
- Depressive illness
- Generalised anxiety disorders
- Panic disorders

DOSE IN NORMAL RENAL FUNCTION

- 37.5–187.5 mg twice daily
- XL: 75–375 mg daily
- Generalised anxiety disorder: 75–225 mg once daily
- Panic disorders: 37.5–225 mg daily

PHARMACOKINETICS

Molecular weight (daltons)	277; (313.9 as hydrochloride)
% Protein binding	27
% Excreted unchanged in urine	5
Volume of distribution (L/kg)	7.5
Half-life – normal/ESRF (hrs)	5/6–8 XL: 9–21

METABOLISM

Venlafaxine undergoes extensive first-pass metabolism in the liver mainly to the active metabolite O-desmethylvenlafaxine; this is mediated by the cytochrome P450 isoenzyme CYP2D6. The isoenzyme CYP3A4 is also involved in the metabolism of venlafaxine. Other metabolites include N-desmethylvenlafaxine and N,O-didesmethylvenlafaxine. Peak plasma concentrations of venlafaxine and O-desmethylvenlafaxine occur about 2 and 4 hours after a dose, respectively.

The majority of venlafaxine is excreted in the urine, mainly in the form of its metabolites, either free or in conjugated form.

DOSE IN RENAL IMPAIRMENT GFR (mL/MIN)

30–50	Dose as in normal renal function.
10–30	Reduce total dose by 50%.
<10	Reduce total dose by 50%.

DOSE IN PATIENTS UNDERGOING RENAL REPLACEMENT THERAPIES

CAPD	Not dialysed. Dose as in GFR<10 mL/min.
HD	Not dialysed. Dose as in GFR<10 mL/min.
HDF/High flux	Unknown dialysability. Dose as in GFR<10 mL/min.
CAV/VVHD	Not dialysed. Dose as in GFR=10–30 mL/min.

IMPORTANT DRUG INTERACTIONS

Potentially hazardous interactions with other drugs
- Analgesics: increased risk of bleeding with aspirin and NSAIDs; possibly increased serotonergic effects with tramadol.
- Anticoagulants: effects of warfarin possibly enhanced; possibly increased risk of bleeding with dabigatran.
- Antidepressants: avoid concomitant use with MAOIs and moclobemide (increased risk of toxicity); possibly enhanced serotonergic effects with duloxetine, mirtazapine and St John's wort.
- Antimalarials: avoid concomitant use with artemether/lumefantrine and piperaquine with artenimol.
- Antipsychotics: increases concentration of clozapine and haloperidol.
- Dopaminergics: use entacapone with caution; increased risk of hypertension and CNS excitation with selegiline – avoid concomitant use.
- Methylthioninium: risk of CNS toxicity – avoid if possible.

ADMINISTRATION

RECONSTITUTION
–
ROUTE
- Oral
RATE OF ADMINISTRATION
–
COMMENTS
–

OTHER INFORMATION

- Withhold dose until after haemodialysis to minimise nausea and any other side effects.
- May be used to treat peripheral diabetic neuropathy in haemodialysis patients; dose is up to 75 mg daily. www.medscape.com/viewarticle/440202
- An ECG is required before treatment.

Verapamil hydrochloride

CLINICAL USE

Calcium-channel blocker:
- Supraventricular arrhythmias
- Angina
- Hypertension

DOSE IN NORMAL RENAL FUNCTION

Oral:
- Supraventricular arrhythmias: 40–120 mg 3 times daily
- Angina: 80–120 mg 3 times daily
- Hypertension: 240–480 mg daily in 2–3 divided doses

IV:
- 5–10 mg followed by 5 mg, 5–10 minutes later if required

PHARMACOKINETICS

Molecular weight (daltons)	491.1
% Protein binding	90
% Excreted unchanged in urine	<4
Volume of distribution (L/kg)	3–6
Half-life – normal/ ESRF (hrs)	4.5–12/Increased

METABOLISM

Verapamil undergoes considerable first pass loss and is extensively metabolised in the liver. Twelve metabolites have been identified. Of these only norverapamil has any significant activity (approximately 20% that of the parent compound).

Norverapamil represents about 6% of the dose eliminated in urine and reaches steady-state plasma concentrations approximately equal to those of verapamil. About 70% of a dose is excreted by the kidneys in the form of its metabolites but about 16% is excreted in the bile into the faeces. Less than 4% is excreted unchanged.

DOSE IN RENAL IMPAIRMENT GFR (mL/MIN)

20–50	Dose as in normal renal function. Monitor carefully
10–20	Dose as in normal renal function. Monitor carefully.
<10	Dose as in normal renal function. Monitor carefully.

DOSE IN PATIENTS UNDERGOING RENAL REPLACEMENT THERAPIES

CAPD	Not dialysed. Dose as in GFR<10 mL/min.
HD	Not dialysed. Dose as in GFR<10 mL/min.
HDF/High flux	Unknown dialysability. Dose as in GFR<10 mL/min.
CAV/ VVHD	Dialysability minimal. Dose as in GFR=10–20 mL/min.

IMPORTANT DRUG INTERACTIONS

Potentially hazardous interactions with other drugs
- Anaesthetics: increased hypotensive effect.
- Anti-arrhythmics: increased risk of amiodarone-induced bradycardia, AV block and myocardial depression; increased risk of myocardial depression and asystole with disopyramide and flecainide; increased risk of bradycardia and myocardial depression with dronedarone.
- Antibacterials: metabolism increased by rifampicin; metabolism possibly inhibited by erythromycin, clarithromycin and telithromycin (increased risk of toxicity).
- Anticoagulants: possibly increases dabigatran concentration – reduce dabigatran dose.
- Antidepressants: enhanced hypotensive effect with MAOIs; concentration of imipramine and possibly other tricyclics increased; concentration significantly reduced by St John's wort.
- Anti-epileptics: effect probably reduced by barbiturates, phenytoin and primidone; enhanced effect of carbamazepine.
- Antifungals: negative inotropic effect possibly increased with itraconazole.
- Antihypertensives: enhanced hypotensive effect, increased risk of first dose hypotensive effect of post-synaptic alpha-blockers.
- Antivirals: concentration possibly increased by atazanavir and ritonavir; use telaprevir with caution.
- Beta-blockers: enhanced hypotensive effect; risk of asystole, severe hypotension and heart failure if co-prescribed with beta-blockers.

- Cardiac glycosides: increased levels of digoxin. Increased AV block and bradycardia.
- Ciclosporin: variable reports of decreased nephrotoxicity and potentiated effect; may also increase ciclosporin levels.
- Colchicine: possibly increased risk of colchicine toxicity – suspend or reduce colchicine, avoid concomitant use in renal or hepatic failure.
- Cytotoxics: possibly increased doxorubicin concentration; possibly increased risk of bradycardia with crizotinib; concentration of both drugs may be increased in combination with everolimus.
- Fingolimod: increased risk of bradycardia.
- Grapefruit juice: concentration increased – avoid concomitant use.
- Ivabradine: concentration of ivabradine increased – avoid concomitant use.
- Sirolimus: concentration of both drugs increased.
- Statins: increased myopathy with simvastatin – do not exceed 20 mg of simvastatin.[1]
- Tacrolimus: may increase tacrolimus levels.
- Theophylline: enhanced effect of theophylline.

ADMINISTRATION

RECONSTITUTION
–

ROUTE
- Oral, IV

RATE OF ADMINISTRATION
- Over 2 minutes (3 minutes in elderly)

COMMENTS
–

OTHER INFORMATION

- Monitor BP and ECG.
- Active metabolites may accumulate in renal impairment.

Reference:
1. MHRA. *Drug Safety Update*. Statins: interactions and updated advice. August 2012; **6**(1): 2–4.

Vigabatrin

CLINICAL USE

Anti-epileptic agent

DOSE IN NORMAL RENAL FUNCTION

1–3 g daily in single or divided doses

PHARMACOKINETICS

Molecular weight (daltons)	129.2
% Protein binding	Negligible
% Excreted unchanged in urine	60–80
Volume of distribution (L/kg)	0.8
Half-life – normal/ ESRF (hrs)	5–8/13–15

METABOLISM

Vigabatrin is not significantly metabolised. About 60–80% of an oral dose is excreted in urine as unchanged drug.

DOSE IN RENAL IMPAIRMENT GFR (mL/MIN)

50–80	Give 75% of normal dose and titrate to response.
30–50	Give 50% of normal dose and titrate to response.
10–30	Give 50% of normal dose and titrate to response.
<10	Give 25% of normal dose and titrate to response.

DOSE IN PATIENTS UNDERGOING RENAL REPLACEMENT THERAPIES

CAPD	Unknown dialysability. Dose as for GFR<10 mL/min.
HD	Dialysed. Dose as for GFR<10 mL/min.
HDF/High flux	Dialysed. Dose as for GFR<10 mL/min.
CAV/ VVHD	Dialysed. Dose as for GFR=10–30 mL/min.

IMPORTANT DRUG INTERACTIONS

Potentially hazardous interactions with other drugs
- Antidepressants: anticonvulsant effect antagonised, convulsive threshold lowered; avoid with St John's wort.
- Anti-epileptics: concentration of phenytoin reduced.
- Antimalarials: mefloquine antagonises anticonvulsant effect.
- Antipsychotics: anticonvulsant effect antagonised.
- Orlistat: increased risk of convulsions.

ADMINISTRATION

RECONSTITUTION

–

ROUTE
- Oral

RATE OF ADMINISTRATION

–

COMMENTS

–

OTHER INFORMATION

- UK SPC advises to use with caution if GFR<60 mL/min, doses in monograph are taken from US data sheet.

Vildagliptin

CLINICAL USE

Dipeptidyl peptidase 4 inhibitor:
● Treatment of type 2 diabetes mellitus in combination with other antidiabetic drugs

DOSE IN NORMAL RENAL FUNCTION

● 50 mg twice daily
● With a sulphonylurea: 50 mg in the morning

PHARMACOKINETICS

Molecular weight (daltons)	303.4
% Protein binding	9.3
% Excreted unchanged in urine	23
Volume of distribution (L/kg)	71 litres
Half-life – normal/ ESRF (hrs)	3/Increased

METABOLISM

About 69% of a dose of vildagliptin is metabolised, mainly by hydrolysis in the kidney to inactive metabolites. About 85% of a dose is excreted in the urine (23% as unchanged drug), and 15% in the faeces.

DOSE IN RENAL IMPAIRMENT GFR (mL/MIN)

20–50	50 mg daily.
10–20	50 mg daily.
<10	50 mg daily.

DOSE IN PATIENTS UNDERGOING RENAL REPLACEMENT THERAPIES

CAPD	Not dialysed. Dose as in GFR<10 mL/min.
HD	Not dialysed. Dose as in GFR<10 mL/min.
HDF/High flux	Not dialysed. Dose as in GFR<10 mL/min.
CAV/ VVHD	Not dialysed. Dose as in GFR=10–20 mL/min.

IMPORTANT DRUG INTERACTIONS

Potentially hazardous interactions with other drugs
● None known

ADMINISTRATION

RECONSTITUTION
–
ROUTE
● Oral
RATE OF ADMINISTRATION
–
COMMENTS
–

OTHER INFORMATION

● Cases of hepatic dysfunction have occasionally been reported.
● There is limited experience in patients with end-stage renal disease; use with caution.
● Oral bioavailability is 85%.
● Vildagliptin AUC increased on average 1.4, 1.7 and 2-fold in patients with mild, moderate and severe renal impairment, respectively, compared to normal healthy subjects. AUC of the metabolites LAY151 (the main metabolite) and BQS867 increased on average about 1.5, 3 and 7-fold in patients with mild, moderate and severe renal impairment, respectively. LAY151 concentrations were approximately 2–3-fold higher than in patients with severe renal impairment.
● 3% of vildagliptin is removed after a 3–4 hour haemodialysis session.
● The main metabolite (LAY 151) is also removed by haemodialysis.

Vinblastine sulphate

CLINICAL USE

Antineoplastic agent

DOSE IN NORMAL RENAL FUNCTION

$5.5-7.4\,mg/m^2$ (maximum of once a week)
Or consult relevant local protocol.

PHARMACOKINETICS

Molecular weight (daltons)	909.1
% Protein binding	99
% Excreted unchanged in urine	14
Volume of distribution (L/kg)	13–40
Half-life – normal/ ESRF (hrs)	25/–

METABOLISM

Vinblastine is extensively metabolised mainly in the liver by the CYP3A group of isoenzymes to desacetylvinblastine, which is more active than the parent compound.

Thirty-three per cent of the drug is slowly excreted in the urine and 21% in the faeces within 72 hours.

DOSE IN RENAL IMPAIRMENT GFR (mL/MIN)

20–50	Dose as in normal renal function.
10–20	Dose as in normal renal function.
<10	Dose as in normal renal function.

DOSE IN PATIENTS UNDERGOING RENAL REPLACEMENT THERAPIES

CAPD	Unlikely to be dialysed. Dose as in normal renal function.
HD	Unlikely to be dialysed. Dose as in normal renal function.
HDF/High flux	Unknown dialysability. Dose as in normal renal function.
CAV/ VVHD	Unlikely to be dialysed. Dose as in normal renal function.

IMPORTANT DRUG INTERACTIONS

Potentially hazardous interactions with other drugs
- Aldesleukin: avoid concomitant use.
- Antibacterials: toxicity increased by erythromycin – avoid concomitant use.
- Anti-epileptics: phenytoin levels may be reduced.
- Antifungals: metabolism possibly inhibited by posaconazole (increased risk of neurotoxicity).
- Antimalarials: avoid with piperaquine with artenimol.
- Antipsychotics: avoid concomitant use with clozapine (increased risk of agranulocytosis).

ADMINISTRATION

RECONSTITUTION
- Add 10 mL of diluent to 10 mg vial. May be administered into fast-running drip of sodium chloride 0.9%.

ROUTE
- IV

RATE OF ADMINISTRATION
- 1 minute

COMMENTS
- Do not dilute with large volumes (e.g. 100–250 mL) or give over long periods (30–60 minutes) as thrombophlebitis and extravasation may occur.

Vincristine sulphate

CLINICAL USE

Antineoplastic agent

DOSE IN NORMAL RENAL FUNCTION

- IV: 1.4–1.5 mg/m^2 weekly; maximum 2 mg
- Consult relevant local protocol.

PHARMACOKINETICS

Molecular weight (daltons)	923
% Protein binding	75
% Excreted unchanged in urine	10–20
Volume of distribution (L/kg)	5–11
Half-life – normal/ ESRF (hrs)	15–155/Unchanged

METABOLISM

Vincristine is metabolised in the liver by the cytochrome P450 isoenzymes CYP3A4 and CYP3A5 and excreted mainly in the bile; about 70–80% of a dose is found in faeces, as unchanged drug and metabolites (40–50%), while 10–20% appears in the urine.

DOSE IN RENAL IMPAIRMENT GFR (mL/MIN)

20–50	Dose as in normal renal function.
10–20	Dose as in normal renal function.
<10	Dose as in normal renal function.

DOSE IN PATIENTS UNDERGOING RENAL REPLACEMENT THERAPIES

CAPD	Unlikely to be dialysed. Dose as in normal renal function.
HD	Unlikely to be dialysed. Dose as in normal renal function.
HDF/High flux	Unknown dialysability. Dose as in normal renal function.
CAV/ VVHD	Unlikely to be dialysed. Dose as in normal renal function.

IMPORTANT DRUG INTERACTIONS

Potentially hazardous interactions with other drugs
- Anti-epileptics: phenytoin levels may be reduced.
- Antifungals: metabolism possibly inhibited by itraconazole and posaconazole (increased risk of neurotoxicity).
- Antimalarials: avoid with piperaquine with artenimol.
- Antipsychotics: avoid concomitant use with clozapine (increased risk of agranulocytosis).

ADMINISTRATION

RECONSTITUTION
–
ROUTE
- IV
RATE OF ADMINISTRATION
- Slow bolus
COMMENTS
- May be administered into fast running drip of sodium chloride 0.9% or glucose 5%.

OTHER INFORMATION

- Most of an IV dose is excreted into the bile after rapid tissue binding.

Vindesine sulphate

CLINICAL USE

Antineoplastic agent

DOSE IN NORMAL RENAL FUNCTION

3–4 mg/m² weekly

PHARMACOKINETICS

Molecular weight (daltons)	852
% Protein binding	65–75
% Excreted unchanged in urine	13
Volume of distribution (L/kg)	8
Half-life – normal/ ESRF (hrs)	20–24

METABOLISM

Vindesine is metabolised by cytochrome P450 (in the CYP 3A subfamily). Elimination is primarily via the biliary route, but 13% is excreted in urine in 24 hours.

DOSE IN RENAL IMPAIRMENT GFR (mL/MIN)

20–50	Dose as in normal renal function.
10–2	Dose as in normal renal function.
<10	Dose as in normal renal function.

DOSE IN PATIENTS UNDERGOING RENAL REPLACEMENT THERAPIES

CAPD	Unlikely to be dialysed. Dose as in normal renal function.
HD	Unlikely to be dialysed. Dose as in normal renal function.
HDF/High flux	Unknown dialysability. Dose as in normal renal function.
CAV/ VVHD	Unlikely to be dialysed. Dose as in normal renal function.

IMPORTANT DRUG INTERACTIONS

Potentially hazardous interactions with other drugs
- None known

ADMINISTRATION

RECONSTITUTION
- 5 mL sodium chloride 0.9% per 5 mg vial
ROUTE
- IV
RATE OF ADMINISTRATION
- 1–3 minutes
COMMENTS
- Can be injected into the tubing of a fast running infusion of sodium chloride 0.9%, glucose 5% or glucose/saline solutions, or directly into a vein.
- Reconstituted solution is stable for 24 hours if stored in a fridge.

OTHER INFORMATION

- Nadir of the WCC occurs 3–5 days after dose with recovery after another 4–5 days.

Vinflunine

CLINICAL USE

Antineoplastic agent (vinca alkaloid):
- Treatment of advanced or metastatic bladder cancer

DOSE IN NORMAL RENAL FUNCTION

IV: 320 mg/m^2 every 3 weeks; consult relevant local protocol.

PHARMACOKINETICS

Molecular weight (daltons)	816.9 (1117.1 as tartrate)
% Protein binding	66.1–68.3
% Excreted unchanged in urine	33
Volume of distribution (L/kg)	35
Half-life – normal/ ESRF (hrs)	40/Increased

METABOLISM

Metabolised by the cytochrome CYP3A4 isoenzyme, except for 4-O-deacetylvinflunine (DVFL), the only active metabolite and main metabolite in blood which is formed by multiple esterases.

Excretion occurs via the faeces (about two-thirds) and the urine (about one-third).

DOSE IN RENAL IMPAIRMENT GFR (mL/MIN)

40–60	280 mg/m^2 every 3 weeks.
20–40	250 mg/m^2 every 3 weeks.
<20	250 mg/m^2 every 3 weeks. Use with care.

DOSE IN PATIENTS UNDERGOING RENAL REPLACEMENT THERAPIES

CAPD	Unlikely to be dialysed. Dose as in GFR<20 mL/min.
HD	Unlikely to be dialysed. Dose as in GFR<20 mL/min.
HDF/High flux	Unknown dialysability. Dose as in GFR<20 mL/min.
CAV/ VVHD	Unlikely to be dialysed. Dose as in GFR=20–40 mL/min.

IMPORTANT DRUG INTERACTIONS

Potentially hazardous interactions with other drugs
- Antibacterials: concentration possibly reduced by rifampicin – avoid concomitant use.
- Antidepressants: concentration possibly reduced by St John's wort – avoid concomitant use.
- Antifungals: concentration increased by ketoconazole and possibly itraconazole (increased risk of neurotoxicity) – avoid.
- Antimalarials: avoid with piperaquine with artenimol.
- Antipsychotics: avoid concomitant use with clozapine (increased risk of agranulocytosis).
- Antivirals: concentration possibly increased by ritonavir – avoid concomitant use.
- Grapefruit juice: concentration of vinflunine increased – avoid.

ADMINISTRATION

RECONSTITUTION
–
ROUTE
- IV infusion
RATE OF ADMINISTRATION
- Over 20 minutes
COMMENTS
- Add to 100 mL of sodium chloride 0.9% or glucose 5%.
- Protect from light.

OTHER INFORMATION

- Vinflunine is eliminated following a multi-exponential concentration decay, with a terminal half-life close to 40 hours. DVFL is slowly formed and more slowly eliminated than vinflunine (half-life of approximately 120 hours).

Vinorelbine

CLINICAL USE

- Treatment of advanced breast cancer (where other anthracyclines have failed)
- Non-small cell lung cancer

DOSE IN NORMAL RENAL FUNCTION

- Oral: 60–80 mg/m^2 once weekly
- IV: 25–30 mg/m^2 once a week
- Maximum 60 mg per dose

PHARMACOKINETICS

Molecular weight (daltons)	1079.1 (as tartrate)
% Protein binding	13.5 (78% bound to platelets)
% Excreted unchanged in urine	18.5
Volume of distribution (L/kg)	>40
Half-life – normal/ ESRF (hrs)	28–44/–

METABOLISM

Metabolism of vinorelbine appears to be hepatic. All metabolites of vinorelbine are formed by the CYP3A4 isoform of cytochrome P450, except 4-O-deacetylvinorelbine which is likely to be formed by carboxylesterases. 4-O-deacetylvinorelbine is the only active metabolite and the main one observed in blood.

Excretion is mainly by the biliary route (18.5% appears in the urine).

DOSE IN RENAL IMPAIRMENT GFR (mL/MIN)

20–50	Dose as in normal renal function and monitor closely.
10–20	Dose as in normal renal function and monitor closely.
<10	Dose as in normal renal function and monitor closely.

DOSE IN PATIENTS UNDERGOING RENAL REPLACEMENT THERAPIES

CAPD	Unlikely to be dialysed. Dose as in normal renal function and monitor closely.
HD	Unlikely to be dialysed. Dose as in normal renal function and monitor closely.
HDF/High flux	Unknown dialysability. Dose as in normal renal function and monitor closely.
CAV/ VVHD	Unknown dialysability. Dose as in normal renal function and monitor closely.

IMPORTANT DRUG INTERACTIONS

Potentially hazardous interactions with other drugs

- Antibacterials: increased risk of neutropenia with clarithromycin.
- Antifungals: metabolism possibly inhibited by itraconazole, increased risk of neurotoxicity.
- Antimalarials: avoid with piperaquine with artenimol.
- Antipsychotics: avoid concomitant use with clozapine (increased risk of agranulocytosis).

ADMINISTRATION

RECONSTITUTION
–
ROUTE
- Oral, IV bolus, infusion
RATE OF ADMINISTRATION
- Bolus: 5–10 minutes
- Infusion: 20–30 minutes
COMMENTS
- Dilute bolus in 20–50 mL with sodium chloride 0.9%.
- Dilute infusion in 125 mL with sodium chloride 0.9%.
- Stable for 24 hours at 2–8°C.

OTHER INFORMATION

- Widely distributed in the body, mostly in spleen, liver, kidneys, lungs, thymus; moderately in heart, muscles; minimally in fat, brain, bone marrow. High levels are found in both normal and malignant lung tissues, with slow diffusion out of tumour tissue.
- Flush line with saline after infusion.
- Dose-limiting toxicity is mainly neutropenia.
- In patients where >75% of the liver volume has been replaced by metastases, it is empirically suggested that the dose be reduced by a third, with close haematological follow-up.

Vitamin B and C preparations

CLINICAL USE

Vitamin B and C supplementation

DOSE IN NORMAL RENAL FUNCTION

- Vitamin B Compound Strong: 1–2 tablets one to 3 times daily
- Pabrinex: Ampoules No 1 and No 2 every 8–12 hours depending on indication
- Post dialysis for vitamin supplementation: 1 pair every 2 weeks.

PHARMACOKINETICS

Molecular weight (daltons)	N/A
% Protein binding	N/A
% Excreted unchanged in urine	N/A
Volume of distribution (L/kg)	N/A
Half-life – normal/ ESRF (hrs)	N/A

METABOLISM

Metabolism is as per normal vitamin handling by the body.

DOSE IN RENAL IMPAIRMENT GFR (mL/MIN)

20–50	Dose as in normal renal function.
10–20	Dose as in normal renal function.
<10	Dose as in normal renal function.

DOSE IN PATIENTS UNDERGOING RENAL REPLACEMENT THERAPIES

CAPD	Dialysed. Dose as in normal renal function.
HD	Dialysed. Dose as in normal renal function.
HDF/High flux	Dialysed. Dose as in normal renal function.
CAV/ VVHD	Dialysed. Dose as in normal renal function.

IMPORTANT DRUG INTERACTIONS

Potentially hazardous interactions with other drugs
- None known

ADMINISTRATION

RECONSTITUTION

–

ROUTE
- Oral, IV, IM

RATE OF ADMINISTRATION
- Bolus: Max volume of 10 mL over 10 minutes
- Infusion: 15–30 minutes

COMMENTS
- Dilute in 50–100 mL sodium chloride or glucose 5%

OTHER INFORMATION

- NOT PRESCRIBABLE ON FP10 PRESCRIPTION
- Supplement in HD patients due to loss on dialysis and poor diet.
- Available as Nephrovite® (Kimal) and Dialyvit® (Vitaline), Renavit® (Stanningley Pharma) – each tablet contains:
  Vitamin B1 (thiamine) 1.5 mg (Renavit 3 mg)
  Vitamin B2 (riboflavin) 1.7 mg
  Vitamin B3 (niacinamide) 20 mg
  Vitamin B6 (pyridoxine) 10 mg
  Vitamin B12 (cyanocobalamin) 6 mcg
  Vitamin C 60 mg (Renavit 120 mg)
  Biotin 300 mcg
  Pantothenic Acid 10 mg
  Folic Acid 800 mcg (Renavit 1 mg)
- Ketovite®, each tablet contains:
  Vitamin B1 (thiamine) 1 mg
  Vitamin B2 (riboflavin) 1 mg
  Acetomenaphthone 500 mcg
  Vitamin B6 (pyridoxine) 330 mcg
  Nicotinamide 3.3 mg
  Vitamin C 16.6 mg
  Biotin 170 mcg
  Pantothenic Acid 1.16 mg
  Alpha tocopheryl acetate 5 mg
  Inositol 50 mg
  Folic Acid 250 mcg
- Pabrinex:
  Vitamin B1 (thiamine) 250 mg
  Vitamin B2 (riboflavin) 4 mg
  Vitamin B6 (pyridoxine) 50 mg
  Vitamin C 500 mg
  Nicotinamide 160 mg

Voriconazole

CLINICAL USE

Antifungal:
- Invasive aspergillosis
- Fluconazole-resistant serious invasive fungal infections
- Immunocompromised patients with progressive, possibly life-threatening infections

DOSE IN NORMAL RENAL FUNCTION

IV:
- 6 mg/kg 12 hourly for 24 hours, then 3–4 mg/kg 12 hourly

Oral:
- <40 kg, 200 mg 12 hourly for 24 hours, then 100–150 mg twice daily
- >40 kg, 400 mg 12 hourly for 24 hours, then 200–300 mg twice daily

PHARMACOKINETICS

Molecular weight (daltons)	349.3
% Protein binding	58
% Excreted unchanged in urine	<2
Volume of distribution (L/kg)	4.6
Half-life – normal/ ESRF (hrs)	6 (depends on dose)/ Unchanged

METABOLISM

Voriconazole is metabolised by hepatic cytochrome P450 isoenzyme CYP2C19; the major metabolite is the inactive N-oxide. Metabolism via isoenzymes CYP2C9 and CYP3A4 has also been shown *in vitro*. Voriconazole is eliminated via hepatic metabolism with less than 2% of the dose excreted unchanged in the urine. After administration of a radiolabelled dose of voriconazole, approximately 80% of the radioactivity is recovered in the urine as metabolites. The majority (>94%) of the total radioactivity is excreted in the first 96 hours after both oral and intravenous dosing

DOSE IN RENAL IMPAIRMENT GFR (mL/MIN)

20–50	Dose as in normal renal function. See 'Other information'.
10–20	Dose as in normal renal function. See 'Other information'.
<10	Dose as in normal renal function. See 'Other information'.

DOSE IN PATIENTS UNDERGOING RENAL REPLACEMENT THERAPIES

CAPD	Probably dialysed. Dose as in normal renal function.
HD	Dialysed. Dose as in normal renal function.
HDF/High flux	Dialysed. Dose as in normal renal function.
CAV/ VVH/HD/ HDF	Dialysed. Dose as in normal renal function.

IMPORTANT DRUG INTERACTIONS

Potentially hazardous interactions with other drugs
- Analgesics: concentration of diclofenac, ibuprofen, alfentanil, methadone and oxycodone increased, consider reducing alfentanil & methadone dose; concentration of fentanyl possibly increased.
- Anti-arrhythmics: avoid concomitant use with dronedarone.
- Antibacterials: concentration reduced by rifabutin; increase dose of voriconazole from 200 to 350 mg and from 100 to 200 mg (depends on patient's weight), and increase IV dose to 5 mg/kg if used in combination – avoid concomitant use if possible; increased rifabutin levels – monitor for toxicity; concentration reduced by rifampicin – avoid concomitant use.
- Anticoagulants: avoid with apixaban and rivaroxaban; enhanced effect of coumarins.
- Antidepressants: avoid concomitant use with reboxetine; concentration reduced by St John's wort – avoid.
- Antidiabetics: possibly increased concentration of sulphonylureas.
- Anti-epileptics: concentration possibly reduced by carbamazepine and phenobarbital – avoid concomitant use; phenytoin reduces voriconazole concentration and voriconazole increases phenytoin concentration – double oral voriconazole dose and increase IV to 5 mg/kg dose if using with phenytoin; avoid concomitant use if possible.
- Antimalarials: avoid concomitant use with artemether/lumefantrine and piperaquine with artenimol.

- Antipsychotics: increased risk of ventricular arrhythmias with pimozide – avoid concomitant use; possibly increased quetiapine levels – reduce dose of quetiapine.
- Antivirals: concentration reduced by efavirenz and ritonavir; also concentration of efavirenz increased – avoid concomitant use with ritonavir; with efavirenz reduce dose by 50% and increase dose of voriconazole to 400 mg twice daily; concentration possibly affected by telaprevir – increased risk of ventricular arrhythmias; possibly increased saquinavir levels.
- Benzodiazepines: may inhibit metabolism of diazepam and midazolam.
- Ciclosporin: AUC increased – reduce ciclosporin dose by 50% and monitor closely.
- Clopidogrel: possibly reduced anti-platelet effect.
- Cytotoxics: possibly increases crizotinib and everolimus concentration – avoid; avoid with lapatinib, nilotinib, pazopanib and cabazitaxel; reduce dose of ruxolitinib.
- Ergot alkaloids: risk of ergotism – avoid concomitant use.
- Lipid-lowering drugs: possibly increased risk of myopathy with atorvastatin or simvastatin.
- Ranolazine: possibly increased ranolazine concentration – avoid.
- Retinoids: possibly increased risk of tretinoin toxicity.
- Sirolimus: increased sirolimus concentration – avoid concomitant use.
- Tacrolimus: AUC increased – reduce tacrolimus dose to a third and monitor closely.
- Ulcer-healing drugs: esomeprazole and omeprazole concentration increased – reduce omeprazole dose by 50%.

ADMINISTRATION

RECONSTITUTION
- 19 mL water for injection

ROUTE
- Oral, IV

RATE OF ADMINISTRATION
- 1–2 hours (3 mg/kg/hour)

COMMENTS
- Not compatible with sodium bicarbonate or TPN solutions.
- Dilute to a concentration of 2–5 mg/mL with sodium chloride 0.9%, Hartmann's solution or glucose 5%.

OTHER INFORMATION

- Haemodialysis clearance is 121 mL/min.
- Oral bioavailability is 96%.
- Only use IV in renal patients if patient is unable to tolerate oral, as intravenous vehicle (SBECD) accumulates in renal failure. The vehicle is dialysed at a rate of 55 mL/min.
- Take oral dose 1 hour before or an hour after meals.
- Monitor renal function as can enhance nephrotoxicity of other drugs and concurrent conditions.
- Rare reports of acute renal failure and discoid lupus erythematosus occurring.
- Also reports of haematuria, nephritis and tubular necrosis.
- In clinical trials, 30% of patients developed visual problems, usually with higher doses.

Warfarin sodium

CLINICAL USE

Anticoagulant

DOSE IN NORMAL RENAL FUNCTION

Depends on INR

PHARMACOKINETICS

Molecular weight (daltons)	330.3
% Protein binding	99
% Excreted unchanged in urine	0
Volume of distribution (L/kg)	0.14
Half-life – normal/ ESRF (hrs)	37/Unchanged

METABOLISM

The R- and S-isomers are both metabolised in the liver. The S-isomer is metabolised more rapidly than the R-isomer, mainly by the cytochrome P450 isoenzyme CYP2C9, which shows genetic polymorphism. Other isoenzymes are also involved in the metabolism of the R-isomer.

The metabolites, which have negligible or no anticoagulant activity, are excreted in the urine following reabsorption from the bile.

DOSE IN RENAL IMPAIRMENT GFR (mL/MIN)

20–50	Dose as in normal renal function.
10–20	Dose as in normal renal function.
<10	Dose as in normal renal function.

DOSE IN PATIENTS UNDERGOING RENAL REPLACEMENT THERAPIES

CAPD	Not dialysed. Dose as in normal renal function.
HD	Not dialysed. Dose as in normal renal function.
HDF/High flux	Unknown dialysability. Dose as in normal renal function.
CAV/ VVHD	Not dialysed. Dose as in normal renal function.

IMPORTANT DRUG INTERACTIONS

Potentially hazardous interactions with other drugs

There are many significant interactions with warfarin. Prescribe with care with regard to the following:

- Anticoagulant effect enhanced by: alcohol, amiodarone, anabolic steroids, aspirin, aztreonam, bicalutamide, cephalosporins, chloramphenicol, cimetidine, ciprofloxacin, clopidogrel, cranberry juice, danazol, danshen, dipyridamole, dronedarone, disulfiram, entacapone, esomeprazole, exenatide, ezetimibe, fibrates, fluconazole, flutamide, fluvastatin, glucosamine, grapefruit juice, itraconazole, ketoconazole, levamisole, levofloxacin, macrolides, methylphenidate, metronidazole, miconazole, mirtazapine, nalidixic acid, neomycin, norfloxacin, NSAIDs, ofloxacin, omeprazole, pantoprazole, paracetamol, penicillins, proguanil, propafenone, rosuvastatin, saquinavir, SSRIs, simvastatin, sulfinpyrazone, sulphonamides, tamoxifen, testosterone, tetracyclines, thyroid hormones, tigecycline, toremifene, tramadol, trimethoprim, valproate, venlafaxine, vitamin E and voriconazole.
- Anticoagulant effect decreased by: acitretin, atorvastatin, azathioprine, barbiturates, carbamazepine, eslicarbazepine, ginseng, griseofulvin, oral contraceptives, phenobarbital, phenytoin, rifamycins, St John's wort (avoid concomitant use), sucralfate, vitamin K.
- Anticoagulant effects enhanced/reduced by: anion exchange resins, atazanavir, corticosteroids, dietary changes, disopyramide, efavirenz, fosamprenavir, nevirapine, ritonavir, telaprevir, tricyclics, trazodone.
- Analgesics: increased risk of bleeding with IV diclofenac and ketorolac – avoid concomitant use.
- Anticoagulants: increased risk of haemorrhage with apixaban, dabigatran and rivaroxaban – avoid concomitant use.
- Antidiabetic agents: enhanced hypoglycaemic effect with sulphonylureas; also possible changes to anticoagulant effect.
- Camomile: enhanced anticoagulation.
- Ciclosporin: there have been a few reports of altered anticoagulant effect; decreased ciclosporin levels have been seen rarely.
- Cytotoxics: increased risk of bleeding with erlotinib and imatinib; enhanced effect with etoposide, fluorouracil, ifosfamide,

gefitinib, gemcitabine, sorafenib and vemurafenib; reduced effect with mercaptopurine and mitotane.
- Melatonin: possibly enhanced INR.

ADMINISTRATION

RECONSTITUTION

–

ROUTE
- Oral

RATE OF ADMINISTRATION

–

COMMENTS

–

OTHER INFORMATION

- Reduced protein binding in renal impairment.

Xipamide

CLINICAL USE

Thiazide diuretic:
- Hypertension
- Oedema

DOSE IN NORMAL RENAL FUNCTION

- Oedema: 40–80 mg in the morning
- Maintenance: 20 mg in the morning
- Hypertension: 20 mg in the morning

PHARMACOKINETICS

Molecular weight (daltons)	354.8
% Protein binding	99
% Excreted unchanged in urine	50
Volume of distribution (L/kg)	10–21 litres
Half-life – normal/ ESRF (hrs)	5–8/9–32

METABOLISM

Xipamide is excreted in the urine, partly unchanged and partly in the form of the glucuronide metabolite. In patients with renal impairment excretion in the bile becomes more prominent.

DOSE IN RENAL IMPAIRMENT GFR (mL/MIN)

20–50	Dose as in normal renal function.
10–30	Dose as in normal renal function.
<10	Dose as in normal renal function.

DOSE IN PATIENTS UNDERGOING RENAL REPLACEMENT THERAPIES

CAPD	Unknown dialysability. Dose as in normal renal function.
HD	Dialysed. Dose as in normal renal function.
HDF/High flux	Dialysed. Dose as in normal renal function.
CAV/ VVHD	Unknown dialysability. Dose as in normal renal function.

IMPORTANT DRUG INTERACTIONS

Potentially hazardous interactions with other drugs
- Analgesics: increased risk of nephrotoxicity with NSAIDs; antagonism of diuretic effect.
- Anti-arrhythmics: hypokalaemia leads to increased cardiac toxicity; effects of lidocaine and mexiletine antagonised.
- Antibacterials: avoid administration with lymecycline.
- Antidepressants: increased risk of hypokalaemia with reboxetine; enhanced hypotensive effect with MAOIs; increased risk of postural hypotension with tricyclics.
- Anti-epileptics: increased risk of hyponatraemia with carbamazepine.
- Antifungals: increased risk of hypokalaemia with amphotericin.
- Antihypertensives: enhanced hypotensive effect; increased risk of first dose hypotension with post-synaptic alpha-blockers like prazosin; hypokalaemia increases risk of ventricular arrhythmias with sotalol.
- Antipsychotics: hypokalaemia increases risk of ventricular arrhythmias with amisulpride; enhanced hypotensive effect with phenothiazines; hypokalaemia increases risk of ventricular arrhythmias with pimozide – avoid concomitant use.
- Atomoxetine: hypokalaemia increases risk of ventricular arrhythmias.
- Cardiac glycosides: increased toxicity if hypokalaemia occurs.
- Ciclosporin: increased risk of nephrotoxicity and possibly hypomagnesaemia.
- Cytotoxics: increased risk of ventricular arrhythmias due to hypokalaemia with arsenic trioxide; increased risk of nephrotoxicity and ototoxicity with platinum compounds.
- Lithium excretion reduced (increased toxicity).

ADMINISTRATION

RECONSTITUTION
–
ROUTE
- Oral
RATE OF ADMINISTRATION
–
COMMENTS
–

OTHER INFORMATION

- Monitor for hypokalaemia.
- Diuresis starts within 1–2 hours, peaks at 4–6 hours and lasts for almost 24 hours.

- Manufacturer advises to avoid in severe renal impairment due to reduced clearance.
- Dose in severe renal impairment from Knauf H, Mutschler E. Pharmacodynamics and pharmacokinetics of xipamide in patients with normal and impaired kidney function. *Eur J Clin Pharmacol.* 1984; **26**: 513–20.

Zafirlukast

CLINICAL USE

Leukotriene receptor antagonist
● Prophylaxis of asthma

DOSE IN NORMAL RENAL FUNCTION

20 mg twice daily

PHARMACOKINETICS

Molecular weight (daltons)	575.7
% Protein binding	99
% Excreted unchanged in urine	0 (10% as metabolites)
Volume of distribution (L/kg)	70 litres
Half-life – normal/ ESRF (hrs)	10/Possibly unchanged

METABOLISM

Zafirlukast is extensively metabolised in the liver, mainly by the cytochrome P450 isoenzyme CYP2C9.

Following a radiolabelled dose the urinary excretion accounts for approximately 10% of the dose and faecal excretion for 89%. The metabolites identified in human plasma were found to be at least 90-fold less potent than zafirlukast in a standard *in vitro* test of activity.

DOSE IN RENAL IMPAIRMENT GFR (mL/MIN)

20–50	Dose as in normal renal function.
10–20	Dose as in normal renal function, but use with care.
<10	Dose as in normal renal function, but use with care.

DOSE IN PATIENTS UNDERGOING RENAL REPLACEMENT THERAPIES

CAPD	Unlikely to be dialysed. Dose as in normal renal function, but use with care.
HD	Unlikely to be dialysed. Dose as in normal renal function, but use with care.
HDF/High flux	Unlikely to be dialysed. Dose as in normal renal function, but use with care.
CAV/ VVHD	Unlikely to be dialysed. Dose as in normal renal function, but use with care.

IMPORTANT DRUG INTERACTIONS

Potentially hazardous interactions with other drugs
● Analgesics: concentration increased by aspirin.
● Antibacterials: concentration reduced by erythromycin.
● Anticoagulants: may enhance the effects of warfarin.
● Theophylline: possibly increases theophylline concentration; zafirlukast concentration reduced.

ADMINISTRATION

RECONSTITUTION
–
ROUTE
● Oral
RATE OF ADMINISTRATION
–
COMMENTS
–

OTHER INFORMATION

● UK SPC advises to use with caution due to lack of experience, no dose reduction is suggested in US data sheet or *Drug Prescribing in Renal Failure*, 5th edition, by Aronoff *et al.*
● Do not take with food as it reduces bioavailability.

Zanamivir

CLINICAL USE

- Treatment of influenza A and B within 48 hours after onset of symptoms
- Post exposure prophylaxis, up to 28 days during an epidemic

DOSE IN NORMAL RENAL FUNCTION

- Treatment: 10 mg twice daily for 5–10 days
- Prophylaxis: 10 mg once daily for 10 days

PHARMACOKINETICS

Molecular weight (daltons)	332.3
% Protein binding	<10
% Excreted unchanged in urine	100
Volume of distribution (L/kg)	No data
Half-life – normal/ ESRF (hrs)	2.6–5/Increased

METABOLISM

Zanamivir is renally excreted as unchanged drug, and does not undergo metabolism.

DOSE IN RENAL IMPAIRMENT GFR (mL/MIN)

20–50	Dose as in normal renal function.
10–20	Dose as in normal renal function.
<10	Dose as in normal renal function.

DOSE IN PATIENTS UNDERGOING RENAL REPLACEMENT THERAPIES

CAPD	Unknown dialysability. Dose as in normal renal function.
HD	Unknown dialysability. Dose as in normal renal function.
HDF/High flux	Unknown dialysability. Dose as in normal renal function.
CAV/ VVHD	Unknown dialysability. Dose as in normal renal function.

IMPORTANT DRUG INTERACTIONS

Potentially hazardous interactions with other drugs
- None known

ADMINISTRATION

RECONSTITUTION
–
ROUTE
- Inhalation
RATE OF ADMINISTRATION
–
COMMENTS
–

OTHER INFORMATION

- 10–20% of dose is systemically absorbed.

Ziconotide (unlicensed)

CLINICAL USE
Analgesia for intrathecal use

DOSE IN NORMAL RENAL FUNCTION
2.4–21.6 mcg daily; majority require <9.6 mcg/day

PHARMACOKINETICS

Molecular weight (daltons)	2639.1 (2699.2 as acetate)
% Protein binding	53
% Excreted unchanged in urine	<1
Volume of distribution (L/kg)	30
Half-life – normal/ESRF (hrs)	1.3/Unchanged

METABOLISM
Ziconotide is a peptide consisting of 25 naturally occurring amino acids and does not appear to be metabolised in the CSF. Once in the systemic circulation, ziconotide is expected to be mainly susceptible to proteolytic cleavage by various peptidases/proteases present in most organs (e.g. kidney, liver, lung, muscle, etc.), and then degraded to peptide fragments and its individual constituent free amino acids. These amino acids are expected to be taken up by cellular carrier systems and either subjected to normal intermediary metabolism or used as substrates for constitutive biosynthetic processes. Due to the wide distribution of these peptidases it is not expected that hepatic or renal impairment would affect the systemic clearance of ziconotide.

The biological activity of the various proteolytic degradation products has not been assessed although they are unlikely to have significant activity.

DOSE IN RENAL IMPAIRMENT GFR (mL/MIN)

20–50	Dose as in normal renal function.
10–20	Dose as in normal renal function.
<10	Dose as in normal renal function. Use with caution.

DOSE IN PATIENTS UNDERGOING RENAL REPLACEMENT THERAPIES

CAPD	Unknown dialysability. Dose as in GFR<10 mL/min.
HD	Unknown dialysability. Dose as in GFR<10 mL/min.
HDF/High flux	Unknown dialysability. Dose as in GFR<10 mL/min.
CAV/VVHD	Unknown dialysability. Dose as in normal renal function.

IMPORTANT DRUG INTERACTIONS
Potentially hazardous interactions with other drugs
- Contraindicated with IT chemotherapy.
- Can increase neuropsychiatric events with IT morphine.

ADMINISTRATION
RECONSTITUTION
–

ROUTE
- Intrathecal

RATE OF ADMINISTRATION
- Over 24 hours

COMMENTS
- Dilute with preservative-free sodium chloride 0.9%; concentration should be no lower than 5 mcg/mL in an external pump and 25 mcg/mL in an internal pump.

OTHER INFORMATION
- Use with caution in renal impairment due to lack of studies – start with the lower dose range.
- Has rarely caused rhabdomyolysis, myositis, acute kidney injury and urinary retention.

Zidovudine

CLINICAL USE

Nucleoside reverse transcriptase inhibitor
- Treatment of HIV in combination with other antiretroviral drugs
- Prevention of maternal-foetal HIV transmission

DOSE IN NORMAL RENAL FUNCTION

- Oral: 200–300 mg twice daily
- IV: 0.8–1 mg/kg every 4 hours
- Prevention of maternal-foetal HIV transmission: 500 mg daily in divided doses

PHARMACOKINETICS

Molecular weight (daltons)	267.2
% Protein binding	34–38
% Excreted unchanged in urine	8–25
Volume of distribution (L/kg)	1.6
Half-life – normal/ESRF (hrs)	1.1/1. 4–3

METABOLISM

Zidovudine is metabolised intracellularly to the antiviral triphosphate. It is also metabolised in the liver, mainly to the inactive glucuronide, and is excreted in the urine as unchanged drug and metabolite.

The 5'-glucuronide of zidovudine is the major metabolite in both plasma and urine, accounting for approximately 50–80% of the administered dose eliminated by renal excretion. There is substantial accumulation of this metabolite in renal failure.

Renal clearance of zidovudine greatly exceeds creatinine clearance, indicating that significant tubular secretion takes place.

DOSE IN RENAL IMPAIRMENT GFR (mL/MIN)

20–50	Dose as in normal renal function.
10–20	Dose as in normal renal function.
<10	Give 50% of normal dose every 8 hours, i.e. 300–400 mg daily in divided doses.[1]

DOSE IN PATIENTS UNDERGOING RENAL REPLACEMENT THERAPIES

CAPD	Not dialysed. Dose as in GFR<10 mL/min.
HD	Not dialysed. Dose as in GFR<10 mL/min. Give post dialysis.
HDF/High flux	Unknown dialysability. Dose as in GFR<10 mL/min. Give post dialysis.
CAV/ VVHD	Not dialysed. Dose as in normal renal function.

IMPORTANT DRUG INTERACTIONS

Potentially hazardous interactions with other drugs
- Antibacterials: absorption reduced by clarithromycin; avoid concomitant use with rifampicin.
- Anti-epileptics: phenytoin levels may be raised or lowered; concentration possibly increased by valproate (increased risk of toxicity).
- Antifungals: concentration increased by fluconazole.
- Antivirals: profound myelosuppression with ganciclovir – avoid if possible; increased risk of anaemia with ribavirin – avoid; effects of stavudine inhibited – avoid concomitant use; concentration reduced by tipranavir.
- Probenecid: excretion reduced by probenecid, increased risk of toxicity.

ADMINISTRATION

RECONSTITUTION
–
ROUTE
- IV, oral
RATE OF ADMINISTRATION
- 1 hour
COMMENTS
- Dilute with glucose 5% infusion to give a final concentration of 2 mg/mL or 4 mg/mL.

OTHER INFORMATION

- Dialysis has little effect on zidovudine, presumably because of rapid metabolism. The glucuronide metabolite (half-life =1 hour) has no antiviral activity and will be significantly removed by dialysis.
- Patients with severe renal failure have 50% higher maximum plasma concentrations.
- Main risk in renal impairment is haematological toxicity.
- Oral bioavailability is 60–70%.

Reference:
1. Izzedine H, Launay-Vacher V, Baumelou A, *et al.* An appraisal of antiretroviral drugs in haemodialysis. *Kidney Int.* 2001; **66**: 821–30.

Zoledronic acid

CLINICAL USE

- Hypercalcaemia of malignancy
- Reduction of bone damage in advanced malignancies
- Paget's disease
- Osteoporosis

DOSE IN NORMAL RENAL FUNCTION

Zometa
- Hypercalcaemia of malignancy: 4 mg as a single dose
- Reduction of bone damage in advanced malignancies: 4 mg every 3–4 weeks

Aclasta
- Paget's disease: 5 mg as a single dose
- Osteoporosis: 5 mg yearly

PHARMACOKINETICS

Molecular weight (daltons)	272.1
% Protein binding	56
% Excreted unchanged in urine	39 +/− 16
Volume of distribution (L/kg)	6.1–10.8
Half-life – normal/ESRF (hrs)	146/Increased

METABOLISM

Zoledronic acid is not metabolised and is excreted unchanged via the kidney. Over the first 24 hours, 39±16% of the administered dose is recovered in the urine, while the remainder is principally bound to bone tissue.

DOSE IN RENAL IMPAIRMENT GFR (mL/MIN)

>60	Dose as in normal renal function.
50–60	Zometa: 3.5 mg; Aclasta: Dose as in normal renal function.
40–45	Zometa: 3.3 mg; Aclasta: Dose as in normal renal function.
30–39	Zometa: 3 mg; Aclasta: avoid if GFR<35 mL/min.
<29	Avoid. Unless benefit outweighs risk.

DOSE IN PATIENTS UNDERGOING RENAL REPLACEMENT THERAPIES

CAPD	Unknown dialysability. Dose as in GFR<29 mL/min.
HD	Unknown dialysability. Dose as in GFR<29 mL/min.
HDF/High flux	Unknown dialysability. Dose as in GFR<29 mL/min.

IMPORTANT DRUG INTERACTIONS

Potentially hazardous interactions with other drugs
- Other nephrotoxic drugs: use with caution as can enhance nephrotoxicity.

ADMINISTRATION

RECONSTITUTION
- Add 5 mL of water for injection to each 4 mg vial.

ROUTE
- IV

RATE OF ADMINISTRATION
- 15 minutes

COMMENTS
- Add to 100 mL sodium chloride 0.9% or glucose 5%.
- Reconstituted solutions are stable for 24 hours at room temperature.

OTHER INFORMATION

- Also administer a calcium supplement of 500 mg daily plus 400 IU of vitamin D daily with zometa and 50 000 to 125 000 IU of vitamin D with Aclasta in patients with recent hip fractures. Renal impairment has been observed following the administration of Aclasta, especially in patients with pre-existing renal impairment. Other risk factors are: increasing age, repeated cycles of bisphosphonates, concomitant nephrotoxic medication, diuretic therapy or dehydration occurring after Aclasta administration.
- A small number of cases of renal failure requiring dialysis or with a fatal outcome have been reported.
- Increased risk of renal impairment in older patients, smokers, previous pamidronate therapy and renal failure. (Oh WK, Proctor K, Nakabayashi M. The risk of renal impairment in hormone-refractory prostate cancer patients with bone metastases treated with zoledronic acid. *Cancer*. 2007 Mar 15; **109**(6): 1090–6.)
- Incidence of acute kidney injury is 10.7%, usually due to acute tubular necrosis. (Chang JT, Green L, Beitz J. Renal failure with the use of zoledronic acid. *N Engl J Med*. 2003; **349**(17): 1679–9.)
- May cause osteonecrosis of the jaw.

Zolmitriptan

CLINICAL USE

5HT$_1$ receptor agonist:
- Acute treatment of migraine
- Cluster headache

DOSE IN NORMAL RENAL FUNCTION

- Oral: 2.5–5 mg, repeated after 2 hours if required; maximum 10 mg in 24 hours
- Intranasally for cluster headaches: 5 mg into 1 nostril as soon as possible after onset, repeated after not less than 2 hours, max 10 mg in 24 hours

PHARMACOKINETICS

Molecular weight (daltons)	287.4
% Protein binding	25
% Excreted unchanged in urine	60 (as metabolites)
Volume of distribution (L/kg)	2.4
Half-life – normal/ESRF (hrs)	2.5–3/3–3.5

METABOLISM

Zolmitriptan is eliminated largely by hepatic biotransformation followed by urinary excretion of the metabolites. There are three major metabolites: the indole acetic acid (the major metabolite in plasma and urine), the N-oxide and N-desmethyl analogues. Only the N-desmethylated metabolite is active. The primary metabolism of zolmitriptan is mediated mainly by the cytochrome P450 isoenzyme CYP1A2 while monoamine oxidase type A is responsible for further metabolism of the N-desmethyl metabolite. Over 60% of a dose is excreted in the urine, mainly as the indole acetic acid, and about 30% appears in the faeces, mainly as unchanged drug.

DOSE IN RENAL IMPAIRMENT GFR (mL/MIN)

20–50	Dose as in normal renal function.
10–20	Dose as in normal renal function.
<10	Dose as in normal renal function.[1]

DOSE IN PATIENTS UNDERGOING RENAL REPLACEMENT THERAPIES

CAPD	Unknown dialysability. Dose as in normal renal function.
HD	Unknown dialysability. Dose as in normal renal function.
HDF/High flux	Unknown dialysability. Dose as in normal renal function.
CAV/ VVHD	Unknown dialysability. Dose as in normal renal function.

IMPORTANT DRUG INTERACTIONS

Potentially hazardous interactions with other drugs
- Antibacterials: quinolones possibly inhibit metabolism – reduce dose of zolmitriptan.
- Antidepressants: increased risk of CNS toxicity with citalopram – avoid; risk of CNS toxicity with MAOIs and moclobemide – reduce dose of zolmitriptan to max 7.5 mg; SSRIs inhibit metabolism of zolmitriptan, reduce dose with fluvoxamine; possibly increased serotonergic effects with duloxetine and venlafaxine; increased serotonergic effects with St John's wort – avoid concomitant use.
- Cimetidine: inhibits metabolism of zolmitriptan; maximum dose is 5 mg.
- Ergot alkaloids: increased risk of vasospasm.
- Linezolid: risk of CNS toxicity – reduce dose of zolmitriptan.

ADMINISTRATION

RECONSTITUTION
–
ROUTE
- Oral
RATE OF ADMINISTRATION
–
COMMENTS
–

OTHER INFORMATION

- Oral bioavailability is 40%.
- Contraindicated if GFR<15 mL/min in UK SPC but not in US data sheet.
- One study showed that no dose reduction was required in patients not on dialysis. (Gillotin C, et al. No need to adjust the dose of 311C90 (zolmitriptan), a novel anti-migraine treatment in patients with renal failure not requiring dialysis. Int J Clin Pharmacol Ther. 1997; **35**: 522–6).

Reference:
1. Bailie GR, Johnson CA, Mason NA, St Peter WL. (Nephrology Pharmacy Associates). Triptans for migraine treatment: dosing considerations in CKD. *Medfacts*. 2002; **4**(5).

Zolpidem tartrate

CLINICAL USE

Insomnia (short term treatment)

DOSE IN NORMAL RENAL FUNCTION

5–10 mg at night.

PHARMACOKINETICS

Molecular weight (daltons)	764.9
% Protein binding	92.5
% Excreted unchanged in urine	Negligible
Volume of distribution (L/kg)	0.34–0.54 (depends on age)
Half-life – normal/ ESRF (hrs)	Average: 2.4/ Increased

METABOLISM

Zolpidem tartrate is metabolised via several hepatic cytochrome P450 enzymes, the main enzyme being CYP3A4 with the contribution of CYP1A2.

All metabolites are pharmacologically inactive and are eliminated in the urine (56%) and in the faeces (37%).

DOSE IN RENAL IMPAIRMENT GFR (mL/MIN)

20–50	Dose as in normal renal function.
10–20	Dose as in normal renal function.
<10	Dose as in normal renal function.

DOSE IN PATIENTS UNDERGOING RENAL REPLACEMENT THERAPIES

CAPD	Not dialysed. Dose as in normal renal function.
HD	Not dialysed. Dose as in normal renal function.
HDF/High flux	Unknown dialysability. Dose as in normal renal function.
CAV/ VVHD	Not dialysed. Dose as in normal renal function.

IMPORTANT DRUG INTERACTIONS

Potentially hazardous interactions with other drugs
- Antibacterials: metabolism accelerated by rifampicin.
- Antidepressants: increased sedative effects with sertraline.
- Antipsychotics: enhanced sedative effects.
- Antivirals: concentration increased by ritonavir (risk of extreme sedation and respiratory depression) – avoid concomitant use.

ADMINISTRATION

RECONSTITUTION
–
ROUTE
- Oral
RATE OF ADMINISTRATION
–
COMMENTS
–

OTHER INFORMATION

- First-pass metabolism by liver is 35%.
- Clearance is reduced in renal impairment.
- Oral bioavailability is 70%.

Zonisamide

CLINICAL USE

Anti-epileptic agent

DOSE IN NORMAL RENAL FUNCTION

Initially: 25 mg twice daily, increasing to
maintenance dose of 300–500 mg daily in 1
or 2 divided doses

PHARMACOKINETICS

Molecular weight (daltons)	212.2
% Protein binding	40–60
% Excreted unchanged in urine	15–35
Volume of distribution (L/kg)	0.8–1.6
Half-life – normal/ ESRF (hrs)	60–63/Increased

METABOLISM

Zonisamide is metabolised mainly by
reductive cleavage of the benzisoxazole
ring of the parent drug by CYP3A4 to form
2-sulphamoylacetylphenol (SMAP) and also
by N-acetylation. Parent drug and SMAP can
also be glucuronidated.

The metabolites, which could not be
detected in plasma, are inactive. Excretion
is mainly in the urine; about 15–30%
appearing as unchanged drug, 15% as
N-acetylzonisamide, and 50% as the
glucuronide of SMAP.

DOSE IN RENAL IMPAIRMENT GFR (mL/MIN)

20–50	Dose as in normal renal function.
10–20	Dose as in normal renal function, titrate slowly. See 'Other information'.
<10	Dose as in normal renal function, titrate slowly. See 'Other information'.

DOSE IN PATIENTS UNDERGOING RENAL REPLACEMENT THERAPIES

CAPD	Dialysed. Dose as in GFR<10 mL/min
HD	Dialysed. Dose as in GFR<10 mL/min.
HDF/High flux	Dialysed. Dose as in GFR<10 mL/min.
CAV/ VVHD	Probably dialysed. Dose as in GFR=10–20 mL/min.

IMPORTANT DRUG INTERACTIONS

Potentially hazardous interactions with other
drugs
- Antidepressants: anticonvulsant effect
  antagonised; avoid with St John's wort.
- Antimalarials: anticonvulsant effect
  antagonised by mefloquine.
- Antipsychotics: anticonvulsant effect
  antagonised.
- Orlistat: increased risk of convulsions.

ADMINISTRATION

RECONSTITUTION

–

ROUTE
- Oral

RATE OF ADMINISTRATION

–

COMMENTS

–

OTHER INFORMATION

- AUC is increased by 35% in patients with a
  GFR<20 mL/min.
- Bioavailability is 100%.
- Increase dose at 2 weekly intervals in
  people with renal impairment and monitor
  more frequently.

Zopiclone

CLINICAL USE

Hypnotic

DOSE IN NORMAL RENAL FUNCTION

3.75–7.5 mg at night

PHARMACOKINETICS

Molecular weight (daltons)	388.8
% Protein binding	45–80
% Excreted unchanged in urine	<5
Volume of distribution (L/kg)	91.8–104.6
Half-life – normal/ ESRF (hrs)	3.5–6.5/Unchanged

METABOLISM

Zopiclone is extensively metabolised in the liver via the cytochrome P450 isoenzyme CYP3A4 and, to a lesser extent, CYP2C8; the 2 major metabolites, the less active zopiclone N-oxide and the inactive N-desmethylzopiclone, are excreted mainly in the urine. About 50% of a dose is converted by decarboxylation to inactive metabolites, which are partly eliminated via the lungs as carbon dioxide.

DOSE IN RENAL IMPAIRMENT GFR (mL/MIN)

20–50	Dose as in normal renal function.
10–20	Dose as in normal renal function.
<10	Start with 3.75 mg.

DOSE IN PATIENTS UNDERGOING RENAL REPLACEMENT THERAPIES

CAPD	Dialysed. Dose as in GFR<10 mL/min.
HD	Dialysed. Dose as in GFR<10 mL/min.
HDF/High flux	Dialysed. Dose as in GFR<10 mL/min.
CAV/VVHD	Dialysed. Dose as in normal renal function.

IMPORTANT DRUG INTERACTIONS

Potentially hazardous interactions with other drugs
- Antibacterials: metabolism inhibited by erythromycin; concentration significantly reduced by rifampicin.
- Antipsychotics: enhanced sedative effects.
- Antivirals: concentration possibly increased by ritonavir.

ADMINISTRATION

RECONSTITUTION

–

ROUTE
- Oral

RATE OF ADMINISTRATION

–

COMMENTS

–

OTHER INFORMATION

- It is recommended that elderly patients and those with severe renal disease should start treatment with 3.75 mg; however, accumulation has not been observed.

Zuclopenthixol

CLINICAL USE

Antipsychotic for schizophrenia and other psychoses

DOSE IN NORMAL RENAL FUNCTION

Schizophrenia and paranoid psychoses:
- Oral: 20–30 mg daily in divided doses; maximum 150 mg daily
- Maintenance: 20–50 mg daily Deep IM: 200–500 mg every 1–4 weeks Maximum: 600 mg weekly

Acute psychoses: (Clopixol Acuphase)
- Deep IM: 50–150 mg, repeated if required after 2–3 days Maximum 400 mg per course

PHARMACOKINETICS

Molecular weight (daltons)	401 (443 as acetate), (473.9 as hydrochloride), (555.2 as decanoate)
% Protein binding	98
% Excreted unchanged in urine	Minimal (10–20% unchanged drug and metabolites)
Volume of distribution (L/kg)	10–20
Half-life – normal/ESRF (hrs)	20–24/–

METABOLISM

Metabolism of zuclopenthixol is by sulphoxidation, side-chain N-dealkylation and glucuronic acid conjugation.

The sulphoxide metabolites are mainly excreted in the urine while unchanged drug and the dealkylated form tend to be excreted in the faeces.

DOSE IN RENAL IMPAIRMENT GFR (mL/MIN)

20–50	Dose as in normal renal function.
10–20	Dose as in normal renal function.
<10	Start with 50% of the dose and titrate slowly.

DOSE IN PATIENTS UNDERGOING RENAL REPLACEMENT THERAPIES

CAPD	Not dialysed. Dose as in GFR<10 mL/min.
HD	Not dialysed. Dose as in GFR<10 mL/min.
HDF/High flux	Unknown dialysability. Dose as in GFR<10 mL/min.
CAV/ VVHD	Not dialysed. Dose as in normal renal function.

IMPORTANT DRUG INTERACTIONS

Potentially hazardous interactions with other drugs
- Anaesthetics: enhanced hypotensive effects.
- Analgesics: increased risk of convulsions with tramadol; enhanced hypotensive and sedative effects with opioids; increased risk of ventricular arrhythmias with methadone.
- Anti-arrhythmics: increased risk of ventricular arrhythmias with anti-arrhythmics that prolong the QT interval – avoid with amiodarone and disopyramide.
- Antibacterials: increased risk of ventricular arrhythmias with moxifloxacin and parenteral erythromycin – avoid.
- Antidepressants: increased level of tricyclics.
- Anti-epileptics: anticonvulsant effect antagonised.
- Antimalarials: avoid concomitant use with artemether/lumefantrine.
- Antipsychotics: avoid concomitant use of clozapine with depot preparations in case of neutropenia.
- Antivirals: concentration possibly increased with ritonavir.
- Atomoxetine: increased risk of ventricular arrhythmias.
- Anxiolytics and hypnotics: increased sedative effects.
- Beta-blockers: increased risk of ventricular arrhythmias with sotalol – avoid.
- Cytotoxics: increased risk of ventricular arrhythmias with vandetanib – avoid; increased risk of ventricular arrhythmias with arsenic trioxide.

ADMINISTRATION

RECONSTITUTION
–

ROUTE
- Oral, IM

RATE OF ADMINISTRATION
–

COMMENTS
–

OTHER INFORMATION

- May cause hypotension and excessive sedation.
- Increased CNS sensitivity in renally impaired patients – start with small doses as can accumulate.
- Peak levels occur 3–6 hours after oral administration.

Drugs for malaria prophylaxis

The malaria prophylaxis regimens below reflect the guidelines agreed by UK malaria specialists, and are aimed at residents of the UK who travel to endemic areas. Because the drug sensitivities of malaria parasites change with time and place, the most up-to-date information on prophylaxis should always be obtained from an appropriate travel clinic.

MEFLOQUINE (LARIAM®)

- 250 mg (ONE tablet) ONCE a WEEK, starting 2½ weeks prior to travelling and continuing for 4 weeks after returning.
- **NO dose changes are required** for patients with any degree of renal impairment.

DOXYCYCLINE

- 100 mg (ONE capsule) ONCE a DAY starting 1–2 days prior to travelling and continuing for 4 weeks after returning.
- **CAPD or HAEMODIALYSIS patients** – No dose adjustment required.
- **TRANSPLANT patients** – Doxycycline can DOUBLE the blood levels of ciclosporin and tacrolimus. Advise to commence taking the doxycycline at least 1 week prior to travelling to enable ciclosporin or tacrolimus levels to be monitored and adjusted as necessary.

CHLOROQUINE (AVLOCLOR® OR NIVAQUINE®) AND PROGUANIL (PALUDRINE®)

- CHLOROQUINE (base) 310 mg (TWO tablets) ONCE a WEEK, **plus**
- PROGUANIL 200 mg (TWO tablets) ONCE a DAY starting 1 week prior to travelling and continuing for 4 weeks after returning.

Chloroquine:
- Malaria *prophylaxis*: no dose adjustment necessary for renal impairment.
- Malaria *treatment, i.e. full therapeutic dose*: take the following into consideration:
  — **Transplant patients**: chloroquine increases plasma ciclosporin levels – monitor carefully.

Patients with renal insufficiency:

GFR (mL/min)	Dose
20–59	100% dose
10–19	100% dose
<10	50% dose

Proguanil:
- **Transplant patients** dose according to the level of function of the renal transplant.
- CAPD and haemodialysis patients **half a tablet (50 mg) once a week.**
- **Patients with renal insufficiency**

GFR (mL/min)	Dose
≥ 60	200 mg OD
20–59	100 mg OD
10–19	50 mg alt days
<10	50 mg once a week

NB. Patients with renal insufficiency receiving proguanil should also be prescribed folic acid 5 mg daily to minimise side effects.

ATOVAQUONE 250 MG + PROGUANIL 100 MG (MALARONE®)

ONE tablet daily starting 1–2 days before travelling, and continuing for 7 days after returning.

GFR (mL/min)	Dose
>30	Normal dose
<30	Malarone not recommended, because with the combined preparation it is not possible to reduce the dose of proguanil but take the full dose of atovaquone. Use alternative therapy.

Vaccines

Live vaccines should NOT be administered to immunosuppressed patients – this includes both transplant patients, and those on dialysis.

Inactivated vaccines can be administered to immunosuppressed patients, although the response may be reduced, and further booster doses may be required as dictated by measuring antibody titres.

VACCINES THAT ARE NOT RECOMMENDED:

- BCG (Bacillus Calmette-Guerin) vaccine
- INFLUENZA vaccine for **intranasal use** (Fluenz*)
- MEASLES, MUMPS, RUBELLA vaccine (MMRvaxPro*, Priorix*)
- POLIO Oral vaccine (**Sabin**) (OPV*), including household contacts of immunosuppressed patients as transmission of the live virus through faeces is possible.
- ROTAVIRUS vaccine (Rotarix*). For vaccination of children, but the rotavirus is excreted in the stool and may be transmitted to close contacts. However, vaccination of those with **immunosuppressed close contacts** may protect the contacts from wild-type rotavirus disease and outweigh any risk from transmission of vaccine virus.
- TYPHOID Oral vaccine (Vivotif*)
- VARICELLA-ZOSTER vaccine (Varilix*, Varivax*, Zostavax*)
- YELLOW FEVER vaccine (Stamaril*)

VACCINES THAT MAY BE ADMINISTERED:

- ANTHRAX vaccine
- CHOLERA oral vaccine (Dukoral*)
- DIPHTHERIA Adsorbed (low dose), TETANUS and INACTIVATED POLIOMYELITIS vaccine (Revaxis*)
- DIPHTHERIA Adsorbed (low dose), TETANUS, PERTUSSIS and INACTIVATED POLIOMYELITIS vaccine (Repevax*)
- DIPHTHERIA Adsorbed, TETANUS, PERTUSSIS, POLIOMYELITIS (inactivated) and Haemophilus Type b Conjugate (Adsorbed) vaccine (Pediacel*)
- HAEMOPHILUS INFLUENZAE type b & MENINGOCOCCAL Group C conjugate vaccine (Menitorix*)
- HEPATITIS A vaccine (Avaxim*, Epaxal*, Havrix Monodose*)
- HEPATITIS B vaccine (Engerix B*, Fendrix*, HBvaxPRO*)
- HEPATITIS A & B vaccine (Ambirix*, Twinrix*)
- HEPATITIS A & TYPHOID vaccine (Hepatyrix*, ViATIM*)
- HUMAN PAPILLOMAVIRUS vaccine (Cervarix*, Gardasil*)
- INFLUENZA Split Virion and Surface Antigen vaccines (Agrippal*, Enzira*, Fluarix*, Fluvirin*, Imuvac*, Viroflu*, Intanza*)
- JAPANESE ENCEPHALITIS vaccine (Ixiaro*)
- MENINGOCOCCAL Group C Conjugate vaccine (Meningitec*, Menjugate Kit*, NeisVac-C*)
- MENINGOCOCCAL A, C, W135 and Y, Polysaccharide vaccine (ACWY Vax*) and Conjugate vaccine (Menveo*, Nimenrix*)
- PNEUMOCOCCAL Polysaccharide vaccine (Pneumovax II*) and Conjugate vaccine (Prevenar 13*, Synflorix*)
- POLIO Inactivated vaccine (**Salk**) (IPV*)
- RABIES vaccine (Rab*, Rabipur*)
- TICK-BORNE ENCEPHALITIS vaccine (TicoVac*)
- TYPHOID Vi Capsular Polysaccharide vaccine (Typherix*, Typhim Vi*)